BIOMEDICAL ENGINEERING TRENDS IN ELECTRONICS, COMMUNICATIONS AND SOFTWARE

Edited by **Anthony N. Laskovski**

INTECHOPEN.COM

Biomedical Engineering Trends in Electronics, Communications and Software
Edited by Anthony N. Laskovski

CBS, Edition **2017**

Published by InTech
Janeza Trdine 9, 51000 Rijeka, Croatia

Publishing Process Manager Ana Nikolic

Technical Editor Teodora Smiljanic

Cover Designer InTech Design Team

Image Copyright Christian Delbert, 2010. Used under license from Shutterstock.com

Additional hard copies can be obtained from orders@intechopen.com

Biomedical Engineering Trends in Electronics, Communications and Software,
Edited by Anthony N. Laskovski
p. cm.
ISBN 978-953-307-475-7

INTECH

open science | open minds

Contents

Contents

Contents

Contents

Preface

Biological and medical phenomena are complex and intelligent. Our observations and understanding of some of these phenomena have inspired the development of creative theories and technologies in science. This process will continue to occur as new developments in our understanding and perception of natural phenomena continue. Given the complexity of our natural world this is not likely to end.

Over time several schools of specialisation have occurred in engineering, including electronics, computer science, materials science, structures, mechanics, control, chemistry and also genetics and bioengineering. This has led to the industrialised world of the 20th century and the information rich 21st century, all involving complex innovations that improve the quality and length of life.

Biomedical Engineering is a field that applies these specialised engineering technologies and design paradigms to the biomedical environment. It is an interesting field in that these established technologies and fields of research, many of which were inspired by nature, are now being developed to interact with naturally occurring phenomena in medicine. This completes a two-way information loop that will rapidly accelerate our understanding of biology and medical phenomena, solve medical problems and inspire the creation of new non-medical technologies.

This series of books will present recent developments and trends in biomedical engineering, spanning across several disciplines. I am honoured to be editing a book with such interesting and exciting content, written by a selected group of talented researchers. This book presents research involving telemetry, wireless body area networks, sensors, instrumentation, imaging, data processing, computation and information management in biomedical engineering.

Anthony N. Laskovski

The University of Newcastle,
Australia

Part 1

Telemetry and Wireless Body Area Networks

1

Biosignal Monitoring Using Wireless Sensor Networks

Carlos Andres Lozano, Camilo Eduardo Tellez and Oscar Javier Rodríguez
Universidad Sergio Arboleda
Colombia

1. Introduction

The continuous search for people welfare through various mechanisms, has led medicine to seek synergy with other disciplines, especially engineering, among many other developments allowing the application of new techniques to monitor patients through their own body signals. The application of new developments in areas such as electronics, informatics and communications, aims to facilitate significantly the process of acquisition of biomedical signals, in order to achieve a correct approach when developing diagnostic or medical monitoring, to optimize the required care process and sometimes to reduce the cost of such processes.

In some specific situations it is desirable that the patient under monitoring does not lose his mobility by the wire connection to the device that captures any particular signal, since this state may interfere with the study. For example, in case you need to measure the heart effort of a person taking a walk or a sprint. It is in this type of environment where new ICT technologies such as Wireless Sensor Networks (WSN) can support the development of biomedical devices allowing the acquisition of various signals for subsequent monitoring and analysis in real time.

Telemedicine also called e-health is everything related to electronic health data for monitoring, diagnosis or analysis for the treatment of patients in remote locations. Usually this includes the use of medical supplies, advanced communications technology, including videoconferencing systems (Enginnering in Medicine & Biology, 2003).

Telemedicine systems can establish good and emerging technologies such as IEEE standards 802.11, 802.15 and 802.16, which these bases are characterized by the distribution networks for medical information, and provision for life-saving services. These systems have certain restrictions in the sense that when these wireless communications may be affected by a storm, or in conditions where the signal to transmit is not the most appropriate spots, then due to these problems, which solutions were sought resulted in great advances in wireless networking technologies providing vital routes for the restoration of services in telemedicine.

The efficiency of telemedicine systems are widely affected by the design of systems, such as standardization, which in this case would not only rapid deployment, but also easy access for maintenance and renewal future systems that support care services.

The constant study and monitoring of biomedical signals, has been an important tool in the development of new medical technology products. However, these over time begin to see that they are useful and important in industries that formerly had not been implemented but that scientific advances are essential. Over the years, monitoring of such signals have been putting more importance and trust in the medical corps, allowing them to exploit technological advances to benefit human care.

Within each wireless sensor network, sensors are one of the most important components of the network. There are several sensors based on the applications we want to use. An example is the temperature sensor, which is a component that is mostly composed of semiconductor materials that vary with temperature change. In the case of biomedical environments, it senses the temperature of the skin or skin temperature, which enables us to monitor it in the patient, allowing for immediate assistance.

We are not too far from the meaning stated above, to make a comparison, we found that both conditions vary only in the ability to sense, as this requires certain conditions of the system or agency is analysing nevertheless remains a fundamental part at the time to learn about processes that is "easy" observe or with our senses is impossible to understand.

However, biomedical sensors, should be chosen under certain parameters that are vital to the development and smooth operation of the same, they should be able to measure the signal in particular, but also to maintain a single precision and replacement capacity fast enough to monitor living organisms. Additionally, these sensors must be able to adapt to variations in the surface bioelectric be implemented (Bronzino, 1999).

This chapter is organized in the following sections. Section 2 shows the main characteristics of wireless sensor networks. We present the essential information about Body Sensor Networks as a WSN specialization in medical environments in Section 3. Section 4 shows our methodology for the development of applications of biomedical signals acquisition. We conclude this chapter with section V.

2. The wireless sensor networks

The wireless sensor networks are formed by small electronic devices called nodes, whose function is to obtain, convert, transmit and receive a specific signal, which is captured by specific sensors, chosen depending on the sensing environment. This technology, due to its low cost and power consumption is widely used in industrial process control, security in shopping malls, hotels, crop fields, areas prone to natural disasters, transport security and medical environments, among other fields.

A sensor network can be described as a group of nodes called "motes" that are coordinated to perform a specific application, this lead to more accurate measurement of tasks depending on how thick it is the deployment and are coordinated (Evans, 2007).

2.1 General features

In a wireless sensor network, devices that help the network to obtain, transmit and receive data from a specific environment, are classified according to their attributes or specific performance in the network (Cheekiralla & Engels, 2005).

A wireless sensor network consists of devices such as are micro-controllers, sensors and transmitter / receiver which the integration of these form a network with many other nodes, also called motes or sensors. Another item that is extremely important in any classification, is to know the processing capacity, due to its necessary because communication being the main consumer of energy, a system with distributed processing features, meant that some of the sensors need to communicate over long distances This leads us to deduce that higher

energy consumption needed. Hence the rationale for knowing when to be processed locally as much energy to minimize the number of bits transmitted (Gordillo & al., 2007).
A node usually consists of 4 subsystems (See Fig. 1):

- **Computing subsystem:** This is a micro controller unit, which is responsible for the control of sensors and the implementation of communication protocols. The micro controller is usually operated under different operating modes for power management purposes.
- **Communications subsystem:** Issues relating to standard protocols, which depending on your application variables is obtained as the operating frequency and types of standards to be used (ZigBee, Bluetooth, UWB, among others.) This subsystem consists of a short range radio which is used to communicate with other neighboring nodes and outside the network. The radio can operate in the mode of transmitter, receiver, standby, and sleep mode.
- **Sensing subsystem:** This is a group of sensors or actuators and link node outside the network. The power consumption can be determined using low energy components.
- **Energy storage subsystem:** One of the most important features in a wireless sensor network is related to energy efficiency which thanks to some research, this feature has been considered as a key metric. In the case of hardware developers in a WSN, it is to provide various techniques to reduce energy consumption. Due to this factor, power consumption of our network must be controlled by 2 modules: 1) power module (which computes the energy consumption of different components), 2) battery module (which uses this information to compute the discharge of the battery.)

When a network contains a large number of nodes, the battery replacement becomes very complex, in this case the energy used for wireless communications network is reduced by low energy multiple hops (multi-hop routing) rather than a transmission high-tech simple. This subsystem consists of a battery that holds the battery of a node. This should be seen as the amount of energy absorbed from a battery which is reviewed by the high current drawn from the battery for a long time (Qin & Yang, 2007).

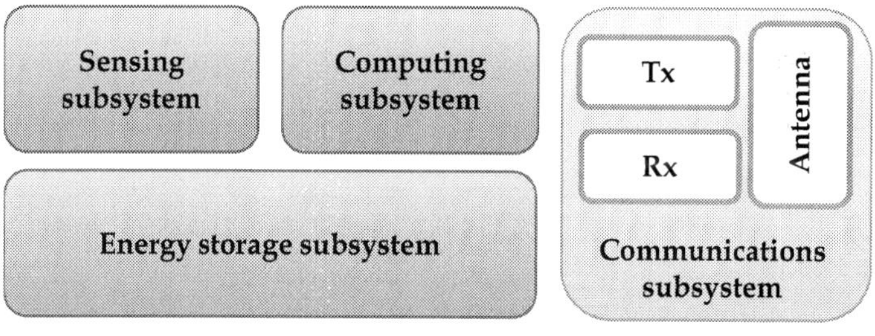

Fig. 1. Wireless Sensor Networks subsystems

2.2 WSN classification and operation mode

A wireless sensor network can be classified depending on their application and its programming, its functionality in the field sensing, among others. In the case of a WSN (Wireless Sensor Networks), is classified as follows:

- **Homogeneous,** refers when all nodes have the same hardware, otherwise it is called heterogeneous.

- **Autonomous** referenced when all nodes are able to perform self-configuration tasks without the intervention of a human.
- **Hierarchical** referenced when nodes are grouped for the purpose of communicating or otherwise shut down, in this classification is common to have a base station that works as a bridge to external entities.
- **Static**, referenced when nodes are static and dynamic otherwise.

A WSN can also be continuous, hybrid, reactive. In the case of the reactive mode, is when the sensor nodes send information about events occurring in the environment and both are scheduled when the information collected under defined conditions or specified for the application that want (Ruiz, Nogueira, & Loureiro, 2003).

A WSN is designed and developed according to the characteristics of the applications to which the design or the environment is implemented, then to which must take into account the following "working models" (Egea-Lopez, Vales-Alonso, Martinez-Sala, Pavon-Mario, & Garcia-Haro, 2006):

- **Flexibility**. In this item, the wireless environment is totally changed due to interference from other microwaves, or forms of materials in the environment, among other conditions, that is why most of the nodes can fail at any time, because should seek new path in real time, must reconfigure the network, and in turn re-calibrate the initial parameters.
- **Efficiency**. This item is very important due to the network to be implemented must be efficient to work in real time, must be reliable and robust to interference from the same nodes, or other signals from other devices. This item is in relation to that should be tightly integrated with the environment where it will work.
- **Scalability**. This item talk about when it comes to wireless sensor network is dynamic, due to its topology or application to use, being a dynamic sensor network, adding nodes is an important factor for the smooth operation of data storage.

2.3 WSN functional levels

WSN network are classified into 3 functional levels: The level of control, the level of Communications Network and the Field Level, as shown in Figure 1.

The field level consists of a sensors set and actuators that interact directly with the environment. The sensors are responsible for obtaining data either thermal, optical, acoustic, seismic, etc. The actuators on the other hand receive orders which are the result of processing the information gathered by the sensors so it can be run later. In the communication network establishing a communication link between the field level and the level of control. Nodes that are part of a communications subsystem WSN are grouped into 3 categories: Endpoints, Routers, and Gateways. Finally found the level of control consists of one or more control and/or monitoring centres, using information collected by the sensors to set tasks that require the performance of the actuators. This control is done through special software to manage network topologies and behaviour of our network in diverse environments (Rodríguez & Tellez, 2009).

One way to consider wireless sensor networks is to take the network to organize hierarchically the nodes of the upper level being the most complex and knowing his location through a transmission technique.

The challenges in hierarchically classify a sensor network is on: Finding relevant quantities monitor and collect data, access and evaluate information, among others. The information

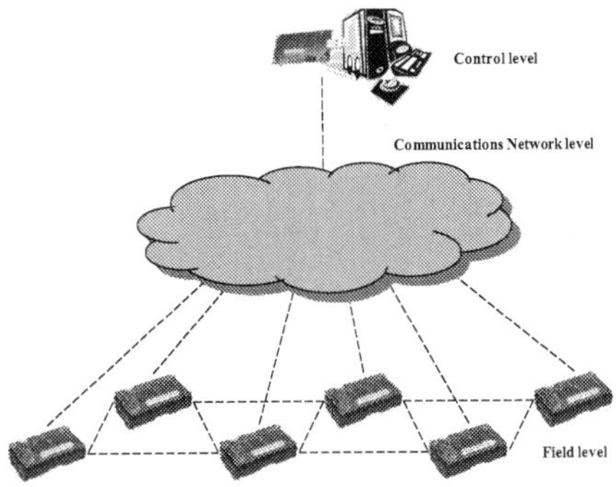

Fig. 2. Architecture of a WSN (Roldán, 2005)

needed for intelligent environments or whose variables are complex to obtain, is provided by a distributed network of wireless sensors which are responsible for detecting and for the early stages of the processing hierarchy (Cao & Zhang, 1999).

2.4 Communications protocols

At the National Institute of Standards and Technology (United States of America) was established as the main task in 2006, set standards that would allow both researchers and doctors to be clear about identifying the quality characteristics of the system to develop, creating an atmosphere of trust between medicine and engineering. Based on the principle of ubiquitous connectivity that seeks to facilitate the connection of different wireless communication standards to establish a wider range of possibilities when biomedical transmit a signal without being affected by the lack of coverage of a particular system (Rodríguez & Tellez, 2009).

In a wireless sensor network, the communication method varies depending on the application either at the medical, industrial or scientific. One of the most widely used communication protocols is the ZigBee protocol, which is a technology composed of a set of specifications designed for wireless sensor networks and controllers. This system is characterized by the type of communication conditional; it does not require a high volume of information (just over a few kilobits per second) and also have a limited walking distance (Roldán, 2005).

ZigBee was designed to provide a simple and easy low-cost wireless communication and also provide a connectivity solution for low data transmission applications such as low power consumption, such as home monitoring, automation, environmental monitoring, control of industries, and emerging applications in the area of wireless sensors. The IEEE 802.15.4 standard, as it is called ZigBee, can work at 3 different frequency bands. This protocol is divided into layers according to the OSI model, where each layer has a specific function depending on the application of our network. The physical layer and the medium access control (MAC) are standardized by the IEEE 802.15 (WPAN) which is a working group under the name of 802.15.4; where the higher layers are specified by ZigBee Alliance. Some characteristics of the layers are given below:

- Physical Layer ZigBee / IEEE 802.15.4: The IEEE 802.15.4 physical layer supports unlicensed industrial, scientific and medical radio frequency bands including 868 MHz, 915 MHz and 2.4 GHz.

- MAC Layer ZigBee / IEEE 802.15.4: At the MAC layer, there are 2 options to access the medium: Beacon-based (based on orientation) and non-beacon (based on non-guidance). In a non-oriented, there is no time for synchronization between ZigBee devices. The Devices can assess to the channel using (CSMA / CA).
- Protocol to the network layer / IEEE 802.15.4: ZigBee got a multi-hop routing and help the capabilities designed as an integral part of the system. This function is implemented within the network layer.

2.5 Topology

The performance of a wireless sensor network is measured depending on the ability to manage energy consumption of all nodes and also the effectiveness in real-time transmission of data from the time of sensing to the display of such signs. Depending on the type of environment and resources in a network of wireless sensors, you can define multiple architectures, among the best known are Star, mesh and cluster tree network (See Fig. 2) (Tellez, Rodriguez, & Lozano, 2009). The nodes have no knowledge of the topology of the network must "discover".

A star topology network is characterized by a base station which can send and receive a Message to a number of router nodes. The advantage of this type of network for a WSN is the ease and ability to maintain energy consumption of a router node to a very low level. The disadvantage of this type of topology is the coordinator node (or base station), as it must be within transmission range of all nodes.

Mesh network topology or is characterized by allowing any node in the network, can transmit to any other node on the network that is within transmission range. This type of topology has an advantage which is the redundancy and scalability compared to a situation of failure. If the router node gets out of service, other nodes can communicate with each other without depending on the node unusable. The disadvantage of this type of network, power consumption for nodes that implement a multi-hop communication, which generally results in the life of the battery consumption, is too short.

Finally, a cluster tree network (union of a star and mesh topology), is one network that provides versatility to a communications network, while it maintains the ability to have low power consumption of wireless sensor nodes. This feature allows the power consumption of the entire network remains.

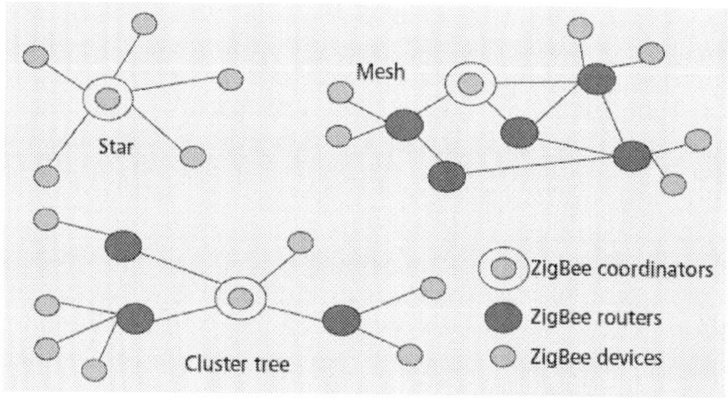

Fig. 3. Network Topology (W., Sohraby, Jana, J., & Daneshmand, 2008)

The position of the sensor nodes in a given area is not predetermined in some situations; this means that the protocols and algorithms used must be capable of self-organization (is the case of a changing field). Some designs have protocols for specific design features the main energy saving and management of the interference signal which is caused by the microwaves.

A wireless sensor network experience some interference in the setting of transmission and reception of data, depending on the type of technologies like the IEEE PAN / LAN / MAN, or some other technology that uses radio frequency. These technologies are deployed mainly in commercial and scientific aspects of WSN environments. They are currently showed a variety of wireless protocols, which focuses more innovation in the communications field.

2.6 Models for power consumption

A wireless sensor network functions depending on the energy consumption of total lifetime of the devices in the network of sensors, instead of relying only on the process of transmitting and receiving data. Energy consumption varies significantly from state to state on which the device is running. Some studies suggest 4 states to optimize our network, one of states or types most used and implemented are those that contain the following steps: transmitting, receiving, listening on hold, and idle. Due to the continued use of networks have been proposed or levels that contain more than 4 states, it is clear that this depends on the application you want to do, and our network energy dissipated.

Energy consumption is one of the most important factors in determining the life of a sensor network, because nodes are usually powered by a battery and because of that have few energy resources. This makes the optimization of energy becomes complex in a sensor network because not only involves the reduction of energy consumption, but also prolongs the life of a network (Raghunathan, Schurgers, Park, & Srivastava, 2002).

2.7 Simulators

Currently there are several simulators for sensor networks, which plays an key role in processing and in turn facilitate easy configuration of the network depending on the application to use. Among the most redeemable find (Bharathidasan & Sai Ponduru):

1. **NS-2**: It was one of the first simulations, which facilitates simulations carried out by both wireless and wired. It is written in C + + and oTCL (Information Sciences Institute).
2. **GloMoSim**: Your initials translate (Global Mobile Information Systems Simulator) is a scalable simulation device for network systems both wired and wireless. This simulator is written in C and Parsec. GloMoSom currently supports protocols for purely wireless network environment (Bajaj, Takai, Ahuja, Tang, Bagrodia, & Gerla, 1999).
3. **SensorSim**: This simulation framework provides channel sensing and sensor models, as models of battery, battery light wide protocols for wireless micro sensors (Park, Savvides, & Srivastava, 2000).

In many software projects are used to acquire data from a WSN by Tiny OS operating system and NESC. This software is well known in the sensor networks and more so in systems that use wireless sensors, is a system that does not use much energy and is small compared to other networking platforms. The system is very useful because its network operation is based on responses, more colloquial, the pot, as is known in Tiny OS; only works when you are authorized to make any transfer of rest is kept in standby.

2.8 Applications

The signal monitoring does not focus only on the medical area also find that developments in the search for home automation and control of enclosed spaces such applications are useful in projects such as houses or indoor intelligent, capable of having a autonomy. Another area of research that is taking shape every day, is the use of sensors in the automotive field, nationally the development of such projects is in its infancy, the development of a small network of sensors that seeks to solve small problems such as system capacity to meet their own needs and those of their neighbors in case of damage, and the ability to work with minimum energy expenditure without altering the quality of service or affect the information transmitted.

It consider finally found another area of application in monitoring signals applied real needs such as caring for the forests to preserve them; systems which can control all kinds of variables in this environment (Estrin, Govindan, Heidemann, & Kumar, 1999).

Sensor networks can have a wide variety of applications:

- Monitoring of habitat,
- Monitoring the environment, soil or water observation,
- The maintenance of certain physical conditions (temperature, light, pressure, etc.),
- Control parameter in agriculture,
- Detection of fires, earthquakes or floods,
- Traffic control,
- Civil or military assistance,
- Medical examination, among others.

3. Body Sensor Networks (BSN)

One of the most interesting areas for the implementation of the WSN is in the medical field because there are different challenges which are associated with monitoring the human body. The human body responds to its environment, as well as external conditions its live every day. Thus in order to monitor all these features, we apply the monitoring and sensor networks in order to get a really diagnose what gets the sensors on the body surface, as may be the frequency of monitoring (Yang, 2006). The name associated with this implementation is Body Sensor Networks (BSN).

The work in BSN has existed for several years and search provides guarantees and confidence to a mass deployment. This technology may offer the possibility of developing a detailed diagnosis of the patient, because the network would be able to monitor all vital signs and synthesize all relevant information for the more effectively patient care.

How Yang say in his book *"BSN patient monitoring systems will provide information that is likely to be as important, dramatic and revolutionary as those initial observations made by Hippocrates himself"* (Yang, 2006).

3.1 Differences between wide-scale WSN and WBSN

Practically the differences between the BSN and the WSN are very few, but it is very important to note that it is these small differences that allow BSN face the challenges posed in the medical field. Table 1 present a summary of the differences between WSN and BSN.

Challenges	WSN	BSN
Scale	As large as the environment being monitored (metres/kilometres)	As large as human body parts (millimetres/centimetres)
Node Number	Greater number of nodes required for accurate, wide area coverage	Fewer, more accurate sensors nodes required (limited by space)
Node Function	Multiple sensors, each perform dedicated tasks	Single sensors, each perform multiple tasks
Node Accuracy	Large node number compensates for accuracy and allows result validation	Limited node number with each required to be robust and accurate
Node Size	Small size preferable but not a major limitation in many cases	Pervasive monitoring and need for miniaturisation
Dynamics	Exposed to extremes in weather, noise, and asynchrony	Exposed to more predictable environment but motion artefacts is a challenge
Event Detection	Early adverse event detection desirable; failure often reversible	Early adverse events detection vital; human tissue failure irreversible
Variability	Much more likely to have a fixed or static structure	Biological variation and complexity means a more variable structure
Data Protection	Lower level wireless data transfer security required	High level wireless data transfer security required to protect patient information
Power Supply	Accessible and likely to be changed more easily and frequently	Inaccessible and difficult to replace in implantable setting
Power Demand	Likely to be greater as power is more easily supplied	Likely to be lower as energy is more difficult to supply
Energy Scavenging	Solar, and wind power are most likely candidates	Motion (vibration) and thermal (body heat) most likely candidates
Access	Sensors more easily replaceable or even disposable	Implantable sensor replacement difficult and requires biodegradability
Biocompatibility	Not a consideration in most applications	A must for implantable and some external sensors. Likely to increase cost
Context Awareness	Not so important with static sensors where environments are well defined	Very important because body physiology is very sensitive to context change
Wireless Technology	Bluetooth, Zigbee, GPRS, and wireless LAN, and RF already offer solutions	Low power wireless required, with signal detection more challenging
Data Transfer	Loss of data during wireless transfer is likely to be compensated by number of sensors used	Loss of data more significant, and may require additional measures to ensure QoS and real-time data interrogation capabilities

Table 1. Different challenges faced by WSN and BSN (Yang, 2006).

3.2 Topology of a BSN

The application design is based BSN regularly in the Star topology, this topology has the main advantage of optimizing the energy consumption of the network due to internal nodes called "slaves" only have the function of the coordinator will transmit information received by the sensors but as a great disadvantage has the high possibility of network failure due to the fall of the coordinator node.

3.3 Relevant applications, prototypes and projects

The importance of being able to identify the concept, functionality and applicability of the BSN, begins to identify the most important projects developed that gave rise to the medical applications. These projects are being used to develop a feedback process to strengthen knowledge and thus build a proposal that offers more input into health care.
Some of the most important research projects in this field include the technological development of the following fields: Miniaturization of hardware, systems integration, sensor integration to clothing, quality of service, information security, communication protocols and new biocompatible materials, amongst others. Here are some little bit references made to identify the progress and knowledge when deploying BSN in the medical field.

3.3.1 WearIT@work

The WearIT@work Project was set up by the European Commission as an Integrated Project to investigate "Wearable Computing" as a technology dealing with computer systems integrated in clothing (wearIT@work).
One of the possible applications of this project is the rapid availability of patient medical information at any time; this may mean an interesting reduction in medical examination fees, also the power to perform medical reviews in the daily circumstances of patients and in extreme cases could save the life of a patient.

3.3.2 SWAN: System for Wearable Audio Navigation

The department of psychology at Georgia Institute of Technology, specifically the Sonification Lab, researchers has created the SWAN project. This project is a practical device, portable whose characteristics are in navigation software for people with vision loss or even in places where the vision of the place is limited, and this emphasized the need for which to avoid obstacles or to obtain characteristics of the environment quickly, where they are using.
This device consists of a small computer, which contains various guidance devices such as GPS, inertial sensors, RFID antennas, RF sensors, among others. When all devices are synchronized and identify the exact location, SWAN through an audio device, sound guidance through the person using the device, which also indicate in real time the location of other characteristics of the sensing environment (GT Sonification Lab).

3.3.3 SESAME (SEnsing in Sport And Managed Exercise)

The SESAME project is development by a consortium of research groups. They base their work in creating several wireless sensor networks for high performance athletes from around the world. Among its features are that can sense both in idle mode and real time variables continued progress of the athlete.
The goals of the project lie in enhancing performance, improving coach education, and advancing sports science using a range of both hardware and software technologies to achieve this (Computer Laboratory & Engineering Dept. University of Cambridge).

3.3.4 Advanced Soldier Sensor Information System and Technology (ASSIST)

It is well known that any technological development is linked to advances in the military. Within these advances, we emphasize the ASSIST program, which is a program that integrates information on the battlefield (location, time, group activities, among others). Where the main tool of the program is based on the soldier to collect, disseminate and display key information, without risking the life or physical integrity (Information Processing Techniques Office). This project is funded by DARPA of the United States of America.

3.3.5 HeartCycle

A consortium with more than 18 entities between which we can highlight research groups, hospitals and industry. The research objective is to improve the quality of life of patients suffering from heart disease. This consortium focuses on developing devices which monitors and prescribes the history to the doctor to know which therapies or recommendations must follow the patient during treatment (Heartcycle).

The system will contain:

- A patient loop interacting directly with the patient to support the daily treatment. It will show the health development, including treatment adherence and effectiveness. Being motivated, compliance will increase, and health will improve.
- A professional loop involving medical professionals, e.g. alerting to revisit the care plan. The patient loop is connected with hospital information systems, to ensure optimal and personalised care.

4. Methodology for development of biomedical signals acquisition and monitoring using WSN

Taking into account the previous considerations, we propose a three phase methodology for the development of applications of biomedical signals acquisition (See Fig. 4). The first phase is the acquisition of biomedical signals, whose main objective is to establish a set of features for the proper selection of sensors that will accurately capture the required signal, and at the same time, allow the correct transduction of signals sent. The second stage concerns to the correct choice of communication protocol to use and to additional features to the network settings such as topology. Finally, we must determine the relevant elements to design the platform for visualization and monitoring of the sensed signals.

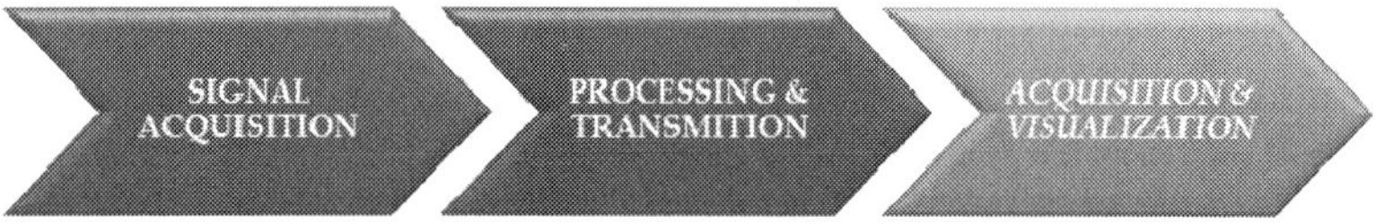

Fig. 4. Methodology for Development of Biomedical Signals Acquisition and Monitoring using WSN (Tellez, Rodriguez, & Lozano, 2009)

4.1 Signal acquisition

The monitoring of biomedical signals, requires mechanisms to strengthen, substantiate and legitimize the information captured by sensors, to try to understand these mechanisms, it should be noted that the acquisition of biomedical signals, you must meet certain

characteristics that do not interfere or alter the information gained, taking into account that the sensor components that are responsible for trapping that generate changes in the captured signals.
The concept of biomedical signals, focuses on the acquisition of data common phenomena of the human body, which can reach diagnoses and predicting diseases in the short and medium term, and a biomedical signal a signal becomes more complex and useful that capture a common signal, this allows to argue the importance of establishing and using elements that provide as much information for the analysis of the signal. Define and translate these signals, set parameters requires special handling and use of biomedical signals, as these because of their complexity and accuracy should have low error rates and sensors that have the ability to capture slight variations in depth to obtain the behaviour of the human body.
To acquiring a biomedical signal surface, such as the humidity or temperature, it should be noted that the structure has characteristics that do not alter sensor data collected by the sensors, may be the case limit or standard level moisture or temperature not met, may yield inaccurate data, or oxidation of the sensor to a more advanced level. However, as the environments are not extreme in relation to an industrial environment where sensors may be exposed to hostile areas, only know the following types of sensors and their respective form of measurement (See Fig. 5).

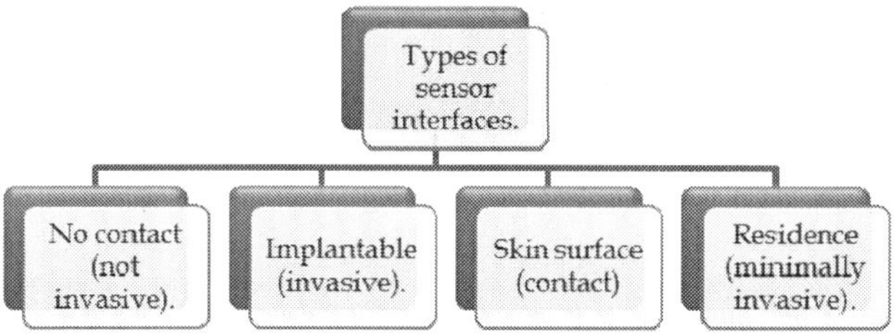

Fig. 5. Type of sensor interfaces (Bronzino, 1999)

The sensors can be used in diagnosis of medical diseases or for therapeutic purposes, which requires that the sensors respond positively to the demands of an analysis of diagnosis of this type are needed. Must also have high accuracy and in case of a touch sensor or implantable, alter the body (negatively affect the functioning of the body by the presence of an external agent as in this case a sensor).
If the sensor must be contact or implantable and this is closely affected by the presence of high humidity or temperature, is chosen for the design and implementation of protective sensor packages, these are intended to protect the sensor the presence of moisture or temperature at the points where the sensor can be affected, leaving only found the part where the sensor makes the sampling. This will protect both the information gathered as the prevention of possible damage to the body to place or deploy foreign agents in the body.
There are some kind of sensors that have direct contact with the body, there may be complications on the replacement of these components, although to deploy sensors should be a prior investigation and documentation on the reliability and accuracy of the sensor, is very complex to make changes or sensor calibration in real time or "in vivo", so you must design a protocol for internal sensor is at least the ability to calibrate itself, or rely on technology to which it is connected to maintain proper operation, all this must be properly

fulfilling predefined maximum quality standards taking into account that is not stopping the functioning of the body.

4.2 Processing & transmition

For optimum performance of a wireless sensor network, it must take certain variables or characteristics such as: Design the network topology sensing environment, energy consumption, distribution, formation of the network, which provide work a detailed selection of elements for optimum performance.

To get a sensing stability, we must be accurate when analysing signals, must turn to decipher and error-free data set give us a straight answer and correct what is a translation of a real situation. For this analysis, must take count that when handling and rely on signals, the noise and signals that alter our report as we may find situations where these noises are not important, as there spaces so. To overcome this obstacle, should be taken into account all types of filters that can regenerate the signal for the system to obtain an adequate response and follow the specifications with which the sensor reported the state of our system.

The next step is the routing of data, that we must consider how we get all this data, and network protocols that we use that are appropriate, including some that are feasible to use are the following: Internet, LAN, Bluetooth, RF, etc.

Can configure the data so that we know the environmental status according to the location of it and thus be able to see your progress. To have a comprehensive approach to what we see, we have three types of messages when creating a virtual environment that allows me to see the real situation. These three types of messages are control messages, which maintain stability in the system to monitor, we have messages of interest, which can give us an overall picture of what happens in reality and finally we have the data messages we give an independent report of the situation as external changes and variations as shown in control (Wassim & Zoubir, 2007).

The functionality of a wireless sensor network occurs in large part on the correct and accurate operation of the nodes that comprise it. For the acquisition of signals in a given environment using specific sensors, these sensors as was seen in the first objective, depending on the application and the environment in which you want sensing.

Based on the basic principles for designing a system for acquiring and processing of biomedical signals (Bronzino, 1999), the text provides 6 phases with which it must have the design of the data acquisition phase and later emphasizes the hardware design. The diagram is proposed as follows:

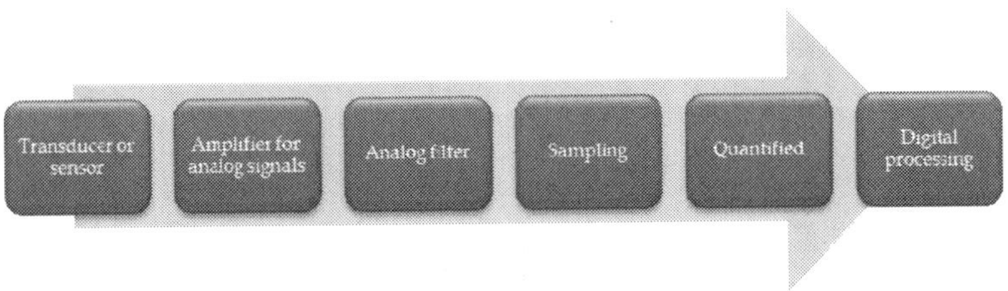

Fig. 6. General block diagram of a procedure analogue to digital (Bronzino, 1999)

The function of a node is to sense, process and communicate data from the signal for a more detailed study as the application that the network administrator requires. Depending on the topology of the network, each node has a specific function, is the case router node, which can only send or receive a message, but cannot send messages or data to other router nodes. On the other hand there is the coordinator node which has a dependency on other nodes for the complete management of a network, unlike router node; this node can send data to different nodes regardless of their classification.

The components that make up a sensor node, are mostly very small devices made by MEMS (Micro Electromechanical Systems), which each plays a vital role in the performance of each node in the network. Some of these components are:

1. Sensing unit and unit performance
2. Processing Unit
3. Communications Unit
4. Power Unit
5. Other

These hardware components should be organized to conduct a proper and effective work without generating any kind of conflict in support of specific applications for which they were designed. Each sensor node needs an operating system (OS) operating system operates between the application software and hardware and is regularly designed to be used in workstations and PCs.

In the market there are several manufacturers of nodes. Currently there are 3 companies that excel in developing this technology. These are: CROSSBOW, MOTEIV, Shockfish. In the Table 2 shows some characteristics of the nodes of the manufacturers of this technology (Serna, 2007).

	Micaz	**Mica2**	**Mica2dot**	**Tmote**	**TinyNode**
Distributed by	Crossbow			Moteiv	Shcokfish
Clock frequency	7.37 MHz		4 MHz	8 MHZ	8 MHz
RAM	4 KB			10 K bytes	10k bytes
Battery	2 AA Battery		Coin cell	2 AA Battery	Solar
Microcontroller	Atmel	Atmega	128 L	Texas Instruments	MSP430 microcontroller

Table 2. WSN Nodes characteristics

Among the key parts of the performance of a WSN, it should detail the minimum consumption for the network. So for the design of a wireless sensor network have focused on the biomedical field to consider the following items (Melodia, 2007):

1. The collisions should be avoided whenever possible, since the relay produces unnecessary energy consumption and other potential delays associated. Must find an optimal solution to avoid overloading the network and avoid the maximum power consumption.
2. The delay of transmission sent data packets is very important because you are working in a biomedical signal, it should be broadcasting continuous time and with the highest possible quality.
3. The receptor of our network must always be in constant operation (On), for it provides an ideal or hypothetical situation where our network only mode when you need to send or receive packets, and minimize the monitoring efforts of our spots.

4. There are points in the design of our wireless system such as: efficient use of bandwidth, delay, channel quality and power consumption.
5. The adaptability and mobility of our network.

4.2.1 Design coordinators and Router nodes

Some new technologies in the design and manufacturing of communications devices, smaller devices and better yields have been able to develop more complete nodes to the field of sensing, transmission and reception of signals obtained. Currently there are several devices that meet the requirements demanded for the development of a wireless sensor network.

The use of communication modules, have helped to design the networks, both in reducing devices included in a node, and the integration of several functions at a level both hardware and software (i. e. Security Protocols) in a single device.

On the other hand a form of management and efficient use for the acquisition of signals and their subsequent communication can be handled through the use of communication modules and modem devices. This solution is temporary and that the management and programming of micro-controller installed in the module, you can get a bit complex due to the type of software from the manufacturer and type of programming. The stage design software, you must set the proper display and lots of useful information necessary for a proper analysis of the situation and a diagnosis of what is sensed.

4.3 Acquisition & visualization

In order to develop a software application that allows the correct visualization of the acquired signals, it must take into account multiple factors to identify the basic features to implement it.

One of the first tasks is the selection of the platform for software development, the parameters to consider are:

- A platform that has the ability to receive a high volume of data
- A platform that allows easy synchronization between hardware and software.
- A platform with virtual instrumentation tools.

After selecting the development platform begins the design phase of the application. This stage should establish the visual and information to be submitted for a proper medical diagnosis. In order to visualize the acquired biomedical signals must be designed the following modules:

- **Acquisition Module**: This module is responsible for taking the BSN biomedical signals gateway.
- **Separation Module**: This module is responsible for recovering the received frame, the different signals transmitted (if more than one)
- **Processing Module**: This module each signal must translate the information received in units of voltage to the unit required by the signal such as temperature and relative humidity among others.
- **Display Module**: Determine the way in which the signal must be represented.
- **Graphical User Interface**: This module is integrated display modules to facilitate the analysis of information by the end user.

Finally completed the respective designs, the following steps are implementing the software and then testing to check its proper functioning (See Fig. 8).

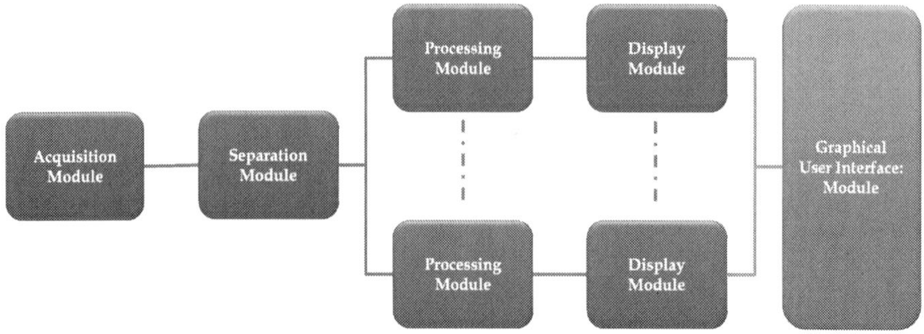

Fig. 7. General block diagram of biomedical signals visualization software

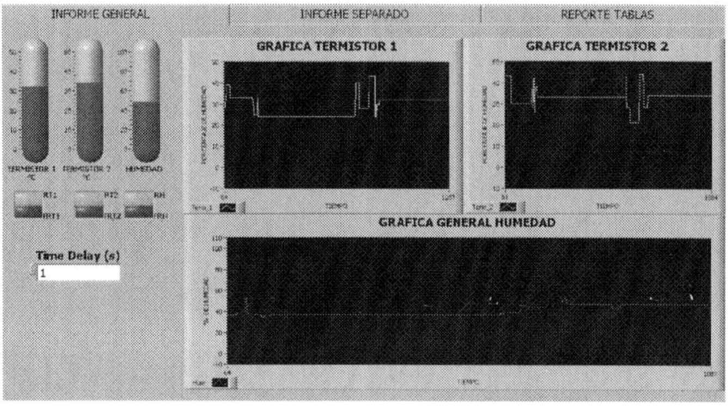

Fig. 8. Temperature and Humidity visualization software (Rodríguez & Tellez, 2009)

5. Conclusion

The impact generated by the use of wireless sensor networks in the quality of patient care is very high. The use of these devices in home care systems can reduce hospitalizations, health professionals timely interventions can extend patients life, and in some cases the use of biofeedback techniques in psychological treatments may overcome difficult phobias.

The development of such systems implies challenges to be faced in the area of engineering, such as minimizing energy consumption, since you want nodes lifetime in the network to be as long as possible. Another challenge is assuring the reliability of the information transmitted, since any slight variation may generate erroneous diagnosis. Finally, one of the biggest concerns is related to the potential impact of electromagnetic radiation to human bodies subject to the use of such devices.

6. References

Aymerich de Franceschi, M. (2009). *Performance Analysis of the Contention Access Period in the slotted IEEE 802.15.4 for Wireless Body Sensor Networks*. Leganés, Spain: Universidad Carlos III de Madrid.

Bajaj, L., Takai, M., Ahuja, R., Tang, K., Bagrodia, R., & Gerla, M. (1999). *GloMoSim: A scalable network simulation environment.* Los Angeles: University of California, Los Angeles.

Bharathidasan, A., & Sai Ponduru, V. A. (s.f.). *Sensor Neoworks: An overview.* Recuperado el 17 de June de 2010, de University of California, Davis: http://wwwcsif.cs.ucdavis.edu/~bharathi/sensor/survey.pdf

Bronzino, J. D. (1999). *Biomedical Engineering Handbook.* CRC Press.

Cao, J., & Zhang, F. (1999). Optimal configuration in hierarchical network routing. *IEEE Canadian Conference onElectrical and Computer Engineering* (págs. 249 - 254). Edmonton, Alta. Canada: IEEE.

Cheekiralla, S., & Engels, D. (2005). A Functional Taxonomy of Wireless Sensor Devices. *2nd International Conference on Broadband Networks, 2005.* (págs. 949-956). Boston, MA : IEEE.

Computer Laboratory & Engineering Dept. University of Cambridge. (s.f.). *SESAME.* Recuperado el 17 de March de 2010, de SEnsing in Sport And Managed Exercise: http://sesame-wiki.cl.cam.ac.uk/twiki/bin/view/Sesame

Cook, D., & Das, S. (2004). *Smart Environmets: Technologies, protocols and Applications.* Wiley-Interscience.

Egea-Lopez, E., Vales-Alonso, J., Martinez-Sala, A., Pavon-Mario, P., & Garcia-Haro, J. (2006). Simulation Scalability Issues in Wireless Sensor Networks. *IEEE Communications Magazine*, 64- 73.

Enginnering in Medicine & Biology. (2003). *Designing a Career in Biomedical Engineering.* Recuperado el 23 de July de 2010, de Enginnering in Medicine & Biology: http://www.embs.org/docs/careerguide.pdf

Estrin, D., Govindan, R., Heidemann, J., & Kumar, S. (1999). Next Century Challenges: Scalable Coordination in Sensor Networks. *Proceedings of the Fifth Annual International Conference on Mobile Computing and Networks (Mobicom '99)* (págs. 263 - 270). Seattle, Washington: ACM.

Evans, J. J. (2007). Undergraduate Research Experiences with Wireless Sensor Networks. *Frontiers In Education Conference - Global Engineering: Knowledge Without Borders, Opportunities Without Passports, 2007. FIE '07. 37th Annual* (págs. S4B-7 - S4B-12). Milwaukee, WI: IEEE.

Gordillo, R., & al., e. (2007). *Deploying a Wireless Sensor Network for Temperature Control.*

GT Sonification Lab. (s.f.). *SWAN: System for Wearable Audio Navigation.* Recuperado el 17 de March de 2010, de SWAN: System for Wearable Audio Navigation: http://sonify.psych.gatech.edu/research/SWAN/

Heartcycle. (s.f.). *HeartCycle Project.* Recuperado el 18 de March de 2010, de HeartCycle: http://heartcycle.med.auth.gr/

Information Processing Techniques Office. (s.f.). *ASSIST.* Recuperado el 17 de March de 2010, de Advanced Soldier Sensor Information System and Technology (ASSIST): http://www.darpa.mil/ipto/programs/assist/assist_obj.asp

Information Sciences Institute. (s.f.). *The Network Simulator - ns-2.* Recuperado el 17 de June de 2010, de The University of Southern California: http://www.isi.edu/nsnam/ns/.

Li, H., & J., T. (2005). An Ultra-low-power Medium Access Control Protocol for Body Sensor Network. *Conference Procceding IEEE Engineering in Medicine & Biology Society.* IEEE.

Melodia, T. (2007). *Future Research Trends in Wireless Sensor Networks.* Bogotá: IEEE Colombia.

Mode Dx Ltd. (s.f.). *Mode Diagnostic.* Recuperado el 15 de March de 2010, de Mode Diagnostic: http://www.modedx.com/

Park, S., Savvides, A., & Srivastava, M. B. (2000). SensorSim: A Simulation Framework for Sensor Networks. *Proceedings of the 3rd ACM International Workshop on Modeling Analysis and Simulation of Wireless and Mobile System* (págs. 104 - 111). ACM.

Qin, W., & Yang, W. (2007). Energy Consumption Model for Power Management in Wireless Sensor Networks. *4th Annual IEEE Communications Society Conference on Sensor, Mesh and Ad Hoc Communications and Networks, 2007.* (págs. 142-151, 18-21). San Diego, CA: IEEE.

Raghunathan, V., Schurgers, C., Park, S., & Srivastava, M. (2002). Energy-aware wireless microsensor networks. *Signal Processing Magazine, IEEE* , 40 - 50 .

Rodríguez, O., & Tellez, C. (2009). *Implementación de un prototipo funcional de un sistema de adquisición y visualización de temperatura y humedad en seres humanos utilizando redes de sensores inalámbricas.* Bogota: Universidad de San Buenaventura.

Roldán, D. (2005). *Comunicaciones inalámbricas: Un enfoque aplicado.* Mexico D.F.: Alfaomega.

Ruiz, L., Nogueira, J., & Loureiro, A. (2003). MANNA: A Management Architecture for Wireless Sensor Networks. *IEEE Communications Magazine*, 116 - 125 .

Serna, J. (2007). *Redes de Sensores Inalámbricas.* Valencia, Spain: Universidad de Valencia.

Tellez, C., Rodriguez, O., & Lozano, C. (2009). Biomedical signal monitoring using wireless sensor networks. *IEEE Latin-American Conference on Communications, 2009.* (págs. 1 - 6). Medellin: IEEE.

W., C., Sohraby, K., Jana, R., J., L., & Daneshmand, M. (2008). Voice communications over zigbee networks. *IEEE Communications Magazine*, 121-127.

Wassim, M., & Zoubir, M. (2007). Middleware for Wireless Sensor Networks: A Comparatvive Analysis. *International Conference on Network and Parallel Computing* (págs. 1 - 8). Dalian, China: IEEE.

wearIT@work. (s.f.). *wearIT@work Project Overview.* Recuperado el 17 de March de 2010, de The Project WearITatWork : http://www.wearitatwork.com/home/the-project/the-project/

Yang, G. (2006). *Body Sensor Networks.* London, UK: Springer.

2

Wireless Telemetry for Implantable Biomedical Microsystems

Farzad Asgarian and Amir M. Sodagar
Integrated Circuits & Systems (ICAS) Lab.,
Department of Electrical & Computer Eng.,
K. N. Toosi University of Technology,
Iran

1. Introduction

Rapid development of microelectronics during the past years allowed the emergence of high-performance *implantable biomedical microsystems* (IBMs). Nowadays, these systems share many features and basic components, and are being used in different applications such as neural signal recording, functional muscular stimulation, and neural prostheses. Due to implant size limitations in a wide range of applications, and the necessity for avoiding wires to reduce the risk of infection, wireless operation of IBMs is inevitable. Hence, an IBM is usually interfaced with an external host through a wireless link. In order to minimize the complexity and size of an implant, most of the signal processing units are kept outside the body and embedded in the external host. Moreover, the power needed for the implant modules including a central processing and control unit, stimulators and sensors is transmitted by the external host via wireless interfacing. The wireless link is also used for bidirectional data transfer between the implanted device and the outside world. Thus, as shown in Fig. 1, the wireless interface on the implant needs to contain a power regulator, a demodulator for receiving control/programming data (*forward data telemetry*), and a modulator for sending the recorded signals and implant status to the external host (*reverse data telemetry*).

Daily increase in the complexity of IBMs leads to demand for sending higher power and data rates towards the implants. This is more obvious in high-density stimulating microsystems such as visual prostheses. Therefore, forward telemetry, which is the main focus of this chapter, has an important role in today's high-performance IBMs.

Design of RF links for power and data telemetry is usually performed based on both system-level aspects (i.e., functional architecture and physical structure), and power transfer efficiency and data rate requirements. This includes physical design of the link, carrier frequency and power of the RF signal, data rate, and also modulation scheme considered for forward and reverse data telemetry. It should be added that there are other important concerns that need to be studied in this area, such as safety levels for the exposure of the human body to electromagnetic waves.

This chapter begins with a discussion on limitations in the design of wireless links due to electromagnetic safety standards. Then, different types of wireless links are introduced and compared, following which, the trend towards multiple carrier links is highlighted. In

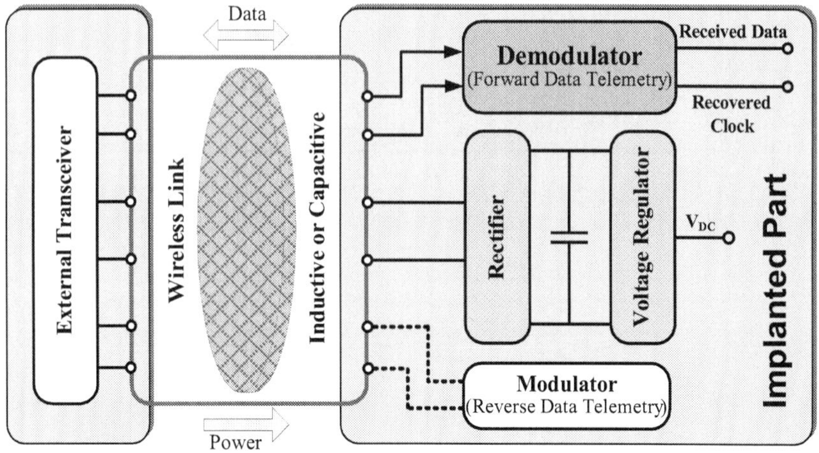

Fig. 1. General block diagram of the wireless interface.

forward data telemetry, commonly-used modulation schemes along with their pros and cons are studied. Finally, recent works on clock recovery and demodulator circuits are presented in detail.

2. Biological concerns

2.1 IEEE standard C95.1-2005

Electromagnetic fields generated by telemetry systems can potentially lead to power dissipation in living tissues and consequently cause damages to the tissue that are sometimes irreversible. Hence, when designing a device capable of wireless data exchange with the external world, it is an inseparable part of the designer's responsibility to make sure that the RF energy generated by the device fulfills the safety levels enforced by the standards for the exposure of human body to RF energy. This is a major concern in the design of wireless portable devices such as laptops and cell phones, and IBMs are not exceptions. Designer of a wireless link needs to make sure that potentially hazardous fields are not exceeded, as indicated in some electromagnetic safety standards. One of the well-known resources in this area is the IEEE standard for safety levels with respect to human exposure to radio frequency electromagnetic fields, 3 KHz to 300 GHz (IEEE Std C95.1-2005). This standard emphasizes that *radio frequency* (RF) exposure causes adverse health effects only when the exposure results in detrimental increase in the temperature of the core body or localized area of the body. For frequencies between 100 KHz and 3 GHz (which are used in most telemetry applications), *basic restrictions* (BRs) are expressed in terms of *specific absorption rate* (SAR) in the standard. This is, indeed, the power absorbed by (dissipated in) unit mass of tissue (Lazzi, 2005). At any point of the human body, SAR is related to the electric field as

$$\mathrm{SAR}(x,y,z) = \frac{\sigma(x,y,z)\,E^2(x,y,z)}{2\rho(x,y,z)} \tag{1}$$

where σ is the tissue conductivity (in S/m), ρ is the tissue density (Kg/m^3), and E is the electric field strength (V/m) at point (x,y,z). Consequently, the SI unit of SAR is Watt per kilogram (W/Kg). In Table 1, BRs for whole-body and localized exposure for both the people in *controlled environments* and the *general public* when an RF safety program is unavailable (*action level*), are shown. The localized exposure BRs are expressed in terms of *peak spatial-average SAR* which is the maximum local SAR averaged over any 10-grams of tissue in the shape of a cube.

<table>
<tr><td colspan="3" rowspan="2"></td><td colspan="2">SAR (W/Kg)</td></tr>
<tr><td>General public</td><td>Persons in controlled environments</td></tr>
<tr><td colspan="2">Whole-body exposure</td><td>Whole-Body Average (WBA)</td><td>0.08</td><td>0.4</td></tr>
<tr><td rowspan="2">Localized exposure</td><td>Localized</td><td rowspan="2">Peak spatial average</td><td>2</td><td>10</td></tr>
<tr><td>Extremities* & pinnae</td><td>4</td><td>20</td></tr>
<tr><td colspan="5">* The extremities are the arms and legs distal from the elbows and knees, respectively.</td></tr>
</table>

Table 1. BRs for frequencies between 100 KHz and 3 GHz (IEEE standard C95.1-2005).

It should be noted that due to the difficulty in calculation of SAR values and for convenience in exposure assessment, *maximum permissible exposures* (MPEs), which are sometimes called *investigation levels*, are provided in this IEEE standard (Table. 2). However, two issues must be kept in mind. First, compliance with this standard includes a determination that the SAR limits are not exceeded. This means that if an exposure is below the BRs, the MPEs can be exceeded. Second, in some exposure conditions, especially when the body is extremely close to an RF field source and in highly localized exposures (which is the case in IBMs), compliance with the MPEs may not ensure that the local SARs comply with the BRs. Therefore, for IBMs, SAR evaluation is necessary and the MPEs cannot be used.

Frequency range (MHz)	**RMS electric field strength (V/m)**	**RMS magnetic field strength (A/m)**
0.1-1.34	614	$16.3/f_M$
1.34-3	$823.8/f_M$ *	$16.3/f_M$
3-30	$823.8/f_M$	$16.3/f_M$
30-100	27.5	$158.3/f_M{}^{1.668}$
100-400	27.5	0.0729
* f_M is the frequency in MHz.		

Table 2. MPE for general public (IEEE standard C95.1-2005).

2.2 SAR calculation

In order to estimate the electric field and SAR in the human body, numerical methods of calculation can be used. One of the most commonly used numerical techniques for electromagnetic field dosimetry, is the *finite-difference time-domain* (FDTD) method, which is a direct solution of Maxwell's curl equations in the time domain. Most of electromagnetic simulators (e.g., SEMCAD X by SPEAG and CST Microwave Studio), in conjunction with computational human-body models, can perform FDTD and SAR calculations. In recent years, *three-dimensional* (3-D) whole body human models have been developed based on high-resolution *magnetic resonance imaging* (MRI) scans of healthy volunteers (Dymbylow, 2005; Christ et al., 2010). Providing a high level of anatomical details, these models play an important role in optimizing evaluation of electromagnetic exposures, e.g. in the human body models presented in (Christ et al., 2010) more than 80 different tissue types are distinguished.

3. Wireless links

3.1 Inductive links

The wireless link for forward power and data telemetry is mostly implemented by two closely-spaced, inductively coupled coils (Fig. 2). The secondary coil is implanted in the human body and the primary coil is kept outside. Usually these coils are a few millimeters apart, with thin layers of living tissues in between. In this approach, normally both sides of the link are tuned to the same resonant frequency to increase the power transmission efficiency (Sawan et al., 2005; Jow & Ghovanloo, 2009). This frequency is known as the carrier frequency and is limited to a few tens of megahertz for transferring relatively large amounts of energy to the implant. This is due to the fact that power dissipation in the tissue, which results in excessive temperature rise, increases as the carrier frequency squared (Lin, 1986). Employing low-frequency carriers is also supported by recent SAR calculations, e.g. in the telemetry link of an epiretinal prosthesis reported in (Singh et al., 2009), the SAR limit of the IEEE standard would be crossed around 16 MHz for a normalized peak current of 0.62 A in the primary coil. Thus, for power transmission, carrier frequencies of inductive links are typically chosen below 15 MHz (Jow & Ghovanloo, 2007 & 2009; Simard et al., 2010).

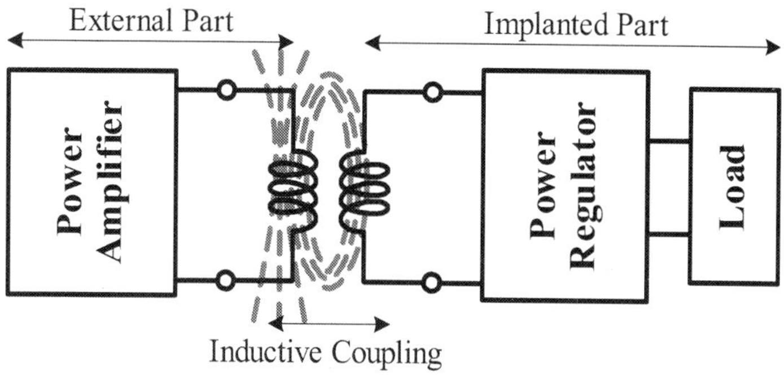

Fig. 2. General block diagram of an inductive power link

In order to convert the dc voltage of an external DC power supply (or battery) to a magnetic field, the primary coil is driven by a power amplifier, as illustrated in Fig. 3(a). In these biomedical applications, usually a class-E amplifier is used because of its high efficiency which is theoretically near 100% (Socal, 1975). As the coils are mutually coupled, magnetic field in the *primary coil* (L_1) induces an ac voltage on the *secondary coil* (L_2). This voltage is then rectified and regulated to generate the dc supply voltages required to operate the implanted electronics. To simplify the efficiency equations, usually the *mutual inductance* (M) of the coils is normalized with respect to L_1 and L_2 by defining K as the *coils coupling coefficient* (Jow and Ghovanloo; 2007)

$$K = \frac{M}{\sqrt{L_1 L_2}}. \tag{2}$$

Moreover, the rectifier, the regulator and the power consumption of all implanted circuits are modeled with an equivalent ac resistance R_L (Kendir et al., 2005; Van Schuglenbergh & Puers, 2009). A simplified schematic for an inductive link is shown in Fig. 3(a) for efficiency calculations. The resistor R_1 is a combination of *effective series resistance* (ESR) of L_1 (used to estimate coil losses) and the output resistance of the power amplifier, while R_2 is the ESR of L_2 (Liu et al., 2005; Harrison, 2007). The capacitors C_1 and C_2 are used to create a resonance on the primary and secondary sides of the link, respectively at

$$\omega_0 = \frac{1}{\sqrt{L_1 C_1}} = \frac{1}{\sqrt{L_2 C_2}}. \tag{3}$$

It is worth noting that C_2 is in fact a combination of the added capacitor and the parasitic capacitance of the secondary coil.

Efficiency of the secondary side of the link (η_2) can be calculated by transforming R_2 to its parallel equivalent at resonance, R_{P2} (Fig. 3(b))

$$R_{P2} = R_2 (1+Q_2^2) \approx Q_2^2 R_2 \tag{4}$$

where $Q_2=\omega_0 L_2/R_2$ is the *quality factor* of the unloaded-secondary circuit. In this case, R_L and R_{P2} both receive the same voltage and η_2 is given by

$$\eta_2 = \frac{R_{P2}}{R_{P2}+R_L} = \frac{Q_2}{Q_2+Q_L} \tag{5}$$

where $Q_L=\omega_0 R_L C_2=R_L/\omega_0 L_2$ is named as the *effective Q of the load network* (Baker & Sarpeshkar, 2007).

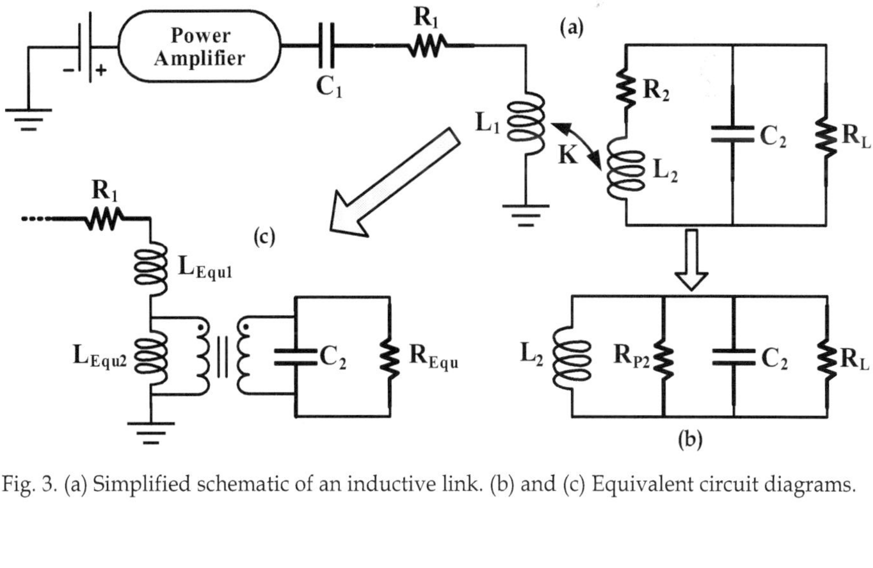

Fig. 3. (a) Simplified schematic of an inductive link. (b) and (c) Equivalent circuit diagrams.

To find the efficiency of the primary side of the link (η_1), first the coupling between the coils is modeled as an ideal transformer, and two inductances $L_{Equ1}=L_1\ (1-K^2)$ and $L_{Equ2}=K^2\ L_1$ (Fig. 3(c)) (Harrison, 2007). Then, C_2 and $R_{Equ}=R_L \| R_{P2}$ are reflected through the ideal transformer, resulting in values of $C_{Reflect}=(C_2/K^2)(L_2/L_1)$ and $R_{Reflect}=(K^2L_1/K_2)\ R_{Equ}$. As $C_{Reflect}$ and L_{Equ2} resonate at ω_0, η_1 can be defined as

$$\eta_1 = \frac{R_{Reflect}}{R_{Reflect}+R_1} = \frac{K^2Q_1Q_2}{1+K^2Q_1Q_2+\frac{R_{P2}}{R_L}} = \frac{K^2Q_1Q_2}{1+K^2Q_1Q_2+\frac{Q_2}{Q_L}} \quad (6)$$

where $Q_1=\omega_0L_1/R_1$ is the quality factor of the primary circuit in the absence of magnetic coupling. Therefore, total power efficiency for an inductive link is defined as:

$$\eta = \eta_1\eta_2 = \frac{K^2Q_1Q_2}{1+K^2Q_1Q_2+\frac{Q_2}{Q_L}} \times \frac{1}{1+\frac{Q_L}{Q_2}}. \quad (7)$$

Equation (7) shows that besides the loading network, η is affected by the coupling coefficient and the quality factors of the coils which are dependent on the coils' geometries, relative distance, and number of turns. For high efficiencies, both η_1 and η_2 should be maximized. This occurs when

$$1 << \frac{Q_2}{Q_L} = \frac{L_2}{R_L}\frac{1}{R_2C_2} << K^2Q_1Q_2 = \frac{K^2L_1}{L_2}\frac{1}{R_2C_2}. \quad (8)$$

However, in IBMs the coils are weakly coupled and K is typically below 0.4 (Kendir et al., 2005; Jow & Ghovanloo, 2009; Simard et al., 2010). Thus, depending on the application, the above conditions might not be satisfied and the overall link efficiency should be maximized with a different method. From equations (5) and (6), increasing Q_L decreases η_1 and increases η_2. This means that there is an optimum value for Q_L, for which the total efficiency is maximized (Baker & Sarpeshkar, 2007; Van Schuylenbergh &. Puers, 2009). In other words, one can determine an optimum loading condition that maximizes the total efficiency. By differentiating (7) with respect to Q_L, the optimum Q_L can be found as

$$Q_{L,opt} = \frac{Q_2}{\sqrt{1+K^2Q_1Q_2}}. \quad (9)$$

Consequently, maximum achievable efficiency is given by

$$\eta_{Max} = \frac{K^2Q_1Q_2}{(1+\sqrt{1+K^2Q_1Q_2})^2} \quad (10)$$

and is plotted as a function of $K^2Q_1Q_2$ in Fig. 4.

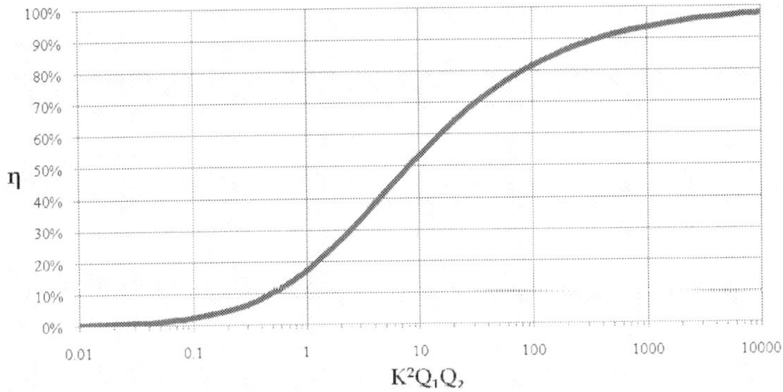

Fig. 4. Maximum achievable link efficiency as a function of $K^2Q_1Q_2$

Wire wound coils have been employed in IBM inductive links for many years. These coils are made of filament wires in the form of a single or multiple individually insulated strands twisted into circular shapes (Litz wires) which reduce the coil losses at high frequencies (Jow & Ghovanloo, 2007). To achieve higher efficiencies, mutual inductance between the primary and secondary coils can be increased by utilizing ferrite cores (Sodagar et al., 2009b). However, as illustrated in Fig. 5(a), with both air cores and ferromagnetic cores, the use of regular coils has a major drawback: Magnetic flux lines are formed around the primary coil as a result of the flow of current through it. They close their paths through the air and spread all around the coil. Therefore, the implanted sensitive analog circuitry is exposed to a major portion of the electromagnetic energy radiated by the primary coil. To reduce the electromagnetic interferences caused by inductive coupling, use of E-shape cores is proposed in (Sodagar et al., 2009b). As shown in Fig. 5(b), primary and secondary coils are wrapped across the cores' middle fingers. This method helps confine the electromagnetic flux within the ferrite cores by forming a closed magnetic circuit through which it can flow. The flux can only radiate some energy to the outside when it passes through the inevitable gap between the two coils. Fig. 5(c) shows a photograph of the coils used to power up a multichannel neural recording system utilizing this technique, which is presented in (Sodagar et al., 2009b). The E-shape ferrite coils are 5.4 mm × 2 mm × 2.7 mm (L×W×H) with the middle finger and the side fingers 1.5 mm and 0.7 mm thick, respectively.

Inductive links can also be implemented by employing *printed spiral coils* (PSCs). As wire-wound coils cannot be batch-fabricated or shrunk down in size without the use of sophisticated machinery (Jow & Ghovanloo, 2007), PSCs have drawn a lot of attention in recent years. Such planar coils are produced using standard photolithographic and micro fabrication techniques on flexible or rigid substrates. Thus, the geometrics of PSCs, which are important factors in the link power efficiency, can be accurately defined. A typical square-shaped PSC is shown in Fig. 6, in which D_o and D_i are the outer and inner diameters of the coil, W is the width of the tracks, and S is the track spacing. Because of size constraints, usually the outer diameter of implanted coils is limited to 10 mm, while the external coils might have larger diameters, depending on the application (Shah et al., 1998; Jow & Ghovanloo, 2007). Classically, in IBMs power and data are transferred through the same wireless link, with the data modulated on the same carrier used for power transfer. However, power transfer is more efficient with high-Q coils, while in many applications

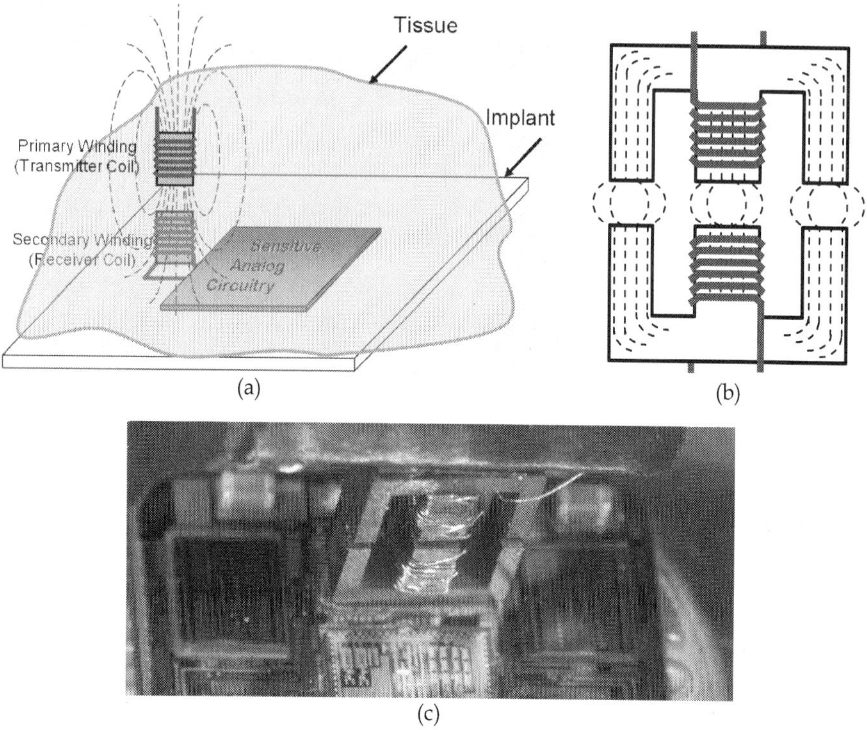

Fig. 5. (a) Problem of magnetic flux with regular coils. (b) Confining the magnetic flux by forming a closed magnetic circuit. (c) Implementation of the idea in (b) on the implantable device presented by (Sodagar et al., 2009b).

such as retinal implants, wideband data transfer is needed, demanding for low quality factors of the coils. Due to contradictory requirements of power and data transfer, there is a trend towards utilizing multiple carrier links in which separate coils are designed for power and data (Ghovanloo & Alturi, 2007; Jow & Ghovanloo, 2008; Simard et al., 2010). These links typically take advantage of PSCs for power transmission. As the data carrier amplitude is much smaller than the power carrier, crosstalk becomes an important issue in multiple carrier links design. Different geometries and orientations of data coils have been reported for solving this problem. In (Jow & Ghovanloo, 2008) vertical and figure-8 data coils are proposed to reduce the cross coupling between power and data coils. Vertical coils are wound across the diameter of the power PSCs, while figure-8 types are implemented as PSCs in the same substrate of the power PSCs and parallel to them. Results show that vertical coils attenuate the power carrier interference more, when the coils are perfectly aligned. On the other hand, figure-8 coils are less sensitive to horizontal misalignments. In (Simard et al., 2010) another geometry named coplanar geometry is presented. Based on the results, in comparison with vertical and figure-8 coils, this approach provides better immunity to crosstalk under misalignments. However, as the total area of the wireless link is increased, it might not be usable in some applications.

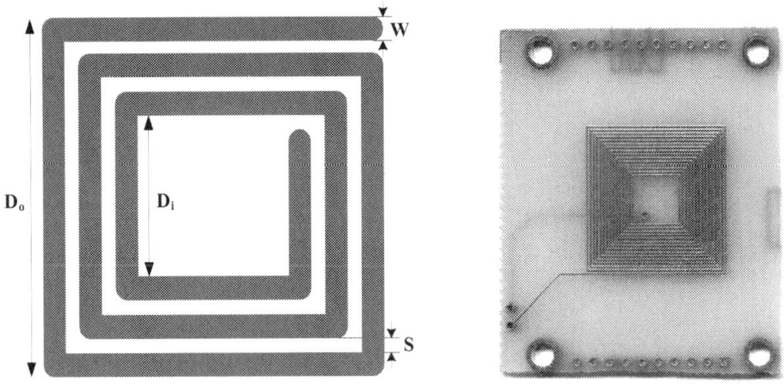

Fig. 6. Typical squared-shaped PSCs. (a) Important geometrical parameters. (b). A prototype fabricated on a *printed circuit board (PCB).*

Multiple carrier architectures allow designing and optimizing power and data links separately and based on their own specific requirements. As a result, optimized data links for different modulation techniques have been reported (Ghovanloo & Alturi, 2007; Simard et al., 2010). Furthermore, by increasing the quality factors of the power coils, efficiencies as high as 72% has been achieved (Jow & Ghovanloo, 2009).

3.2 Capacitive links

Although capacitive coupling has been already used for inter-chip data communication (Canegallo et al., 2007; Fazzi et al., 2008) and even for power transfer (Culurciello & Andreou, 2006), it was studied for implantable biomedical applications in (Sodagar & Amiri, 2009) for the first time. This method is based on capacitive coupling between two parallel plates. One of the plates is placed on the implant side and the other is attached to the skin on the external side. The plates are aligned to have maximum overlapping, while the skin and thin layers of tissue act as dielectric. In this approach, electric field is used as the carrier for power and data, contrary to the traditional inductive approach where magnetic field plays the key role. As illustrated in Fig. 7, the field lines defining the RF energy conveying power and data in capacitive links are well confined within the area considered for this purpose. This helps extremely reduce or even eliminate the relatively large electromagnetic interference on the sensitive analog circuitry in the system. A significant side benefit of this energy confinement is that several power, data and clock signals can be exchanged between the implant and the external setup without interfering with each other even at the same frequencies. Moreover, another important advantage of capacitive links is that they are naturally compatible with standard *integrated circuit* (IC) fabrication technologies.

A simplified schematic of a capacitive link is shown in Fig. 8, where V_{ext} is the input voltage, C_{Body1} and C_{Body2} are the capacitances between the implanted and external plates, C_{in} is the equivalent input capacitance of the circuits directly connected to the link, and R_L is the equivalent ac resistance of the loading network. The voltage received on the implant side, V_{int}, is determined as

$$V_{int} = V_{ext}\left[\frac{R_L^2(1+P)}{R_L^2(1+P)^2 + X_{Ceq}^2} + j\frac{R_L X_{Ceq}}{R_L^2(1+P)^2 + X_{Ceq}^2}\right] \tag{11}$$

where X_{Ceq} is the reactance of $C_{eq}=C_{Body1}+C_{Body2}$, and $P=C_{in}/C_{eq}$. Assuming $C_{in}<<C_{eq}$, equation (11) becomes

$$V_{int} = V_{ext}\left(\frac{R_L^2}{R_L^2 + X_{Ceq}^2} + j\frac{R_L X_{Ceq}}{R_L^2 + X_{Ceq}^2}\right), \tag{12}$$

and the voltage transfer rate is given by

$$\left|\frac{V_{int}}{V_{ext}}\right| = \sqrt{\frac{R_L^2}{R_L^2 + X_{Ceq}^2}}. \tag{13}$$

Thus, V_{int} is maximized when $X_{Ceq}<<R_L$.

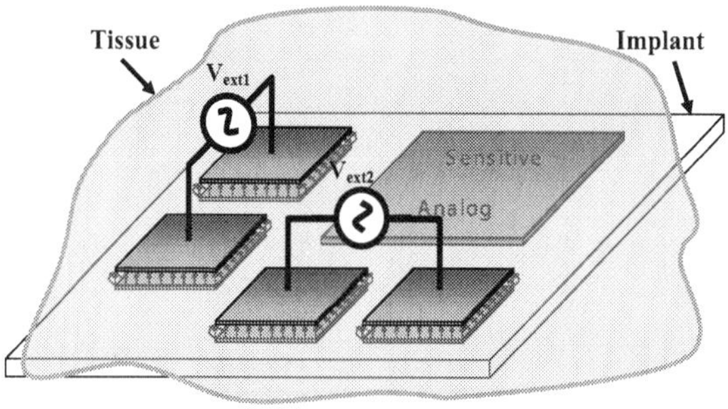

Fig. 7. Energy confinement in the capacitive coupling approach.

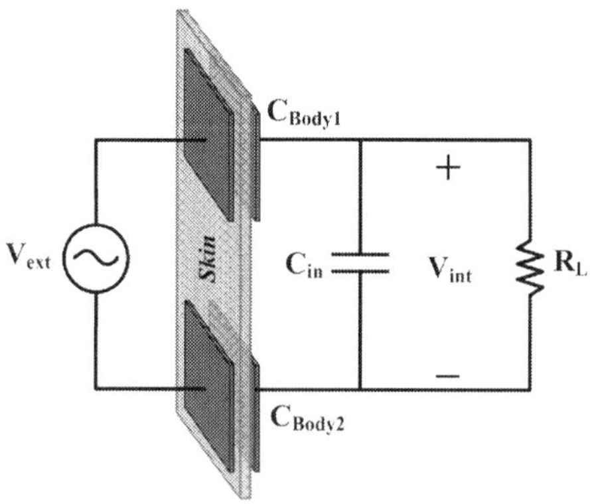

Fig. 8. Simplified schematic of a capacitive link.

Unit capacitances and reactance of 1 mm × 1 mm parallel plates 1 mm apart from each other are calculated and plotted in Figs. 9 and 10 for frequencies between 100 kHz and 10 MHz. Calculations are based on the dielectric properties of biological tissues at RF and microwave frequencies reported in (Gabriel et al., 1996a, b & c), which are also available as an internet resource by the *Italian National Research Council, Institute for Applied Physics* (IFAC). Fig. 9 shows that, in general, unit capacitances of the skin and muscle decrease with the frequency. However, as illustrated in Fig. 10, unit reactance of dry skin decreases as the frequency increases, while unit reactances of wet skin and muscle are almost constant and only change about 20% over the frequency range 1 MHz - 10 MHz.

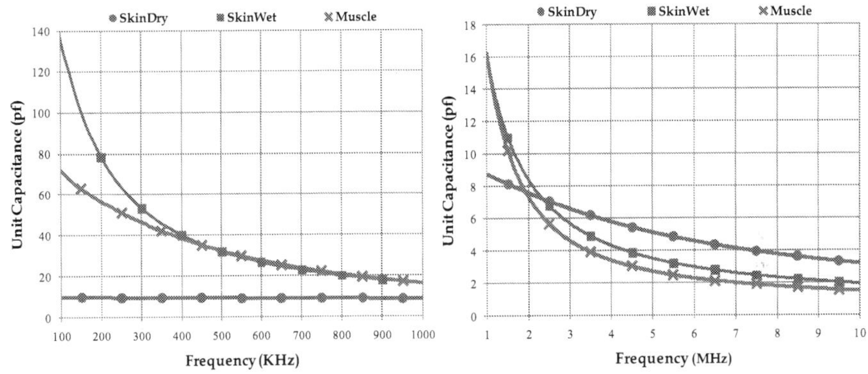

(a) (b)

Fig. 9. Unit capacitance of 1 mm × 1 mm plates 1 mm apart from each other for frequencies between (a) 100 kHz and 1 MHz, and (b) 1 MHz and 10 MHz

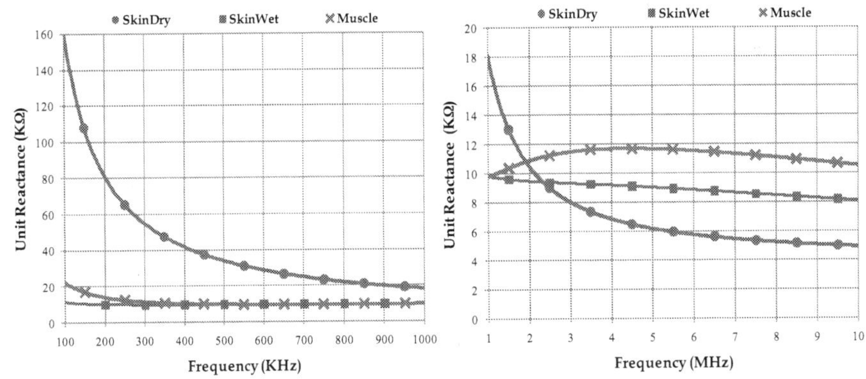

(a) (b)

Fig. 10. Unit reactance of 1 mm × 1 mm plates 1 mm apart from each other for frequencies between (a) 100 kHz and 1 MHz, and (b) 1 MHz and 10 MHz

According to Equation (13) R_L plays a key role in the voltage transfer rate of a capacitive link. Hence, it is of crucial importance to note that the value of R_L for power transfer through a telemetry link is completely different from the case where the link is used for data telemetry. Thus, similarly to inductive links, it is more practical to use the multiple carrier approach, and design each link separately. In data links, C_{Body1} and C_{Body2} are connected to high-impedance nodes, such as inputs of voltage buffers or comparators (Asgarian & Sodagar, 2010). This implies that even with small plates, voltage transfer rates close to 1 can be achieved. For instance, 2 mm × 2 mm plates 3 mm apart from each other result in a X_{Ceq} less than 4 kΩ (assuming dry skin as the dielectric), which is relatively much smaller than R_L in data links. On the other hand, in power transmission R_L is typically below 10 kΩ modeling substantial current draw from the power source. To optimize the voltage gain, X_{Ceq} should be kept as low as possible. This is achieved by choosing larger plates, while still complying with the implant size constraints. As an example, with dry skin as the dielectric and 5 mm × 5 mm plates 3 mm apart from each other, X_{Ceq} and voltage transfer rate are about 0.6 kΩ and 95%, respectively, for R_L=2 kΩ.

4. Data transfer to biomedical implants

4.1 Modulation schemes

Regardless of the type of the telemetry link, data needs to be modulated onto a carrier for wireless transmission. Forward data telemetry should be capable of providing a relatively high data rate, especially in applications where the implant interfaces with the central nervous system such as visual prostheses (Ghovanloo & Najafi, 2004). On the other hand, as discussed before, there are limitations on increasing the carrier frequency for implantable devices. Therefore, *data-rate-to-carrier-frequency (DRCF) ratio* is introduced as an important measure, indicating the amount of data successfully modulated on a certain carrier frequency. From among the different types of modulation schemes available for wireless data transfer, digital modulation techniques including *amplitude shift keying* (ASK), *frequency shift keying* (FSK), and *phase shift keying* (PSK) are more commonly used in IBMs. These modulations are illustrated in Fig. 11.

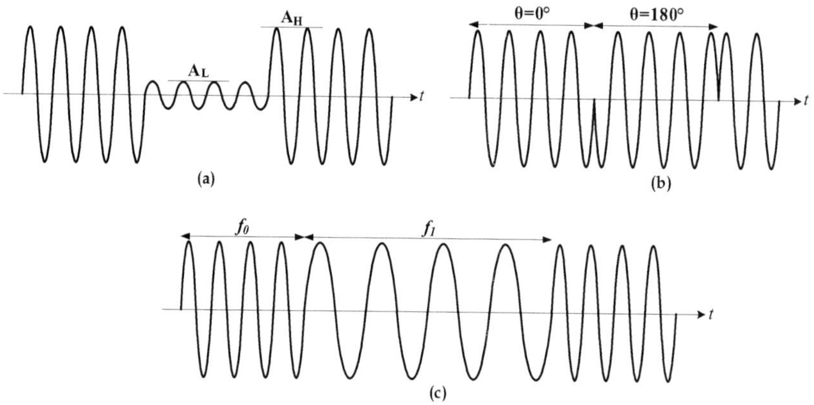

Fig. 11. Digital modulation schemes: (a) ASK, (b) PSK, and (c) FSK.

Although ASK has been used in some early works due to its simple modulation and demodulation circuitry, it suffers from low data rate transmission and high sensitivity to amplitude noise (Sodagar & Najafi, 2006; Razavi, 1998). In FSK, employing two different carrier frequencies limits the data rate to the lower frequency and consequently decreases the DRCF ratio. In contrast with FSK, PSK benefits from fixed carrier frequency and provide data rates as high as the carrier frequency (DRCF=100%).

In terms of *bit error rate* (BER), PSK exhibits considerable advantage over FSK and ASK at the same amplitude levels. This can be easily shown by plotting signal constellations or signal spaces for different modulation techniques (Fig. 12), and considering the fact that BER is mostly affected by the points with the minimum Cartesian distance in a constellation (Razavi, 1998). Additionally, a detailed analysis of two types of PSK modulation, *binary PSK* (BPSK) and *quadrature PSK* (QPSK) is given in (Razavi, 1998), which shows that they have nearly equal probabilities of error if the transmitted power, bit rate, and the differences between the bit energy and symbol energy are taken into account.

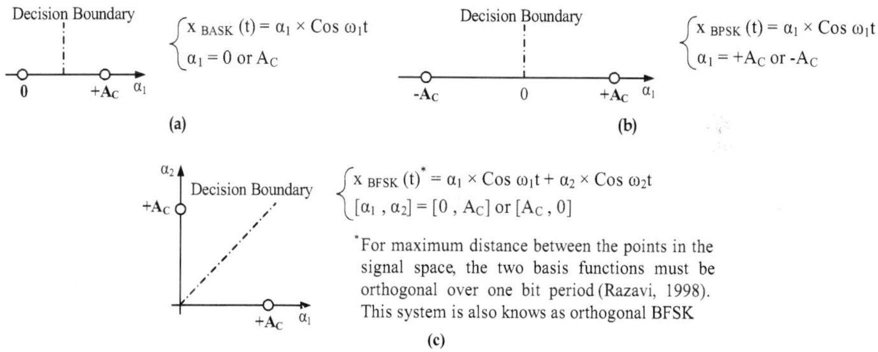

Fig. 12. Signal constellation of binary (a) ASK, (b) PSK, and (c) FSK modulations.

4.2 Data and clock recovery circuits

4.2.1 Amplitude Shift Keying (ASK)

One of the first techniques employed for digital data modulation in IBMs is ASK. In this technique, two carrier amplitude levels are assigned to logic levels "0" and "1", as illustrated in Fig. 11(a). Perhaps it was the straightforward implementation of both modulators and demodulators for ASK that attracted the interest of designers to this modulation scheme. To facilitate detection of ASK-modulated data on the receiver end and reduce the possibility of having errors in data transfer, there should be enough distinction between the two amplitude levels associated with 0's and 1's, A_L and A_H, respectively. *Modulation index (depth)* is a measure for this distinction, which is defined for ASK as:

$$m\% = \frac{A_H - A_L}{A_H} \times 100\% \tag{14}$$

It is, however, the nature of amplitude modulation techniques, e.g., AM for analog and ASK for digital, that makes them susceptible to noise. To overcome this weakness, modulation index is chosen as high as possible.

When used only for data telemetry (not for power telemetry), whether from the implant to the outside world or vice versa, ASK modulation index can be increased to even 100%. This extreme for ASK, also referred to as *On-Off Keying* (OOK), obviously exhibits the best robustness against noise in ASK. A side benefit for increasing the modulation index to 100% is the power saving achieved by not spending energy to transmit logical 0's to the outside. Examples of using OOK only for data telemetry are (Yu & Bashirullah, 2006; Sodagar, et al, 2006 & 2009a).

Early attempts in designing IBM wireless links for both power and data telemetry employed ASK technique for modulation. The functional neuromuscular stimulator microsystem designed by (Akin & Najafi, 1994) is an example of a complete system that wirelessly receives power and data from the outside and returns backward data to the outside all using ASK modulation. Although ASK was successfully used for both power and data telemetry in several works (Von-Arx & Najafi, 1998; Yu & Najafi, 2001; Coulombe et al., 2003), it could not satisfy the somehow conflicting requirements for efficient telemetry of power and data at the same time. One of such conflicts can be explained as follows: The power regulator block needs to be designed to work desirably even when the amplitude received through the link is at A_L. For this purpose, A_L should be high enough to provide sufficient overhead voltage on top of the regulated voltage. On the other hand, it was explained before that A_H needs to be well above A_L in order to result in a high-quality data transfer, i.e., a low BER. This leads to two major problems:

- From the circuit design viewpoint, the regulator needs to be strong enough to suppress the large amplitude fluctuations associated with switchings between A_L and A_H. Not only these fluctuations are large in amplitude, they are also low in frequency as compared to the carrier frequency. This makes the design of the regulator challenging, especially if it is expected to be fully integrated.
- A_H values much higher than A_L are not welcomed from the standpoint of tissue safety either. This is because at A_H the amount of the power transferred through the tissue is much higher than what the system needs to receive (already guaranteed by the carrier energy at A_L).

Although ASK technique is a possible candidate for reverse data telemetry in the same way as the other modulation techniques are, it is a special choice in passive reverse telemetry. In this method, also known as *Load-Shift Keying* (LSK), reverse data is transferred back to the external host through the same link used for forward telemetry. While the forward data is modulated on the amplitude, frequency, or phase of the incoming carrier, backward data is modulated on the energy drawn through the link. The backward data is simply detected from the current flowing through the primary coil on the external side of the inductive link. What happens in the LSK method is, indeed, ASK modulation of the reverse data on the energy transferred through the link or on the current through the primary coil.

4.2.1 Frequency Shift Keying (FSK)

Three FSK demodulators are studied in (Ghovanloo & Najafi, 2004) that employ two carrier frequencies f_1 and $f_0=2f_1$ to transmit logic "1" and "0" levels, respectively. As a result, the minimum bit-time is $1/f_1$ and data rates higher than f_1 cannot be achieved. Moreover, by considering the average frequency as $(f_1+f_0)/2$, the DRCF ratio is limited to 67%. In all three circuits, FSK data is transmitted using a phase-coherent protocol, in which both of the carrier frequencies have a fixed phase at the start of each bit-time (Fig. 13). Whether a zero or 180° phase offset is chosen for sinusoidal FSK symbols, data bits are detected on the receiver side by measuring the period of each received carrier cycle. In this case, every single long period (a single cycle of f_1) represents a "1" bit and every two successive short periods (two cycles of f_0) indicate a "0" bit. As illustrated in Fig. 14, in the demodulators reported by (Ghovanloo & Najafi, 2004), the received FSK carrier first passes through a clock regenerator block, which squares up the analog sinusoidal carrier. For period or, in general, time measurement in FSK demodulation, both analog and digital approaches have been examined.

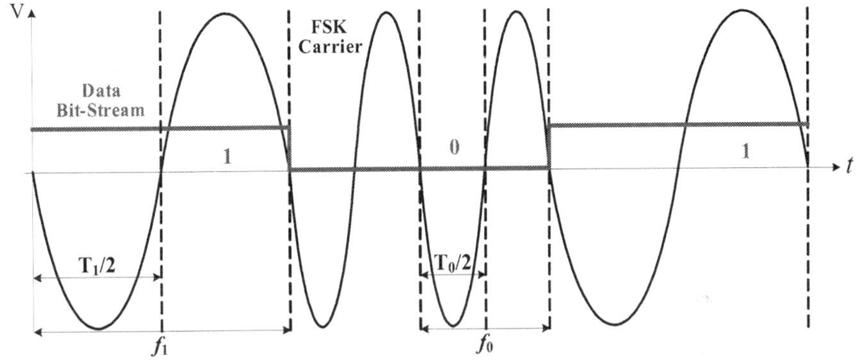

Fig. 13. Phase-coherent BFSK Modulation.

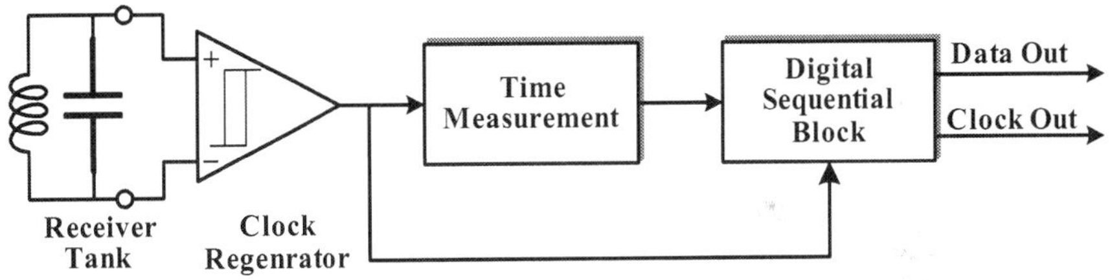

Fig. 14. General block diagram of the demodulators presented in (Ghovanloo & Najfi, 2004)

The analog approach is based on charging a capacitor with a constant current to examine if its voltage exceeds a certain threshold level (logic "1" detection) or not (logic "0" detection). In this method, charging and discharging the capacitor should be controlled by the logic levels of the digitized FSK carrier. The demodulator, in which the capacitor voltage is compared with a constant reference voltage, is known as *referenced differential FSK* (RDFSK) demodulator. On the other hand, in *fully differential FSK* (FDFSK) demodulator, two unequal capacitors are charged with different currents, and their voltages are compared by a Schmitt trigger comparator.

In the *digital FSK* (DFSK) demodulator scheme, duration of carrier cycles is measured with a 3-bit counter, which only runs at the first halves of the carrier cycles (i.e., during $T_1/2$ and $T_0/2$). The final count value of the counter is then compared with a constant reference number to determine whether a short or long period cycle has been received. The counter clock, which is provided by a 5-stage ring oscillator, is several times higher than f_0, and should be chosen in such a way that the counter can discriminate between $T_1/2=1/(2f_1)$ and $T_0/2=1/(4f_1)$ time periods.

In all the three demodulators, the output of the comparator is fed into a digital block to generate the received data bit-stream. Additionally, detection of a long carrier cycle or two successive short carrier cycles in every bit-time is used along with the digitized FSK carrier to extract a constant frequency clock.

Measurement results of the three circuits in (Ghovanloo & Najafi, 2004) indicate that with 5 and 10 MHz carrier frequencies over a wideband inductive link, the DFSK demodulator has the highest data rate (2.5 Mbps) and the lowest power consumption. At lower carrier frequencies, however, since the current required to charge the capacitor in the RDFSK method can be very small, the RDFSK circuit might be more power efficient. On the other hand, due to the fact that the FDFSK demodulator benefits from a differential architecture, it is more robust against process variations. It should be noted that the inductive link used in (Ghovanloo & Najafi, 2004) was designed for both power and data transfer. Hence, data rate for the DFSK demodulator was limited to 2.5 Mbps in order to comply with the limited wireless link bandwidth set for efficient power transfer. In other words, the DFSK method would be capable of providing data rates as high as 5 Mbps (equal to the lower carrier frequency) if the link was designed merely for data telemetry.

4.2.3 Phase Shift Keying (PSK)

Recently, PSK modulation with constant amplitude symbols and fixed carrier frequency has attracted great attention in designing wireless links for IBMs (Zhou & Liu, 2007; Asgarian & Sodagar, 2009b; Simard et al., 2010). Demodulators based on both coherent and noncoherent schemes have been reported. In coherent detection, phase synchronization between the received signal and the receiver, called carrier recovery, is needed (Razavi, 1998). Therefore, noncoherent detectors are generally less complex and have wider usage in RF applications in spite of their higher BERs (Razavi, 1998). Coherent BPSK demodulators are mostly implemented by the COSTAS loop technique (Fig. 15), which is made up of two parallel *phase-locked-loops* (PLL). In Fig. 15, *d(t)* represents the transmitted data ("1" or "-1"), θ_1 is the received carrier phase, θ_2 is the phase of the oscillator output, and the upper and lower branches are called *in-phase* and *quadrature-phase* branches, respectively. In this method the goal is to control the local oscillator with a signal that is independent of the data stream (d(t)) and is only proportional to the *phase error* (θ_1-θ_2). In the locked state, phase error is approximately zero and the demodulated data is the output of the in-phase branch.

In order to reduce the complexity of conventional COSTAS-loop-based BPSK demodulators, nowadays, they are mainly designed by digital techniques such as filtering, phase shifting, and digital control oscillators (Sawan et al., 2005). Employing these techniques and inspiring from digital PLLs, a coherent BPSK demodulator is proposed in (Hu & Sawan, 2005). It is shown that the circuit behaves as a second-order linear PLL, and its natural frequency and damping factor are also calculated. Maximum data rate of the demodulator depends on the lock-in time of the loop which is determined by the natural frequency (Hu & Sawan, 2005). Increasing the natural frequency may decrease the damping factor and affect the dynamic performance of the system. Therefore, the maximum data rate measured for a 10-MHz carrier frequency is 1.12 Mbps, which results in a DRCF ratio of only 11.2% for this circuit. This idea is then evolved into a QPSK demodulator in (Deng et al., 2006) to achieve higher data rates. Moreover, improved version of the QPSK demodulator is studied in (Lu &

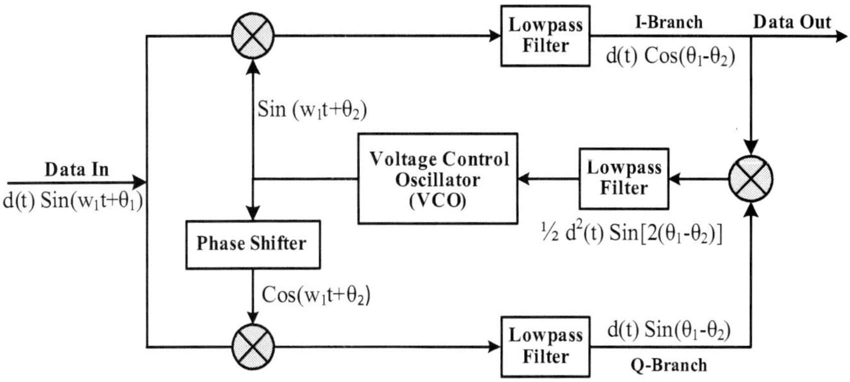

Fig. 15. COSTAS loop for BPSK demodulation.

Sawan, 2008) and is tested with a multiple carrier inductive link and a carrier frequency of 13.56 MHz in (Simard et al., 2010). According to the experimental results, maximum data rate and DRCF ratio for this circuit are 4.16 Mbps and about 30%, respectively.

Noncoherent BPSK demodulators can be implemented much simpler than coherent ones. Fig. 16 shows the general block diagram of two types of these demodulators presented in (Gong et al., 2008) and (Asgarian & Sodagar, 2009a). The received analog carrier first passes through a 1-bit *analog-to-digital converter* (ADC). Then, the *digitized carrier* (*BPSK*) is fed into the edge detection block, which contains two D flip-flops. By defining two sinusoidal waveforms with 180° phase difference associated with "0" and "1" symbols, this block can easily detect the received data based on either rising (logic "1") or falling (logic "0") edges of the digitized signal. Additionally, as both rising and falling edges occur in the middle of the symbol time ($T_{BPSK}/2$), detection of either edge can be used as a reference in the clock and data recovery unit in order to extract a clock signal from the received carrier and reconstruct the desired bit stream. Obviously, it is necessary to reset the D flip-flops after each detection, but it should also be noted that between any two (or more) consecutive similar symbols an edge occurs that should not be detected as a change in the received data. Hence, for proper operation of the demodulator, a reset signal is needed after each symbol time is over and before the edge of the next symbol (which takes place in the middle of it). For this purpose, in (Gong et al., 2008) a capacitor is connected to a Schmitt trigger comparator, whose output is the required reset signal. After each edge detection, this capacitor is charged towards the switching point of the comparator. Thus, its voltage rise time, which should have a value greater than $0.5T_{BPSK}$ and smaller than T_{BPSK}, is chosen to be $0.75T_{BPSK}$ in (Gong et al., 2008).

Another method of generating the reset signal is proposed by (Asgarian & Sodagar, 2009a), in which a 3-bit asynchronous counter has been designed in such a way that it starts counting after the detection of each edge. The *most significant bit* (MSB) of the counter goes high between $0.5T_{BPSK}$ and T_{BPSK}, and resets the D flip-flops. A free running 5-stage ring oscillator generates a *clock signal* (f_{osc}), which is used to prepare the clock of the counter. The oscillator frequency range is determined by the required activation time of the reset signal. As shown in Fig. 17, considering the two worst cases, the following conditions should be met

$$3T_{osc} > 0.5T_{BPSK}, \tag{14a}$$

and

$$4T_{osc} < T_{BPSK}\,. \tag{14b}$$

Therefore, frequency of the oscillator can be chosen between $4f_{BPSK}$ and $6f_{BPSK}$, which is set to $5f_{BPSK}$ in (Asgarian & Sodagar, 2009a).

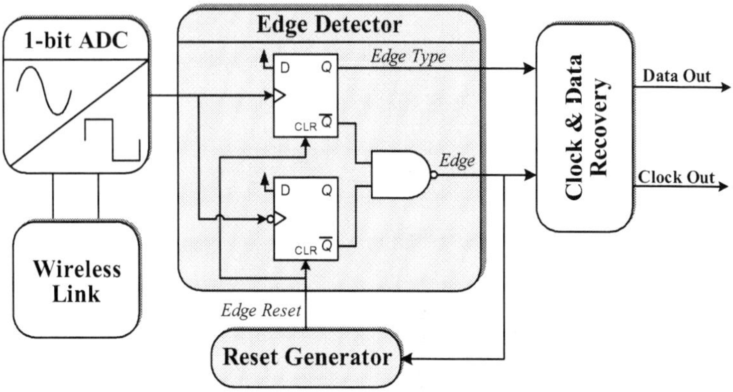

Fig. 16. General block diagram of two noncoherent demodulators presented in (Gong et al., 2008) and (Asgarian & Sodagar, 2009a).

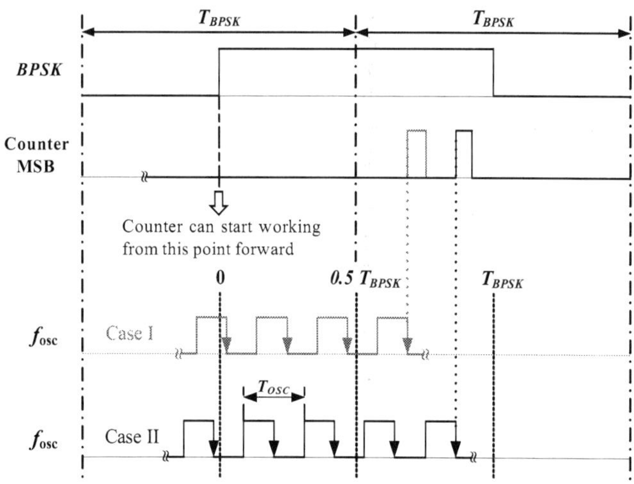

Fig. 17. Two worst cases for determining the range of f_{osc} in (Asgarian & Sodagar, 2009a)

Both of the described noncoherent BPSK demodulators have much lower power consumption than their coherent counterparts. Moreover, they can provide data rates equal to the carrier frequency provided that phase shifts are propagated through the wireless link quickly. In inductive links, this usually requires a low quality factor for the resonant circuits on the primary and secondary sides of the link (Fig. 3), which leads to higher power dissipation. In (Wang et al., 2005) a PSK transmitter with Q-independent phase transition time is reported. The circuit, however, only modulates the phase of the carrier within two carrier cycles. Due to these limitations, experimental results of the demodulator studied in (Gong et al., 2008) with an inductive link, shows a DRCF ratio of only 20%. Similarly to the DFSK demodulator, this again emphasizes that in order to take advantage of the maximum demodulator speed, optimization of the data link in multiple carrier topologies is essential.

Most of the demodulators designed for IBMs can only operate with a specific carrier frequency, while their DRCF ratio is constant. In other words, at least one part of these circuits is dependent to the frequency of the modulated signal. For instance, in analog FSK demodulators (Ghovanloo & Najafi, 2004) and (Gong et al., 2008) the values of capacitors are determined based on the carrier frequency, or in (Hu & Sawan, 2005; Simard et al., 2010) the voltage controlled oscillator (VCO) is designed to work with a modulated carrier of 13.56 MHz. In (Asgarian & Sodagar, 2010) a *carrier-frequency-independent BPSK* (CFI-BPSK) demodulator is presented (Fig. 18). Similarly to (Asgarian & Sodagar, 2009a), the received data are detected based on rising or falling edge of the digitized carrier, while a new reset mechanism is proposed. As shown in Fig. 19, the required *reset signal* (*EdgeReset*) is generated by employing two *different digitized waveforms* (*BPSK+* and *BPSK-*) of the received analog carrier. In this method, *EdgeReset* is activated after a falling edge occurs in both *BPSK+* and *BPSK-* signals, and disabled with the first rising edge (or high level) of either *BPSK+* or *BPSK-*. In order to fulfill these requirements, the reset generator is composed of a clipping circuit, and a control and edge detection block (Fig. 18). Experimental results of a prototype in (Asgarian & Sodagar, 2010) indicate that this circuit can achieve a DRCF ratio of 100% with capacitive links, while all of its components are independent of the carrier frequency.

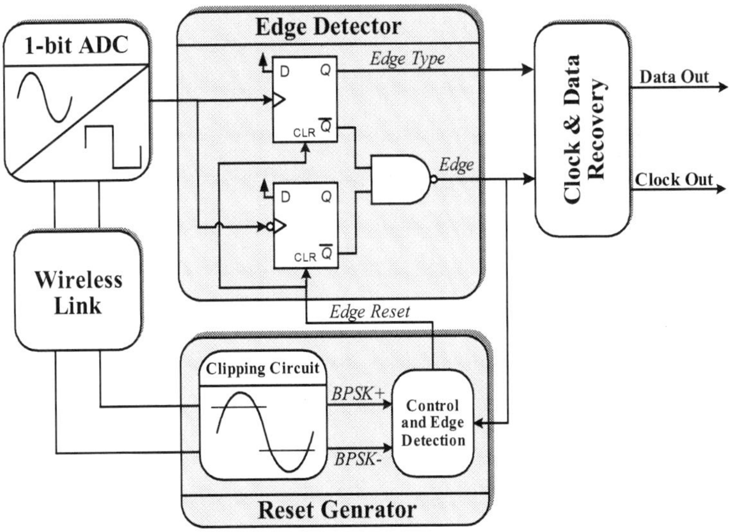

Fig. 18. Block diagram of the CFI-BPSK demodulator (Asgarian & Sodagar, 2010).

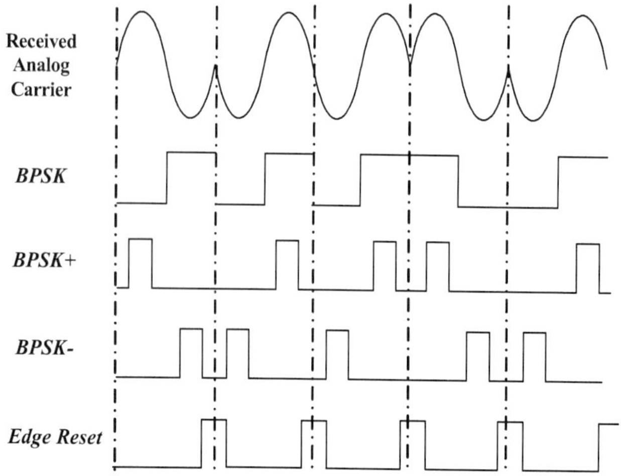

Fig. 19. Generating *EdgeReset* from the sinusoidal carrier in CFI-BPSK demodulator.

5. Conclusion

Wireless telemetry is one of the most important parts of IBMs, as it provides them with the power they require to operate, and also enables them to communicate with the external world wirelessly. Traditionally, wireless interfaces are implemented by inductive links. However, recently, employing capacitive links has been introduced as an alternative. Additionally, due to conflicting requirements of power and data telemetry, researches are mainly focused on utilizing multiple carrier or multiband links in both inductive and capacitive approaches. Besides size constraints, power dissipation in the human body is a key issue, especially in power telemetry where it may lead to excessive temperature increase in biological tissues. Hence, RF energy absorptions resulted from electromagnetic fields available in telemetry systems, should be evaluated by taking advantage of 3-D human body models and computational methods. In regards with forward data telemetry, recent works indicate that noncoherent BPSK demodulators are among the best choices for high data rate biomedical applications. These circuits are capable of providing DRCF ratios of up to 100%, provided that the link propagates phase shifts rapidly. This implies that the main speed limiting factor is going to be the wireless link and not the demodulator circuitry. Therefore, further optimization is needed in designing data links, where the capacitive method can potentially be a good solution.

6. References

Akin, T. & Najafi, K. (1998). A telemetrically powered and controlled implantable neural recording system with CMOS interface circuitry, *Proceedings of 7th Mediterranean Electrotechnical Conf.*, Vol. 2, pp. 545-548, Antalya, Apr. 1994.

Asgarian, F. & Sodagar, A.M. (2009a). A high-data-rate low-power BPSK demodulator and clock recovery circuit for implantable biomedical devices, *Proceedings of 4th Int. IEEE/EMBS Conf. Neural Eng.*, pp. 407-410, Antalya, Apr. 29–May 2, 2009.

Asgarian, F. & Sodagar, A.M. (2009b). A low-power noncoherent BPSK demodulator and clock recovery circuit for high-data-rate biomedical applications, *Proceedings of 31st Int. Conf. IEEE/EMBS*, pp. 4840-4843, Minnesota, Sep. 2009.

Asgarian, F. & Sodagar, A.M. (2010). A carrier frequency independent BPSK demodulator with 100% data-rate-to-carrier-frequency ratio, *Proceedings of IEEE Bio. Circuits and Systems Conf. (BioCAS)*, pp. 29-32, Paphos, Nov. 2010.

Baker, M.W. & Sarpeshkar, R. (2007). Feedback analysis and design of RF power links for low-power bionic systems, *IEEE Trans. Bio. Circuits and Systems*, Vol. 1, No. 1, Mar. 2007, pp. 28-38.

Canegallo, R.; Fazzi, A.; Ciccarelli, L.; Magagni, L.; Natali, F.; Rolandi, P.L.; Jung, E.; Di Cioccio, L. & Guerrieri, R. (2007). 3D capacitive interconnections for high speed interchip communication, *Proceedings of IEEE Custom Integrated Circuits Conf. (CICC)*, pp. 1-8, San Jose, Sept. 2007.

Christ, A.; Kainz, W.; Hahn, E.G.; Honegger, K.; Zefferer, M.; Neufeld, E.; Rascher, W.; Janka, R.; Bautz, W.; Chen, J.; Kiefer, B.; Schmitt, P.; Hollenbach, H.P.; Shen, J.; Oberle, M.; Szczerba, D.; Kam, A.; Guag, J.W. & Kuster, N. (2010). The Virtual Family—development of surface-based anatomical models of two adults and two children for dosimetric simulations, *Phys. Med. Biol.*, Vol. 55, No. 2, Jan. 2010, pp. 23-38.

Coulombe, J.; Gervais, J.-F. & Sawan, M. (2003). A cortical stimulator with monitoring capabilities using a novel 1 Mbps ASK data link, *Proceedings of IEEE Int. Symp. Circuits and Systems (ISCAS)*, Vol. 5, pp. 53-56, Bangkok, May 2003.

Culurciello, E. & Andreou, A. G. (2006). Capacitive inter-chip data and power transfer for 3-D VLSI, *IEEE Trans. Circuits and Systems-II*, Vol. 53, No. 12, Dec. 2006, pp. 1348-1352.

Deng, S.; Hu, Y. &. Sawan, M. (2006). A high data rate QPSK demodulator for inductively powered electronics implants, *Proceedings of IEEE Int. Symp. Circuits and Systems (ISCAS)*, pp. 2577-2580, Island of Kos, May 2006.

Dimbylow, P. (2005). Development of the female voxel phantom, NAOMI, and its application to calculations of induced current densities and electric fields from applied low frequency magnetic and electric fields, *Phys. Med. Biol.*, Vol. 50, No. 6, Mar. 2005, pp. 1047-1070.

Fazzi, A.; Canegallo, R.; Ciccarelli, L.; Magagani, L.; Natali, F.; Jung, E.; Rolandi, P. & Guerrieri, R. (2008). 3-D capacitive interconnections with monoand bi-directional capabilities, *IEEE J. Solid-State Circuits (JSSC)*, Vol. 43, No. 1, Jan. 2008, pp. 275-284.

Gabriel, C.; Gabriel, S. & Corthout, E. (1996a). The dielectric properties of biological tissues: I. Literature survey, *Phys. Med. Biol.*, Vol. 41, No. 11, Nov. 1996, pp. 2231-2249.

Gabriel, S.; Lau. R.W. & Gabriel, C. (1996b). The dielectric properties of biological tissues: II. Measurements in the frequency range 10 Hz to 20 GHz, *Phys. Med. Biol.*, Vol. 41, No. 11, Nov. 1996, pp. 2251-2269.

Gabriel, S.; Lau. R.W. & Gabriel, C. (1996c). The dielectric properties of biological tissues: III. Parametric models for the dielectric spectrum of tissues, *Phys. Med. Biol.*, Vol. 41, No. 11, Nov. 1996, pp. 2271-2293.

Ghovanloo, M & Najafi, K. (2004). A wideband frequency-shift keying wireless link for inductively powered biomedical implants, *IEEE Trans. Circuits and Systems-I*, Vol. 51, N0. 12, Dec. 2004, pp. 2374-2383.

Ghovanloo, M. & Alturi, S. (2007). A wide-band power-efficient inductive wireless link for implantable devices using multiple carriers, *IEEE Trans. Circuits and Systems-I*, Vol. 54, No. 10, Oct. 2007, pp. 2211-2221.

Gong, C.-S.A.; Shiue, M.-T.; Yao, K.-W. & Chen, T.-Y. (2008). Low-power and area-efficient PSK demodulator for wirelessly powered implantable command receivers, *Electronics Letters*, Vol. 44, No. 14, Jul. 2008, pp. 841-842.

Harrison, R.R. (2007). Designing efficient inductive power links for implantable devices, *Proceedings of IEEE Int. Symp. Circuits and Systems (ISCAS)*, pp. 2080-2083, New Orleans, May 2007.

Hu, Y. & Sawan, M. (2005). A fully-integrated low-power BPSK demodulator for implantable medical devices, *IEEE Trans. Circuits and Systems-I*, Vol. 52, No. 12, pp. 2552-2562, Dec. 2005.

IEEE Standard C95.1-2005. *IEEE standards for safety levels with respect to human exposure to radio frequency electromagnetic fields, 3 KHz to 300 GHz.*

Jow, U.-M. & Ghovanloo, M. (2007). Design and optimization of printed spiral coils for efficient transcutaneous inductive power transmission, *IEEE Trans. Bio. Circuits and Systems*, Vol. 1, No. 3, Sep. 2007, pp. 193-202.

Jow, U.-M. & Ghovanloo, M. (2008). Optimization of a multiband wireless link for neuroprosthetic implantable devices, *Proceedings of IEEE Bio. Circuits and Systems Conf. (BioCAS)*, pp. 97-100, Baltimore, Nov. 2008.

Jow, U.-M. & Ghovanloo, M. (2009). Modeling and optimization of printed spiral coils in air, saline, and muscle tissue environments, *IEEE Trans. Bio. Circuits and Systems*, Vol. 3, No. 5, Oct. 2009, pp. 339-347.

Kendir, G.A.; Liu, W.; Wang, G.; Sivaprakasam, M.; Bashirullah, R.; Humayun, M.S. & Weiland, J.D. (2005). An optimal design methodology for inductive power link with class-E amplifier, *IEEE Trans. Circuits and Systems-I*, Vol. 52, No. 5, pp. 857-866, May 2005.

Lazzi, G. (2005). Thermal effects of implants, *IEEE Eng. Med. Bio. Mag.*, Vol. 24, No. 5, Oct. 2005, pp. 75-81.

Lin, J.C. (1986). Computer methods for field intensity predictions, In: *CRC Handbook of Biological Effects of Electromagnetic Fields*, C. Polk and E. Postow, Eds., Ch. 2, pp. 273-313, CRC, Boca Raton, FL.

Liu, W.; Sivaprakasam, M.; Wang, G.; Zhou. M.; Granacki, J.; Lacoss, J. & Wills, J. (2005). Implantable biomimetic microelectronic systems design, *IEEE Eng. Med. Bio. Mag.*, Vol. 24, No. 5, Oct. 2005, pp. 66-74.

Lu, Z. & Sawan, M. (2008). An 8 Mbps data rate transmission by inductive link dedicated to implantable devices, *Proceedings of IEEE Int. Symp. Circuits and Systems (ISCAS)*, pp. 3057-3060, Seattle, May 2008.

Razavi, B. (1998). *RF Microelectronics*, Prentice-Hall Inc., 0-13-887571-5, USA.

Sawan, M.; Hu, Y. & Coulombe, J. (2005). Wireless smart implants dedicated to multichannel monitoring and microstimulation, *IEEE Circuits and Systems Mag.*, Vol. 5, No. 1, 2005, pp. 21-39.

Shah, M.R.; Phillips, R.P. & Normann, R.A. (1998). A study of printed spiral coils for neuroprosthetic transcranial telemetry applications, *IEEE Trans. Bio. Eng.*, Vol. 45, No. 7, Jul. 1998, pp. 867-876.

Simard, G.; Sawan, M. & Massicotte, D. (2010). High-Speed OQPSK and efficient power transfer through inductive link for biomedical implants, *IEEE Trans. Bio. Circuits and Systems*, Vol. 4, No. 3, Jun. 2010, pp. 192-200.

Singh, V.; Qusba, A.; Roy, A.; Castro, R.A.; McClure, K.; Dai, D.; Greenberg, R.J.; Weiland, J.D.; Humayun, M.S. & Lazzi, G. (2009). Specific absorption rate and current densities in the human eye and head induced by the telemetry link of an epiretinal prosthesis, *IEEE Trans. Antennas and Propagation*, Vol. 57, No. 10, part 2, Oct. 2009, pp. 3110-3118.

Sodagar, A.M. & Najafi, K. (2006). Wireless interfaces for implantable biomedical microsystems, *Proceedings of IEEE Int. Midwest Symp. Circuits and Systems (MWSCAS)*, Vol. 2, pp. 265-269, Aug. 2006.

Sodagar, A.M.; Wise, K.D. & Najafi, K. (2006). An interface chip for power and bidirectional data telemetry in an implantable cochlear microsystem, *Proceedings of IEEE Bio. Circuits and Systems Conf. (BioCAS)*, pp. 1-4, London, Nov. 29 2006-Dec. 1 2006.

Sodagar, A.M. & Amiri, P. (2009). Capacitive coupling for power and data telemetry to implantable biomedical microsystems, *Proceedings of 4th Int. IEEE/EMBS Conf. Neural Eng.*, pp. 411-414, Antalya, April 29–May 2, 2009.

Sodagar, A.M.; Perlin, G.E.; Yao, Y.; Najafi, K. & Wise, K.D. (2009a). An implantable 64-channel wireless microsystem for single-unit neural recording, *IEEE J. Solid-State Circuits (JSSC)*, Vol. 44, No. 9, Sep. 2009, pp. 2951-2604.

Sodagar, A.M.; Wise, K.D. & Najafi, K. (2009b). A wireless implantable microsystem for multichannel neural recording, IEEE *Trans. Microwave Theory and Techniques*, Vol. 57, No. 10, Oct. 2009, pp. 2565-2573.

Sokal, N.O. & Sokal, A.D. (1975). Class E-A new class of high-efficiency tuned single-ended switching power amplifiers, *IEEE J. Solid-State Circuits (JSSC)*, Vol. 10, No. 3, Jun. 1975, pp. 168-175.

Van Schuglenbergh, K. & Puers, R. (2009). *Inductive Powering, Basic Theory and Application to Biomedical Systems*, Springer, 978-90-481-2411-4.

Von-Arx, J.A. & Najafi, K. (1999). A wireless single-chip telemetry-powered neural stimulation system, *Technical Digest, IEEE Int. Solid-State Circuits Conf. (ISSCC)*, pp. 214-215, San Francisco, Feb. 1999.

Wang, G.; Liu, W.; Sivaprakasam, M.; Zhou, M.; Weiland, J.D. & Humayun, M.S. (2005). A wireless phase shift keying transmitter with Q-independent phase transition time, *Proceedings of 27th Int. Conf. IEEE/EMBS*, pp. 5238-5241, Shanghai, Sep. 2005.

Yu, H. & Najafi, K. (2001). Circuitry for a wireless microsystem for neural recording microprobes, *Proceedings of 23rd Int. Conf. IEEE/EMBS*, Vol. 1, pp. 761-764, Istanbul, Oct. 2001.

Yu, H. & Bashirullah, R. (2006). A low power ASK clock and data recovery circuit for wireless implantable electronics, *Proceedings of IEEE Custom Integrated Circuits Conf. (CICC)*, pp. 249-252, San Jose, Sept. 2006.

Zhou, M. & Liu, M. (2007). A non-coherent PSK receiver with interference-canceling for transcutaneous neural implants, *Technical Digest, IEEE Int. Solid-State Circuits Conf. (ISSCC)*, pp. 156-593, San Francisco, Feb. 1997.

3

Microsystem Technologies for Biomedical Applications

Francisco Perdigones, José Miguel Moreno,
Antonio Luque, Carmen Aracil and José Manuel Quero
University of Seville
Spain

1. Introduction

Microsystems, also often known as microelectromechanical systems (MEMS), are miniaturized devices fabricated using techniques called "micromachining", and that are common in different application areas, such as automotive, consumer electronics, industrial measurements, and recently biomedical too Dean & Luque (2009). The typical definition states that a microsystem is any device which has at least one feature size in the order of micrometers (1:1000 of a mm).

Historically, silicon has been used as the material of choice for fabricating microsystems, due to the processing equipment which was already available in microelectronics foundries, and the thorough understanding of the properties that the impressive development of electronics in the 1950s and 60s made possible. Another advantage derived from microelectronics is the low cost associated when fabricating devices at very large production volume. It was then natural to try to integrate other devices with the microelectronic chips, and so the first microsystems were born. Initially, the market was driven by automotive applications, and accelerometers for stability control and airbag deployment were one of the first commercial successes of microsystems technology. Other typical examples from this age are pressure sensors and inkjet printer nozzles. Since then, the global MEMS market has not ceased to grow, and their applications are more diverse now. It is expected that by 2010 more than 8000 million MEMS devices will be sold yearly *Status of the MEMS industry* (2008).

As explained before, due to the importance of the microelectronics foundries, silicon is nowadays a widely available material, with a relatively low cost. Its mechanical and electrical properties have been very well known for decades, a fact which still makes it an ideal choice for many microsystems. Silicon is nearly as strong as steel, but with a much lower fracture toughness Petersen (1982). It is usually sold in circular wafers of varying diameters, from 100 to 500 mm. In microsystems, the final devices are sometimes built by removing part of the material in the substrate, in a process called bulk micromachining, while in other occasions, thin films are deposited on top of the wafer and then parts of them are etched away to form the device, which is known as surface micromachining Kovacs et al. (1998). The actual micromachining of silicon is performed using etchants, which can be liquid (wet etching) or in gas or plasma form (dry etching). Both types can etch the silicon isotropically or anisotropically, depending on the etchant composition and operating parameters. Other materials are commonly present in silicon-based microsystems, most of which also derive from silicon, such as polycrystalline silicon, silicon dioxide, or silicon nitride. Thin or thick films of other materials can be deposited on top of the substrate using chemical vapor deposition (CVD), sputtering, thermal evaporation, or spin coating, among other techniques. All the mentioned process are complemented by photolithography, by means of which a particular area of the wafer where to etch or deposit a material can be selected. This is done using a photosensitive resist which is exposed to light (usually ultraviolet) through a mask with opaque and transparent areas. The resist is then developed and the exposed areas are removed (if the photoresist is positive). The remaining photoresist protects the wafer and avoid that area to be etched away, or a material to be deposited on top of it.

Silicon has been used successfully to fabricate devices such as microfluidic control valves, blood micropumps and microneedles for drug delivery through the skin Henry et al. (1998), but other materials are of more importance for biomedical applications. These materials are usually polymers, which offer the advantage of being cheap and fast to process, especially for small-scale production. Many of the polymers used are biocompatible.

Two of the most common used polymers are PMMA (poly-methyl-metacrylate) and PDMS (poly-dimethyl-siloxane). PMMA is available in solid form, and thermal casting or molding are used to shape it Huang & Fu (2007). PDMS is available as two liquid products (prepolymer and curing agent), which should be mixed together, poured over a mold, and cured at moderately high temperatures. Then it becomes solid and can be demolded. This process has been widely adopted by the microfluidics and biomedical communities since it was developed in 2000 Duffy et al. (1998). Another material used in rapid prototyping is the negative photoresist called SU-8. Examples of actual devices built using PDMS and SU-8 will be showcased below.

The measurement of substances in the blood was one of the first biomedical applications of MEMS devices. Nowadays, personal glucometers are inexpensive, and some of them are starting to include an insulin pump, also built with MEMS technology, which is able to deliver insulin to the patient when the measured glucose level is too high.

One of the most important goals of the research in BioMEMS is the fabrication of a lab-on-chip (LOC) device, where all the needed components to perform extraction, movement, control, processing, analysis, etc. of biological fluids are present. This LOC device would be a truly miniaturized laboratory, which would fulfill many of today's needs in portable medicine.

To accomplish a task like building a LOC, many smaller parts must be considered. In the rest of the sections of this chapter, these parts will be discussed. Section 2 will discuss in detail the fabrication processes for the materials described above, which are the most commonly used now. In Section 3, the issue of power supply will be considered, and some solutions to integrate the microfluidic power in the microsystem will be presented. Section 4 will deal with control and regulation of biological fluids inside the chip. In Section 5, the integration of the different components will be discussed, giving some examples of actual devices, and finally in Section 6, some conclusions will be remarked.

2. Fabrication processes for biocompatible materials

2.1 Introduction

In this section the basis of fabrication processes using the most commonly biocompatible polymers used in MEMS are reported. These materials are Glycidyl-ether-bisphenol-A novolac (SU-8) Lorenz et al. (1997) and polydimethilsiloxane (PDMS) McDonald & Whitesides (2002).

Regarding SU-8 fabrication processes, the typical fabrication process and multilayer technique Mata et al. (2006) are presented in this introduction. Then, in section 2.3 a new process to

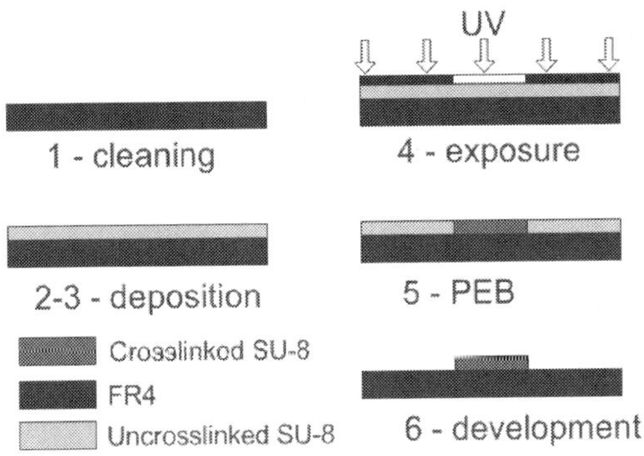

Fig. 1. Typical SU-8 process

transfer SU-8 membranes are commented in order to achieve closed structures. The PDMS material is also presented in this introduction together with the facilities used to process both materials. Neither applications nor functionality of the fabricated devices are presented in this section, only the materials, equipment and processes are reported.

SU-8 is a negative epoxy photoresist widely used in MEMS fabrication, above all in microfluidics and biotechnology due to its interesting properties such as biocompatibility, good chemical and mechanical resistance, and transparency. The typical fabrication process of SU-8 Lorenz et al. (1997) has the following steps as is shown in Fig. 1.

1. Cleaning: The substrate is cleaned using the appropriated substances.
2. Deposition: Deposition by spin coating. The equipment in this step is a spin coater thanks to the thickness of deposited layer can be controlled.
3. Softbake: Softbake in a hot plate, in order to remove the solvent and solidified the deposited layer.
4. Exposure: The SU-8 layer is exposed to ultraviolet UV light using an appropriate mask. The exposed SU-8 will crosslink whereas not exposed SU-8 will be removed. In this step a mask-aligner is necessary in order to align the different masks and expose.
5. Post exposure bake (PEB): The layer is baked using a hot plate in order to crosslink the exposed SU-8.
6. Development: The uncrosslinked SU-8 is developed by immersion and agitation using a developer, e.g., PGMEA.

Times, exposing doses and temperatures are proposed by the SU-8 manufacturer, e.g., MicroChem Corporation or Gersteltec Engineering Solutions.

The SU-8 multilayer technique is used to achieve different thickness in the fabricated structure. This procedure of fabrication consists of performing the previous steps 2 to 5 and them these steps are carried out as many times as additional different thicknesses are required. The final step is a development of the whole structure. In Fig. 2 a multilayer process (two layers) is depicted.

Polydimethylsiloxane (PDMS) is an elastomer material with Low Young modulus. In this respect, PDMS is more flexible material than SU-8. PDMS is also widely used in microfluidic

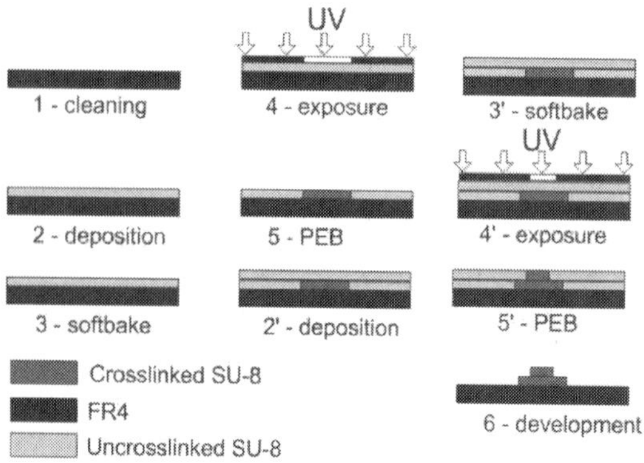

Fig. 2. Multilayer SU-8 process

circuits and biotechnology as base material. It is composed by a prepolymer and a curing agent that must be mixed in order to obtain the PDMS. Depending on the ratio of both substances the PDMS will require a certain time of curing for a fixed temperature. The equipment necessary to process PDMS includes a vacuum chamber to remove the bubbles that appear during mixing and an oven to cure the PDMS. The fabrication of PDMS device is preceded by molds fabrication. These molds are necessary to define the PDMS structure as it will be explained.

2.2 PDMS fabrication processes

The fabrication using PDMS elastomer is based on soft lithography McDonald & Whitesides (2002). The procedure starts with the fabrication of molds. There are several techniques to fabricate these molds, among others, photolithography or micromachining. The substrate widely used for photolithography is silicon, and the material to define the structures is SU-8. The molds are fabricated using the typical process of SU-8 or using more complex techniques as multilayer fabrication. The low adherence of PDMS to SU8 and silicon facilitates the demolding process. We propose Flame Retadant 4 (FR4) of Printed Circuit Board (PCB) as substrate due to its low cost and good adherence with SU-8, Perdigones, Moreno, Luque & Quero (2010). However this material presents more roughness than silicon or pyrex but no problems have been observed due to this issue. A mold fabricated performing the typical process with FR4 as substrate and SU-8 can be seen as an example in Fig. 3. As it is explained later, the PDMS will be poured over it, achieving the negative pattern of the mold.

Once the molds have been produced, a mixture of prepolymer and curing agent is performed with a commonly used ratio in weight percent of 10:1. This mixture is performed by agitation using a stirring bar, and then is degassed in order to remove the bubbles that appear during mixing. Once the mixture has been degassed, it is poured over the mold and put into an oven at 65 °C during 1 h approximately until PDMS is crosslinked and solidified. Finally, the PDMS is peeled off the mold. Using this method only opened structures or microchannels can be fabricated.

There are several techniques of PDMS to PDMS bonding in order to complete the fabrication and achieve the closed structures Eddings et al. (2008). Among these techniques, Partial

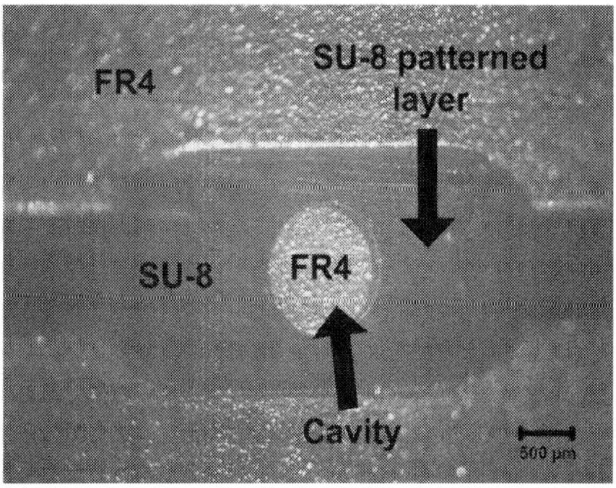

Fig. 3. Fabricated mold using FR4 as substrate and SU-8 to define the structure. The SU-8 patterned layer defines a microchannel with an internal column due to the central cavity.

Curing, Uncured PDMS adhesive and Varing Curing Ratio are the most interesting ones due to their high average bond strengths. In literature, authors propose different temperatures, baking times and ratios to perform the bonding using these techniques. In this respect, our group uses a combination of Partial Curing and Varing Curing Ratio with successful results in multilayer fabrication. We use a ratio 20:1 and 10:1 alternatively, i.e., 20:1 for the first layer, 10:1 for the second one, for the third layer 20:1, etc. The baking times can be selected in a range of 30-45 min for 10:1 ratio, and 50-60 min for 20:1 ratio, at 65 °C in an oven. Finally, the bonding is performed at 65 °C during 2 h in the oven. In Fig. 4, the PDMS part of an extractor of liquid for submicroliter range Perdigones, Luque & Quero (2010b) can be seen.

In order to fabricate the PDMS structure shown in Fig. 4 only one mold is necessary. The procedure of fabrication is very simple, where two PDMS pieces are bonded. This process can be seen in Fig. 5 and it starts with the fabrication of the mold using the SU-8 typical procedure. Once the mold has been done, a PDMS with a ratio of 10:1 is poured over it (layer 1), step (a),

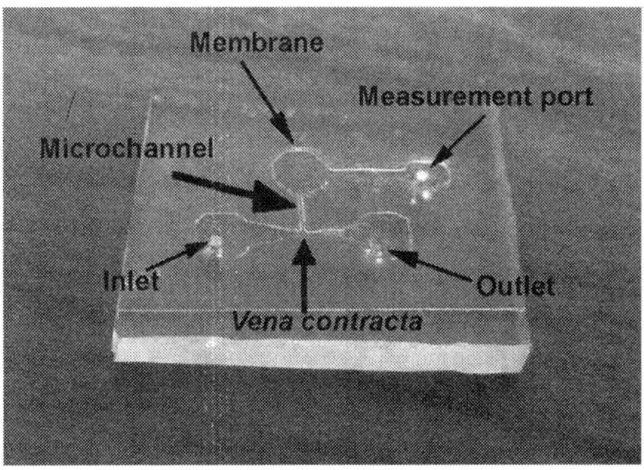

Fig. 4. PDMS extractor of liquid for submicroliter range.

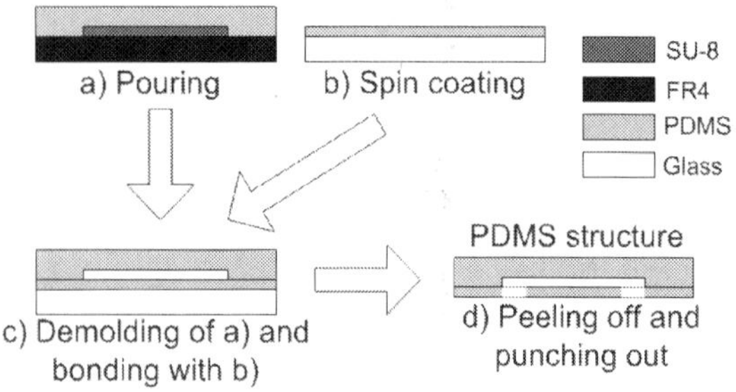

Fig. 5. Fabrication process for the structure in Fig. 4

and other mixture of 20:1 is spin coated over a glass substrate (layer 2), step (b). The layers are put into an oven at 65 °C during 45 min for the first one and 1 h for the second one. Then, the layer 1 is demolded and put into contact to layer 2, (step c), as can be seen in Fig. 5 and the bonding is performed in an oven at 65 °C during 2 h. Once the bonding has been performed, the final structure is peeled off the glass substrate and the layer 2 is punched out.
A more complex PDMS three dimensional structure with three different layers and fabricated using the presented process is shown in Fig. 6. This is a cross section of a PDMS flow regulator with positive gain as will commented in section 4.
The process to fabricate the structure in Fig. 6 requires two molds and is shown in Fig. 7. The first one (mold 1) is made using the typical process and the second one (mold 2) using the multilayer technique. The procedure starts performing three mixtures with a ratio 10:1 for the intermediate layer (layer 2) and 20:1 for the rest. Once the mixtures have been degassed, the mixture 10:1 is spin coated over the mold 1 in order to achieve a structure (layer 2) with a membrane on top (step a). Next, one of 20:1 mixture is poured over the mold 2 (step b) defining the layer 1, and the other is spin coated over a glass substrate (step c) defining the layer 3. All layers are put into an oven at 65 °C during 30 min for layer 2 and 1 h for the rest. Once the PDMS layers are partially curing, layer 1 is demolded and put into contact with layer 2 as can be seen in step d. Both layers are put into an oven at 65 °C during 5 min in order to achieve a initial bonding. This bonding is necessary to demold layer 2 without breaks that might appear due to its low thickness. Once this initial bonding is performed, the structure is

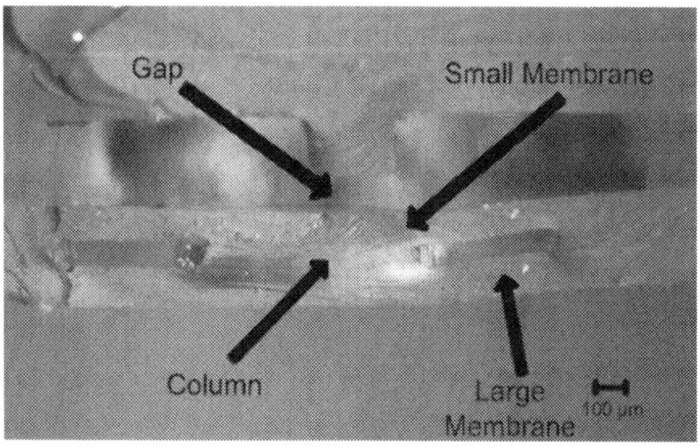

Fig. 6. Three dimensional PDMS structure with three layers

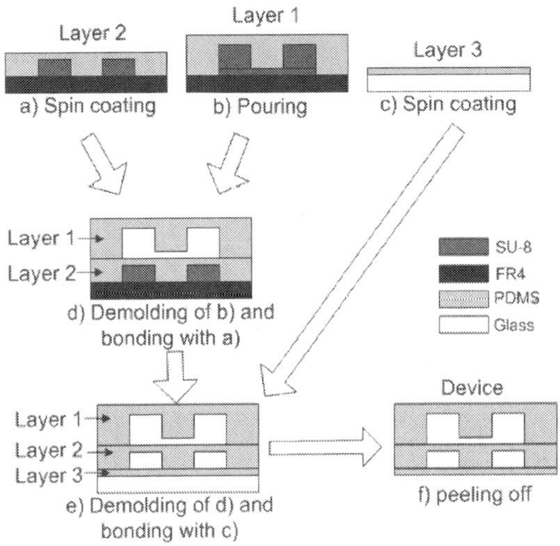

Fig. 7. Fabrication process for the structure in Fig. 6

demolded from mold 1, and put into contact with layer 3 as can be seen in step e. Next, these three layers are bonding at room temperature during 24 h because the air in the cavities could expand and lead the separation between layer 2 and 3. After this step, the final structure is put in a hot plate at 50 °C during 5 min to ensure a good bonding and then the device is peeled off the glass substrate.

2.3 SU-8 closed structures

A special effort is associated to processes which achieve 3D structures to fabricate microchannels and microreservoirs, taking into account that SU-8 typical process is focused for the fabrication of open structures.

Different ways to achieve SU-8 closed structures have been reported but mainly we can find two trends. The first approach employs sacrificial layers, where uncrosslinked SU-8 is used as base to obtain upper layers and afterwards it is removed. A microchannel fabricated by this method is shown in Fig.8. The significant disadvantages of this approach are the limitation of the design of structures with an aperture to strip off the uncrosslinked SU-8, and an excessive development time for the required multilayer deposition Chung & Allen (2005). However, in recent years there is an evolution in various aspects of this approach improving the mask-process Guerin et al. (1997), embedding the masks Haefliger & Boisen (2006), and controlling the exposure, Chuang et al. (2003).

The second trend widely used, consists in sealing the SU-8 structure by means of transferring SU-8 layers. In this way, the use of removable films to transfer SU-8 layers obtaining monolithic devices by lamination has been broadly reported. Many different materials are used as removable layer, among others, PDMS Patel et al. (2008), PET Abgrall et al. (2008), kapton Ezkerra et al. (2007). Besides from using different materials, there are plenty of flow processes based in the transfer of the SU-8 layers as well. An important requirement in the development of processes is the compatibility with previous processes to be able to improve the complexity and integration with other devices.

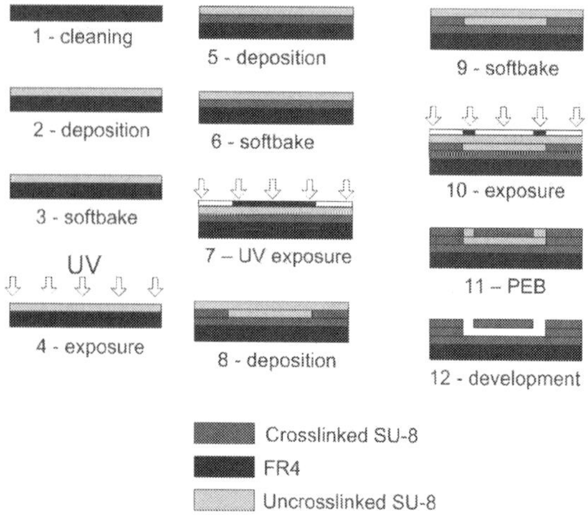

Fig. 8. Flow of fabrication process of a sacrificial layer process.

A particular example of this approach is the transferring process has been named BETTS Aracil, Perdigones, Moreno & Quero (2010) (Bonding, UV Exposing and Transferring Technique in SU-8). The key step of this process is the use of the layer substrate not only to transfer the SU-8 layer, but also to act as a mask to pattern the SU-8 layer and to allow peeling off the transferred film easily. Therefore, bonding, UV exposing and transferring processes are carried out in a single step. The process flow of BETTS can be seen in Fig. 9. The transfer process can be achieved over different kind of substrates, like glass, silicon, SU-8 or FR4, what extends the number of applications that can use of it. The thickness of the transferred layer is variable according to the application. Its value is very closed linked to the height of the microchannel. The shallowest microchannel fabricated corresponds to 40μm, for a thickness of the transferred layer of 5μm. The compatibility with others fabrication processes allows the integration with other electronic devices wire bonded to the substrate. 3D structures are easily manufactured by means of the repetition of the flow of process. An example of 3D multichannel network is shown in Fig. 10.

3. Autonomous microdevices

3.1 Pressure chambers

Nowadays, an important challenge still to be overcome in the field of Lab on Chip devices is the improvement of portability and fluid flow generation. Although there is a wide range of methods to develop fluid flow in microfluidic devices such as electroosmotic flow, electrokinetic pumps or by centrifugal force or capillary action, Laser & Santiago (2004); Lim et al. (2010), on-chip pumping is in general externally generated by traditional macroscale syringe or vacuum pumps. This limitation makes LOC devices encapsulation and portability a very difficult task when developing miniaturized autonomous microfluidic systems. Moreover, MEMS packaging results more expensive compared to the microsystem itself when considering vacuum or pressure sealing, being indispensable to find simple and low cost encapsulation methods fully compatible and easy to integrate with former fabrication processes and materials.

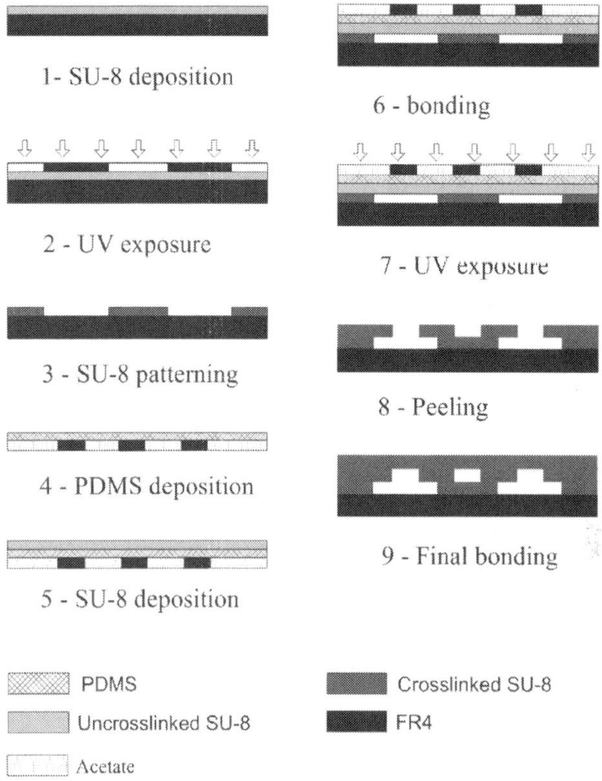

Fig. 9. Flow of fabrication process of a transferring process named BETTS.

Peristaltic micropumps have been widely used for LOC fluid flow generation, allowing the transport of a controlled fluid volume in clinical diagnosis and drug delivery applications Koch et al. (2009). Nevertheless, this alternative presents some disadvantages such as the large area required in the LOC device and the high power consumption to impulse the fluid. The solution presented in this chapter to minimize these limitations is the use of disposable microfluidic devices, based on a single use thermo-mechanical microvalve activation which releases a stored pressure to achieve a controlled fluid flow impulsion. This system can be easily integrated in a small area of the LOC, providing a portable reservoir of pneumatic energy.

The mechanism of differential pressure is a well known method in microfluidic fluid flow impulsion, where the use of epoxy resins such as SU-8 opens up new possibilities for the implementation of pressure-driven flow on-chip. Although polymers are typically several orders of magnitude more permeable to gas leakages than glass or metals, epoxy resins are characterized by a low gas permeability and thus can be used for simple and low-cost sealing of packages Murillo et al. (2010). In addition to this, SU-8 epoxy shows a decrease in gas permeability when the level of crosslinking is increased, being a suitable and interesting alternative for pressurized or vacuum microchambers fabrication Metz et al. (2004).

In this section two portable pressure driven flow devices for LOC applications are presented: vacuum and pressurized chambers.
The pressurized system consists in a monolithical SU-8 structure composed by a sealed microchamber connected to a valve that will be introduced in section 3.2. The chamber structure is connected to a microfluidic channel to seal it at a fixed and controlled pressure by an extra UV isolation step compatible with the traditional SU-8 fabrication process. The pressurized portable system SU-8 layout is shown in Fig. 11. To seal the chamber and store a fluid at a fixed pressure, low-viscous SU-8 is externally injected in the chamber hole through the control serpentine microchannel by means of a compressed air supply connected to a pressure transducer. The viscosity of the SU-8 supplied by Microchem is determined by the manufacturer by means of a code number (2005, 2025, 2150, etc.), where the lower number means lower SU-8 viscosity. Thus, to seal the chamber SU-8 2005 is employed. The dimensions of the microchannel are previously calculated according to the isothermal process for an ideal gas and the Boyle's law:

$$PV = k \rightarrow P_1V_1 = P_2V_2, \tag{1}$$

Where P_1 is the desired final pressure in the microchamber, V_1 is its volume, P_2 is the initial pressure before sealing process (atmospheric pressure), $V2$ the total air volume inside the structure and k is a constant. When the SU-8 2005 is injected through the inlet, the air volume entrapped inside the control channel at atmospheric pressure pushes the air in the chamber, proportionally increasing its pressure depending on the expression (1). As an example, the control microchannel area in the layout is calculated to be the same than the chamber area, in order to obtain 2 bar absolute pressure inside the chamber. Then, an UV exposure step polymerizes the liquid SU-8 inside the control channel to seal hermetically the chamber which is pressurized and ready for use. The stored pneumatic energy of the gas inside the chamber is expressed as follows, Hong et al. (2007).

$$E = \int PdV = P_1V_1 ln\left(\frac{P_1}{P_F}\right) \tag{2}$$

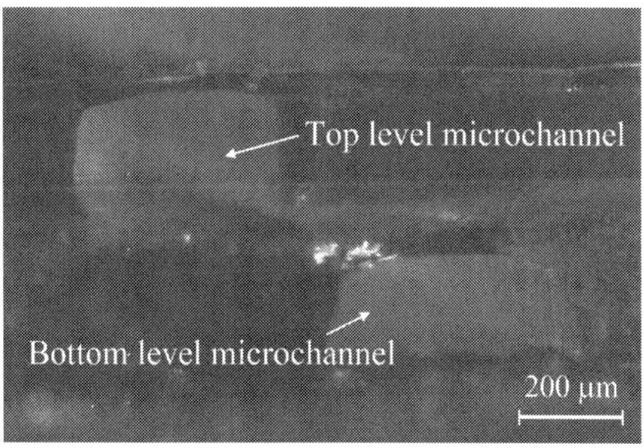

Fig. 10. Fabrication of three dimensional micro-channels network using BETTS process. The height of the walls is 200 μm while the thickness of the transferred layer is 40 μm. The width of the microchannels are 400 μm.

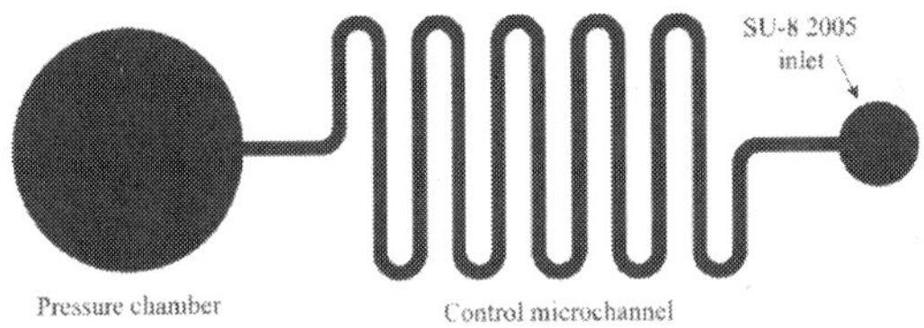

Fig. 11. Layout SU-8 mask for a pressurized chamber.

where P_1 is the absolute pressure of the gas in the chamber, V_1 is the volume of the gas in the chamber and P_F is the final pressure after the opening process (normally, it will be ambient pressure). This stored energy will be used to pump the working fluids in LOCs.

3.1.1 Fabrication of a pressurized chamber

The device implementation is simple to be carried out employing a traditional SU-8 fabrication process and PCB-based technology already explained in section 2. The first step is the consideration of a suitable and inexpensive substrate for the structure, where FR4 is chosen. A SU-8 2150 layer is deposited over the substrate by a spin coater and then soft baked for 15 min at 65°C and 90 min at 95°C. The result is a planar 200 μm thickness layer over the FR4, ready for a UV exposure step to transfer the structure shown in the layout of Fig. 11 in the SU-8. After a PEB step for 5 min at 65°C and 10 min at 95°C which polymerizes the SU-8, the board is immersed in SU-8 developer for 5 min and the final device structure patterned. Then, the board is carefully rinsed in isopropyl alcohol (IPA).

After this, the cover bonding process is carried out to close hermetically the structure by BETTS: A thin PDMS layer is spin coated over a transparent acetate film, cured by temperature and then a 40 μm thickness SU-8 2025 layer is deposited over the PDMS. This thin SU-8 layer is transferred placing the acetate film over the structure and exposing it to UV light during 2 min. This step produces a strong crosslinking between the SU-8 device structure and the SU-8 of the acetate, sealing completely the patterned layout. Then, the acetate with the PDMS is easily removed due to the low adhesion between the crosslinked SU-8 of the cover and the PDMS.

Once the SU-8 microchamber and control channel is finished and sealed by BETTS, a thin orifice is performed over the beginning of the microchannel in order to create the SU-8 2005 inlet. This fluid port is externally connected to a syringe pump than impulses the liquid SU-8 2005 through the microchannel and gradually increases the pressure of the air entrapped inside the chamber. The syringe flow rate is selected to pump 1 mL/min and the microchannel shape of a serpentine provides an easy method to precisely control the pumping time in order not to fill the chamber. With this method, the syringe is stopped when the SU-2005 reached the end of the channel before entering into the chamber, which would produce an undesired increment on its pressure. The SU-8 2005 is chosen as the pumping liquid due to its low viscosity, making easier the flow from the syringe through the control microchannel.

Then, with the syringe pump fixed and the microchannel filled with SU-8, the board is exposed to UV light for 5 min in controlled steps of 1 min in order to avoid an increment of the chamber temperature which would produce a pressure increment as well due to the ideal gas law. After the UV exposure step, the device is soft baked for 10 min at 95°C, achieving a strong crosslinking between the injected SU-8 and the microchannel SU-8 walls. Finally, the

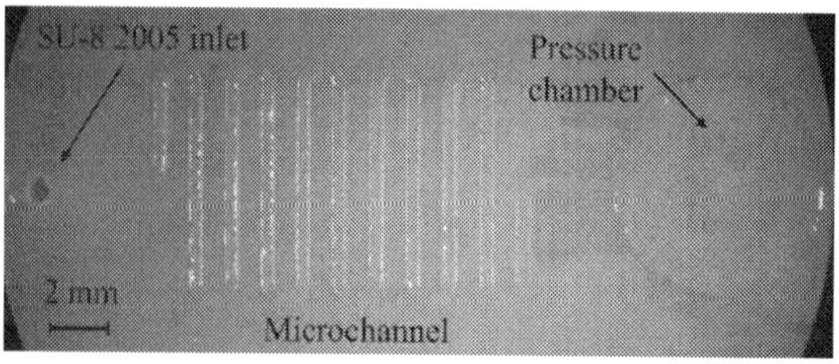

Fig. 12. Photograph of the pneumatic impulsion device.

syringe pump is disconnected from the device, and a 2 bar pressurized chamber hermetically sealed is obtained. The fabricated pneumatic impulsion device is show in Fig. 12. The total dimensions of the device are 10x35x1,75 mm^3, with a microchamber internal volume of 11 μL. Following this fabrication process, the manufacturing of a multiple array of pneumatic microdevices is easy to be carried out with the SU-8 layout mask shown in Fig. 13. The SU-8 2005 is distributed from a common inlet through the different microchannels in order to set a fixed pressure on each chamber. The dimensions of the distribution microchannels shown in the figure are calculated to push an identical volume of air into the chambers, in order to fabricate eight independent pressurized reservoirs fixed at the same pressure value. Moreover, it is easy to design the system with different stored pneumatic energies on each chamber just by changing the dimensions for every distribution channel. The white parts inside the microchambers shown in Fig. 13 are designed to work as pillars for the SU-8 chamber structure, supporting the cover fixed to the SU-8 walls during pressurizing step in order to avoid leakages or device breakages.

With the multiple structure presented, a microvalve could be easily added on each pressure chambers just by adding few fabrication steps in the manufacturing process, as is described in 5, developing a multi-pneumatic flow generator device capable of supplying eight different and independent fluid impulsions. From this point, the next step is to minimize the layout area of each device in order to copy the structure and to develop an array platform with tens of disposable pressurized chambers for complex LOC microfluidic systems.

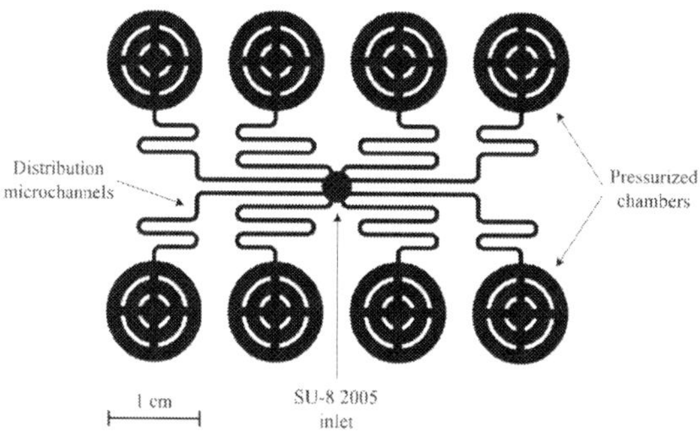

Fig. 13. Layout SU-8 mask of a multiple pressurized portable device

3.1.2 Fabrication of a vacuum chamber

Once the method and fabrication process for pressurizing SU-8 microstructures has been described, the manufacturing steps to develop vacuum chambers is explained as follows. In this case, the device layout just consists of the vacuum chamber without the need of using the control microchannel. The chamber dimensions are selected in order to calculate the volume of air displaced into the chamber when an activation is performed, according to ideal gas law equation (1). The initial fabrication steps to create the SU-8 microchamber are identical to the explained before with the pressurized system until cover layer is bonded to the structure. Now, a small orifice is drilled in the chamber in order to provide an air outlet for vacuum process. The FR4 board with the microchamber is placed inside a macro-vacuum chamber in the laboratory, which contains a syringe dispenser manually controlled from the outside. The SU-8 microchamber is then carefully placed underneath the dispenser, which is filled with SU-8 2025.

Then, the macro-vacuum chamber is sealed and starts to pump out the air contained inside the microchamber until a pressure of 0.1 bar is reached and observed by a pressure transducer externally connected to the vacuum pump. At this point, the dispenser is activated, releasing a droplet of SU-8 2025 over the cover orifice of the microchamber. The SU-8 2025 formulation plays a fundamental role due to its medium viscosity, which completely covers the lid orifice without filling the microchamber inside. Once the droplet has slightly entered into the orifice, a UV lamp illuminates the device, crosslinking the SU-8 droplet with the SU-8 cover of the chamber and thus sealing completely the microchamber at vacuum pressure.

Pressurized and vacuum portable systems explained above represent two inexpensive, fast prototyping and easy to fabricate alternatives for fluid flow generation. Moreover, the working fluids pressurized in the chambers could be either gas or liquid due to the low gas permeability of the SU-8 used in the device fabrication. As it is shown in section 5, the integration of these systems with other basic microfluidic components described throughout the chapter will lead in a portable and small LOC for fast microfluidic handling.

3.2 3D impulsion devices

Respect to the propulsion of fluid there are two main methods for driving the flow of fluids in microchannels: pressure-driven and electrokinetic. In the first case the propulsion is due to a difference of pressure between the ends of the microchannels, while in the second one the movement of charged molecules is due to an electric field. Both methods are effective, but the pressure-driven can be used for a wider range of solvents, even the not electrically conductive ones. On the other hand, the pressure driven uses to include an external pump or vacuum source, making non autonomous its operation.

One strategy of design to solve this disadvantage is to integrate microdevices that produces the difference of pressure. Furthermore, the disposability of many applications sets the trend to integrate one-shot devices. A simple way to obtain the difference of pressure is to open a chamber with an internal overpressure. With this approach there is no need of external impulsion so the connections and the complexity of the setup of the system is reduced. As example of this kind of devices, an autonomous microdevice for the impulsion in microfluidic applications is explained in detail in Aracil, Quero, Luque, Moreno & Perdigones (2010). The one-shot pneumatic impulsion device (OPID) is composed by a chamber and a single-use microvalve that connects its output port to the external microfluidic circuit where the fluid is propelled, Fig. 14. Due to the in-plane structure, a high integration with microfluidic and electronic components can be achieved. The activation is based in the combination of

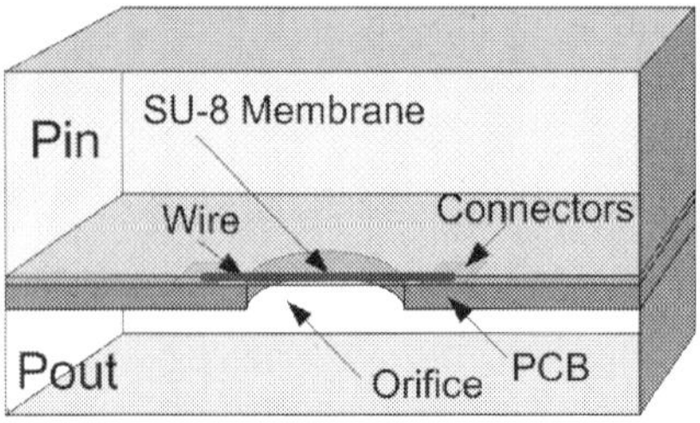

Fig. 14. Cross section of the 3D pneumatic impulsion device.

mechanical to thermal phenomena. The thermal effect is produced by making an electrical current flow through a resistor, implemented by a wire bonded gold filament, and the mechanical one by a differential pressure stored in the chamber. The combination of these phenomena at the time of activation produces a reduction of the required electrical energy with respect to other devices. The impulsion can be produced in the two directions, making a positive or negative difference pressure respect to external pressure. The fabrication of an array of devices can be easily implemented allowing the propulsion of fluid sequentially and in different directions. The device working can be seen in Fig. 15. These photos show three consecutive moments on the activation of the microdevice. Firstly, in (a), the microdevice is on repose. In (b), the current is applied, and changes on the membrane can be seen by the light changes. Finally, (c) shows the fluid coming into the chamber.

3.3 2D impulsion devices

An alternative to the 3D impulsion devices has been developed, consisting in a planar structure with the membrane acting as a vertical wall between the pressurized chamber and a microchannel Moreno & Quero (2010). The hybrid thermo-mechanical operating principle is similar: a gold microwire acting as a resistor crosses the SU-8 membrane that withstands the pressure difference between both sides. When an electric current is supplied to the wire the membrane heats up, drastically decreasing its fracture strength and causing the valve activation. The schematic of the 2D impulsion device design is shown in Fig. 16 and Fig. 17: According to the mathematical approximation reported by Roark et al. (2001), the maximum bending stress σ_{max}, generated by a uniform pressure P on a clamped rectangular plate with a height Ly, a length Lx and a thickness h can be expressed as:

$$\sigma_{max} = cP\left(\frac{L_y}{h}\right)^2, \tag{3}$$

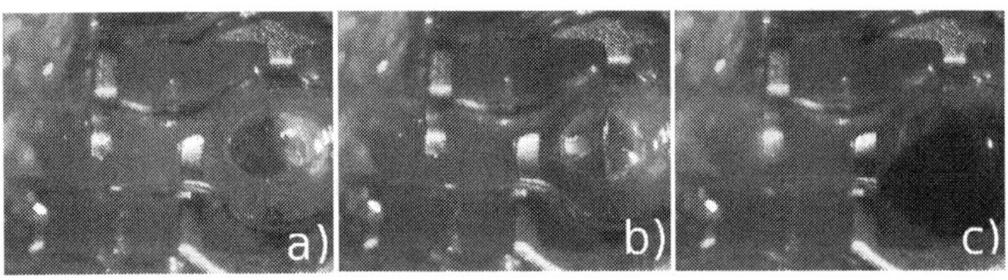

Fig. 15. Sequence of different frames of the device activation.

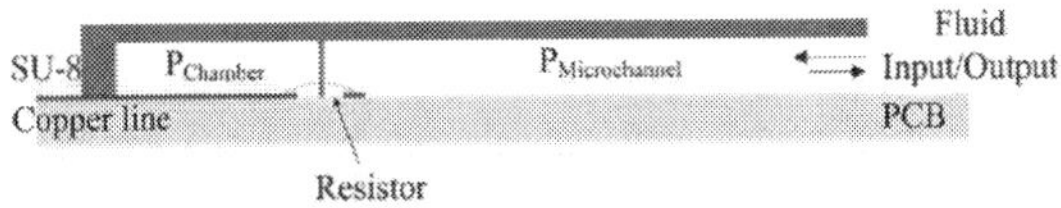

Fig. 16. Cross-section view of the 2D micro impulsion device. Pressure in the chamber is regulated through a PCB orifice.

where c is calculated by the polynomial least-squares curve fitting as a function of Ly and Lx. It is interesting to highlight that σ_{max} is thickness-to-width aspect ratio quadratic dependent, establishing the membrane aspect ratio and the pressure applied as main parameters involved in mechanical actuation. This fact determines that membrane fabrication is a critical step in the microvalve fabrication process.
The implementation of the microvalve employs SU-8 and PCB, integrating microfluidics with classical PCB electronic connections in a common substrate. The fabrication process starts with a photolithography and wet etching step of the copper layer on top of PCB, obtaining the connections to bond the gold wire. A flat bonding and a high accuracy in the gold microwire alignment are crucial tasks in order to heat the membrane on its mechanical weakest point, which is in the bottom center surface on the substrateMoreno et al. (2008). The next step is the deposition of a thick SU-8 layer over the board, making a softbake stage, a UV exposure, a post exposure bake and finally developing the SU-8 to pattern the final structure of the valve. Membranes with widths near to 45 μm and aspect ratios of 11 are achieved with nearly perfect vertical profiles. Two orifices are drilled on the PCB in the pressure chamber and in the right end of the microchannel to connect an external pump with the working pressure and to provide an inlet or outlet for the fluid flow, depending on the valve operation mode. Pressure on chamber will determine the fluid flow direction, establishing a reversible device operation bearing in mind that the microchannel is opened to outside air and consequently set at atmospheric pressure. If chamber pressure is higher than atmospheric, the device will operate as a microinjector, whereas with lower pressure than atmospheric the valve will work in microextractor mode, forcing the fluid contained in the inlet/outlet port through the channel towards the chamber.
Finally, the SU-8 cover is bonded to the structure by BETTS, sealing the chamber to avoid pressure leakages. The total dimensions of the device re 4x12x5 mm^3, with a microchannel length of 8 mm and a square section of 500x500 μm^2. A photograph of the microvalve is illustrated in Fig. 18:

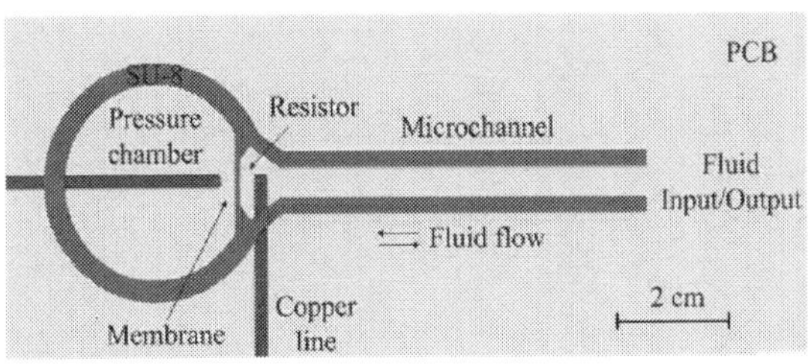

Fig. 17. Layout of the 2D micro impulsion device.

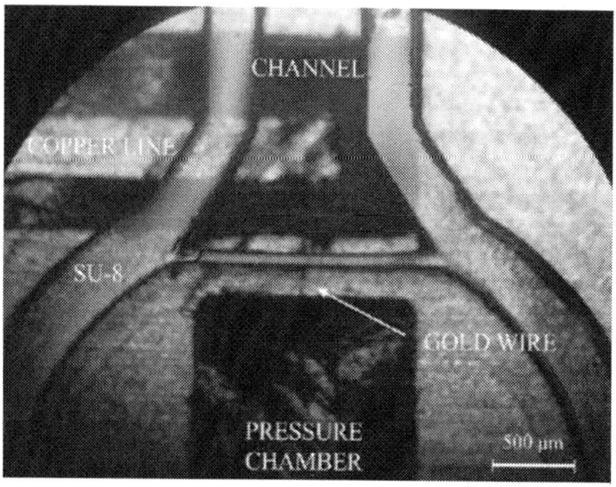

Fig. 18. Photograph of the SU-8 membrane crossed by the gold wire.

4. Flow regulation

4.1 Introduction

The control of fluids is an important issue when considering LOC devices and their applicability in biotechnology as is commented in section 1. Regarding microdevices to control or regulate the flow rates, there are many of them Oh & Ahn (2006) with different actuations. Among these devices, the most interesting ones are those which actuation is pneumatic due to the damage can be avoided in biological flows when through the devices. On this respect, there are many devices, for instance, the microvalves reported by Takao & Ishida (2003); Baek et al. (2005), all of them present negative gain, G, defined as

$$G = \left.\frac{\partial Q}{\partial P_1}\right|_{P_2} \leq 0, \tag{4}$$

where Q is the working flow rate, P_1 and P_2 are the control and working pressure, respectively.

4.2 Positive gain device

A recent publication Perdigones, Luque & Quero (2010a) demonstrates how the positive gain can be achieved. Thanks to the positive gain device a pneumatic microvalve can be fabricated. A simple cross section sketch of the microvalve is depicted in Fig. 19, which includes a control and a working channel. In the control channel is included the positive gain device, which is composed by two circular membranes with different diameters and a column linking them.

When positive pressure is applied in the control channel, the difference of membrane areas makes possible the aperture of the working channel, decreasing the fluidic resistance and increasing the flow rate. The behavior depends on the membrane and column diameters as is explained in Perdigones, Luque & Quero (2010a). If low Young modulus materials are used, i.e., PDMS, the shape of the large membrane must be chosen to be pseudo-elliptical Perdigones et al. (In press).

These kind of devices has been fabricated using the SU-8 technology in a FR4 substrate and using a combination of typical SU-8 process and BETTS (Fig. 20). On the other hand, the PDMS device has also been fabricated using the bonding technique commented above, Fig. 21 which

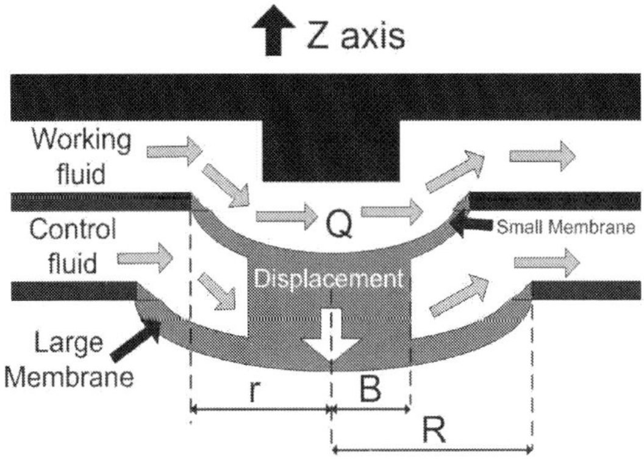

Fig. 19. Cross section of microvalve

section is Fig. 6 , in this case the device has pseudo-elliptical shape for the large membrane, unlike SU-8 device which membrane has circular shape.
The graphic which relates the working flow rate and the control pressure demonstrates the positive gain behavior. The slope of these curves is the gain of the microdevice, Perdigones, Luque & Quero (2010a). This slope is positive so the behavior of the device is governed by the positive gain, mathematically,

$$G = \left.\frac{\partial Q}{\partial P_1}\right|_{P_2} \geq 0, \tag{5}$$

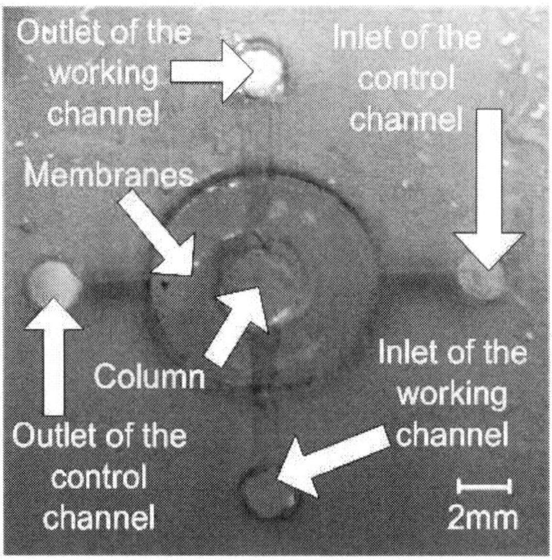

Fig. 20. Positive gain flow regulator fabricated using SU-8.

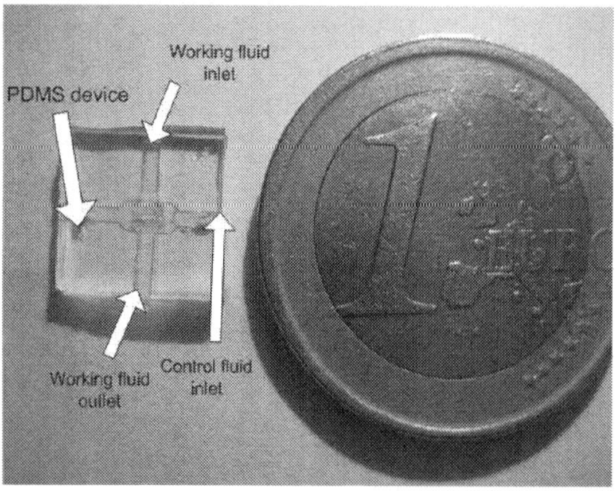

Fig. 21. Positive gain flow regulator fabricated using PDMS.

where Q is the working flow rate, P_1 and P_2 are the control and working pressure, respectively. The positive gain behavior provides improvement to the fluidic circuits, e.g., all pneumatic microvalves (positive and negative gain) can be controlled using positive pressure sources leaving out the vacuum systems. In addition, if a negative pressure is applied to the control channel, the microdevice is converted to a normally open microvalve because the control channel closes when that negative pressure is applied.

5. Integration

The final aim of this chapter is the integration of the previous components to achieve more complex devices. Therefore, an fundamental objective is to find compatible materials and fabrication processes in order to develop a monolithic, functional and autonomous fluidic microdevice without many manufacturing steps. In this task we will principally focus on SU-8 polymer and Printed Circuit Board (PCB) technology, taking advantage of the possibilities that these materials offer. A combination of the fabrication techniques commented before, such as BETTS, and new devices, such as pneumatic fluid impulsion devices, is essential to achieve this purpose. To illustrate this, next are detailed the design and fabrication steps involved in the fabrication of a portable microfluidic platform capable of storing, injecting, mixing and heating a chemical reagent and a human blood sample to finally analyze its glucose concentration.

The proposed design consists in a pressurized chamber connected to a single use microvalve in charge of driving the fluid flow through a microfluidic circuit. When the valve is activated, the pressure in the chamber pushes the fluid stored in two independent reservoirs, flowing towards a serpentine micromixer to finally reach a detection chamber where the mixture is heated and finally analyzed photometrically. A chemical reagent which contains enzyme glucose-oxidase is stored in one microreservoir, whereas a solution with a given glucose concentration is placed in the other reservoir. Both are connected by a microchannel to the entrance of a serpentine that mixes both fluids to finally reach the detection chamber, where the reaction takes place accelerated by the temperature supplied by the microheater. The chemical reaction results in a colored solution that can be measured in terms of optical

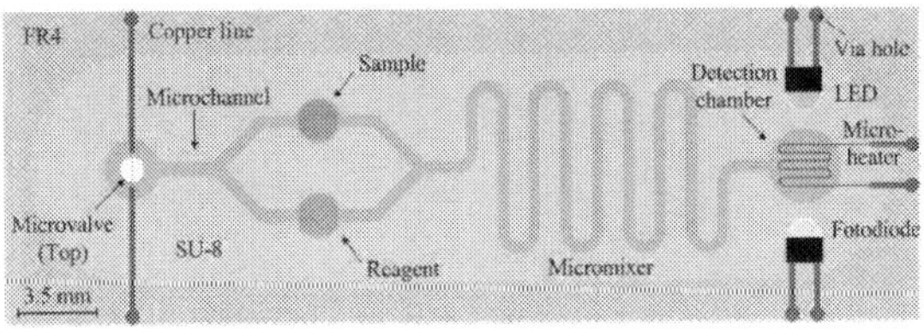

Fig. 22. Top layer of the microfluidic platform design, describing a potential integration of an optical sensor and heater.

absorbance by means of a light emitting diode and a photodetector. The commented design, developed in a two layer structure is illustrated in Fig. 22 and Fig. 23.
An interesting theoretic modeling for a pressure driven microfluidic design is the assumption of equivalent circuit theory (EC) in the context of microfluidics Bruus (2001). It derives its name from the 1:1 mathematical similarity between microfluidic components and the equivalent electronic components, with the basic assumption that the flow is incompressible and pressure driven with $Re < 1$. These low order models result very effective in describing the observed fluid dynamic effects and in addition have very attractive mathematical properties and highly intuitive applicability. The table 1 summarizes the equivalent circuit elements for microfluidic and electric circuits Vedel (2009).

Fluidic circuits	Electric circuits
Pressure drop = ΔP	Voltage = ΔV
Resistance = R_{hyd}	Resistance = R_{el}
Compliance = C_{hyd}	Capacitance = C_{el}
Inertance = L_{hyd}	Inductance = L_{el}

Table 1. Summary of equivalent circuit elements for microfluidic and electric circuits

With this method is possible to design the microchambers and microchannels dimensions of the microfluidic device in order to assure to entry of the mixed fluids in the detection chamber, avoiding the need of using complex fluid mechanics simulation software. Following the table above, the microchannels where replaced by fluidic resistances, R_{hyd}, comparing the linear relationship between an applied constant pressure difference ΔP and the resultant flow rate Q with the Ohm's law which describes the drop in electrical potential, ΔV across a resistor with resistance R in which a current I is running:

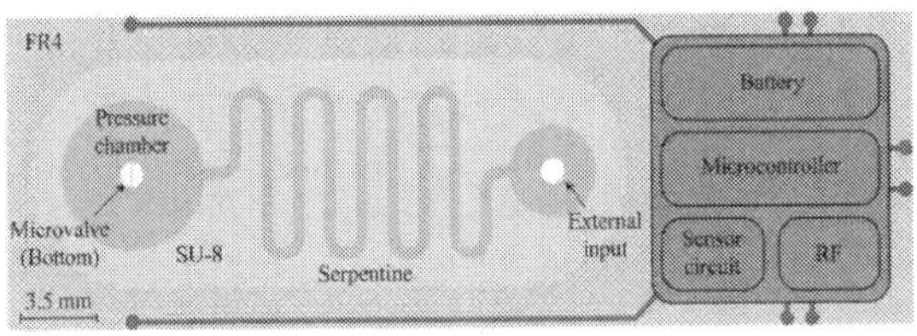

Fig. 23. Bottom layer of the microfluidic platform design, describing a potential integration of an electronic system.

$$\Delta P = \frac{128\mu L}{\pi D_H^4} Q = R_{hyd} Q \Longleftrightarrow \Delta V = RI \tag{6}$$

where μ is the fluid viscosity, L is the length of the microchannel and D_H the hydraulic diameter. In common microfabrication technology the microchannels are normally rectangular or square shaped, being necessary to add a relation between the microchannel height and width with the equivalent hydraulic diameter.

$$D_H = \frac{4S}{P_{wet}} = \frac{2wh}{w+h} \tag{7}$$

where S is the microchannel cross sectional area, P_{wet} is the wetted perimeter, w is the microchannel width and h is the microchannel height. According to the similarities shown between electric and fluidic principles, hydraulic compliance can be thought as a storage of volume in the hydraulic circuit since change in pressure will cause a change in volume, just as capacitance is a storage of electric charge. In this manner, the solution for the gas pressure $P(t)$ trapped in a chamber when it opens is easily seen to be analogous to the voltage across a discharging capacitor with a characteristic RC time. Moreover, if fluid flow branches off (e.g. in a T-junction) the total flow rate leaving and entering the junction must be identical because of the assumption of incompressible flow and mass conservation equation. These simple arguments illustrate the EC framework: understanding a microfluidic system as a network of parameters. The two arguments for series and parallel coupling are identical to Kirchhoff's laws from electric circuits, so electric network analysis is applied to EC models of microfluidics. With this method, the microfluidic device presented in this section can be designed and analyzed as a network of interconnected elements, as is shown in Fig. 24.

Once the device is theoretically studied and characterized, the next step is the fabrication process based on the integration of the different microdevices and fabrication techniques presented in previous sections.

The device is fabricated over a two-layer common PCB substrate, with the pneumatic impulsion system on the bottom layer connected through the microvalve to the top layer where the reagent and sample reservoirs with the microfluidic circuitry and detection chamber are placed. A photograph of the top and bottom SU-8 structures are shown in Fig. 25. A microhole is performed on top of the detection chamber to avoid air entrapment during device activation, as well as on the top of the pressure chamber to be used as an inlet for the air injection. To seal a fixed pressure in the chamber, low-viscous SU-8 2005 is externally injected in the chamber hole through the serpentine by means of a compressed air supply connected to a pressure transducer. When the desired pressure is reached in the chamber, the system is exposed to UV light in order to polymerize the liquid SU-8 entrapped inside the microchannel, closing hermetically the chamber. Finally, the sample and reagent fluids are injected and sealed inside the top layer reservoirs.

The microfluidic circuitry of the device has been successfully tested in the laboratory, achieving a controlled filling of the detection chamber. When an electric current is supplied to the gold wire embedded in the membrane, the pressure contained inside the chamber accelerates the valve activation, bringing the impulsion of the air and thus the fluid contained in the reservoirs almost instantly. The sample and reagent (e.g. glucose with its respective reagent) flows through the microchannel to the mixer, taking place the chemical reaction that makes the mixture to change its colour intensity, which is linearly proportional to the glucose concentration. When the colored mixture reaches the detection chamber and is heated up by

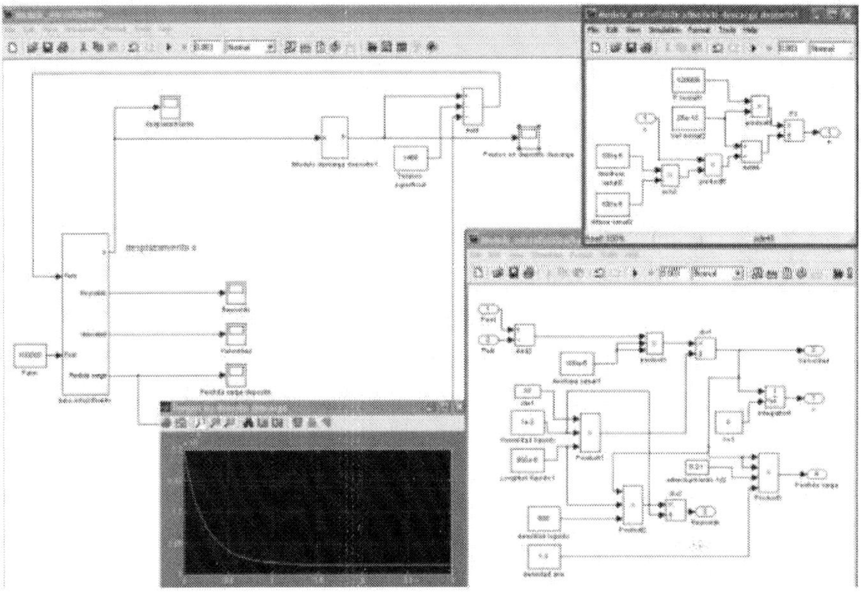

Fig. 24. Design of the microfluidic network using Matlab (Simulink)

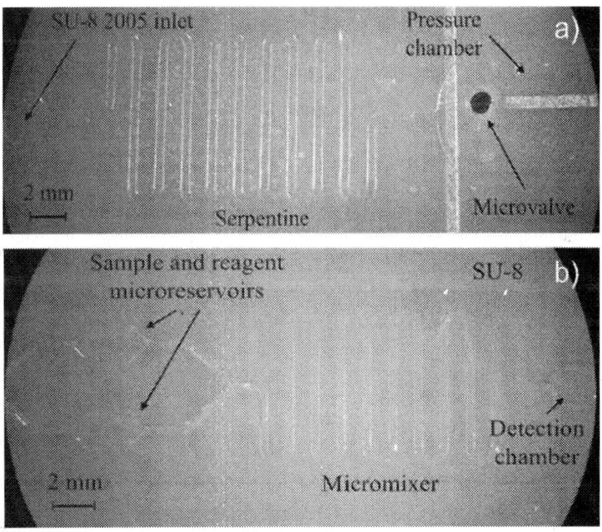

Fig. 25. Bottom and top layers, a) and b) respectively, of the SU-8 microfluidic platform, composed by the sample and reagent microreservoirs, the micromixer and the detection chamber.

the copper microlines, the photodiode will receive the light emitted by the LED through the detection chamber, generating a measurable electric current proportional to the intensity of the light.

6. Summary

This chapter has summarized design concepts, manufacturing processes and integration of MEMS devices for the realization of complex microfluidic systems. These implementations are based on polymer technology that enables the low cost and rapid prototyping of biomedical applications. The initial introduction has described the overall objectives and includes a comparison between the standard silicon MEMS technology and the polymeric one, remarking the facility of use and low cost of the latter. A review of standard processes using the most common materials, PDMS and SU-8, has been described in detail in section 2. The basic steps include deposition, photolithography, baking, and development. The machinery needed for the described processes are a photoplotter to print acetate masks, a spin-coater, a photolithography machine with mask aligner, a hot-plate and a chemical bank for polymer development. This machinery is available to the scientific community at a very reasonable cost compared to the significantly more expensive silicon technologies. Based on the previous basic manufacturing processes, a set of microfluidic devices have been introduced. A one-shot pneumatic impulsion device has been studied in section 3 due to its relevance in microfluidic systems, because it avoids the use of external pumps and complex microfluidic interfaces. Other devices, such as valves and flow regulators are also described in section 5. All these devices make use of a PCB as substrate to facilitate its integration with complementary electronic circuitry. These devices, together with many other that are found in literature, can be integrated to perform more complex microfluidic systems. Modeling a new fluidic design by means of the EC theory and simple simulation software allows the fast design of autonomous pneumatic microfluidic systems, also providing an easy design tool for a wide variety of pressure driven LOC devices, considerably reducing the prototyping and development time. An example of a microfluidic system modeling has been developed in section 5. Finally, an example of a basic LOC including an impulsion device, a mixer and a reaction chamber has been fabricated. The final device requires 0.35J of electrical energy supplied to activate the impulsion device, with a pressure of 3 bar stored in the chamber in order to assure the complete filling of the detection chamber by the fluid to be analyzed. The total time to implement such a system is only one day, thus facilitating a fast improvement of the designs. This example can be easily generalized to implement much more complex microfluidic systems.

7. References

Abgrall, P., Charlot, S., Fulcrand, R., Paul, L., Boukabache, A. & Gue, A. (2008). Low-stress fabrication of 3d polymer free standing structures using lamination of photosensitive films, *Microsyst. Technol.* 14(8): 1205–1214.

Aracil, C., Perdigones, F., Moreno, J. M. & Quero, J. M. (2010). BETTS: bonding, exposing and transferring technique in SU-8 for microsystems fabrication, *Journal of Micromechanics and Microengineering* 20: 035088.

Aracil, C., Quero, J. M., Luque, A., Moreno, J. M. & Perdigones, F. (2010). Pneumatic impulsion device for microfluidic systems, *Sensors and Actuators A: Physical* vol. 163, issue 1: pp. 247–254.

Baek, J. Y., Park, J. Y., Ju, J. I., Lee, T. S. & Lee, S. H. (2005). A pneumatically controllable flexible and polymeric microfluidic valve fabricated via in situ development, *Journal of Micromechanics and Microengineering* 15(5): 1015.

Bruus, H. (2001). *Theoretical Microfluidics*, McGraw-Hill.

Chuang, Y.-J., Tseng, F.-G., Cheng, J.-H. & Lin, W.-K. (2003). A novel fabrication method of embedded micro-channels by using SU-8 thick-film photoresists, *Sens. Actuators A, Phys.* 103(1-2): 64 – 69.

Chung, C. & Allen, M. (2005). Uncrosslinked SU-8 as a sacrificial material, *J. Micromech. Microeng.* 15(1): 113–121.

Dean, R. N. & Luque, A. (2009). Applications of microelectromechanical systems in industrial processes and services, 56: 913–925.

Duffy, D., McDonald, J. C., Schueller, O. & Whitesides, G. M. (1998). Rapid prototyping of microfluidic systems in poly(dimethylsiloxane), *Anal. Chem.* 70(23): 4974 – 4984.

Eddings, M. A., Johnson, M. A. & Gale, B. K. (2008). Determining the optimal PDMS PDMS bonding technique for microfluidic devices, *Journal of Micromechanics and Microengineering* 18: 067001.

Ezkerra, A., Fernandez, L. J., Mayora, K. & Ruano-Lopez, J. M. (2007). Fabrication of SU-8 free-standing structures embedded in microchannelsfor microfluidic control, *J. Micromech. Microeng.* 17(11): 2264–2271.

Guerin, L., Bossel, M., Demierre, M., Calmes, S. & Renaud, P. (1997). Simple and low cost fabrication of embedded micro-channels by using a new thick-film photoplastic, *TRANSDUCERS '97. International Conference on Solid State Sensors and Actuators, Chicago*, Vol. 2, pp. 1419–1422.

Haefliger, D. & Boisen, A. (2006). Three-dimensional microfabrication in negative resist using printed masks, *J. Micromech. Microeng.* 16(5): 951–957.

Henry, S., McAllister, D. V., Allen, M. G. & Prausnitz, M. R. (1998). Micromachined needles for the transdermal delivery of drugs, *Proceedings of the IEEE Eleventh Annual International Workshop on Micro Electro Mechanical Systems, Heidelberg, Germany*, pp. 494–498.

Hong, C. C., Choi, J. W. & Ahn, C. H. (2007). An on-chip air-bursting detonator for driving fluids on disposable lab-on-a-chip systems, *Journal of Micromechanics and Microengineering* 17: 410–417.

Huang, H. & Fu, C. (2007). Different fabrication methods of out-of-plane polymer hollow needle arrays and their variations, *J. Micromech. Microeng.* 17: 393–402.

Koch, C., Remcho, V. & Ingle, J. (2009). Chemical,pdms and tubing-based peristaltic micropumps with direct actuation, *Sensors and Actuators B: Chemical* 135(2): 664–670.

Kovacs, G. T. A., Maluf, N. I. & Petersen, K. E. (1998). Bulk micromachining of silicon, 86(8): 1536–1551.

Laser, D. J. & Santiago, J. G. (2004). A review of micropumps, *Journal of Micromechanics and Microengineering* 14: R35–R64.

Lim, Y. C., Kouzani, A. Z., & Duan, W. (2010). Lab-on-a-chip: a component view, *Microsyst. Technol.* 16:1995-2015.

Lorenz, H., Despont, M., Fahrni, N., LaBianca, N., Renaud, P. & Vettiger, P. (1997). SU-8: a low-cost negative resist for MEMS, *Journal of Micromechanics and Microengineering* 7: 121–124.

Mata, A., Fleischman, A. J. & Roy, S. (2006). Fabrication of multi-layer su-8 microstructures, *Journal of Micromechanics and Microengineering* 16: 276–284.

McDonald, J. C. & Whitesides, G. M. (2002). Poly(dimethylsiloxane) as a material for fabricating microfluidic devices, *Accounts of Chemical Research* 35(7): 491 – 499.

Metz, S., Jiguet, S., Bertsch, A., & Renaud. (2004). Polyimide and SU-8 microfluidic devices manufactured by heat-depolymerizable sacrificial material technique, *Lab Chip* 4:114-120.

Moreno, J. M. & Quero, J. M. (2010). A novel single-use SU-8 microvalve for pressure-driven microfluidic applications, *Journal of Micromechanics and Microengineering* 20: 015005.

Moreno, M., Aracil, C. & Quero, J. (2008). High-integrated microvalve for lab-on-chip biomedical applications, pp. 313 –316.

Murillo, G.,Davis, Z. J., Keller, S., Abadal, G., Agusti, J., Cagliani, A., Noeth, N., Boisen, A. & Barniol, N. (2010). Novel SU-8 based vacuum wafer-level packaging for MEMS devices,*Microelectronic Engineering* 87:1173-1176.

Oh, K. W. & Ahn, C. H. (2006). A review of microvalves, *Journal of Micromechanics and Microengineering* 16: R13–R39.

Patel, J. N., Kaminska, B., Gray, B. L. & Gates, B. D. (2008). Pdms as a sacrificial substrate for SU-8-based biomedical and microfluidic applications, *J. Micromech. Microeng.* 18(9): 095028 (11pp).

Perdigones, F., Luque, A. & Quero, J. M. (2010a). Novel structure for a pneumatically controlled flow regulator with positive gain, *Journal of Microelectromechanical Systems.* 19(5): 1070 – 1078.

Perdigones, F., Luque, A. & Quero, J. M. (2010b). PDMS microdevice for precise liquid aspiration in the submicroliter range based on the Venturi effect, *Microelectronic Engineering* 87(11): 2103 – 2109.

Perdigones, F., Moreno, J. M., Luque, A. & Quero, J. M. (2010). Characterisation of the fabrication process of freestanding SU-8 microstructures integrated in printing circuit board in microelectromechanical systems, *Micro and Nano Letters* 5: 7–13.

Perdigones, F., Luque, A. & Quero, J. M. (In press). Highly integrable flow regulator with positive gain, *Journal of Microelectromechanical Systems* In press.

Petersen, K. E. (1982). Silicon as a mechanical material, 70(5): 420–457.

Roark, R. J., Budynas, R. G. & Young, W. C. (2001). *Roark's Formulas for stress and strain*, McGraw-Hill.

Status of the MEMS industry (2008). Yole Dveloppement.

Takao, H. & Ishida, M. (2003). Microfluidic integrated circuits for signal processing using analogous relationship between pneumatic microvalve and MOSFET, *Journal of Microelectromechanical Systems* 12(4): 497–505.

Vedel, S. (2009). *Millisecond dynamics in microfluidics: Equivalent circuit theory and experiment*, PhD thesis, DTU Nanotech, Department of Micro and Nanotechnology.

4

A Low Cost Instrumentation Based Sensor Array for Ankle Rehabilitation

Samir Boukhenous and Mokhtar Attari
Laboratory of Instrumentation, Faculty of Electronics and Computers USTHB, Bab-Ezzouar, Algiers Algeria

1. Introduction

Tactile sensing technology has made significant progress towards the development of devices where robot fingers must have the ability of multi-dimensional tactile sensing in order to perform grasping and manipulating tasks (Chi & Shida, 2004); (Webster, 1998); (Nicholls & Lee, 1989); (Tarchanidis & Lygouras, 2001); (Da Silva et al., 2000). Therefore, many researchers have tried to develop various types of tactile sensors by applying MEMS technologies which usually rely on the measurement of pressure or force on a sensing element (Hasegawa et al, 2007). A variety of different types of sensors have been used, including resistive strain gauges, piezoelectric film, infrared displacement sensors, capacitive sensors, sensors detecting conductance, magnetic, magnetoelectric and ultrasonic sensors. Frequently large numbers of sensing elements are built into an array and the outputs of those sensors are processed, often in conjunction with a mathematical model, to give an assessment of the contacting object. Nowadays, force sensing becomes an important component for diver applications in biomedical applications and orthopedic rehabilitation. Thus, tactile sensors have been used in hand clinical evaluations and foot rehabilitation (Da Silva et al., 2000); (Mascaro & Asada, 2001); (Boukhenous & Attari, 2007); (Attari & Boukhenous, 2008). Human tactile sensing is achieved by means of at least four different types of receptor cells (Jayawant, 1989); (Cowie et al., 2007) and is used to feel, grasp and manipulate objects, and to assess attributes such as shape, size, texture, temperature, hardness, discontinuities such as holes or edges, and movement, including vibration. Reston and Kolesar (Reston et al., 1990) described a robotic tactile sensor manufactured from piezoelectric polyvinylidene fluoride (PVDF) film. It was not the best choice for finger mounted tactile sensors due to its limited load range and inability to measure static forces. Beebe and al (Beebe et al., 1989) developed a force sensor based on a silicon diaphragm structure instrumented with piezoresistors in Wheatstone bridge configuration. The applied force is distributed across the diaphragm via a grasping solid dome and mounted on rigid substrate with an excellent performance characteristic. In this paper a low cost tactile sensors array for the measurement of hand grasping forces is described in a first step. A second step is dedicated to the study of two-dimensional reaction forces distribution of foot during rehabilitation in the case of ankle sprain. The sensor element of the array is an easy structure based on the use of low cost Hall device and a general purpose polymer (polysiloxanes). First the elastic polymer is studied to show its ability in building such sensing element. After mounting the sensors, the outputs signals are conditioned, filtered and then digitized with a high resolution data acquisition card. A static calibration test has been fulfilled to estimate the degree of linearity. Preliminary measurement has been carried out concerning the fingertip forces grasping of hand during holding objects and the distribution of impacts forces during foot contact.

2. Principe and sensor design

For the design of the sensor element, a Hall Effect sensor UGN3503 from Allegro Micro-Systems was selected. This sensor is used for measuring magnetic flux densities with extreme sensitivity and operates well in the temperature range from -20°C to +85°C and in the frequency range from DC to 23 kHz. This device is widely used for measuring linear position, angular position, velocity and rotational speed. Hall sensors are also commonly incorporated into CD-ROM drive, hard disk drives, automotive ignition, electrical current sensing and ABS braking systems as they are robust, unaffected by dirty environments and low-cost (Ripka & Tipek, 2007). In contrast to other magnetic sensors, the manufacture of Hall magnetic sensors does not require special fabrication techniques as they are compatible with microelectronics technology. Most of the sensors are low-cost discrete devices but an increasing proportion now come in the form of integrated circuits. The integrated Hall magnetic sensors usually incorporate circuits for biasing, offset reduction, temperature compensation, signal amplification and signal level discrimination. The most advanced Hall sensors incorporate digital signal processing and are programmable such as HAL800 from Micronas (Bushbaum & Plassmeier, 2007). The considered sensor element is constructed by placing a magnet which produces a constant magnetic field nearby the selected Hall sensor. The layer of thickness *d* between the magnet and the Hall sensor is realized with an elastic polymer materiel (Fig.1). Special care was dedicated to the positioning of magnet in the direction of the surface area of sensing in order to reduce the nonlinearity of the tactile sensor (Ehrlich, 2000); (Kyberd & Chappel, 1993). After the placement of the different layers composing the whole sensor element, a thin twisted pair wire is soldered to the Hall sensor as the voltage produced is at low level and need low noise amplification.

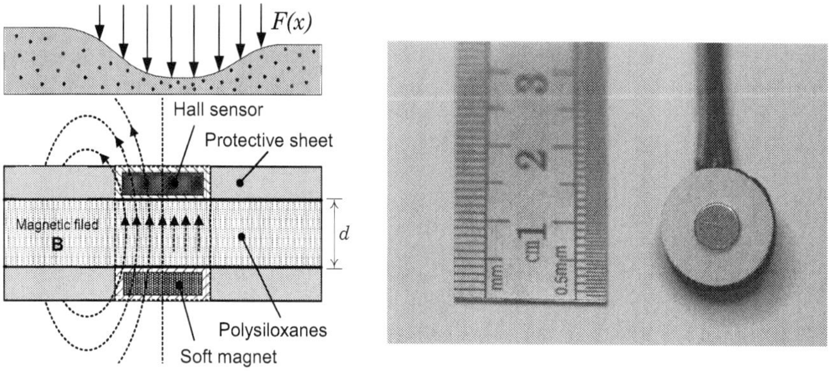

Fig. 1. The sensor element principle and realization

First, the elastic polymer (polysiloxanes) and a piece taken from mouse mat were studied to show the possibility of using this material in building the sensing element. A test bed with Lutron FG-5000A was performed for this purpose and experimental data are reported in Fig.2 for the two chosen materials.

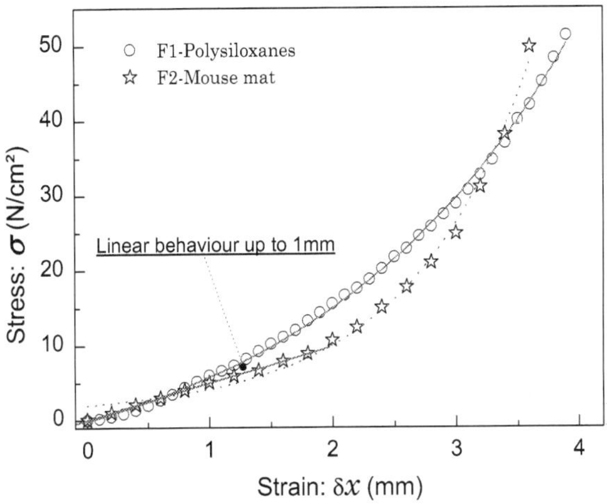

Fig. 2. Characteristics of the materials

For the second material (mouse mat) a strong nonlinear behavior was observed for strain greater than 2 mm. For strain up to 2 mm, the characteristic was quasi linear. The second material exhibits a better monotony with soft nonlinearity. As a calibration curve the following exponential growth was found with a correlation coefficient of about 0.997:

$$F = \beta + \alpha \times \exp(\delta x / k) \tag{1}$$

A more precise calibration curve was obtained with a third-order polynomial with a correlation coefficient of about 0.999, thus:

$$y = F(\delta x) = a_0 + a_1.\delta x + a_2.(\delta x)^2 + a_3.(\delta x)^3 \tag{2}$$

As a nonlinear property is found for the studied material, a software routine was implemented after digital signal acquisition to perform nonlinearity correction. From the calibration curve of the sensor an equi-spaced 1-D look-up table is created and a quadratic interpolation was used (Attari, 2004); (Dias Pereira et al., 2001) whose curve passes through three points $(y_{k-1},\ \delta x_{k-1})$, $(y_k,\ \delta x_k)$, $(y_{k-1},\ \delta x_{k+1})$,

$$\begin{aligned} \delta x = \delta x_k + (y - y_k) f[y_{k-1}, y_k] + \\ + (y\text{-}y_{k-1})(y - y_k) f[y_{k-1}, y_k, y_{k+1}] \end{aligned} \tag{3}$$

with the second divided difference given by,

$$f[y_k, y_{k+1}] = \frac{\delta x_{k+1} - \delta x_k}{y_{k+1} - y_k}$$
$$f[y_{k-1}, y_k, y_{k+1}] = \frac{f[y_k, y_{k+1}] - f[y_{k-1}, y_k]}{y_{k+1} - y_{k-1}} \quad (4)$$

3. Signals conditioning and experimental

The outputs signals issued from the sensors elements are carried onto a low level instrumentation amplifier (AD622, *Analog Devices*) with low offset voltage, low noise and high CMRR. After analog conditioning, these signals are filtered with a second order Butterwoth active filter and sampled and digitalized with a commercial National Instrument data acquisition card (*DaqBoard 1005*) and then fed a PCI PC bus. Fig.3. show the analog and digital part of the prototype circuit which is directly connected to each sensor element where the output signals are multiplexed with the circuit included in the data acquisition card. First step is to perform the static calibration characteristics by applying a variable force from 1 to 10N provided by a test bed (*Lutron FG-5000A*). Fig.4 shows outputs signals from five sensors elements. Least squares linear regression were performed to compute the estimated linear calibrating curves and to determine the sensor sensitivity for each sensor. After analyzing the sensors data, a linearity was observed for the range [0-10N] with a correlation coefficient greater than 0.99. For forces up to 10N the responses become less accurate against linearity shape and correction based on the method described above (Sec.2) was performed for further investigation, for instance in 2D stress measurement for foot reaction forces distribution. For dynamic experimentation two tests in real environment have been realized.

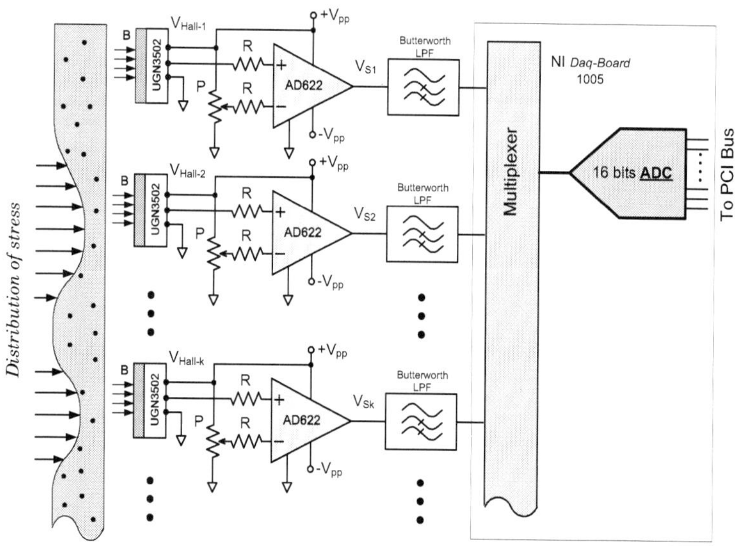

Fig. 3. Conditioning circuit array and data acquisition

3.1 Test during holding objects

For the test five sensors element are bonded onto the fingertips of human hand (Fig. 5). Outputs signals are observed and a software program is developed to analyze the fingertips movement during holding objects. Fig.6 shows the response corresponding to grasping of the thumb, index, middle, ring and little fingertips during holding a bottle of mineral water. The experimental results show that the changes of dynamic fingertips force affects the transducers in the contact phase measurement. The thumb, index and middle are the fingers that give the highest signal level as they exert high pressures regarding the two other fingers. This observation is in concordance with the biomechanics of hand which verify the feasibility of the proposed sensors arrays.

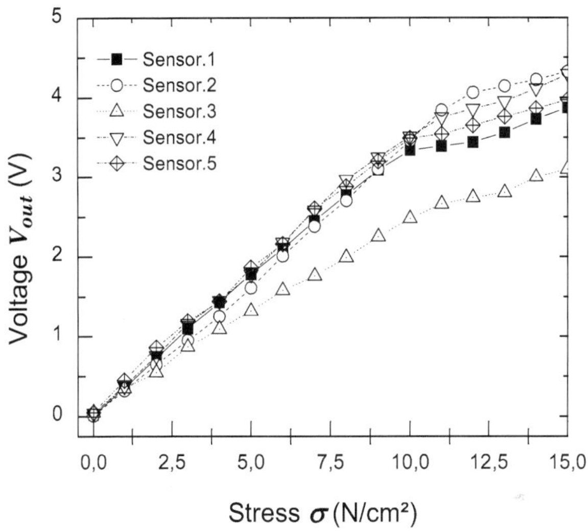

Fig. 4. Static calibration

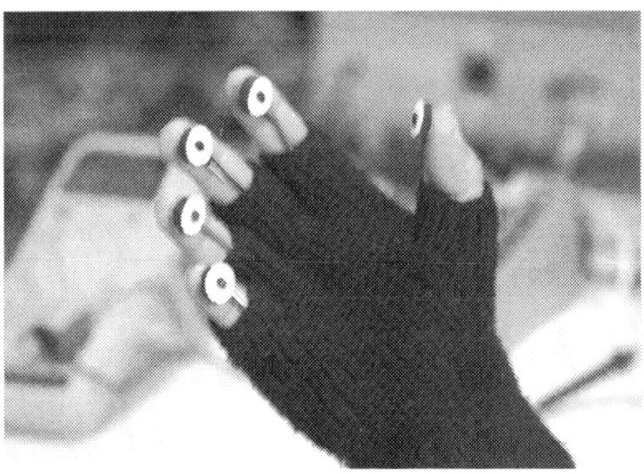

Fig. 5. Tactile sensors bounded on fingers hand

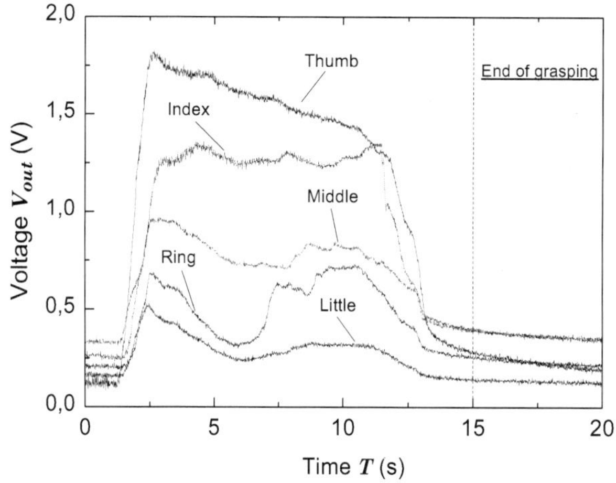

Fig. 6. Outputs signals of transducers during holding

3.2 Test for ankle rehabilitation

Second dynamic measurement in real environment has been carried out with eight realized sensors which are bonded onto a flexible material as foot shape (Fig. 7). Fig. 8 shows the apparatus constructed with wood beech dedicated for the rehabilitation of ankle. Fig.9 shows the response corresponding to eight tactile sensors distributed on the insole surface during an experiment of ankle rehabilitation. The experimental results for 30s recording show clearly the frequency swing of the wood substrate. Also, a delay time is observed for example between sensors S1 and S8 during foot swing where the whole body is maintained stable with one foot. This observation is in concordance with the geometry of the placement of sensors and it is obvious to show that the time delay is approximately half time the time of swinging, thus,

$$T_{Delay} \approx \frac{1}{2} T_{Swing} \tag{5}$$

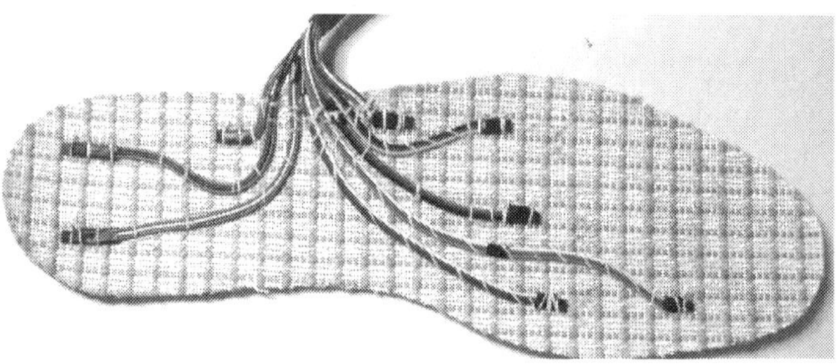

Fig. 7. Placement of eight tactile sensors

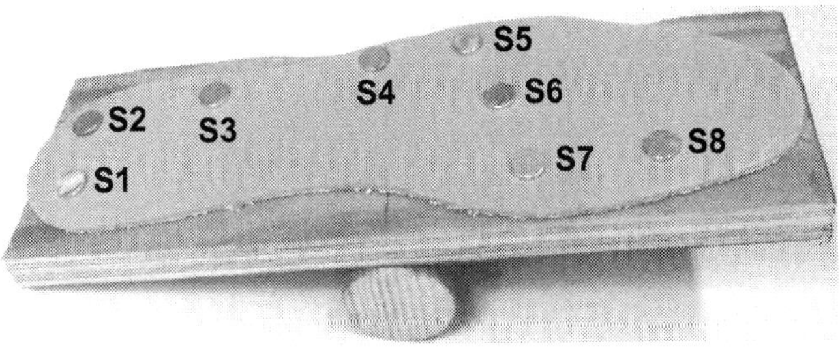

Fig. 8. Apparatus for ankle rehabilitation

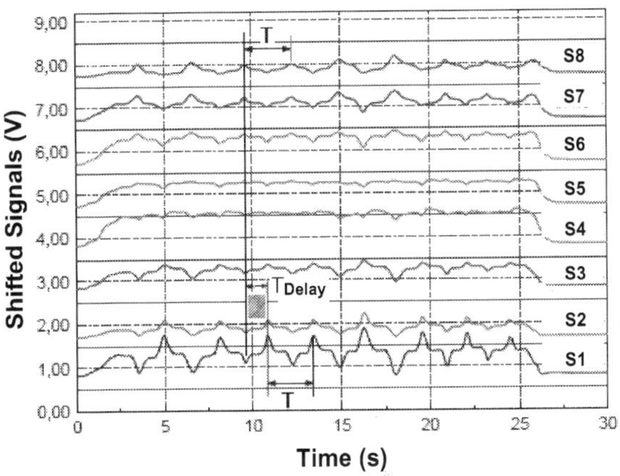

Fig. 9. The eight recorded signals

Futures investigations are oriented toward the realization of embedded bioinstrumentation system for the measurement of foot reaction forces for a dedicated balanced platform. This one will be the essential part of the test bed system for the determination of force shape of foot during the rehabilitation of ankle. Fig. 10 shows the principle part of the whole system which consists on positioning a numbers of sensors elements on a special platform fit with dimension of a standard foot. The number of sensors will be determined with resolution required for the foot reaction forces study (Boukhenous et al., 2006). For better flexibility of data acquisition with high special resolution, the HAL800 digital programmable Hall Effect device is preferred. The proposed printed circuit board (PCB) for the realizing of the whole 2D sensing system is shown in Fig. 11. Notice that the number of signals outputs pads is equal to the number of sensors elements. Also, a special care will be considered in positioning precisely the Hall devices with taken into account shielding and grounding of the whole PCB. An epoxy resin will be deposited carefully on the sensors array in order to standardize the first layer against the elastic material.

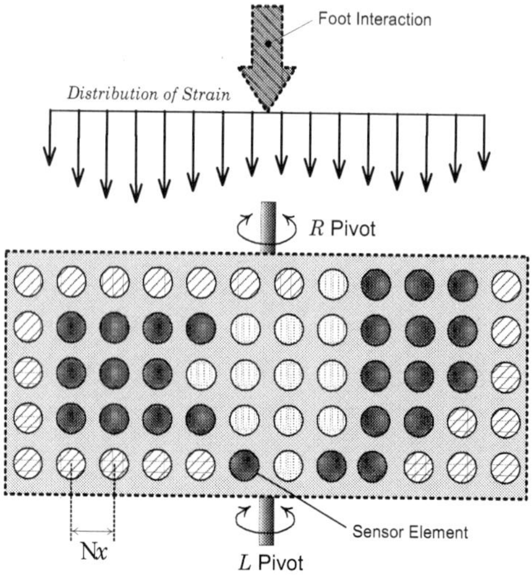

Fig. 10. Tactile sensors array for ankle rehabilitation

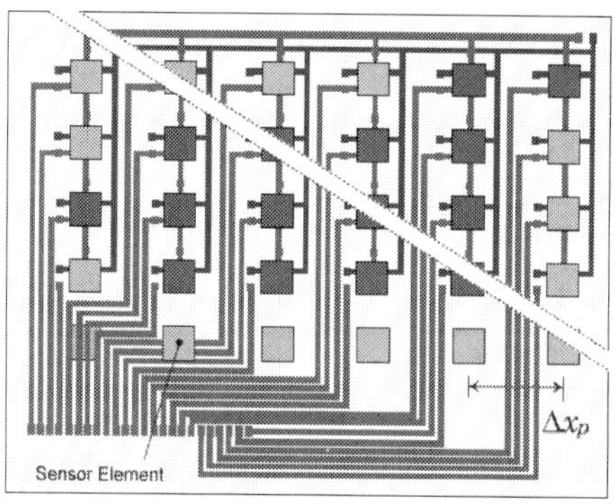

Fig. 11. Placement of sensors elements in a rigid PCB

4. Conclusion

In this paper a low cost tactile sensors array for biomedical applications are presented. Each sensor element was constructed separately and based on the use of Hall sensor devices. The sensors were calibrate and trimmed before proceeding to the experimental tests. A dedicated analog signal processing was designed and realized according to the specificity of the realized sensor. Accurate settings have been achieved by offset and gain trimming for zero crossing and required sensitivity. Outputs signals from the conditioning circuit of the eight transducers are coupled to a high resolution data acquisition card. The software program developed analyzes and calibrates the multisensors signals. Dynamic experimentation for fingertips grasping of the hand during holding an objects and the distribution of impacts forces during foot contact for ankle rehabilitation shows a satisfactory response and verify the feasibility of the proposed sensors array. After analyzing the sensors, the data found in the range [0-10N] is the optimized interval for best linearties. Future works are focused toward an intelligent calibration and processing of the acquired signals using dedicated analog processor and FPGA implementation of a matrix of sensors elements for the monitoring of ankle rehabilitation.

5. References

Attari, M. & Boukhenous, S. (2008). A Tactile Sensors Array for Biomedical Applications, *Proceeding of 5th International Multi-Conference on Systems, Signals and Devices, IEEE-SSD'08,* ISBN: 978-1-4244-2206-7, Amman, Jordanie, Juillet 20-23, 2008

Attari, M. (2004). Correction Techniques for Improving Accuracy in Measurements, State of the Art, *Proceeding of International Conference on Computer Theory and Applications, ICCTA/2004,* Alexandria, Egypt, September 2004

Beebe, D.J. & Denton, D.D. (1998). A silicon-based tactile sensor for finger-mounted applications. *IEEE Trans. Biomed. Eng.,* Vol. 45, pp. 151-159, Feb. 1998

Boukhenous, S. & Attari, M. (2007). A Low Cost Grip Transducer Based Instrument To Quantify Fingertip Touch Force, *Proceedings of IEEE Engineering in Medicine and Biology Society,* Science and Technologies for Health, EMB'2007, pp. 4834-4837, ISBN: 1-4244-0788-5, ISSN: 1557-170X, , Lyon, France, Vol. 4, August 21-24, 2007

Boukhenous, S.; Attari, M. & Ababou, N. (2006). A Dynamic Study of Foot-to-Floor Interaction During a Vertical Jumping. *AMSE Journals, Modeling B,* Vol.75, N°1, April 2006, pp. 41-49, ISSN: 1259-5969

Buschbaum, A & Plassmeier,V.P. (2007). Angle measurement with a Hall effect sensor, *Smart Mater. Structl.,* Vol. 16, 2007, pp. 1120-1124

Chi, Z. & Shida, K. (2004). A New Multifunctional Tactile Sensor for Three-Dimensional Force Measurement. *Sensors and Actuators,* Vol. A111, 2004, pp. 172-179

Cowie, B.M.; Webb, D.J.; Tam, B.; Slack, P. & Brett, P.N. (2007). Fibre Bragg gratting sensors for distributive tactile sensing. *Journal of Meas. Sci. Technol.;* Vol. 18, 2007, pp. 138-146

Da Silva, J.G.; Carvalho, A. A. & Silva, D. D. (2000). A strain gage tactile sensor for finger-mounted applications, *Proceeding of IEEE Instrum. Meas. Technol.* Conf., IMTC/2000, Baltimore, MD, May 1–4, 2000

Da Silva, J.G.; Carvalho, A. A. & Rodrigues, R. O. (2000). Development of a dynamometer for hand clinical evaluation, *Proceedings of Iberdiscap Conf.,* pp. 429-434, Portugal, 2000

Dias Pereira, J.M.; Silva Girão, P.M.B. & Postolache, O. (2001). Fitting Transducer Characteristics to Measured Data. *IEEE Instrumentation and Measurement Magazine,* pp. 26-39, December 2001

Ehrlich, A.C. (2000). The Hall Effect, In : The Electrical Engineering Handbook Ed. Richard C. Dorf Boca Raton: CRC Press LLC, 2000

Hasegawa, Y.; Shikida, M.; Sasaka, H.; Itoigawa, K. & Sato, K. (2007). An active tactile sensor for detecting mechanical charactyeristics of contacted objects. *Journal. Micromech. Microeng.,* Vol. 16, 2007, pp. 1625-1632

Jayawant, B.V. (1989). Tactile Sensors in Robotics. J. Phys. E: Sci. Instrum., Vol. 22, 1989, pp. 684-692

Kyberd, P.J. & Chappell, P.H. (1993). A Force Sensor for Automatic manipulation Based on the Hall Effect. *Journal of Meas. Sci. Technol.*, Vol. 4, 1993, pp. 281-287

Mascaro, S. & Asada, H. H. (2001). Photoplethysmograph fingernail sensors for measuring finger forces without haptic obstruction. *IEEE Trans. Robot. Automat.*, Vol. 17, pp. 698–708, Oct. 2001

Nicholls, H.R. & Lee, M.H. (1989). A Survey of Robot Tactile Sensing Technology. *Int. Journal. Robotics Res*, Vol. 8, N. 3, 1989, pp.3-30

Reston, R.R.; Kolesar, J.E. & Mascaro, S. (1990). Robotic tactile sensor array fabricated from piezoelectric polyvinilidene fluoride film, *Proceedings of Nat. Aerospace Electron. Conf. (NAECON)*, pp. 1139-1144, 1990

Ripka, P. & Tipek, A. (2007). *Modern Sensors Handbook*, ISTE Ltd, UK, 2007, 536 p

Tarchanidis, G.K.N. & Lygouras, J. N. (2001). Data glove with a force sensor, *Proceedings of IEEE Instrum. Meas. Technol*, Budapest, Hungary, May 21-23, 2001

Webster, J.G. (1998). *Tactile Sensors for robotics and Medicine*, J.G. Webster, Ed. Wiley, New York

5

New Neurostimulation Strategy and Corresponding Implantable Device to Enhance Bladder Functions

Fayçal Mounaïm and Mohamad Sawan
Polystim Neurotechnologies Laboratory, Department of Electrical Engineering
École Polytechnique de Montréal
Canada

1. Introduction

Spinal cord injury (SCI) is one of the most complex and devastating medical conditions. Its worldwide incidence ranges from 11 to 112 per 100,000 Population (Blumer & Quine, 1995; DeVivo, 1997). SCI leads to different degrees of dysfunction of the lower urinary tract due to a large variety of possible lesions. Immediately after SCI, flaccid paralysis sets in, followed by the absence of reflexes and a complete loss of sensory and motor control below the level of lesion, rendering the urinary bladder areflexic and atonic. This period, termed spinal shock, can extend from a few days to several months (Chai & Steers, 1996). Most patients with suprasacral SCI suffer from detrusor over-activity (DO) and detrusor sphincter dyssynergia (DSD) (Blaivas et al., 1981). DSD leads to high intravesical pressure, high residual urine, urinary tract infection, and deterioration of the upper urinary tract. In order to recover the voluntary control of micturition, functional electrical stimulation (FES) has been investigated at different sites of the urinary system: the bladder muscle (detrusor), the pelvic nerves, the spinal cord and the sacral nerve roots. Among these, sacral nerve root stimulation is considered the most efficient technique to induce micturition and has been prevalent in clinical practice over the last two decades (Elabaddy et al., 1994). Using cuff-electrodes, this technique offers the advantages of a safe and stable fixation of electrodes as well as confinement of the spread of stimulation current within the targeted nerves. However, the detrusor and the external urethral sphincter (EUS) muscles share the sacral nerves as common innervations pathways, and stimulation of the entire sacral root induces contraction of both. Thus, the efficiency of micturition by means of sacral neurostimulation depends on the capability to contract the detrusor without triggering EUS contraction. In order to improve this neurostimulation selectivity, several techniques have been proposed, among which are rhizotomy, and EUS blockade using high-frequency stimulation.

Dorsal rhizotomy consists of selectively severing afferent sacral nerve roots that are involved in pathological reflex arc in suprasacral SCI patients. Rhizotomy abolishes DO, reduces DSD, and prevents autonomic dysreflexia. As a beneficial result, the uninhibited bladder contractions are reduced, the bladder capacity and compliance are increased, urine flow is improved, and consequently the upper urinary tract is protected from ureteral reflux and hydronephrosis. In case of a complete SCI, dorsal rhizotomy is combined with an implantable sacral ventral root stimulator such as the Finetech-Brindley Bladder System (also known as the VOCARE in North America) (Kutzenberger, 2007). In fact, this neurostimulation system is the only commercialized and FDA-approved solution aiming for micturition in SCI patients (Jezernik et al., 2002). Unfortunately, rhizotomy being irreversible, it has a fundamental disadvantage which is the abolition of sexual and defecation reflexes, as well as sacral sensations if still present in case of incomplete SCI.

High-frequency stimulation can be used to inhibit the contraction of the EUS muscle. However, the mechanism by which the EUS inhibition is obtained is not well understood and three explanations are possible: high-frequency stimulation may stop the propagation of nerve action potentials, may maintain the motor end-plate (neuromuscular junction) in a refractory status, or may fatigue the aimed muscle (Kilgore & Bhadra, 2004; Tai et al., 2005; Williamson & Andrews, 2005). Frequencies from 300 Hz to 30 kHz can be used to achieve a complete and reversible nerve conduction block depending on the stimulation amplitude (Solomonow, 1984; Sievert et al., 2002; Schuettler et al., 2004; Bhadra et al., 2006). However, below 1 kHz, a sinusoidal stimulation can generate action potentials at the same or a submultiple rate. Increasing the frequency has the advantage of lowering the amount of injected charge per-phase needed for a complete blockade. A graded blockade can also be achieved as blockade of each axon within the nerve is influenced by its diameter and the stimulation amplitude (Tai et al., 2005). If a graded blockade is applied distally in combination with low-frequency stimulation, selectivity with respect to axon diameter can be obtained by adjusting stimulation amplitude (Williamson & Andrews, 2005). Finally, combining sacral root stimulation with bilateral high-frequency pudendal nerve block led to effective micturition in male cats (Boger et al., 2008).

The efficiency of high-frequency blockade was studied with dog experiments using a neurostimulator designed by Polystim Neurotechnologies Laboratory (Robin et al., 1998; Shaker et al., 1998; Ba et al., 2002; Sawan et al., 2008b). The Polystim's stimulator generated a rectangular waveform combining two frequencies (e.g. 600 Hz and 30 Hz). It is important to point out in this case, that stimulation and blockade are both applied simultaneously at the same nerve site, with the same bipolar electrode. According to Kilgore et al. (Kilgore & Bhadra, 2004), blockade at 600 Hz frequency with less than 2 mA current is probably due to a muscle fatigue mechanism rather than nerve conduction blockade. The same neurostimulator was also implanted in paraplegic dogs for chronic experiments where it was demonstrated that the combination of low and high frequency stimuli resulted in 45 % reduction in EUS activity and that urine evacuation improved up to 91 % of the mean bladder capacity during the six months of chronic stimulation (Abdel-Gawad et al., 2001). The latest Polystim's neurostimulation prototypes using that stimulation strategy were UroStim6 and UroStim7 presented in (Mounaim et al., 2006; Mounaim & Sawan, 2007) respectively.

This chapter first describes a new sacral neurostimulation strategy to enhance micturition, based on nerve conduction blockade using high frequency stimulation as an alternative to rhizotomy. In order to test this strategy in chronic animal experiments, an implantable neurostimulation device is required. Thus, this chapter presents the design, test, prototyping and encapsulation of such neurostimulator (UroStim8) implementing the proposed stimulation strategy and using only commercially available discrete components.

2. New stimulation strategy

The proposed multi-site sacral neurostimulation strategy is illustrated in Fig. 1 and based on the following: High-frequency stimulation with an alternating waveform (such as sinusoidal or rectangular) and optimum parameters, induces a blockade of the nerve (motor and/or sensory) activity, that may be complete (all axons) or partial (large diameter axons only). With a complete nerve blockade, the effect would be equivalent to that of rhizotomy while being controlled and totally reversible. With a partial blockade, selective stimulation can be achieved by blocking large axons only.

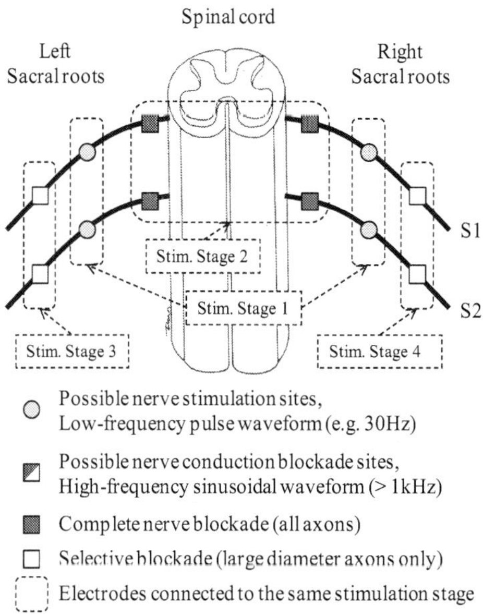

Fig. 1. Proposed multi-sites sacral neurostimulation strategy (dog model)

In order to induce a contraction of the detrusor, a low-frequency (e.g. 30 Hz) pulse current stimulation is applied to S2 sacral nerve(s) (or S1 eventually), unilaterally or bilaterally. Adjusting the stimulation pulse amplitude and width, the degree of contraction can be modulated. In most cases, the EUS contracts as well. The stimulation-evoked EUS contraction may be explained by direct and/or reflex mechanisms due to efferent and/or afferent fibers activation respectively. Both types of EUS activation can be avoided by blocking axons innervating the EUS muscle with high-frequency (> 1 kHz) stimulation. A selective blockade can be applied distally (between the low-frequency stimulation site and the EUS) to inhibit direct EUS activation, while a complete blockade can be applied proximally (between the low-frequency stimulation site and the spinal cord), to inhibit reflex EUS activation. However, reflex EUS activation may involve sacral root(s) other than the one(s) stimulated by the low-frequency waveform. In such case, they should be blocked as well. Anatomically, the lower urinary tract innervations are the same from one animal to another but there is a functional variability. It is possible that one type of EUS activation mechanisms is dominant. For illustration purposes, Fig. 1 shows all possible blockade sites, but it is also possible that one blockade site prove to be sufficient. In case of incomplete SCI, conventional sacral nerve stimulation may lead to pain perception. Rhizotomy can be a way to abolish the stimulation-evoked pain but will probably not be considered at the cost of losing important reflexes and sensations if still present. With the proposed stimulation strategy, a complete proximal high-frequency blockade of sensory activity during low-frequency stimulation can inhibit pain sensation as well. Polystim Lab. recently presented preliminary results obtained with this strategy based on a dog model. Acute dog experiments were carried out and EUS blockade has been achieved in 8 animals after spinal cord transection (Mounaim et al. 2008; 2010). However, such experiments are not sufficient to validate the strategy especially that spinal shock generally lasts several weeks after SCI. Chronic experiments are mandatory in order to evaluate the long-term efficiency. This obviously requires a custom implantable neurostimulator that implements the proposed strategy, and will be capable of generating conventional stimulation waveforms as well as high-frequency sinusoids simultaneously over multiple channels.

3. Discrete implantable neurostimulator

3.1 Neurostimulator architecture

The block diagram of Fig.2 illustrates the architecture of the implantable neurostimulator UroStim8 dedicated to the new stimulation strategy. The neurostimulator has been designed with commercially available off-the shelf components. The control unit is one of the latest generation of Field Programmable Gate Arrays (FPGA) that presents advantageous low-power and small-scale features (Igloo, ACTEL). This FPGA also offers an In-Sytem Programming (ISP) feature that would allow (wired) subsequent code updates even after encapsulation of the neurostimulator. Such option was not possible with anti-fuse FPGAs used in previous prototypes (Ex, ACTEL) leading to the assembly of a new prototype for each new code to be tested. With near-field inductive coupling of spiral antennas, energy and data are wirelessly transmitted through the skin to the implanted stimulator using an external controller. The inductive coupling frequency used in previous prototypes was 20 MHz, but to comply with the Industrial, Scientific and Medical (ISM) radio band, it is reduced to 13.56 MHz. This frequency is chosen taking into account the coupling attenuation through the skin tissues and the spiral inductors characteristics. The Power Recovery stage rectifies and filters the inductive carrier signal to provide different regulated power supplies to the stimulator. The Data Recovery stage demodulates the 600 kHz On-Off Keying (OOK) modulated carrier to provide Manchester-coded data to the FPGA. As soon as the inductive energy is present and the power supply sufficient, the FPGA starts Manchester decoding to extract data at 300 Kbps and a synchronized clock at 300 kHz. Transmission data frames are sent cyclically until the FPGA acknowledges that a valid one is received without errors using a low power and short-range 1 kbps RF uplink at 433 MHz. Depending on the received instruction and parameters, a specific mode is executed. This could be a stimulation mode where one or multiple Stimulation Stages outputs can be activated with chosen parameters, or a telemetry mode where impedance module and phase of each electrode-nerve interface (ENI) can be measured at a chosen frequency. Even though all stimulation stages are similar and can generate any waveform to a certain extent, Stimulation Stage 1 is dedicated to the low-frequency pulse waveform while Stages 2 to 4 are dedicated to the high-frequency sinusoidal waveform. The stimulation frequency is common to Stages 2 to 4 but the stimulation current amplitude can be adjusted independently. The synchronized clock extracted from the Manchester-coded data was used as a time base for stimuli generation in previous neurostimulators. However, this clock suffers from time jitter due to inductive noise during data demodulation. Timing is very important as for conventional biphasic stimulation for example, positive and negative phases must have the same duration so that total charge injection into the ENI is null. The oscillator in Fig. 2 is a low power component that brings a simple solution to this problem. Frequency of oscillation is adjusted with one resistance and an internal divider setting. The oscillator is activated for stimuli generation only and provides a stable clock of 300 kHz that can be eventually increased or decreased (hardware modification, not through the FPGA) depending on the available inductive power and the desired stimulation parameters.

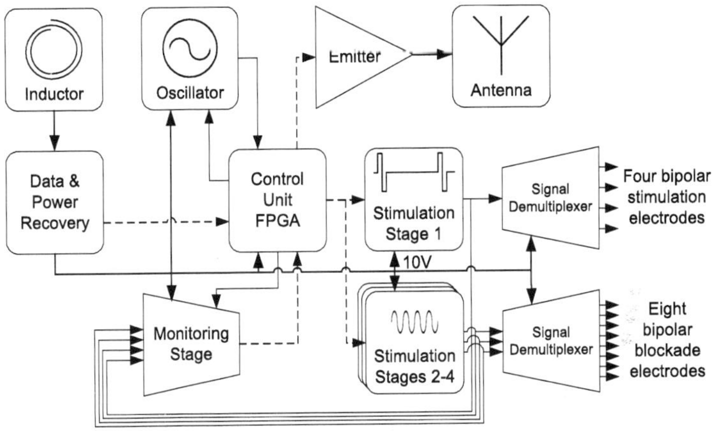

Fig. 2. Architecture of the UroStim8 neurostimulator dedicated to the new strategy

3.2 Power and data recovery

The neurostimulator front-end is responsible for power and data recovery as shown in Fig.3. Inductive energy transmitted by the external controller is recovered by the implanted stimulator using a parallel LC network resonating at the same frequency. Inductance L is a 3-turn spiral antenna that is printed on a thin and flexible PCB with external diameter of less than 4 cm and a trace width of 1 mm to reduce the series resistance. Capacitance C is made of parallel combinations of ceramic NPO capacitors that offer high Q and high temperature stability. The capacitors are also specified for 100 V in order to maintain acceptable values at high voltages and high frequency. C_{tune} is a miniature variable capacitor that allows fine tuning of the resonant frequency to recover maximum energy with respect to the average power consumption of the implant. The voltage across the resonating LC network is an alternating signal that may exceed 60 V peak-to-peak in case of a high inductive coupling and a weak load. This signal is rectified with diodes (D1, D2) and filtered with the capacitor C_{filter} which can be seen as the energy storage for the implant. Because of such high voltage, this capacitor has been chosen with a compromise between voltage specification (50 V), capacitance value (6.8 μF), and physical dimensions. When inductive coupling is suddenly interrupted, reverse currents may occur, leading to negative voltages at the input of the first regulator (Fig.3). Diode D4 protects the circuit from such situations.

As shown in Fig.3, three linear regulators provide different power supply voltages to the neurostimulator. The first one is adjusted between 5 and 12 V for the supply of current sources and the analog supply of CMOS switches in the Stimuli Stages (Fig.4). This regulator

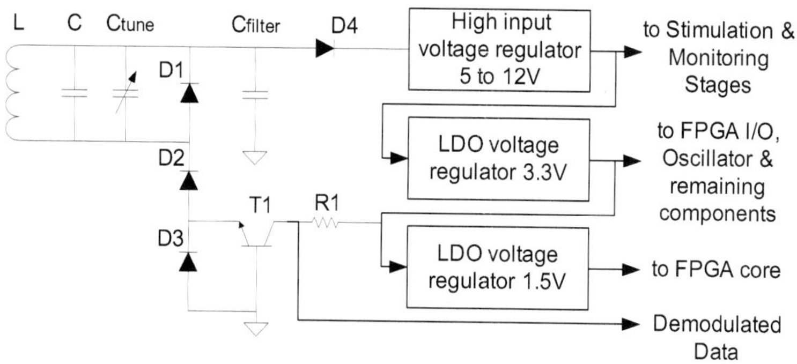

Fig. 3. Power and data recovery in UroStim8

can tolerate high input voltages up to 80 V. The second regulator provides 3.3 V that is the main supply used by the FPGA Input/Outputs buffers, the DAC, the logic supply of CMOS switches in the Stimuli Stages, and the remaining components. This regulator provides a Power-OK (POK) signal that indicates to the FPGA that the 3.3V supply is available and well regulated. No stimulation will be started unless the POK signal is high. Finally, the third supply of 1.5 V is used by the FPGA core only to reduce its power consumption.

To protect the system from a high induced voltage, power recovery circuits use voltage clipping, Zener diodes or shunt regulators (Schneider, 2001; Ba et al., 2002; Ba, 2004; Yunlei & Jin, 2005; Balachandran & Barnett, 2006). In previous neurostimulators, a shunt regulator was adjusted to be able to provide the required voltage supply in the worst case that is maximum stimulator current consumption and minimum available inductive energy. However, except in this case, it is not an efficient solution because the shunt regulator simply short-cuts the excess current. With the high input voltage of the first regulator, there is no need for voltage limiting, and the excess of inductive energy translates to voltage instead of current. Voltage is indirectly limited by the maximum available inductive energy and the minimum stimulator current consumption. Compared to the zener shunt regulator, it is a more efficient solution that also allows recovering high voltage supply for stimulation without using step-up DC/DC converters. For data recovery, the OOK demodulator is a simple envelope detector which is implemented as an amplification of small variations across diode D3 that is stacked in series between the rectifier diodes (D1, D2) and the common ground. These variations are due to the carrier modulation and are amplified with the NPN transistor T1 in a common-base configuration. A pull-up resistor R1 limits the current when the demodulated data signal is low but also limits its rising time. The design simplicity of this demodulator is the reason behind the choice of such modulation scheme for data transmission. However, the OOK modulation turns-off the coupling carrier with a duty cycle of around 50 % for each Manchester-coded bit. Consequently, inductive energy is wasted because of the simultaneous data transfer. Now that an oscillator provides a stable clock, the recovered clock is not needed anymore for stimuli generation. Thus, as soon as the FPGA acknowledges to the external controller a valid transmission, the downlink data transfer is stopped while keeping the inductive coupling. That way, more inductive energy is available for stimulation or telemetry.

3.3 Stimulation stages

UroStim8 neurostimulator has 4 stimulation stages. As presented in Fig.4, Stage 1 is dedicated to the low-frequency pulse stimulation, offers 4 bipolar outputs, and includes an 8-bit Digital to Analog Converter (DAC), an Operational Amplifier (OpAmp) used as a current source, as well as CMOS analog switches for biphasic stimulation and outputs multiplexing.

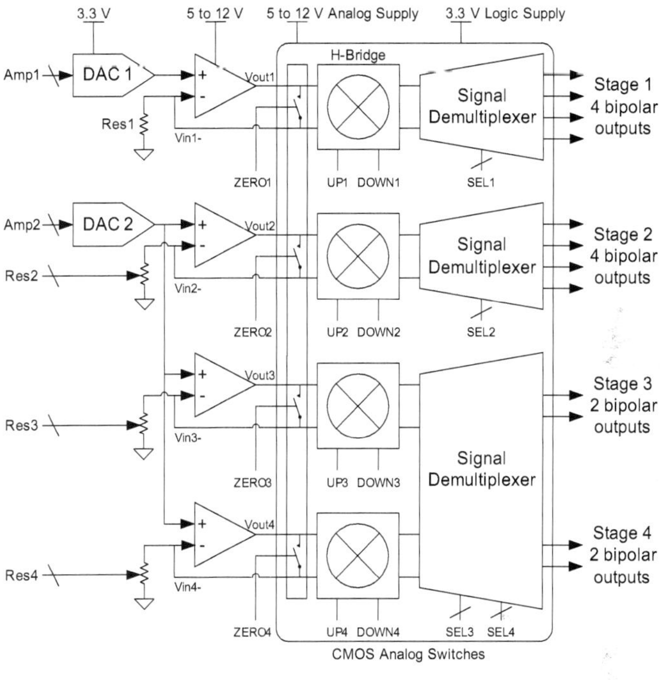

Fig. 4. Stimulation stages in UroStim8

The four outputs of Stage 1 share the same frequency and can be activated individually or in any combination. Even though meant for simultaneous stimulation, the four low-frequency pulse outputs are sequentially activated with a small delay to avoid cumulative power consumption load peaks. Thus, pulse amplitude can be programmed independently which is important because the impedance of the cuff-electrodes may be different. Before each stimulation pulse, the FPGA sends the amplitude code to the DAC that provides a proportional voltage V_{DAC} between 0 and a reference voltage of 1.2 V. This voltage is then converted into current by the OpAmp and resistance Res1 that operates as a current source. Constant current is injected into the nerve via CMOS analog switches that enables reversing the current for biphasic stimulation. The stimulation current is equal to Istim=V_{DAC1} /Res1, as long as the OpAmp is not saturated. Resistance Res1 has been chosen equal to 600 Ω to provide a maximum current of 2 mA (1.2 V/600 Ω). For an ENI impedance of 1 kΩ, a voltage supply of 3.3 V would have been sufficient for the OpAmp. However, previous chronic animal experiments proved that the ENI impedance may become higher than 4 kΩ leading to lower stimulation currents because of the OpAmp saturation. Hence, its voltage supply can be increased up to 12 V so that a current of 2 mA could be injected into an ENI impedance up to 5.4 kΩ. Stimulation Stages 2 to 4 share the same DAC that will generate the sinusoidal waveform required for nerve conduction blockade. They offer 8 bipolar outputs that are grouped according to the stimulation strategy (Fig.1). For the three groups of outputs, the blockade amplitude can be adjusted independently through digital potentiometers Res2 to 4. The stimulation stages are controlled by the FPGA similarly but separately. Signals UP and DOWN sets the current direction with an H-Bridge that is made of four switches mounted as a mixer. Signal ZERO controls a fifth switch that shortcuts the OpAmp output with its negative input before activating one of the UP or DOWN signals. That way, before and after each pulse, the same voltage is applied on both electrodes (of each bipolar output) before releasing the ZERO switch (Mounaim & Sawan, 2007). The output CMOS analog switches are critical elements. If they must transmit currents under voltages as high as 12 V, they still need to be controlled by 3.3 V signals directly from the FPGA. Thus, they have been chosen with dual power supplies: a logic supply of 3.3 V and an analog supply up to 12 V.

3.4 Telemetry

The goal of the implemented telemetry is to verify the capacity of the implant to stimulate each connected nerve. Thus, it is important to monitor the load impedance presented by each ENI as it must not be too high for the desired stimulation current (Sawan et al., 2007, 2008a).

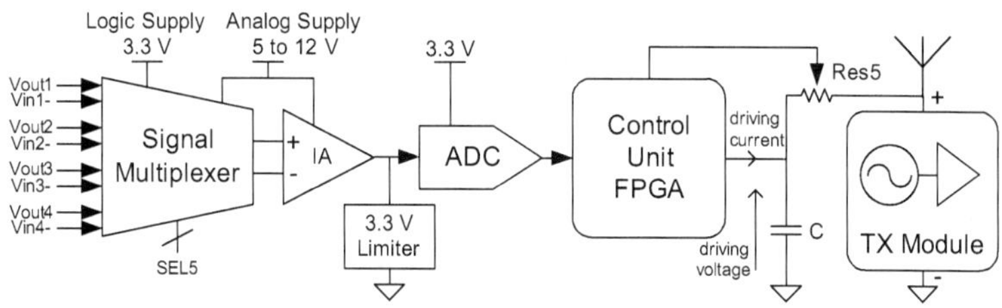

Fig. 5. Telemetry in UroStim8

The neurostimulator has a total of 12 bipolar outputs. Making use of the demultiplexers already present in the stimulation stages, monitoring can be done at the current source OpAmp output of each stage by activating one single bipolar output at a time. As shown in Fig.5, the four differential OpAmp outputs voltages are multiplexed, differentially measured with an instrumentation amplifier and then sampled with an Analog to Digital Converter (ADC) before being sent to the FPGA. The stimulus used for AC impedance measurement is a sinusoidal waveform that each stimulation stage is capable of generating. After a programmable number of cycles, the maximum amplitude and zero-crossing time of the voltage difference across the ENI, are used with the programmed stimulation parameters to estimate the impedance module and phase respectively. Once these measurements are ready, they are sent to the external controller thanks to a miniature transmission module. It is an RF emitter oscillating at 433 MHz and OOK modulated at 1 kHz. The transmission range can be adjusted with a digital potentiometer (Res5) that limits the driving current.

5. Results

The complete UroStim8 neurostimulator prototype has been assembled on a large breadboard for design and tests. Table 1 presents the achieved stimulation parameters and Fig. 6 presents different oscilloscope screen captures. Fig. 6a shows the low-frequency pulse stimulation waveform generated by Stimulation Stage 1. Single-end outputs are probed by oscilloscope channels Ch1 and Ch2 respectively. The differential output (Ch1-Ch2) is shown by the Math curve (M). Control signals ZERO1 and UP1 (according to Fig. 4) are probed by channels Ch3 and Ch4 respectively. The waveform is not a conventional biphasic one but rather an alternating monophasic waveform as proposed in (Mounaim & Sawan, 2007). Fig. 6b shows the Stimulation Stage 1 OpAmp's output Vout1 (Ch1) when all four bipolar outputs are activated. Ch2 to 4 probe three of them (single-ends only). Stimulation on the four outputs is not "truly" simultaneous but rather alternated with a small delay between pulses. This has the advantage of avoiding large current consumption peaks but also allowing different pulse amplitudes for each output. Fig. 6c and 6d show the high-frequency sinusoidal waveform at the minimum and maximum achieved frequencies respectively. For both figures, single-end outputs are probed by Ch1 and Ch2, control signals UP and DOWN (according to Fig. 4) by channels Ch3 and Ch4 respectively, while the differential output is shown by the Math curve (M).

<table>
<tr><th>Waveform</th><th colspan="3">Pulse</th><th colspan="2">Sinusoid</th></tr>
<tr><th>Parameters</th><th>Amp.</th><th>Width</th><th>Frequency</th><th>Frequency</th><th>Amp.</th></tr>
<tr><td>Max</td><td>2 mA</td><td>217 μs</td><td>8.9 kHz (with min width)
1 kHz (with max width)</td><td>8.6 kHz</td><td>2 mA</td></tr>
<tr><td>Min</td><td>0</td><td>3.39 μs</td><td>18 Hz</td><td>1 kHz</td><td>0</td></tr>
<tr><td>Resolution</td><td>8 μA</td><td colspan="3">Time resolution = 3.39 μs (clock = 295 kHz)</td><td>8 μA</td></tr>
</table>

Table 1. UroStim8 measured stimulation parameters

A normalized half-period of the waveform is stored as a map table of 1024 amplitude samples. To change the frequency of stimulation, the map table is read with a memory address step as it is scanned with the 300 kHz clock. The general equation determining the digitally programmed sinusoidal frequency is given by equation (1).

$$Frequency = 300kHz * \left(\frac{2*1024}{F+7} + 5 \right)^{-1} \quad (1)$$

where F is the decimal equivalent of a programmable 6-bit binary code. As the frequency is increased, the resulting total number of amplitude steps is reduced from more than 256 (=2*1024/8) to less than 32 (=2*1024/64). Any other stimulation waveform and/or mapping strategy can be easily implemented by reprogramming the FPGA. Table 2 presents the measured system total current consumption at different conditions. With all stimulation stages and all their outputs activated, total system current consumption is 4.54 mA (rms) at 30 Hz pulse (2 mA, 217 μs) and 1 kHz sinusoidal frequencies. For Stimulation Stages 2-4, 1 mA current is distributed over outputs of each stage. Thus, stimulation parameters must be adjusted taking into account the available inductive power energy. The FPGA core current consumption in this prototype is less than 100 μA.

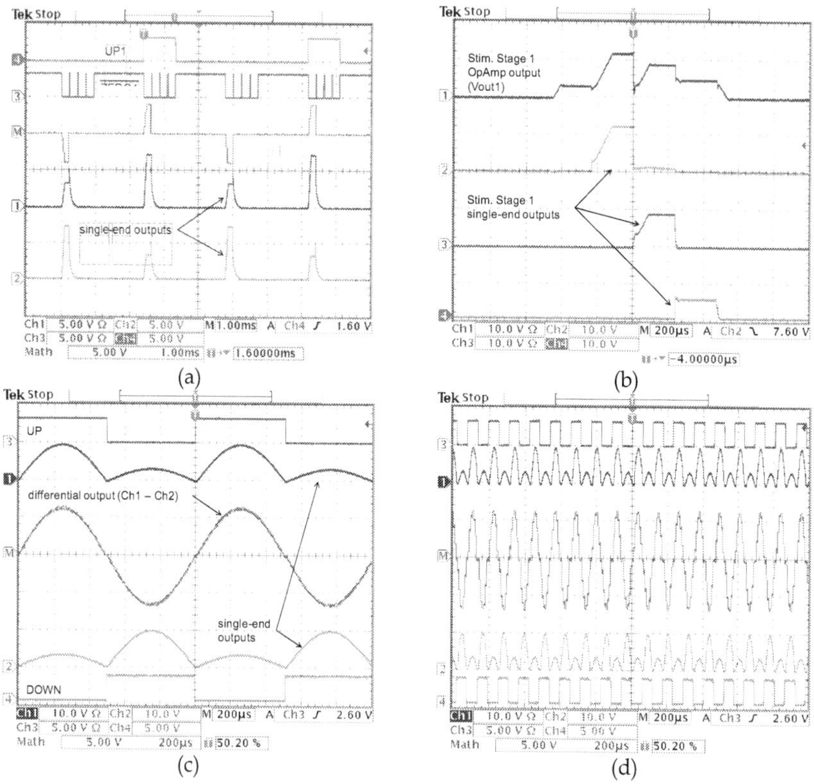

Fig. 6. Oscilloscope captures showing (a) alternating monophasic stimulation waveform and control signals, (b) Stimulation Stage 1 OpAmp output and three single-ends outputs, and sinusoidal waveform at (c) 1 kHz and (d) 8.6 kHz frequencies

Conditions		**Current consumption mA (rms)**
Stimulation Stage 1	**Stimulation Stages 2-4**	
OFF	OFF	1.83
30 Hz	OFF	2.12
1 kHz	OFF	4.59
30 Hz	1 kHz	4.54
30 Hz	8.6 kHz	5.33
1 kHz	8.6 kHz	7.80

Table 2. UroStim8 measured system total current consumption (rms) with following stimulation conditions: Stage 1 (2 mA, 217 μs); Stages 2-4 (1 mA each, current is distributed over outputs of each stage)

UroStim8 neurostimulator's printed circuit board have been designed, fabricated and assembled as shown in Fig. 7. UroStim8's PCB is 38 mm diameter and can host a FPGA in

12x12 Fine Pitch Ball Grid Array (FBGA) of 13x13 mm dimensions and 1 mm pitch. Because of the relatively large number of discrete components and the limited space, the design of such PCB is challenging. It required eight PCB layers and numerous blind vias for a complete routing of the system. For chronic animal implantation, the prototype will be encapsulated in two layers of different materials. The first layer is a rigid epoxy that protects the implant from infiltration of fluids and offers a reliable isolation for the electronic components. The second layer is a biocompatible silicone that offers a soft contact for corporal tissues. Encapsulation is done using custom made Teflon or aluminum moulds. Fig. 8 shows the targeted encapsulation dimensions for the neurostimulator. The encapsulated UroStim8 will be thinner than previous prototypes that had embedded batteries (10 mm compared to 16 mm).

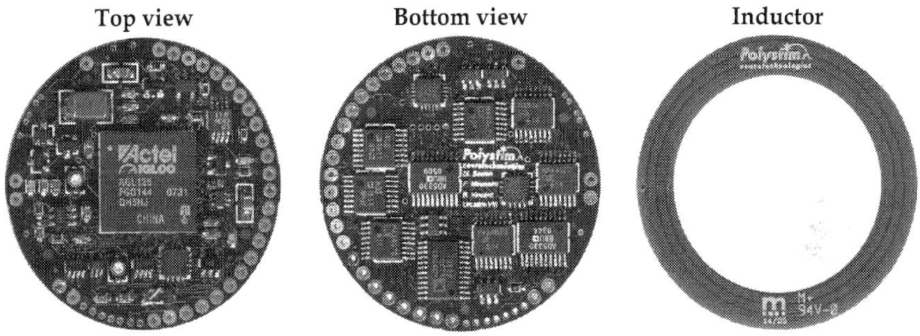

Fig. 7. UroStim8 printed circuit board

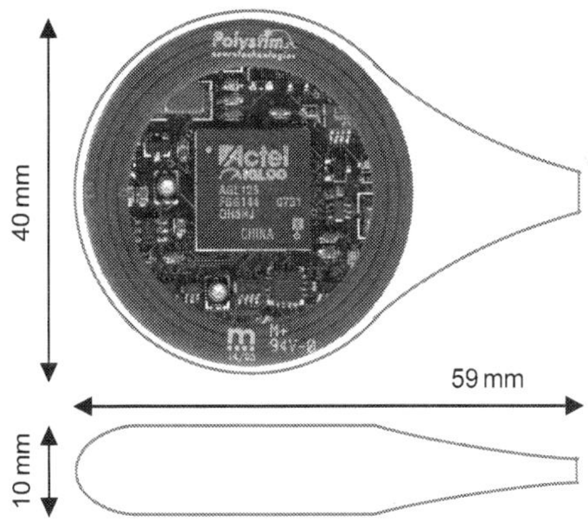

UroStim8

Fig. 8. UroStim8 encapsulation dimensions

6. Conclusion

This chapter presented a new sacral neurostimulation strategy to enhance micturition in spinal cord injured patients. In order to carry-on chronic animal experiments, a discrete implantable neurostimulator has been designed implementing the proposed stimulation strategy and using commercially available discrete components. Measurements and prototyping results were presented. The discrete prototype is capable of generating a low frequency pulse waveform as low as 18 Hz with a simultaneous high frequency alternating waveform as high as 8.6 kHz, and that over different and multiple channels. With all stimulation stages and all their outputs activated, total system current consumption is around 4.5 mA (rms) at 30 Hz pulse (2 mA, 217 μs) and 1 kHz sinusoidal frequencies. In the same conditions, using a sinusoidal stimulation at the highest frequency of 8.6 kHz, increases current consumption up to 7.8 mA. With 50 mW of available inductive power for example and 4.5 mA current consumption, the high voltage regulator can be set to 10 V allowing 2 mA stimulation of 4.4 kΩ electrode-nerve impedance. However, with 7.8mA current consumption, the high voltage regulator will have to be set to 6 V reducing the maximum possible stimulation current to 1 mA for a 4.4 kΩ electrode-nerve impedance. Thus, the effective number of activated outputs and the maximum achievable stimulation parameters are limited by the available energy provided by the inductive link and the impedance of the electrode-nerve interfaces. Future developments will include chronic animal experiments after full characterization of the encapsulated and implanted neurostimulation prototype, taking into account the resulting inductive link efficiency.

7. Acknowledgement

Authors would like to acknowledge the financial support from the Natural Sciences and Engineering Research Council of Canada (NSERC), the Mycrosystems Strategic Alliance of Quebec (ReSMiQ), and the Canada Research Chair on Smart Medical Devices. Also, thanks are due to all Polystim's members and students that have participated in the design of the UroStim8 prototype and to Laurent Mouden for its assembly.

8. References

Abdel-Gawad, M.; Boyer, S.; Sawan, M. & Elhilali, M.M. (2001). Reduction of bladder outlet resistance by selective stimulation of the ventral sacral root using high frequency blockade: a chronic study in spinal cord transected dogs, *Journal of Urology*, Vol. 166, No.2, Aug. 2001, pp.728-733, 0022-5347

Ba, A.; Schneider, E.; Abdel-Karim, A.; Sawan, M. & Elhilali, M. M. (2002) Implantable dual stimulator to recuperate the bladder functions: Chronic experiments in dogs, *Int'l Functional Electrical Stimulation Society Conf.*, June 2002, IFESS, Ljubljana

Ba, A. (2004). Stimulations combinées dédiées au rétablissement de l'évacuation chez les patients souffrant de dysfonctions urinaires, M.Sc.A. dissertation, Ecole Polytechnique, Montreal (Canada), 2004.

Balachandran G. K. & Barnett, R. E. (2006). A 110 nA Voltage Regulator System With Dynamic Bandwidth Boosting for RFID Systems, *IEEE Journal of Solid-State Circuits*, Vol.41, No.9, Sept. 2006, pp.2019-2028, 0018-9200

Bhadra, N.; Kilgore, K. & Gustafson, K.J. (2006) High frequency electrical conduction block of the pudendal nerve, *Journal of Neural Engineering*, Vol.3, No.2, June 2006, pp.180-187, 2006, 1741-2560

Blaivas, J.G.; Sinha, H.P.; Zayed, A.A. & Labib, K.B. (1981). Detrusor-external sphincter dyssynergia, *Journal of Urology*, Vol.125, No.4, 1981, pp.542-544, 0022-5347

Blumer, C.E. & Quine, S. (1995). Prevalence of spinal cord injury: an international comparison, *Neuroepidemiology*, Vol.14, No.5, 1995, pp.258-68, 0251-5350

Boger, A.; Bhadra, N. & Gustafson, K.J. (2008). Bladder voiding by combined high frequency electrical pudendal nerve block and sacral root stimulation, *Neurourology and Urodynamics*, Vol.27, No.5, 2008, pp.435-439, 0733-2467

Chai, T.C. & Steers, W.D. (1996). Neurophysiology of micturition and continence, *Urologic Clinics of North America*, 1996, Vol.23, pp.221-236, 0094-0143

DeVivo, M.J. (1997). Causes and costs of spinal cord injury in the United States," *Spinal Cord*, 1997, Vol.35, No.12, pp.809-813, 1362-4393

Elabaddy, A.A.; Hassouna, M. & Elhilali M.M. (1994) Neural stimulation for chronic voiding dysfunction, *Journal of Urology*, Vol.152, 1994, pp.2076-2080, 0022-5347

Jezernik, S.; Craggs, M.; Grill, W.M.; Creasey, G. & Rijkhoff, N.J. (2002). Electrical stimulation for the treatment of bladder dysfunction: current status and future possibilities, *Neurological Research*, Vol.24, No.5, 2002, pp.413-430, 1743-1328

Kilgore, K.L. & Bhadra, N. (2004). Nerve conduction block utilising high-frequency alternating current," *Medical & Biological Engineering & Computing*, Vol.42, No.3, 2004, pp.394-406, 0140-0118

Kursun, V.; Narendra, S.G.; De, V.K. & Friedman, E.G. (2004). High input voltage step-down DC-DC converters for integration in a low voltage CMOS process, *Int'l Symp. on Quality Electronic Design*, pp.517-521, 0-7695-2093-6, Aug. 2004, IEEE, San Jose

Kutzenberger, J. (2007). Surgical therapy of neurogenic detrusor overactivity (hyperreflexia) in paraplegic patients by sacral deafferentation and implant driven micturition by sacral anterior root stimulation: methods, indications, results, complications, and future prospects, *Acta neurochirurgica Supplement*, Vol.97, No.1, 2007, pp.333-339, 0065-1419

Mounaim, F.; Sawan, M. & Bedard, S. (2006). Implantable neuro-monito-stimulation system dedicated to enhance the bladder functions, *Biomedical Circuits and Systems Conf.*, pp.198-201, 978-1-4244-0436-0, Nov. 2006, IEEE, London

Mounaim, F. & Sawan, M. (2007). Miniature Implantable System Dedicated to Bi-Channel Selective Neurostimulation, *Int'l Symp. on Circuits and Systems*, pp.2072-2075, 1-4244-0920-9, May 2007, IEEE, New Orleans

Mounaim, F.; Elzayat, E.; Sawan, M.; Corcos, J.; & Elhilali, M.M (2008). New sacral neurostimulation strategy to enhance micturition in paraplegics: Acute dog experiments, *Int'l Functional Electrical Stimulation Society Conf.*, pp.22-24, Sep. 2008, IFESS, Freiburg

Mounaim, F.; Elzayat, E.; Sawan, M.; Corcos, J.; & Elhilali, M.M (2010). New neurostimulation and blockade strategy to enhance bladder voiding in paraplegics, accepted for publication in *Contemporary Engineering Sciences*, Hikari Ltd, 1313-6569

Robin, S.; Sawan, M.; Abdel-Gawad, M.; Abdel-Baky, T.M. & Elhilali, M.M. (1998). Implantable stimulation system dedicated for neural selective stimulation, *Medical & Biological Engineering & Computing*, Vol. 36, No.4, 1998, pp.490-492, 0140-0118

Sawan, M.; Laaziri, Y.; Mounaim, F.; Elzayat, E. & Elhilali, M.M. (2007). Electrode-tissues interface: Modeling and experimental validation, *Biomedical Materials*, Vol. 2, No.1, 2007, 1748-6041

Sawan, M.; Mounaim, F. & Lesbros, G. (2008a). Wireless monitoring of electrode-tissues interfaces for long-term characterization, *Analog Integrated Circuits & Signal Processing*, Vol.55, No.1, April 2008, 0925-1030

Sawan, M.; Ba, A.; Mounaim, F.; Corcos, J. & Elhilali, M.M. (2008b). Biomedical Circuits and Systems Dedicated for Sensing and Neurostimulation: Case study on Urinary Bladder dysfunctions, *Turkish Journal of Electrical Engineering & Computer Sciences*, Vol. 16, pp.171-187, 2008, 1300-0632

Schneider, E. (2001). Conception et évaluation d'un système de stimulation électrique neurale dédié à la réhabilitation des fonctions vésicales, M.Sc.A. dissertation, Ecole Polytechnique, Montreal (Canada), 2001.

Schuettler, M.; Andrews, B.J. & Donaldson, N. de N. (2004). Blocking of Peripheral Nerve Conduction Using AC Signals: Which Frequency is Best? *Int'l Functional Electrical Stimulation Society Conf.*, pp.324-326, Sep. 2004, IFESS Bournemouth

Shaker, H.S.; Tu, L.M.; Robin, S.; Arabi, K.; Hassouna, M.; Sawan, M. & Elhilali, M.M. (1998). Reduction of bladder outlet resistance by selective sacral root stimulation using high-frequency blockade in dogs: an acute study, *Journal of Urology*, Vol.160, No.3, 1998, pp.901-907, 0022-5347

Sievert, K.D.; Gleason, C.A.; Jünemann, K.P.; Alken, P. & Tanagho, E.A. (2002). Physiologic bladder evacuation with selective sacral root stimulation: sinusoidal signal and organ-specific frequency, *Neurourology and Urodynamics*, Vol.21, No.1, 2002, pp.80-91, 0733-2467

Solomonow, M. (1984). External Control of the Neuromuscular System, *IEEE Transactions on Biomedical Engineering*, Vol.31, No.12, 1984, pp.752-763, 0018-9294

Tai, C.; de Groat, W.C. & Roppolo, J.R. (2005) Simulation analysis of conduction block in unmyelinated axons induced by high-frequency biphasic electrical currents, *IEEE Transactions on Biomedical Engineering*, Vol.52, No.7, 2005, pp.1323-1332, 0018-9294

Williamson R.P. & Andrews, B.J. (2005). Localized electrical nerve blocking, *IEEE Transactions on Biomedical Engineering*, Vol.52, No.3, 2005, pp.362-370, 0018-9294

Yunlei L. & Jin, L. (2005). A 13.56 MHz RFID transponder front-end with merged load modulation and voltage doubler-clamping rectifier circuits, *Int'l Symp. on Circuits and Systems*, Vol.5, pp.5095-5098, 0-7803-8834-8, May 2005, IEEE, Kobe

6

Implementation of Microsensor Interface for Biomonitoring of Human Cognitive Processes

E. Vavrinsky[1], P. Solarikova[2], V. Stopjakova[1], V. Tvarozek[1] and I. Brezina[2],
[1]*Department of Microelectronics, Slovak University of Technology,*
[2]*Department of Psychology, Comenius University,*
Slovakia

1. Introduction

Miniaturization of biomedical sensors has increased the importance of microsystem technology in medical applications, particularly microelectronics and micromachining. This work presents a new approach to biomedical monitoring and analysis of selected human cognitive processes. The system is based on our preliminary described theory and experiments (Vavrinsky et al. 2010). We are primarily interested in biomonitoring of human cognitive processes and psychophysiological conditions of car drivers in order to enhance road safety.

Actually often used method is evaluation of abnormal car driver actions (sudden changes of direction with no direction indicators or too hard cornering). Main disadvantage of such a system is that they offer no prediction. More effective are prediction systems, which offer enough reaction time before undesirable situations, and so they can minimize human error factors and improve road-traffic safety.

Our present research is focused on sensing, processing and analysis of selected physiological signals for mental and medical condition recognition. They are known some studies describing interface between emotional condition and physiological responses, and we want also present some, since new ideas and research in psychological recognition and biomonitoring are very welcome. It is also proved that human decisions and reactions are affected by emotional and physical comfort. Emotional reconnoiter of a car driver conditions is influenced by many cognitive processes, such as mind organization, vigilance, planning or fatigue. Nervous and angry people can be very dangerous for traffic road safety.

In our experiments, we have monitored:

- psycho-galvanic reflex (PGR) - skin conductivity changes,
- heart rate + electrocardiogram (ECG),
- body temperature,
- respiration frequency,
- emotions.

To improve the reliability of our measurements, these parameters have been monitored often by duplicate methods, sometimes at macro level, sometimes by local microsystems technologies. In first step, we implemented our technology to the virtual reality driving simulator but preparations for real implementation have been already started, and the final car implementation will follow.

Two following experiments were performed:
- Divided Attention "DA" experiment - psychological monitoring of human cognitive processes,
- Car Driver Monitoring System "CDMS" - biomonitoring on a car simulator.

Both experiments are similar, since they are based on several common principles. Preliminary psychological experiment was focused on monitoring of selected psycho-physiological parameters (vigilance test, memory test, alcohol influence) possibly useful in road-traffic safety, and achieved results were applied in the following experiment "Car Driver Monitoring System".

2. Developed multipurpose microsensor

Successful development of high integrated and miniaturized electronic instrumentation and sensors needs to overcome a wide dimension-scale of mezo-micro-nano structures. This leads to the convergency and complementarity of microsystem technology and nanotechnology, and it demands an interdisciplinary scientific/technical collaboration also in basic research. Thin films serve as both: the source of new compound materials (particularly in optoelectronics) as well as well-defined and reproducible micro-/nano-interfaces between sensing, recognition and bio-chemical-physical-electrical transductions of signals in sensors (Tvarozek et al. 2007).

From electrical model of IDA (interdigital array) microelectrode/skin interface and simulations, the important outcome has arisen: the electric field distribution and depth of penetration into the outer skin layers (epidermis laminar structures) depend mainly on the configuration and size of an electrode system (Ivanic. 2003). This knowledge provides the possibility to examine different layers of epidermis by electrical impedance method, and this was used for the analysis of electrophysiological processes in the human skin when a person is under the stress influence.

Recently, new thin microsensors (IDAT), depicted in Fig. 1, have been developed, where:
- an interdigital array (IDA) of microelectrodes is integrated together with
- temperature sensor (T) on a single chip.

The developed microsensor allows measurement of psychogalvanic reflex (PGR) by IDA structure and body temperature by T meander, locally from "one place". Moreover, it can be found in previous experiments on the heart rate monitor. Therefore, the microsensor allows continual monitoring and analysis of complex physiological, pathophysiological, and therapeutic processes.

The microelectrodes were fabricated by a standard thin film technology: Pt (Au) films (150 nm in thickness) underlaid by Ti film (50 nm) were deposited by rf sputtering on Al_2O_3 substrates, and microelectrodes were lithographically patterned by lift-off technique. However, in electro-optical research, transparent conductive oxide of ZnO doped by Al (ZnO:Al) can be also utilized (Tvarozek et. al., 2007). The total size of the microelectrode chip is 10 x 13 mm. IDA structure was made in symmetric configuration: 100 μm / 100 μm and 200 μm / 200 μm (finger/gap) dimensions. Total resistance of thermal resistive meander by using Pt is between 530 and 540 Ω. Pt thin film is used to minimize the polarization effect. In all experiments described later, 200 μm / 200 μm symmetric structure was used.

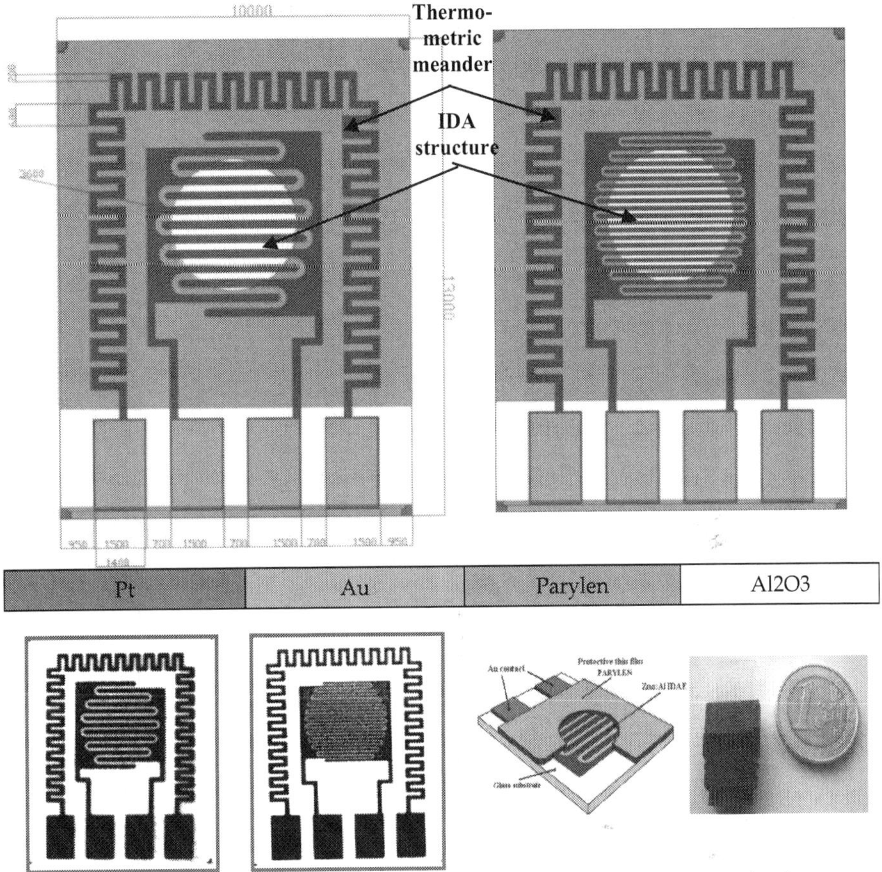

Photo snapshots

Transparent thin films technology - ZnO:Al

Fig. 1. IDAT microelectrodes

3. Divided attention experiment

Presented experiment was carried out in the laboratory of cognitive processes at Department of Psychology, Comenius University, in cooperation with Department of Microelectronics, Slovak University of Technology. This experiment has been performed on a group of 63 probands (all university students) in age between 18 and 29 (average = 20) years (48 female, 15 male). The experiment was focused on analysis of relations between cognitive processes, psychophysiological correlatives and human personality parameters at different activation levels. Secondarily, we have mapped also relations of psychophysiological correlatives to emotional reflex (face mimic) and alcohol intoxication (Fig. 2).

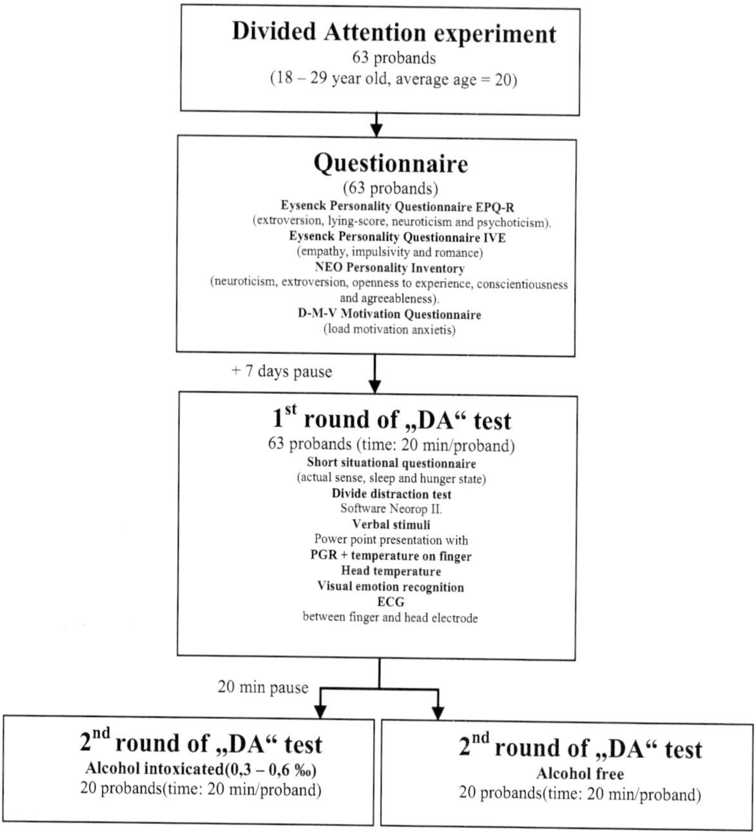

Fig. 2. Divided Attention experiment

Divided attention "DA" test was separated into three rounds:

- Questionnaire,
- 1st round of "DA" test, and
- 2nd repeat round of "DA" test with alcohol influence monitoring.
    - (Blood alcohol concentration: 0,3 – 0,6 ‰)

Each round of the "DA" test itself was divided into four time phases:

1st – Relaxation time (3 - 4 minutes): self concentration, relaxation music, etc.

2nd - Advice listening (3 – 5 minutes): listening to spoken words

3th – Distraction stress (5 - 6 minutes): solving two tasks at same time:

- Vigilance task:
    - Software Neurop II – SPEED test (measurement of reaction time - image and sound stimuli). (Gaal. 2002)
- Memory task:
    - Power Point presentation with verbal stimuli (numerical tasks and words remembering (10 negative, 10 positive, 10 neutral types of words)).

4th – Memory task (2 minutes): Writing of remembered words from 3th phase.

3.1 Technical set-up

The complete measurement set-up used in "DA" experiment is depicted in Figure 3. The developed IDAT sensor was first used in "Divide Attention" psychoexperiment.

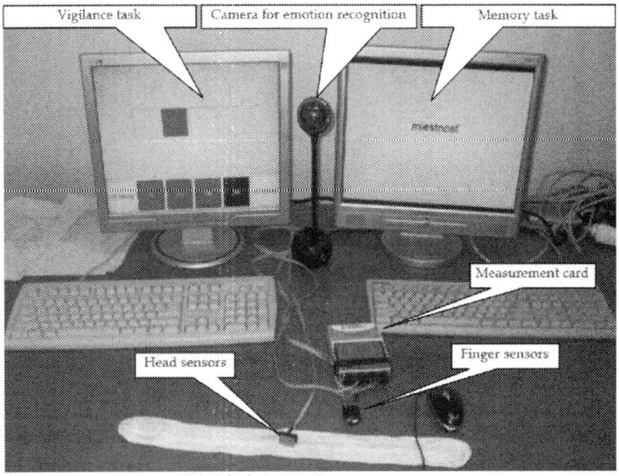

Divided Attention test set-up

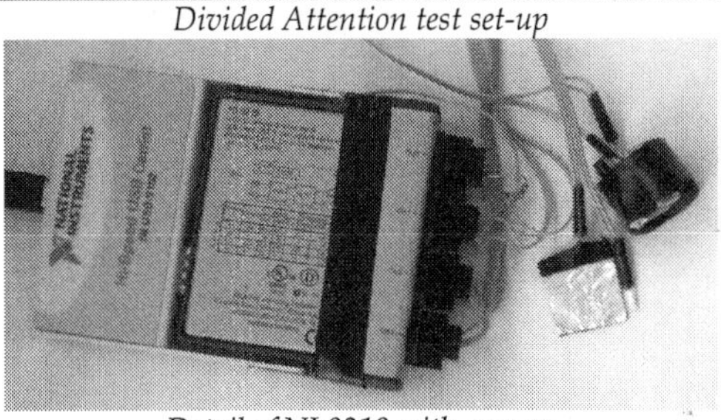

Detail of NI 9219 with sensors

Fig. 3. Divided Attention test - measurement equipment

During this cognitive test, four electro-physiological parameters were monitored:

- psychogalvanic reflex (PGR) and body temperature sensed by the designed IDAT integrated microsensor on the ring-finger of non-dominant hand,
- head temperature sensed by a standard Pt100 sensor,
- Electrocardiograph (ECG) sensed between head and the ring-finger.

Additionally, the face mimic representing different psychological emotions were recorded by a camera (Logitech, 2009), and visually recognized and diagnosed using software "eMotion" (eMotion, 2009). "eMotion" was designed in "ISLA Laboratory at the Universiteit van Amsterdam" for real-time visual (face mimic) emotional recognition. The program allows recognition of these emotions, "Neutral", "Happy", "Surprise", "Angry", "Disgust", "Fear" and "Sad", from saved video files or online video source (camera).

Experiment was controlled by a personal computer (PC) with new programmed software "Psychoprogram" (Fig. 4). "Psychoprogram" was designed in Labview 8.6 environment, and has built up software interfaces for the camera, "eMotion" program and NI 9219 measurement card with sensors. NI 9219 has measured resistances from IDAT sensor (PGR + temperature),

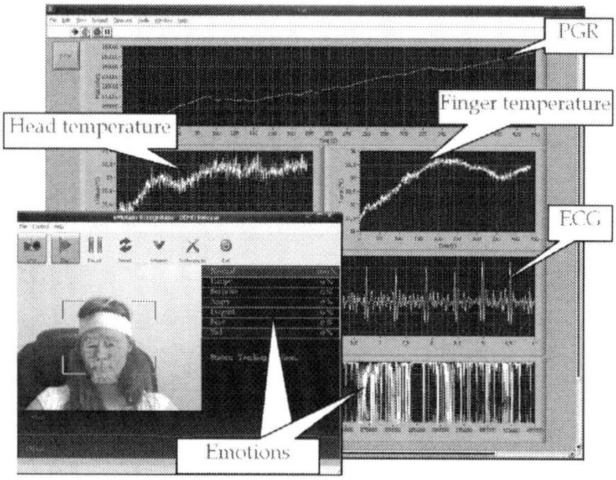

Fig. 4. Divided Attention test - Control computer print screen

resistance from Pt100 head sensor and ECG voltage at 100 samples/s and 24-bit resolution (Fig. 3 bottom). For ECG signal we applied software IIR Bandpass filter (Cutoff frequencies: 7 - 40 Hz, Order: 7, Topology: Bessel). Other signals were only resampled down to 2 S/s.

3.2 Results and discussion

The achieved results have confirmed several previously obtained observations (Vavrinsky et. al, 2010), shown in Fig. 5:

- The psycho-galvanic reflex causes a change of the skin impedance during periods of stress, excitement or shock. Under these conditions, skin conductivity increases, whereas during periods of relaxation the conductivity declines to a minimum (Olmar. 1998, Weis et al. 1995, Brezina. 2007)
- Psychological activation results in human body temperature decreasing and increasing of the skin conductivity (PGR) at the same time.
- The amplitude of a particular parameter depends on the stress activation level, and it is individual for each proband.
- The temperature response shows also more integral character.
- Activation phase of the parameters' response is followed by the relaxation phase.
- Memory task (4th phase of "DA" test) decreases the body temperature more significantly than observed for phases 2 and 3.
- The conductivity (PGR) in 4th phase is decreasing in contrast to phase 2 and 3.

In 3rd phase of "DA" test - "Distraction stress" (activation) phase the following observations were registered:

- Heart rate grows up approximately by 11 beats, in comparison to 1st relaxation phase. This result observed for all probands is very reliable (Fig. 6).
- Visual emotions are changed from "Neutral" emotion in 1st phase to "Happy" or "Angry" emotions in 3rd phase. The intensity of "Happy" and "Angry" emotions is more than doubled (Fig. 7). We also found that emotion "Angry" can by often reflected as "Concentration" emotion, which was not reckoning in "eMotion" software.
- Emotion "Disgust" corresponds to faster reaction times in "Vigilance task".
- Emotion "Fear" causes increased heart rate.
- Sleepiness from questionnaire decrease total performance in "Vigilance task".

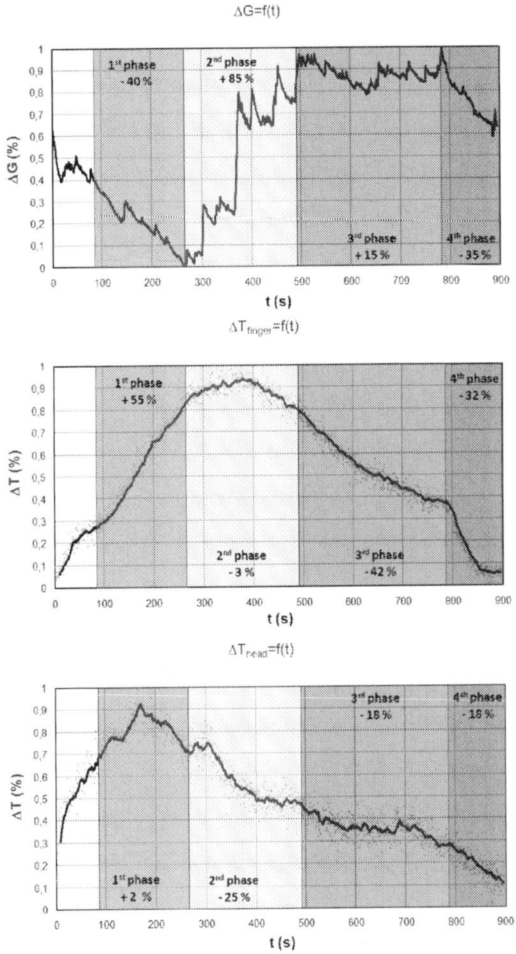

Fig. 5. Conductivity and temperature results of "DA" Test over respective phases (typical example)

In 2nd round of "DA" test we divided 40 probands in 2 groups to monitor alcohol influence on test effectivity and heart rate changes.

We had:

- 20 slightly alcohol intoxicated probands (0,3 – 0,6 ‰),
- 20 normal probands.

They are existing scientific findings, that alcohol has negative influence on learning and memory processes. Principally alcohol decrease remembering of new information. The visual memory falls rapidly, but semantic memory is not influenced. The efficiency of recognition tasks decrease, even though the number of right answers is increased, but the accuracy falls rapidly (Nociar. 1991, Snel. 1999).

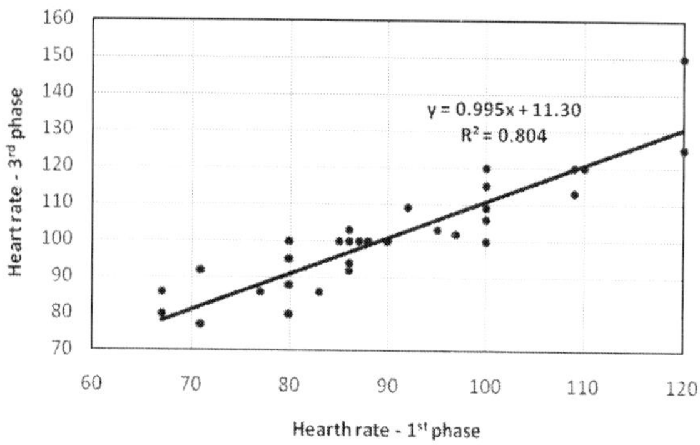

Fig. 6. Divide Attention test – Increasing of the heart rate in distraction stress

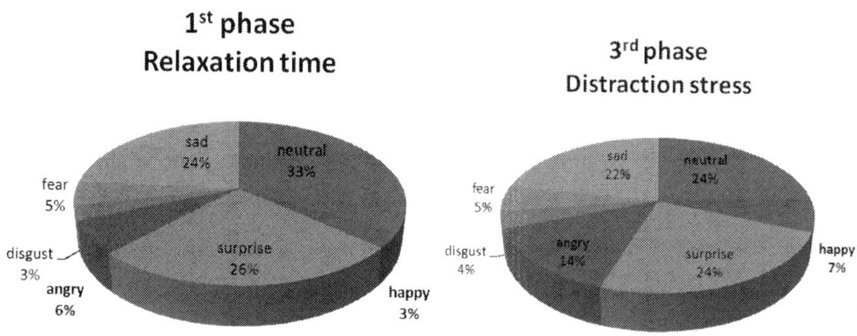

Fig. 7. Divide Attention test – Emotion changes

It is also known: If alcohol concentration in blood is in range 0,3 – 0,5 ‰ (our case), the probands are more relax, open - mind, self-confidence, but motoric reactions are slower. On 1‰ concentration start decreasing of sensor and talking functions and some people are more aggressive or retiring and crabbed (Atkinson. 2003).

We found that in 2nd round of "DA" test:

- Probands perform better than in 1st round, which is caused by better preparation on repeated task.
- Slightly "alcohol intoxicated" probands can achieve better results in vigilance task (3rd phase of distraction test), however, in memory task (4th phase) their performance was worse compared to "alcohol free" probands (Fig. 9). The difference was +7 % in vigilance task and – 3 % in memory task. The result corresponds to literature knowledge (Snel. 1999, Nociar. 1991).
- Heart rate of slightly "alcohol intoxicated" probands decrease comprised to normal state (Fig. 8). The literature knowledge was verified.
    - We calculated formula for alcohol intoxication influence on heart rate:

      Alcohol intoxicated heart rate = 0,63 * Normal heart rate + 29,5

    - For more precise formula estimation is possible to perform experiments with variable values of alcohol concentrations in blood.

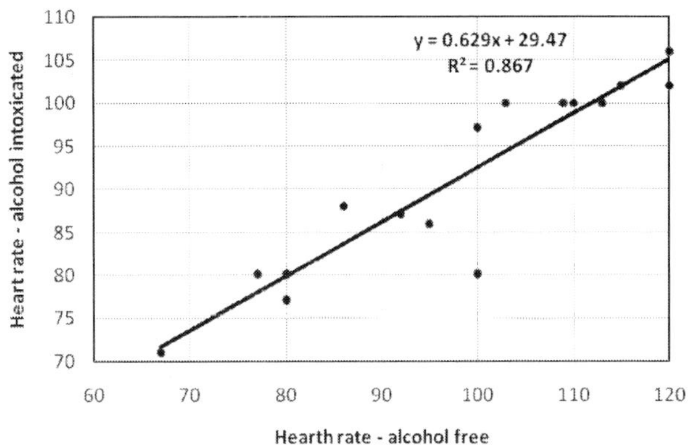

Fig. 8. Divide Attention test – Decreasing of the heart rate under alcohol intoxication

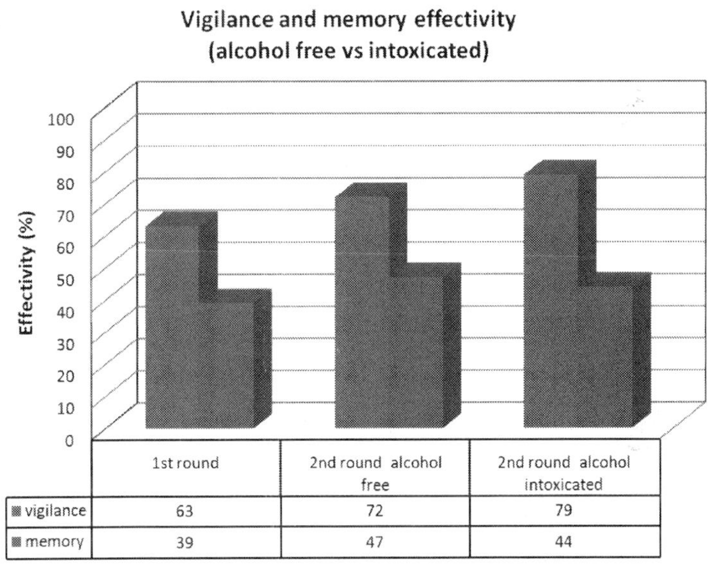

Fig. 9. Divide Attention test – Influence of alcohol intoxication on vigilance and memory

4. Car driver monitoring system

Obtained results and tested set-up configurations of "Divided Attention experiment" were used in next "Card Driver Monitoring System" (CDMS).

4.1 Technical set-up

The proposed and designed Car Driver Monitoring System (CDMS), depicted in Fig. 10, consists of:

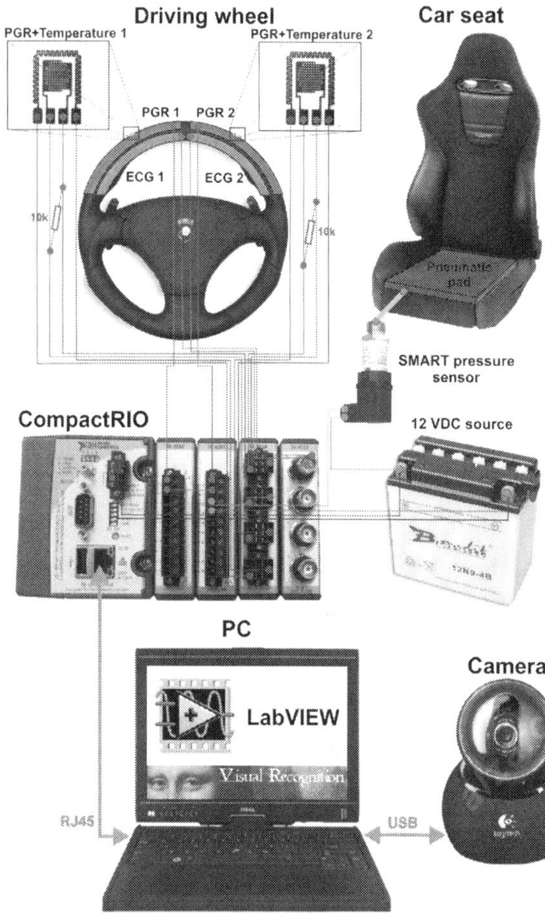

Fig. 10. Car Driver Monitoring System (CDMS)

- 2 local micro PGR + temperature (left and right hands)IDAT sensors on a driving wheel
- 1 global macro PGR sensor and 1 global macro ECG sensor for monitoring of conductivity and ECG between left and right hand placed on driving wheel
- 1 smart pressure sensor, placed in the driver seat, for heart rate and respiration frequency monitoring (Partin et. al, 2006). It can be partially used for the driver weight measurement too.
- The system also includes an infrared (IR) modified camera with several tested optical filters to minimize shadows and glitters in real conditions, for visual emotion recognition. The camera can be also used in the eye position system or in the safety system for driver identification.
- "Compact RIO system" (National Instruments, 2009) controlled by NI Labview 8.6, with implemented mathematical apparatus for signal processing, filtering and analysis:

- NI 9263:
  - 4-Channel, 100 kS/s, 16-bit, ±10 V, Analog Output Module
- NI 9219:
  -24-bit, 100S/s, Ch-Ch Isolated Universal Analog Input Module (±125 mV to ±60 V, ±25 mA, TC, 3 and 4-wire RTD, ¼, ½, and Full-Bridge)
- NI 9203:
  -8-Ch ±20 mA, 200 kS/s, 16-Bit Analog Current Input Module
- NI 9234:
  -4-Channel, ±5 V, 51.2 kS/s per Channel, 24-Bit IEPE
- 12 VDC power supply

- Control PC with camera software connected over RJ45 net

The design of measurement unit is based on the modular programmable automation controller CompactRIO (NI 9014), low-cost reconfigurable control, and acquisition system designed for applications that require high performance and reliability. The system combines an open embedded architecture, small size, extreme ruggedness, and hot-swappable industrial I/O modules. Because we want to make a low-cost final product, finally, only a classical web-camera, not high precision cameras or thermal cameras will be used, and the final electronic part of the system will be placed on a single board.

4.2 Results and discussion

4.2.1 Driving wheel sensors

4.2.1.1 ECG and PGR by macroelectrodes

For global monitoring of ECG and PGR by driving wheel we used:

- Aluminum macro electrodes
- ECG electrodes were connected to NI 9234.
  - Sample frequency: 25,6 kHz (can be reduced to about 100 Hz)
  - Software IIR filters:
    -Bandpass filter: (Cutoff frequencies: 1 - 130 Hz, Order: 10, Topology: Bessel)
    -Bandstop filter: (Cutoff frequencies: 48 - 52 Hz, Order: 10, Topology: Bessel)
- Conductivity (PGR) electrodes were serial connected to NI 9263 (±10 V Analog Output Module: V_{OUT} = 3V, f = 1 kHz) and NI 9203 (Analog Current Input Module, Sample frequency: 100 Hz)

Typical result for ECG monitoring is shown in Fig. 11.

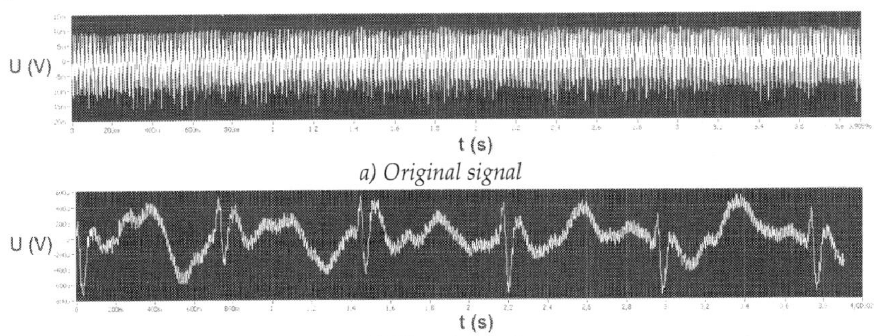

a) Original signal

b) Filtered signal

Fig. 11. ECG signal from a driving wheel

The PGR response of macroelectrodes (skin conductivity) corresponds to typical signal of commercial PGR sensors like in old results (Vavrinsky, 2010).
Macroelectrodes offer very fixed contact between human skin and electrodes and the total reliability is very good.

4.2.1.2 PGR, body temperature and heart rate by multipurpose microsensor

In this set-up we used multipurpose IDAT microelectrodes (Fig. 1) placed up on driving wheel and connected to NI 9219 card (Sample frequency: 100 Hz).
Electrical experiments led to a very important result: the developed microelectrode probes are able to monitor PGR, temperature as well as heart rate simultaneously. The PGR and temperature output signal corresponds to preliminary experiment (Fig. 5) and the heart rate was easily read out by derivation of the measured skin conductivity waveform (Fig. 12).
Standard psychotests also showed that the response signals of IDAT microelectrodes and macroelectrodes were similar. IDAT microelectrodes signals were more stabile with shorter response time, but for better reliability in real praxis, we need to place microsensors on several positions of driving wheel - to obtain more fixed contact.
In real praxis is ideal to combine macro and micro-sensors results.

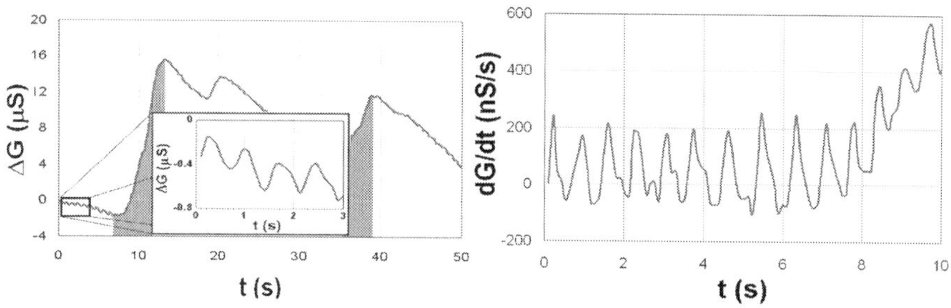

Fig. 12. CDMS - Heart rate by IDA microstructure

4.2.2 Seat sensor

For biomonitoring seat sensor was proved. In this set-up, the pressure sensor Treston DMP 331 converts mechanical (pressure) force from air filled seat cushion (modified medical pressure cuff XXL) (Medihum. 2008) to the output current that is then, measured via a serially connected National Instruments 9219 card (24-bit, 100 Hz sample frequency). As power supply we used 12 DC batteries. Treston DMP 331 is a smart sensor with the following features (Treston. 2010):

- Hybrid integrated technology
- Pressure range 0 - 0,6 bar
- Output current 4 - 20 mA
- Input voltage 12 - 36 V
- Excellent long service life and linearity
- Negligible temperature effect on output signal
- Long service life
- Gas and liquid pressure measurement

Typical measured signal is shown in Fig. 13a. Period designated as T_{heart} corresponds to heart pulse signal, and period $T_{respiration}$ corresponds to the respiration frequency. For better

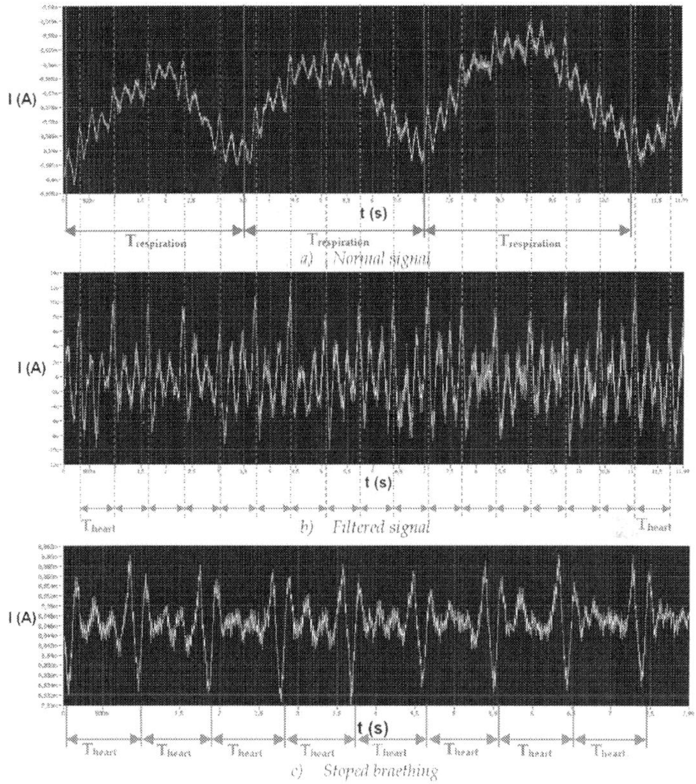

Fig. 13. Heart pulse and respiration frequency measured by the seat sensor

readability and reliability of heat rate, we can use mathematical filter IIR Highpass filter (Topology: Butterworth, Cutoff: 700 mHz, Order: 7) implemented in LabView (Fig. 13b). Fig. 13c shows output signal if you stop breathing.

Additionally, this system can be used also for measurement of a driver weight and then, his/her identification. We tested also fill seat cushion with water, but there was significant difference to air filling.

4.2.3 Visual emotion recognition

For visual emotional recognition we used like in first "DA" experiment cameras and eMotion software, but to improve reliability in real conditions (daylight, night), and to minimize the influence of unwanted optical effects like shadows and reflex from the outer sources, we used an infrared (IR) modified (active method) and thermal camera (passive method).

4.2.3.1 Active method

In first method (Fig. 14), to keep cost of the system down and make the system widely shareable, we have modified web camera for near IR spectra (0,8 - 1,3 μm). In front of the camera, optical filters to filter the visible light have been placed.

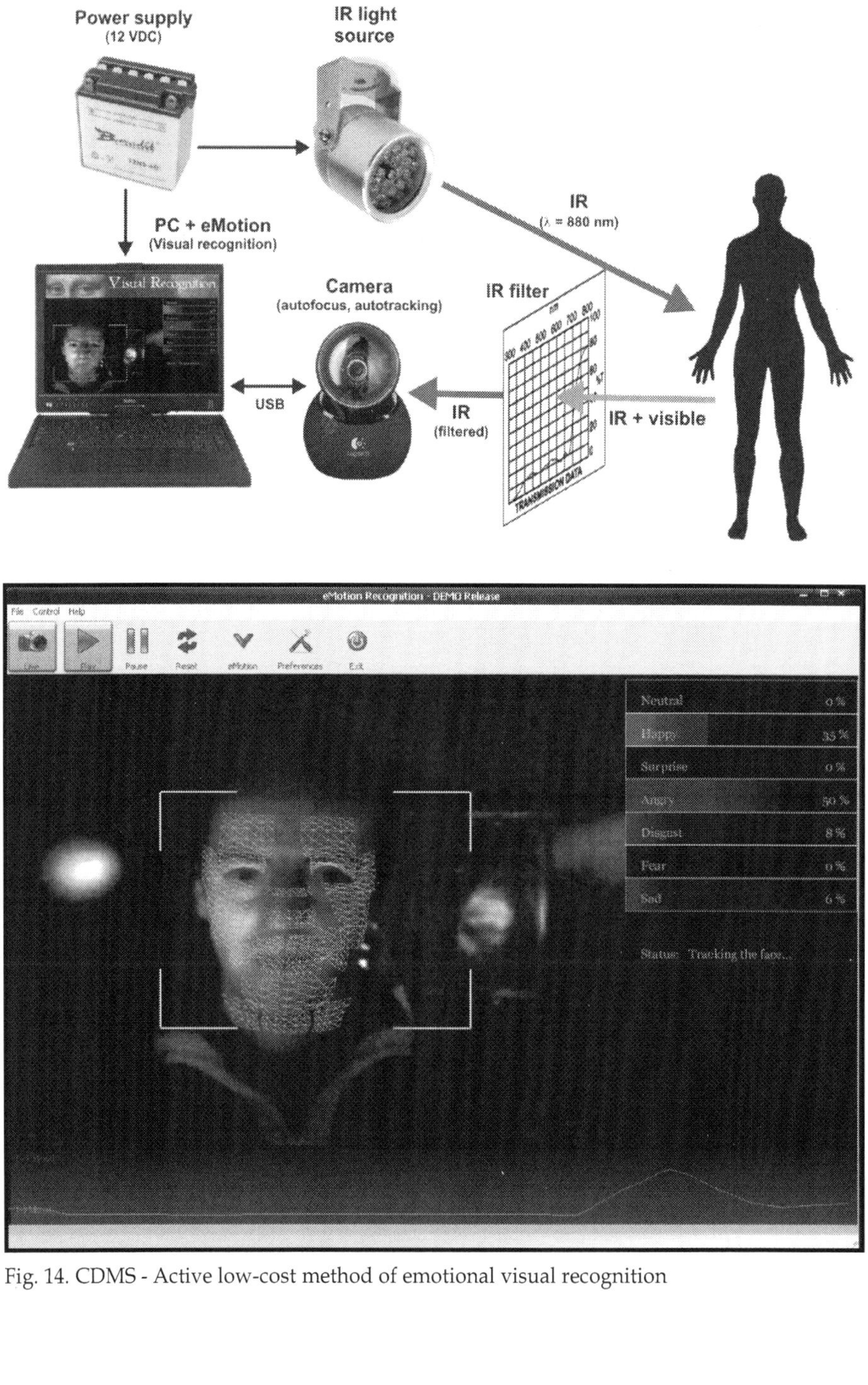

Fig. 14. CDMS - Active low-cost method of emotional visual recognition

Test set-up consist of:

- IR light source (λ = 880 nm)
- Camera: Logitech QuickCam® Orbit AF (Logitech. 2009)
    - Focused on a driver: With motorized tracking and autofocus, the spotlight is always on a driver's face, even when the driver moves around.
- Optical filters (Apollo Design Technology. 2008) (Fig. 15)
    - AP5300 - Apollo Green:
    - AP2330 - .9 Neutral Density:

Using this system we can read a driver mimic and obtain his/her real-time emotions in real road traffic conditions. The system of optical filters can be also easily modified.

AP5300

- Made of double coated, heat-resistant polyester
- %T = 4.4
- Pantone Match: 341
- RGB Match: 0 - 130 - 101
- CMYK Match: 100 - 0 - 67 - 29

AP2330

- Made of double coated, heat-resistant polyester
- %T = 12.7
- Pantone Match: 70% of black
- RGB Match: 109 - 111 – 113
- CMYK Match: 0 - 0 - 0- 70

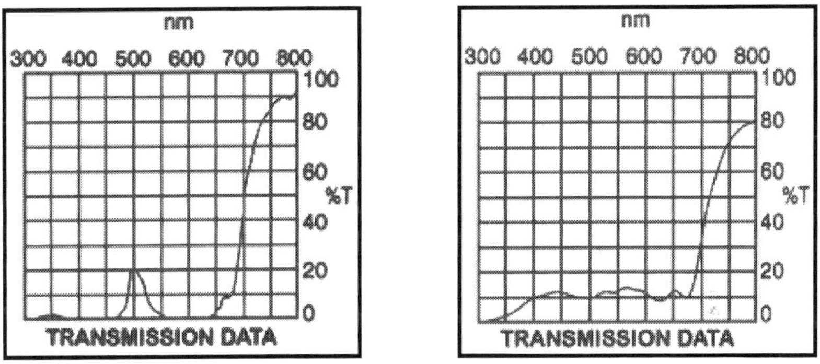

Fig. 15. CDMS - Transmission spectra of used optical filters

4.2.3.2 *Passive method*

In this set-up thermal camera EasIR 4 for far IR (8 - 14μm) was connected to a personal computer via S-Video (NTSC norm) input of AVerTV USB2.0 lite card. For visual recognition we used again eMotion software. This experimental equipment is not one of the low-cost versions, however, it can be additionally used for "contact-free stress monitoring for drivers divided attention" like in (Shastri et al. 2008). One disadvantage over previous active set-up is lower resolution of captured video (160x120 versus 1600x1200 pixels).

We found, that visual recognition software "eMotion" is able to work in near IR (B&W) (Fig. 14) and also in middle IR (Thermal) (Fig. 16) mode.

Thermal camera EasIR 4 - parameters (Guide Infrared, 2009):

- Detector Type: Microbolometer UFPA 160×120 pixels, 25μm
  Spectral range: 8 - 14μm

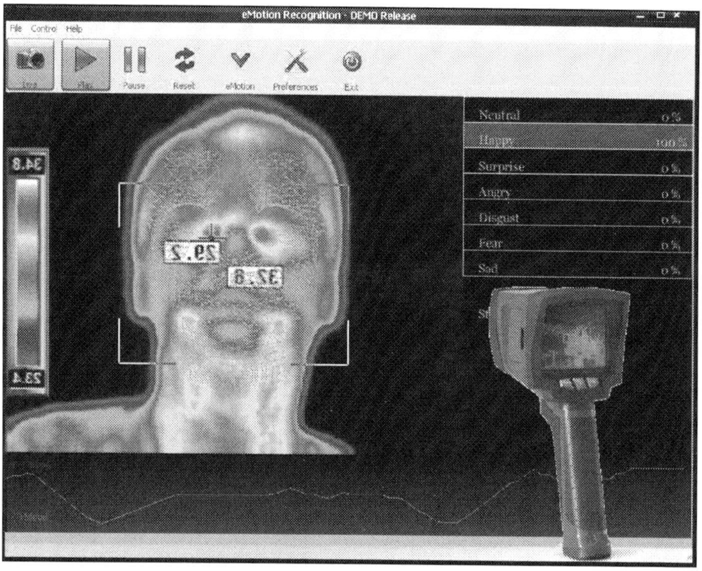

Fig. 16. CDMS – Using of passive thermal camera for emotional recognition

5. Next opportunities

Using of ZnO:Al materials for IDAT microelectrodes allows simultaneous optical (light reflectance of human skin in the 545 nm - 575 nm wave length ranges) and electrical (skin conductivity, temperature and heart rate) measurements. This method can measure the quantity and oxygenation of hemoglobin in top layers of the human skin (based on pulse-oximetry principle), that might offer another very important input factor in monitoring some psychosomatic processes. The advantage of the optical method is also in the contactless manner of monitoring, which is independent on the contact quality variations due to the possible physical activity of the respondent during testing (Vavrinsky et al. 2010).

Implemented camera can be used not only for biomonitoring of car driver psychical state. We can use traditional or skin texture analyzing face recognition (Bonsor et al. 2008) in car security system, where digital image of yourself, your face could replace your car key (password). They exists several free software products (KeyLemon. 2010, Banana Security. 2010).

One of the negative aspects of driving is also "lack of events" on the road and instant driver's drowsiness. To minimize this effect, a driver's head, eye-lid and papilla movement might be sensed by a camera. Several software methods exist. The testing of these methods is prepared and will be included in our future experiments.

At last, car driver monitoring system can by enhanced by electromyography EMG analyzer, Doppler sensors for respiration frequency and driver movement measurement, or online alcohol sensors.

6. Conclusion

The achievements from „DA" experiment were implemented into a driving simulator "CDMS". Used set-up offers continuous biomonitoring and analysis of different electrophysiological aspects of human physiology in a completely safe and non-invasive manner. This technique also has no undesired influence on natural physiological processes. Motivated by the promising results achieved so far, the research will go on by the next step that is integration of the whole biomonitoring system into a real car conditions. We prove that ideal and reliable car monitoring system needs often using multiple measurements methods and the final product will need very robust and smart programmed analyzing software.

7. Acknowledgement

Presented work was supported by the Excellence Centre „CENAMOST", project VEGA grant 1/0220/09, V-10-025-00 and Project ENIAC No. 120 228 (Project MAS - Nanoelectronics for Mobile Ambient Assisted Living).

I would like thank to Dr. I. Novotny and Dr. S. Flickyngerova for production and analysis of microelectrodes.

8. References

Apollo Design Technology. (2008). http://www.internetapollo.com

Atkinson, R. L.; Atkinson, R. C. ; Smith, E. E. ; Bem, D. J. ; Nolen-Hoeksema, S. (2000). *Hilgard's introduction to psychology (13th ed.)*, Fort Worth, TX: Harcourt Brace.

Bonsor, K.; Johnson, R. (2008). How Facial Recognition Systems Work,
http://electronics.howstuffworks.com/gadgets/high-tech-gadgets/facial-recognition.htm

Brezina, I. (2007). Simultaneous performance of double controlled tasks and their impact of psychophysiological processes, *X. European congress of psychology, Book of papers*, Prague, Czech Republic

eMotion. (2009). Faculty of Science, University of Amsterdam, Netherlands
http://www.visual-recognition.nl/eMotion.html.

Gaal, L. (2002). Operation manual to Neurop II test, *Stimul*, FiFUK, Bratislava, Slovakia

Guide Infrared. (2010). Thermal camera EasIR 4.
http://www.wuhan-guide.com/Content.aspx?lang=en&id=195

Ivanic, R.; Novotny, I.; Rehacek, V.; Tvarozek, V.; Weis, M. (2003). Thin film non-symmetric microelectrode array for impedance monitoring of human skin, *Thin Solid Films 433*, pp. 332-336

KeyLemon. (2010). http://www.keylemon.com/

Logitech. (2009). Logitech Quickcam Sphere AF, http://www.logitech.com/en-in/webcam-communications/webcams/devices/3480

Medihum. (2008). http://www.medihum.sk/items.aspx?cat=47&Menu=6

National Instruments, (2009). NI CompactRIO Embedded Design Platform. www.ni.com

National Instruments, (2009). NI Labview 8.6. www.ni.com

Nociar, A. (2005). *Alcohol, Drugs and Personality*, Universitas Tyrnaviensis, Trnava, Slovakia

Olmar, S. (1998). *Bioelectrochemistry and Bioenergetics, 45. 2*, pp. 157-160

Partin, D. L.; Sultan, M. F.; Trush, Ch. M.; Prieto, R.; Wagner, S. J. (2006). Monitoring Driver Physiological Parameters for Improved Safety, *SAE World Congress*, Detroit, USA, ISBN 0-7680-1633-9

Shastri, D. (2008). Contact-free Stress Monitoring for User's Divided Attention, *Human Computer Interaction*, IN-TECH, Vienna, Austria, ISBN 978-953-7619-19-0, pp. 127-134

Snel, J. (1999). *Psychology of ban fruit*, Psychoprof, ISBN 80-968083-2-X, Nove Zamky, Slovakia

Treston. (2010). Pressure sensors with internal transmitter, http://www.treston.cz

Tvarozek, V.; Novotny, I. ; Sutta, P. ; Flickyngerova, S. ; Shtereva, K. ; Vavrinsky, E. (2007) Influence of Sputtering Parameters on Crystalline Structure of ZnO Thin Films. *Thin Solid Films*, Vol. 515, 2007, pp. 8756-8760, ISSN 0040-6090.

Vavrinsky, E.; Stopjakova, V.; Brezina, I.; Majer, L.; Solarikova, P.; Tvarozek, V. (2010). Electro-Optical Monitoring and Analysis of Human Cognitive Processes, *Semiconductor Technologies*, IN-TECH, Vienna, Austria, ISBN 978-953-307-080-3, pp. 437-462

Weis, M.; Danilla, T.; Matay, L.; Hrkut, P. , Kakos, J. (1995). Noninvasive Biomedical Sensors on the Biology - Interface of Human Skin, *7th International Conference on Measurement in Clinical Medicine*, pp. 89-91, Stara Lesna, Slovakia

7

Wireless Communications and Power Supply for *In Vivo* Biomedical Devices using Acoustic Transmissions

Graham Wild and Steven Hinckley
Edith Cowan University
Australia

1. Introduction

Acoustic transmissions are investigated for use in the wireless transmission of digital communications signals and power supply for *in vivo* biomedical devices. The acoustic transmissions are intended to be used for fixed implanted biomedical devices, such as pacemakers, but more importantly, neural implants were wired and wireless radio frequency communications cannot be used. The acoustic transmissions can be used for both wireless communications and to recharge the device, *in vivo*, using conventional piezoelectric power harvesting techniques.

Current research in biomedical engineering is looking at implantable devices to regulate conditions such as Parkinson's and other neuromuscular conditions (Varadan, 2007). Transient devices, such as those used in the gastrointestinal track, make use of high frequency RF, were the permittivity of the human body begins to decrease (Kim et al., 2007). However, significant power is still required. This results in local tissue heating, due to the absorption of the electromagnetic radiation. This heating has side effects that limit the exposure times for safe practices (Gabriel, 1996a; b; c). For neural implants, were the goal is to have the product implanted for long periods of time, without complications and minimal side effects, radio frequency communications cannot currently be used. Acoustic transmissions represent an ideal low power method of communicating with *in vivo* biomedical devices, and for recharging them through the use of piezoelectric based power harvesting. Acoustic transmissions have previously been demonstrated as a means of communicating through elastic solids, with applications to NDT and structural health monitoring (Wild & Hinckley, 2010).

In this work, results presented show the general performance of the acoustic communications channel and sample digital communications signals, through a biological specimen, *in vivo*. The frequency response, transfer function, and transient response (at resonance) of the communications channel were measured. Due to the frequency response of the communications channel, phase shift keying has the best signal performance. To show this, the three basic digital encoding methods were tested. Successful communication was achieved through the communications channel using all three methods. The results support the hypothesis that phase shift keying would be the best encoding method to utilise, particularly in terms of signal robustness.

Results of harvesting acoustic signals to provide power for recharging *in vivo* biomedical devices are also presented. For the piezoelectric transducer used, we show the current-voltage, and voltage-power characteristic curves. These are compared with theoretical models of the power generation. Power requirements for pacemakers are discussed, and how acoustic power harvesting could be successfully used to recharge the devices over their respective lives.

2. Background

Biomedical devices implanted within the human body have been used since last century, starting with the cardiac pacemaker. Cardiac pacemakers are a ubiquitous technology, with over 3 million implanted worldwide (Wood & Ellenbogen, 2002). Since then, *in vivo* biomedical devices have been utilised for further applications. The "pacemaker", a term now used as a general device that generates electrical pulses within the human body, has been applied to the regulation of a number of conditions beyond their primary application for cardiac arrhythmia. When used in the brain, the technique of alleviating the symptoms of neurological disorders with electrical signals is called deep brain stimulation. Although the use of direct brain stimulation began as early as 1947 (Hariz et al., 2010), the use of a permanent pacemaker for deep brain stimulation is a much more recent development (Varadan, 2007). These pacemakers for neurological conditions have been developed recently primarily as a result of improve surgical and imaging techniques associated with neurology (Elias & Lozano, 2010).

Elias and Lozano (2010), give an overview of the current applications of deep brain stimulation. Neurological pacemakers have been applied in the brain for movement disorders, including Parkinson's disease, tremors, and dystonia. Also, they have been used for the treatment of psychological problems such as depression and obsessive-compulsive disorder. Current research on the topic is investigating the use of neurological pacemakers for epilepsy, cluster headache, impaired consciousness, and morbid obesity. Pacemakers have also been used for pain management, particularly pain associated with severe back problems (Blain, 2009).

Currently, pacemakers have their batteries replaced after a five year period. Typically, the entire pacemaker is removed, leaving the electrodes implanted. The battery life of a cardiac pacemaker can be assessed using magnet electrocardiographic assessment. This can even be performed over the telephone using transtelephonic monitoring (Schoenfeld, 2009). For implantable cardioverter-defibrillators, radiofrequency transmissions are used in their assessment, which has proven more effective than transtelephonic monitoring (Crossley et al., 2009). However, the primary advantage of acoustic transmission is not only the ability to safely conduct device follow-up for history taking, physical examination, electrocardiography, radiography, interrogation, and reprogramming (Schoenfeld & Blitzer, 2008). Acoustic transmissions will allow for *in vivo* recharging of the battery, reducing the number of surgeries associated with pacemaker replacement, ideally down to zero, depending on the battery itself.

3. Theory

3.1 Piezoelectric transducer

For a complete understanding of piezoelectric materials and transducers, see Silk's Ultrasonic Transducers for Nondestructive Testing (1984). A brief overview is included here for completeness.

The term piezoelectric means electricity from pressure. So as a force, either in the form of a pressure or a stress (both measured in force per unit area), is applied to the transducer, an electric signal is generated. Specifically, a charge dipole is generated within the crystal structure of the material, which when used inside of a capacitor, results in the generation of a voltage drop across the transducer.

In linear elastic solids, the strain (*S*) and stress (*T*) are related by the elastic stiffness (*c*). In the same material, the electric displacement (*D*) is related to the electric field (*E*) by the permittivity (ε_r) of the material. These equations are referred to as the constitutive equations. In a piezoelectric linear elastic material, the constitutive equations are coupled. Hence, a change in stress or strain corresponds to a change in the charge distribution within the material. The constitutive equations for a piezoelectric material are,

$$\begin{aligned} T &= cS + hE \\ D &= \varepsilon_r E + hS, \end{aligned} \tag{1}$$

where *h* is the piezoelectric coupling coefficient.

Fig. 1(a) shows the crystal lattice structure of lead zirconate titanate (PZT), a peizoceramic material. As a force is applied to the crystal, the lattice is strained, and a charge dipole is produced, similar to that seen in Fig. 1(b).

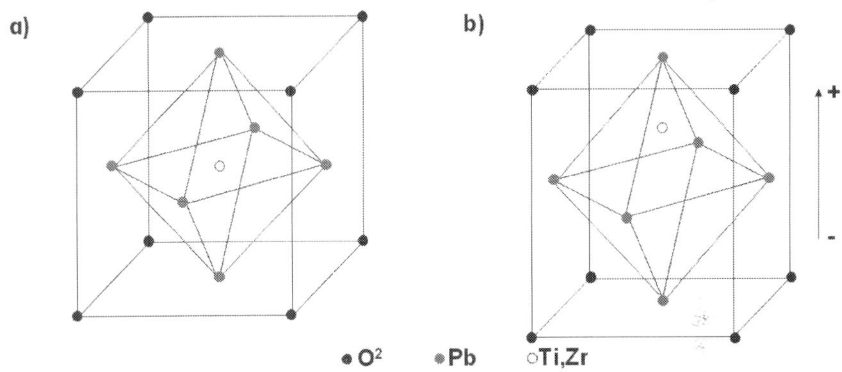

Fig. 1. Principle behind the use of a piezoelectric material, both before (a) and after (b) strain.

3.2 Digital communications

Due to the properties of the communications channel, only digital encoding methods have been investigated. The primary benefit of digital encoding is improved fidelity. The three basic digital encoding methods used include amplitude shift keying, frequency shift keying, and phase shift keying. For the purpose of concept demonstration, only binary keying methods were utilized.

3.2.1 Amplitude shift keying.

In amplitude shift keying, the digital information is encoded onto the analogue carrier as a time varying signal of the amplitude. The simplest form of amplitude shift keying is on-off keying, where a '1' is represented by the amplitude function being maximum (on), and a '0' is represented by the amplitude function being zero (off). The on-off keying signal will have the form,

$$f(t) = A(t)\cos(2\pi f_c t), \tag{2}$$

where f_c is the carrier frequency, and,

$$A(t) = \begin{cases} 0 & for\ data = 0 \\ A & for\ data = 1. \end{cases} \tag{3}$$

On-off keying is decoded by using a rectifier and a low-pass filter that has a cut-off frequency above the data rate, but below the carrier frequency. This removes the carrier wave component ($\cos(2\pi f_c t)$) and recovers the amplitude function which is the digital signal ($A(t)$).

Fig. 2 shows the decoding process for an amplitude shift keying signal. Fig. 2 (a) shows the data to be transmitted defined by (3); Fig. 2 (b) shows the on-off keying signal defined by (2). The received signal is then rectified and low-pass filtered, to remove the carrier frequency, shown in Fig. 2 (c). This also results in some distortion of the information signal due to the removal of higher harmonics. Hence, the signal is passed through a comparator to recover the digital information as shown in Fig. 2 (d).

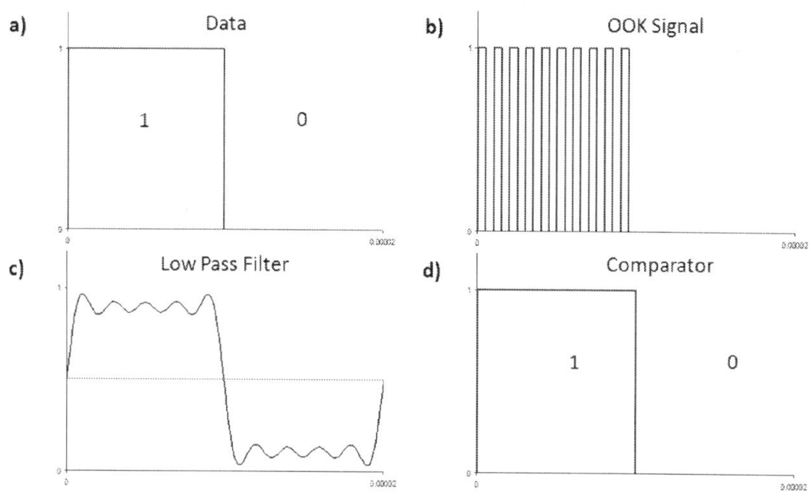

Fig. 2. Decoding an amplitude shift keying signal, a) the digital data to be transmitted, b) the on-off keying signal, c) the rectified low-pass filtered signal, d) digital information recovered after a comparator.

3.2.2 Frequency shift keying.

In frequency shift keying the digital information is encoded onto the analogue carrier as a time varying signal of the frequency. In binary frequency shift keying, two frequencies are used; one frequency represents a digital '1' and the second represents a digital '0'. Frequency shift keying can be thought of as two interweaved on-off keying signals with different carrier frequencies. This means that a similar non-coherent decoding method can be used to recover the digital information. However, the advantage frequency shift keying has over amplitude shift keying is lost in this way. To maintain the independence of the signal from amplitude variations, a coherent detection method is used. Here, the received signal is split into two separate, but identical signals; each of the form,

$$f(t) = A_0 \cos\left(2\pi f_c(t)t\right), \tag{4}$$

where,

$$f_c(t) = \begin{cases} f_1 & \text{for } data = 0 \\ f_2 & \text{for } data = 1. \end{cases} \tag{5}$$

The two signals are each multiplied with a synchronous sinusoid, one with frequency f_1, the other with frequency f_2. This shifts the signal to zero and $2f_n$. A low pass filter is used to remove the $2f_n$ component from each signal. The two filtered signals are then compared to each other to recover the digital information.

In Fig. 3 we see the stages involved in the decoding of a frequency shift keying signal. The data transmitted, Fig. 3 (a), is encoded as two separate frequencies in the signal, defined by (4). The received signal is then split into two identical signals, each mixed with a sinusoid at one of the two frequencies, shown in Fig. 3 (c). Here one of the data bits has no offset, while the second bit has an offset. When filtered, the lack of an offset will result in a zero, while an offset will give a one. The recovered signal after the filter and comparator is shown in Fig. 3 (d).

3.2.3 Phase shift keying.

In phase shift keying, the digital information is encoded onto the analogue carrier as a time varying signal of the phase. Decoding phase shift keying uses some simple mathematics to retrieve the phase information. The phase shift keying signal,

$$f(t) = A_0 \cos\left(2\pi f_c t + \phi(t)\right), \tag{6}$$

where,

$$\phi(t) = \begin{cases} -90 & \text{for } data = 0 \\ 90 & \text{for } data = 1, \end{cases} \tag{7}$$

is multiplied by a synchronous sine and cosine, giving,

$$\begin{aligned} h(t) &= A_0 \cos(2\pi f_c t + \phi(t)) \times \sin(2\pi f_c t) \\ &= \frac{A_0}{2}[\sin\left(\left(4\pi f_c t + \phi(t)\right)\right) + \sin\left(\phi(t)\right)], \end{aligned} \tag{8}$$

and,

$$\begin{aligned} g(t) &= A_0 \cos(2\pi f_c t + \phi(t)) \times \cos(2\pi f_c t) \\ &= \frac{A_0}{2}[\cos(\phi) + \cos\left(\left(4\pi f_c t + \phi(t)\right)\right)]. \end{aligned} \tag{9}$$

These two components are called the in-phase (I) and quadrature (Q) components. Both the in-phase and quadrature components contain high and low frequency components, where the low frequency component is the sine or cosine of the time dependent phase. Using a low pass filter the high frequency components are removed, leaving only the phase component,

$$
\begin{aligned}
h'(t) &= \frac{A_0}{2}\sin\left(\phi(t)\right), \\
g'(t) &= \frac{A_0}{2}\cos\left(\phi(t)\right).
\end{aligned}
\tag{10}
$$

Then by taking the arc-tangent of I on Q, the time dependent phase information is recovered,

$$
\begin{aligned}
y(t) &= \arctan\left(\frac{h'(t)}{g'(t)}\right) \\
&= \arctan\left(\frac{\sin(\phi(t))}{\cos(\phi(t))}\right) \\
&= \arctan\left(\tan(\phi(t))\right) \\
&= \phi(t).
\end{aligned}
\tag{11}
$$

Fig. 4 shows the decoding process for a phase shift keying signal. The digital information, Fig. 4 (a), is encoded onto the carrier as a 180 degree phase shift, as shown in Fig. 4 (b). The resultant in-phase and quadrature components after the signal mixing are shown in Fig. 4 (c). When filtered, the mixed signals show that the in-phase component has a positive value for the first bit, then a negative value for the second bit, while the quadrature component has a value of zero. The arc-tanagent of this ratio will then recover the digital information.

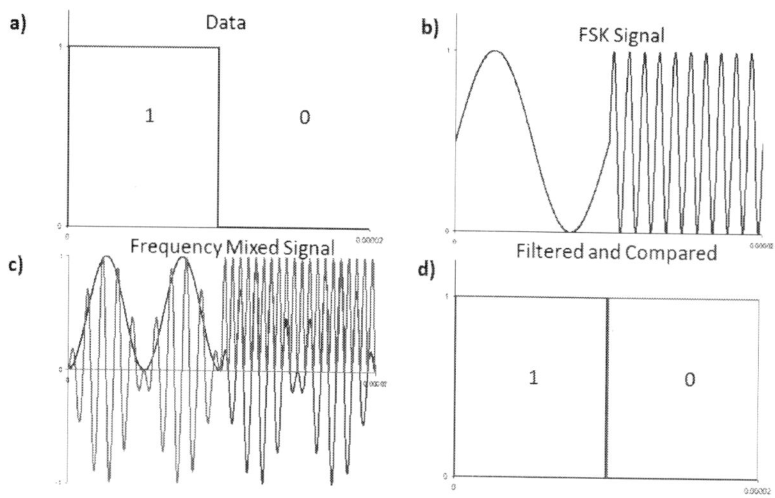

Fig. 3. Decoding a frequency shift keying signal, a) the digital data to be transmitted, b) the frequency shit keying signal, c) the frequency mixed signal, d) digital information recovered after filtering and comparing.

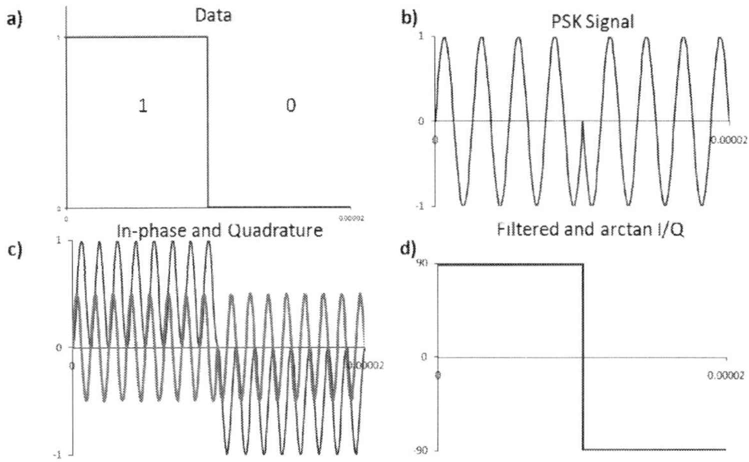

Fig. 4. Decoding a phase shift keying signal, a) the digital data to be transmitted, b) the phase shift keying signal, c) the in-phase and quadrature components, d) digital information recovered after filtering and taking the arc-tangent.

3.3 Power harvesting

For the power harvesting, the piezoelectric receiver is modelled as a current source, i_P, in parallel with a capacitor, C_P. The source current can be written as (Ottman, et al., 2002),

$$i_P(t) = I_P \sin(\omega t), \tag{12}$$

where I_P is the peak current, also referred to as the short circuit current, and ω is the angular frequency of the alternating current signal. The open circuit voltage, V_{OC}, can then be defined in terms of the short circuit current and the reactance of the capacitor (X_C) (Guan & Liao, 2004), that is,

$$V_{OC} = I_P X_C = \frac{I_P}{\omega C_P}. \tag{13}$$

To harvest power, the piezoelectric element needs to be connected across a load. In the case of the alternating current analysis, this is simply a load resistance. There is a 90 degree phase shift between the current flowing through the load resistor (R) and the current flowing through the capacitor. The total power can be expressed as the geometric sum of the power stored in the capacitor, and the power dissipated through the resistor. That is,

$$\begin{aligned} P_T &= \sqrt{P_R^2 + P_C^2} \\ &= \sqrt{I_R^2 R + I_C^2 X_C}. \end{aligned} \tag{14}$$

Since the circuit is an alternating current current divider, the short circuit current can be expressed as,

$$I_P = \sqrt{I_R^2 + I_C^2}. \tag{15}$$

The peak power will then occur when the current flow through the capacitor and the resistor is equal. That is, the load resistance is equal to the capacitor's reactance,

$$R = \frac{1}{\omega C}. \quad (16)$$

The resistor current at peak power is then,

$$I_R = \frac{I_P}{\sqrt{2}}. \quad (17)$$

The voltage at peak power is then,

$$V_{max} = I_R X_C = \frac{I_P}{\sqrt{2}\omega C_P}. \quad (18)$$

We can also express the voltage out as a function of the resistance. From (15) we see that,

$$V = RI_P = R\sqrt{I_P^2 - I_C^2}, \quad (19)$$

The capacitor current is also a function of the voltage, so with a little algebra we see (Ottman, et al., 2002),

$$V = \frac{I_p R}{\sqrt{1 + \left(\omega C_p R\right)^2}}. \quad (20)$$

The power as a function of the load resistance can then be expressed as,

$$P = \frac{V^2}{R} = \frac{I_P^2 R}{1 + \left(\omega C_p R\right)^2}. \quad (21)$$

4. Method

4.1 Acoustic channel configuration

The acoustic transmissions channel is shown in Fig. 5. The setup consists of a PZT transducer as the transmitter, coupled to one side of the forearm using acoustic coupling gel, and a second transducer on the opposite side as a receiver. The ultrasonic signals were generated by an arbitrary waveform generator, an Agilent 33120A. The received signals were recorded on a digital storage oscilloscope, an Agilent 54600A. The piezoelectric transducers used were Steiner and Martins SMQA PZTs, and were unbacked. They had a thickness of 2.1 millimetres, corresponding to a resonant frequency of 1 megahertz, and a radius of 10 millimetres.

4.2 Acoustic communications

Testing the communications involved looking at a number of different quantities. These included,

- the transfer function,
- the frequency response,

- the transient response,
- the digital encoding method, and,
- the data rate.

First, the transfer function of the communications channel was measured. The waveform generator was set to give a continuous sine wave at the resonant frequency of the PZT transducers, 1 megahertz. The amplitude was then varied from 1 volt to 10 volts. Values were recorded at 1 volt increments. This process was repeated several times to give an average and statistical uncertainty.

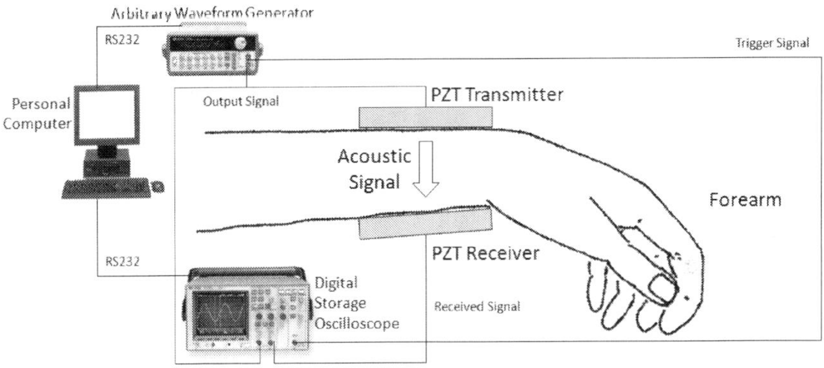

Fig. 5. The configuration of the acoustic transmissions channel through a forearm.

Next, the frequency responses of the communications channel were determined. The function generator was set to give a continuous sine wave at maximum voltage, 10 Volts peak. The frequency was then varied from 10 kilohertz to 1 megahertz. Values were recorded every 10 kilohertz.

Finally, the transient response of the communications channel was investigated, using a low rate sine wave burst at 1 megahertz with 100 cycles. The trailing signal was also examined to determine if it would have any adverse effects on the performance of the communications channel.

The communications signals were generated on the arbitrary waveform generator. Amplitude shift keying (specifically on-off keying) signals were generated using the burst function of the arbitrary waveform generator. A 1 megahertz sine wave carrier was used with a data rate of 40 kilobits per second. The waveform generator used had a built-in frequency shift keying function. This was used to generate the signals, with frequencies of 440 kilohertz and 880 kilohertz at a data rate of 14.5 kilobits per second. The phase shift keying signals were generated in the Waveform Editor software for the arbitrary waveform generator. The signals were then downloaded to the device via the computer interface. The generated waveform consisted of a sine wave carrier, with a data rate of 1/100 the carrier frequency (the software does not generate time so the frequency is set and varied on the generator, and hence a ratio is used for reference). Hence, for the carrier wave frequency of 1 megahertz, the data rate was 10 kilobits per second.

All of the communications signals were recorded on the digital oscilloscope, and downloaded to a personal computer. The demodulation of the signals was then implemented in Matlab™ (The Mathwork Inc). The filter used was a raised cosine filter (Proakis & Salehi, 1994).

4.3 Acoustic power transmission

For the preliminary acoustic power harvesting, the alternating current performance was analysed. In the alternating current circuit experiments, first the capacitance of the piezoelectric element was measured using a capacitance meter. After calculating the reactance at the resonant frequency, the output of the piezoelectric receiver was applied to a variety of suitable load resistors. The voltage drop across the load resistor was measured using a 1 megaohm digital storage oscilloscope. To compare the experimental results to the theoretical analysis, the alternating current circuit was also simulated in PSpice (Cadance Design Systems). The value of I_P was obtained using (13), with the measured values of C_P and V_{OC}. A parametric analysis was performed, varying the value of the load resistance in a frequency domain analysis. The load value was swept from 10 ohms to the value of the digital storage oscilloscope, 1 megaohm, at 10 points per decade. For the practical experiments, a decade resistance box was included, in parallel with the digital storage oscilloscope, as the load resistor. Fig. 6 shows the modified experimental setup for the acoustic power harvesting, and the circuit used in the simulations.

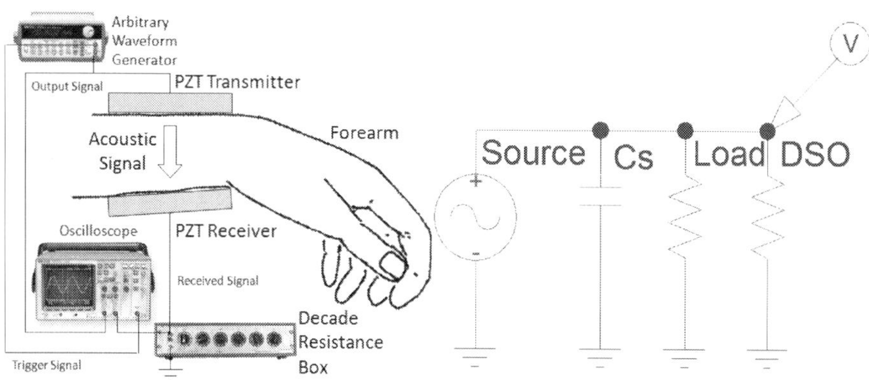

Fig. 6. The modified experimental setup for the acoustic power harvesting, shown left, and the circuit used in the simulation of the power harvesting, shown right.

5. Results

5.1 Transfer function

Fig. 7 shows the transfer function of the acoustic-communications channel at 1 megahertz. The relationship between the input signal strength and the output signal strength is linear, with a correlation coefficient of 1. The noise (and hence, error bars) in the curve is due to small movements in the transmission medium.

5.2 Frequency response

The frequency response of the acoustic-communications channel is shown in Fig. 8. As expected, a strong peak in the frequency spectrum occurs at the resonant frequency of the piezoelectric transducers, that is, 1 megahertz. A secondary peak is noticeable at 100 kilohertz.

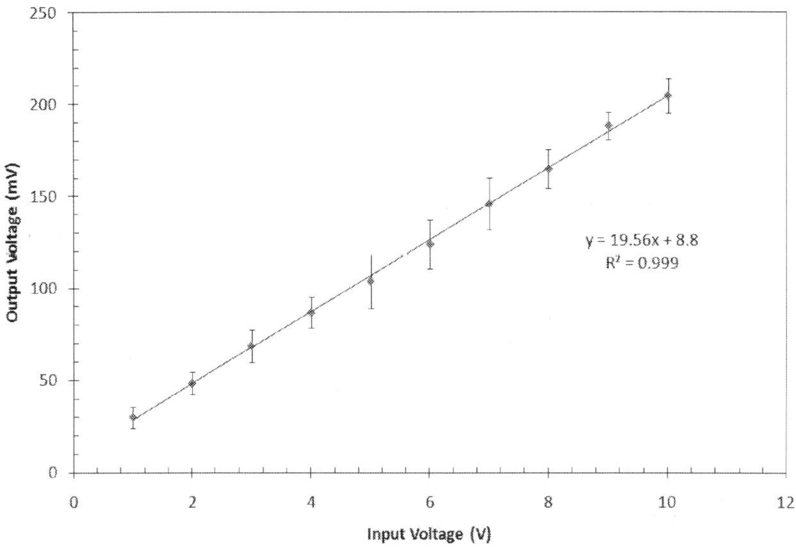

Fig. 7. The transfer function of the acoustic transmissions channel at resonance.

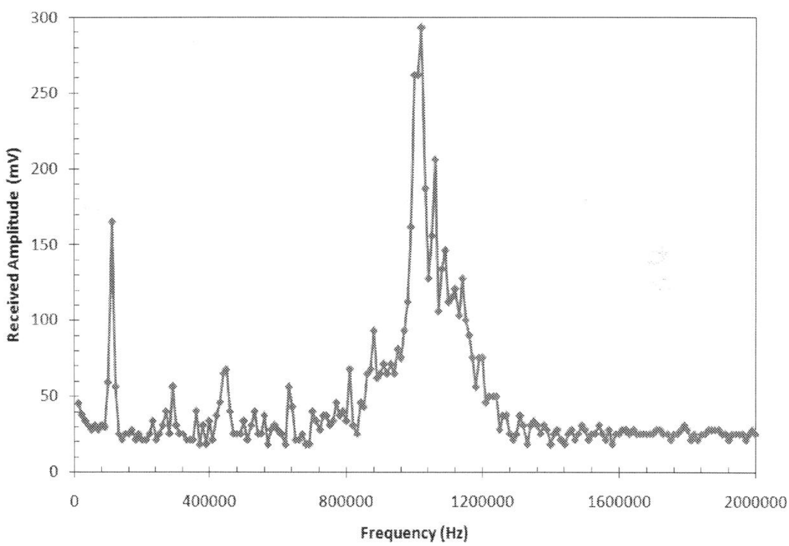

Fig. 8. The frequency response of the acoustic transmissions channel.

5.3 Transient response

Fig. 9 shows the transient response of the acoustic-communications channel for several cycles at 1 megahertz. The received tone burst is relatively compact, with a short transient period, and only a small amount of signal in the tail. Fig. 10 shows the transient response with enough cycles to achieve steady-state. The rise time is then given by approximately 25 cycles, at 1 megahertz, giving 25 microseconds.

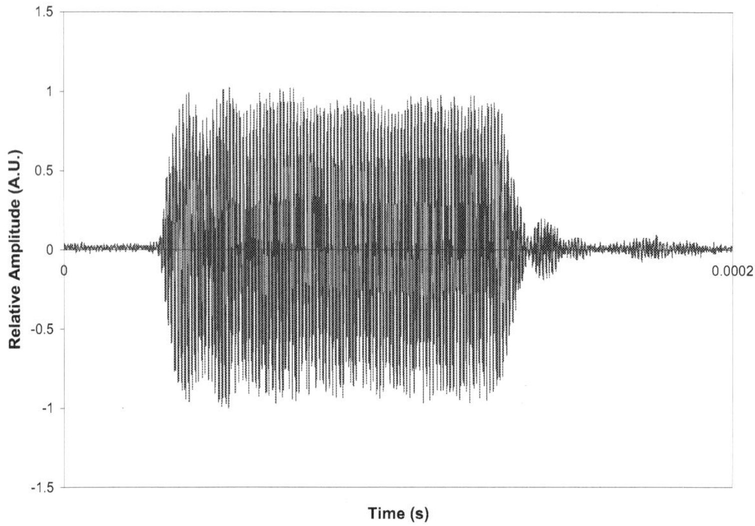

Fig. 9. The transient response of the acoustic transmissions channel at resonance with maximum amplitude, showing the full 100 cycle tone burst.

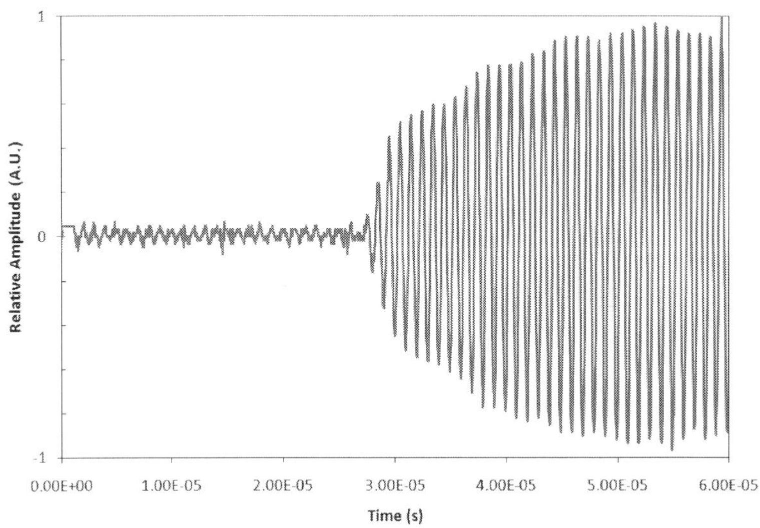

Fig. 10. The transient response of the acoustic transmissions channel at resonance with maximum amplitude, showing the number of cycles required to achieve steady state.

5.4 Communications signals

Fig. 11 shows the transmitted amplitude shift keying signal. Ringing is noticeable as the signal is switched off. Fig. 12 shows the received amplitude shift keying signal. A rectifier and a low pass filter above the data rate, but below the carrier frequency, will recover the envelope, and the use of a comparator with a suitable compare level will enable the digital information to be recovered. This step is not shown, as it simply recovers the four bits that corresponds exactly to the transmitted information.

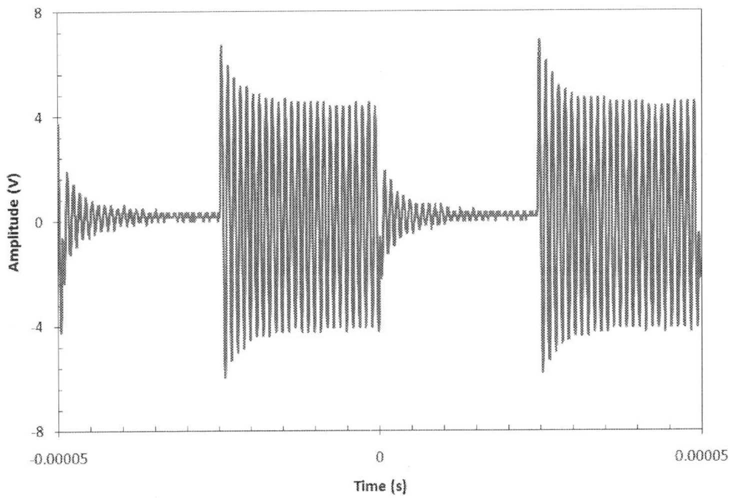

Fig. 11. The transmitted amplitude shift keying/on-off keying signal.

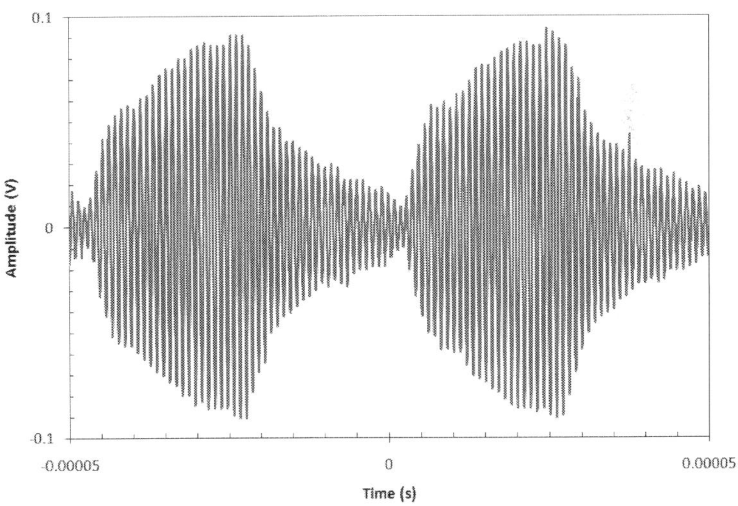

Fig. 12. The received amplitude shift keying/on-off keying communications signal.

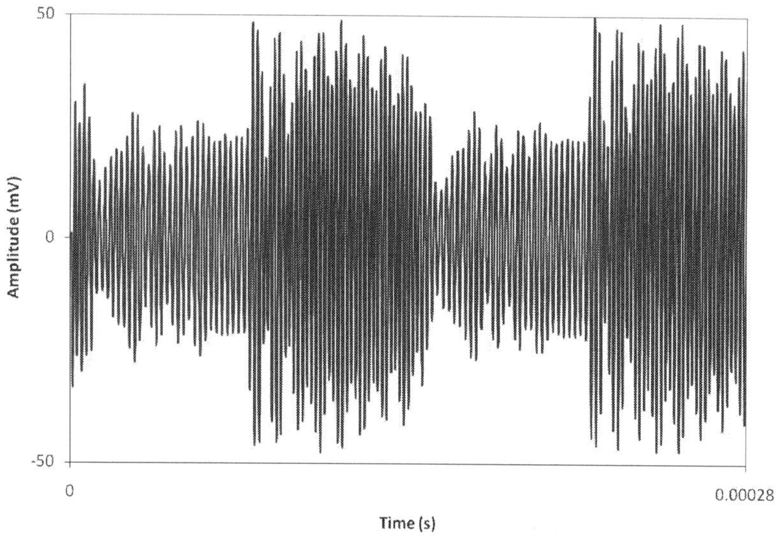

Fig. 13. The received frequency shift keying signal, showing the two frequency signals mixed together.

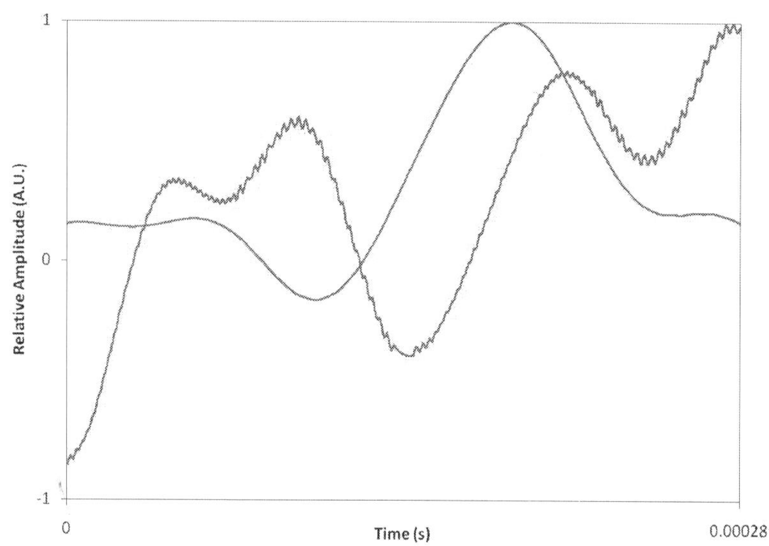

Fig. 14. The received frequency shift keying signal after signal mixing and filtering.

Fig. 13 shows the received frequency shift keying signal. A clear difference between the two frequency components can be seen. As expected, the 880 kilohertz signal has a larger amplitude, as a result of the improved channel response over the 440 kilohertz. Fig. 14 shows the signals after the frequency mixing and filtering. From here, there are four separate sections.

The first starts with the 880 kilohertz signal on top. From here, the signals cross over as expected, enabling the original digital information to be recovered by comparing the two signals to each other. An interesting point occurs around a quarter of the way in, where the two components nearly cross over again, which could result in a bit error. Hence, it is safe to assume that the data rate is almost at a maximum with frequency shift keying.

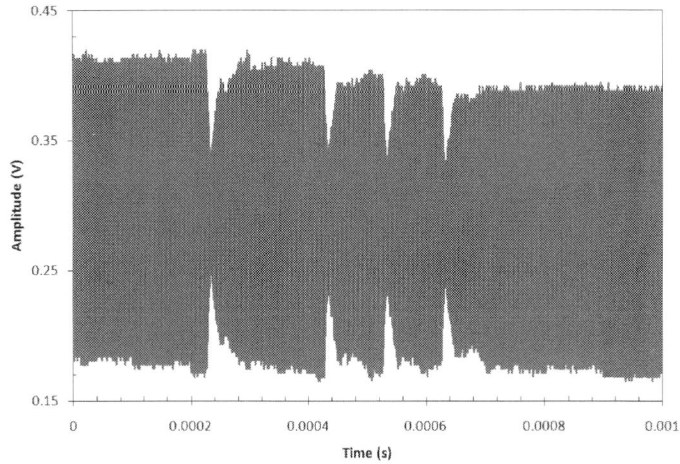

Fig. 15. The received phase shift keying signal, where the change in phase appears as a transient signal similar to the on-off keying of the signal.

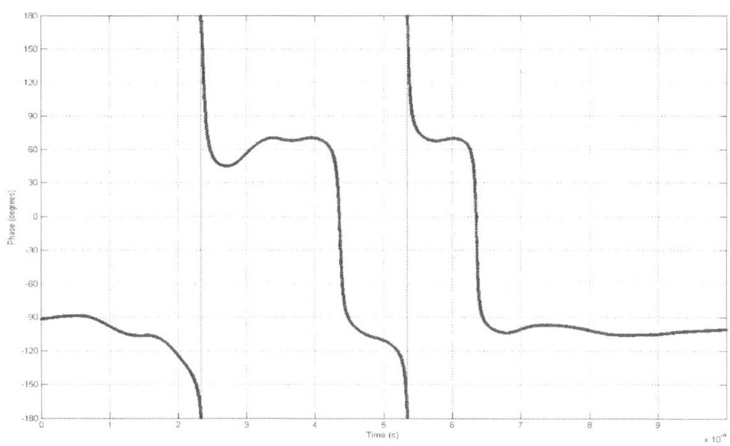

Fig. 16. The recovered phase information decoded from the received phase shift keying communications signal.

Fig. 15 shows the received phase shift keying signal, which contains the data stream [1 1 0 0 1 0 1 1 1 1]. The decoded phase shift keying signal is then shown in Fig. 16. The original digital information can be recovered by selecting a digital 1 as a phase less than 0 degrees, and a digital 0 as a phase greater than 0 degrees. Note that the transmitted phase shift keying signal is not shown, as no information is visible on the time scale of the entire signal.

5.5 Power transmission

The capacitance of the piezoelectric receiver was measured to be 1.086 nanofrads. At the resonant frequency of 1.035 megahertz, this gives a reactance of 141 ohms. With an open circuit voltage of 570 millivolts, (13) gives a short circuit current of 4 milliamps. These values where then used in the PSpice simulation of the alternating current circuit.

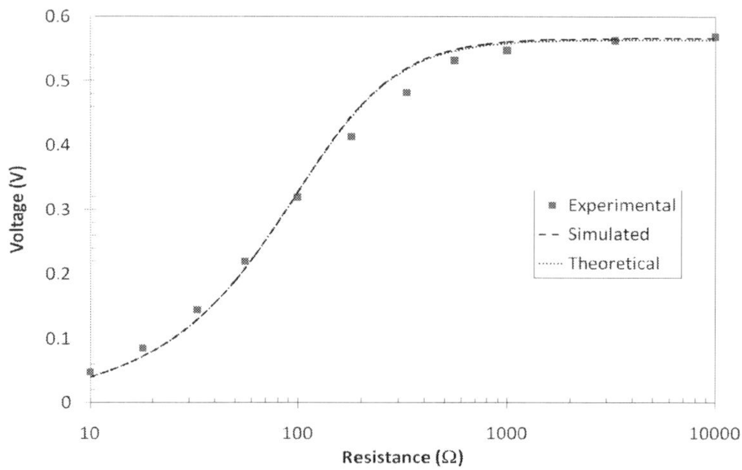

Fig. 17. Voltage as a function of load resistance for the power harvesting.

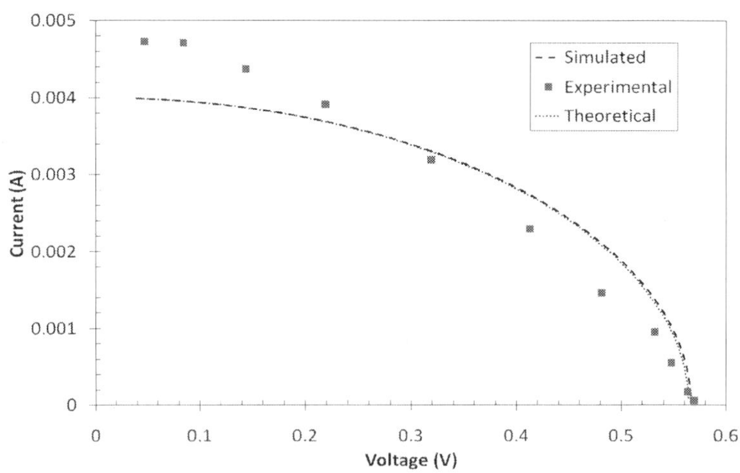

Fig. 18. Load current as a function of the voltage, current-voltage curves.

Fig. 17 shows the comparison between the applied load and the voltage drop across it, for both the experimental values and the simulated results. As expected, as the load resistance decreases in size, the output voltage also decreases.

Fig. 18 shows the load current as a function of the output voltage (current-voltage curves), and Fig. 19 shows the power delivered to the load as a function of the output voltage (power-voltage curves), for the experimental, theoretical and simulated results. The power-voltage curves shows a measured peak power of 1 milliwatt, while theory and simulation give peak power values of 1.121 milliwatts and 1.125 milliwatts, respectively.

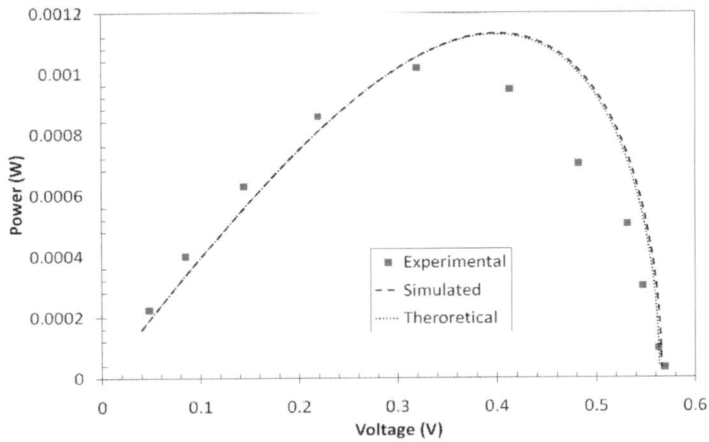

Fig. 19. Power delivered to the load as a function of the voltage, power-voltage curves.

6. Discussion

Another important advantage of acoustic communications is security. With implantable cardioverter-defibrillators utilising wireless radiofrequency communications, the security of the signal needs to be considered. A commercially avilable implantable cardioverter-defibrillator was easily attacked in a recent study (Halperin, et al., 2008). As a contact wireless communications method, acoustic transmissions are inherently secure, in that someone needs to touch you to be able to communicate with the *in vivo* biomedical device. From here, an encryption method could be utilised for communications if necessary. Halperin et al. suggest that encryption is expensive in the power budget. However, the use of acoustic power harvesting means that the power required for encryption would not be an issue.

6.1 Transmissions channel

As expected, the transfer function is linear. Some randomness is noticeable in the signal, hence the uncertainty. It is worth noting that a similar uncertainty would be expected on all other results. The experiments were performed with the arm as immobile as possible. A significant variation was noticed when the arm/hand was allowed to articulate. When deliberately trying to alter the output voltage, the peak value varied from around 140 millivolts to 280 millivolts, a factor of 2. This fluctuation may be an issue, in particular if amplitude shift keying is used as the encoding method. This is one of the reasons that phase shift keying would be a more robust encoding method for the communications signals.

The frequency response shows a strong primary resonance at the through thickness resonance of the transducer, 1 megahertz, and a secondary resonance at 100 kilohertz, corresponding to the radial resonance of the transducer. Overall, the frequency response of the transmissions channel suggests that frequency shift keying would not be suitable. However, there is a small resonance at 440 kilohertz, and another tertiary resonance at 880 kilohertz. Hence, these two frequencies were ideal to test frequency shift keying.
The transient response of the transmission channel is relatively neat. The compact form of the tone burst only has a minor tail effect, elongating the signal in time. One of the main reasons for this is due to the composite nature of the communications channel. The various materials which the body is made up of all have different acoustic velocities. The result of this is that the various paths travelled by the ultrasound in the medium will result in significant temporal dispersion, and then interference.

6.2 Acoustic communications

The result of the amplitude shift keying communications signal tests suggests that relatively high data rates could be achieved for the sort of information that needs to be transmitted. The amplitude shift keying signal is limited primarily by the transient response of the transmissions channel. That is, with a transient response time of 25 micro seconds, a data rate of 40 kilobits per second is possible when using a 1 megahertz carrier frequency. By utilising a transducer with a high resonant frequency, and a larger bandwidth, the achievable data rate could be significantly increased. However, amplitude shift keying has a limited effectiveness, particularly as the coupling efficiency varies with movement of the transmission medium (the forearm).
The frequency shift keying results suggest that the data rate may not be able to be improved much further. This is illustrated by the relative closeness of the two mixed signals in Fig. 14, approximately a quarter of the way through. The most likely cause of this is the frequency response. Since the 880 kilohertz signal is close to the resonant frequency of 1 megahertz, this could lead to a stronger amplitude in the 880 kilohertz signal, which is seen as the consistently higher signal strength of the corresponding mixed and filtered signal (Fig. 14, red trace). The resultant "steady state" frequency will also be affected by the resonant frequency of the transducer, which will be given as a combination of the driving frequency, and the resonant frequency. This explains the drift shown in Fig. 14, where the curves both steadily increase.
The recovered phase information, from the phase shift keying signal, suggests that a relatively high data rate is possible. The phase transitions indicate that a data rate up to that of the amplitude shift keying signal (40 kilobits per second) could be used. However, unlike the amplitude shift keying signal, the phase shift keying has robustness relative to the amplitude variation in the received signal. The phase transitions are not as quick as those shown in previous work (Wild & Hinckley, 2010), when communicating through an aluminium panel, but as previously mentioned, the data rate is relatively high for the intended application. The primary advantage of a high communications rate would be to reduce the effect of fluctuations due to motion of the communications medium.

6.3 Power harvesting

The preliminary results for the power harvesting are promising. The value of 1 milliwatt was significant compared to values expected. However, in the attempt to implement an alternating-current to direct-current converter circuit, the very high frequency (1 megahertz) appears to be limiting the ability to successfully rectify the output of the transducer. This is mainly due to the high junction capacitance of the rectifier diodes. In the conversion from alternating-current to direct-current, the capacitance is an important consideration to achieve peak power output (Ottman et al., 2002). To resolve this issue, transducers with a lower resonant frequency, in the kilohertz range, need to be utilised. Ideally, broadband transducers could be used to quantify the performance of the power conversion as a function of frequency, as (13) indicates that the higher the frequency, the less power that can be generated. In addition to this, the overall output voltage needs to be a larger amplitude. This is required due to the loss associated with the use of the diode rectifier circuit to convert the alternating-current to direct-current, which is required to power the actual biomedical device. This could be achieved in two ways; according to the transfer function the input voltage could be increased. However, it would be more effective if the efficiency of the channel could be improved. This could be achieved by selecting a transducer with a resonant frequency equal to the resonant frequency of the channel, which is related to the thickness of the channel, and the acoustic velocity.

Overcoming the two limitations encountered here with these preliminary results, could yield relatively large power generation. That is, with the successful implementation of an alternating-current to direct-current converter circuit, using a lower frequency, and a more efficient transfer of acoustic energy through the channel, the measured power levels could easily be utilised for the *in vivo* recharging of a device such as a pacemaker, which have relatively lower power consumptions (Mallela et al., 2004).

7. Conclusion

Successful communication was achieved through the communications channel. We also show the result of harvesting acoustic signals to provide power for recharging *in vivo* biomedical devices. In future work, we will optimise the transducers used to maximise the amplitude of the received acoustic transmissions. This is primarily a concern for the acoustic power harvesting, which will also include the implementation of adaptive direct current to direct current power converters to track the peak power point, to ensure efficient power transfer.

8. References

Blain, L. (2009). Spinal Cord Stimulators - the 'pacemaker' for chronic pain, *Gizmag*, (12 August 2009), viewed 8 September 2010, < http://www.gizmag.com/eon-mini-spinal-cord-stimulator/12486/>

Crossley, G.H., Chen, J., Choucair, W., Cohen, T.J., Gohn, D.C., Johnson, W.B., Kennedy,E.E., Mongeon, L.R., Serwer, G.A., Qiao, H. & Wilkoff, B.L. (2009). Clinical Benefits of Remote Versus Transtelephonic Monitoring of Implanted Pacemakers, *Journal of the American College of Cardiology*, Vol. 54, No. 22, (November 2009) 2012–2019, ISSN 0735-1097

Elias, W.J. & Lozano, A.M. (2010). Deep brain stimulation: the spectrum of application, *Neurosurgical Focus*, Vol. 29, No. 2, (August 2010) Introduction, ISSN 1092-0684

Gabriel, C., Gabriely, S. & Corthout, E. (1996a). The dielectric properties of biological tissues: I. Literature survey, *Physics in Medicine and Biology*, Vol. 41, No. 11, (November 1996) 2231–2249, ISSN 1361-6560

Gabriely, S., Lau, R. W. & Gabriel, C. (1996b). The dielectric properties of biological tissues: II. Measurements in the frequency range 10 Hz to 20 GHz," *Physics in Medicine and Biology*, Vol. 41, No. 11, (November 1996) 2251–2269, ISSN 1361-6560

Gabriely, S., Lau, R. W. & Gabriel, C. (1996c). The dielectric properties of biological tissues: III. Parametric models for the dielectric spectrum of tissues," *Physics in Medicine and Biology*, Vol. 41, No. 11, (November 1996) 2271–2293, ISSN 1361-6560

Guan, M. & Liao, W.H. (2005). Comparative analysis of pie-zoelectric power harvesting circuits for rechargeable batteries, *Proceedings of the 2005 IEEE International Conference on Information Acquisition*, pp. 243-246, ISBN 0-7803-9303-1, Hong Kong and Macau China, June 2005, IEEE Press, Washington DC

Halperin, D., Heydt-Benjamin, T.S., Ransford, B., Clark, S.S., Defend, B., Morgan, W., Fu, K., & Kohno, T., (2008). Pacemakers and Implantable Cardiac Defibrillators: Software Radio Attacks and Zero-Power Defenses, *Proceedings of the 2008 IEEE Symposium on Security and Privacy*, pp. 129-142, ISBN 978-0-7695-3168-7, Oakland, Ca, May 2008, IEEE Press, Washington DC

Hariz, M.I., Blomstedt, P. & Zrinzo, L. (2010). Deep brain stimulation between 1947 and 1987: the untold story, *Neurosurgical Focus*, Vol. 29, No. 2, (August 2010) E1, ISSN 1092-0684

Kim, C., Lehmanna, T. & Nooshabadib, S. (2007). An Ultra-Wideband Transceiver for Biotelemetry Systems, *Proceedings of SPIE Microelectronics: Design, Technology, and Packaging III*, ISBN 9780819469694, Canberra, December 2007, SPIE, Bellingham

Mallela, V.S., Ilankumaran, V. & Rao, N.S. (2004). Trends in cardiac pacemaker batteries, *Indian Pacing Electrophysiology Journal*, Vol. 4, No. 4, (October 2004) 201–212, ISSN 0972-6292

Ottman, G.K., Hofmann, H.F., Bhatt, A.C. & Lesieutre, G.A. (2002). Adaptive piezoelectric energy harvesting circuit for wireless remote power supply, *IEEE Transactions on Power Electronics*, Vol. 17, No. 5, (September 2002) 669-676, ISSN 0885-8993

Proakis, J., Salehi, M. (1994). *Communication Systems Engineering*, Prentice Hall, ISBN 978-0131589322, New Jersey, USA,

Schoenfeld, M.H. (2009). Transtelephonic Versus Remote Monitoring of Cardiovascular Implantable Electronic Devices, *Journal of the American College of Cardiology*, Vol. 54, No. 22, (November 2009) 2020–2022, ISSN 0735-1097

Schoenfeld, M.H., & Blitzer, M,L. (2008). Follow-up assessments of the pacemaker patient, In: *Cardiac Pacing and ICDs, 5th edition*, Ellenbogen K.A. & Wood M.A. (Eds.), 498 - 545, Wiley-Blackwell, ISBN 978-1-4051-6350-7, Hoboken, NJ

Silk, M.G. (1984). *Ultrasonic Transducers for Nondestructive Testing*, Adam Hilger Ltd, ISBN 0852744366, Bristol, UK.

Varadan, V.K. (2007). The role of Nanotechnology and Nano and Micro-Electronics in monitoring and control of Cardiovascular Diseases and Neurological Disorders, *Proceedings of SPIE Nanosensors, Microsensors, and Biosensors and Systems 2007*, ISBN 9780819466495, San Diego, March 2007, SPIE, Bellingham

Wild, G. & Hinckley, S. (2010). PSpice Simulation of an Electro-Acoustic Communications Channel, *IEEE Transactions on Ultrasonics, Ferroelectrics and Frequency Control*, Vol. 57, No. 4, (April 2010) 981-985, ISSN 0885-3010

Wood, M.A. & Ellenbogen, K.A. (2002). Cardiac Pacemakers From the Patient's Perspective, Circulation, Vol. 105, No. 18, (May 2002) 2136-2138, ISSN 1524-4539

8

Power Amplifiers for Electronic Bio-Implants

Anthony N. Laskovski and Mehmet R. Yuce
The University of Newcastle
Australia

1. Introduction

Healthcare systems face continual challenges in meeting their aims to provide quality care to their citizens within tight budgets. Ageing populations in the developed world are perhaps one of the greatest concerns in providing quality healthcare in the future. Figure 1 shows projections from the United Nations, indicating that the median age of citizens in economically developed regions is set to approach 40 years by the year 2050, and reach as high as 55 years in Japan. This trend is likely to lead to strained economies caused by less revenue raised by smaller workforces. Another effect of ageing populations is the need of further care in order to remain healthy. This care varies from frequent check-ups to condition monitoring, compensation for organ malfunction and serious surgical operations. As a result of these trends, healthcare systems will face the task of servicing more people with more serious and expensive health services, all using less available funds. Effort is being focused on running cheaper and more effective healthcare systems and the development of technology to assist in this process is a natural research priority.

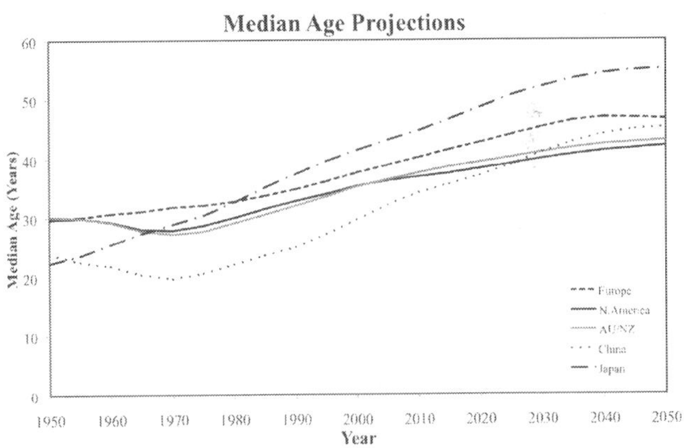

Fig. 1. UN Median Age Statistics (UN, 2010)

1.1 Technology in medicine

Archaeological evidence shows the application of technology to medicine for rehabilitative, functional and aesthetic purposes as far back as 5000 years ago in ancient Egypt, where prosthetic devices were designed engineered and constructed with basic materials such as leather and wood. The earliest written evidence exists from ancient India, mentioning a prosthetic iron leg (Thurston, 2007). These materials formed the basics of prosthetics until recently, the only variations being in manufacturing techniques.

The application of titanium alloys to medicine was a significant advance due to their ability to form biological bonds with human tissue (Long and Rack, 1998). Developments in polymer technology led to biocompatible polymers, allowing more precise, detailed and finer implants to be made such as blood vessel reinforcements (Ramakrishna et al., 2001). The latest developments in biomaterial research is in fact designing polymers to allow the body to heal itself (Hench and Polak, 2002).

1.2 Electrical and electronic technology

The field of electronics has been a relatively recent technological advance in history, and it has seen an escalating rate of sophistication. After the renaissance, serious curiosity in the phenomenon of electrical charge developed, and several fundamental developments were made such as the discovery in 1791 by Galvani, that electricity was the medium through which information was passed to muscles in the body. The voltaic pile was developed in 1800 by Volta, which provided the first reliable source of electrical energy, and other major developments happened such as the recognition of electromagnetism by Orsted and Ampere, and Faraday's electric motor.

Tesla's achievements in the transmission of low frequency wireless power were significant. He proposed to apply the concept of resonance to electrical energy in order to transmit energy wirelessly. Hertz used spark gaps to generate high frequency power and detect it at a receiving end, using parabolic reflectors at the transmitting and receiving ends. These developments were further built upon in the late 1930s with the availability of higher energy microwave power generators. Developments in microwave power transmission escalated during the 20th century due to World War II and the Cold War, resulting in sophisticated satellite communication technologies (Brown, 1984).

The development of quantum theory and semiconductor electronics laid the foundations for rapid technological development in what is now being called `The Age of Silicon' (Jenkins, 2005). They allowed for the rapid development of integrated circuit technology characterised by Moore's Law, which states that the number of transistors in a given surface area increases exponentially with time (Łukasiak and Jakubowski).

Computer networks developed in the 1970s and led to the eventual creation of internet (Kleinrock, 2008). This has led to a technological and sociological revolution characterising the 21st century as `The Information Age', with omnipresent networks, small sensors, constant and cheap access to information on increasingly intelligent personal devices that are modestly called `phones'.

1.3 Electronics in medicine

Galvani's frog experiment showed biology as one of the original phenomena through which human understanding of electricity was developed. Interestingly, knowledge in the field of electronic engineering has since advanced to a stage where it is being used to understand, monitor and even treat biological and medical systems.

Medical imaging is fundamental to the understanding of the human body and diagnosing medical problems. X-Ray technology is widely used to capture two-dimensional details for orthopaedic applications. The rays are created by rapidly decelerating electrons to produce high frequency electromagnetic radiation, which is diffracted and penetrated differently by bones and flesh, allowing the resultant radiation to be recorded on X-ray sensitive polymers to show internal details of the body. Ultrasound is commonly use to provide a real-time image of the body's internal operations, being a popular and safe technology in monitoring various stages of pregnancy. Computed Tomography (CT) scanning and Magnetic Resonance Imaging (MRI) provide three-dimensional images of the body's internal organs, allowing fine differentiation between different types of body tissue. Such types of scans involve powerful computing capability to reconstruct models of internal organs, and have been invaluable to the understanding of the human body in a non-destructive way (Seligman, 1982).

Robotics in medicine has become another exciting field in which the application of intelligent electronics is contributing greatly, to the point where they are used to conduct complex surgery, which is remotely controlled by surgeons. Their ability to move accurately without shaking hands or unstable movements allows minute and delicate operations to take place, while still being controlled by a doctor. The application of robotics to medical prosthesis is another significant advance since the first pneumatically powered hand in 1915 (Childress, 1985). So advanced is this field, that robotic prosthetic arms are being developed and controlled by electrical signals sent by the brain through the body's nervous system.

The cardiac pacemaker is the oldest and perhaps best known implantable prosthetic electronic device. It was first used externally on a patient in 1952 and as the first semiconductor transistors were developed, the possibility to implant led to the first human implant in 1960 (Greatbatch and Holmes, 1991). This was the beginning of several exciting developments in the area of medical prosthetics.

Cochlear implants, popularly termed `Bionic Ears' were a major breakthrough in medical prosthesis. The Cochlea is a part of the ear that converts sound vibrations to electrical signals that are sent via the audio nerve to the brain where they are interpreted. In deaf patients where the Cochlea does not operate properly and the auditory nerve does, cochlear implants are possible. A system was designed and created to replace the Cochlea with an electronic prosthetic device, such that the sound recorded by a microphone is processed by an implanted device and sent to the brain on the audio nerve.

Retinal prostheses, popularly termed 'Bionic Eyes' have been the focus of much research. The concept is similar to Cochlear prosthesis, however this electronic prosthetic device aims to substitute the retina, which is the part of the eye which converts light to electrical signals and sent to the brain via the optic nerve. For patients that have suffered blindness due to macular degeneration, this prosthetic device has the potential to re-introduce sight.

Patient monitoring is an important part of medicine in that it assists doctors in understanding the condition of their patients, be it for known issues or as a means of diagnosis. Condition monitoring of patients is also conducted after serious surgical operations, in order to ensure that no complications arise. This is often a major reason for a patient's long stay in hospital after an operation.

Prevention is preferable to treatment, and the ability to monitor vital health indicators such as the electrocardiogram (ECG), body temperature and blood pressure information via medical telemetry may offer adequate tools to view logged or real time data for vulnerable patients, especially the elderly. Growing telecommunications infrastructure with increasing sophistication is opening the possibilities with regards to medical telemetry, making it theoretically possible for patients to carry out their daily tasks while being monitored remotely by doctors. Implantable medical telemetry is in fact becoming an increasingly important field of research, with the potential to reduce medical risks, lower medical costs and cater for ageing populations.

2. Telemetry

Telemetry is a significant element of health care, involving the measurement and communication of a patient's biological information for interpretation by medical professionals. It is mostly conducted by external medical equipment, however medical telemetry is making its way into the body in the form of implantable monitoring devices, which will potentially be able to measure very detailed body signals. Figure 2 shows a general block diagram of most implantable telemetry systems.

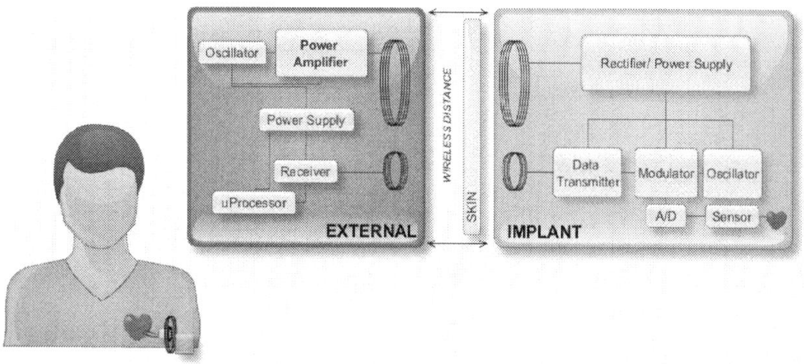

Fig. 2. General architecture of telemetry systems

One important factor to consider when dealing with implantable devices is the supply of power. In order to send power to implantable devices, wireless links are usually employed in the form of inductive links. Inductive power transfer is more efficient at lower frequencies (Vaillancourt et al., 1997). However, lower transmission frequencies use larger circuit components, especially transmission coils. From the perspective of implantable devices, space is important and this has led to a need to design highly efficient transmission circuits at higher frequencies.

Switching power amplifiers have been a popular choice for the transmission of wireless power (Raab et al., 2002). While the most popular choice has been the Class-E amplifier, it is also useful to gain an understanding of other power amplifiers, Class-F and Class-D.

3. Class-F amplifier

The Class-F power amplifier may be seen as a development from the Class-A and Class-B power amplifier, with a 50% conduction time and the use of harmonic resonators on the load network (Reynaert and Steyaert, 2006). An example of the Class-F amplifier is shown in Figure 3 comprising a transistor, choke inductor and an input source.

The network attached to the output of the transistor is manipulated by harmonics such that the voltage and current are manipulated. The voltage is shaped by odd harmonics of the fundamental frequency such that the voltage appears as a square-wave. The current is 180^0 out of phase and shaped to appear as a half sine-wave (Raab, 1997).

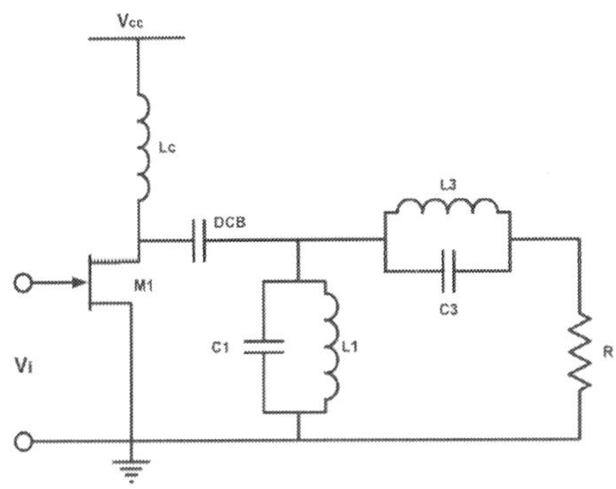

Fig. 3. Class-F Amplifier

The more harmonic frequencies are used to shape the voltage and current curves, the higher the efficiency of the Class-F amplifier. The theoretical efficiency of the amplifier with the use of third harmonics is 88.4%, while the additional use of fifth harmonic resonators produces an efficiency of 92% (Reynaert and Steyaert, 2006).
Inverse Class-F amplifiers also exist where the current curve is shaped to be a square-wave, while the voltage is shaped as a half sine-wave (Young, 2006).

4. Class-D amplifier

Like the Class-F power amplifier, the Class-D power amplifier is a non-linear amplifier in that the transistors of the amplifier behave as switches such that the output of the transistors is related to the supply or reference voltage, depending on which transistor is turned on at the time. The fact that the output signal of the amplifier is determined by the switching of the amplifier's transistors means that the Class-D power amplifier may be described as a switching power amplifier (Reynaert and Steyaert, 2006).

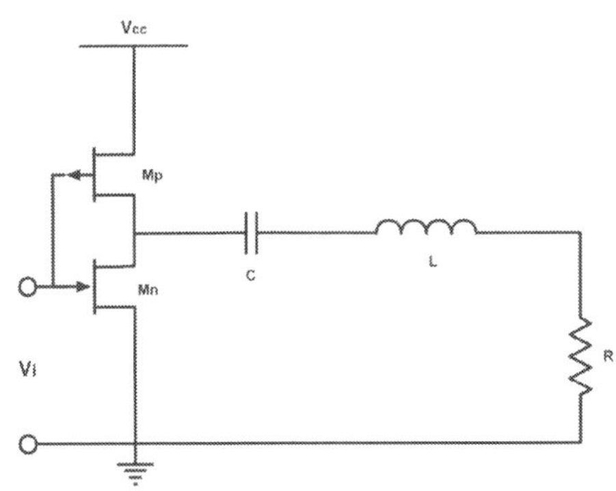

Fig. 4. The Class-D amplifier

Figure 4 shows an example of a Class-D switching power amplifier. It comprises an inverter, which switches two transistors on and off alternatively to generate a square wave. The output of the inverter is connected to a series RLC network as shown in Figure 4, which is resonant at the fundamental frequency of the square-wave, producing a sinusoidal signal at this frequency. Assuming that the series L and C network only allows sinusoidal current to reach the load R, the theoretical efficiency of the Class-D amplifier is 100%.
In reality, circuit elements are not ideal and several losses have been analysed with a focus on parasitic drain-source capacitance in each of the transistors, which becomes significant in higher frequency RF designs. The drain-source capacitance, C_{ds} actually introduces a capacitor where an open circuit should ideally exist. At high frequencies, typical capacitor values are in the order of pico Farads, which means that parasitic capacitance C_{ds} becomes a significant circuit element, which dissipates energy during switching cycles thus decreasing the amplifier's efficiency (El-Hamamsy, 1994, Kiri et al., 2009, Raab et al., 2002).

5. Class-E amplifier

The Class-E power amplifier was introduced by Sokal et al., shown in Figure 5 (Sokal and Sokal, 1975). Like the Class-D amplifier it is also a switching power amplifier driven by a square-wave input, however rather than two transistors it comprises one transistor and a choke inductor. As a result the signal seen by the load is not hard-switched.
Similar to the Class-D amplifier, the series LC network of the Class-E amplifier only allows a sinusoidal voltage and current to pass to the load. The Class-E amplifier also includes a capacitor C_1 across the transistor terminals and forms a key component of the circuit's high efficiency operation at high frequencies as well as absorbing C_{ds}. The amplifier's high efficiency operation lies in the shape of the voltage across C_1. Circuit elements are chosen such that the voltage at this point is zero when the transistor is switched on such that no stored energy is dissipated from the capacitor. The voltage is shaped such that the rate of change of voltage (dv_{C1}/dt) across this point is also zero. This feature enables robustness to phase or frequency irregularities in practice.

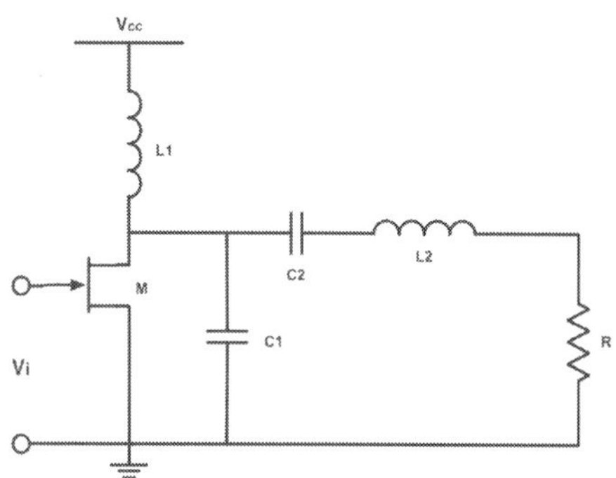

Fig. 5. The Class-E amplifier

Since the amplifier's introduction several analyses have been presented to enhance the design processes of the Class-E amplifier such that it includes more practical considerations. One of the original assumptions of the Class-E amplifier design process was that it has an infinitely loaded quality factor (Q). Kazimierczuk et al. presented a design procedure in which the amplifier can be designed at a specific Q and switch duty cycle (Kazimierczuk and Puczko, 1987). Suetsugu et al. presented a design procedure to handle off-nominal operation where the voltage across C_1 is zero but its derivative is not, concluding that a higher C_1 capacitance is required for such conditions (Suetsugu and Kazimierczuk, 2006).

The Class-E amplifier has been applied to a number of applications, however its relevance to biomedical engineering came to light with Troyk et al.'s proposal to use the Class-E amplifier as a transmitter to transfer inductive power and data for micro implants, with L_2 representing the primary inductive coil (Troyk and Schwan, 1992).

A number of design procedures have been presented in literature, however it is interesting to consider the amplifier in the frequency domain. Given that L_1 is considered to be large, the transfer function for the output voltage (across R) is given by (1). This transfer function is a second order system, which implies that it has a resonant frequency ω, damping factor ζ and Q factor, indicated in (2)-(4).

$$\frac{V_{out}(s)}{V_{in}(s)} = \frac{g_m R C_2}{s^2 L_2 C_1 C_2 + sRC_1 C_2 + C_1 + C_2} \tag{1}$$

$$\omega = \frac{1}{\sqrt{L_2 C_1 \,||\, C_2}} \tag{2}$$

$$\zeta = \frac{R}{2}\sqrt{\frac{C_1 \,||\, C_2}{L_2}} \tag{3}$$

$$Q = \frac{1}{2\zeta} \tag{4}$$

If a Class-E amplifier design was to be conducted for a practical application where the inductive coil's properties (L_2) are known as is the load R and resonant frequency ω, equations (2)-(4) can be re-arranged to select the unknown parameters. Combining (2) and (3) gives (5) and (6).

$$\zeta = \frac{R}{2\omega L_2} \tag{5}$$

$$C_1 \,||\, C_2 = \frac{2\zeta}{R\omega} \tag{6}$$

Where:

$$C_1 \,||\, C_2 = \frac{C_1 C_2}{C_1 + C_2} \tag{7}$$

The damping factor ζ (and therefore Q) is determined in the first step by substituting the known values of R, L_2 and ω into (5). This essentially implies that the quality factor of the amplifier is highly dependant on the coil inductor's quality factor. The ζ value is then used in (6), along with R and ω, which determines the capacitor combination $C_1 \,||\, C_2$.

Determining the individual capacitor values C_1 and C_2 is the more complicated step and requires care, given that the voltage between the two capacitors is vital to the circuit's Class-E operation. Generally speaking, if C_1 is smaller than C_2, charge across C_1 is dissipated quickly into C_2 prior to the transistor's next half-cycle switch. This implies that the voltage and voltage derivative of the capacitor junction is zero during switching.

6. Oscillators

Power amplifiers require square-wave clock signal inputs, so while they are known to operate efficiently at high frequencies they require a high frequency square-wave input in order to operate effectively, which is often not included in the determination of the efficiency of the amplifiers. These input signals are produced by oscillator circuits.
Oscillators are frequently used to generate high frequency signals, using resonant elements and a form of feedback. The Colpitts oscillator is a popular oscillator topology, which involves an LC network with feedback to a transistor. Other oscillators use crystals as the resonant feedback network rather than inductors and capacitors.
The idea of feeding an oscillated output signal back to the input of the amplifier implies that the circuit becomes self-oscillating- similar to the Colpitts oscillator- while operating with zero switching conditions. This is the concept behind the Class-E Oscillator shown in Figure 6 (Ebert and Kazimierczuk, 1981).

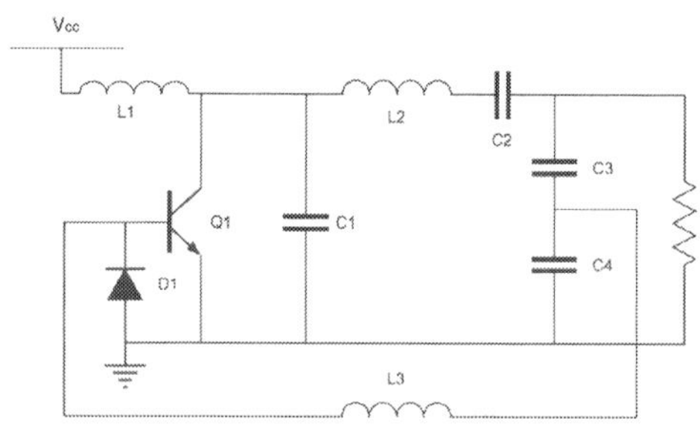

Fig. 6. Class-E Oscillator (Ebert and Kazimierczuk, 1981).

Additional circuit elements are added to form the Class-E oscillator, namely feedback elements C_3, C_4 and L_3. It was designed by Ebert et al. to constructively shift the phase of the feedback point of the oscillator. The diode D_1 is placed at the input of the transistor in order to clip the input signal such that it appears as a square wave, satisfying the requirement of the Class-E circuit to have a square-wave input.
Given that low power consumption is advantageous in biomedical systems, it is useful to consider a self-oscillating Class-E oscillator as a wireless power transmitter rather than a Class-E power amplifier. Similar to the power amplifier, the oscillator would transmit energy through L_2. This idea is currently being explored.

7. Wireless power links

The next module of an implanted telemetry system is the wireless power link. As previously mentioned, inductive power transfer has been the most popular means to transfer power wirelessly to implants. Inductive power transfer may be understood by considering two inductive coils L_1 and L_2 shown as the power transmission coils in Figure 2. A time-varying current i_1 in L_1 produces a linearly proportional magnetic flux, which passes through L_2 inducing an e.m.f. v_2 in that coil as shown in (8). The symbol M is a combination of the magnetic flux flowing between the two inductors and proportional to the number of turns in L_1 and L_2, and is referred to as the mutual inductance between the coils. A pair of inductors is considered to be strongly coupled if the mutual inductance between them is high in comparison to the respective inductances, as shown in (9), where k is referred to as the coupling coefficient.

$$v_2(t) = M\frac{di_1(t)}{dt} \tag{8}$$

$$k = \frac{M}{\sqrt{L_1 L_2}} \tag{9}$$

In the application of inductively powering implantable medical devices, one inductor of the power transmitter circuit forms the primary coil, and a receiving inductor implanted in the body forms the secondary coil. This essentially describes a weakly coupled transformer, the core of which is a combination of air and the layers of human tissue that exist between the two coils (Schuylenbergh and Puers, 2009). Typical coupling coefficients for power transfer in air are 0.17 (Ghovanloo and Atluri, 2007).

It is more efficient to transmit wireless power at lower frequencies (Vaillancourt et al., 1997), and as the complexity of implants increases, data rates are also required to increase. Wang et al. proposed the advantages of biomedical implants operating in dual frequency bands to send power and data, and it has since been the basis of further work in the area (Wang et al., 2006).

Transmission coils are an obvious point of focus, as their design holds the key to how well power is transmitted from the external device and received by the implant. Many biomedical implants employ traditional wire-wound cylindrical inductors for the power transmitting and receiving coils. In some scenarios such as retinal prosthesis wire-wound coils are preferred. Best results are usually obtained with the use of Litz wire, which reduces eddy currents caused by the skin-effect (Yang et al., 2007).

In situations such as pre-clinical monitoring, the issues related to wireless power transfer for implanted devices become more difficult to manage, mainly due to random movement by the subject of the implant. A common pre-clinical scenario involves an enclosure in which the subject is free to move. Zimmerman et al. (Zimmerman et al., 2006) investigated the optimisation of wireless power transfer in such a situation, monitoring the overall transfer efficiency by varying transmission frequency and the number of turns on the secondary coil, which was a distance of 1cm from the primary coil. The system produced 3V at 1.3mA in the implant itself, accounting for a tilting angle of 600. The primary coil was a cylindrical wire-wound coil, wrapped around the circumference of the base of the enclosure.

Zeirhofer et al. (Zierhofer and Hochmair, 1996) investigated the enhancement of magnetic coupling between coils using a geometric approach. It was concluded that coupling is enhanced when turns of the coil are distributed across the radii rather than concentrating them at the outer radius of the inductors. A number of subsequent papers have been presented analysing and using planar spiral coils for implantable applications (Harrison,

2007, Jow and Ghovanloo, 2010, Silay et al., 2008, Simons et al., 2004). The theory used to design planar spiral coils is quite involved, with most designers opting for simplified and sometimes empirically derived equations such as (10), where L is the inductance calculated by the surface area A of a square spiral and the number of turns n within the area (Liao, 1987, Wadell, 1991).

$$L = 8.5\sqrt{A}n^{5/3} \tag{10}$$

Work is being implemented in the use of stacked spiral coils for use in implantable devices. Stacking spiral coils together allows the advantages of spiral shapes to be combined with space efficiency. An increase in coil capacitance also reduces the self-resonant frequency of these coils making them compact and optimised for lower frequency transmission, which is advantageous for the inductive transfer of power (Laskovski et al., 2009).

8. Data carrier generation

Implantable biomedical telemetry schemes are moving towards a dual-band approach, meaning that power and data are sent at different frequencies, power at a lower frequency and data at a higher frequency. There are several methods used to generate data carrier frequencies for implantable devices.

Many systems involve the generation of data carrier signals on the external side of the system, leaving only the data recovery, modulation and transmission to the implantable circuitry (Mandal and Sarpeshkar, 2008, Zhou et al., 2006). Ziaie et al. presented a dual band implantable neuromuscular stimulator, the 2MHz data clock of which is recovered from 2MHz power supply (Ziaie et al., 1997), while Wise et al. operated at 4MHz (Wise et al., 2004) as did Sauer et al.'s (Sauer et al., 2005). Generating data carrier signals external to the implanted device allows for the reduction of device complexity and power consumption, however such a system requires a synchronised send/receive protocol as well as an accurate data recovery block.

The other option popularly used is to generate a data carrier frequency from within the implantable device itself. Kocer et al. presented an on-chip LC oscillator for general non-implantable non-medical telemetry, and other options for implantable devices involve ring oscillators (Ghovanloo and Najafi, 2004).

One idea currently being developed for implantable involves the generation of a data carrier signal within the implant. However, this signal is generated without the use of a dedicated oscillator block. It is generated by using an inverter to turn the incoming power signal into a non-sinusoidal square-wave signal in order to generate harmonics. One of these harmonics is then filtered and used to transmit data (Laskovski and Yuce, 2008).

9. Modulation techniques

The majority of modulation techniques used to encode biological signals are digital in that the signals are digitised within the implants. Some common forms of modulation include Frequency Shift Keying (FSK), Load Shift Keying (LSK), Amplitude Shift Keying (ASK), Phase Shift Keying (PSK).

FSK involves allocating different frequencies for different bit values. For example, binary FSK translates to bit `0' transmitting at a frequency $f_1$ and bit `1' transmitting at a different frequency f_2. Modulating a signal using FSK involves a switch and the generation of two different carrier frequencies, and bits are usually decoded by bandpass filters (Ghovanloo and Najafi, 2004).

Impedance modulation or LSK involves altering a load in the transmitting circuit according to digital information. Since it usually involves switching one part of the load on and off, the frequency of transmission is varied with each bit, making this scheme very similar to FSK. A number of medical devices make use of this scheme (Chaimanonart and Young, 2006, Mandal and Sarpeshkar, 2008, Wang et al., 2005).

Shifting a carrier frequency's phase occurs to achieve PSK. Depending on the number of symbols in the scheme, the phase shift varies. A popular PSK scheme is Binary PSK (BPSK), where a 180^0 phase shift is implemented in order to indicate a particular bit. A number of biomedical and non-biomedical telemetry systems use this scheme (Kocer and Flynn, 2006, Zhou et al., 2006)

ASK modulation is achieved by producing a different amplitude for different bits. A typical and simple example of ASK is called On-Off Keying (OOK), where bits are distinguished by either sending data at a carrier frequency to represent bit `1', or no no signal to represent bit `0'. This type of modulation is very straightforward to implement, being as simple as implementing a data controlled switch in series with an RF transmitter. It can be decoded by rectification and/or a lowpass filter (Ziaie et al., 1997). For low-power implantable circuits, OOK is a simple and space efficient method of modulation.

10. Conclusion

This chapter provided a broad background in the development of biomedical engineering, and the recent contribution of electronics to this field. The role of power amplifiers was explained in the form of three switching power amplifiers, specifically the Class-E amplifier, which included a simple design process. A new idea to use Class-E oscillators was highlighted and is being developed. Basic theory of wireless power transfer was explained and methods in data carrier generation explained. A new method of generating carrier frequencies was briefly explained, which simplifies and reduces the power use of implantable devices. The meaning behind the acronyms of major data modulation schemes were explained, with the features of each described.

11. References

BROWN, W. (1984) The History of Power Transmission by Radio Waves. *Microwave Theory and Techniques, IEEE Transactions on,* 32, 1230 - 1242.

CHAIMANONART, N. & YOUNG, D. (2006) Remote RF powering system for wireless MEMS strain sensors. *IEEE Sensors Journal,,* 6, 484-489.

CHILDRESS, D. (1985) Historical aspects of powered limb prostheses. *Clinical prosthetics and orthotics.*

EBERT, J. & KAZIMIERCZUK, M. (1981) Class E high-efficiency tuned power oscillator. *IEEE Journal of Solid-State Circuits,,* 16, 62 - 66.

EL-HAMAMSY, S.-A. (1994) Design of high-efficiency RF Class-D power amplifier. *IEEE Transactions on Power Electronics,,* 9, 297-308.

GHOVANLOO, M. & ATLURI, S. (2007) A Wide-Band Power-Efficient Inductive Wireless Link for Implantable Microelectronic Devices Using Multiple Carriers. *IEEE Transactions on Circuits and Systems I: Regular Papers,,* 54, 2211 - 2221.

GHOVANLOO, M. & NAJAFI, K. (2004) A wideband frequency-shift keying wireless link for inductively powered biomedical implants. *IEEE Transactions on Circuits and Systems I: Regular Papers,* , 51, 2374 - 2383.

GREATBATCH, W. & HOLMES, C. (1991) History of implantable devices. *IEEE Engineering in Medicine and Biology Magazine,* , 10, 38 - 41.

HARRISON, R. (2007) Designing Efficient Inductive Power Links for Implantable Devices. *IEEE International Symposium on Circuits and Systems, 2007. ISCAS 2007.* , 2080 - 2083.

HENCH, L. & POLAK, J. (2002) Third-generation biomedical materials. *Science's STKE.*

JENKINS, T. (2005) A brief history of... semiconductors. *Physics education.*

JOW, U. & GHOVANLOO, M. (2010) Optimization of Data Coils in a Multiband Wireless Link for Neuroprosthetic Implantable Devices. *IEEE Transactions on Biomedical Circuits and Systems,* , PP, 1 - 1.

KAZIMIERCZUK, M. & PUCZKO, K. (1987) Exact analysis of class E tuned power amplifier at any Q and switch duty cycle. *IEEE Transactions on Circuits and Systems,* , 34, 149 - 159.

KIRI, A., OHARA, K., TOMITA, Y., SHUKURI, S., YASUKOUCHI, T. & SUETSUGU, T. (2009) Class D and class E selectable power amplifier. *31st International Telecommunications Energy Conference, 2009. INTELEC 2009.* , 1 - 4.

KLEINROCK, L. (2008) History of the Internet and its flexible future. *IEEE Wireless Communications,* , 15, 8 - 18.

KOCER, F. & FLYNN, M. (2006) A new transponder architecture with on-chip ADC for long-range telemetry applications. *IEEE Journal of Solid-State Circuits,*, 41, 1142 - 1148.

LASKOVSKI, A. N. & YUCE, M. R. (2008) Harmonics-based bio-implantable telemetry system. *30th Annual International Conference of the IEEE Engineering in Medicine and Biology Society, 2008. EMBS 2008.* , 3196 - 3199.

LASKOVSKI, A. N., YUCE, M. R. & DISSANAYAKE, T. (2009) Stacked spirals for use in biomedical implants. *Asia Pacific Microwave Conference, 2009. APMC 2009.*, 389 - 392.

LIAO, S. Y. (1987) *Microwave Circuit Analysis and Amplifier Design,* Englewood Cliffs, NJ USA, Prentice-Hall.

LONG, M. & RACK, H. (1998) Titanium alloys in total joint replacement-a materials science perspective. *Biomaterials.*

ŁUKASIAK, L. & JAKUBOWSKI, A. History of Semiconductors. *itl.waw.pl.*

MANDAL, S. & SARPESHKAR, R. (2008) Power-Efficient Impedance-Modulation Wireless Data Links for Biomedical Implants. *IEEE Transactions on Biomedical Circuits and Systems,* , 2, 301 - 315.

RAAB (1997) Class-F power amplifiers with maximally flat waveforms. *IEEE Transactions on Microwave Theory and Techniques,* , 45, 2007 - 2012.

RAAB, F., ASBECK, P., CRIPPS, S., KENINGTON, P., POPOVIC, Z., POTHECARY, N., SEVIC, J. & SOKAL, N. (2002) Power amplifiers and transmitters for RF and microwave. *IEEE Transactions on Microwave Theory and Techniques,* , 50, 814 - 826.

RAMAKRISHNA, S., MAYER, J. & WINTERMANTEL, E. (2001) Biomedical applications of polymer-composite materials: a review. *Composites Science and ....*

REYNAERT, P. & STEYAERT, M. (2006) *RF Power Amplifiers for Mobile Communications,* P.O. Box 17, 3300 AA Dordrecht, The Netherlands, Springer.

SAUER, C., STANACEVIC, M., CAUWENBERGHS, G. & THAKOR, N. (2005) Power harvesting and telemetry in CMOS for implanted devices. *IEEE Transactions on Circuits and Systems I: Regular Papers,*, 52, 2605-2613.

SCHUYLENBERGH, K. V. & PUERS, R. (2009) *Inductive Powering. Basic Theory and Application to Biomedical Systems,* P.O. Box 17, 3300 AA Dordrecht, The Netherlands, Springer.

SELIGMAN, L. J. (1982) Physiological Stimulators: From Electric Fish to Programmable Implants. *IEEE Transactions on Biomedical Engineering,* , BME-29, 270 - 284.

SILAY, K., DEHOLLAIN, C. & DECLERCQ, M. (2008) Improvement of power efficiency of inductive links for implantable devices. *PRIME 2008. Ph.D. Research in Microelectronics and Electronics, 2008.* , 229 - 232.

SIMONS, R., HALL, D. & MIRANDA, F. (2004) Spiral chip implantable radiator and printed loop external receptor for RF telemetry in bio-sensor systems. *IEEE Radio and Wireless Conference, 2004.*

SOKAL, N. & SOKAL, A. (1975) Class E-A new class of high-efficiency tuned single-ended switching power amplifiers. *IEEE Journal of Solid-State Circuits,*, 10, 168-176.

SUETSUGU, T. & KAZIMIERCZUK, M. K. (2006) Design procedure of class-E amplifier for off-nominal operation at 50\% duty ratio. *IEEE Transactions on Circuits and Systems I: Regular Papers,* , 53, 1468 - 1476.

THURSTON, A. (2007) Pare and prosthetics: the early history of artificial limbs. *ANZ Journal of Surgery.*

TROYK, P. & SCHWAN, M. (1992) Closed-loop class E transcutaneous power and data link for MicroImplants. *IEEE Transactions on Biomedical Engineering,* 39, 589-599.

UN (2010). United Nations.

VAILLANCOURT, P., DJEMOUAI, A., HARVEY, J. & SAWAN, M. (1997) EM radiation behavior upon biological tissues in a radio-frequency power transfer link for a cortical visual implant. *Proceedings of the 19th Annual International Conference of the IEEE Engineering in Medicine and Biology Society, 1997.* .

WADELL, B. C. (1991) *Transmission Line Design Handbook,* 685 Canton Street Norwood, MA 02062 USA, Artech House.

WANG, G., LIU, W., SIVAPRAKASAM, M. & KENDIR, G. (2005) Design and analysis of an adaptive transcutaneous power telemetry for biomedical implants. *IEEE Transactions on Circuits and Systems I: Regular Papers,* , 52, 2109-2117.

WANG, G., LIU, W., SIVAPRAKASAM, M., ZHOU, M., WEILAND, J. & HUMAYUN, M. (2006) A Dual Band Wireless Power and Data Telemetry for Retinal Prosthesis. *28th Annual International Conference of the IEEE Engineering in Medicine and Biology Society, 2006. EMBS '06.* .

WISE, K., ANDERSON, D. J., HETKE, J. F., KIPKE, D. R. & NAJAFI, K. (2004) Wireless implantable microsystems: high-density electronic interfaces to the nervous system. *Proceedings of the IEEE,* 92, 76 - 97.

YANG, Z., LIU, W. & BASHAM, E. (2007) Inductor Modeling in Wireless Links for Implantable Electronics. *IEEE Transactions on Magnetics,* 43, 3851-3860.

YOUNG (2006) Analysis and experiments for high-efficiency class-F and inverse class-F power amplifiers. *IEEE Transactions on Microwave Theory and Techniques,*, 54, 1969 - 1974.

ZHOU, M., LIU, W., WANG, G., SIVAPRAKASAM, M., YUCE, M., WEILAND, J. & HUMAYUN, M. (2006) A Transcutaneous Data Telemetry System Tolerant to

Power Telemetry Interference. *28th Annual International Conference of the IEEE Engineering in Medicine and Biology Society, 2006. EMBS '06.* , 5884 - 5887.

ZIAIE, B., NARDIN, M. & COGHLAN (1997) A single-channel implantable microstimulator for functional neuromuscular stimulation. *Biomedical Engineering, IEEE Transactions on,* 44, 909 - 920.

ZIERHOFER, C. & HOCHMAIR, E. (1996) Geometric approach for coupling enhancement of magnetically coupled coils. *IEEE Transactions on Biomedical Engineering,* , 43, 708 - 714.

ZIMMERMAN, M., CHAIMANONART, N. & YOUNG, D. (2006) In Vivo RF Powering for Advanced Biological Research. *Engineering in Medicine and Biology Society, 2006. EMBS '06. 28th Annual International Conference of the IEEE.*

Part 2

Sensors and Instrumentation

9

Subthreshold Frequency Synthesis for Implantable Medical Transceivers

Tarek Khan and Kaamran Raahemifar
Ryerson University, Department of Electrical & Computer Engineering
Canada

1. Introduction

Implantable medical devices (IMDs) have evolved greatly since the first pacemaker was designed in the 1950s. The current generation of IMDs are capable of replacing damaged or malfunctioning organs, and are designed for long-term patient care. Cochlear implants, which differ greatly from hearing aids, convert received audio signals to electrical impulses and are capable of bypassing damaged parts of the ear and interfacing directly with auditory nerves. Microstimulators for neuromuscular stimulation can restore functionality to paralysed limbs. Implantable drug administration devices can deliver precise amounts of a drug, such as insulin for diabetics, at particular intervals, replacing the need for regular injections. Wireless IMDs designed for biotelemetry applications include implantable ECG and EEG recording, intra-ocular pressure sensing and wireless endoscopy capsules. In order to address the unique design requirements of wireless IMDs, namely ultra-low power consumption to extend battery life, small form factor to make the device suitable for implantation, and reliability to ensure correct operation once implanted, circuit designers must use new topologies and design techniques when conventional designs fail to address these requirements. In this work, we propose several novel circuits for an integer-N frequency synthesizer operating in the 402 MHz to 405 MHz Medical Implant Communication Service (MICS).

2. Design specifications

The designs presented in this work consist of novel circuits for an ultra-low power CMOS integer-n frequency synthesizer for use in a wireless implantable medical device operating the the 402 MHz to 405 MHz Medical Implant Communication Service spectrum. The architecture of an integer-n frequency synthesizer is shown in Fig. 1. In order to be suitable for use in an implantable device, the synthesizer should utilize as few off chip components as possible (ideally none) to achieve the required specifications and functionality, and to decrease its physical size and cost, be as insensitive as possible to process variations and temperature in order to provide accurate and stable carrier frequencies for data transmission under all conditions, and consume minimal power resulting in maximum lifetime of the device.

Frequency synthesizers and phase-locked loops have been covered extensively in literature (Gardner, 2005), (Lee, 2004), (Razavi, 2001), (Razavi, 1998), and the reader is encouraged to review those references for a thorough treatment of frequency synthesis. The main components of the frequency synthesizer are the phase/frequency detector, charge pump, loop filter, voltage-controlled oscillator and programmable frequency divider. For the

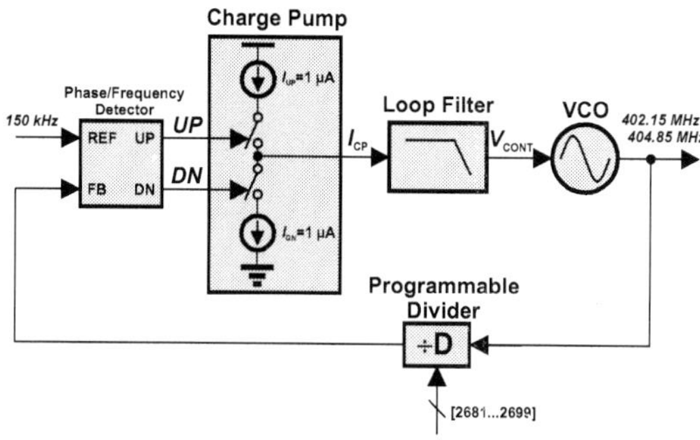

Fig. 1. Proposed integer-n frequency synthesizer.

purposes of this work, it is enough to say that frequency synthesizers generate a multitude of frequencies from a fixed reference frequency. The relationship between the output frequency and input frequency is $f_{OUT} = D \times f_{IN}$, and by changing the control word of the programmable divider, different output frequencies can be generated which satisfy this relationship. For integer-n frequency synthesizers, f_{IN} must be equal to the channel spacing.
The application for the proposed frequency synthesizer is the Medical Implant Communication Service frequency band, which was established in 1999 for use by implantable medical devices. Favourable propagation characteristics, international availability and low probability of interference are the reasons for choosing the 402 MHz to 405 MHz spectrum for the MICS band. Although there is no fixed channel arrangement for the MICS band, an MICS channel is permitted to have an emission bandwidth between 25 kHz and 300 kHz. In the proposed frequency synthesizer, we will use the maximum bandwidth of 300 kHz per channel, resulting in 10 channels (Fig. 2).
In this work, novel designs for the main components of the integer-n frequency are proposed to address the design constraints of implantable medical devices. The proposed designs are implemented using a 130 nm CMOS process from IBM and simulated using Cadence Spectre circuit simulator.

3. The proposed current-reuse quadrature voltage-controlled oscillator

Since the first quadrature LC-tank VCO was proposed (Rofougaran et al., 1996), a number of modified topologies have been presented which improve RF performance metrics such as phase noise and quadrature accuracy. These include the disconnected-source QVCO (DS-QVCO) (Mazzanti et al., 2006), the series QVCO (SQVCO) (Chamas & Raman, 2007b), the phase-tunable QVCO (PT-QVCO) (Chamas & Raman, 2007a), and the transformer-coupled

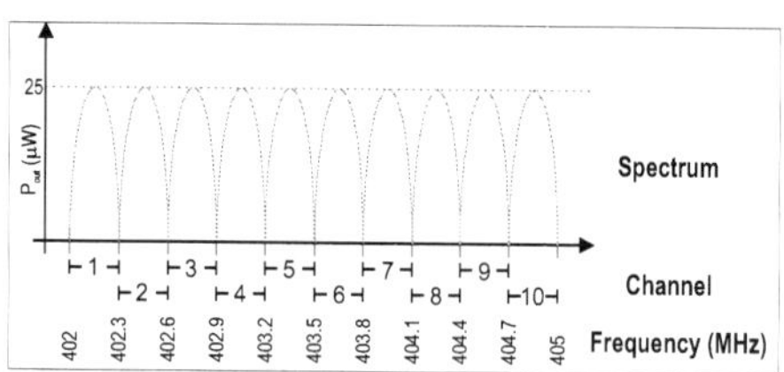

Fig. 2. Allocated frequency spectrum for Medical Implant Communication Service.

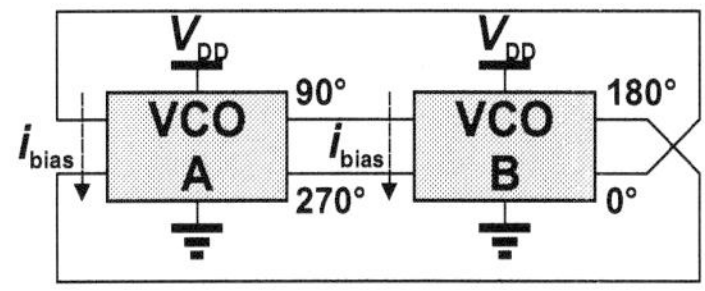

(a) Conventional QVCO.

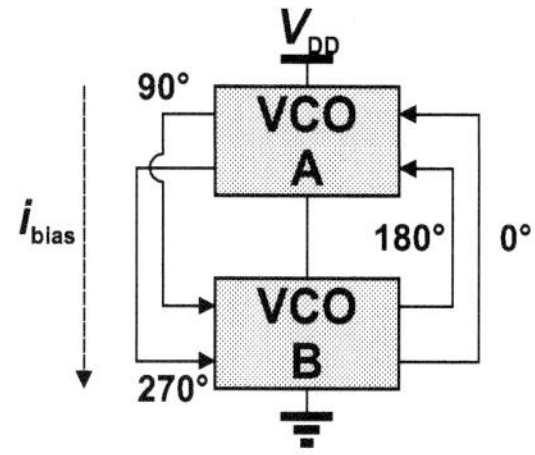

(b) Proposed QVCO with current-reuse.

Fig. 3. Quadrature VCO block diagram.

QVCO (TC-QVCO) (Ng & Luong, 2007). However there have not been many attempts to reduce the power consumption of the QVCO. In order to make the *LC* QVCO a viable choice for ultra-low power applications, such as implantable medical devices, we propose a novel QVCO topology utilizing three design principals to lower the power consumption: current-reuse, supply voltage scaling and weak inversion operation.

3.1 Circuit design

Existing QVCO topologies consume significant amounts of power, making them unsuitable for ultra-low power applications such as IMDs. Increasing the quality factor of the tank to achieve high oscillation amplitude for small bias currents has it's limits, since the quality factor of inductors in CMOS processes is typically between 10 to 20. Therefore, it is necessary to explore other means to reduce power consumption of the QVCO. One of the salient properties of the QVCO is that its power consumption is double that of the standard *LC* VCO, as shown in Fig. 3(a). When stacking two different circuits, the performance of one circuit may be compromised because it may have better performance when biased independently. However in the QVCO both oscillator cores are ideally identical, thus current reuse is viable and will provide a 50% improvement in power consumption. The conceptual QVCO with current-reuse (CR-QVCO) is shown in Fig. 3(b), where two coupled *LC* tank oscillators are stacked between the supply rails.

The circuit implementation of the CR-QVCO is shown in Fig. 4. In this topology, the oscillator nodes for both cores are at the same DC level (ignoring the losses across the inductors), eliminating the need for DC level shifting of the coupling transistor inputs and the use of a frequency tuning circuit for the varactors. The capacitor, C_{GND}, at the intermediate node provides AC ground for both oscillators, and allows the cores to be decoupled for analytical purposes. An expression for the QVCO oscillation amplitude was given in (Andreani et al., 2002), however the equation requires modification due to the loading effect of the coupling transistors (Rofougaran et al., 1998) and the use of a differential spiral inductor:

$$\hat{V}_0 = \frac{1}{\sqrt{2}\pi}(1-\delta)I_{bias}R_p. \tag{1}$$

When the CR-QVCO is to be designed for weak inversion (subthreshold) operation the supply voltage can be approximated as

$$V_{DD} = V_{thn} + \left|V_{thp}\right| + V_{DSAT}, \tag{2}$$

where V_{thn} and V_{thp} are the threshold voltages of the NMOS and PMOS transistors respectively, and V_{DSAT} is the saturation voltage of the current source transistor. Since the transistors are biased in the subthreshold region, the supply voltage can be lower than this value because the DC bias points of the switching transistors will be less than $V_{thn,p}$.

To reduce the current drawn by the CR-QVCO, an inductor with high inductance and quality factor was used. The inductors provided with the PDK did not provide high quality factors at low frequencies (> 1 GHz), which required the use of a custom spiral inductor. Cadence Virtuoso Passive Component Designer was used to synthesize a symmetrical octagonal inductor with high inductance and quality factor at the center frequency of the MICS band. The inductor was formed over an M1 groundplane to decrease substrate coupling and raise the quality factor (Yue & Wong, 1998). The layout of the synthesized inductor and its simulated inductance and quality factor are shown in Fig. 5.

The bias current was provided using the PMOS transistor. The upconversion of flicker noise generated by the current source transistor is a known contributor to the phase noise of the oscillator. To combat this effect, the PMOS bias current transistor was sized to have long channel length and width as flicker noise is inversely proportional to the area of the active device. NMOS varactors were used as the frequency tuning element in the tank, and a fixed metal-insulator-metal (MIM) capacitor was used to set the tuning range around the frequency band of interest. Existing CR-QVCOs require the use of a frequency tuning circuit that accounted for the different DC voltages between the differential output nodes, which resulted in different voltage drops across the varactors in each tank. By designing the CR-QVCO such that the top tank is PMOS only and the bottom tank is NMOS only, a frequency tuning circuit was not necessary as the DC voltage of the quadrature outputs was the same. A small DC offset can be attributed to series resistance of the inductors. Omitting the frequency tuning circuit also improves the phase noise as the thermal noise generated by biasing resistors is not present.

3.2 Results

Voltage-controlled oscillators are subjected to variations due to process, supply voltage and temperature which cause the oscillation frequency to drift from the nominal value. In order to ensure the CR-QVCO can operate on across the MICS frequency band, simulations were

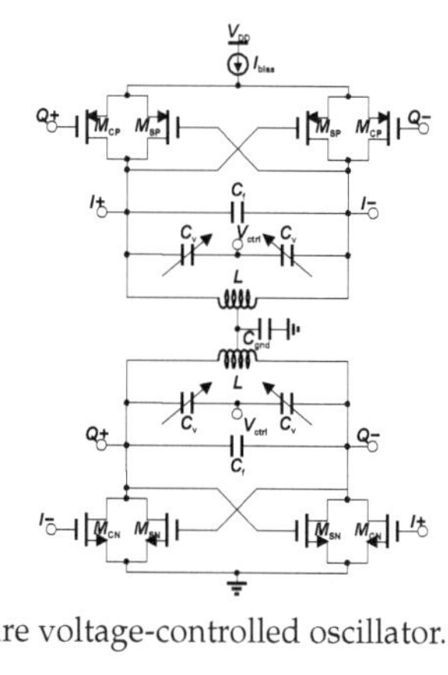

Fig. 4. Current-reuse quadrature voltage-controlled oscillator.

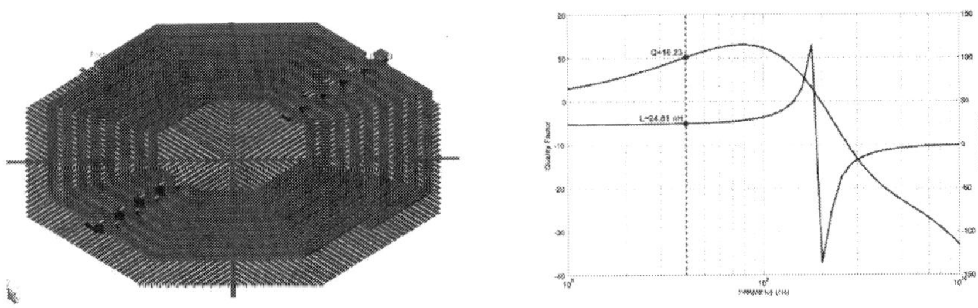

(a) Three dimensional view. (b) Simulated inductance and quality factor

Fig. 5. Synthesized spiral inductor for current-reuse quadrature VCO.

performed to verify its oscillation frequency. The results of corner analysis and supply voltage sensitivity are shown in Fig. 6 and Fig. 7 respectively (biasing adjusted for each simulation to achieve same oscillation amplitude).

As per the requirements of the MICS frequency band, the IMD must be tested over temperature variations from 0° C to 55° C (Federal Communications Commission, 1999).

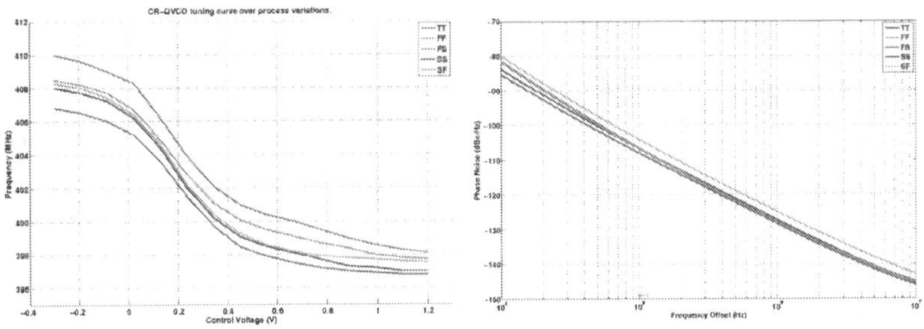

(a) Tuning range. (b) Phase noise.

Fig. 6. CR-QVCO simulated over process variations.

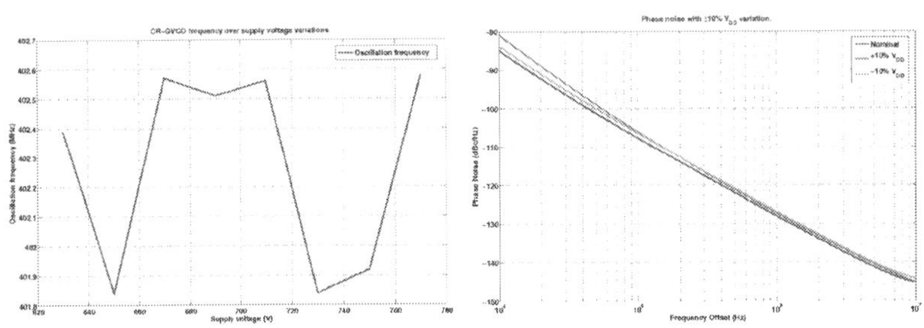

(a) Free-running frequency. (b) Phase noise.

Fig. 7. CR-QVCO simulated over $\pm$ 10% supply voltage variations.

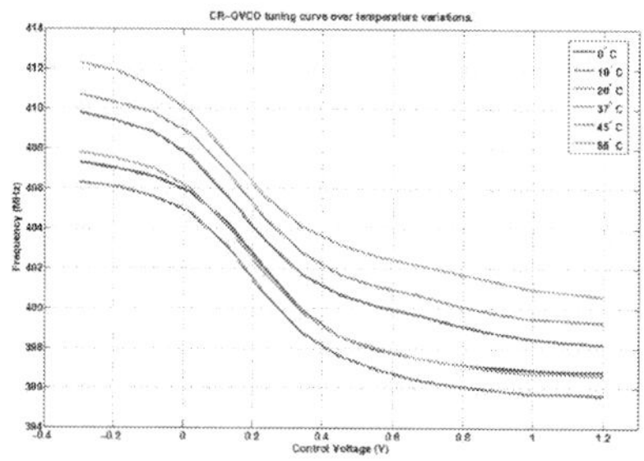

(a) Tuning range.

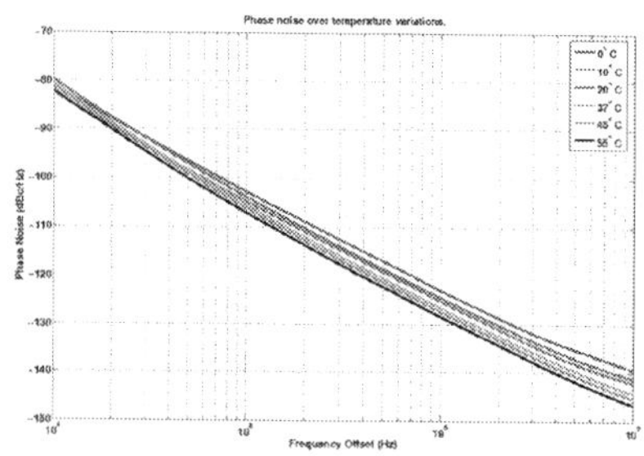

(b) Phase noise.

Fig. 8. CR-QVCO simulated over temperature variations.

Although the proposed work is not a complete IMD, the CR-QVCO performance at different temperatures in the required range was simulated to ensure the operating frequency and phase noise do not degrade significantly. The graphs in Fig. 8 show the tuning curves and phase noise plots for simulations at 0° C, 10° C, 20° C, 37° C, 45° C and 55° C.
The CR-QVCO consumed 600 μW from a 0.7 V supply, and the phase noise was -127.2 dBc/Hz. The simulation results of the proposed CR-QVCO were compared with existing VCOs designed to operate in the MICS band, and are summarized in Table 1.
As shown in the comparison results, the proposed CR-QVCO demonstrates improved power consumption and phase noise performance. Although both (Bae et al., 2009) and (Ryu et al., 2007) have lower power consumption, it is important to note that these designs do not produce quadrature signals. If the VCOs in these works were used to implement a PQVCO to produce quadrature signals, the power consumption would at least double. Furthermore the VCOs use off-chip inductors with high Q values. Although off-chip inductors are a valid method

Reference (Technology)	Tuning Range [MHz]	V_{DD} [V]	Power [mW]	Phase Noise [dBc/Hz]	Topology
This work (0.13 μm)	**398 to 410**	**0.7**	**0.42**	**-127.2 @ 1 MHz**	**Current-reuse quadrature oscillator**
(Carrara et al., 2009) (0.13 μm)	401 to 406	1.2	0.72	-96 @ 1 MHz	LC tank VCO
(Tekin, Yuce, Shabani & Liu, 2006) (TSMC 0.18 μm)	—	1.5	1.11	—	Differential ring VCO
(Liu et al., 2009) (TSMC 0.18 μm)	402	1.3	0.78	—	6-bit digitally controlled oscillator
(Bae et al., 2009) (0.18 μm)	398 to 408	0.7	0.21	-118 @ 1 MHz	7-bit digitally controlled oscillator
(Bohorquez et al., 2009) (0.09 μm)	391 to 415	0.7	0.46	-108 @ 100 kHz	Digitally controlled oscillator
(Liu et al., 2006) (TSMC 0.18 μm)	—	1.5	—	—	Dual band LC tank VCO
(Tekin, Yuce & Liu, 2006) (TSMC 0.18 μm)	—	1.5	1.2	-98 @ 160 kHz	LC tank VCO
(Li et al., 2009) (0.13 μm)	380 to 440	1.2	1.2	-107 @ 100 kHz	Injection-locked oscillator
(Ryu et al., 2007) (0.18 μm)	440	1.5	0.231	-103 @ 100 kHz	Single-ended cross-coupled oscillator

Table 1. Comparision of existing MICS VCOs

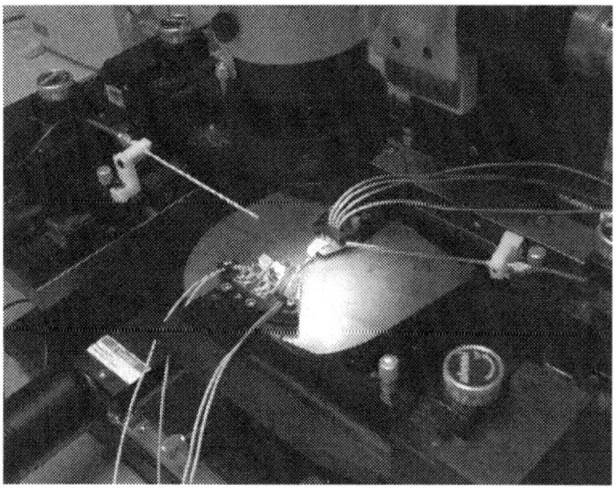

Fig. 9. Wafer probe station

of reducing power consumption, their use violates one of the objectives of this work in this thesis which is to eliminate the need for off-chip components to lower the size and cost of the frequency synthesizer.

The proposed CR-QVCO was fabricated using a 130 nm CMOS process from IBM through MOSIS Integrated Fabrication Service to provide validation of the design beyond simulation results. Testing of the integrated circuit was performed using wafer probing on a Cascade Microtech IC probe station. Each of the four positioners on the probe station is capable of holding a different set of probes for applying and measuring signals to and from the device under test. The available probe configurations were Ground-Signal-Ground (GSG) operating at up to 40 GHz, Signal-Ground-Signal-Signal-Ground-Signal (SGSSGS) "wedge" operating up to 100 MHz, and a DC needle. The wafer probe station and probe pad configuration diagrams are shown in Fig. 9 and Fig. 10 respectively. The square probe pads have side lengths of 100 μm and a pitch of 150 μm.

The CR-QVCO had four RF outputs (I+, I-, Q+, Q-) and four DC bias voltages (core V_{DD}, V_{cont}, V_{bias}, and buffer V_{DD}). To implement the required input and output configuration four sets of probe pads for the GSG probes were used (only two could be probed at a time), a DC needle was used for the output buffer supply voltage and the SGSSGS wedge was used for

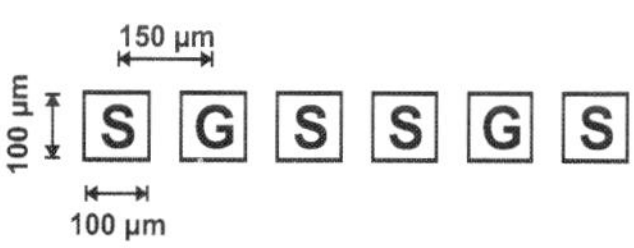

(a) SGSSGS

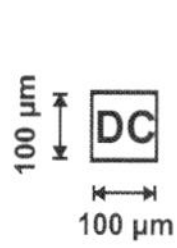

(b) DC needle

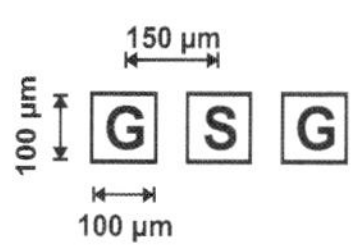

(c) GSG

Fig. 10. Probe configurations

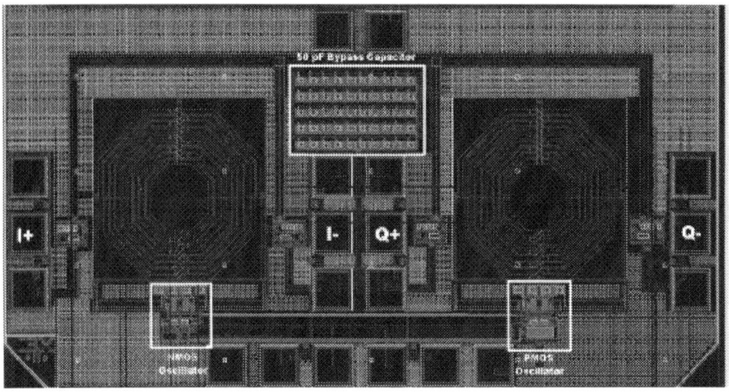

(a) CR-QVCO layout.

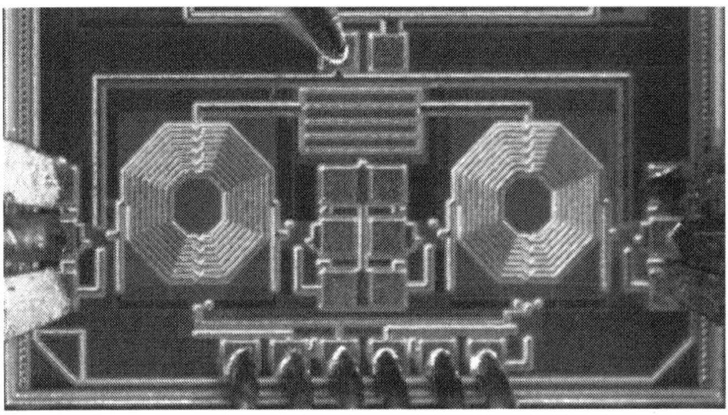

(b) CR-QVCO die photo.

Fig. 11. Physical implementation of current-reuse quadrature VCO.

the remaining DC signals. The layout and die photo of the CR-QVCO are shown in Fig. 11. The total silicon area occupied by the CR-QVCO including bond pads was 2 mm $\times$ 1 mm. Measurement results were obtained using an Agilent 4407B spectrum analyser, and power and bias voltages were provided using two high precision DC sources. The measured output spectrum and control voltage are shown in Fig. 12. The tuning curve was obtained by adjusting the control voltage across the desired range and observing the change in the output spectrum. It can be observed that although the frequency range of the MICS is covered, the total tuning range is narrower than the desired range due to parasitics and other variations in the fabrication process such as increased capacitance density of the MIM capacitors or smaller tuning range of the varactors.

4. The proposed source-coupled logic clear/preset D-latch

D-type latches and flip-flops are important components of the frequency synthesizer. The conventional phase/frequency detector, which consists of two resettable D flip-flops and an

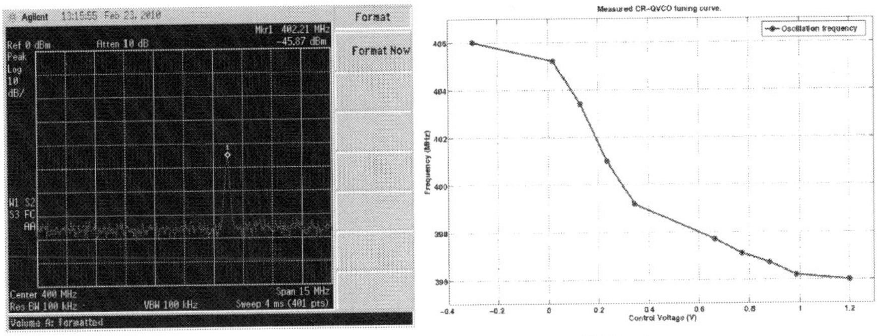

(a) Output spectrum.

(b) Tuning range.

Fig. 12. Measurement results of CR-QVCO.

AND gate, has its UP and DN outputs cleared when $UP \cdot DN = 1$. The Pulse and Swallow counters in the programmable frequency divider are programmed to their initial value by clearing and presetting the D flip-flops, each corresponding to a bit in the control word. Previously proposed low power programmable frequency dividers and phase/frequency detectors were implemented using true single-phase clocked (TSPC) logic (Lee et al., 1999), (Kuo & Wu, 2006), (Kuo & Weng, 2009), (Lei et al., 2009). Although TSPC logic occupies small silicon area, it suffers from drawbacks such as generation of switching noise, charge leakage at low frequencies, and requires rail-to-rail input signal swing (Luong, 2004). These drawbacks can be avoided by using source-coupled logic (SCL) at the expense of increased silicon area. Additionally these implementations were designed for saturation region operation and therefore their power consumption is high relatively compared to ultra-low power requirements. These reasons provide the motivation for choosing the SCL logic family for implementing the programmable frequency divider and phase/frequency detector.

Existing SCL latches presented in literature are not suitable for applications such as implantable medical devices because they required too many stacked transistors (Cong et al., 2001), (Desikachari et al., 2007) or do not perform both clear and preset functions (Cheng & Silva-Martinez, 2004), (Dai et al., 2004). To this end, we present a SCL D latch with clear and preset capability which is suitable for low power, low voltage applications.

4.1 Circuit design

The proposed D-latch is shown in Fig. 13. It consists of two stages and requires an additional input to enable the clear and preset circuit. The first stage is a latch where the sensing pair $(M1, M2)$ is active while CLK is high and the latching pair $(M3, M4)$ is active while CLK is low. Instead of cross coupling the outputs of the sensing pair via the latching pair as in a conventional SCL D-latch, the intermediate outputs $(X, \overline{X})$ are routed to the second stage. Devices $M5, M6$ act as a buffer when EN is low, and the outputs are fed back to the latching pair. When EN is high, the Set/Reset latch $(M7, M8)$ is active and the latch is initialized according to the state of CLR and PRE. The complementary enable signals can be generated by

$$EN = CLR \oplus PRE, \tag{3a}$$

$$\overline{EN} = \overline{CLR \oplus PRE}. \tag{3b}$$

This comes at the cost of an additional XOR/XNOR gate, since SCL gates produce complementary outputs. However in this application EN can be obtained from the $RELOAD$ signal generated by the pulse counter in the programmable frequency divider or by the AND gate output in the phase/frequency detector, eliminating the need for the additional logic gate. The clear/preset circuit in the D-latch avoids the $S = R = 1$ state since when CLR and PRE are both high, EN is low and the D-latch continues to operate normally.

In (Tajalli et al., 2008), the authors demonstrated that a high resistance load device can be obtained by shorting the bulk of a minimum sized PMOS transistor to its drain, reducing the amount of bias current required to achieve an output voltage sufficient to drive subsequent gates. By exploiting this result in the design of the proposed clear/preset D-latch, the power consumption can be significantly reduced when compared with conventional SCL logic.

4.2 Results

The proposed D-latch was simulated along with an ideal D-latch written in Verilog-A to verify that the proposed design produces the correct output. The latch was simulated for two cases to verify that it can operate over the required frequency range. In Fig. 14(a), the frequency of the data and clock inputs are 250 kHz and 120 kHz respectively, and in Fig. 14(b) they are 20 MHz and 15 MHz respectively.

To demonstrate the clear and preset functionality, the proposed D-latch was connected in a master-slave D flip-flop divide-by-two configuration and alternating PRE and CLR signals were applied every 20 ns. As shown in Fig. 15 the output signal (V_{CLKOUT}) is pulled high when V_{PRE} is applied, and pulled low when V_{CLR} is applied.

5. A subthreshold source-coupled logic pulse/swallow programmable divider

The pulse-swallow frequency division architecture shown in Fig. 16 is used in the proposed design. It consists of a dual-modulus prescaler and two programmable counters, referred to as the Pulse counter and Swallow counter. The DMP divides by M when MC is logic 0 and by $M + 1$ when MC is logic 1, and the programmable counters are initialized by N-bit control words and count down from that value, then reload from zero to the value of the control

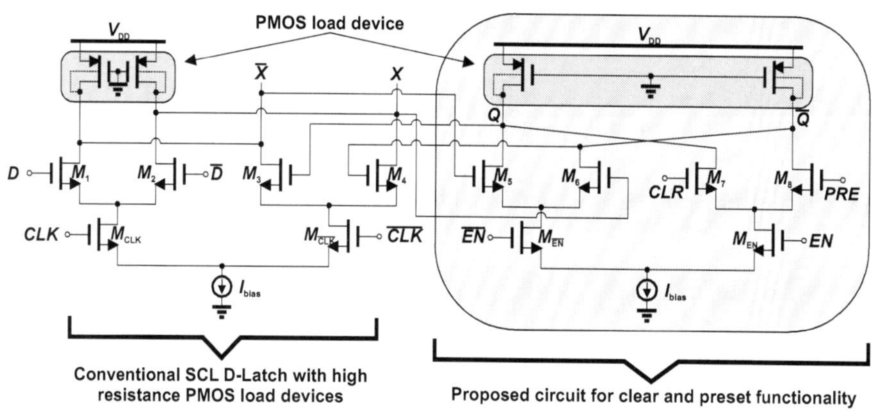

Fig. 13. Proposed D-latch with clear and preset.

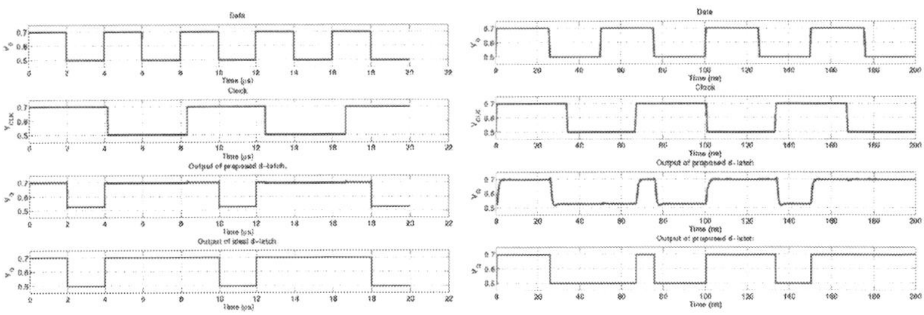

(a) D=250 kHz, CLK=120 kHz. (b) D=20 MHz, CLK=15 MHz.

Fig. 14. Transient simulation of proposed D-latch and ideal D-latch.

word. The programmable divider operates as follows: When a CLK_{OUT} pulse is generated by the Pulse counter, both counters reload to their initial states and the MC signal goes high. The initial states are determined by the S and P control words. The DMP divides CLK_{IN} by $(M+1)$ until the swallow counter has counted down to 0. The Swallow counter generates a CLK_{OUT} pulse which changes the MC to low and the DMP divides CLK_{IN} by M until the Pulse counter has counted down to 0. The Pulse counter generates a CLK_{OUT} pulse and the process repeats. Since the DMP divides by $(M+1)$ S times and by M $(P-S)$ times, the division ratio, D, of the programmable divider is given by

$$D = (M+1)S + (P-S)M, \tag{4}$$

$$= MP + S. \tag{5}$$

5.1 Circuit design

The synthesizer must be able to operate on one of the 10 channels in the 402 MHz to 405 MHz spectrum, with each channel spaced 300 kHz apart. Intuitively one would design the divider so that the output frequency is the center frequency of the ith channel,

$$f_{OUT} = 402.15 \text{ MHz} + \text{(i-1)}300 \text{ kHz}. \tag{6}$$

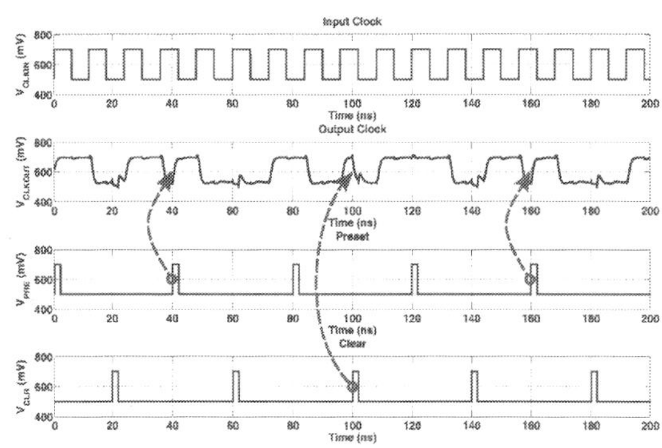

Fig. 15. Simulation of D-flip flop with clear and preset.

Channel #	f_{out}	D
1	402.15 MHz	2681
2	402.45 MHz	2683
3	402.75 MHz	2685
4	403.05 MHz	2687
5	403.35 MHz	2689
6	403.65 MHz	2691
7	403.95 MHz	2693
8	404.25 MHz	2695
9	404.55 MHz	2697
10	404.85 MHz	2699

Table 2. Division ratios for integer-n frequency synthesizer with 150 kHz reference frequency.

However, the corresponding divider moduli calculated by $D = \frac{f_{OUT}}{f_{IN}}$ and $f_{IN} = 300$ kHz result in non-integer values. Integer value of the division ratio by changing the synthesizer reference frequency from 300 kHz to 150 kHz. Table 2 summarizes the required division ratios for the integer-n frequency synthesizer.

Now that an integer value of D has been obtained, the dual-modulus divider, pulse counter and swallow counter values must be obtained to satisfy (5). By using a divide-by-32/33 dual-modulus divider (M=32), the values of the pulse (P) and swallow (S) counters can be obtained by assuming a value for P and solving for the range of values for S. If we assume P=83,

$$
\begin{aligned}
S &= D - MP && (7)\\
&= 2699 - (32)(83) && (8)\\
&= 2699 - 2656 && (9)\\
&= 43, && (10)
\end{aligned}
$$

and so on for the remaining values of D. Using these values, the range of S is [25, 27, ... 43], therefore the P counter must be 7-bits and the S counter can be a 6-bit counter. The pulse counter has a fixed modulus and its control bits can be set on-chip, but the swallow counter must be programmable – either off-chip or by separate control logic. Consider the control word $S[5:0] = S_5S_4S_3S_2S_1S_0$, the control bits are assigned as shown in Table 3.

By analysing the truth table of Fig. 3 we can observe that $S_5 = \overline{S_4}$ and $S_0 = 1$. The number of inputs for the Swallow counter can be reduced to four by inverting S_5 to obtain S_4 and forcing

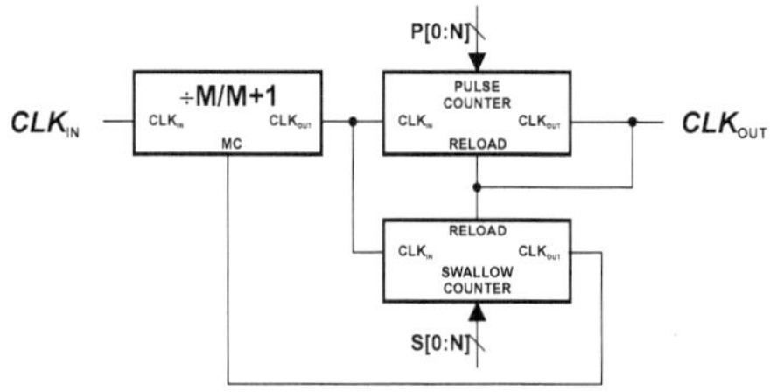

Fig. 16. Block diagram of programmable frequency divider.

Decimal	S_5	S_4	S_3	S_2	S_1	S_0	Division Ratio
25	0	1	1	0	0	1	2681
27	0	1	1	0	1	1	2683
29	0	1	1	1	0	1	2685
31	0	1	1	1	1	1	2687
33	1	0	0	0	0	1	2689
35	1	0	0	0	1	1	2691
37	1	0	0	1	0	1	2693
39	1	0	0	1	1	1	2695
41	1	0	1	0	0	1	2697
43	1	0	1	0	1	1	2699

Table 3. Control bits for the swallow counter.

the state of S_0 to a logic 1. The gate-level diagrams of the 7-bit pulse counter, the 6-bit swallow counter and divide-by-32/33 DMP are shown below.

5.2 Results

The divide-by-32/33 dual modulus prescaler in Fig. 18 was implemented Using subthreshold source-coupled logic gates. Since clear and preset functionality were not needed for the DMP, the conventional SCL D-latch was used, and the load resistors were replaced with the PMOS load device proposed in (Tajalli et al., 2008). The divide-by-32 and divide-by-33 operations were simulated using a 990 MHz input signal, and the results are shown in Fig. 19. As shown in the figure the divider output frequency is 30.9375 MHz when dividing by 32, and 30 MHz when dividing by 33.

Transient simulations of the 6-bit and 7-bit programmable counters were performed to verify the desired behaviour of the down counters. Since clear and preset functionality were necessary for correct operation of the programmable counters, the D-latch proposed in Section 4was used. The control word for the 6-bit counter was set to $S[5:0] = S_5S_4S_3S_2S_1S_0 = 011001$, corresponding to a count-down starting from 25. In Fig. 20 the input frequency was 12 MHz and an output pulse was produced from the counter every 25 pulses, resulting in an output frequency of 480 kHz. For the 7-bit counter the control word was $P[6:0] = P_6P_5P_4P_3P_2P_1P_0 =$

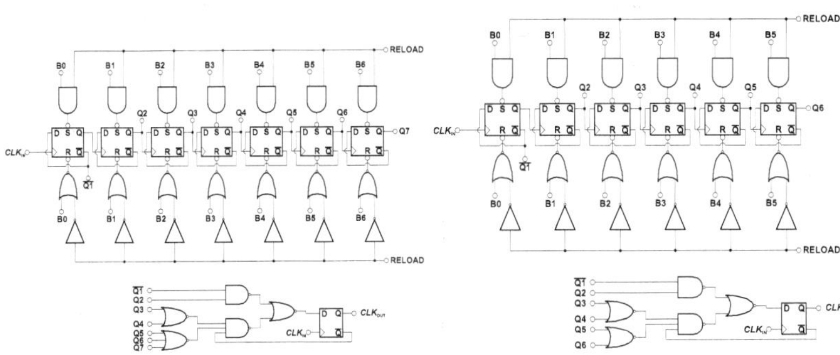

(a) Pulse counter. (b) Swallow counter.

Fig. 17. Block diagram of programmable counters.

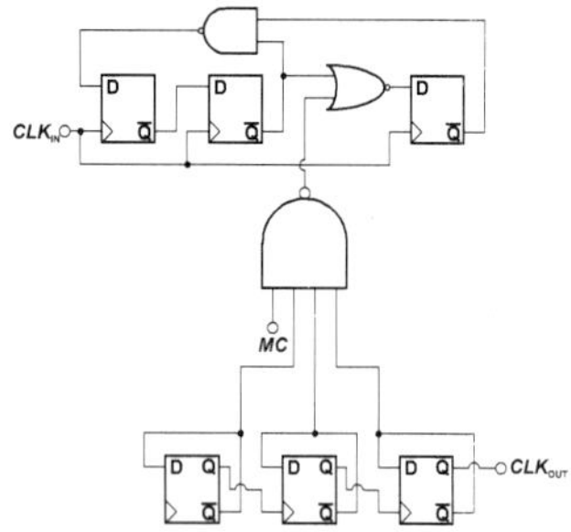

Fig. 18. Block diagram of dual modulus prescaler.

1010011, or 83 in decimal. In Fig. 21 the input frequency was 50 MHz and an output pulse was produced from the counter every 83 pulses, resulting in an output frequency of 602.4 kHz.
Once the major blocks of the proposed programmable divider were simulated, the divider itself was implemented and simulated to ensure it can produce the correct output frequency which would serve as the FB input for the phase/frequency detector. The frequency for each MICS channel was used as the input for the divider, and the control word of the Swallow Counter was adjusted so that the corresponding division ratio was used. It was verified that for each channel, the corresponding division ratio produced an output frequency of 150 kHz. The simulation waveforms in Fig. 22 and Fig. 23 show the input waveform, output waveform and output frequency of the programmable divider when the input frequency is 402.15 MHz (channel 1) and 404.85 MHz (channel 10) respectively.
A comparison between the proposed subthreshold programmable divider and recently published programmable dividers is given in Table 4. The figure of merit used to compare the results is the power consumption at the operating frequency, given in μW/MHz.
The programmable divider was submitted for fabrication as part of an MICS band frequency synthesizer. The layout of the programmable divider is shown in Fig. 24. Measurement results were not available as the design was still being fabricated. The total simulated power consumption of the proposed programmable divider was 200 μW. A summary of the power consumption for each of the major blocks is given in Table 5.

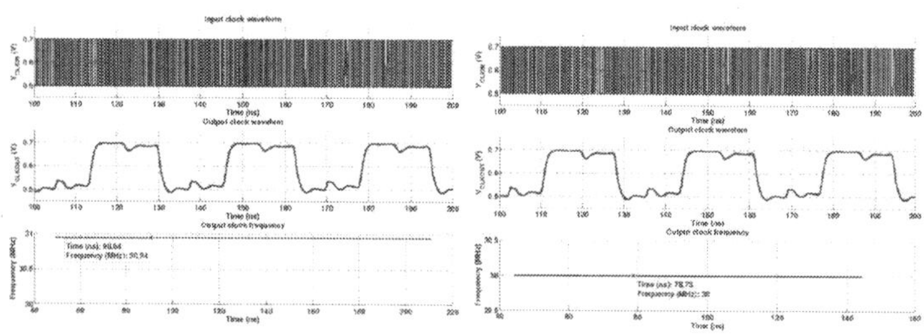

(a) Divide by 32. (b) Divide by 33.

Fig. 19. Transient simulation of dual-modulus prescaler.

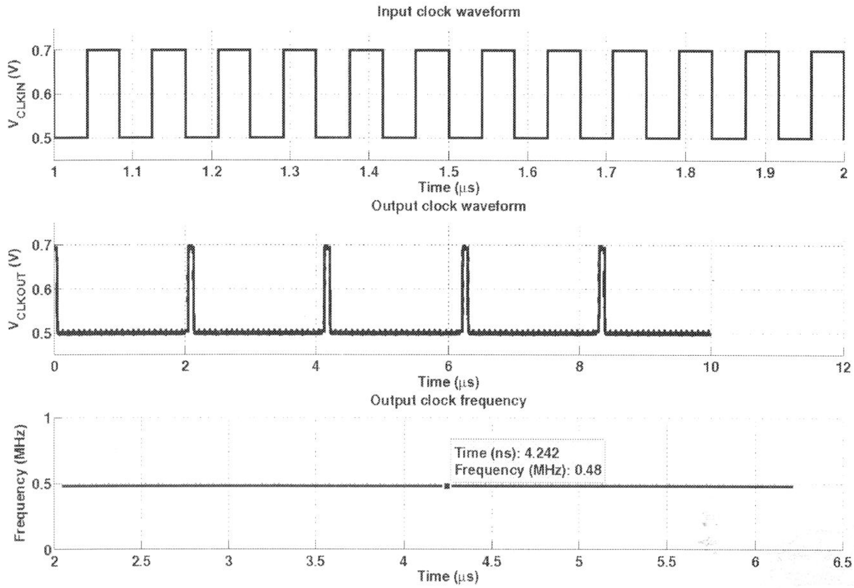

(a) Input and output waveforms.

Fig. 20. Transient simulation of 6-bit down counter.

Reference (Technology)	Frequency [MHz]	V_{DD} [V]	Power [mW]	FOM [μW/MHz]
This Work (0.13μm)	**200 to 1000**	**0.7**	**0.21**	**0.247**
(Kuo & Wu, 2006) (0.18μm)	2400 and 5000	1.8	2.6	1.08
(Kuo & Weng, 2009) (0.18μm)	5141 to 5860	1.5	4.8	0.934
(Lei et al., 2009) (0.18μm)	500 to 3500	1.8	3.01	0.86
(Pan et al., 2008) (0.18μm)	1600	1.2	0.475	0.296
(Kim et al., 2008) (0.18μm)	3000	1.5	3.58	1.19
(Zhang et al., 2009) (0.18μm)	1700	1.5	3.2	1.88
(Zhang et al., 2006) (0.18μm)	440	1.8	0.54	1.23

Table 4. Comparison of low power programmable dividers

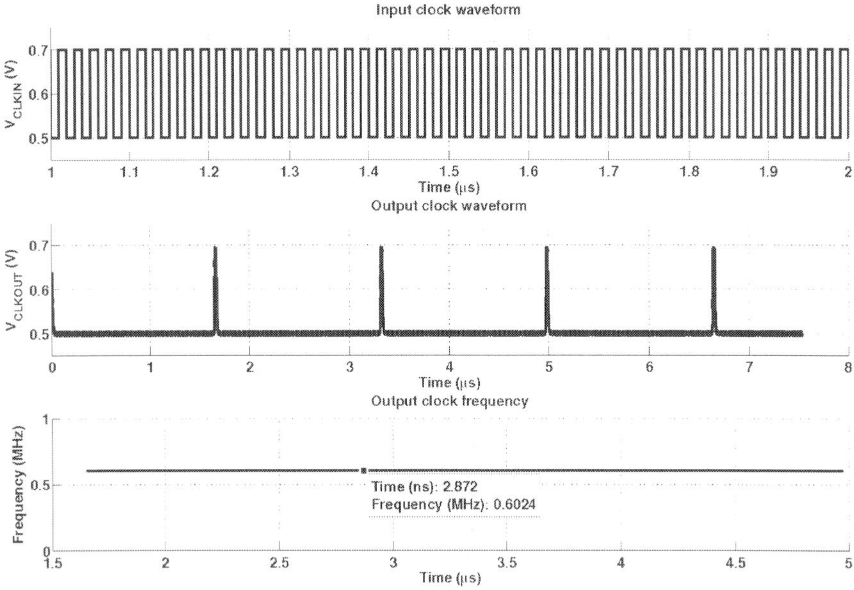

(a) Input and output waveforms.

Fig. 21. Transient simulation of 7-bit down counter.

6. A subthreshold source-coupled logic phase/frequency detector, current-steering charge pump, and loop filter

The phase/frequency detector (PFD) uses the architecture of Fig. 25(a). The proposed D-latch with clear preset is used to implement the master-slave D flip-flops in the PFD. The outputs of the 2-input SCL AND/NAND gate drives the *EN* and $\overline{EN}$ signals in the proposed D-latch. In order to perform the required function, the *CLR* signal is tied to the positive supply and the *PRE* signal is tied to the negative supply. The block diagram of the PDF is shown in Fig. 25(b) The charge-pump used in this work is a modification of the low voltage charge pump circuit proposed in (Chang & Kuo, 2000) shown in Fig. 26.

Block	Power consumption [μW]
Dual modulus prescaler	30
6-bit programmable counter	76
7-bit programmable counter	89
Pulse-swallow programmable divider	200

Table 5. Power consumption of programmable divider components.

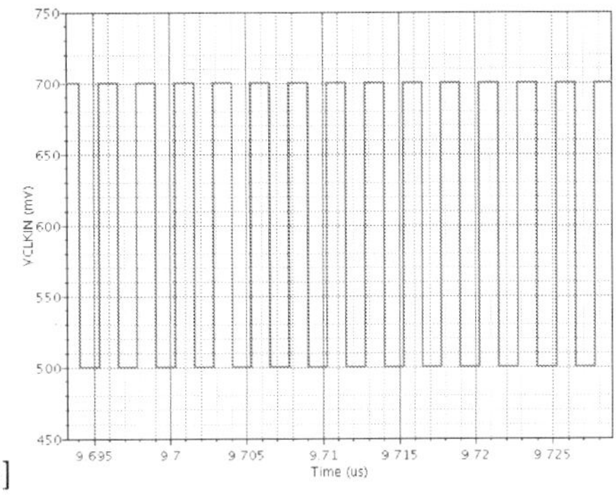

p!]

(a) Input voltage waveform

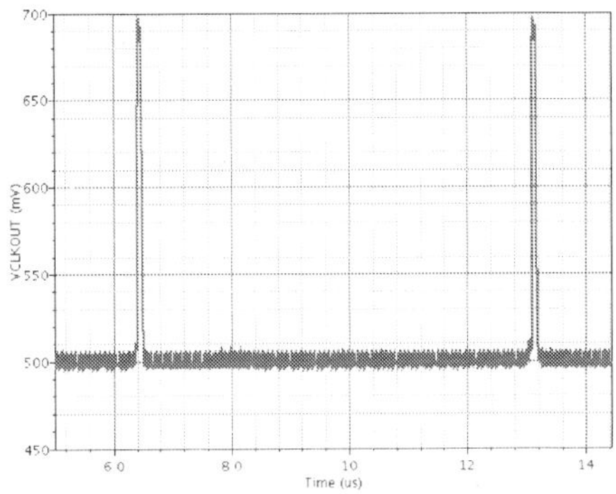

(b) Output voltage waveform

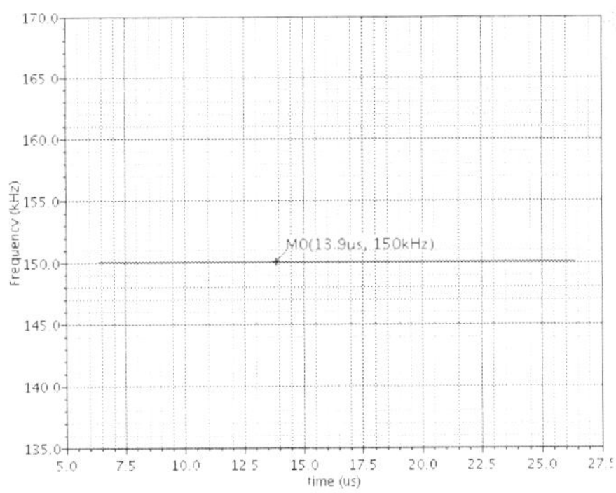

(c) Output frequency

Fig. 22. Programmable divider output when f_{in} = 402.15 MHz

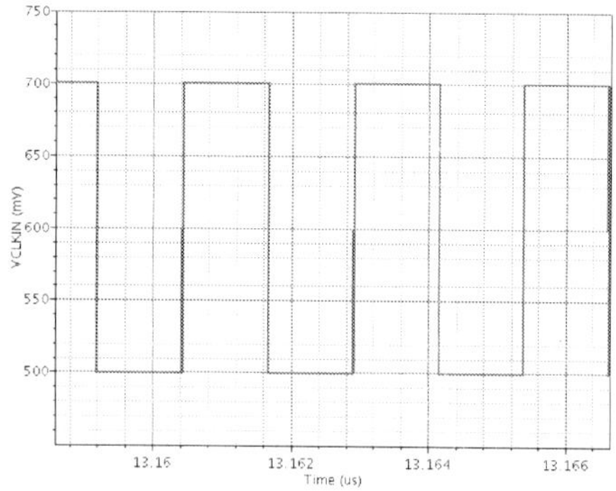

(a) Input voltage waveform

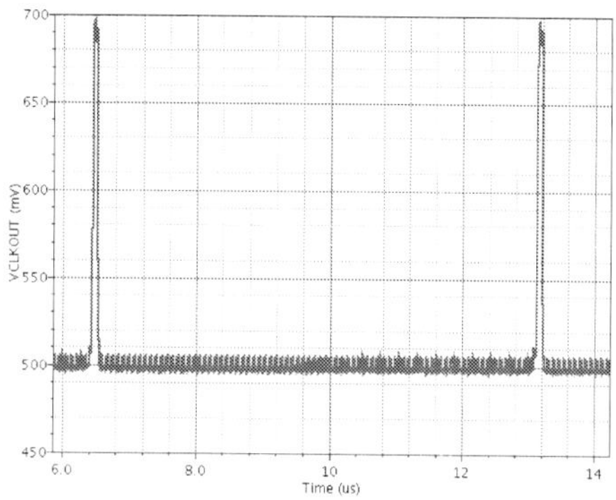

(b) Output voltage waveform

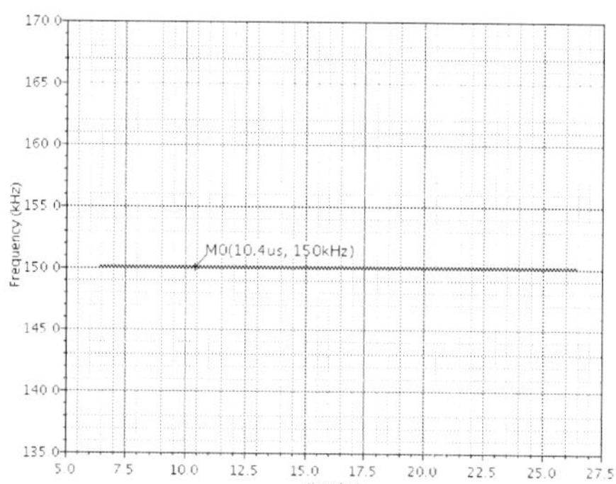

(c) Output frequency

Fig. 23. Programmable divider output when f_{in} = 404.85 MHz

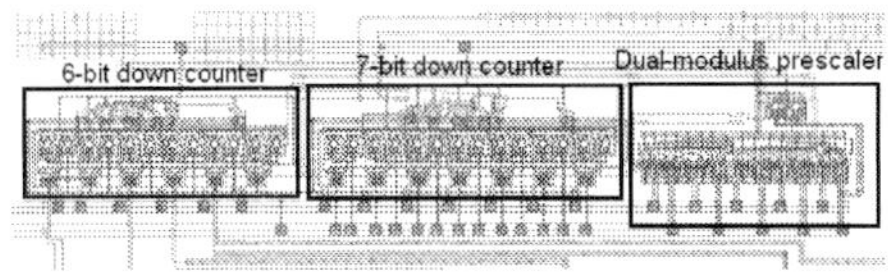

Fig. 24. Programmable frequency divider layout.

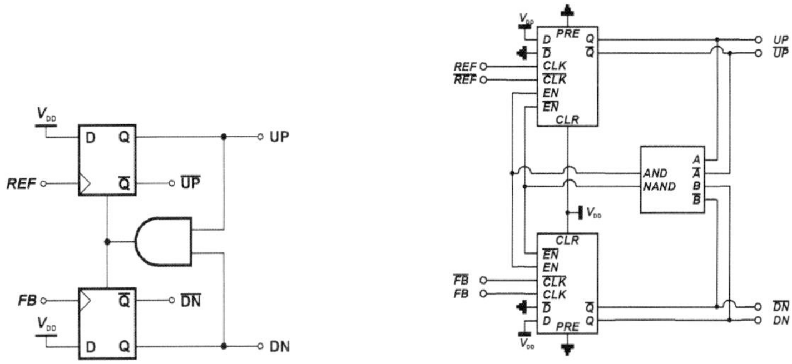

(a) Conventional architecture.

(b) Adapted architecture.

Fig. 25. Phase/frequency detector.

The circuit consists of a wide-swing current mirror and symmetric charge pumps to provide I_{UP} and I_{DN}. Each charge pump is controlled by a differential input pair biased with a tail current source, a current mirror load and a diode connected load. In the "pump up" circuit, when UP is high the bias current flows through M_1 and is mirrored to the output through the current mirror $M_{5,16}$. A pull-up transistor M_9 is added to immediately bring the gate of the current mirror transistors to V_{DD} when UP is low in order to shut off the current mirror and prevent any current from leaking into the output. The "pump down" circuit can be analysed in the same fashion. The wide-swing current mirror M_{11-14} mirrors the pump down current to the output of the charge pump. The loop filter is a 3rd order passive filter and the components were chosen to have a loop bandwidth of approximately 15 kHz to reduce reference spurs.

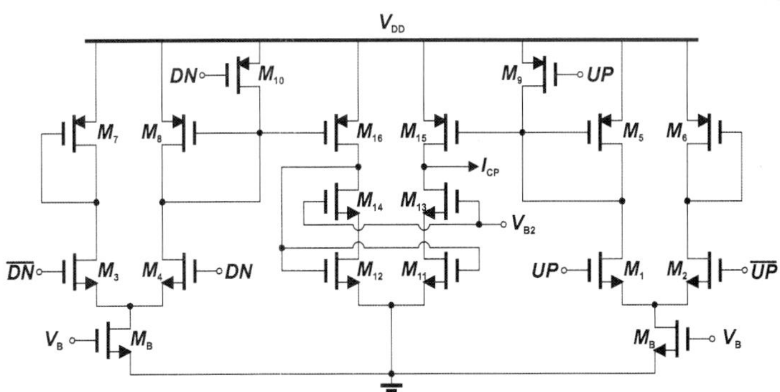

Fig. 26. Current-steering charge pump.

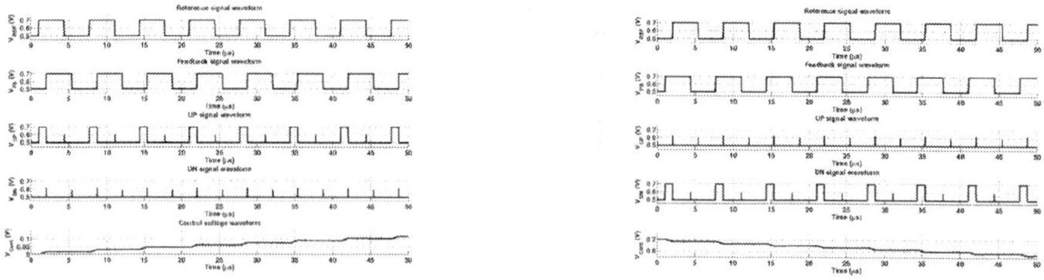

(a) Reference leads feedback. (b) Reference lags feedback.

Fig. 27. Transient simulation of PFD/CP/LF.

The simulation results of the proposed subthreshold source-coupled logic phase/frequency detector, current-steering charge pump and loop filter are presented in Fig. 27. In Fig. 27(a), the reference signal phase leads the feedback signal phase and the control voltage increases as expected. Similarly in Fig. 27(b), the reference signal phase lags the feedback signal phase and the control voltage decreases. It should be noted that an initial voltage was placed on the loop filter capacitor for the simulation in Fig. 27(b) because when the simulator starts the initial control voltage would be zero and the charge pump cannot remove any more charge from the capacitor.

The PFD/CP/LF was submitted for fabrication as part of the previously mentioned MICS band frequency synthesizer, and measurement results are not currently available. The layout of the PFD/CP/LF is shown in Fig. 28. The CP was designed to have I_{UP}=I_{DN}=1 μA. The entire PFD/CP/LF consumes under 20 μW of power, most of which is consumed by the PFD.

7. The proposed ultra-low power integer-n frequency synthesizer

Using the proposed proposed CR-QVCO, subthreshold SCL programmable frequency divider and PFD implemented using the proposed clear/preset D latch, the modified current-steering charge pump and third order loop filter, a 402 MHz to 405 MHz integer-n frequency synthesizer was implemented.

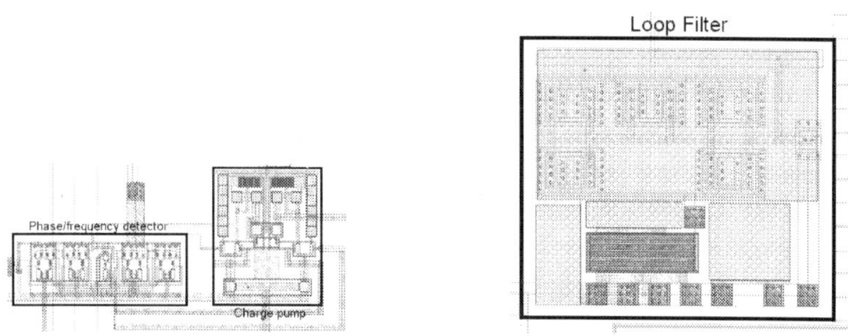

(a) Phase/frequency detector and charge pump. (b) Loop filter.

Fig. 28. Phase/frequency detector, charge pump and loop filter layouts.

Block	Power consumption [μW]
Current-reuse quadrature voltage-controlled oscillator	420
Pulse-swallow programmable divider	200
Charge pump, phase/frequency detector and loop filter	20
Total	640

Table 6. Power consumption of programmable divider components.

7.1 Results

The frequency synthesizer in Fig. 1 was simulated to verify the locking behaviour, and simulation results show that the synthesizer reaches the lock stated in 250 μs. The total power consumption is 700 μW. A summary of the power consumption for all the blocks of the proposed frequency synthesizer is presented in Table 6.

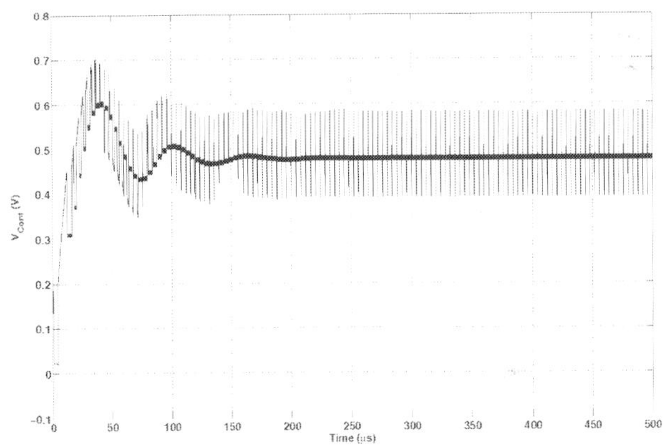

Fig. 29. Frequency synthesizer control voltage.

The chip layout of the entire subthreshold integer-n frequency divider is shown in Fig. 30. The total silicon area including probe pads is 2 mm × 1.5 mm. At the time of publication, the synthesizer was still in fabrication thus measurement results were not available.

8. Conclusion

In this research, novel circuits and design methodologies were presented for the design and implementation of an ultra-low power integer-n frequency synthesizer operating in the 402 MHz to 405 MHz Medical Implant Communication Service band of frequencies. The principal design concepts to achieve ultra-low power operation were introduced, namely current reuse, supply voltage scaling and subthreshold operation. Using these techniques, several novel circuits for use in the ultra-low power integer-n frequency synthesizer were proposed, namely:

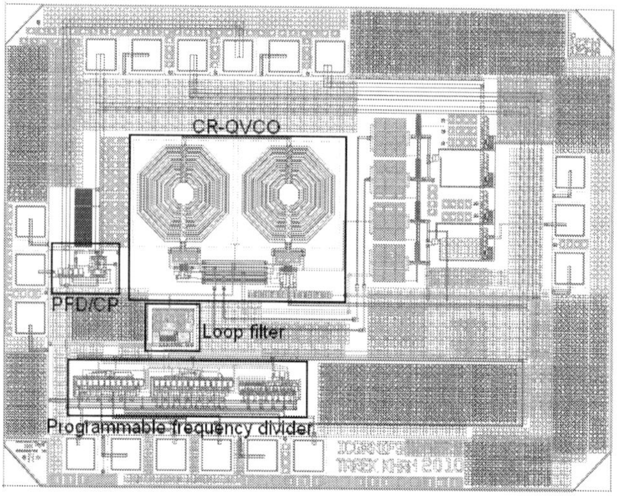

Fig. 30. Frequency synthesizer layout.

- A current reuse quadrature voltage-controlled oscillator.
- A novel clear/preset SCL D-latch.
- A subthreshold SCL programmable divider and phase/frequency detector based on the proposed clear/preset SCL D-latch.

Using IBM CMRF8SF 130 nm CMOS technology, the proposed circuits were used to implement an integer-n frequency synthesizer. Simulations and preliminary silicon measurements confirmed that the proposed CR-QVCO, ST-SCL programmable divider and ultra-low power frequency synthesizer achieve better performance than existing designs.

9. References

Andreani, P., Bonfanti, A., Romano, L. & Samori, C. (2002). Analysis and design of a 1.8-GHz CMOS LC quadrature VCO, *IEEE Journal of Solid-State Circuits* 37(12): 1737–1747.

Bae, J., Cho, N. & Yoo, H.-J. (2009). A 490uW fully MICS compatible FSK transceiver for implantable devices, *2009 Symposium on VLSI Circuits*, pp. 36–37.

Bohorquez, J., Chandrakasan, A. & Dawson, J. (2009). A 350 μW CMOS MSK Transmitter and 400 μW OOK Super-Regenerative Receiver for Medical Implant Communications, *IEEE Journal of Solid-State Circuits* 44(4): 1248–1259.

Carrara, F., Italia, A., Palmisano, G. & Guerra, R. (2009). A 400-MHz CMOS radio front-end for ultra low-power medical implantable applications, *2009 European Solid-State Circuits Conference*, pp. 232–235.

Chamas, I. R. & Raman, S. (2007a). A 5 GHz I/Q Phase-tunable CMOS LC Quadrature VCO (PT-QVCO) for Analog Phase Calibrated Receiver Architectures, *2007 Topical Meeting on Silicon Monolithic Integrated Circuits in RF Systems*, Long Beach, CA, pp. 269–272.

Chamas, I. R. & Raman, S. (2007b). A Comprehensive Analysis of Quadrature Signal Synthesis in Cross-coupled RF VCOs, *IEEE Transactions on Circuits and Systems I: Regular Papers* 54(4): 689–704.

Chang, R. C. & Kuo, L.-C. (2000). A new low-voltage charge pump circuit for PLL, *2000 IEEE International Symposium on Circuits and Systems*, Vol. 5, Geneva, pp. 701–704 vol.5.

Cheng, S. & Silva-Martinez, J. (2004). 6.8 mW 2.5 Gb/s and 42.5 mW 5 Gb/s 1:8 CMOS demultiplexers, *2004 IEEE International Symposium on Circuits and Systems*, Vol. 4, pp. IV – 209–12 Vol.4.

Cong, H.-I., Logan, S. M., Loinaz, M. J., O'Brien, K. J., Perry, E. E., Polhemus, G. D., Scoggins, J. E., Snowdon, K. P. & Ward, M. G. (2001). A 10-Gb/s 16:1 multiplexer and 10-GHz clock synthesizer in 0.25-μm Sige BiCMOS, *IEEE Journal of Solid-State Circuits* 36(12): 1946–1953.

Dai, F. F., Chimakurthy, L. S. J., Yang, D., Huang, J. & Jaeger, R. C. (2004). A low power 5 GHz direct digital synthesizer designed in Sige technology, *2004 Topical Meeting on Silicon Monolithic Integrated Circuits in RF Systems*, pp. 21–24.

Desikachari, R., Steeds, M., Huard, J. & Moon, U. (2007). An Efficient Design Procedure for High-speed Low-power Dual-modulus CMOS Prescalers, *2007 IEEE International Conference on Electronics, Circuits and Systems*, Marrakech, pp. 645–648.

Federal Communications Commission (1999). Amendment of Parts 2 and 95 of the Commission's Rules to Establish a Medical Implant Communication Service in the 402-405 MHz Band, *Technical Report FCC 99-363*, Federal Communications Commission.
URL: *http://www.fcc.gov/*

Gardner, F. M. (2005). *Phaselock techniques*, Wiley-Interscience, Hoboken, N.J.

Kim, K.-Y., Lee, W.-K., Kim, H. & Kim, S.-W. (2008). Low-power programmable divider for multi-standard frequency synthesizers using reset and modulus signal generator, *IEEE Asian Solid-State Circuits Conference*, pp. 77–80.

Kuo, K.-C. & Wu, F.-J. (2006). A 2.4-GHz/5-GHz Low Power Pulse Swallow Counter in 0.18-μm CMOS Technology, *2006 IEEE Asia Pacific Conference on Circuits and Systems*, Singapore, pp. 214–217.

Kuo, Y. F. & Weng, R. M. (2009). 5 GHz low power frequency synthesiser with dual-modulus counter, *IET Circuits, Devices & Systems* 3(6): 365–375.

Lee, T. H. (2004). *The design of CMOS radio-frequency integrated circuits*, Cambridge University Press, New York.

Lee, W.-H., Cho, J.-D. & Lee, S.-D. (1999). A high speed and low power phase-frequency detector and charge-pump, *Design Automation Conference, 1999. Proceedings of the ASP-DAC '99. Asia and South Pacific*, pp. 269–272.

Lei, X., Wang, Z., Wang, K. & Wang, X. (2009). A high speed low power pulse swallow frequency divider for DRM/DAB frequency synthesizer, *2009 International Conference on Wireless Communications & Signal Processing*, Nanjing, pp. 1–4.

Li, K. W., Leung, L. & Leung, K. N. (2009). Low power injection locked oscillators for MICS standard, *2009 IEEE Biomedical Circuits and Systems Conference*, pp. 1–4.

Liu, Y.-H., Liu, H.-H. & Lin, T.-H. (2009). A super-regenerative ASK receiver with $\Delta\Sigma$ pulse-width digitizer and SAR-based fast frequency calibration for MICS applications, *2009 Symposium on VLSI Circuits*, pp. 38–39.

Liu, Y.-H., Tung, C.-J. & Lin, T.-H. (2006). A low-power asymmetrical MICS wireless interface and transceiver design for medical imaging, *2006 IEEE Biomedical Circuits and Systems Conference*, pp. 162–165.

Luong, H. C. (2004). *Low-voltage CMOS RF frequency synthesizers*, Cambridge University Press, New York, NY.

Mazzanti, A., Svelto, F. & Andreani, P. (2006). On the amplitude and phase errors of quadrature LC-tank CMOS oscillators, *IEEE Journal of Solid-State Circuits* 41(6): 1305–1313.

Ng, A. W. L. & Luong, H. C. (2007). A 1-V 17-GHz 5-mW CMOS Quadrature VCO Based on Transformer Coupling, *IEEE Journal of Solid-State Circuits*, Vol. 42, pp. 1933–1941.

Pan, J., Yang, H. & wu Yang, L. (2008). A high-speed low-power pulse-swallow divider with robustness consideration, *9th International Conference on Solid-State and Integrated-Circuit Technology*, pp. 2168–2171.

Razavi, B. (1998). *RF microelectronics*, Prentice Hall, Upper Saddle River, NJ.

Razavi, B. (2001). *Design of analog CMOS integrated circuits*, McGraw-Hill, Boston, MA.

Rofougaran, A., Chang, G., Rael, J. J., Chang, J. Y. C., Rofougaran, M., Chang, P. J., Djafari, M., Ku, M. K., Roth, E. W., Abidi, A. A. & Samueli, H. (1998). A single-chip 900-MHz spread-spectrum wireless transceiver in 1-μm CMOS. I. Architecture and transmitter design, *IEEE Journal of Solid-State Circuits* 33: 515–534.

Rofougaran, A., Rael, J., Rofougaran, M. & Abidi, A. (1996). A 900 MHz CMOS LC-oscillator with quadrature outputs, *1996 IEEE International Solid-State Circuits Conference*, San Francisco, CA, pp. 392–393.

Ryu, J., Kim, M., Lee, J., Kim, B.-S., Lee, M.-Q. & Nam, S. (2007). Low Power OOK Transmitter for Wireless Capsule Endoscope, *2007 IEEE/MTT-S International Microwave Symposium*, pp. 855–858.

Tajalli, A., Brauer, E. J., Leblebici, Y. & Vittoz, E. (2008). Subthreshold Source-coupled Logic Circuits for Ultra-low-power Applications, *IEEE Journal of Solid-State Circuits* 43(7): 1699–1710.

Tekin, A., Yuce, M. & Liu, W. (2006). Integrated VCO Design for MICS Transceivers, *2006 IEEE Custom Integrated Circuits Conference*, pp. 765–768.

Tekin, A., Yuce, M., Shabani, J. & Liu, W. (2006). A low-power FSK modulator/demodulator for an MICS band transceiver, *2006 IEEE Radio and Wireless Symposium*, pp. 159–162.

Yue, C. P. & Wong, S. S. (1998). On-chip spiral inductors with patterned ground shields for Si-based RF ICs, *IEEE Journal of Solid-State Circuits* 33(5): 743–752.

Zhang, H., gang Yang, H., Zhang, J. & Liu, F. (2009). High-speed programmable counter design for PLL based on a delay partition technique, *IEEE International Symposium on Radio-Frequency Integration Technology*, pp. 100–103.

Zhang, L., Chi, B., Wang, Z., Chen, H. & Wu, E. (2006). A Low Power 440-MHz Pulse-Swallow-Divider Combination Synchronization-Asynchronism-Hybrid Frequency Divider, *IEEE International Midwest Symposium on Circuits and Systems*, Vol. 2, pp. 566–568.

10

Power Efficient ADCs for Biomedical Signal Acquisition

Alberto Rodríguez-Pérez, Manuel Delgado-Restituto and Fernando Medeiro
Institute of Microelectronics of Seville (IMSE-CNM) and University of Seville Spain

1. Introduction

In the last years, there has been a growing interest in the design of biomedical wireless sensors (Harrison et al., 2007; Zou et al., 2009). These sensors can be used for online monitoring, detection and prevention of many diseases with a minimum disturbance to the patient and reducing the hospital expenses, so they are having a big acceptance in the medical community.

Most biomedical signals are characterized by their low voltage amplitude (in the range of mili-volts) and their low frequency ranges (few tens of kHz) (Northrop, 2001; Northrop, 2004). Also, due to the electrode used to sense them, they usually present a high DC offset that needs to be suppressed. A typical biomedical sensor interface consists on a band-pass filter, a low-noise programmable amplifier and an Analog-to-Digital Converter (ADC). The digitalization of the sensed biosignals is usually done with 8 or 12-bits of resolution (depending on the kind of signal) and with sampling frequencies between 1kS/s and 100kS/s (Scott et al., 2003; Verma and Chandrakasan, 2007; Zou et al., 2009).

Due to their isolation from any kind of external supply source, one of the most important design constraints of these wireless sensors is the minimization of their power consumption. Because of that, most of the works about biomedical sensor designs have been focused on low-power and low-voltage techniques and architectures.

For the design of the ADCs, many authors choose the SAR architecture with capacitive-based DACs due to their suitability for low-power and low-voltage needed requirements (Agnes et al., 2008; Hong and Lee, 2007; Saurbrey et al., 2003; Scott et al., 2003; Verma and Chandrakasan, 2007; Zou et al., 2009).

However, this architecture present some problems when the needed resolution growths. They become more area consumer, present high sensitivity to parasitic capacitances and demand more power from the supply source.

In this chapter we will present two different architectures, the most-known SAR and a new one based on a Switched Capacitor (SC) implementation of a Binary Search Algorithm, which solves many of the limitations of the SARs and present higher reconfigurability, a very important fact in these kinds of applications. The chapter will focus on the most relevant design constraints and the study of the effect of the different non-idealities, in order to get an area and power optimized design.

Two real implementations will be presented at the end of the chapter to illustrate the given theory through experimental and simulation results.

2. Low-power ADC architectures

2.1 Successive approximation architecture

The successive approximation algorithm performs the A/D conversion over multiple clock periods by exploiting the knowledge of previously determined bits to determine the next significant bit. The method aims to reduce the circuit complexity and power consumption using a low conversion rate by allowing one clock period per bit (plus one for the input sampling).

Fig. 1a shows the typical block diagram of an n-bit SA ADC. It consists of a Sample-and-Hold (S&H) circuit followed by a feedback loop composed by a comparator, a Successive Approximation Register (SAR) logic block, and an n-bit DAC. Circuit operation is controlled by a clock signal with frequency f_{clk}. The SAR block captures the data from the comparator at each clock cycle and assembles the words driving the DAC bit by bit, from the most- to the least-significant bit, using a binary search algorithm, as Fig. 1b illustrates (Maloberti, 2007). After n cycles, the digital counterpart, d_{out}, of the analog sampled voltage, v_{sh}, is obtained. Besides, the S&H clock uses m clock periods for the sampling of the input signal, v_{in}. Therefore, a total of $n+m$ clock intervals are required for completing an n-*bit* conversion.

At the start of the next conversion, while the S&H is sampling the next input, the SAR provides the n-bit output and resets the registers.

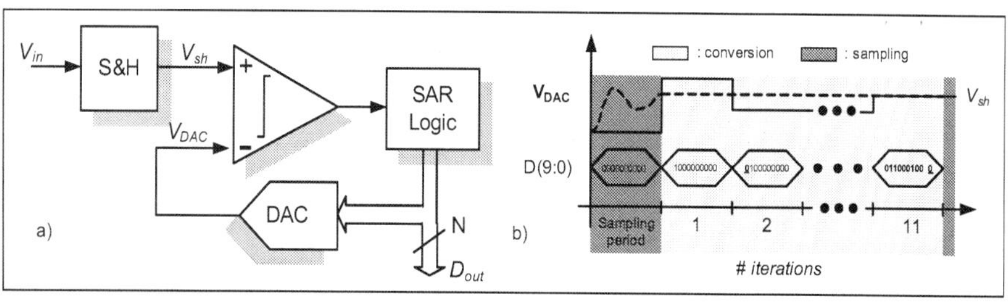

Fig. 1. a) SAR ADC architecture, b) Timing diagram

Among the very different existing architectures to perform the Analog-to-Digital Conversion, the Successive Approximation one have been chosen by many authors as the most efficient in terms of power consumption to digitalize biomedical signals. As it has been explained above, a minimum number of analog blocks and a very simple digital logic are needed to perform the complete conversion. Therefore, the overall power consumption presented by these solutions is very low.

2.2 Capacitive-based DAC

One of the most critical blocks of these solutions in terms of power consumption reduction is the Digital-to-Analog Converter. To implement it, many authors choose a capacitive-based solution (Agnes et al., 2008; Hong and Lee, 2007; Saurbrey et al., 2003; Scott et al., 2003; Verma and Chandrakasan, 2007; Zou et al., 2009) due to their low power consumption characteristics and because they can also be used as a passive S&H. As they are based on the charge

redistribution principle, they only consume power at the beginning of the conversion, when the matrix is loaded. Therefore, they are really suitable for the biomedical devices.
One of the main problems of these capacitive DACs is that their performance is in many cases strongly affected by the parasitic capacitances (Cong, 2001; Rodriguez-Perez et al., 2010). We will present an exhaustive study about the effect of the parasitic capacitances on the performance of the capacitive-based DACs.
Depending on their structure, the capacitive-based DACs can be divided in different sub-types.

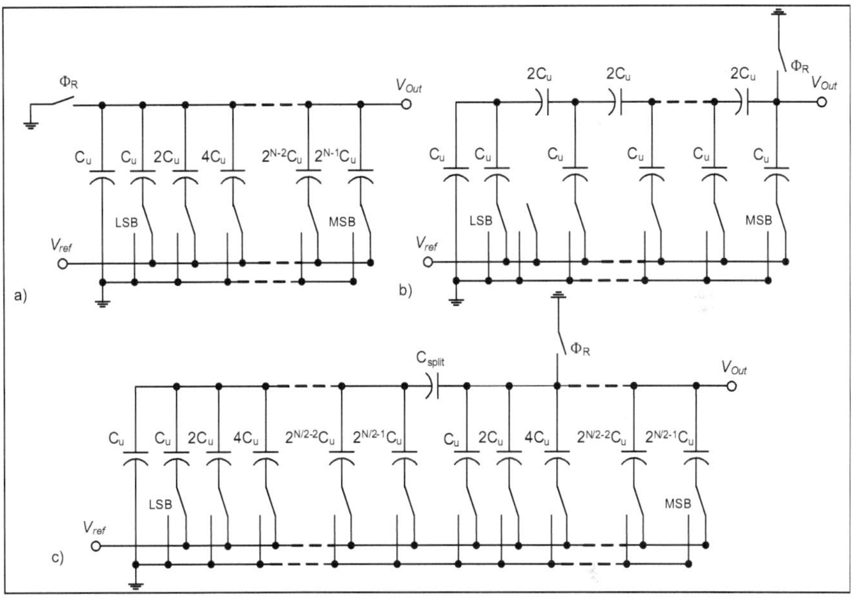

Fig. 2. Capacitive DACs architectures: a) Binary Weighted Array (BWA), b) C-2C, c) Binary Weighted Array with an attenuation Capacitor (BWAC)

Binary Weighted Arrays (BWA)

This structure is used by many authors in their works. It consists on a binary scaled array of capacitors, as Fig. 2a shows. The top of the capacitors are shorted and constitute the analog output of the DAC, while the bottoms are connected to different switches controlled by the digital input bits. The MSB is connected to the biggest capacitor while the LSB is connected to the smallest one. Then, the voltage output of the DAC will be given by:

$$V_{out} = \frac{\sum_{i=0}^{N-1} D_i \cdot 2^i}{2^N} \quad (1)$$

where N is the resolution of the DAC and D_i is the i-th input bit.
The power of these capacitive DACs is essentially due to the switching activity of the capacitive matrix, which will be given by:

$$P_{ADC} = \frac{1}{2} \cdot f_S \cdot 2^N C_u \cdot V_{DAC}^2, \tag{2}$$

where f_s is the sampling frequency, N the resolution and C_u the unitary capacitance.
The area occupied by the DAC will be proportional to $2^N \cdot A_{cu}$, where A_{cu} is the area occupied by an unitary capacitance.
Considering that the equivalent parasitic capacitance at the top of the capacitive matrix is given by C_p (which groups parasitic capacitances at the top of the capacitors and parasitic capacitances due to the routing), the output voltage will be given by:

$$V_{out} = \frac{C_u 2^N}{C_u 2^N + C_p} \cdot \frac{\sum_{i=0}^{N-1} D_i \cdot 2^i}{2^N} \tag{3}$$

As can be extracted from the given equation, parasitic capacitances in the BWA structure produce a gain error in the final result.
The main drawback of this solution is that its power consumption and area occupation increase binarily with the resolution. Therefore, for more than 8-bits of resolution DACs, this architecture is not recommended due to the difficulty of doing a proper matched array and the huge increase in terms of area and power consumption.

Binary Weighted Arrays with an attenuation capacitor (BWAC)

As the former architectures are not suitable for medium-high resolutions because their increase in terms of power consumption, area occupation and complexity, many authors prefer to divide the BWA into two using a capacitive divider for the less significant part of the matrix (Agnes et al., 2008). The schematic of the architecture is shown in Fig. 2c), where the value of the attenuation capacitor, C_{att}, is given by:

$$C_{att} = \frac{2^{\frac{N}{2}}}{2^{\frac{N}{2}-1}}, \tag{4}$$

where N is the resolution of the converter. Then, the output voltage of the capacitive DAC is given by:

$$V_{out} = \frac{\left(2^{\frac{N}{2}} \cdot m\right) + n}{2^N}, \tag{5}$$

where m is the number of capacitors placed on the most significant part of the matrix, while n is the number in the Least Significant one. The optimum configuration in terms of area and power consumption is when m and n are the same, that is, there is the same number of capacitors in the most significant part of the matrix as in the least one.
The switching power of these architectures is given by:

$$P_{DAC} = \frac{1}{2} \cdot f_S \cdot 2^{\frac{N}{2}+1} \cdot C_u \cdot V_{DAC}^2, \tag{6}$$

being the area occupation of these structures proportional to $2^{\frac{N}{2}+1} \cdot A_{cu}$.

It is obvious at first glance that this architecture can reduce the number of unitary elements of the BWA solutions. This reduction helps in the optimization of the power consumption and area occupation, which is one of the main objectives in the design of devices for biomedical purposes.

However, these attenuation capacitor-based architectures present higher sensitivity towards parasitic capacitances than the BWA ones. While in the second ones parasitic capacitances only induce an offset error, in this case they cause a non linearity error, which degrades the performance and the effective resolution of the DAC.

To evaluate the effect of the parasitic capacitances in these architectures, we have to distinguish between the parasitic capacitances at the top of the most significant part of the matrix, which will be named as C_{pA} and those at the least significant one, C_{pB}. Considering that the two parts of the matrix are equal and that the attenuation capacitor is almost an unitary one, the output voltage of the DAC will be given by:

$$V_{out} = \frac{V_{ref}\cdot\sum_{i=\frac{N}{2}}^{N-1} D_i \cdot 2^{i-\frac{N}{2}}\cdot C_u}{C_{eqMSB}+\left(C_{eqLSB}\,//\,C_{att}\right)} + \frac{V_{ref}\cdot\sum_{i=0}^{\frac{N}{2}-1} D_i\cdot 2^i\cdot C_u}{C_{eqLSB}+\left(C_{eqMSB}\,//\,C_{att}\right)}\cdot\frac{C_{att}}{C_{att}+C_{eqMSB}}, \quad (7)$$

where C_{eqMSB} is the equivalent capacitance of the MSB part the array, and C_{eqLSB} is the equivalent capacitance of the LSB part of the matrix.

$$V_{out} = \frac{V_{ref}\cdot\sum_{i=\frac{N}{2}}^{N-1} D_i \cdot 2^{i-\frac{N}{2}}\cdot C_u}{\left(2^{\frac{N}{2}}-1\right)C_u + \dfrac{\left(2^{\frac{N}{2}}C_u + C_{pB}\right)\cdot C_{att}}{2^{\frac{N}{2}}C_u + C_{pB} + C_{att}} + C_{pA}} + \frac{V_{ref}\cdot\sum_{i=0}^{\frac{N}{2}-1} D_i\cdot 2^i\cdot C_u}{2^{\frac{N}{2}}C_u + \dfrac{\left(\left(2^{\frac{N}{2}}-1\right)C_u + C_{pA}\right)\cdot C_{att}}{\left(2^{\frac{N}{2}}-1\right)C_u + C_{pA} + C_{att}} + C_{pB}}\cdot\frac{C_{att}}{C_{att}+\left(2^{\frac{N}{2}}-1\right)C_u + C_{pA}} \quad (8)$$

Fig. 3 shows the best straight line INL for different parasitic capacitances per unit capacitances ratio for a 10-bit DAC. When the parasitic per unitary capacitance ratio rises above 3%, the non-linearity introduced by the parasitic capacitances is so high that the equivalent resolution is affected.

Then, although the architecture is better in terms of area and power consumption than the BWA one, it is more affected by the parasitic capacitances and its design must be carefully studied, as will be described later.

C-2C Structures

The schematic of the C-2C structures are shown in Fig. 2b. This kind of structures is an extension of the BWAC ones, in which the matrix is divided as many times as bits to be converted, using attenuation capacitors to divide the different unitary capacitances. The value of these attenuation capacitors is given by the expression (4), where N is two. Then,

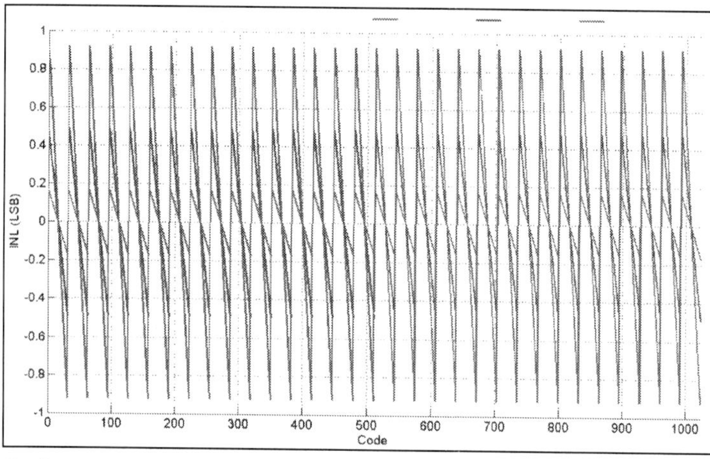

Fig. 3. INL of parasitic capacitances effect on 10-bit BWAC DAC

the value of these attenuation capacitors must be twice higher than the unitary capacitance, building the C-2C structures.
The switching power dissipated will be given by:

$$P_{DAC} = \frac{1}{2} \cdot f_S \cdot (N+1) \cdot C_u \cdot V_{DAC}^2 , \quad (9)$$

and the area occupation is proportional to $(N+1) \cdot A_{cu}$.
The area and power consumption of these architectures are drastically reduced if compared with the other solutions. However, they are rarely employed due to their extremely high sensitivity towards the parasitic capacitances, which completely degrades its performance unless they were very low, which is not feasible in standard technologies.
To study the effect of the parasitic capacitances in the C-2C structures, we have to consider the parasitic capacitances shown in Fig. 4, where $C'_{pA} = 2 \cdot (C_{put} + C_{pub})$, while $C_{pA} = 3 \cdot C_{put} + 2 \cdot C_{pub}$. As the bottom parasitic capacitances are usually bigger than those of the top, we can consider that $C'_{pA} \approx C_{pA}$ for simplicity.

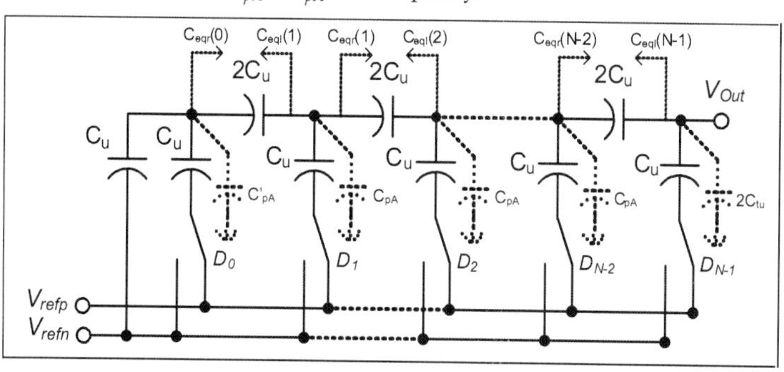

Fig. 4. Parasitic capacitances on C-2C structure

The output of the DAC can be calculated as:

$$V_{out} = \sum_{i=0}^{N-1} D_i \cdot V_{DAC}(i) \,, \tag{10}$$

where D_i will be the i-th digital input bit (with a digital value of '1' or '0'), and $V_{DAC}(i)$ is the equivalent voltage at the output of the DAC if only the bit i-th is activated. These voltages will be given by:

$$V_{DAC}(i) = \begin{cases} \dfrac{V_{ref} \cdot C_u}{\alpha + C_{eql}(i) + C_{eqr}(i)} \cdot \dfrac{2 \cdot C_u}{2 \cdot C_u + \beta} \cdot \prod_{n=i+1}^{N-2} \dfrac{2 \cdot C_u}{2 \cdot C_u + \alpha + C_{eqr}(n)} & 0 < i < N-1 \\ \dfrac{V_{ref} \cdot C_u}{\alpha + C_u + C_{eqr}(0)} \cdot \dfrac{2 \cdot C_u}{2 \cdot C_u + \beta} \cdot \prod_{n=1}^{N-2} \dfrac{2 \cdot C_u}{2 \cdot C_u + \alpha + C_{eqr}(n)} & i = 0 \\ \dfrac{V_{ref} \cdot C_u}{\beta + C_{eql}(N-1)} & i = N-1 \end{cases} \tag{11}$$

where $\alpha = C_u + 3 \cdot C_{put} + 2 \cdot C_{pub}$ and $\beta = C_u + 2 \cdot C_{put}$. $C_{eqr}(i)$ and $C_{eql}(i)$ are the equivalent capacitance at the right and left of the i-th bit, respectively. To calculate these equivalent capacitances, the following expression can be employed:

$$C_{eqr}(i) = \begin{cases} \dfrac{2C_u \cdot \left[C_{eqr}(i+1) + \alpha \right]}{C_{eqr}(i+1) + 2C_u + \alpha} & 0 \le i < N-2 \\ \dfrac{2C_u \cdot \beta}{2C_u + \beta} & i = N-2 \end{cases} \tag{12}$$

$$C_{eql}(i) = \begin{cases} \dfrac{2C_u \cdot \left[C_{eqr}(i+1) + \alpha \right]}{C_{eqr}(i+1) + 2C_u + \alpha} & 0 \le i < N-1 \\ \dfrac{2C_u \cdot (\alpha + C_u)}{3C_u + \alpha} & i = N-2 \end{cases} \tag{13}$$

These expressions allow us to build the INL figure shown in Fig. 5, where it is clear that the parasitic capacitances induce a complete degradation in the linearity and, consequently, the performance of the DAC, even if they are small.

Although there are some solutions which try to solve the parasitic capacitance sensitivity of these ladders (Cong, 2001), they are not really implementable as they are based on non-integer scaling of the reference voltages. Also, there are some solutions which implement these structures in Silicon-Over-Insulator (SOI) technologies, where substrate parasitic capacitances are dramatically reduced due to the bulk isolation.

As a consequence, these solutions are rarely employed in real implementations.

2.3 Binary search algorithm

Although the SAR ADC architectures based on capacitive DAC matrix are widely used on biomedical sensor interfaces, they present some drawbacks which usually difficult their design:

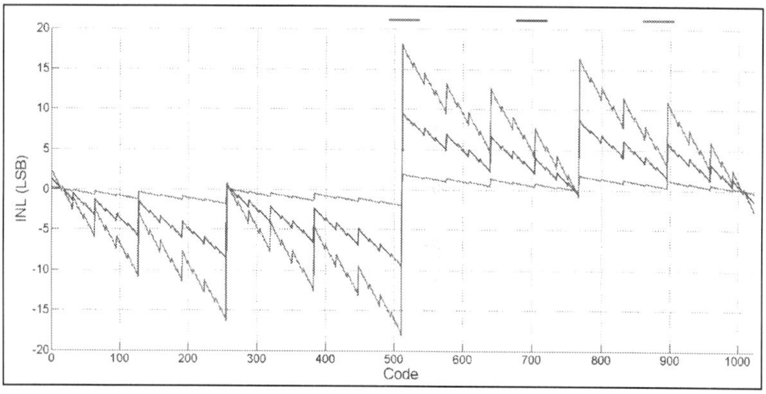

Fig. 5. INL of parasitic capacitances effect on 10-bit C-2C DAC

- **Large area occupation.** Capacitive-based DACs, and especially in the case of the BWA structures, usually require a huge area to be implemented (even more if the resolution is high), because they need many unitary capacitors. This high number of elements also complicates the routing and their proper matching.
- **Large switching power consumption.** Although one of the benefits of the capacitive DACs is that they are based on the charge redistribution principle and they don't have static power consumption is zero, the peaks of current from the supply voltage can be large, which can complicate the correct working of the circuit as they are usually supplied by unstable sources.
- **High equivalent input capacitance.** Due to the fact that the capacitive matrix is usually employed as a passive Sample & Hold in order to save power consumption, the input signal has to be load in the capacitive matrix at the beginning of the conversion. As this input signal has to be amplified and filtered by a previous active block, this latter has to load a very high capacitance, which means an increase in the power consumption.
- **High sensitivity towards parasitic capacitances.** As it has been previously studied, parasitic capacitances can affect the performance of the capacitive-based DACs, so their proper design can be complicated.

Due to the listed problems related to the design of the capacitive DACs for the SAR ADC architectures, we introduce another architecture implemented using Swithed-Capacitor Circuits (SC) and based on the Binary Search Algorithm.

The Binary Search Algorithm, which Flow Diagram is shown in Fig. 6a, is really the basis of the Successive Approximation conversion principle. It begins with the sampled of the input signal, which is compared with a certain threshold value. The result of this first comparison will set the Most Significant Bit (MSB), and we will add or subtract (depending on the result of the comparison) to the input value a certain reference voltage V_{ref}. Then we will perform again a new comparison, which will set the next bit, and after that we will add or subtract the reference voltage divided by two. This iteration is successively repeated as many times as bits to be converted, dividing by two the residual reference voltage each time. Then, after n iterations, the residual value of the reference voltage that we add or subtract will be $V_{ref} / 2^n$.

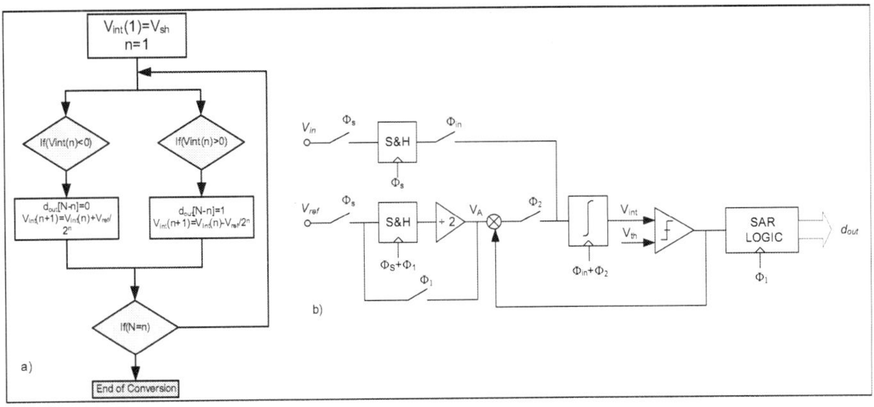

Fig. 6. Binary Search Algorith: a) Flow Diagram, b) Block Diagram schematic

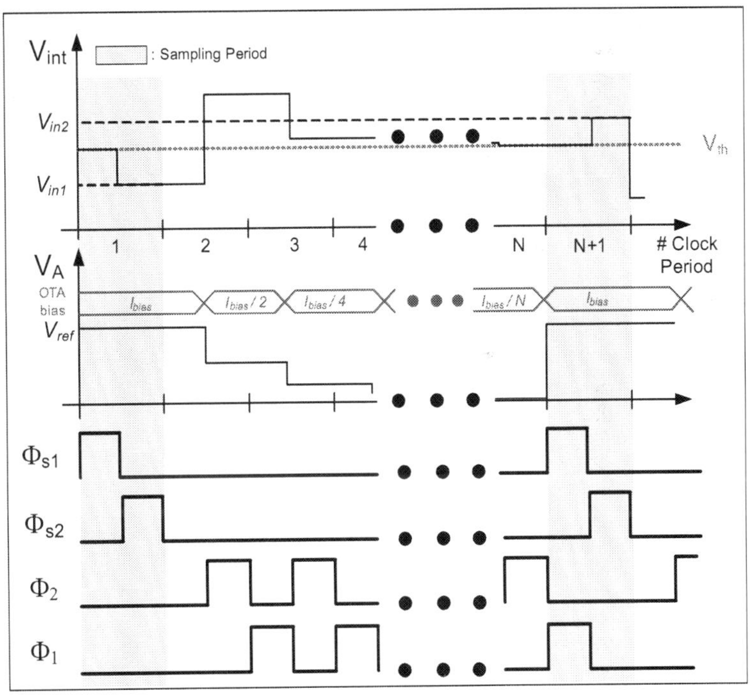

Fig. 7. Waveform of the Binary Search Algorithm implementation

Based on this algorithm, the block diagram of the proposed solution is presented in Fig. 6b. It consists on a Sample&Hold, an integrator, a divider-by-two and some logic to implement the Binary Search Algorithm. The evolution of the signals during a conversion for a certain input V_{in} is shown in Fig. 7.

2.4 Reconfigurable ADC based on SC techniques

Based on the block diagram of Fig. 6b, a Switched-Capacitor solution to implement the desired ADC in presented in Fig. 8a. The proposed solution only uses one operational amplifier in order to minimize as much as possible the power consumption (Rodriguez-Perez el al., 2009).

Fully-Differential operation reduces charge injection errors, makes easier the sum and subtraction operations and allows rail-to-rail input swing. The scheme is reconfigurable in terms of input gain (through programmable input capacitances C_{var}), resolution (controlling the number of performed iterations) and sampling frequency (through the frequency of the input clock).

The current bias of the operational amplifier is also programmed depending on the chosen configuration for the ADC in order to optimize the overall power consumed. Once a configuration has been selected, this current is also dynamically controlled during the conversion operation in order to adapt it to the residual reference voltage, which is smaller each time. Fig. 7 illustrates how the bias current is successively adapted along the conversion.

The schematic of the S&H operation is shown in Fig. 8c. This operation is performed during the first three cycles of the conversion. During the first one, the fully-differential input signal is stored on the programmable capacitor C_{var}. The next two cycles are used to transfer the stored charge on the integrator. This configuration is insensitive to parasitic capacitances (Johns and Martin, 1997).

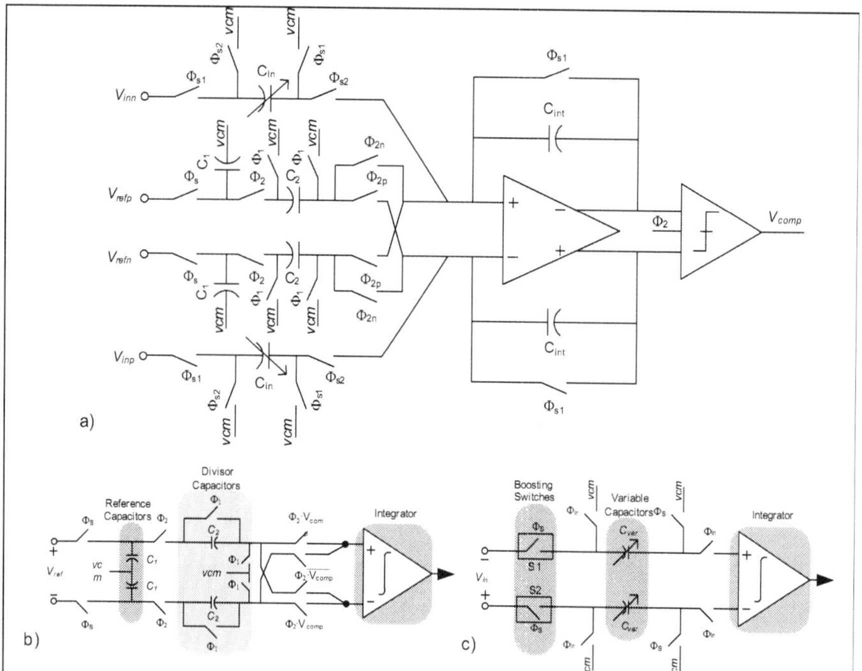

Fig. 8. Reconfigurable SC-based ADC: a) Schematic, b) Division-by-two, c) Programmable Gain Amplifier S&H

As the value of the capacitor C_{var} is reconfigurable, this architecture can be used as a Programmable Gain Amplifier, which is very useful for the biomedical interfaces as the amplitude of the input signal can vary along time.

The reference voltage division is made capacitively as Fig. 8b shows. During the first periods, the reference voltage is stored on the capacitor C_1. After that, during phase Φ_2, half of the charge is transferred to capacitor C_2 and it is either summed or subtracted to the integrated value depending on the value of the signal V_{comp}. During the phase Φ_1, capacitor C_2 is reset.

The schematic of the fully differential operational amplifier is shown in Fig. 9a. It follows a folded-cascode architecture where the transistors M2 and M3 of the input differential pair are biased in weak inversion in order to get the best g_m / I_D ratio (Enz et al., 1995). Transistors M1, M4, M5, M10 and M11, which are current mirrors, are biased in the saturation region of strong inversion in order to improve their mismatch. The width of these transistors can be programmed in order to get the dynamic bias control.

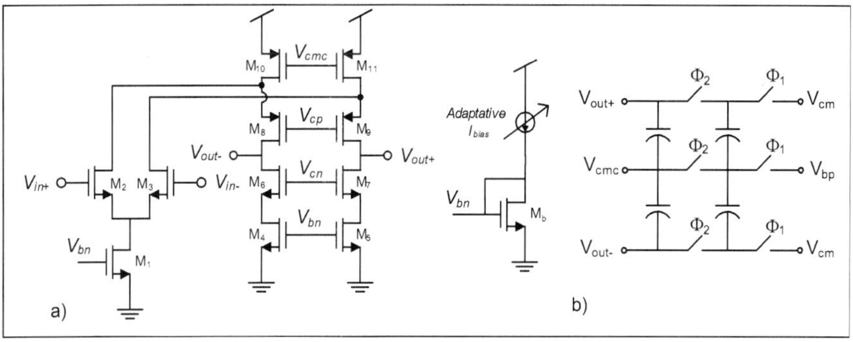

Fig. 9. a) Schematic of the folded-cascode opamp, b) SC common-mode feedback

The schematic of the capacitive common-mode control circuit in presented in Fig. 9b. This circuit controls the common-mode voltage through the control of the gate voltage of transistors M10 and M11 (Gray et al., 2001). The use of a capacitive-based configuration allows the minimization of the power consumption.

3. Basic building blocks design

3.1 Comparator

The comparator is a key block in any of the presented ADCs and one of the biggest power consumers, so its design must be carefully done in order to optimize the power consumption without a degradation in the performance of the ADC.

Many published SAR ADCs use a simple current-controlled dynamic latch as a comparator (Scott et al., 2003, Zou et al., 2009). Although these solutions are very attractive because of their low power consumption, they can present a DC offset of around 10mV due to the mismatch of their input differential pair, which imply an offset error in the performance of the ADC too. Considering that the circuit operates from rail-to-rail, this error means a loss in the input range of the converter.

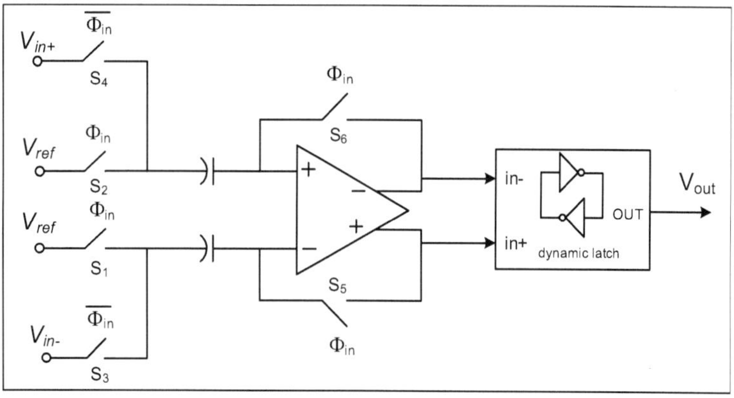

Fig. 10. Schematic of the comparator with an autozeroed pre-amplifier

Fig. 10 shows the schematic of the proposed comparator, which solves the offset problem. The comparator consists on a fully differential pre-amplifier stage with a cancellation offset scheme followed by a current-controlled dynamic-latch that boosts the pre-amplified difference to the rails. The auto-zeroing is achieved by closing a unity gain loop around it and storing the offset voltage on the input capacitors (Rodriguez-Perez et al., 2009). The gain of the pre-amplifier should be high enough in order to save the input voltage offset of the dynamic-latch.

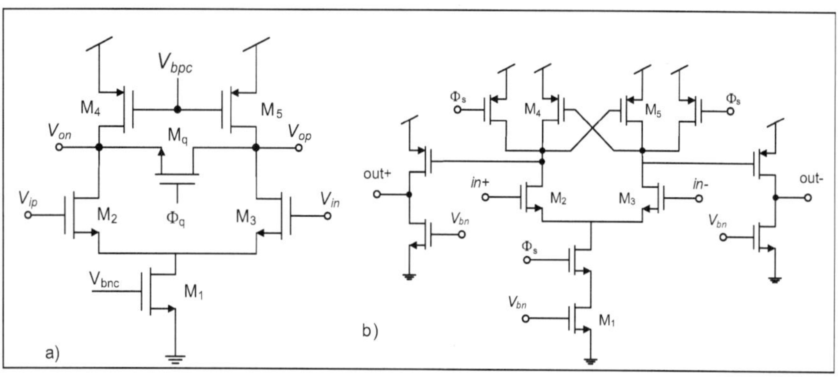

Fig. 11. a) Schematic of the pre-amplifier, b) Schematic of the dynamic-latch

The schematic of the pre-amplifier is shown in Fig. 11a. It is a single differential pair with a SC-based common-mode control circuit. In order to maximize the transconductance of the input differential pair and their matching, transistors M2 and M3 work in weak inversion. The rest of the transistors, which work as current mirrors, are in the saturation region to improve their matching.

The schematic of the dynamic-latch is presented in Fig. 11b. It is formed by an input differential pair which imbalances a pair of cross-coupled inverters, creating a positive feedback that boost the outputs to the rails. Current-controlled digital buffers are connected

at the outputs before an RS latch that gives the digital single-ended output of the comparator.
In order to optimize the power consumption of the comparator, the minimum required bias current for the pre-amplifier has to be evaluated. The design of the pre-amplifier will depend on the minimum input voltage needed at the input of the dynamic latch to counteract the offset voltage. It means that the dynamic gain of the pre-amplifier must be:

$$A_{pre} > \frac{V_{off_{latch}}}{\frac{LSB}{2}} = 2^{N+1} \cdot V_{off_{latch}}, \tag{14}$$

where $V_{off_{latch}}$ is the offset voltage of the dynamic latch and N is the required resolution. Considering that the dynamic gain of the pre-amplifier for a period T_S is approximated by:

$$A_{pre} = g_m \cdot \frac{T_S}{C_p} \tag{15}$$

where C_p represents the parasitic capacitance at the output of the pre-amplifier, and g_m the transconductance of the input transistors.
Following the *EKV* model (Enz et al., 1995), the g_m / I_D expression for MOS transistors valid for all regions is given by:

$$\frac{g_m}{I_D} = \frac{1}{n \cdot U_T} \cdot \frac{2}{1+\sqrt{1+4 \cdot IC}}, \tag{16}$$

where n is the slope factor, U_T is the thermal voltage and IC is the inversion coefficient, given by:

$$IC = \frac{I_D}{2n\mu C'_{ox}\left(\frac{W}{L}\right)U_T}. \tag{17}$$

Depending on the value of this coefficient, the transistor will work in weak inversion ($IC < 0.1$), moderate inversion ($0.1 < IC < 10$), or strong inversion ($IC > 10$). To obtain the optimum g_m / I_D ratio, we will dimension the transistors to work in weak inversion.
Then, considering equations (14)-(16) we have that:

$$I_D > \frac{2^{N+1} \cdot V_{offset} \cdot nU_T\left(1+\sqrt{1+4 \cdot IC}\right)}{2 \cdot T_S} \tag{18}$$

For a standard technology, normal values are n=7, U_T=27mV, C_p=250fF and IC=0.1. Using this values and the needed sampling frequency in equation (18) gives us the minimum required bias current for the pre-amplifier.

3.2 Boosted switch

In order to get rail-to-rail input voltage swing, the input switch must be boosted in order to avoid a degradation of the signal due to the dependence of the switch resistance with the input voltage, especially when the input frequency is near to Nyquist.

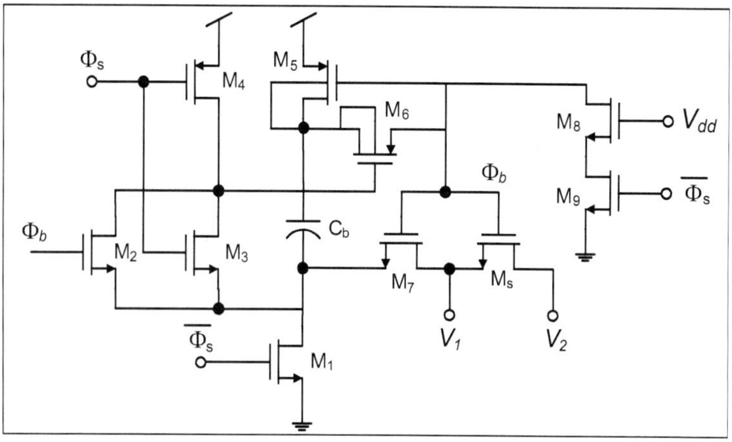

Fig. 12. Schematic of the boosting switch

The schematic of the boosted switch is shown in Fig. 12 (Dessouky and Kaiser, 1999). The circuit works as follows. When $\Phi_{sw}=0$, the supply capacitor C_b is charged to V_{DD}-V_{thp}. In the next phase, when Φ_{sw} switches on, this stored value is added to the input voltage to set the gate voltage Φ_{sw} of the input switch, M_S, which ensures a constant conductance of the input transistor during the sampling phase.

3.3 SAR logic

The Successive Approximation algorithm starts with the activation of the MSB while the others remain to zero. While the conversion is running, the rest of the bits are successively activated, while the value of the one who was activated just before will depend on the result of the comparator.

The schematic of the logic that implements the Successive Approximation operation is shown in Fig. 13a.

This architecture is based on the dependency of the state of each bit with the others bits state (Rossi and Fucili, 1996). Each bit evaluates the state of the others and in function of the result, it decides either it has to be activated, keeps its value, or take the value of the comparator.

The logic is implemented using a cascade of N+1 multiple input shift registers (Fig. 13b). Through a multiplexer and a decoder, each register (k^{th}) can choose three data inputs coming from: the output of the $(k+1)^{th}$ flip-flop, the output of the comparator or itself output. This selection will depend on itself state and the state of the following registers states.

With only 11 flips-flops to complete a 10-bits conversion, this architecture consumes nearly a forty percent less than others more popular (Anderson, 1972), which need 22 flip-flops to perform the same operation.

3.4 Current reference generator circuit

In order to generate on-chip the bias current needed for the active blocks, some current reference generator cell is needed. The non-resistance Oguey based cell shown in Fig. 14 is a good solution.

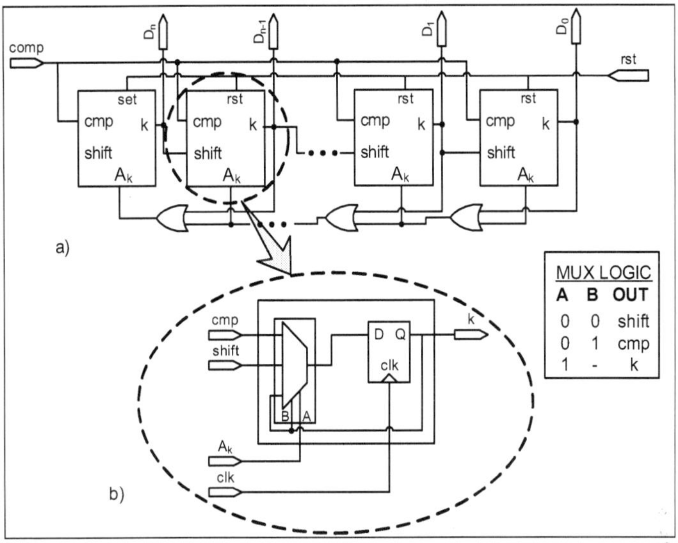

Fig. 13. Schematic of the Succesive Approximation Logic

The cell is based on the circuit presented in (Oguey and Aebischer, 1997), where the resistor has been replaced by an nMOS transistor working below saturation. The added transistors M2 and M1 provide the gate voltage for M3.

The generated current reference Iref is given by:

$$I_{ref} = n^2 \cdot \beta_{n3} \cdot V_T^2 \cdot K_{eff} \,, \quad K_{eff} = \left[K_2 - \frac{1}{2} + \sqrt{K_2 (K_2 - 1)} \right] \cdot \left(\ln (K_1) \right)^2 \tag{19}$$

where $K_1 = \dfrac{S_{M4} \cdot S_{M7}}{S_{M6} \cdot S_{M5}}$ and $K_2 = \dfrac{S_{M3} \cdot S_{M2}}{S_{M1} \cdot S_{M5}}$, being S_{Mx} the *W/L* ratio of the transistor M_x.

It is also important to include a start-up circuit to the current reference circuit in order to bring out the reference circuit from a zero current operation point to its normal operation point, like the presented in Fig. 14. It also provides the possibility of leaving the circuit on a standby mode (Mandal et al., 2006).

4. Simulation and experimental results

In order to validate the theoretical study done along the chapter, two different designs have been implemented and validated.

4.1 A 1-V, 10-bit, 2kS/s SAR ADC with a BWAC architecture capacitive DAC

The SAR ADC was implemented in a 0.35um CMOS standard technology with a resolution of 10-bit, 2kS/s of sampling frequency and 1-V of voltage supply. It uses a BWAC architecture for the implementation of the capacitive-based DAC.

The layout of the ADC can be seen in Fig. 15.

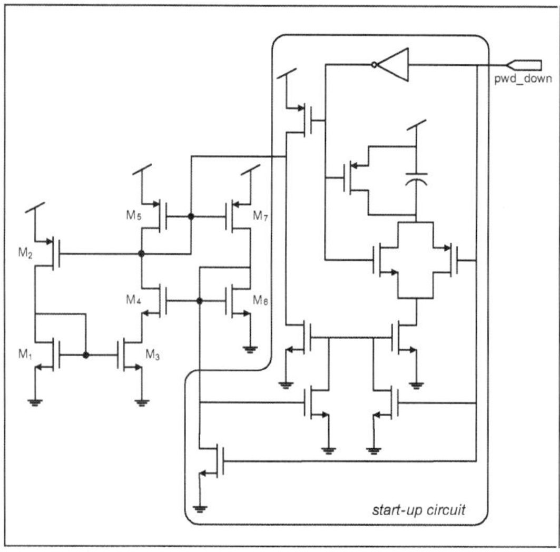

Fig. 14. Schematic of the current reference and start-up circuit

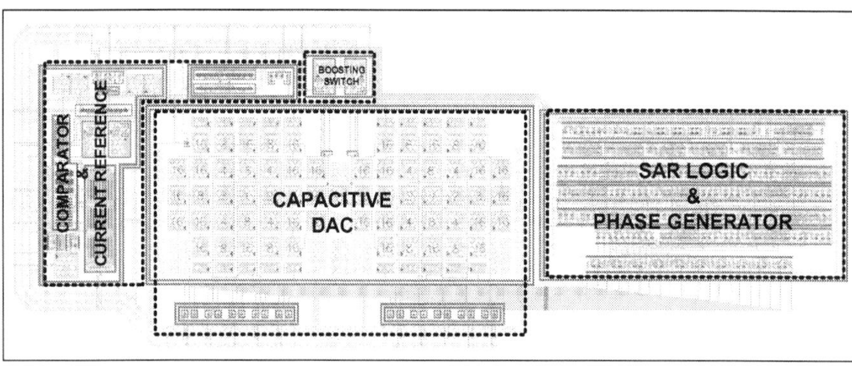

Fig. 15. Layout of the SAR ADC with capacitive DAC

Table 1 summarises the measured results of the integrated SAR ADC for the nominal conditions. The Equivalent Number of Bits (ENOB) is defined as:

$$ENOB = \frac{SNDR - 1.76}{6.02} \tag{20}$$

Fig. 16 shows the 8192-samples FFT of the ADC output response for a 140-Hz sinusoidal input signal of 1-V amplitude sampled at 2kHz at 1-V supply. The Signal to Noise Distorsion Ratio (SNDR) of 58.39dB, which gives a ENOB of 9.41-bits.

Fig. 16a compares the performance of the circuit for different input frequencies, supply voltages and sampling frequencies configurations. As can be extracted from the given graph, the ADC can work under a high range of supply voltages. This is extremely

Technology	CMOS 0.35μm
Nominal Voltage Supply	1-V
Input Voltage Range	Rail-to-Rail
Nominal Resolution	10-bits
Sampling Frequency	2kS/s - 8kS/s
SNDR (300Hz Input tone)	58.40dB
ENOB (300Hz Input tone)	9.4-bits
INL	< ±0.8LSB
DNL	-0.7<*DNL*<0.2 LSB
Power consumption (2kS/s mode) Without Current Reference With Current Reference	 130nW 250nW
Area occupation	0.212mm^2

Table 1. Measured Results of the SAR ADC

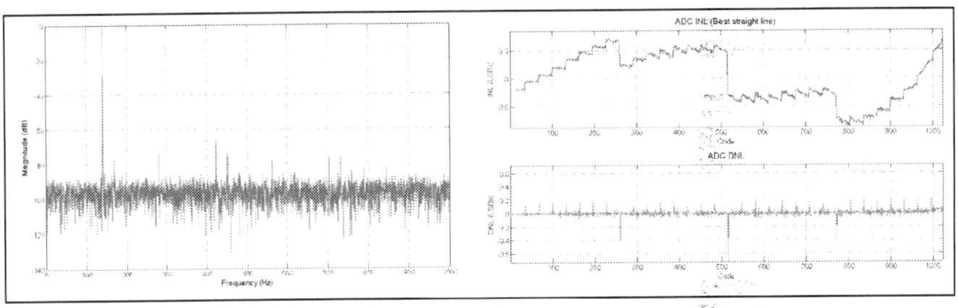

Fig. 16. a) FFT-response of the SAR ADC, b) DNL and INL response of the SAR ADC

important in biomedical wireless sensors, which voltage supply sources are weak and can present high variations. The frequency of the input signals can vary through the entire Nyquist band with a minimum loss of resolution. The ADC can be programmed to work under different sampling frequencies with a similar performance.

The integral nonlinearity (INL) and differential nonlinearity (DNL) plots are shown in Fig. 16b. The major errors in the INL and DNL curves are in the codes 256, 512 and 768, where the MSBs change. These linearity errors are due to the mismatch because of the lack of dummy capacitors. The measured INL and DNL are within $\pm 0.8LSB$ and $-0.7 < DNL < 0.2$, respectively.

The power consumption was measured using a 10fA-resolution picoamperimeter. These measures showed that the power consumption of the complete system including the current generation cell and the clock generation circuitry is 250nW for 1-V supply and 2kS/s sampling mode, while the consumption of the ADC without the current generation cell is 130nW.

An interesting study comes from the comparison of the two different designs included in the integration, the one with dummy capacitors and the other without them. Following post-layout simulations, the parasitic capacitances introduced by the dummy capacitors

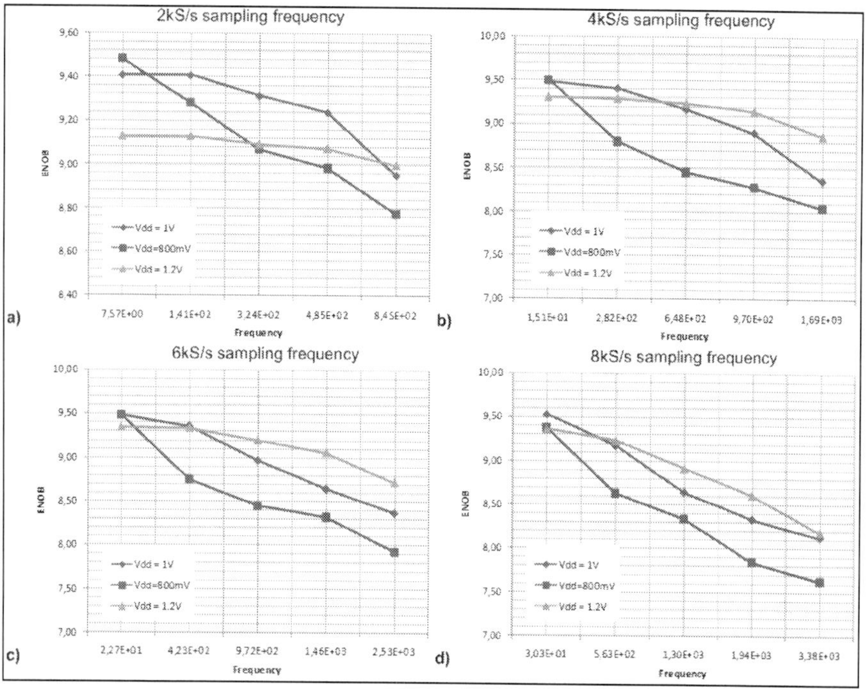

Fig. 17. Evolution of the resolution of the ADC with the input frequency for different voltage supplies under different sampling frequencies: a) 2kS/s, b) 4kS/s, c) 6kS/s, d) 8kS/s

should affect the behaviour of the ADC, degrading its resolution and linearity. This was validated in the experimental measurements, as Fig. 18 illustrate. The solution that included dummies presented higher harmonics than the other. Also, the parasitic capacitances introduced by the dummies capacitors induce higher errors in the INL and DNL than those due to the mismatch of the unitary capacitors of the capacitive array.

These linearity errors induce losses of more than 0.2-bits ENOB, as was predicted by the post-layout simulation results.

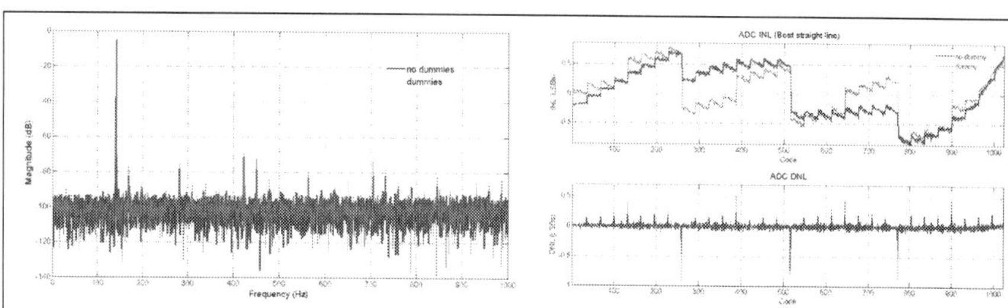

Fig. 18. Comparison of performance of the SAR ADC with and without dummies: a) FFT-response, b) INL and DNL

4.2 A 1.2-V, 10-bit reconfigurable SC-based ADC

The Reconfigurable ADC based on a Binary Search Algorithm with SC techniques was designed in a standard CMOS 130nm technology. The ADC is reconfigurable in terms of input gain (from 0.5 to 4 by means of 2-bits) and sampling frequency (from 10kS/s to 100kS/s). The power consumption is adapted to the chosen configuration in order to optimize it, and varies between 200nW to 2uW.

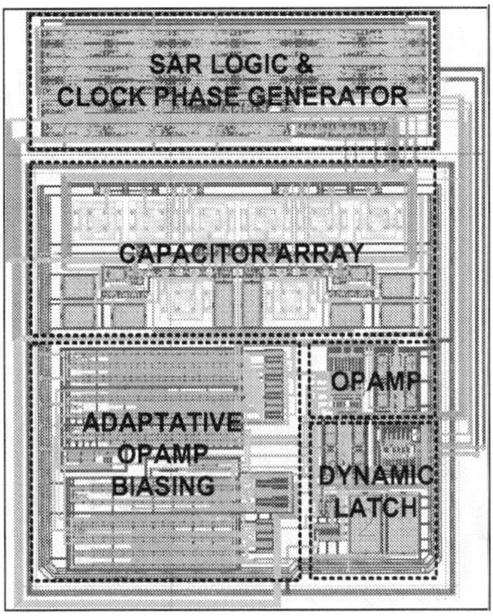

Fig. 19. Layout of the SC-based ADC

The layout of the complete ADC is presented in Fig. 19. It occupies an area of 190um x 225um.

Technology	CMOS 0.13μm
Nominal Voltage Supply	1.2-V
Input Voltage Range	Rail-to-Rail
Nominal Resolution	10-bits
Sampling Frequency	10kS/s - 100kS/s
SNDR	60.76dB
ENOB	9.8-bits
Power consumption 10kS/s 100kS/s	 200nW 2uW
Area occupation	0.043mm^2

Table 2. Performance summary of the SC-based ADC

Post-layout simulations with Process, Voltage and Temperature (PVT) variations were performed to validate the design. Table 2 summarises the main characteristics of the ADC, while Fig. 20a and Fig. 20b present the FFT-spectrum response for small and Nyquist sinusoidal inputs frequencies sampled at 20kS/s and 90kS/s, respectively. Simulation results show a SNDR of 60.76dB, which gives an ENOB of 9.8-bits.

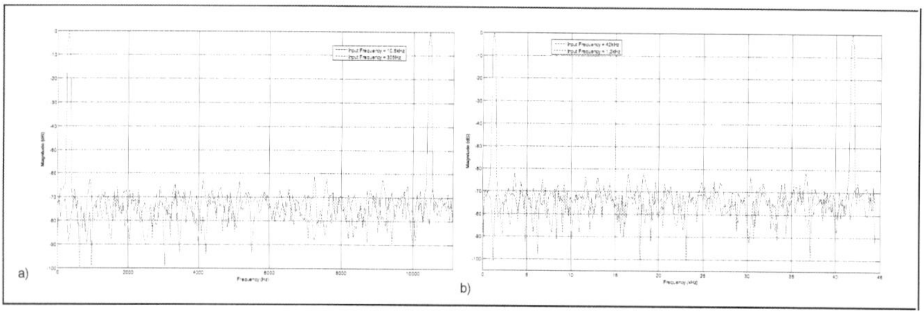

Fig. 20. FFT-response of the SC-based ADC for small and Nyquist frequency sinusoidal inputs sampled at: a) 20kS/s, b) 90kS/s.

5. Conclusions

This chapter have introduced the main concepts concerning to the design of ADC for biomedical interfaces, where two main architectures have been studied, concluding with the presentation and results of some real implementations.

The chapter has studied the most important design concerns of the Successive Approximation Architecture with capacitive DACs, one of the most popular ones. This architecture is very useful in a biomedical contest due to its low area and low power consumption. However, the implementation of this structures can derivate some problems related to their high sensitivity to parasitic capacitances and their high area and switching energy demand, especially when the resolution became higher than 8-bits.

The presented example includes a 10-bit SAR ADC with a capacitive-based DAC using a Binary Weighted Array with an attenuation capacitor to reduce the size of the matrix. The importance of the parasitic capacitances effect over other non-idealities was shown by means of two different implementations, one using a capacitive array with dummies an another one without them. As the first one presented more parasitic capacitances, experimental results showed that its performance was more degraded than in the case of the second one implementation without dummies, unless the mismatch of this latter was worse.

Due to some of the drawbacks of the of the SAR architecture, we have introduced in this chapter another proposal based on the Binary Search Algorithm too, but using an implementation based on SC-techniques. This architecture results highly flexible as it can be easily reconfigured in terms of resolution, sampling frequency and input gain. Also, the area occupation and switching power demand is dramatically reduced due to the elimination of the big capacitive arrays needed in the SAR capacitive DACs based architectures.

6. References

Anderson, T. O. (1972). Optimum control logic for successive approximation A-D converters. *Computer Design,* vol. 11, no. 7, July 1972, pp. 81-86.

Agnes, A.; Bonizzoni, P. ; Malcovati, P. and Maloberti, F. (2008). A 9.4-ENOB 1V 3.8uW 100kS/s SAR ADC with Time-Domain Comparator, *Proceedings of International Solid-State Circuits Conference*, pp. 246-247, San Francisco, February 2008.

Cong, L. (2001). Pseudo C-2C Ladder-Based Data Converter Technique. *IEEE Transactions on Circuits and Systems II*, vol. 48, no. 10, October 2001, pp. 927-929.

Dessouky, M. and Kaiser, A. (1999). Input switch configuration suitable for rail-to-rail operation of switched opamp circuits. *Electronic Letters*, vol. 35, January 1999, pp. 8-10.

Enz, C. C. ; Krummernacher, F. and Vittoz, E. A. (1995). An Analytical MOS Transistor Model Valid for All Regions of Operation and Dedicated to Low-Voltage Low-Current Applications. *Analog Integrated Circuits and Signal Processing Journal*, vol. 8, July 1995, pp. 83-114.

Gray, P. R. ; Hurst, P. J. ; Lewis, S. L. and Meyer, R. G. (2001). *Analog Design of Analog Integrated Circuits, 4th Edition*. John Wiley & Sons, ISBN 0-471-32168-0, New York, USA.

Harrison, R. R. ; Watkins, P. T. ; Kier, R. J. ; Lovejoy, R. O. ; Black, D. J. ; Greger, B. and Solzbacher (2007). A Low-Power Integrated Circuit for Wireless 100-Electrode Neural Recording System. *IEEE Journal of Solid-State Circuits*, vol. 42, no. 1, January 2007, pp. 123-132.

Hong, H. C. and Lee, G. M. (2007). A 65fJ/Conversion-Step 0.9-V 200kS/s Rail-to-Rail 8-bit Successive Approximation ADC. *IEEE Journal of Solid-State Circuits*, vol. 42, October 2007, pp. 2161-2168.

Johns, D. and Martin, K. (1997). *Analog Integrated Circuit Design*. John Wiley & Sons, ISBN 0471144487, New York, USA.

Maloberti, F. (2007). *Data Converters*. Springer Publishers, ISBN 0-387-32485-2, Dordrecht, The Netherlands.

Mandal, S. ; Arfin, S. and Sarpeshkar, R. (2006). Fast Startup CMOS Current References, *Proceedings of International Symposium on Circuits and Systems*, pp. 2845-2848, Greece, May 2006.

Northrop, R. B. (2001), *Non-Invasive Instrumentation and Measurements in Medical Diagnosis*. CRC Press LLC, ISBN 0-8493-0961-1, Boca Raton, Florida.

Northrop, R. B. (2004), *Analysis and Application of Analog Electronic Circuits to Biomedical Instrumentation*. CRC Press LLC, ISBN 0-8493-2143-3, Boca Raton, Florida.

Oguey, H. J. and Aebischer, D. (1997). CMOS Current Reference Without Resistance. *IEEE Journal of Solid-State Circuits*, vol. 32, no. 7, July 1997, pp. 1132-1135.

Rodriguez-Perez, A. ; Delgado-Restituto, M. ; Medeiro, F. and Rodriguez-Vazquez, A. (2009). A low-power Reconfigurable ADC for Biomedical Sensor Interfaces, *Proceedigns of Biomedical Circuits and Systems Conference*, pp. 253-256, Beijing, November 2009.

Rodriguez-Perez, A. ; Delgado-Restituto, M. and Medeiro, F. (2010). Impact of parasitic capacitances on the performance of SAR ADCs based on capacitive arrays, *Proceedings of Latin-American Symposium on Circuits and Systems*, Iguazú, February 2010.

Rossi, A. and Fucili, G. (1996). Nonredundant successive approximation register for A/D converters. *Electronic Letters*, vol. 32, no. 12, June 1996, pp. 1055-1057.

Sauerbrey, J. ; Schmitt-Landsiedel, D. and Thewes, R. (2003). A 0.5-V 1-uW Successive Approximation ADC. *IEEE Journal of Solid-State Circuits*, vol. 38, July 2003, pp. 1261-1265.

Scott, M. D. ; Boser, B. E. and Pister, K. S. J. (2003). An ultralow-energy ADC for smart dust. *IEEE Journal of Solid-State Circuits*, vol. 38, July 2003, pp. 1123-1129.

Verma, N. and Chandrakasan, A. P. (2007). An Ultra Low Energy 12-bit Rate-Resolution Scalable SAR ADC for Wireless Sensor Nodes. *IEEE Journal of Solid-State Circuits*, vol. 42, June 2007, pp. 1196-1205.

Zou, X. ; Xu, X. ; Yao, L. and Lian, Y. (2009). A 1-V 450-nW Fully Integrated Programmable Biomedical Sensor Interface Chip. *IEEE Journal of Solid-State Circuits*, vol. 44, no. 4, April 2009, pp. 1067-1077.

11

Cuff Pressure Pulse Waveforms: Their Current and Prospective Application in Biomedical Instrumentation

Milan Stork[1] and Jiri Jilek[2]
[1]*University of West Bohemia, Plzen*
[2]*Carditech, Culver City, California*
[1]*Czech Republic*
[2]*USA*

1. Introduction

Use of the arterial pulse in the evaluation of disease states has a long history. Examination of the arterial pulse is recorded by historians as being an essential part of ancient Chinese, Indian, and Greek medicine. Palpation of the pulse was very much a part of the "art" of medicine with a bewildering array of terminologies. The first accurate recording of the arterial pulse in man was performed by Etienne Jules Marey in the nineteenth century. Marey (Marey, 1881) developed a series of mechanical devices used to noninvasively record the radial pulse in humans for physiological and clinical studies. His device for the recording the peripheral arterial pulse, the sphygmogram, was soon taken up by leading clinicians of the day, who considered the contours of the arterial pulse waveform to be important for diagnosing clinical hypertension. Interest developed in detecting the onset of hypertension in asymptomatic individuals. The principal means of doing this in the late nineteenth century was using a variety of types of sphygmographs to record the arterial pulse in a wide range of asymptomatic individuals. For the first time in history, the range of contours of the human arterial pulse was recorded and interpreted.

In 1886, Marey placed the forearm and hand in a water-filled chamber to which a variable counter-pressure was applied. The counter-pressure for maximum pulse wave amplitude detected in the chamber determined that the vessel walls were maximally relieved of tension at that counter-pressure. When counter pressure was increased or decreased, the amplitudes of pulsations in the chamber decreased. This process was called *vascular unloading*.

In the early twentieth century the Italian physician Riva-Rocci invented the cuff sphygmograph (Riva-Rocci, 1896). Riva-Rocci used palpation to determine the systolic pressure. The cuff sphygmograph was later improved by the use of Korotkoff sounds that were discovered by Korotkov (Korotkov, 1956). The use of Korotkoff sounds made the sphygmomanometer much simpler to use and allowed the clinician to base diagnosis and treatment on just two numbers, the systolic and diastolic pressures, rather than requiring the rigors of arterial waveform interpretation. The cuff sphygmomanometer was rapidly introduced into clinical practice and replaced the sphygmogram as part of the evaluation of hypertension. The reliance on the maximum and minimum values of arterial pressure, with the abandonment of interpretation within these two limits, occurred just at the time when interpretation of electrocardiographic waveforms as an important part of clinical assessment was increasing in popularity. The application of arterial pressure wave to clinical hypertension languished until the 1980s. Recordings of the ascending aortic pressure wave in individuals of varying ages and levels of blood pressures were made by Murgo in 1980 (Murgo et al, 1980) and Takazawa in 1986 (Takazawa, 1987). Such studies have led to a reawakening of interest in pressure wave contour analysis in essential hypertension. Until this recent reemergence of interest in waveform contours, pressure data obtained invasively was still largely interpreted in terms of the systolic and diastolic pressures between which the pressure wave fluctuated. There have, however, been some instances where the pressure wave contour has been utilized in the clinical evaluation. In the Framingham Study, plethysmographic volume waveforms were recorded noninvasively, using a cuff placed around the finger. In this study in over 1,000 individuals, the investigators focused their attention on the descending part of the waveform. They showed that with increasing age there was a decreasing prevalence of the diastolic wave with a less clearly defined dicrotic notch than in young individuals. In addition to an age relationship, the investigators also noted a correlation between waveform contour and the clinical incidence of coronary heart disease.

In the late twentieth century, a noninvasive method called *applanation tonometry* (Kelly et al, 1989) was used by increasing number of researchers interested in pressure waveform contours. The method uses a pencil-shaped tonometer to obtain pressure waveforms. Skilled application of the tonometer is required to obtain correct waveforms. Most published studies have used waveforms obtained from the radial artery at the wrist. By mathematical manipulation of the waveforms, it was possible to obtain an approximation of the aortic pressure (Cameron et al, 1998). O'Rourke found alterations in the tonometric waveforms with age similar to the findings of the Framingham Study.

Pulsations in the blood pressure cuff were first observed by Riva-Rocci. He called them *oscillations*. They were much later used to develop a simple, noninvasive method for the determination of blood pressures. Vascular unloading first noted by Marey became the basis for the *oscillometric* method of automatic blood pressure determination. Posey and Geddes showed in 1969 (Posey & Geddes, 1969) that the maximum amplitude of cuff pulse waveforms corresponded to true mean arterial pressure (MAP). When pressure in the cuff was increased above MAP and then decreased below MAP, the waveform amplitudes decreased. Cuff pressure (CP) and wrist cuff waveforms (WW) acquired during a gradual CP deflation procedure are shown in Fig. 1. The waveforms appear at the beginning of the procedure and reach maximum amplitude at the point of MAP. From MAP to the end of the procedure the WW amplitudes decrease.

Electronic oscillometric instruments capable of determining the systolic (SBP), mean (MAP), and diastolic arterial pressure (DBP) started appearing on the market in the 1970s. Microprocessors facilitated algorithmic methods for the determination of SBP and DBP. One of the first descriptions of a microprocessor-based device appeared in 1978 (Looney, 1978) and many more automatic BP devices have been introduced since. The exact nature of their algorithmic methods is mostly unknown because the algorithms are considered proprietary and are kept secret. The few published algorithms are based on processing the amplitudes rather than contours of the cuff pressure pulsations. One could speculate that the misleading term *oscillations* caused the lack of attention to their contours. The term oscillations first used by Riva-Rocci appears to have been accepted without much investigation into the true nature of cuff pulsations.

Periodic waveforms usually generated by an oscillator are normally called oscillations. Pulsations generated by a beating heart are not oscillations. The terms arterial waveforms and pulse waveforms are standard terms used when contours of arterial pulsations along the arterial tree are described. Arterial waveforms acquired by several noninvasive methods have been accepted into the family of hemodynamic waveforms. The above mentioned finger cuff, finger plethysmograph, and aplanation tonometer waveforms have been analyzed more comprehensively than brachial or wrist cuff waveforms.

In the course of past several years we studied cuff pulse waveforms and noticed that under certain conditions they are similar to arterial waveforms acquired by other methods. With the aid of specially designed experimental data acquisition and processing systems we were able to gain more understanding of the cuff pressure pulse waveforms.

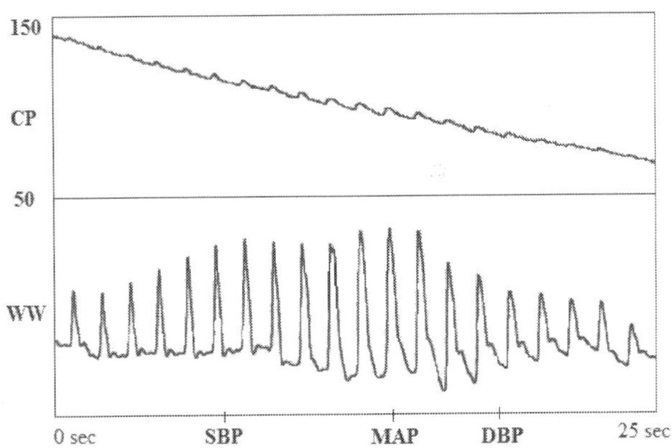

Fig. 1. Cuff pressure (CP) and wrist waveforms (WW) derived from CP. Systolic blood pressure (SBP) and diastolic pressure (DBP) reference points were determined by auscultation.

2. Description of the data acquisition and processing systems

The original wrist cuff system (Jilek & Stork, 2003) was conceived ten years ago. The system consists of a compact, battery powered module, a wrist cuff, and a notebook computer. Fully automatic operation of the system is controlled by the computer and a test takes less than one minute. Block diagram of the module and the cuff is in Fig. 2. The module's microcontroller (Intel 87C51) communicates with the notebook via serial interface (USB). The notebook controls inflation and deflation of the cuff and acquisition of data. Operation of the system starts with cuff inflation to about 30 mmHg above expected SBP. Cuff pressure is converted to analog voltage by pressure sensor (piezoresistive bridge type, range 0-250 mmHg). The analog voltage is amplified by an instrumentation amplifier (Burr-Brown INA118) and filtered by a low-pass filter with cutoff frequency of 35 Hz. The pressure voltage is digitized by a 12-bit A/D converter with serial output (MAX1247). The A/D converter operation is controlled by the microcontroller.

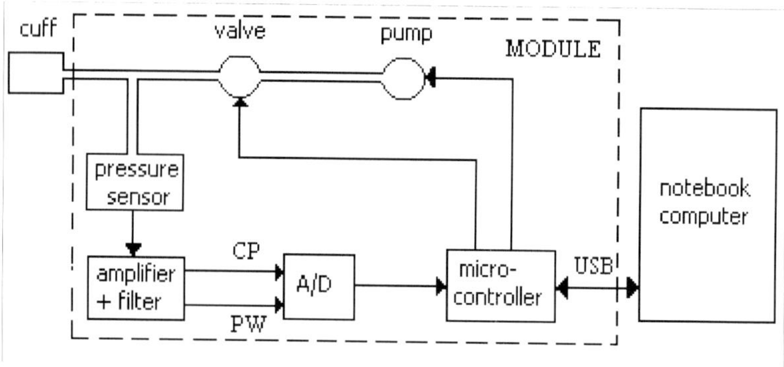

Fig. 2. Block diagram of single cuff system for acquisition and processing of wrist cuff waveforms.

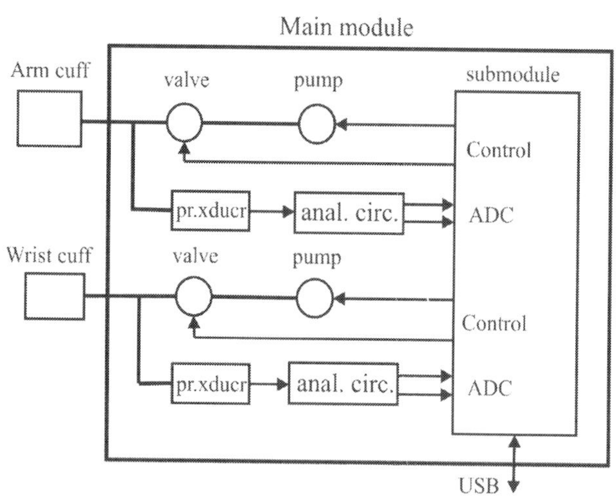

Fig. 3. Block diagram of the dual cuff system.

Sampling rate is 85 samples per second. The digitized samples are sent to the notebook at 11.6 ms intervals. The deflation of the cuff is controlled by a current controlled air-flow valve (Omron 608). Deflation rate is controlled by notebook software.

When cuff pressure drops below diastolic pressure, the valve opens and the cuff is rapidly deflated. Computation of blood pressures and hemodynamics takes place next. All functions and computations are performed by special software.

The need to improve the system led to the development of dual cuff system. The system consists of a compact module with pneumatic and electronic circuits, two detachable cuffs (arm and wrist), and a notebook computer that is connected to the module via a USB cable.

Block diagram of the module with two cuffs is in Fig. 3. The two pneumatic and analog circuits for the cuffs are similar. Pumps inflate the cuffs and cuff deflation is controlled by the valves. Piezoelectric pressure transducers (pr.xducr) provide analog signal that is amplified, filtered, and separated into two channels. One channel provides cuff pressure and the other channel provides amplified cuff-pressure waveforms. The analog circuits are close approximation of the single cuff system's circuit. The resulting analog signals are digitized in the ***submodule***. Analog-to-digital conversion is 12-bit, 85 conversions/ sec operation. The digitized data are converted into USB format and made available to the notebook. The notebook contains special software that controls the module's functions and receives four channels of digitized data. We designed the specialized software as Windows-based multifunction system that performs the following functions:

- **Dual-cuff test** - uses both the upper-arm and wrist cuffs. The arm cuff is used to acquire brachial cuff pressure pulses and the wrist cuff is used in a manner similar to a stethoscope; appearance of wrist-cuff pulses indicates SBP. SBP, MAP and DBP values are also determined by a commonly used ratiometric method from the arm cuff pulses.
- **Wrist-cuff test** - uses only wrist cuff pulses in a manner similar to the single cuff system. Blood pressures and hemodynamics are determined from wrist waveforms and body area.
- **Show waveforms** - shows waveforms from both cuffs (dual-cuff system) or only from wrist cuff. Each individual sample can be examined visually and numerically.
- **Show Quadrant** (wrist-cuff test only) - shows hemodynamics numerically and graphically (see Fig. 12 and Fig. 13).
- **Store test** - stores all raw data and subject name in a numbered file.
- **Get test** - gets raw data from disc file and performs computations.
- **Variables** - shows important computed variables.
- **Test directory** - shows test (file) numbers and subject names.

3. Characteristics of the cuff-pulse waveforms

Waveforms acquired from blood pressure cuffs exhibit characteristics that are similar to, but not the same as arterial waveforms acquired by other methods. Even waveforms acquired simultaneously, but from different anatomical sites are not identical. The brachial cuff and wrist cuff waveforms in Fig. 4 illustrate this assertion. The top trace shows the wrist waveforms (WW) and the bottom trace shows arm (brachial) waveforms (AW) acquired simultaneously with the dual cuff system from an adult volunteer in the sitting position. The waveforms were acquired at the cuff pressure (CP) just below the point of DBP. The wrist waveforms have more sharply defined contours when compared with the brachial waveforms. The dicrotic notches on the descending part of the waveforms are well defined on the wrist waveforms. The brachial waveforms are more rounded and the dicrotic notches are barely visible. We believe that larger volume of air in the brachial cuff and larger amount of soft tissue on the upper arm cause the substantial damping of brachial cuff waveforms. Smaller volume of air and relatively low amount of soft tissue make the wrist cuff waveforms better suited for waveform analysis. It is important to acquire the waveforms at CP lower than the point of DBP. The waveforms shown in Fig 5 illustrate the need for appropriate cuff pressure. The waveforms were acquired during a gradual cuff deflation as is done during automatic BP measurement.

The waveforms at cuff pressures above DBP are distorted because the radial artery is fully or partially occluded by the wrist cuff and blood flow under the cuff is turbulent. Turbulent blood flow is the source of Korotkoff sounds that are used in manual BP determination. When CP is lowered to pressures equal to or below DBP, the artery is no longer occluded, the waveforms are not distorted and Korotkoff sounds are no longer heard.

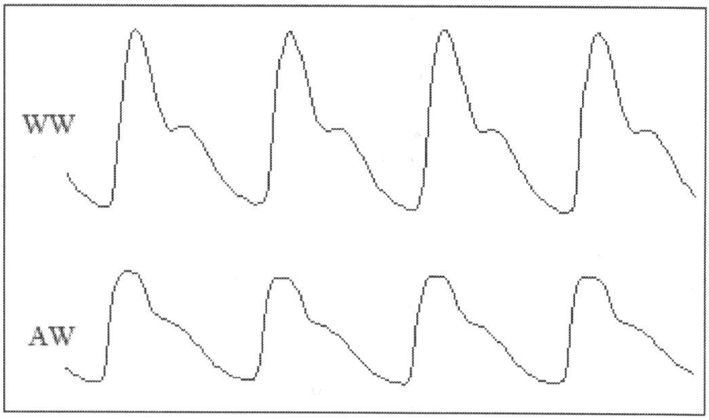

Fig. 4. Wrist waveforms (WW) and arm waveforms (AW) were acquired simultaneously.

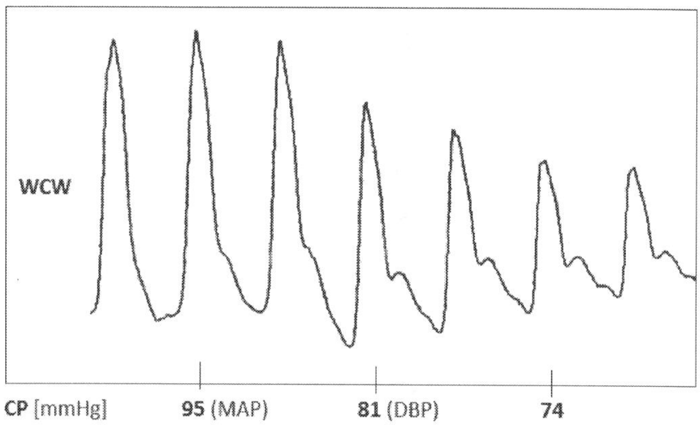

Fig. 5. Wrist cuff (WCW) waveforms acquired during a gradual cuff deflation. Cuff pressure decreases from left to right. The DBP reference point of 81 mmHg was determined by the manual method.

Wrist cuff waveforms acquired at DBP or lower CP are similar to waveforms obtained by other noninvasive methods. Fig. 6 shows wrist cuff waveforms (WCW) and finger photoplethysmograph (PPG) waveforms acquired simultaneously. Another example of noninvasive waveforms is in Fig. 7. The waveforms were acquired by applanation tonometry from the radial artery (wrist).

The waveforms shown in Fig. 6 and 7 are not identical but their contours are similar and they share some important characteristics. The important arterial waveform segments are rapid systolic upstroke, late-systolic downturn, dicrotic wave, and diastolic segment. Rapid systolic upstroke lasts approximately from the onset to the peak of the waveform. Late-systolic downturn lasts approximately from the peak to the dicrotic wave. Diastolic segment lasts from the dicrotic wave to the onset of the next systolic upstroke.

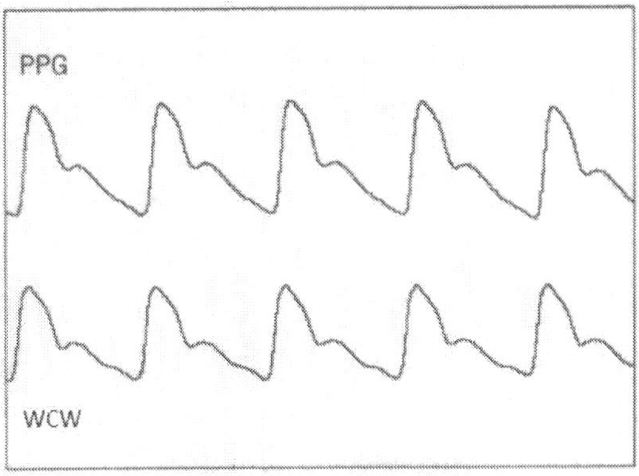

Fig. 6. Wrist cuff (WCW) and photoplethysmographic (PPG) waveforms were acquired simultaneously.

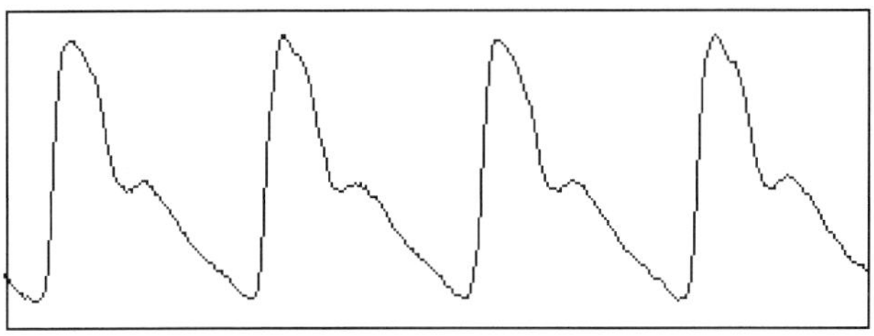

Fig. 7. Radial (wrist) waveforms acquired from the wrist by applanation tonometry.

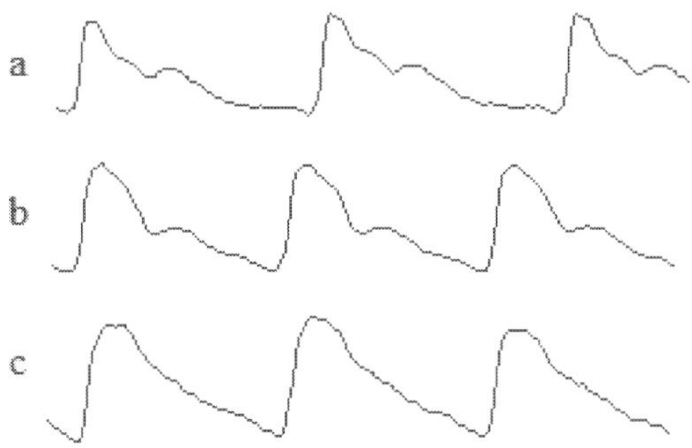

Fig. 8. Wrist cuff waveforms reflecting age differences.

Systolic upstroke, late-systolic downturn, dicrotic wave, and diastolic segment can be easily identified on all of the waveforms in Fig. 6-7. The waveforms are not, however, identical.

The reasons for differences in contour shapes are numerous and they include location on the arterial tree, arterial compliance, wave reflections, and subject's age. Age differences can be observed on the wrist cuff waveforms in Fig. 8. Waveforms from a young subject (a) have steeper systolic upstroke and more pronounced dicrotic wave than those of middle age (b) and elderly (c) subjects. Similar age-related changes were observed in tonometric radial waveform contours (Kelly et al, 1998).
The comparisons of wrist cuff waveforms with waveforms acquired by other methods led us to the conviction that the cuff waveforms are suitable for applications beyond blood pressure measurement.

4. Current and new methods using cuff pressure waveforms

Cuff pressure waveforms have been used almost exclusively in automatic BP monitors, where their amplitudes are the basis for algorithmic computations of SBP, MAP, DBP, and heart rate (HR). Cuff pressure waveforms contours have been largely ignored.

4.1 Current automatic blood pressure measurement

Automatic oscillometric BP monitors are the dominant types of noninvasive BP devices. There are many models on the market, ranging from professional monitors used in health care facilities to inexpensive monitors used in homes. Most home monitors are the upper-arm (brachial) type, but wrist monitors are gaining popularity. Finger cuff monitors are not recommended by professionals because of the accuracy issues. The main advantage of oscillometric BP monitors is their ease of use. Only the cuff must be applied to the appropriate physiological site. A typical automatic oscillometric device uses an air pump to inflate the cuff and cuff pressure is then slowly deceased. A pressure transducer is used to convert the cuff pressure into electronic signal. The signal is then amplified, filtered and the cuff pulsations are separated from the cuff pressure. The resulting cuff pulsation waveforms (see Fig. 1) are then used to algorithmically determine the pressures. Published algorithmic methods for the determination of SBP and DBP present differing approaches. Geddes makes certain empirical assumptions about algorithmic determination. His proposed algorithm is based on the ratio of waveform amplitudes. According to Geddes (Geddes, 1982), SBP corresponds to the point of 50% of maximum amplitude (MAP); for DBP, the ratio is 80%. Another proposed ratio algorithm (Sapinsky, 1992) uses the point of SBP at 40% of maximum amplitude and 75% of max. amplitude for DBP. Other algorithms for the determination of blood pressure are based on the change of slope in the waveform amplitude envelope. An article describing the function of an oscillometric BP device (Borow, 1982) claims that the device determines SBP as the point of the initial increase of the cuff pulsations. Another author (Ng, 1999) puts SBP on the minimal ascending slope of the amplitude envelope and DBP on the maximum slope of the descending envelope. The above algorithmic approaches result in differing SBP and DBP values. Furthermore, the approaches do not offer physiological explanation for their assertions. The only commonly recognized and physiologically verified variable is the MAP. Common to the published algorithms is that they use amplitudes of cuff pulsations. Little attention has been paid to the contours of these pulsations. Algorithms used in commercial monitors are generally considered intellectual property and are kept secret. This makes verification of accuracy difficult. There are several test instruments on the market, but they can perform only static tests, such as static pressure accuracy, leakage test, cuff deflation test, and overpressure test.

They cannot, however, perform dynamic algorithmic accuracy tests. No regulatory agency has put forth a standard as to how oscillometric pulse amplitudes should be interpreted to determine BP values. Because there are no reliable instruments for testing the dynamic accuracy of BP monitors, performance testing protocols for device validations have been developed. The Association for the Advancement of Medical Instrumentation, the British Hypertension Society, and the European Society of Hypertension recommend validation of NIBP devices against auscultation or against intra-arterial methods. Validation studies require recruitment of large number of volunteers with varied blood pressures, ages, and arm circumferences. These requirements inevitably make validation studies expensive.

Many validation studies have been conducted and some reviews of validation results have been published. Their findings indicate that the accuracy of BP determination is problematic for many NIBP devices. Validation protocols are not without problems either. A recently published study (Gerin et al, 2002) exposed limitations of current validation protocols. The study concludes that the existing protocols are likely to pass devices that can be systematically inaccurate for some patients. Disappointing validation results, lack of information from device manufacturers and errors observed in healthcare institutions have led to warnings issued by experts in the field of BP measurements. The American Heart Association issued an advisory statement from the Council for High Blood Pressure Research (Jones et al, 2001). The Council cautioned healthcare professionals not to abandon mercury sphygmomanometers until adequate replacement instruments are available. A recent report by a group of leading experts (Jones et al, 2003) stressed the importance of accurate BP measurements. The report called for additional research to assess accuracy of NIBP devices and concluded that mercury sphygmomanometer remains the gold standard for noninvasive BP measurement.

The above issues led us to investigations into prospective improvements of the cuff pulse based BP measurement and into applications reaching beyond BP measurement.

4.2 Database of physiological cuff pressure waveforms

Cuff pressure BP waveforms are indispensable for noninvasive determination of BPs and they may contain other useful information. An investigator or a device developer who wants to study cuff pressure waveforms needs a reasonably large database of waveforms and reference blood pressure measurements. Manufacturers of oscillometric BP devices must have such databases in order to conduct their development efficiently. These databases are, however, proprietary. There are no publicly accessible databases of cuff waveforms at the present time. On the other hand, public databases for some physiologic waveforms do exist, mainly for interpretation of electrocardiograms. General principles of acquisition and use of physiological waveforms are described in the Association for the Advancement of Medical Instrumentation Technical Information Report (AAMI, 1999). The report stresses the necessity to test algorithmic functions of digital devices with real physiologic data. Properly documented databases are needed for such testing. The waveforms can then be used to test devices repeatedly and reproducibly. A wide-ranging, publicly available database of oscillometric BP waveforms could advance the field of oscillometric BP measurement in the following ways:

- New research into the largely unknown physiological basis of oscillometric BP measurement. The research could result in the development of a generic algorithmic method for the determination of SBP and DBP.

- Device developers would enjoy the advantage of not having to develop their own proprietary databases, as the past and present manufacturers had to do. Costs of development and time to market could be decreased. A standardized, public database would serve as a common knowledge base and it should produce devices performing in a similar, predictable manner.
- Repeatable, reproducible performance testing of oscillometric BP devices could become possible. The expensive, time consuming testing as performed today could eventually be eliminated.
- Determination of hemodynamic variables. It may be possible to derive cardiac output (CO), total peripheral resistance, and arterial compliance from cuff pulse waveform contours and blood pressures. Several contour methods for CO determination already exist.

A specialized data acquisition system such as the dual cuff system we have developed could be used to build a database of cuff pressure waveforms.

	SBP [mmHg]	DBP [mmHg]
Reference BP	122	78
Geddes method	135	88
Sapinsky method	144	81

Table 1. Results of 2 algorithmic methods applied to data acquired for this study

The acquired cuff pulse and reference BP data can be used to test algorithms for BP determination (Jilek & Stork, 2005). The data acquired for this study were applied to 2 published algorithms. According to Geddes and Sapinsky, SBP and DBP can be determined as fixed ratios of OMW amplitudes. Geddes specifies 50 % of maximal OMW amplitude as the point of SBP; for DBP, the ratio is 80 %. Sapinsky specifies the ratio for SBP as 40 % of maximal OMW amplitude; for DBP the ratio is 55%. The results are shown in Table 1. Different SBP and DBP values obtained by reference measurement by auscultation and by the algorithmic methods are indicative of problems that exist in the field of oscillometric BP measurement.

Another important prospective database application is performance testing of oscillometric BP monitors. There are several commercial testing instruments on the market but they can perform only static tests of pressure sensors and amplifiers. Proper dynamic BP accuracy testing can be performed only by applying real physiological waveforms. Monitors equipped with suitable interfaces could be tested for dynamic accuracy. Such monitors do not exist today but in the future the interfaces could be incorporated reasonably easily. A BP monitor test system could be implemented with a notebook computer, a USB interface, a special software for CP and cuff pulse waveform processing, and the database stored on a CD-ROM. Monitor testing could be performed quickly and reproducibly.

The concept of a database of physiological cuff waveforms has two major advantages over currently used validations of automatic BP monitors: (1) the database needs to be developed only once and it can then be used quickly and repeatedly to test BP algorithms and to develop new ones; (2) automatic BP monitors could be equipped with interfaces allowing database waveforms to bench-test performance of monitors. Such testing is not presently possible. Expensive, time consuming monitor validations as performed today could be eventually eliminated.

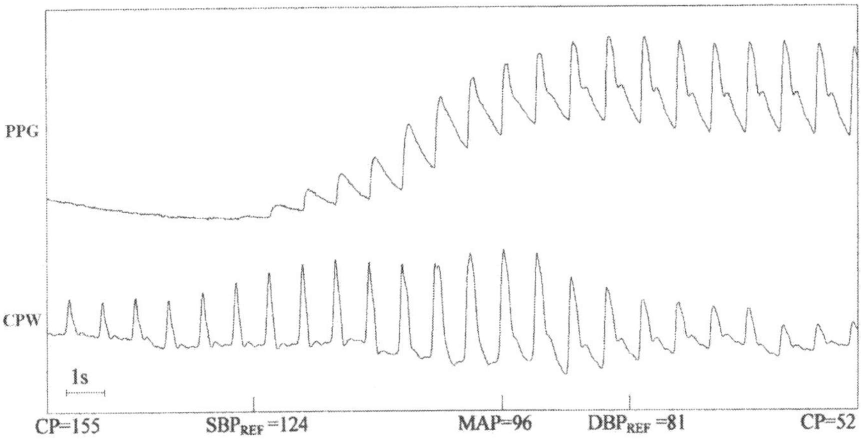

Fig. 9. Cuff pressure waveforms (CPW) and photoplethysmographic (PPG) waveforms were acquired simultaneously. Reference points SBP_{REF} and DBP_{REF} were determined manually.

4.3 Automatic BP determination based on physiological principles

A gradual wrist cuff deflation procedure was divided into four segments (Jilek & Fukushima, 2007). The following section contains description of CPW and PPG amplitude and shape changes and explanation of each phase in terms of vascular unloading and blood flow. The phases of Korotkoff sounds are mentioned where appropriate.

The first segment lasts from cuff pressure approximately 30 mmHg above SBP_{REF} to SBP_{REF} (Fig. 9). Cuff pressure waveforms (CPWs) are present because arterial pulsations are transmitted to the upper edge of the cuff. The CPW amplitudes increase according to vascular unloading as cuff pressure is deflated toward SBP_{REF}. No blood flows past the cuff and no Korotkoff sounds are heard. The PPG trace is flat because no flow signal passes past the cuff. The second segment lasts from SBP_{REF} to MAP. Turbulent blood flow starts passing under the cuff into the distal vasculature. The vasculature initially exhibits low resistance (R) to the flow (Q). The low R lowers the pressure (P) according to

$$P = Q * R \qquad \text{[mmHg, ml/min, mmHg]} \tag{1}$$

Low P counteracts vascular unloading and the slope of CPW amplitude envelope is decreased. As flow starts passing past the cuff, volume and pressure in the distal vasculature increase and PPG waveforms appear. As more flow passes past the cuff, volume and pressure in the distal vasculature increases due to blocked venous return. The PPG reflects this by rising baseline and amplitude increase. When CP and arterial wall pressures are equal, the CPWs reach maximal amplitudes. The CP at this point is equal to MAP according to vascular unloading. The CPW shapes are distorted because of the continuing partial occlusion of the artery. The flow is still turbulent and Phase II Korotkoff sounds are heard. The third segment lasts from MAP to DBP_{REF}. The CPW amplitudes start decreasing with cuff pressure deflation according to vascular unloading. Continuing blood outflow into the vasculature enhances the rate of amplitude decreases. The CPW shapes continue to be distorted because the artery is still partially occluded. Blood flow under the cuff is still turbulent, but the blood flow velocity is decreased and Korotkoff sounds are muffled (Phase 4). When cuff pressure reaches DBP_{REF}, the flow becomes laminar and the Korotkoff sounds are no longer heard (Phase V). The artery under the cuff is free from partial occlusion and the CPWs are no longer distorted.

The fourth segment lasts from DBP_{REF} to the end of procedure. When cuff pressure is further deflated below DBP_{REF}, the artery under the cuff is free from partial occlusion, blood flow is laminar and CPWs are not distorted. Korotkoff sounds are not heard. Further cuff pressure lowering decreases CPW amplitudes according to vascular unloading. At some arbitrary cuff pressure below DBP_{REF}, the cuff is quickly deflated and the cuff deflation procedure is terminated.

Observations of the effects of blood flow under the cuff and in the hand on the CPW amplitude envelope resulted in the following hypothesis: The slope of CPW waveform amplitude envelope at cuff pressures higher than the reference systolic pressure and the slope at cuff pressures between mean pressure and reference diastolic pressure are steeper than the slope between reference systolic pressure and mean pressure. Based on the above observations we conducted a study of 32 volunteers (Jilek & Fukushima, 2007). To test the hypothesis, 3 slopes (S1-S3) on the waveform amplitude envelope were computed and compared. S1 is the slope from cuff pressure 30 mm higher than reference systolic pressure to the cuff pressure equal to the reference systolic pressure. S2 is the slope from cuff pressure equal to the reference systolic pressure to the cuff pressure equal to mean pressure. S3 is the slope from cuff pressure equal to mean pressure to cuff pressure equal to reference diastolic pressure.

$$S1 = (WA_{HSBP} - WA_{SBP}) / (CP_{HSBP} - CP_{SBP}) \qquad (2)$$

$$S2 = (WA_{SBP} - WA_{MAP}) / (CP_{SBP} - CP_{MAP}) \qquad (3)$$

$$S3 = (WA_{MAP} - WA_{DBP}) / (CP_{MAP} - CP_{DBP}) \qquad (4)$$

WA_{HSBP} is the wave amplitude at cuff pressure about 30 mmHg higher (CP_{HSBP}) than cuff pressure at reference systolic pressure. WA_{SBP} is the wave amplitude at cuff pressure equal to the reference systolic pressure (CP_{SBP}). WA_{MAP} is the wave amplitude at cuff pressure equal to the computed mean pressure (CP_{MAP}). WA_{DBP} is the wave amplitude at cuff pressure equal to the reference diastolic pressure (CP_{DBP}).

The tabulated mean values are shown in Table 2. The slopes S1, S2 and S3 were computed according to the formulas (1-3).

N=32	SBP	MAP	DBP	S1	S2	S3
Mean	132	102	85	-0.065	-0.025	0.114
SD	17	13	12	0.022	0.012	0.035

Table 2. Mean values of SBP, MAP, DBP, and amplitude envelope slopes S1, S2, and S3 of 32 volunteers.

Our observations and the experimental results supported the central hypothesis. All the S1 and S3 slopes were steeper than the S2 slopes. The inter-subject variability suggests that the

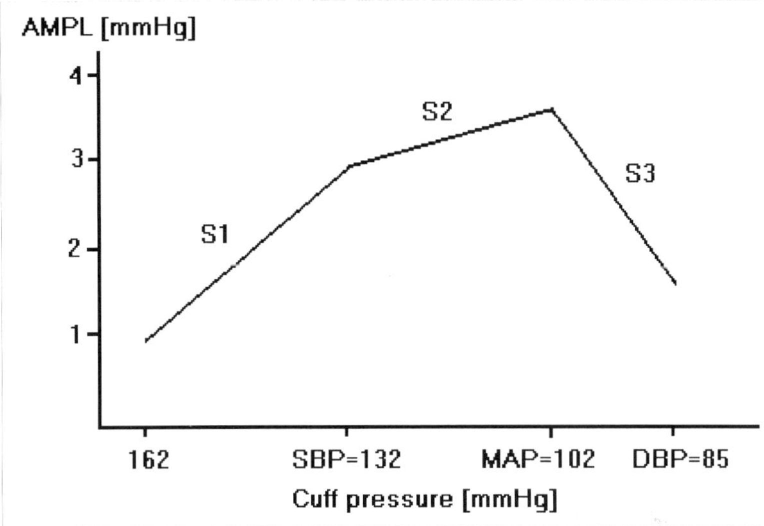

Fig. 10. Graphic representation of the amplitude envelope slopes S1, S2 and S3. AMPL (vertical axis) are mean values of waveform amplitudes.

slopes are affected by a number of variables. Arterial compliance, mean pressure, heart rate, stroke volume, and blood viscosity have been cited as factors affecting the slopes. These factors do not change substantially during a single gradual cuff deflation. Our study suggested that the blood flow under the cuff and in the hand is an important physiological variable decreasing S2 during a gradual cuff deflation procedure.

Graphic representation of amplitude envelope constructed from the mean values in Table 1 is in Fig. 10. Transition point from S1 to S2 in the vicinity of SBP has implications for a prospective development of a new type of algorithmic method based on physiology. A method capable of detecting the transition from S1 to S2 could improve the accuracy of SBP determination. High level of accuracy may be, however, difficult to achieve with manipulation of the cuff pressure pulse amplitudes. The slopes are not very steep and they may be difficult to determine without reference BP values. Furthermore, cuff waveform amplitudes are affected by a number of factors, such as movement artifacts, arrhythmias, tremors and deep breathing. Arrhythmias present especially difficult problems because their nature and frequency of occurrence are not always apparent.

4.4 Dual cuff method for the determination of systolic blood pressure

Cuff pressure waveform amplitude methods have been widely used in electronic BP monitors, but their accuracy has been questioned. The manual method using a sphygmomanometer and a stethoscope is still the gold standard of noninvasive BP determination. Improvement in automatic noninvasive methodology is desirable.

We previously studied the use of a finger photoplethysmographic (PPG) waveforms for improved determination of the SBP (Jilek & Stork, 2004). As illustrated in Fig. 9, the cuff waveforms appear at cuff pressures well above the SBP. This is in contrast to the auscultatory method. At CPs higher than SBP no sounds are heard. When CP drops to below SBP the Korotkoff sounds can be heard. Similarly, the PPG waveforms appear just below the level of SBP. Observation of the waveforms in Fig. 9 makes it obvious that it is easier to detect SBP with PPG signal than with just the cuff pressure waveforms. The PPG method has, however, some shortcomings. A PPG transducer must be attached to a finger and adjusted to detect usable waveforms. When the patient's fingers are cold, it becomes difficult to obtain usable waveforms.

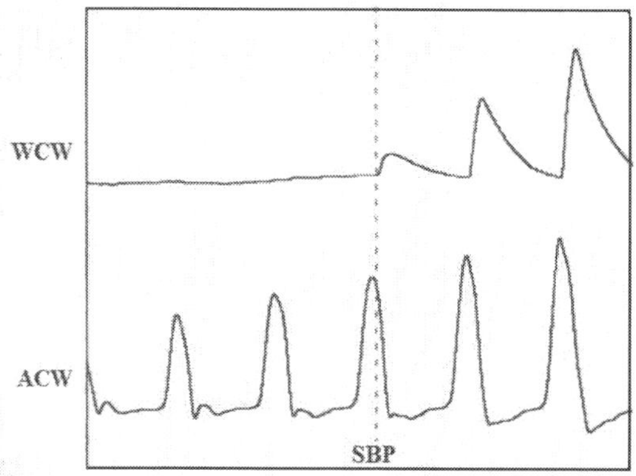

Fig. 11. Wrist cuff waveforms (WCW) and arm cuff waveforms (ACW) obtained simultaneously. Systolic pressure (SBP) is the point of WCW appearance.

A better method is the use of two cuffs. We used the dual cuff system to study the method. The arm cuff is used for the determination of MAP and DBP, and the wrist cuff is used to detect pulsations that appear at CPs lower than SBP. Waveforms acquired during dual-cuff test are shown in Fig. 11. The upper trace shows waveforms from the wrist cuff (WCW) and the lower trace shows waveforms from the arm cuff (ACW). The appearance of WCW indicates SBP. In the test shown in Fig. 11 the SBP measured by WCW appearance was 174 mmHg and the SBP determined by amplitude ratio method was 159 mmHg. The amplitude ratio method erroneously determined the SBP because of uneven slope S1.

4.5 Determination of hemodynamics from cuff pressures and waveforms

As shown in section 3, cuff pressure waveforms obtained at CPs at or below DBP level exhibit properties similar to arterial waveforms obtained by other methods. We have previously investigated the use of wrist cuff pressures and waveforms for the determination of hemodynamics (Jilek & Stork, 2003). The waveforms are used principally to compute stroke volume (SV). Since the SV is not obtained by estimating the actual left ventricular volume, the SV computed from the radial artery must be adjusted for body surface area (BSA) (formula 5).

$$BSA = (weight + height - 60)/100 \qquad [m^2, kg, cm] \tag{5}$$

Cardiac output is then computed by multiplying stroke volume by heart rate:

$$CO = SV * HR \quad [L/min, mL, bpm] \tag{6}$$

Total peripheral resistance (TPR) is obtained by dividing mean arterial pressure by cardiac output:

$$TPR = 80 * MAP/CO \qquad [dyn, mmHg, L/mi] \tag{7}$$

Systemic arterial compliance (SAC) is computed according to the formula (8), where

$$SAC = SV/PP = SV / (SBP - DBP) \qquad [mL, mL, mmHg] \tag{8}$$

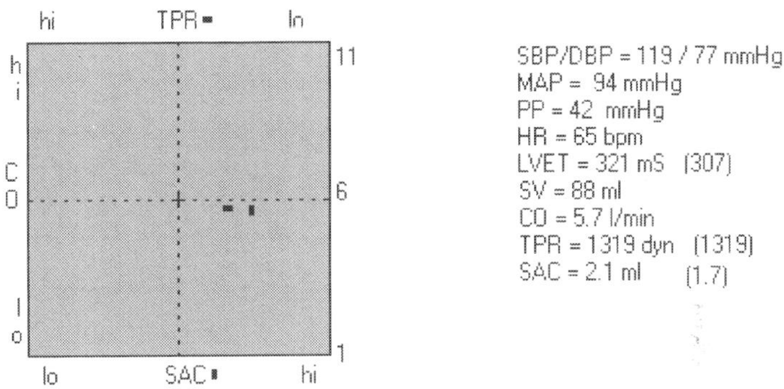

Fig. 12. Graphic and numeric results of a "normal" test.

This measure of compliance was used because both of the variables used (SV, PP) are already available. Moreover, pulse pressure is recognized as surrogate measure of arterial compliance. The computed blood pressure and hemodynamic variables are displayed on the computer screen as numeric values and as a "quadrant" graphic format (Fig. 12). The quadrant shows the relationships of cardiac output (CO), total peripheral resistance (TPR), and systemic arterial compliance (SAC). TPR and SAC are graphically represented by small rectangles and they move together on the vertical (CO) axis according to the value of CO. TPR and SAC rectangles are positioned on the horizontal axis according to their values. Higher SAC and lower TPR values move the rectangles to the right. Normal values of TPR and SAC are displayed graphically in the right half of the quadrant. Abnormal values (usually accompanied by hypertension) are located in the left half.

The values displayed in Fig. 12 are typical values of a normotensive, middle-age male. TPR and SAC values are graphically represented in the right "good" half of the quadrant.

Fig. 13. shows hemodynamic values corresponding to chronic hypertension in an elderly woman. Blood pressures are elevated, cardiac output is within normal range and total peripheral resistance (TPR) is high. Systemic arterial compliance (SAC) is substantially reduced. Both TPR and SAC are graphically represented in the left "bad" half of the quadrant.

Data from the system's developmental database were used to compute and compare hemodynamic values estimated by the system with values obtained from a study conducted by De Simone et al (De Simone et al, 1997). Our data from a group of 41 male and female volunteers (age 17 -76) were computed. The comparative values are displayed in table 3. This informal comparison shows good agreement between our HR, SV, CO values and the values obtained by De Simone.

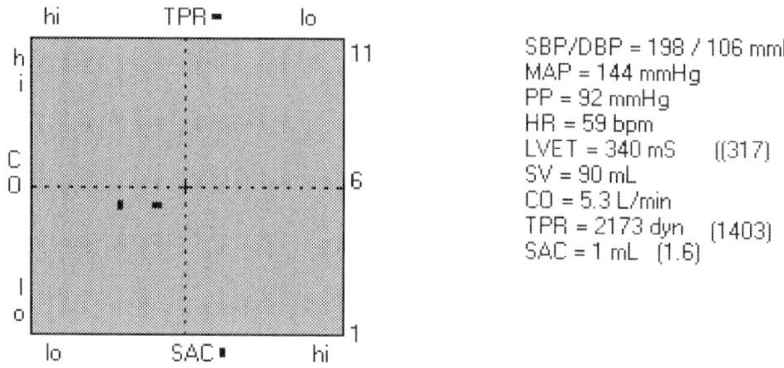

Fig. 13. Test results of a hypertensive woman.

	HR [bpm]	SV [ml]	CO [l/min]
System (n=41)	70	76	5.3
De Simone (n=544)	68	81	5.5

Table 3. Comparison of hemodynamic variables

5. Conclusion and future work

Our preliminary investigation into the nature of cuff pressure waveforms resulted in promising future possibilities for their practical applications:

- A comprehensive database of cuff pulse waveforms and reference BP values could lead to improved BP determination and to improved testing of automatic BP monitors.
- Improved determination of blood pressures from slope transitions.
- A new method for improving SBP determination is the use of wrist cuff to detect the onset of blood flow past the arm cuff.
- The estimation of blood pressures and hemodynamics promises to improve the diagnosis and treatment of resistant hypertension.
- Wrist cuff waveforms may find applications as surrogates for radial tonometric waveforms.

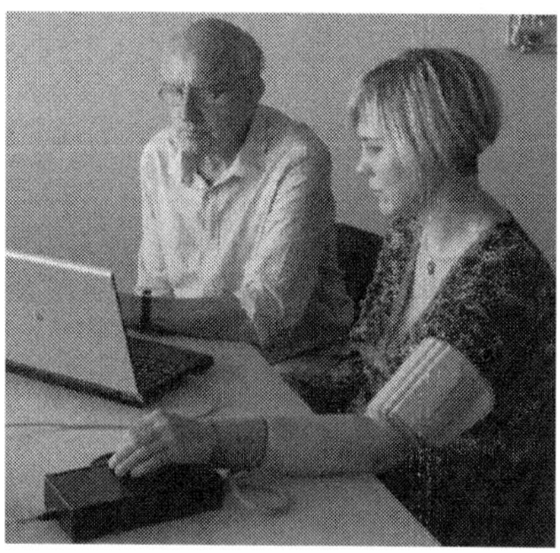

Fig. 14. The blood pressure measuring with dual-cuff method.

It should, however, be noted that the results of our investigation are preliminary and that verification studies will have to be performed before the new methods can be applied in current clinical instrumentation. Example of dual cuff measuring is shown in Fig. 14.

6. References

AAMI, (1999). Acquisition and use of physiologic waveform database for testing of medical devices, *Technical information report AAMI TIR no. 24,* Arlington, VA.

Borow, K.M. & Newburger J.W. (1982). Noninvasive estimation of central aortic pressure using the oscillometric method for analyzing systemic artery pulsatile blood flow; comparative study of indirect systolic, diastolic and mean brachial artery pressure with simultaneous direct ascending aortic pressure measurement, *Am Heart J,* Vol. 103, pp 879-898.

Cameron, JD. et al (1998). Use of radial artery applanation tonometry and a generalized transfer function to determine aortic pressure augmentation in subjects with treated hypertension, *J Am Coll Cardiol,* Vol. 32, pp 1214-1220.

De Simone G., et al (1997). Stroke volume and cardiac output in normotensive children and adults. *Circulation,* Vol. 95, pp 1837-1843.

Geddes, L.A. (1982). Characterization of the oscillometric method for measuring indirect blood pressure. *Ann Biomed Eng,* Vol. 10, pp 271-280.

Jilek, J. & Stork, M. (2003). An experimental system for estimation of blood pressures and hemodynamics from oscillometric waveforms. *Proceedings of AE2003 International Conference,* pp 111-114, ISBN 80-7082-951-6, Pilsen, September 2003.

Gerin, W. et al (2002). Limitations of current validation protocols for home blood pressure monitors for individual patients. *Blood Press Monit,* Vol. 7, pp 313-318.

Jilek, J. & Stork, M. (2004). Improved noninvasive systolic blood pressure detection with finger photoplethysmograph. *Proceedings of AE2004 International Conference,* pp 91-94, ISBN 80-7043-274-8, Pilsen, September 2004.

Jilek, J. & Stork, M. (2005). Data acquisition for a database of oscillometric blood pressure waveforms. *Proceedings of AE2005 International Conference,* pp 151-154, ISBN 80-7043-369-8, Pilsen, September 2005.

Jilek, J. & Fukushima, T. (2007). Blood flow under wrist cuff, in hand alters oscillometric waveforms during blood pressure measurement. *Biomed Instrum Technol,* Vol. 41, pp 238-243.

Jones, D.W. et al (2001). Mercury sphygmomanometers should not be abandonded: an advisory statement from the Council for High Blood Pressure Research, American Heart Association. *Hypertension,* Vol. 37, pp 185-186.

Jones, D.W. et al (2003). Measuring blood pressure accurately. *JAMA,* Vol. 289, pp 1027-1030.

Kelly, R.P. et al, (1998). Non-invasive registration of arterial pressure pulse-waveform using high-fidelity applanation tonometry. *J Vasc Med Bio,* Vol. 1, pp 142-149.l

Korotkov, N.S. (1956). A contribution to the problem of of methods for the determination of the blood pressure. In:Ruskin A, ed. *Classics of Arterial Hypertension,* Thomas, Sprigfield, Ill., pp 127-133.

Looney, J. (1978). Blood pressure by oscillometry. *Med Electron.* Pp 57-63.

Marey, E.J. (1881). La Circulation du sang a l'etat physiologique et dans les maladies, Paris, Masson.

Murgo, J.P. et al (1980). Aortic input impedance in normal man: Relationship to pressure waveforms. Circulation, Vol. 62, pp 105-116.
Ng, K.G. Blood pressure measurement, Med Electron, Vol. 19, pp 61-64.
Posey, J.A. & Geddes, L.A. (1969). The measuring of the point of maximum oscillations in cuff pressure in the indirect measurement of blood pressure. *Cardiovasc Res Bul,* Vol. 8, pp 15-25.
Riva-Rocci, S. (1896). Un sfigmomanometro Nuevo, *Gaz Med Trino.* pp981-996.
Takazawa K. (1987). A clinical study of the second component of left ventricular systolic pressure. *J Tokyo Med Coll.* Vol. 45, pp 256-270.

12

Integrated Microfluidic MEMS and Their Biomedical Applications

Abdulilah A. Dawoud Bani-Yaseen
Department of Chemistry, Faculty of Science Taibah University,
Al-Madinah Al-Munawarah P.O. Box 30002, KSA

1. Introduction

Microfluidic technology has been revolutionizing the landscape of various fields of analytical sciences since its introduction back in the early 1990s [1,2]. This emerging technology offers a variety of advantages over conventional pinch-top chemical instrumentation, such as performing rapid and low cost analysis, integrating various functional elements onto a single platform, consuming minimal amount of reagents and hence producing nominal waste volumes, and being more amenable for portability and automation. Interestingly, such superiority of these advantages has been demonstrated via utilizing various microfluidic systems in performing a wide range of tasks for various applications; this includes biomedical diagnostics [3-6], genomic and proteomics analyses [7-11], drug discovery and delivery [12-14], and environmental investigations [15-18]. On the other hand, integrated microfluidic systems has recently gained a great amount of attention, where the operation process of the microfluidic system is fully controlled via integrated circuit, which in systems defined as microfluidic micro-electro-mechanical-systems (MEMS), i.e. microfluidic MEMS.

While the microfluidic technology can be utilized to perform different functionalities, microfluidic devices that function based on the phenomenon of capillary-electrophoresis (CE) still the main applicability of this technology [2, 19-22]. Practically, the CE-based microfluidic devices are utilized to perform sample injection, separation, and detection of a wide range of analytes. Recently, there has been a great interest in integrating various detection modes, such as electrochemical and optical detectors, onto microfluidic devices of various architectures and designs [23-26]. However, notable attentions toward electrochemical detection (ECD), amperometric detection in particular, have increased. Although laser induced fluorescence (LIF) is considered as the most sensitive detection mode interfaced with various separation methods including the microfluidic technology, LIF is ineffective in detecting molecules that exhibit weak native fluorescence at room temperature, such as DNA adducts. Thus, ECD, amperometry in particular, offers an effective remedy for detecting those molecules that are natively weak fluorescent at room temperature such as Dopamine (DA)-derived DNA adduct (4DA-6-N7Gua) and 8-Hydroxy-2′-deoxyguanosine (8-OH-dG) adduct [26, 27].

Interfacing integrated ECD with CE-based microfluidic devices can fully exploit many advantages of miniaturization. The sensing electrodes can be arranged in two distinctive arrangements, namely in-channel and end-channel detection. However, the influence of the electrophoretic current on the detection current necessitates the introduction of a decoupler for the in-channel detection, whereas optimizing the location of the sensing electrodes near the exit of the separation channel is necessary for end-channel detection. We have shown that introducing a palladium decoupler for in-channel ECD significantly enhanced the stability of the sensing electrode, where the limit of detection (LOD) for sensing 8-OH-dG was lowered one order of magnitude for the in-channel ECD in comparison to the end-channel ECD that was used for sensing 4DA-6-N7Gua [27]. The palladium decoupler was introduced implementing the electroplating technique for depositing nano size palladium particles on the surface of integrated gold microelectrodes. On the other hand, we have reported implementing the electroplating technique for enhancing the coulometric efficiency (C_{eff}) of an integrated gold microelectrode for sensing selected biotargets, such as DA, where C_{eff} was tripled for roughened electroplated sensing gold electrode in comparison to bare electrodes [28].

DNA adducts formation that results from covalent interaction of genotoxic carcinogens with DNA can create various mutations in some critical genes and subsequently development of various diseases, such as cancer [29,30]. There are two general pathways for the formation of the DNA adducts; first, direct binding of some genotoxic carcinogens DNA to create the mutation, the second pathway proceeds via certain metabolic pathways, where some active metabolites can react with the DNA to form the adducts [31,32]. The role of DNA damage and subsequently formation of DNA adducts that can be considered as potential biomarkers are of particular importance in studies involving cancer and other diseases [33-36]. In this chapter, the fabrication and applicability of microfluidic devices with integrated ECD for the analysis of DNA adducts, namely 4DA-6-N7Gua and 8-OH-dG adducts are outlined. In particular, the applicability of the microfluidic device with end-channel and in-channel detections was evaluated for the analysis of 4DA-6-N7Gua and 8-OH-dG DNA adducts, respectively.

2. Principle of operation

In CE-based microfluidic systems, the flow of liquids inside the microchannels is driven according to the electrokinetic phenomenon. On the other hand, electrophoresis is defined as the migration of electrically charged specie under the influence of external electric field. As many details pertaining to this phenomenon can be found in the literature, brief description of this phenomenon is provided here. Wide range of solid materials acquires surface charge upon coming into contact with electrolytes, where this surface charge attracts counter charged species to form a very thin layer, which in turn known as Stern layer and consequently another layer is formed under the influence of Stern layer known as Gouy-Chapman layer. Hence, both layers jointly form the electrical double layer (EDL). It is noteworthy mentioning that the formation of EDL is mandatory to generate a flow inside the microchannels, where upon applying an electric field along the microchannel; charged species as well as solvent molecules migrate toward the counter charged electrodes to generate what is known as the electroosmotic flow (EOF). The speed of EOF (u_{EOF}) is governed according to Helmholtz-Smoluchowski equation [37,38]:

$$u_{EOF} = \frac{\varepsilon E_{el} \xi}{\eta} \tag{1}$$

where, ε is the dielectric constant, η is viscosity of the solution, E_{el} is strength of the electric field, ξ is the zeta potential.
However, as the u_{EOF} concerns the speed of bulk solution, mainly generated by migration of solvent molecules, another parameter that is characteristic for other charged species known as the electro-osmotic mobility (μ_e):

$$\mu_e \frac{q}{6\pi r\eta} \quad (2)$$

where, q is the ion charge, r is the ion radius. Furthermore, it is worth mentioning that CE is one type of electrophoresis with various modes, including Capillary Zone Electrophoresis (CZE), Capillary Isoelectric Focusing (CIEF), Capillary Gel Electrophoresis (CGE), Capillary Isotachophoresis (ITP), Capillary Electrokinetic Chromatography (EKC), Non-Aqueous Capillary Electrophoresis (NACE), and Capillary Electrochromatography (CEC). Hence, the common characteristic of all these modes of CE is the fact that they are electrophoretic processes performed in a capillary tube with usually a diameter that less than 100 μm. Thus, in caparison to the hydrodynamic driven flow inside the same capillary, one can notice that EOF and hydrodynamic driven flow profile flat and laminar flow with broad profile, respectively. Such observation can be attributed to the fact that there is no pressure drop along the capillary operating under EOF due to uniformity of EOF along the capillary, and hence flat profile is observed for the EOF. In addition, CE systems are used frequently for performing separation experiments that is analogous to other separation techniques, such as high performance liquid chromatography (HPLC), where the main task is to separate a mixture of various analytes into its components followed by analyzing these components quantitatively and/or qualitatively. It is noteworthy mentioning that all analytes migrate toward the cathode where a detector is aligned across the end of the capillary regardless their charge, and hence the migration of each analyte is characterized by the apparent electro-osmotic mobility (μ_a) instead of (μ_e), where (μ_a) and (μ_e) are correlated as:

$$\mu_a = \mu_e + \mu_{EOF} \quad (3)$$

On the other hand, various modes of detection have been interfaced with CE systems; this includes electrochemical detection (mainly amperometric and conductometric), laser induced fluorescence (LIF), UV-Vis absorption, Raman spectroscopy, mass spectrometry, H^1-NMR spectroscopy, refractive index spectroscopy, and FT-IR spectroscopy. In principle, all theories and mechanism of flow that govern CE systems can be extended to govern microfluidic systems operating under electrokinetic phenomenon. Commonly, a capillary that is made of silica is used for performing CE, where the double layer is constructed between the ionized hydroxyl groups (Si-O$^-$) and protons (H^+) that correspond to both surface charge and buffer species, respectively. Thus, it is essential to fabricate the microfluidic system from a material that can support the formation of the EDL. Hence, various types of materials have been utilized for fabricating microfluidic devices operating under electrokinetic phenomenon. Among these materials, glass and polymeric materials are the most popular ones. Glass exhibit characteristics, such has optically transparent, well-understood surface characteristics that are analogous to fused silica, chemicals resistant, and electrically insulator. On the other hand various types of polymers have been recently utilized for fabricating microfluidic systems; where among these materials PDMS is considered as the most popular one. However, while glass exhibit physicochemical properties that are more analogous to fused silica than PDMS, its relatively more complicated fabrication procedure in comparison to PDMS renders its application in advanced microfluidic systems, such as integrated microfluidic MEMS. Furthermore, fabricating integrated necessitates the inclusion of detection mode to the microfluidic MEMS. Hence, integrating ECD to the microfluidic MEMS is considered the most practical approach in term ease and expenses of fabrication, which in turn if particular importance when disposability of biomedical Microdevices is needed. Figure 1 exhibits a schematic representation for CE interfaced with amperometric detection mode. As can be noticed, chemical specie in a reduced form migrates with the EOF at μ_a in the direction toward the electrophoretic cathode, where it is oxidized upon coming into contact with surface of the working electrode (WE) to generate a current that is proportional to its concentration. It is noteworthy mentioning herein that similar principle of operation is applied for microfluidic MEMS with EC detection presented in this chapter.

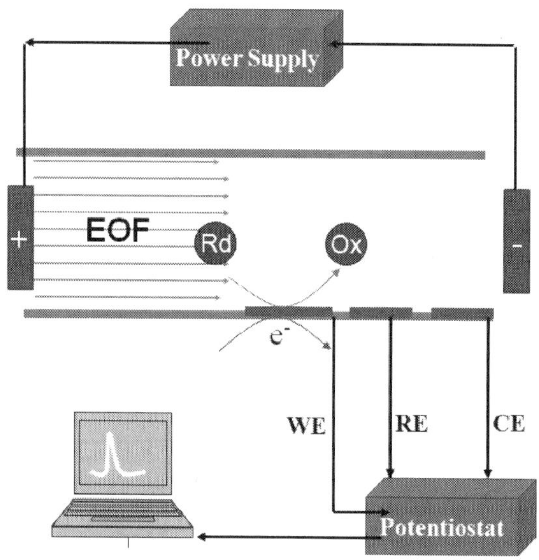

Fig. 1. Experimental setup for CE system interfaced with 3-electrode electrochemical configuration.

3. Experimental

3.1 Chemicals, reagents & materials:

DNA adducts: DA-derived DNA adduct (4DA-6-N7Gua), 2.8-Hydroxy-2′-deoxyguanosine (8-OHdG; neurotransmitters: dopamine, L-tyrosine, L-DOPA; separation buffers (10 mM): boric acid, monosodium phosphate, 2-[N-morpholino] ethanesulfonic acid (MES); Metals: gold, titanium; sodium hydroxide,), deoxyguanosine (dG), catechol; photoresists (SU-8 25, AZ-5214); photoresists developers (Microchem); gold etchant: iodine and potassium iodine (1:4, w:w); organic solvents: acetone, methanol, ethanol; Poly dimethylsiloxane (PDMS) (Sylgard 184); potassium hexachloropalladate (IV) (K_2PdCl_6); sodium tetrachloroaurate (III).

$2H_2O$ ($NaAuCl_4$. $2H_2O$); potassium hexachloroplatinate (IV) (K_2PtCl_6); morphine; codeine; glass microscopic slides; silicon wafers; and photomasks. All materials were purchased from commercial suppliers and were used as received, except for 4DA-6-N7Gua.

3.2 Equipments

Radio frequency (RF) plasma cleaner, resistive evaporation system, spin coater, stream of high purity nitrogen, UV light exposing system, potentiostat, DC power supply, picoammeter.

3.3 Methods

3.3.1 DNA adducts synthesis

Detailed outline for the synthesis of 4DA-6-N7Gua was published previously [39]; in brief:

1. DA is oxidized using silver oxide (Ag_2O) in dry dimethylformamide (DMF) to form the DA quinone.
2. The of solution of DA quinone is filtered onto a solution of dG in CH_3COOH/DMF/H_2O (v:v:v, 1:1:1); the solution is stirred for approximately 10 hr at room temperature.
3. The 4DA-6-N7Gua adduct is purified using preparative HPLC system and can be verified using ^1H NMR and mass spectrometry.

3.3.2 Sample preparation

1. Stock solutions of 1mM of each analytes is prepared in the running buffer and kept frozen at -20 °C until further needed.
2. Analytes' solution with different desired concentrations can be prepared daily by diluting the stock solutions using the running buffer.
3. Various running buffers with a concentration of 10 mM and different pH were prepared by dissolving a desired amount of the buffer sample in highly pure water; adjustment to the desired pH was performed using a solution of 0.5 M NaOH.

3.3.3 Microfluidic devic1 Fabrication

3.3.3.1 PDMS microchannel fabrication

1. The PDMS slabs with microchannels network is prepared implementing the micromolding technique and using a mold that is made of SU-8025 photoresist polymerized on silicon wafer.
2. The mold is prepared by spin coating the photoresist on the surface of the silicon wafer, followed by the necessary drying process.
3. The desired architecture of the microchannels network is transferred onto the mold through exposing the silicon wafer (covered with the photoresist) to UV light through in-house prepared photomask, followed by the curing process.
4. Pre-polymerized PDMS solution is prepared and degassed shortly before starting the micromolding procedure.
5. The PDMS solution is poured onto the mold, followed by a curing process at 65°C for 2 hr.
6. Then the PDMS slab is peeled off the mold gently and kept in clean area until further needed. Optimal microchannels' dimensions that are recommended are 25 and 75 µm for the depth and width, respectively. The length of the separation channel may vary, which depends on the resolution that is expected from the separation process; hence, longer separation channel is needed for better resolution.

3.3.3.2 Metalic microelectrodes fabrication

1. Pre-cleaned glass substrates are loaded inside the resistive evaporation chamber.
2. Two layers of titanium and gold are deposited onto the substrates surfaces with thickness of 10 and 200 nm, respectively.
3. Thin layer of photoresist (AZ-5214) is spun coated on the surface of the substrates then dried at 90°C for 20 min.
4. The pattern of the microelectrodes is transferred to the substrates through exposing the substrates to UV light through a photomask that encloses the structure of the microelectrodes.
5. After the UV exposure, the photoresist is developed, followed by hardening process at 120°C for 20 min.
6. The substrates are immersed inside freshly prepared solution of gold etchant with shaking for approximately 2 minutes.
7. After the etching process, the pattern of the microelectrodes is clear and the remaining photoresist is wiped away through rinsing the substrates with acetone then methanol in order to expose the surface of the gold electrodes.

3.3.3.3 Carbon microelectrodes fabrication

Schematic representation of the fabrication process is presented in Figure 2.

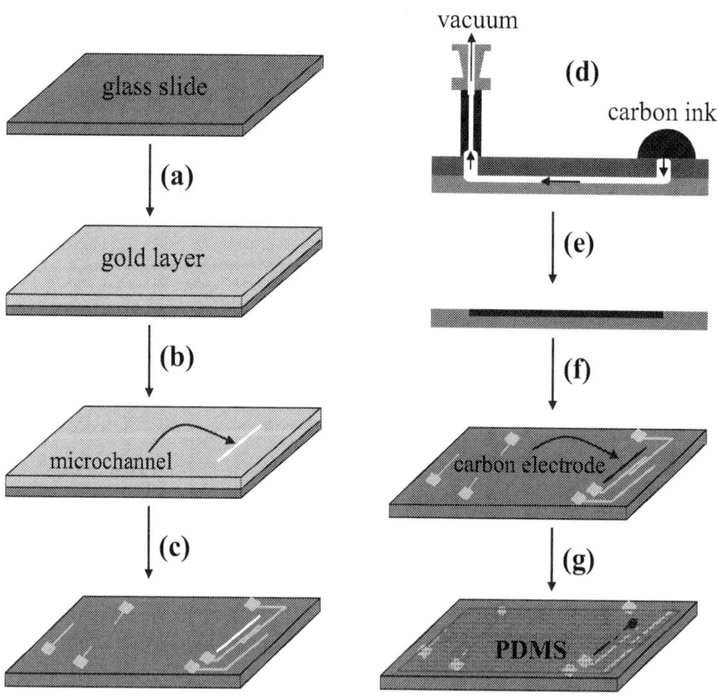

Fig. 2. Step-by-step procedure for microfabrication of carbon microelectrode integrated within microfluidic MEMS

1. Ending with the substrate in the previous section, thin layer of photoresist (AZ-5214) is spun coated on the surface of the substrates then dried at 90°C for 20 min.
2. The pattern of the microchannel, where the carbon ink will be injected, is transferred to the substrates through exposing the substrates to UV light through a photomask that encloses the structure of the microchannel.
3. After the UV exposure, the photoresist is developed, followed by hardening process at 120°C for 20 min.
4. Drops of buffered HF are added over the exposed area that defines the location of the microchannel on the substrate. The depth of the microchannel can measured frequently till reach an optimum depth of approximately 15 μm.
5. After the etching process, the pattern of the microelectrodes is clear and the remaining photoresist is wiped away through rinsing the substrates with acetone then methanol in order to expose the surface of the substrate.
6. Small piece of PDMS with two holes is bonded reversibly to the microelectrodes substrate, where the two holes on the PDMS match the two end of the microchannel.
7. A drop of the carbon ink is loaded into one hole while applying vacuum to the other hole.
8. The carbon ink will fill the microchannel, then the PDMS slab can be removed, and the carbon microelectrode is left for dryness at room temperature for 1 hr.

3.3.3.4 Microdevice assembling

9. The PDMS slab with the microchannels is cut onto the desired size using a lazar blade.
10. Four holes are created at the end of each microchannel using hand-punch holes maker.
11. For cleaning, the PDMS slab is immersed in ethanol and sonicated for 10 min., then dried at 60°C.
12. Assembling the microfluidic device is carried out either reversibly or irreversibly by binding the PDMS slab with the microchannels to the gold-patterned glass substrate.

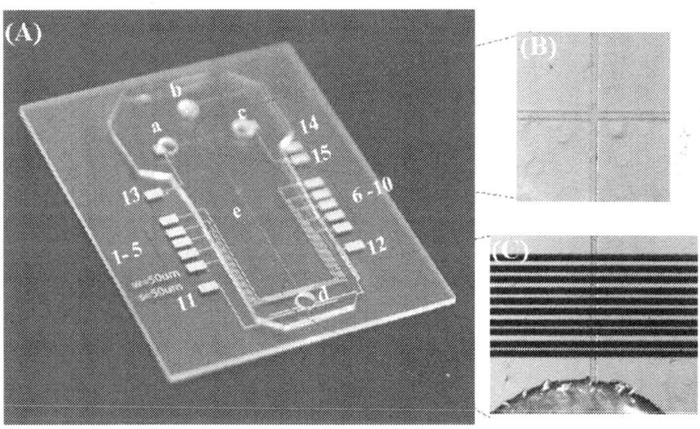

Fig. 3. Integrated microfluidic device with ECD (A): buffer reservoir (a), sample reservoir (b), waste reservoirs (c, d), separation channel (e), an array of working electrodes (1-10), reference electrode (11), auxiliary electrode (12), electrodes for injection and separation (13-15), frame (B): enlarged image for the microchannel where injection is performed; frame (C): enlarged image for the detection zone where the array of the microelectrodes are located. Note: the first electrode serves as decoupler for the in-channel detection.

13. To carry out the reversible binding, the PDMS slab is bound to the glass substrate without any further treatment.
14. For the irreversible binding, the PDMS slab and the glass substrate are subjected to RF-plasma treatment operating with stream of oxygen at 1-Torr for 1 min; then they are brought onto contact tightly. Figure 3 shows detailed image for the integrate microfluidic MEMS.

3.3.4 Electroplating procedure

Schematic representation for experimental setup of electrochemical deposition of metals nanoparticles son the surface of microelectrodes inside microchannels is presented in Figure 4.

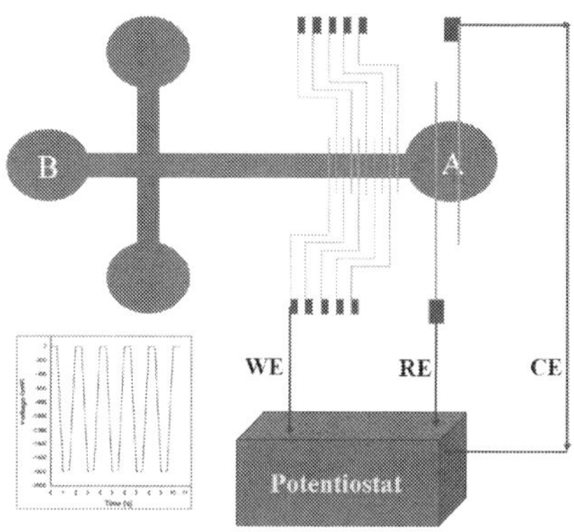

Fig. 4. Experimental setup for electrochemical deposition of metals nanoparticles on the surface of microelectrodes inside a microchannel of microfluidic MEMS

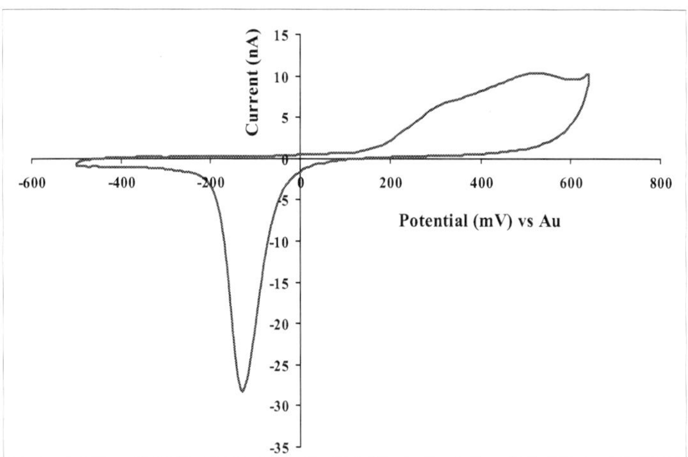

Fig. 5. Typical cyclic voltammogram of gold electrode obtained using 50 mM of $HClO_4$; scan rate: 100 mV/sec

1. The cleanness of the gold electrodes should be checked before performing the electroplating process. Cyclic voltammograms (CVs) in the range -500 - 700 mV and scan rate of 100 mV/cm using an ionic solution (e.g. 50 mM $HClO_4$) is performed. Figure 5 shows typical example of CV for clean gold surfaces, where observing the adsorption/desorption peaks of oxygen are efficient strategy for evaluating the cleanness of the gold electrodes surfaces.
2. Solution of K_2PdCl_6 (10 mM) is loaded into the waste reservoir (labeled as A in Figure 4) while applying vacuum to the waste reservoir (B) in order to fill the microchannel with the depositing solution.
3. Square potential signal is applied between 0 and -1800 mV from a potentiostat with a frequency of 2 Hz, see inset in Figure 4.

3.3.5 Electrophoresis

4. Prior to performing any electrophoresis separation process, the microchannels are flushed with a solution of NaOH (0.1 M) for 10 minutes followed by flushing with deionized water for another 10 min. The flushing is performed by loading the desired solution to the reservoirs a,b, and c while applying vacuum to the reservoir d.
5. After the flushing process, the microchannels are filled with the running buffer.
6. Fresh buffer and sample solutions are added loaded onto reservoirs a and b, respectively.
7. After the sample is injected (see below), a separation voltage is applied in the range 100-300 V/cm. For each separation process, fresh buffer solution is loaded.

3.3.6 Injection

Simplified gated injection is applied, where single power supply is used for injection and separation, via which a variable resistor is connected to the sample reservoir; hence, a relevant voltage is applied to the sample reservoir (e.g. 75% of that is applied to the buffer reservoir). Figure 6 illustrates detailed procedure with real images for the injection process.

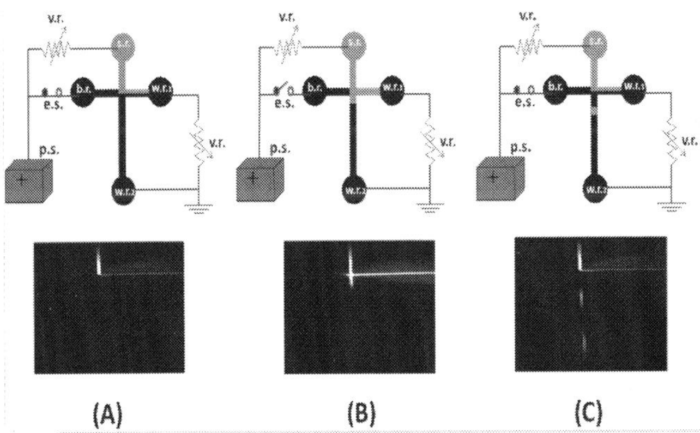

Fig. 6. Illustration of the simplified gated injection process using single power supply. Left column: schematic operation; right column: experimental imaging of real injection process. Frames A, B, and C correspond to the pre-injection, injection, and the post-injection (separation) steps, respectively. Microfluidic labels: buffer reservoir (a), sample reservoir (b), waste reservoirs (c, d), variable resistors (R1, R2); injection time: 1 sec.

The injection process consists of 3 steps:

1. Pre-injection, where voltage is applied between reservoirs "b.r.-w.r.1" and "s.r.-w.r.1"; during this step, the sample solution fills the microchannel that connects reservoirs s.r. and w.r.1 while the flow of the buffer solution between reservoirs b.r. and w.r.1 prevents the sample solution to flow toward the separation channel.

Injection, the electrode in b.r. is floated for approximately 1 sec, which causes the sample solution to flow toward the separation channel.

2. Post-injection (separation), the electrode in b.r. is reconnected, and hence the conditions for the pre-injection are resumed; however, a sample plug is generated and the separation process begins.

3.4 Electrochemical detection

All electrochemical measurements are performed using 3-electrode configuration with in-channel and end-channel detection; in both arrangements the auxiliary and reference electrodes are located inside the waste reservoir d:

3.4.1 End-Channel detection

The working electrode is located at very short distance from the separation channel exit (~ 15 μm) and inside the waste reservoir d. An array of ten microelectrodes that can serve as individual working electrodes is fabricated in order to assure locating the working electrode abruptly after the separation channel exit. The position of the working electrode is optimized using the microelectrodes array that spreads over a total distance of approximately 1 mm, which offers positioning the microelectrodes at different locations from the separation channel exit. Within this arrangement, the working electrode is located before the electrophoretic ground, and hence both electrodes are located inside the waste reservoir d.

3.4.2 In-Channel detection (implementing Pd decoupler)

The working electrode is located inside the separation channel e, after the electrophoretic ground. Within this arrangement, a decoupler is introduced via electrodepositing palladium particles on the surface of the first microelectrode of the array (electrode # 1 in Figure 3). The distance between the decoupler and the working electrode is optimized using the microelectrodes 2 to 10 individually.

After optimizing the location of the working electrode, optimizing the amperometric detection before the separation process is needed for each arrangement. The optimized detection potential for each analyte is determined through constructing the hydrodynamic voltammograms under similar injection and separation conditions. Figure 7 shows typical hydrodynamic voltammograms for various analytes of interests, including the 4DA-6-N7Gua and 8-OH-dG DNA adducts.

4. Discussion and technical notes

Various issues and technical approaches have to be considered upon performing analyses using the microfluidic MEMS. Among these issues, stability of the DNA adducts is critical issue, where leaving the sample solution at room temperature for a long time could lead to oxidizing the DNA adducts and their related analytes, especially at basic pH. Observing

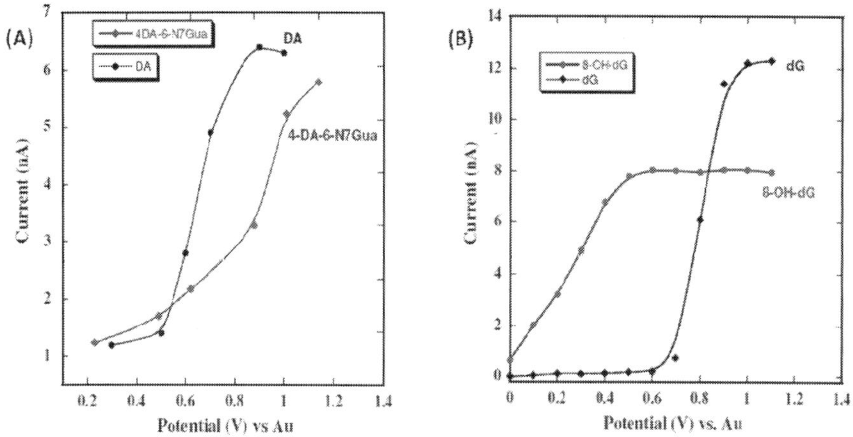

Fig. 7. Hydrodynamic voltammograms of DA (380 μM) and 4DA-6-N7Gua adduct (500 μM), and dG (50 μM) and 8-Oh-dG adduct (75 μM) obtained using end-channel and in-channel with electroplated Pd decoupler ECD, respectively. Operating conditions: 10 mM borate buffer at pH 9.1, injection time: 1 sec; separation electric field: 200 and 300 V/cm for A and B, respectively.

brownish color for the 4DA-6-N7Gua adduct and related neurotransmitters is indication for the formation of the corresponding quinones as a result of the oxidation reaction in solution. Hence, preserving the analytes solutions at low temperature (-20°C) is essential for increasing the lifetime of the analytes under investigation.

The dimensions of the microchannels are controlled by the photomask and the photoresist viscosity; while the length and the width of the microchannels are controlled by the photomask dimensions, the viscosity of the photoresist controls the depth of the microchannels. Importantly, choosing the right photoresist with certain viscosity and following the recipes provided by the photoresist vendor are essential for obtaining the desired microchannels' depth. The microchannels' dimensions are critical for obtaining stable electrochemical signal. Hence, wide and shallow microchannels are recommended for obtaining stable detection current, where deep microchannels exhibit high electrophoretic current, which in turn reduces the stability of the background detection current. In addition, Starting with ultra clean microscopic glass slides is essential for obtaining good adhesion of the metals on the glass surface, which in turn can increase the durability of the microelectrodes. Furthermore, the titanium layer is needed to serve as seed layer for the gold layer. While other metals, such as chromium can be used too, titanium exhibits better adhesion properties toward the glass surface. Titanium layer > 10 nm is not recommended, where thicker layer of titanium requires using special etchant that may etch the upper layer of gold, and hence losing the continuity of the microelectrodes strips. Also, following the instruction that are provided by the photoresist (AZ-5214) vendor for processing the gold payer patterning is recommended for obtaining defined shapes for the gold microelectrodes stripes. The concentration of the gold etchant is critical in obtaining defined shapes for gold microelectrodes stripes, where more concentrated etchant needs shorter etching time. As the iodine-based gold etchant has deep blue color, it is hard to observe the completion of the etching process, and hence checking out the etching process periodically is recommended. Etching for a long time could cause to break the continuity of the gold microelectrodes stripes.

Using different materials for fabrication the microelectrode that serve as working electrode can also be utilized [40,41]. In particular, carbon electrodes can exhibit lower noise current and wider detection window. Such features are of significant importance upon analyzing electrochemically chemical species with large geometrical structures, such as codeine and related metabolites. Figure 8 shows normalized CVs of four related materials of forensic interests, namely codeine, morphine, hydromorphone and normorphine. Interestingly, carbon ink based electrodes exhibit background CV that is comparable to CV observed for commercial glassy carbon electrodes frequently used electrochemical experimentation, which has characteristic importance in analyzing electrochemically chemical species at relatively high potential such as codeine.

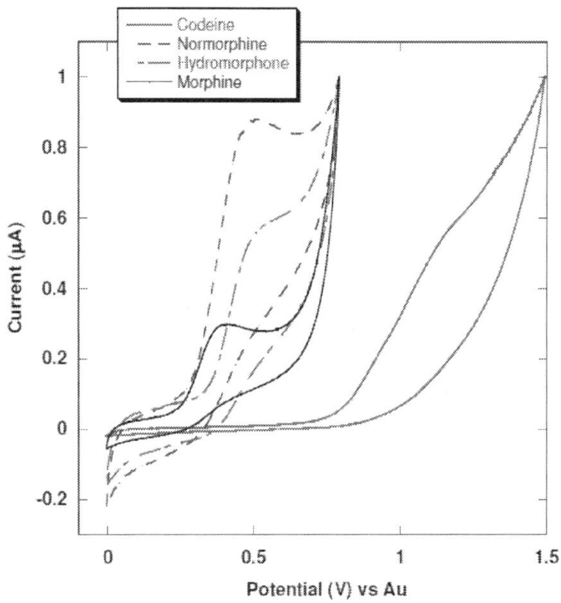

Fig. 8. Normalized CV of codeine, morphine, normorphine, and hydromorphone over CI electrode 10mM MES buffer. Scan rate 100 mV/s.

While the reversible binding of the PDMS slab to the gold-patterned glass substrate is easier to perform than the irreversible binding, microchannels with hydrophobic surfaces are produced, and hence difficulties in filling the microchannels are observed in addition to retarded electroosmotic flow. In addition, reversibly assembled microdevice cannot stand higher pressure that could be developed because of generating air bubbles, which in turn could damage the microdevice. On the other hand, irreversibly assembled microdevice can stand much higher pressure with preferably hydrophilic microchannels. However, it is worth mentioning that the plasma-treated PDMS surfaces have to be assembled within approximately 3 min to obtain strong binding, where the PDMS surfaces notably lose their binding strength after exposing to air for longer time. Furthermore, the hydrophilic microchannels can retain their hydrophilicity for approximately 1 hr upon being exposed to air. Thus, it is highly recommended to keep the microchannels wet using aqueous solutions, e.g. filling the microchannels with the running buffer or water immediately after the assembling process. Interestingly, the array of the microelectrodes over a total distance of approximately 1 mm facilitates the process of the aligning process without using microscopes.

It is noteworthy mentioning that the cleanness of the microelectrodes surfaces is critical issue for obtaining high sensitivity and hence reliable analysis. As it is expected that the gold surface could get contaminated during the fabrication process, it is essential to ensure that the microelectrodes surfaces are ultra cleaned before performing any ECD. Also, clean surfaces are necessary for obtaining stable palladium electrophoretic ground produced using the electroplating technique. The length of the electroplating process strongly depends on the desired density of the palladium electroplated decoupler, which in turn depends on the applied separation electric field and the running buffer. For high density of electroplated palladium, longer deposition time is needed (e.g. 4 min); meanwhile, applying vacuum periodically during the electroplating process to the other end of the microchannel in order to refresh the electroplating solution is recommended for obtaining efficient electroplating process. It is noteworthy that vigorous formation of air bubbles at the electrophoretic ground may cause the electroplated palladium particles to be released from the gold surface, and hence interrupting the separation process.

Obtaining electrophoretic separation with high resolution depends on several factors including the separation channel length, the running buffer, and the applied separation electric field. As longer separation channel is expected to offer better resolution, longer analysis time is observed, which contradicts the advantageous features of using microfluidic devices to perform chromatographic and electrophoretic separation. On the other hand, performing the electrophoretic separation at low separation electric field could lead to diffusion-controlled detection process, and hence reduced sensitivity is observed. However, higher separation electric field has the advantages of observing better sensitivity due to more efficient interaction between the analyte and the electrochemical sensing electrode. Unfortunately, less stable and high level of background detection current is observed for end-channel detection current. However, reduced effect for the higher separation electric field is observed for the in-channel detection with palladium decoupler, and hence notable enhanced sensitivity and stability of the in-channel detection is observed. Figure 9 shows the effect of the applied separation voltage on the capillary electrophoretic separation of 8-OH-dG and dG. For ECD interfaced with capillary electrophoresis, the electrophoretic current strongly affects the detection current; thus, using running buffer with low ionic mobility is recommended. Hence, MES buffer is widely used as running buffer for ECD interfaced with CE. However, using MES buffer as the running buffer for performing an electrophoretic separation of a mixture of 4DA-6-N7Gua, dopamine, L-tyrosine, L-DOPA, and catechol, and a mixture of dG and 8-OH-dG generated electropherograms with only two and one peaks, respectively. Interestingly, although borate buffer exhibit higher ionic mobility than MES buffer, significantly enhanced resolution is observed. Figure 10 shows an electropherogram for the separation of a mixture of 4DA-6-N7Gua, dopamine, L-tyrosine, L-DOPA, and catechol obtained using borate buffer with end-channel ECD arrangement. Generally, optimizing the separation process strongly depends on the nature of the analytes under investigation, where each separation parameter has to be optimized separately.

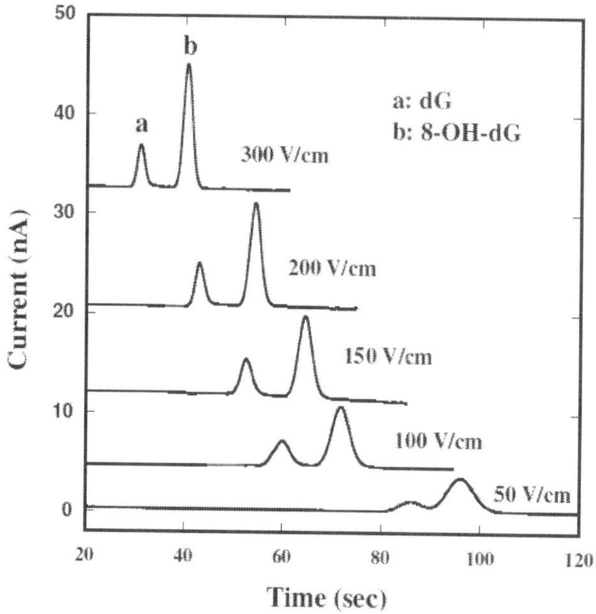

Fig. 9. Separation of dG (50 μM) and 8-OH-dG adduct (75 μM) at various separation electric fields. Operating conditions:10 mM borate buffer (pH 9.5), injection time: 1 sec, EC potential: 900 mV vs Au.

PDMS has weak heat dissipation capability, and hence high Joule's heating that is observed at high electrophoretic current could cause severe damage to the microfluidic device. As can be seen in Figure 3, the variable resister # 2 that is connected in series with waste reservoir (w.r. 1) provides comparable electric field along the injection microchannel to that is observed along the separation channel. Such arrangement is essential while using single power supply for injection and separation. Gated injection offers variable sample plug's size, where more intense signal is observed for long injection time (e.g. 2-5 sec). However, large sample plug's size generates low resolution. Hence, optimizing the injection time is performed depending on the complexity of the mixture to be analyzed, where shorter injection time is recommended for more complex sample. Finally, the durability of the microfluidic device depends mainly on the lifetime of the sensing electrodes. Working electrode passivation during the ECD, which results from the adsorption of some oxidized analytes, could reduce the sensitivity of the working electrode. Thus, applying sinusoidal wave potential regularly and after each injection process is recommended.

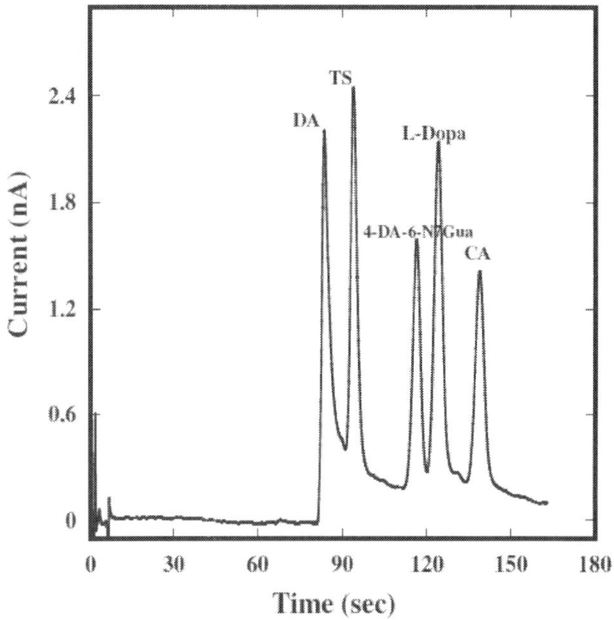

Fig. 10. Electropherogram for the separation of a mixture of 200 μM 4-DA-6-N7Gua adduct and related analytes. Operating conditions: 10 mM Borate buffer (pH 9.1), separation electric field: 140 V/cm, injection time: 1 sec, EC potential: +1000 mV vs Au.

5. Acknowledgement.

The author is grateful to the Strategic Research Unit at Taibah University (Nanotechnology Program Project Grant 08-NANO-22-05) for partial support of the work. The author also is thankful to Dr. Elham Mohammad at Taibah Universuty, Prof. R.Jankowiak at Kansas State University (KS, USA), and Dr. T. Kawaguchi at Hokaido University (Japan) for their valuable discussion and support.

6. Reference

[1] Manz, A., Grabner, N., Widmer, H.M. (1990) Miniaturized total chemical analysis systems: a novel concept for chemical sensing. *Sens. Actuators B* 1, 244–248.

[2] Harrison, D.J., Manz, A., Fan, Z., Lüdi, H., Widmer, H.M. (1992) Capillary electrophoresis and sample injection systems integrated on a planar glass chip. *Anal. Chem.* 64, 1926–1932.

[3] Lenshof A, Ahmad-Tajudin A, Jaras K, Sward-Nilsson AM, Aberg L , Marko-Varga G, Malm J, Lilja H (2009) Acoustic whole blood plasmapheresis chip for prostate specific antigen microarray diagnostics, Anal Chem 81 (15): 6030.

[4] Sollier E, Cubizolles M, Fouillet Y, Achard JLA (2010) Fast and continuous plasma extraction from whole human blood based on expanding cell-free layer devices, Biomed. Microdev 12 (3): 485.

[5] Munro NJ, Snow K, Kant JA, Landers JP (1999) Molecular diagnostics on microfabricated electrophoretic devices: from slab gelto capillary- to microchip-based assays for T- and B-cell lymphoproliferative disorders. Clin. Chem. 45: 1906.

[6] Kartalov EP, Lin DH, Lee DT, Anderson WF, Taylor CR, Scherer AA (2008) Internally calibrated quantification of protein analytes in human serum by fluorescence immunoassays in disposable elastomeric microfluidic devices, Electrophoresis 29 (24): 5010.

[7] Dawoud AA, Saryia H, Lazar IM (2007) Microfluidic platform with mass spectrometry detection for phosphoproteins analysis. Electrophoresis 28: 4645.

[8] House DL Chon CH, Creech CB ,Skaar EP, Li DQ (2010) Miniature on-chip detection of unpurified methicillin-resistant Staphylococcus aureus (MRSA) DNA using real-time PCR. J Biotechn 146: 93.

[9] Armenta JM, Dawoud AA, Lazar IM, Microfluidic chips for protein differential expression profiling. Electrophoresis 30: 1145.

[10] Lee, Park SH, Chung KH, Pyo HB (2008) A disposable plastic-silicon micro PCR chip using flexible printed circuit board protocols and its application to genomic DNA amplification. IEEE Sensors J 8 (6): 558.

[11] Ramalingam N, Rui Z, Liu HB, Dai CC, Kaushik R, Ratnaharika B, Gong HQ (2010) Real-time PCR-based microfluidic array chip for simultaneous detection of multiple waterborne pathogens Gong, Sens. Actuat. B Chem. 145: 543

[12] Sung JH, Kam C, Shuler ML (2010) A microfluidic device for a pharmacokinetic-pharmacodynamic (PK-PD) model on a chip. Lab Chip 10 (4): 446.

[13] Wen Y, Yang ST (2008) The future of microfluidic assays in drug development. Expert Opin Drug Discov 3: 1323

[14] Li X, Huang J, Tibbits GF, Li PCH (2007) Real-time monitoring of intracellular calcium dynamic mobilization of a single cardiomyocyte in a microfluidic chip pertaining to drug discovery, Electrophoresis 28 (24) 4723.

[15] Shen SL, Li Y, Wakida SA (2010) Characterization of dissolved organic carbon at low levels in environmental waters by microfluidic-chip-based capillary gel electrophoresis with a laser-induced fluorescence detector. Environ. Monit Assess 166: 573.

[16] Chen G, Lin Y, Wang J (2006) Monitoring environmental pollutants by microchip capillary electrophoresis with electrochemical detection. Talanta 68: 497.

[17] Wakida S, Fujimoto K, Nagai H, Miyado T, Shibutani Y, Takeda S (2006) On-chip micellar electrokinetic chromatographic separation of phenolic chemicals in waters. J Chromatogr A 1109: 179.

[18] Masadome T, Nakamura K, Iijima D, Horiuchi O, Tossanaitada B, Wakida S, Imato T (2010) Microfluidic polymer chip with an embedded ion-selective electrode detector for nitrate-ion assay in environmental samples Anal Sciences 26: 417.

[19] Woolley, A.T., Mathies, R.A. (1995) Ultra-high-speed DNA sequencing using capillary electrophoresis chips. *Anal. Chem.* 67, 3676–3680.

[20] Burns, M.A., Johnson, B.N., Brahmasandra, S.N., Handique, K., Burke, D.T. (1998) An integrated nanoliter DNA analysis device. *Science* 282, 484–487.

[21] Dolník, V., Liu, S., Vladisl, S.J. (2000) Capillary electrophoresis on microchip. *Electrophoresis* 21, 41–54.

[22] Woolley, A.T., Lao, K., Glazer, A.N., Mathies, R.A. (1998) Capillary electrophoresis chips with integrated electrochemical detection, *Anal. Chem.* 70, 684–688.

[23] Chabinyc, M.L. (2001) An integrated fluorescence detection system in poly (dimethylsiloxane) for microfluidic applications, *Anal. Chem.* 73, 4491–4498.

[24] Malic, L., Kirk, A.G. (2007) Integrated miniaturized optical detection platform for fluorescence and absorption spectroscopy. *Sens. Actuators A* 135, 515-524.

[25] Ro, K.W., Lim, K., Shim, B.C., Hahn, J.H. (2005) Integrated light collimating system for extended optical-path-length absorbance detection in microchip-based capillary electrophoresis. *Anal. Chem.* 77, 5160-5166.

[26] Dawoud, A.A., Kawaguchi, T., Markushin, Y., Porter, M.D., Jankowiak, R. (2006) Separation of catecholamines and dopamine-derived DNA adduct using a microfluidic device with electrochemical detection. *Sens. Actuators B* 120, 42–50

[27] Dawoud, A.A., Kawaguchi, T., Jankowiak, R. (2007) Integrated microfluidic device with an electroplated palladium decoupler for more sensitive amperometric detection of the 8-hydroxy-deoxyguanosine (8-OH-dG) DNA adduct. *Anal. Bioanal. Chem.* 388, 245-252.

[28] Dawoud, A.A., Kawaguchi, T., Jankowiak, R. (2007) In-channel modification of electrochemical detector for the detection of bio-targets on microchip. *Electrochem. Comm.* 9, 1536–1541

[29] Singh, R., Todorovic, R., Devanesan, P., Higginbotham, S., Zhao, J., Gross, M.L., Rogan, E.G., Cavalieri, E.L. (2001) Analysis of potential biomarkers of estrogeninitiated cancer in the urine of Syrian golden hamsters treated with 4-hydroxyestradiol. *Carcinogenesis* 22, 905–911.

[30] Shigenaga, M., Gimeno, C., Ames, B. (1989) Urinary 8-hydroxy-2'-deoxyguanosine as a biological marker of in vivo oxidative DNA damage, *Proc. Natl. Acad. Sci.* 86, 9697-9701.

[31] Hemminki, K. (1983) Nucleic acid adducts of chemical carcinogens and mutagens. *Arch. Toxiocol.* 52, 249-285.

[32] Dipple, A. (1995) DNA adducts of chemical carcinogens. *Carcinogenesis* 16, 437-441.

[33] Wogan, G.N., Hecht, S.S., Felton, J.S., Conney, A.H., Loeb, L.A. (2004) Environmental and chemical carcinogenesis. *Semin. Cancer Biol.* 14, 473-486.

[34] Luch, A. (2005) Nature and nurture lessons from chemical carcinogenesis. *Nat. Rev. Cancer* 5, 113-125.

[35] Markushin, Y., Gaikwad, N., Zhang, H., Kapke, P., Rogan, E.G., Cavalieri, E.L., Trock, B.J., Pavlovich, C., Jankowiak, R (2006) Potential biomarker for early risk assessment of prostate cancer. *Prostate* 66, 1565–1571.

[36] Markushin, Y., Kapke, P., Saeed, M., Zhang, H., Dawoud, A.A., Rogan, E., Cavalieri, E.G., Jankowiak, R. (2005) Development of monoclonal antibodies to 4-hydroxyestrogen-2-N-acetylcysteine conjugates: immunoaffinity and spectroscopic studies. *Chem. Res. Toxicol.* 18, 1520-1527.

[37] Hunter, R.J., *Zeta Potential in Colloid Science: Principles and Applications*, Academic Press, (1981), pp 1-56.

[38] Delgado, A. V., *Interfacial Electrokinetics and Electrophoresis*, Marcel Dekker, New York (2002), pp 1-54.

[39] Cavalieri, E.L., Li, K.-M., Balu, N., Saeed, M., Devanesan, P., Higginbotham, S., Zhao, J., Gross, M.L., Rogan, E.J. (2002), Catechol ortho-quinones: the electrophilic compounds that form depurinating DNA adducts and could initiate cancer and other diseases. *Carcinogenesis* 23, 1071- 1077.

[40] Dawoud Bani-Yaseen, A.A. (2009), Fabrication and Characterization Fabrication of Fully Integrated Microfluidic Device with Carbon Sensing Electrode for the Analysis of Selected Biomedical Targets. IEEE Sensors J. 9 (2), 81-86.

[41] Dawoud Bani-Yaseen, A.A., Kawaguchi, T., Jankowiak, R. (2009), Electrochemically Deposited Metal Nanoparticles for Enhancing the Performance of Microfluidic MEMS in Biochemical Analysis. Int. J. Nanomanufact., 4, 99-107.

13

MEMS Biomedical Sensor for Gait Analysis

Yufridin Wahab and Norantanum Abu Bakar
University Malaysia Perlis
Malaysia

1. Introduction

Gait analysis is the study of lower limb movement patterns and involves the identification of gait events and the measurements of kinetics and kinematics parameters. These include for example, toe-off, landing, stance, swing, displacement, speed, acceleration, force, pressure and the pressure-time-integral. Gait analysis is a very important procedure in assessing and improving many quality of life indicators. In sports, gait analysis can be used to improve athlete's performance and injury prevention. For patients, such as those suffering from diabetes, gait analysis can be used to screen for development of foot ulceration thus preventing them. In term of gait stability, gait analysis is proven to be very helpful in assessing and improving balance among the elderly, patients with diabetes or peripheral neuropathy and many other sicknesses. Gait analysis is also widely used in rehabilitation.

The occurrence of fall is becoming more of a significant health threat recently. This is due to the fact that the worldwide phenomenon of growing population of the elderly is continuously observed in many developed and developing countries. It is estimated that the world's elderly citizen will reach 2 billion in 2050 from current figure of 670 million. To make matters worse, the total number of the world's diabetic sufferers is increasing from 171 million in 2000 to 366 million in 2030, with an obvious trend of surging proportion for the above 65 years group.

In order to further understand the situation that leads to the health hazard, many research groups around the world are seriously looking into the matter. Recently, it is reported that foot plantar pressure can be used to asses gait stability and risk of fall. In addition, foot clearance above ground/floor during gait is also reported to be related to the occurrence of fall among the elderly. This is especially true when the foot is swaying on the air, or also called swing phase. Notably, pressure is measured when the foot is already touching the ground, which is known as stance phase, while clearance is measured during mid-swing to heel strike. If both pressure and clearance parameters of gait analysis are used together in an integrated manner, a better way of fall prediction and prevention can be produced.

In addition to assessing balance, the measurement of foot plantar pressure and foot clearance are also useful in many other gait assessments. This foot pressure measurement has wide applications, for example in screening for high risk diabetic foot ulceration, design of orthotics for diabetes mellitus and peripheral neuropathy, footwear design, sports injury prevention in athletes, study of the development of gait among the children plus many more. It also can be used to identify gait events such as heel strike, toe off, the timing of swing, stance, stride, the double support phase and also cadence. If stride length is known, the horizontal speed and acceleration can also be determined. On the other hand, the foot clearance measurement can also be useful in determining the vertical component of gait kinematics such as maximum vertical displacement, vertical velocity and its acceleration.

At current, the health system is still lacking. While the ratio of medical professional to patients is reducing, such measurements are still mostly conducted in exclusive research facilities, rehabilitation laboratories or hospitals. For example, the use of gait mats, force sensing platforms, motion analysis systems with efficient computer processing and ultrasonic ranging system are used for indoor analysis. Despite their efficiency and reliability, these state-of-the-art measurement systems are still using the bulky old fashioned technology. Considering the global trend of increasing elderly and diabetic population, a major paradigm shift is therefore highly required. As a solution, the advances in the instrumentation technology should be explored and used to its fullest capability. The aim is to enable the measurement to be performed in the patient's real environment with the revolutionary e-health connectivity and supporting pervasive healthcare concept.

While e-health system demands internet application for better management and implementation of healthcare provision, pervasive healthcare promotes wireless interconnection between monitoring devices. In this case, sensors that are part of body sensor network can be used. These sensors should not interfere with the actual movement itself so that the readings are representative of the actual tasks performed. This demands that the devices be small, lightweight and easily attached to the shoes or feet. One possible way of satisfying such exclusive demands is, of course, through the application of the fast developing micro-electro-mechanical system (MEMS) technology. This relatively new but promising instrumentation technology provides a great opportunity to further advance the intended gait measurement system.

This technology is proven to be capable of shrinking the device size, integrating sensors and actuators with their processing and controlling circuitry and lowering the power consumption of the overall system. The fusion of its technology is now covering wide applications across a multitude of disciplines from medical to military and spaces from in-vitro of human body organs to the infinity of aerospace. The great achievement has been due to cheap and easy integration of microelectronic signal processing circuits and MEMS technologies. Thus, the potential of these technologies should be explored in the design of newer generation of gait analysis instruments to ensure greater progress of the gait analysis application with significant impact to society. Therefore, in this thesis, the exploration and realization of micro-sensors for the measurement of gait parameters using MEMS technology is explained.

As roughly mentioned in the previous section, the current status of the development of untethered in-shoe gait stability measurement devices is still lacking behind the reality of technology achievement. In this subsection, the motivation for this research is described. Specifically, with respect to their measurand, the current devices are not fully optimized in many aspects.

Foot Clearance:

- Not suitable for real world or outdoor measurement.
- Not cost effective
- Not enabling efficient signal processing
- Not fully integratable for better reliability and long lasting use

Foot Plantar Pressure:

- Not providing the required pressure range for diabetic related application
- Not supporting efficient signal processing
- Exhibits hysteresis and other weaknesses.

Most interestingly, despite the proven track records, there is no reported innovation that targets gait analysis parameters of clearance and plantar pressure concurrently based on MEMS as yet.

2. Trends in human motion measurement

Gait is simply defined as a style of walking (Curran, 2005). Gait analysis is the study of lower limb movement patterns and involves the measurements of kinetics and kinematics parameters. These include, for example gait events and phases such as toe-off, landing, stance, swing, double support, and kinematics such as foot displacement, speed, acceleration, and kinetics such as force, pressure and the pressure-time-integral (Rodgers, 1988). The understanding of normal gait principles is the basis for understanding the pathologic and compensatory gait deficits. Normal gait for human being is bipedal in nature that distinguishes human from other primates but is often taken for granted until something goes wrong (Curran, 2005). It is achieved by use of the lower limbs that comprise of foot as one of the key parts. The foot is a complex structure that is made of 26 bones, 33 joints and more than 300 soft-tissue structures (Curran, 2005). As the terminal structure in the human kinetic chain, it performs the pivotal roles of dissipator for compressive, tensile and shear forces while performing rotational motions during stance. In other words, from a podiatrics point of view, foot functions as a shock absorber, a mobile adapter and finally a rigid lever (Curran, 2005). Nowadays, the need for the measurement of human motion parameters is getting higher due to the increase in the number of fields requiring it, especially numerous medical specializations (Simon, 2004), activity of daily living (ADL) assesment and sports (Billing et al.,2006; Aminian & Najafi, 2004). In medical field, the use of gait analysis encompasses the tests for central nervous disorders, locomotor disorders, rheumatology, orthopedics, endocrinology and neurology (Simon, 2004). At present, the measurement is mostly performed in specialized facilities such as hospital or laboratories (Best & Begg, 2006). These facilities require very high setting up cost (Simon, 2004). Despite the high cost, it is argued that the performed measurement is not accurate or a true representative of the actual daily activities of the subject as it is claimed to only gauge a person's potential walking ability at a given time (Simon, 2004). In fact, the facilities also limit the space usable for the measurement. It is claimed that the most inconvenient aspects of these systems is the fact that the subject must walk in a closed and restrained space (Aminian & Najafi, 2004). The expanding use of gait analysis is catalyzed by the fact that it is able to evaluate walking "out-of-the lab" where most of the daily living activities are performed (Simon, 2004). As an example, it is reported that the locations where falls occur are 77 % outside of the house (Berg et al., 1997). Even though the recent instruments does not measure the gait in real living condition, the trends is moving towards that direction. In addition to their competitive price, user friendliness, miniaturized for portability, capability of efficiently recording and processing larger number of parameters in less time and space are among the required traits of such devices (Simon, 2004). Obviously, these 'dream' system can only be materialized by adoption of the already practically proven microelectronics and micro-electro-mechanical system technologies.

These technologies are said to bring over a number of significant improvements into biomedical instrumentation realization which includes miniaturization, low power consumption, full integration of system and also low cost of production (Bryzek et al., 2006; Jovanov et al., 2005; Hierold,2003). Miniaturization is a great advantage as it means the devices or systems should require only small volume of space. With low power consumption, only small batteries might be needed as power supply, or maybe even energy scavenging can be enough to power them up, if not a combination of them. As full system integration on single silicon chip is also possible, the signal processing and computation can be performed on the same silicon piece with greatly improved overall system performance. Most interestingly, the low per-unit cost is what business and consumers are looking for in every product and have been an undeniable trend (Grace, 1991). In addition, technologically, it also offers numerous materials that not only excellent mechanically for sensing and actuation (Bryzek et al., 2006), they are also biologically compatible (Kotzar et al., 2002). Undoubtedly, these MEMS based devices are the promising tools for outdoor ambulatory measurement and monitoring (Aminian & Najafi, 2004). More interestingly, biomedical application is considered as one of the key new frontiers of MEMS based device development in the future with the worth of billions of dollars (Ko, 2007; Kotzar et al., 2002). In short, with the integration of elegant engineering, advanced instrumentation technology and continuous development in computing propels the art and science of human movement analysis beyond its basic description towards a more prominent role in surgery decision making, orthosis design, rehabilitation, ergonomics and sports (Curran, 2005).

3. Foot pressure measurement: an overview

Fig. 1 depicts foot plantar pressure pattern during gait. The foot is the key limb in human movement. Without foot, a person's mobility is significantly reduced. As a result, the activities of daily living are limited and quality of life is dropped. One way of determining the foot health is by examining the foot plantar pressure. For example, foot ulceration due to diabetes related excessive foot plantar pressure is estimated to cause over $1 billion per year worth of medical expenses in the United States alone (Mackey & Davis, 2006). Diabetes is now considered an epidemic and the number of patients is expected to increase from 171 million in 2000 to 366 million in 2030 (Wild et al., 2004). It is therefore critical to ensure the availability of an accurate and efficient technique of measuring this type of pressure.

In fact, the interface pressure between foot plantar surface and shoe soles is among the key parameters frequently measured in biomechanical research. This parameter is widely used in various applications, for example, screening for high risk diabetic foot ulceration, design of orthotics for pressure redistribution of diabetes mellitus and peripheral neuropathy patients, design of footwear (Mueller,1999), improvement of balance (Santarmou et al.,2006; Bamberg et al., 2006), sports injury prevention in athletes (Gefen, 2002).

Traditionally, the foot plantar pressure measurement is performed in the specialized settings such as laboratories, hospitals or other clinical premises (Best & Begg, 2006). This includes various gait analysis systems such as foot plantar pressure platforms and foot plantar pressure mats. Due to their sizes and the number of equipments required, these measurement systems require specialized settings.

As the depicted pressure measuring systems measure barefoot pressure, the results are obviously not representing real dynamics of foot-shoe interactions. Due to these two

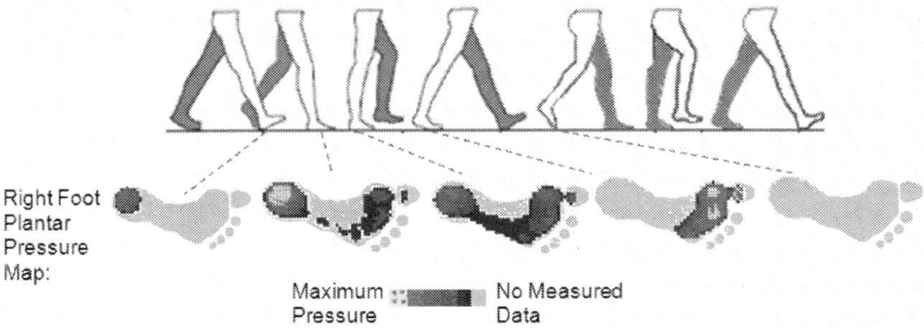

Fig. 1. Foot plantar pressure changes during gait. The foot plantar pressure during stance phase can be measured using many methods and tools.

obvious limitations, a more natural way of measuring pressure is highly required. For that reason, in-shoe pressure measurement devices are more suitable for use in natural living environment.

3.1 In-shoe pressure sensing

Nowadays, a number of foot-shoe pressure sensors are available in the market and many are mentioned in (Urry, 1999). These sensors are made of many different types of material, using different types of manufacturing technologies, made in different sizes, characterized by unique specifications and are operated based on various measurement techniques.

The materials include flexible polymeric layers, dielectrics and also electrical conductors. Some materials used in the sensor development limit the sensor's performance thus creating many issues such as hysteresis, repeatability, accuracy and creep as highlighted in (Lee et al.,2001; Wheeler et al., 2006). Slow response time is among the highlighted weaknesses too (Wheeler et al., 2006). In short, there are obviously many limitations of the currently available sensors in the market as discussed in detail and compiled in the literature (Hsiao, Guan & Weatherly, 2002). Many of the sensors are made as arrays of similarly sized sensor elements. Size of individual sensor affects the efficiency of the measurement system (Urry, 1999). Basically, there are two categories of in-shoe sensors available, the research ones and the commercial ones. Examples of sensor integrated shoes are shown in Fig. 2 which include GaitShoe (Morris, 2004; Bamberg et al, 2008), Smartshoe (Kong & Tomizuka, 2008) and another instrumented (Liedtke et al., 2007). There are also other related works (Abu-Faraj et al., 1997; Tanwar, Nguyen & Stergiou, 2007). Fig. 3 presents some of the available instrumented insoles.

In terms of measurement technique, commonly used techniques are resistive, capacitive, ink-based and others. Each of the techniques offers unique sensitivity and other signal properties. The sensors that are made of polymer or elastomer exhibits some limitations. The resulting issues include repeatability, hysteresis, creep and non-linearity of the sensor output (Lee et al., 2001). In addition to the above weaknesses, some sensors have a relatively large sensor size that may significantly underestimate the pressure, if the arguments in (Urry, 1999) is considered. In fact, this view is supported by another report too (Sarah, Carol & Sharon, 1999).

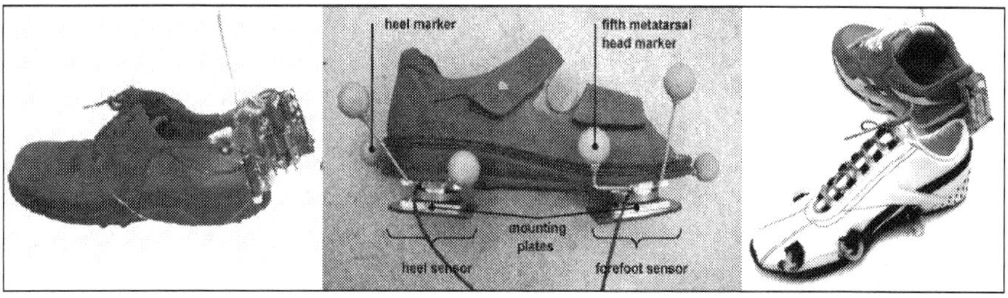

Fig. 2. (Left) The Gaitshoe proposed in MIT (Morris, 2004; Bamberg et al.,2008), (Middle) The instrumented shoe for Ground Reaction Forces determination (Liedtke et al., 2007) and (Right) SmartShoe (Kong & Tomizuka, 2008).

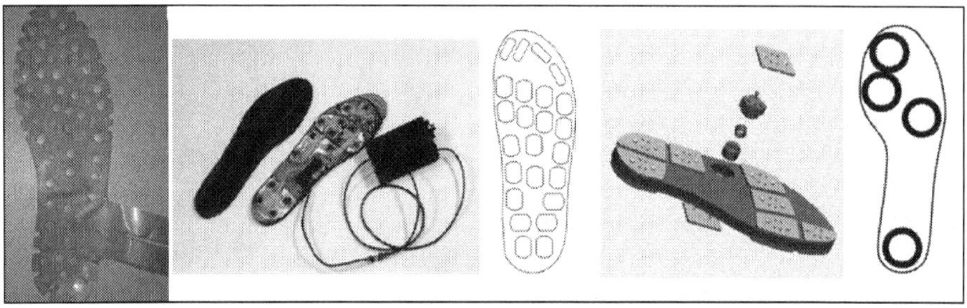

Fig. 3. (Far Left) Bio-foot ® insole with 64 piezoelectric pressure sensors (Martinez-Nova et al., 2007), (Middle Left) the SIMS insole with 32 pressure sensors (Zhang et al., 2004), (Middle) the Parotec insole layout (Chesnin, Selby-Silverstein & Besser, 2000), (Middle Right) the instrumented shoe sole (Faivre et al., 2004) and (Far Right) the SmartShoe sole (Kong & Tomizuka, 2008).

3.2 The application requirement

In performing any measurement, the measuring device must be optimized for that specific application, or else, the observed readings might possibly not accurate. Therefore, a very careful and detail analysis of the specific application requirement must be thoroughly considered before any measurement is performed. Any devices that are to be used in gait analysis must fulfill the requirements such as those explained in detail in (Lee et al.,2001; Urry,1999; Morris, 2004; Bamberg et al.,2008). The required key specifications for a pressure sensor in terms of sensor performance include linearity (linear), hysteresis (low), operating frequency (at least 200 Hz), creep and repeatability (no creep or deformation over repetitive or high cyclic loads), temperature sensitivity (20°C to 37°C), sensing size, pressure range (every 31.2 mm^2 foot plantar area is close to 2.3 MPa), sensing area of the sensor and its placement (micro sized sensors as a dense array sensor).

3.2.1 In-shoe implementation requirement

Nowadays, real-time and in-situ measurement of natural parameters is becoming an unavoidable trend. To catch-up with the fast changing and very demanding trend, also, as gait analysis is about measurement of uninterrupted real parameters, it is very important that the measurement is performed in the real environment. In fact, the effect of daily activities on our health is clearly understood (Urry, 1999). This means the sensor should be very mobile, un-tethered, can be placed in the shoe sole and also can measure effectively in the targeted environment. The detailed requirements are very mobile, limited cabling, shoe placement and also low cost.

3.2.3 Diabetic requirement

In diabetic application, no reports highlight any required additional features other than pressure range. For this reason, the maximum pressure measurable is the only key determining factor. Pressure readings as high as 1900 kPa is reported in the literature (Cavanagh, Ulbrecht & Caputo, 2000). This is obviously a very demanding requirement, as compared to the maximum pressure as obtained in normal people. The pressure ranges of the currently available sensors are very limited. As an example, most of the diabetic sufferers are off the scale as the upper measuring limit of the Emed SF device is approximately 1250 kPa only (Cavanagh, Ulbrecht & Caputo, 2000). Another worrying fact is that, another famous foot plantar pressure product, the F-scan insole, is reported to produce linear pressure reading only up to 1700 kPa (Luo, Berglund & An, 1998). In addition to the above mentioned requirements, a report on diabetic ulceration highlighted that patients measured with foot pressure of ~875 kPa or 87.5 Ncm-2 may be susceptible to ulceration (Lavery et al., 2003). The development of foot plantar ulcer can be visualized as in the Fig. 4.

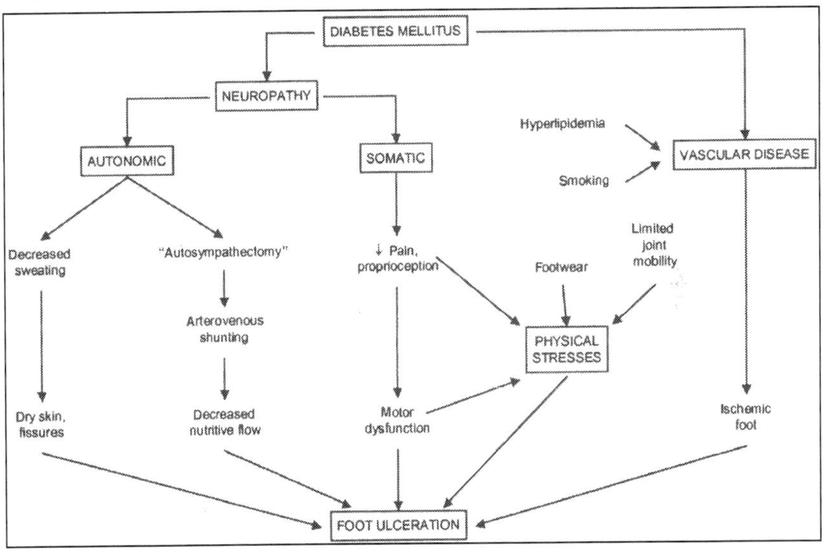

Fig. 4. The factors that lead to foot ulceration among diabetics (Boulton, 2004).

In another report, it is stated that there are three mechanisms that account for the occurrence of ulceration generating pressure (van Schie, 2005). They are: increased duration of exposure to pressures, increased magnitude of pressures and also increased frequency or repetition of exposure to pressure.

Another very important finding from the literature is the fact that for the measurement of foot plantar pressure among the diabetic sufferers, high resolution measurement is required (Urry, 1999).

3.3 Section summary

It is obvious that the need for lower cost in-shoe based pressure sensing devices due to the changing demographics of the world population. Unluckily, the currently available in-shoe sensors are not fully supporting the actual application due to their documented limitations such as limited pressure range, inappropriate sensing area size, hysteresis, linearity, creep and repeatability. Considering all the above requirements and the current limitations, it is obvious that there is a need for an improved design of in-shoe foot plantar pressure measurement device to satisfy the requirements. The great potentials of MEMS technology, which are already proven in other applications, should be explored to achieve this target.

4. The foot clearance measurement: an overview

Gait related healthcare cost continues to increase globally partly due to the surge in occurrence of falls among the elderly population. As higher and higher percentage of the world population, including Australia, is made up of the elderly, more and more occurrence of falls is expected each year. In Australia alone, a total of about $3 billion is reported to be spent as a result of the falls-related injuries in 1999 (Best & Begg, 2006). Among the important gait parameters that directly influence the risk of fall among the elderly is foot clearance. It is the spatial parameter of the foot during the swing phase of the gait cycle representing the distance of shoe sole above the ground. In a recent study involving the analysis of the tripping and falls risks among the elderly individuals during walking (Begg et al., 2007; Best & Begg, 2006; Winter, 1992), it is found that the movement of the foot during mid-swing phase is the most critical event that can initiate the possibility of trip-related fall. This highly important parameter is called minimum foot clearance (MFC). The pattern of foot clearance during gait is depicted in Fig. 5(a) where MFC of below 5 cm and foot trajectory of up to about 17 cm is shown (Begg et al., 2007). Unluckily, the current practice in measuring foot clearance mostly requires laboratory settings with the use of reflective or active markers, as shown in Fig. 5(b)-(d), one or more video cameras, thread-mill or suitable floor and computer software running on suitable computers (Best & Begg, 2006). This type of foot clearance measurement may not be representative of real life ADL based measurement in natural settings (Lai et al., 2008), such as at home or outdoor. Problems such as marker slippage may also occur even during laboratory measurement (Best & Begg, 2006). A more advanced technique is by the use of accelerometers, however, the required calculation that involves double integration of acceleration data yields erratic results due to the effect of drift and errors (Aminian & Najafi, 2004; Lai et al., 2008). The sensing of MFC using accelerometer based measurement on surfaces that are uneven, bumpy or during stair descend or ascend is obviously problematic as it is not directly measuring clearance but rather calculate it using acceleration data.

As current state-of-the-art instruments are mostly requiring exclusive research, clinical or rehabilitation laboratories settings, plus the fact that they are limited in simulating the real world activities of an individual (Best & Begg, 2006; Lai et al., 2008), an in-shoe approach is undoubtedly a better option of implementation.

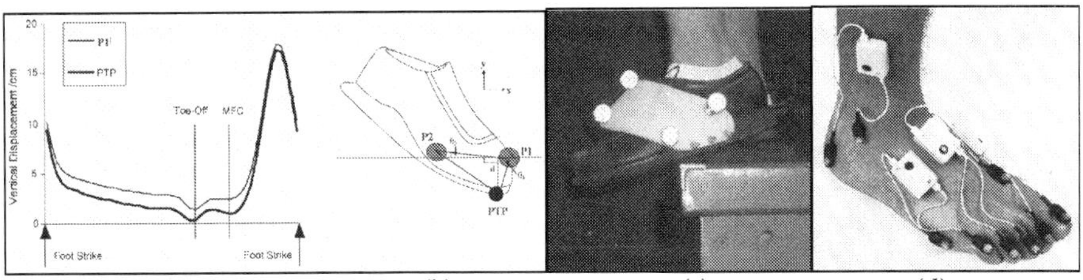

(a) (b) (c) (d)

Fig. 5. (a) Foot trajectory during gait detailing the vertical displacement of foot for one gait cycle showing MFC during mid swing. (b) The markers on the shoe (Begg et al., 2007). (c) A foot clearance measurement during stair decent using passive markers (Hamel et al., 2005). (d) Passive markers (Bontrager, 1998).

4.1 Shoe integrated foot clearance measurement

At current, foot clearance measurement is performed in the laboratories or other clinical settings that use markers, video recorders and other bulky equipments. Only markers are placed on the shoes. Other calculation based measurements, but shoe integrated, are actually accelerometer based system (Aminian & Najafi, 2004; Lai et al., 2008). A shoe integrated direct foot clearance measurement system is the mostly unexplored topic in gait analysis and bio-mechanic research. So far, only one design of shoe integrated direct foot clearance measurement system is reported in the literature (Morris, 2004; Bamberg et.at, 2008). It is as shown in Fig. 6 (a) the sensing walking principle is as detected in fig. 6 (b).

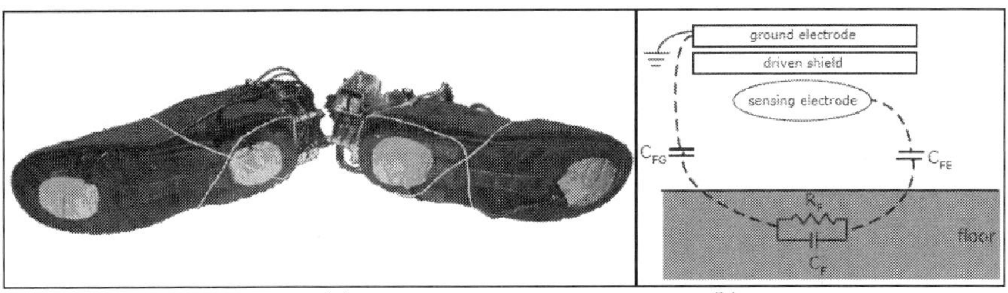

(a) (b)

Fig. 6. (a) Electric field distance sensor electrode attached to the Gaitshoe outsole for foot clearance measurement (Morris, 2004). (b) The working principle of electric field sensing for height determination (Morris, 2004).

Unluckily, the design exhibits several key drawbacks such as follows:

- Low height or clearance measurement range of just up to 5 cm.
- The requirement for minimum 5 layers of electrodes and insulators increases the total thickness of the insole.
- The placement of the conductive electrodes beneath the shoe sole exposes the large area electrode to environmental elements such as water or other materials that may reduce the efficiency and repeatability of the system output.

Due to the obvious limitations, newer systems based on more mobile technology are highly required. As discussed earlier, MEMS offer many great opportunities to close the gap between current requirements and their solutions. Possibility of developing MEMS based devices for clearance measurement is therefore considered. For that reason, various distances measurement techniques need to be analysed and their MEMS applicability needs to be identified. This requires that a better understanding of the requirements of this particular measurement is gained. The knowledge is then compared with the actual strengths and weaknesses of MEMS technology to formulate probably the most suitable and efficient implementation.

4.2 The foot clearance measurement requirement

In order to enable a thorough and effective study, it is crucial that the measurement and monitoring devices are brought into the real environment where the activities are performed. This means, the ability to be attached to the subject's own shoes is the key requirement. Other general requirements for gait analysis are that the device must not affect movement, un-tethered and capable of measuring parameters for both feet (Wahab, et al., 2007a, 2007b, 2008; Morris, 2004). This means that the device should be as small and as light as possible. A measurement range of close to 20 cm is preferable considering maximum toe clearance. However, our current laboratory research suggests minimum foot clearance during the swing phase of walking to be within 3 cm above the walking surface (Begg et al., 2007).
A portable system attached to the lower limb having a mass of 300 g or less has been reported to not affect the normal gait (Morris, 2004). For monolithic CMOS integration, only compatible materials and processes must be used. MEMS device normally fabricated of the size range between 1 μm and 1 cm (Liu, 2006). Considering a 120 steps per minute of adult walking, the sampling rate of 75 Hz, or every 13.4 ms suits well for this application (Morris, 2004). It is reported that the toe clearance above walking surface or ground is minimum around 1.4-1.6 cm during normal walking and around 1.7-2.1 cm during fast walking. On the other hand, the maximum clearance during normal walking is around 5.7-6.9 cm while during fast walking, it is about 6.3-7.8 cm (Elble et al., 1991).

4.3 Distance measurement techniques

Currently, foot clearance measurements are being implemented using electric field sensing technique. However, ultrasound measurement technique is widely used in many other aspect of biomedical and clearance determination application.

4.3.1 Electric Field Sensing (EFS)

The electric field sensing technique developed at the MIT Media Laboratory is proven to be successful in various applications such as gait analysis, entertainment, home automation, automotive etc. In general terms of sensing technique, this technique is basically another type of capacitive sensing. Therefore, this technique is a unique technique. More interestingly, there is a microchip produced by Motorola to support the technique (Morris, 2004), indirectly indicating its capability and commercial value. However, the chip is not fabricated with integrated sensor electrodes so as to enable more flexibility to application designers. An implementation of this technique in gait analysis is also reported in the literature (Morris, 2004; Bamberg et al., 2008). The working principle is shown in Fig. 6(b).
This technique involves electric field sensing between two plates of a capacitor, namely the sensing plate or sensing electrode, and the ground plate or ground electrode. The sensing electrode is connected to the signal transmitting circuitry to generate an electrical field from a sinusoidal AC signal. On the other hand, the ground electrode is connected to

the ground of the circuitry. The floor, as the target of which its distance from the sensing plate is to be measured, contributes to the change in capacitance reading. The change is sensed by the sensing electrode. As the distance between the floor and sensing electrode is varied, the measured capacitance is also varied. Even though this technique is quite simple, it is highly capable of producing quality data for distance measurement. Despite its simplicity and high accuracy, its use is limited by the sensing electrode size requirement. This fact agrees well with the published design guideline (Sieh & Steffen, 2006).

4.3.2 Ultrasonic Sensing (US)

Initially, ultrasound is used for tracking the seabed following the Titanic disaster in 1912 from which it then developed into what is called today as Sound Navigation and Ranging (SONAR) (Smith & Schoenwald, 1984). The application of ultrasound for distance measurement is basically the same with the underwater SONAR, the only difference is the speed of measurement. The speed of ultrasound in air is around 345 ms^{-1}. A number of system level and transducer level design for ultrasonic range measurement realization are reported in the literature such as in automotive and robotic applications (Carullo & Parvis, 2001; Song, Chen & Huang, 2004; Kajita & Tani, 1997). Examples of ultrasonic technique used are such as robotic obstacle avoidance (Bank, 2002), robot height above ground (Kajita & Tani, 1997), car reverse parking assistance (Turner & Austin, 2000), car height above road surface determination (Carullo & Parvis, 2001). It is also used in other assistive technology for the disabled such as assistance for the blind (Ando, 2003) and wheelchair (Simpson et al., 2004; Dutta & Fernie, 2005). Ultrasonic sensing is among the mostly used techniques in biomedical fields, inclusive of several laboratory measurements of gait (Wahab et al., 2008; Begg et al., 2007; Sabatini & Colla, 1998; Weir & Childress, 1997; Abulaffio, Gelernter & Pillar, 1996). Other biomedical applications include therapy, 3D imaging and arterial diameter determination and other biomedical uses (Ling et al., 2007; Coleman et al., 2004). The interest in ultrasound technique is increasing due to its non-ionising or non-electromagnetic characteristic (Smith & Schoenwald, 1984). It is thus a safer method as compared to the ionising ones. Interestingly, it is said that the widespread use of ultrasound for distance measurement is sparked by the famous pocket-sized Polaroid camera developed in the late 1970s. This very portable technology relies on a 5 V battery to produce up to 400 V of pulse-train signal for the excitation of the camera's capacitive ultrasound transducer during auto-focus operation (MacIsaac & Hamaalainen, 2002). With this technology, the camera is able to sense an object 11 m away. Polaroid produces similar ultrasound ranging system for the market and thus enabled development of other ultrasound distance measurement systems for various applications by other companies. It is becoming the precursor for development of ultrasonic ranging systems (Smith & Schoenwald, 1984) and is then considered as one of the enabling technology of the 90's (Grace, 1991).

It is also said that ultrasound signals are used as most of surfaces and objects are good reflectors of ultrasound (Turner & Austin, 2000). Two applications that successfully measure height above ground surface in real outdoor environments are as shown in the Fig. 7. The figure proves that it is highly probable that ultrasound based system is capable of measuring foot clearance above ground.

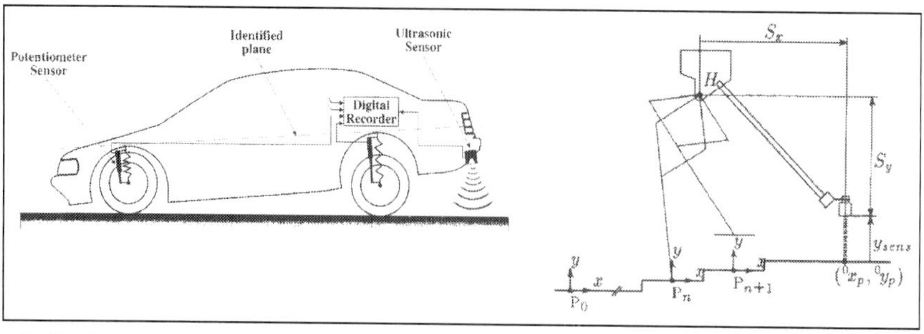

Fig. 7. (Right) Ultrasound sensor is used by robot to measure height (ysens) with resolution of 0.3 mm(Kajita & Tani, 1997), (Left) A 40 kHz Ultrasonic car height measurement for 0°C-40°C operating temperature, 0.1m-0.6m range and better than 1mm resolution (Carullo & Parvis, 2001).

Considering that ultrasound ranging systems are already bearing fruit in mobile ranging application, height above ground application and other gait analysis applications with good distance range, it is therefore a very promising technology for the target application. Several techniques of distance measurement for ultrasound ranging system were proposed in the literature. These include time-of-flight (tof), continuous wave phase-shift method, and also combination of tof and phase (Gueuning et al., 1997). For example, in using tof method as shown in Fig. 8, after an ultrasound signal is transmitted by a transmitting transducer (transmitter), the distance, l, can be calculated based on the time, t, taken by the ultrasound echo to return to the receiver.

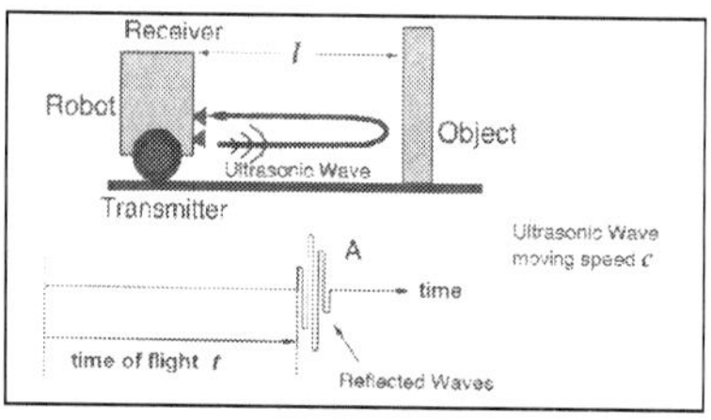

Fig. 8. A simple time of flight concept (Ohya, Ohno & Yuta, 1996).

It is generally understood that increasing ultrasound frequency improves detection resolution (Coleman et al., 2004; Yano, Tone & Fukumoto, 1987) and reduces dead zone length (Bruinsma et al., 2006). However, the high attenuation in air which increases with frequency is a great challenge (Magori, 1994; Yano, Tone & Fukumoto, 1987). It is reported that 1 MHz signal can theoretically measure distance up to 20 cm (Yano, Tone & Fukumoto, 1987), while 2 MHz signal can measure up to few centimeters (Noble et al., 1995). Recently, very high frequency ultrasonic transducers are reported for various high resolution biomedical applications. A more detail discussion on this technology is provided in the next section of the chapter.

4.4 Section summary

From the extensive reference in the literature, it is finally obvious that a direct measurement of foot clearance is highly needed. Unluckily, the instrumentation technology is not paying enough attention to this need for unknown reason. The need for it is increasing due to the changing global population demography. Therefore, this research is trying to close the obviously expanding gap. Two suitable distance measurement techniques are identified for consideration. Each of the technique has its own strength and weaknesses. Therefore, further analysis on the mentioned techniques is warranted. Next, consideration is going to take into account the limitation and strength of MEMS. In this regard, the applicability of the three techniques will again be evaluated after adaptation to suit MEMS technology requirement is made on them.

5. MEMS technology for gait measurement

In evaluating suitability of an identified distance and pressure measurement methods for MEMS realization, a closer look into each of the technologies are necessary. This includes the structural requirement, the operational requirement and the material requirement.

5.1 MEMS clearance sensor

Results from numerical simulations to evaluate the two distance measurement techniques, which include, electric field sensing and also ultrasonic sensing are already presented and discussed. Summary of the results showing some important aspects of the two measurement techniques are presented in Table 1 for comparison.

Key observation	*EFS*	*US*
Sensing range with up to 1 cm^2 sensor area	15 - 20 cm @ 1 cm^2	11 cm @ 1 mm^2 diameter (Kuratli & Huang,2000) ~25cm @ 1 cm^2 using CMUT (Almqvist et al.,2002) 1 m @ 1 MHz, 0.49 cm^2 and 24 cm @ 2 MHz, 0.49 cm^2 (Ergun et al.,2006)
Previously reported as MEMS or micromachined	No	Yes (Kuratli & Huang, 2000; Yaralioglu, 2003)
Ever used in foot clearance measurement	Yes (Morris, 2004)	No
Signal to distance relationship (linearity)	Non-linear	Linear
Remarks based on the analysis results in Section 3	Not suitable due to size	Ultrasound of around 1 MHz may offer good resolution and signal strength
Suitability for MEMS, taking range dependent sensor size as limit	Not suitable	Suitable

Table 1. Comparison of the two techniques.

As presented in Table 1, the comparison between the two techniques shows that high resolution ultrasound ranging is the best choice due to the fact that it is capable of sensing the distance of up to 30 cm, which is the highest range achieved if MEMS size is the key criteria. If the most recently published experimental work by Ergun et al. (2006) is considered, there is no doubt that ultrasound is the best choice for implementation. Obviously, the ultrasonic measurement technique is not only suitable for MEMS, it is also theoretically proven to be able to measure the foot clearance during most of gait related activities too. In MEMS technology, ultrasound sensors are called Capacitive Micromachind Ultrasonic Transducer (CMUT) if it operates on capacitive technique. This result indicates that ultrasound is a very promising technique. Considering those facts, ultrasound is thus selected in this work for the design of a foot clearance measurement sensor.

The target of this work is to design a sensor for use in a portable gait analysis and fall prevention system. To ensure practicality of the design, an application based design specification is developed considering the application requirements. The specifications are:

Operating frequency

The target operating frequency of between 500 kHz and 1 MHz is a good choice. As discussed in the previous section, to eliminate the ultrasound noise, frequencies above 500 kHz is compulsory. On the other hand, frequencies more than 1 MHz may cause significant signal degradation of more than 100 dB. Even though good dynamic range can be realized theoretically, it is better to allow more signals to noise margin (SNR) figure, possibly more up to 30 dB. In the selected frequency range, however, 1 MHz signal may offer higher resolution due to its low wavelength. Nevertheless, if system level algorithm optimization is considered, even low frequency ultrasound can be used to produce sub-millimeter resolutions, as discussed in the preceding section.

Supporting the required sampling frequency

The sensor should be capable of supporting the required 75 Hz distance sampling frequency. Which means, a distance value must be obtained every 13.3 ms. This is not a problem with ultrasonic technique as, consider the worst case scenario where 30 cm foot clearance is measured (ultrasound speed of 340 ms^{-1}) by calculation, the TOF is merely 1.765 ms. In this case, about seven distance measurement can be performed every 13.3 ms, which proves the compliance with the requirement.

Foot clearance range

The sensor must be designed to be able to measure foot clearance above ground/floor of at least 5 cm.

A structural cross-sectional view for CMUT is given in Fig. 9(a) while its electromechanical model is depicted in Fig. 9(b). To understand the CMUT electromechanical behaviour, it is imperative to firstly analyze the fundamental equation for capacitance and then use it together with the electromechanical model.

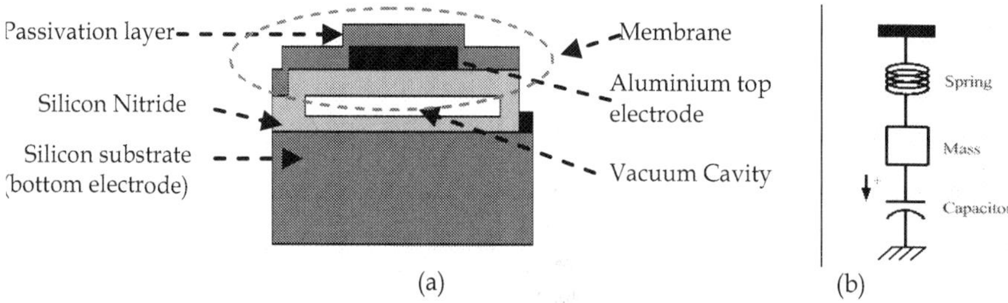

(a) (b)

Fig. 9. (a) A cross-sectional view of a CMUT (adapted from Ergun, Yaralioglu & Khuri-Yakub, 2003). (b) The lumped electromechanical model for CMUT.

The reflected signal activates vibration of the receiver transducer and alters the capacitance value of the transducer structure. The readout circuit detects the capacitance change for appropriate processing of distance information. Considering an ultrasonic measurement technique, a system view of the proposed model is shown in Fig. 10.

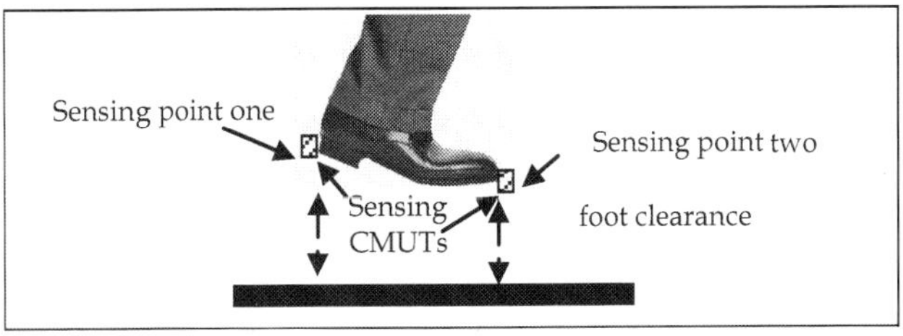

Fig. 10. A possible implementation using two points sensing.

There are two critical measures of a MEMS CMUT. The two are collapse voltage, V_{col} and resonance frequency, f_r. The collapse voltage indicates the possible values of operating voltage while resonance frequency determines the signal characteristic. By referring equation (1), collapse voltage, V_{col} can be determined. In this equation, Y_0 is the young modulus of the membrane material, t_g is a gap/cavity height, t_m is the membrane thickness, ε_0 is the permittivity of free space, 8.854x10^{-12} F/m and r is the membrane radius.

$$V_{col} = \sqrt{\frac{128 Y_0 t_m^3 t_g^3}{27 \varepsilon_0 (1-\sigma^2) r^4}} \quad (1)$$

The deflection of membrane at collapse voltage can be referring to the Fig 11.

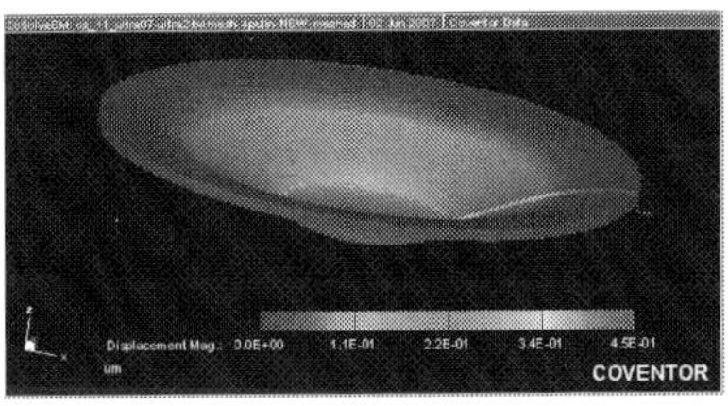

Fig. 11. The deflection of membrane at collapse voltage.

While, for resonance frequency, f_r is shown in equation (2) where ρ_m is the material's density, d_m is its thickness, d_g is a sacrificial layer of thickness, ρ_o is air density, and v_s is sound speed in air. Table 2 shows some good calculation results using (2) and yet it is very simple and fast.

$$f_r = \frac{1}{2\pi}\sqrt{\frac{\rho_o v_s^2}{\rho_m d_m d_g}} \quad (2)$$

All CMUT on silicon design work is performed using the industry standard *Coventorware* tool (Coventor Inc., 2006). As nitride layer is used as the membrane structure material, therefore the top and bottom electrode will never be touched during membrane deflection as it vibrates following the AC voltage excitation.

Membrane Material	Structure dimension	Calculated frequency	Comments
Silicon Nitride,	d_g=0.5μm d_m=0.5μm	2.19 MHz	Comply with calculation in example of (Eccard, Niederer & Fischer, 1997)
Silicon Nitride,	d_g=1.0μm d_m=1.0μm	1.11 MHz	In close agreement with result in (Jones et al., 2001)
Silicon Nitride,	d_g=0.3μm d_m=0.2μm	1.6 MHz	About 10% difference with measured in (Ladabaum et al., 1998)
Al_2O_3	d_g=0.75μm d_m=0.6μm	4.1 MHz	About 5% difference with measured in (Liu et al., 2004)
Silicon Nitride,	d_g=1.0μm d_m=1.1μm	1.05 MHz	Calculation for the optimized frequency

Table 2. Design examples using (2) and comparison with measurements in relevant literature.

Process for developing the transducer is custom sequenced using the available process libraries in *Coventorware Process Editor* module. The sequence starts with a silicon substrate and followed by a nitride deposition of 0.5 μm. A conducting polysilicon of 0.5 μm is then deposited, patterned to form the bottom plate of 45 μm diameter. Following this, the unwanted polysilicon areas are removed by etching.

The release of the membrane structure is performed next where all sacrificial material beneath the structural nitride is removed. This is done through an opening at the side of the wall where the sacrificial layer is exposed. A nitride seal is then deposited in low pressure process to seal the hole left by sacrificial removal leaving cavity in near vacuum.

5.2 MEMS foot presure sensor

Firstly, the shape is determined based on the piezo-resistance sensing requirement. Based on literature, square shape membrane is capable of providing high stress areas, as high as 1.64 times as compared to a circular one (Berns et al., 2006). Mathematical modeling is the first major step of the design with an aim of determining the membrane thickness and side length that can perform pressure measuring task for the specified range. The values of its thickness, length and width must allow linear membrane deflection within the pressure range while ensuring no mechanical damage or fracture.

Silicon as a mechanical material has long being studied and the material characteristics documentations for it have long been published. Silicon is a very promising material in micro-scale sized. These proven facts further boost the exploration activities around silicon based MEMS device realization. Key properties that are important in selection of MEMS materials are such as Yield Strength, Mechanical Hysteresis and Fatigue Failure. Yield Strength is the point when the material starts to exhibit plasticity, which mean, it will elongate un-proportionally the same way a plastic material reacts under external force. This is true in many materials such as steel. In contrast, silicon is a perfect elastic material so that it exhibits a linear or proportional stress-strain relationship. In fact, it yields catastrophically when stress of more than its Yield (or Fracture) Strength figure is applied (Jia & Madou, 2006). Silicon exhibits almost double the Yield Strength as compared to Steel. In addition, perfect elasticity also indicates another great advantage of silicon in sensing performance as it means no Mechanical Hysteresis. As silicon is not exhibiting deformation, it is very insensitive to fatigue and creep (Jia & Madou, 2006). Therefore, in terms of Mechanical

Hysteresis and Fatigue Failure, silicon is showing significant advantages as none of both characteristic being exhibited (Bryzek et al., 2006).
Fig. 12 shows how MEMS pressure sensor is used in Exoskeleton and Parotec insole application.
Fig. 13 shows a crossection of a MEMS pressure sensor.

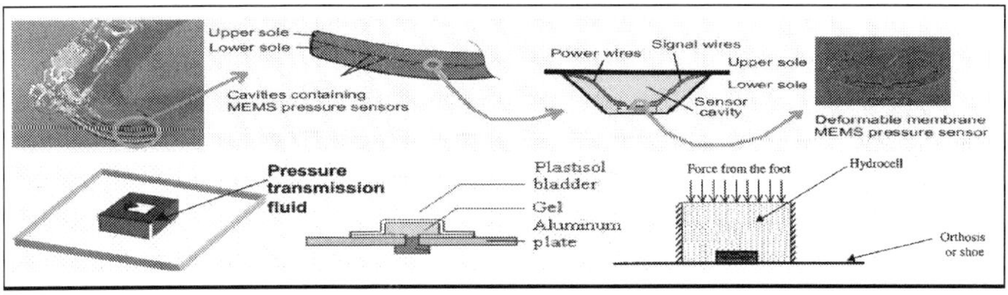

Fig. 12. A Piezoresistive MEMS pressure sensor in action: (Top) the insole of a Robot at University California, Berkeley (Wheeler et al., 2006), (Bottom-Right) The Parotec hydrocell insole (Chesnin, Selby-Silverstein & Besser, 2000), and (Bottom-Left & Middle) a biomechanical pressure sensor (Lee et al., 2001).

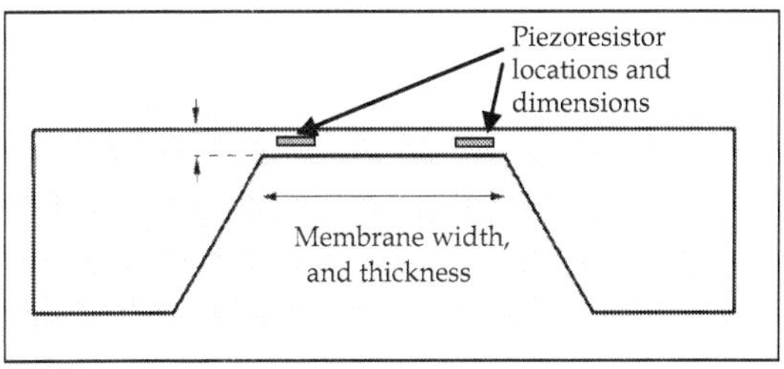

Fig. 13. A conceptual design of a MEMS pressure sensor in a crossectional view.

So, it is highly crucial that the effect of membrane thickness and membrane size on the pressure induced membrane deflection and membrane stress is thoroughly studied at the initial stage. As the output of the sensor is highly dependent on the deflection characteristic parameter and resistance change parameter, the output voltage linearity is thus affected by both parameters too. According to the foundry design guidelines (MultiMEMS, 2007), the piezoresistance change and stress relationship is governed by the linear equation given in (3). On the other hand, equations (4) and (5) relate piezoresistor stresses to the applied pressure in small deflection regime (Gong & Lee, 2001). In these equations, R and R_o are the piezoresistor's resistance value when external pressure is applied and the piezoresistor's resistance without any applied pressure respectively, Π_L and Π_T are the piezoresistance coefficient for longitudinal and transversal directions respectively, h is membrane thickness, L is membrane edge length, e_m is the m-th coefficient as given by Gong & Lee (2001), v is Poisson ratio, l_p is piezoresistor's length, σ_T is the average transversal stress across the piezoresistor and σ_L is the average longitudinal stress along the piezoresistor. The stress components are shown in Fig. 14. Value of e_m coefficients for particulars e_1 is -0.37, while for value of e_m coefficients for particulars e_3 is 0.0379 and for value of e_m coefficients for particulars e_5 is 0.0175.

$$R = R_0(1 + \Pi_L \sigma_L + \Pi_T \sigma_T) \tag{3}$$

$$\sigma_T = \frac{-48}{\pi^4} P\left(\frac{L}{h}\right)^2 \left(\frac{L}{l_p}\right) \sum_{m=1,3,5}^{\infty} \frac{e_m}{m} (-1)^{\frac{m-1}{2}} \sin\left(\frac{m\pi l_p}{2L}\right) \tag{4}$$

$$\sigma_L = v\sigma_T \tag{5}$$

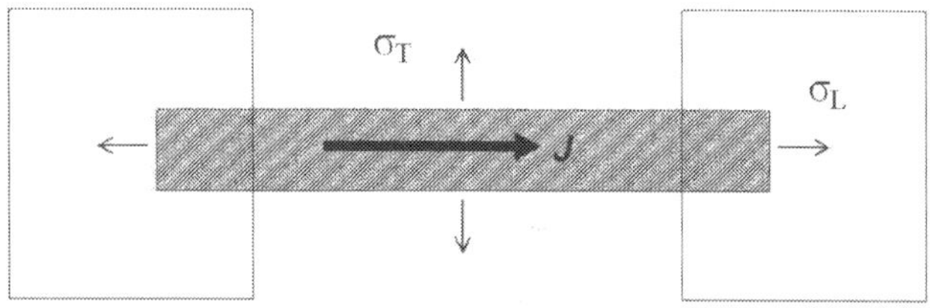

Fig. 14. Transversal and longitudinal stresses acting on a piezoresistor with respect to the current flow direction J (Zamali & Talghader, 2006).

The importance of membrane deflection lies on the fact that since the resistance change due to deflection is already linear in nature, the deflection characteristic therefore becomes the sole determining factor for the linearity of the sensor output. It is reported that the magnitude of membrane deflection is linear with the applied pressure when the deflection is still in the small deflection regime. The membrane is said to operate in this regime as long as the deflection is less than 25 to 50 % of its thickness (Wang et al., 2005, Gong & Lee 2001). For comparison, two equations representing the applied pressure and square membrane deflection are given in equation (6) and (7) (Linlin, Chen & Guangdi, 2006). The former equation is for small deflection regime while the latter represents the large deflection regime. Maier-Schneider, Maibach & Obermeier (1995) also reported large deflection relationship in even more detail, complete with its derivation. As can be seen, the small deflection equation represents a linear relationship, as opposed to the non-linear cubic equation for large deflection. In these equations, in addition to the previously defined symbols, v is Poisson ratio, a is half of edge length, σ_0 is the intrinsic stress of the membrane, E is the Young's Modulus and w_0 are the maximum deflection of the membrane.

$$P = (3.41\frac{h\,\sigma_o}{a^2} + 4.31\frac{Eh^3}{a^4(1-v^2)})w_0 \tag{6}$$

$$P = 3.04\frac{h\,\sigma_o}{a^2} w_0 + 1.88\frac{Eh}{a^4} w_0^{\,3} \tag{7}$$

In addition to the linearity requirement, the mathematical analysis is also important in determining another key design specification, namely maximum pressure measurable. This is due to the fact that the magnitude of total membrane stress determines the maximum pressure value that the membrane may be able to withstand, beyond which the membrane breaks. For that reason, the point of rupture which is also known as Fracture Stress must be taken into account in the determination of suitable membrane dimension. Therefore, the relationship between membrane dimensions and its deflection and stress is extensively analyzed.

After extensive mathematical analysis, the final designs are then determined which consists of only thick membranes. This is due to their compliance with the physical design requirements as identified in the stated foundry maximum size limits, the derived foundry rule based minimum size limit, deflection linearity modelling result and stress withstanding capability modelling result. Finally, only few membrane sizes are chosen to be modeled in silicon.

These selected designs include the ones using 100 μm, 200 μm and 278 μm membranes. Out of the three sensors, the 100 μm sized sensor is the one that can measure wider pressure range, but with less sensitivity and signal magnitude. Whereas, the 200 μm and 278 μm ones are also designed and simulated for comparison and further studies purposes Silicon modeling involving the use of MultiMEMS processes is implemented in Coventorware™ and the three dimensional models are generated for performance analysis.

In using the process steps to model the devices, it is necessary to perform the three model design stages. These stages includes identification of key structural layers required for successful and effective implementation of finite element analysis, layout specifications of the required layers and finally meshing design requirement. Fig. 15 show 3D model and its mesh. In actual design, all four corners of the model are symmetrical.

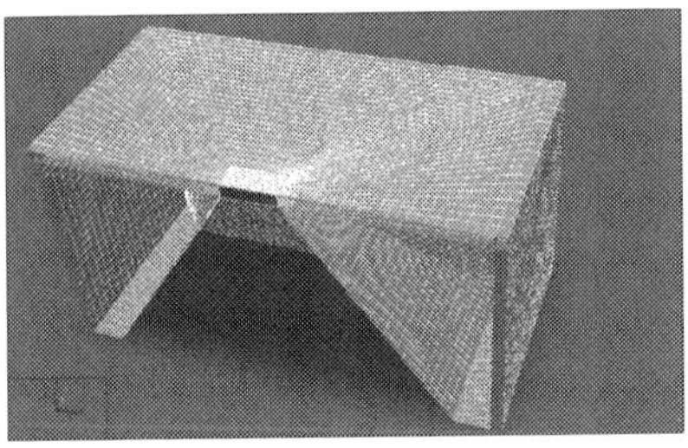

Fig. 15. 3D model and its mesh. In actual design, all four corners of the model are symmetrical.

Supporting the mathematical modeling results are the more computational intensive computer based Coventorware™ results. The Von Mises stress values are considered a good indicator to determine whether a design is suitable or not (Bistue et al., 1997). As the Von Mises stress is the effective stress acting in the membrane, if the membrane Von Mises stress is more than the fracture stress, the material will break (Cardenas et al., 2007). The Von Misses stress is observed at its maximum at the center of the membrane where deflection is at its peak. However, the value for the 100 μm is merely 13 MPa.

The middle of the four sides of the membrane also show significant stress values of about 6 MPa. This much lower stress value shows that the design is very suitable for the targeted range and it is highly probable that in practical, even if a pressure of more than 3 MPa is applied, the membrane is still far from the risk of rupture. In another observation, the resonance frequencies of the membranes as obtained from modal analysis are in the mega-Hertz zones, putting the device in a very safe operation zone, as far as harmonics related error of gait measurement is concerned. These high resonance frequencies are expected considering the membranes thickness. The Von Mises Stress maximum values are given in Table 3. As can be seen, the magnitude of stress is very far from the fracture values for all of the sensors and this observation supports the mathematical analysis. The applied pressure is from 0 to 3 MPa and the observed stresses for the 100, 200 and 278 μm membranes are colour coded for easy observation. The results from FEA simulation, encompassing various membrane stresses is kept in the Coventorware design database. This database can be accessed from other Coventorware modules for further analysis too. In the next section, the database is retrieved to perform a sensor system level analysis.

Sensors	100 μm	200 μm	278 μm
Von Mises Stress	13 MPa	58 MPa	96 MPa

Table 3. The Maximum Von Mises Stress

Using the optimized locations and dimension, the relationship of the output voltage and the applied pressure is obtained. The optimized relationship of the output voltage and pressure when the applied pressure is varied from 0 Pa to 3 MPa on the membrane is superbly linear. The results as presented in the optimization section are hereby verified. The sensor output is again increased 100 times by use of operational amplifier circuit. Another important observation but not directly shown is that, as predicted in the calculation, the deflection is linearly proportional to the pressure magnitude.

The foundry fabrication completes in about six months. Dice in Level 0 Package are shown in a close-up view of the delivered items as shown in Fig. 16(a). Dimensions of the dice are roughly 3 mm X 3 mm X 1.5 mm. It is obvious that the scales on the ruler behind the dice indicate 3 mm die side length. As the holes are drawn for each of the sensors, three holes can be seen on one side of the Level 0 Package (the die on the left of the photograph). On the opposite side of the dice, a cavity is seen above the aluminium interconnection lines. Process variations that may cause thicker than 23.1 μm membranes and also reduced piezoresistance of the piezoresistors are also reported by the foundry (MultiMEMS, 2009b).

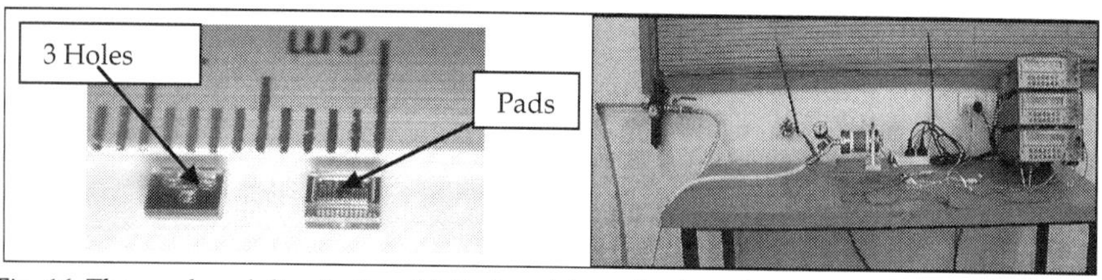

Fig. 16. The produced dice (in Level 0 Package) from the foundry.

The development of custom mechanical set-up which is basically consists of a pressure chamber, its stand, a valve, several steel pipe components (threaded end caps, Y connectors etc) and a pressure gauge is also completed prior to the mechanical laboratory testing. Initially, the design uses RF signal transmission but as metal blocks RF signal and to avoid environmental related attenuation, wired solution is later chosen. Wired connection also provides more direct, accurate and highly reliable readings.

A high pressure industrial grade compressed air system is used to supply pressurized air into the chamber through the valve and the Y connector. To ensure gradual increase of pressure in the chamber, the valve is manually controlled. Air pressure is gauged using the readily fitted pressure gauge as its pressure sensing mechanism is also exposed to the pressurized air in the chamber through the other branch of the Y connector. A photograph showing the complete mechanical testing set-up is given in Fig. 16(b).

Pressure is increased gradually from slightly above the atmospheric pressure up to the maximum pressure allowed by the calibration certificate. Fig. 17 shows the graphs of the output of the three pressure sensors. The measurements begin with 20 psi level, which is equivalent to 137.9 kPa and ends at 135 psi (930.825 kPa) due to calibration limitation. It is clear that the pressure and output voltage relationship of all the sensors are very linear as expected from simulation result. The system is powered by a 9V battery. Most interestingly, the results prove the quality of the designed piezoresistive pressure sensors in producing very linear pressure to voltage relationship, which is the key objective of this research.

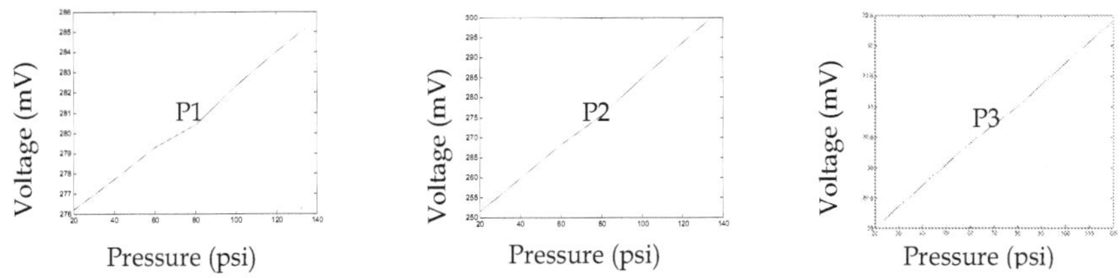

Fig. 17. The graphs produced from the recorded experimental pressure and output voltage relationship. The voltages are not amplified.

6. Chapter summary and discussion

The current state of gait analysis instrumentation is discussed. It is proven that newer generation of gait analysis/biomechanical instrumentation is produced to ensure real time and efficient measurement. Therefore MEMS technology is explored. In this chapter, two MEMS based sensors, one for foot plantar pressure measurement, and the other one for foot clearance measurement are discussed.

In concluding this chapter let us begin with foot clearance measurement. Two most suitable distance measurement techniques are studied and presented for consideration towards realization of a MEMS based foot clearance sensing device. They are firstly optimized for MEMS according to the MEMS technology requirement, in aspects such as structural materials and size. They are then evaluated in terms of suitability for foot clearance measurement application by means of maximum distance and linearity simulations. The requirements for gait analysis application are also presented and used as the guidelines for the selection. The analysis of the simulation results and comparisons with the measured data in literature are also included. Ultrasound-based distance measurement technique is preferred due to its proven practical use in similar other applications and also due to good simulation results in terms of maximum foot clearance that can be measured. In addition, it is also generally showing linear relationship between clearance and tof signal.

Various ultrasound generation and sensing mechanisms such as piezoelectric and capacitive are studied. The selection of sensing mechanism is based on aspects of fulfilment of gait analysis needs, competitiveness of manufacturing cost and capability for total integration with circuitry for performance and system miniaturization. Among the gait analysis needs include small size, light weight and suitable range. In addition to dependency of sensing range on signal frequency, the measureable range is also dependent on signal strength, so, the right choice of elelctromechanical coupling factor is important when biasing the CMUT. This characteristic offers an additional flexibility in terms of range and power management.

As a result, a CMOS compatible CMUT realization is chosen and explored. This includes the design requirement and specification, mathematical analysis, computer simulation and finally design implementation of a CMOS compatible CMUT tailored for ultrasonic foot clearance measurement. All results pertaining to various steps are presented and discussed. Some key parameters of the CMUT are also included.

In addition to the many device related advantages inherited from the use of CMUT technology, the system level strengths, such as signal processing, will be further enhanced due to its CMOS compatibility. The literature proves that CMUT dedicated CMOS circuits such as for signal processing is already studied and developed (Wygant et al., 2004). The inclusion of sensors, signal processing and compensation circuitry, memory and wireless communication capability in one chip as an SoC may produce a high performance ultrasonic system (Svilainis & Dumbrava, 2005; Schweinzer & Elmer, 2005).

In short, the objective of the study which is to explore MEMS applicability for the measurement of foot-to-ground clearance has been achieved and demonstrated. A suitable technique is identified, and as a result, an ultrasonic transducer suitable for foot clearance measurement system is fully designed, modelled, and implemented. The transducer/sensor is optimized for gait analysis application. As it is CMOS compatible, further works on CMOS circuitry will enable system level integration for the realization of an integrated high performance system for foot clearance measurement.

Next, let us recall a discussion on foot plantar pressure. The testing and characterization of a silicon MEMS pressure sensor for biomedical application is also described. Every steps of the project is explained, including the internal pads interconnection, Level 0 Package design, GDS II foundry file generation for tape-out, wirebonding from Level 0 Package pads to Level 1 Package pins, Level 1 Packaging, printed circuit board design, amplifier circuit design, complete circuit integration on printed circuit board, electrical testing system design and testing implementation and finally mechanical testing system design and testing implementation. All the steps are successfully performed. The results of each of the steps are recorded, displayed and discussed in detail. The key findings of the work in this chapter cover the electrical and mechanical testing results.

From the electrical design and testing aspects of the fabricated pressure sensor, the resistance of the piezoresistors are of great importance and are thus is discussed in detail. To verify this, the measured results are compared with the calculated values from the design stage. The comparison shows very acceptable resistance variations across three different sensor designs. The source of variation is identified as resulting from foundry process deviation, according to the fabrication report from the foundry (MultiMEMS, 2009b). The result proves that the layout design stage is very important to ensure achievability of the target specification as outlined during the design and optimization stage.

Further work then includes the study of the sensors' response under varying pressure. This is the final part of the research where the sensing capability is studied and discussed. Due to the nature of the measurand, this final job is also very demanding, especially in the aspects of mechanical preparation. A specialized pressure chamber is designed solely for this purpose with the sensor board size and cabling requirements in mind. Finally, the much awaited sensor characterization results are performed and the recorded results prove that the sensors' responses are very linear.

With the completion of the pressure sensor characterization, the research work is now completed successfully. Results from both finite element analysis and experimental works have proven that the sensors are linear and capable of producing high signal values. Therefore, the mission is now accomplished.

7. References

Abu-Faraj, Z.O., Harris, G.F., Abler, J.H. and Wertsch, J.J. A Holter-type, 1997. 'Microprocessor-based, rehabilitation instrument for acquisition and storage of plantar pressure data', *Journal of Rehabilitation Research and Development*, vol. 34, pp. 187–194.

Abulaffio, D.R., Gelernter, I & Pillar, T., 1996. 'An ultrasonic-operated kinematic measurement system for assessment of stance balance in the clinic', *Clinical Biomechanics*, Vol. 11, pp. 173–175.

Aminian, K. and Najafi, B., 2004. 'Capturing human motion using body-fixed sensors: Outdoor measurement and clinical applications', *Computer Animation and Virtual Worlds*, vol. 15, no. 2, pp. 79-94.

Ando, B., 2003, 'Electronic sensory systems for the visually impaired', *IEEE Measurement Magazine*, vol. 6 No. 2, pp. 62- 67.

Bamberg, S.J.M., Benbasat, A.Y., Scarborough, D.M., Krebs, D.E. and Paradiso, J.A., 2008. 'Gait analysis using a shoe-integrated wireless sensor system', *IEEE Transactions on Information Technlogy in Biomedicine*, July, vol. 12, no 4, pp. 413-23.

Bank, D., 2002. 'A Novel Ultrasonic Sensing System for Autonomous Mobile Systems', *IEEE Sensors Journal*, vol. 2, no. 6, pp.597-606.

Berg, W.P., Alessio, H.M., Mills, E.M. and Tong, C.,1997. 'Circumstances and consequences of falls in independent community-dwelling older adults', *Age Ageing*, Vol. 26 , No. 4, pp. 261–268.

Berns, A., Buder, U., Obermeier, E., Wolter, A. and Leder, A., 2006. 'AeroMEMS sensor array for high-resolution wall pressure measurements', *Sensors and Actuators A:Physical*,vol. 132,pp. 104-111.

Best, R. and Begg, R.K., 2006. 'Overview of Measurement Analysis and Gait Features', in *Computational Intelligence for Movement Sciences: Neural Networks and Other Emerging Techniques*, eds Begg, R.K. and Palaniswami, M., Hershey, PA, USA, pp. 1-69.

Bistue, G., Elizalde, J. G., Garcia-Alonso, S., Castano, E., Gracia, F. J. and Garcia-Alonso, A., 1997. 'A design tool for pressure microsensors based on FEM simulations', *Sensors and Actuators A: Physical*, vol. 62, pp. 591-594.

Bontrager, E.L.1998. 'Instrumented gait analysis systems' in *Gait Analysis in the. Science of Rehabilitation*, ed. De Lisa, J.A., Chapter 2. Department of Veterans Affairs, Washington, DC, USA. pp. 11-32.

Boulton, A., 2004. 'Pressure and the diabetic foot: clinical science and offloading techniques', *The American Journal of Surgery*, Vol. 187, No. 5, pp. S17-S24.

Bruinsma, A.J.A, 2006. *Level sensor lithographic apparatus and device manufacturing method*, Paris,France: European Patent Office, EP1674939A1.

Bryzek, J., Roundy, S., Bircumshaw, B., Chung, C. A. C. C., Castellino, K. A. C. K., Stetter, J. R. and Vestel, M. A. V. M., 2006, 'Marvelous MEMS', *Circuits and Devices Magazine, IEEE*, vol. 22, pp. 8-28.

C. Hierold, 2003. 'Micro- and Nanosystems: Review and Outlook', in *Proceedings of the 14th Micromechanics Europe Workshop (MME03)*, Nov. 2-4, Delft, The Netherlands, pp. 101-104.

Cardenas, M.L., Cardenas-Valencia, A. M., Dlutowski, J., Bumgarner, J. and Langebrake, L., 2007. 'A finite element method modeling approach for the development of metal-silicon nitride MEMS single-use valve arrays', *J. Micromech. Microeng.*, vol. 17, pp 1671-1679.

Carol, M. W., Sarah, M. G. and Sharon, J. D., 1999. 'The shock attenuation characteristics of four different insoles when worn in a military boot during running and marching', *Gait & Posture*, vol. 9, no. 1, pp.31-37.

Carullo, A. and Parvis, M., 2001. 'An Ultrasonic Sensor for Distance Measurement in Automotive Applications', *IEEE Sensors Journal*, vol. 1, no. 2, pp.143-146.

Cavanagh, PR., Ulbrecht, JS. and Caputo, GM., 2000. 'New developments in the biomechanics of the diabetic foot',. Sep-Oct., *Diabetes Metab Res,* Rev. 16, Suppl. 1, pp. S6-S10.

Chesnin, K. J., Selby-Silverstein, L. and Besser, M. P., 2000. 'Comparison of an in-shoe pressure measurement device to a force plate: concurrent validity of center of pressure measurements', *Gait & Posture,* Vol. 12, No. 2, 1 October, pp. 128-133.

Coleman, D.J., Silverman, R.H., Chabi, A., Rondeau, M.J., Shung, K.K., Cannata, J., Lincoff, H. 2004. 'High-resolution Ultrasonic imaging of the posterior segment', *Ophthalmology*, Vol. 111, No 7, pp. 1344-1351.

Coventor Inc.,2006. *CoventorWare® 2006:Master Help*, Coventor Inc., Cary, NC, USA.

Curran, S. A. and Dananberg, H. J. 2005. 'Future of Gait Analysis: A Podiatric Medical Perspective', *Journal of American Podiatry Medical Association,* vol. 95, no 2, pp 130-142.

Elble, R.J., Thomas, S.S., Higgins, C. and Colliver, J.,1991. 'Stride-dependent changes in gait of older people', *Journal of Neurology*, vol. 238, no 1, pp 1-5.

Ergun, A. S., Yaralioglu, G.G., Oralkan, O. and Khuri-Yakub, B. T.,2006. 'Techniques and Applications of Capacitive Micromachined Ultrasonic Transducers', in *MEMS/NEMS Handbook Techniques and Applications*, ed. Cornelius T. Leondes, vol. 1, Springer, New York, USA, pp. 223-285.

Faivre, A., Dahana, M. , Parratteb B. and Monnier, G., 2004. 'Instrumented shoes for pathological gait assessment', *Mechanics Research Communications*, Vol. 31, no. 5, September-October, pp. 627-632.

Gefen, A.,2002. 'Biomechanical analysis of fatigue-related foot injury mechanisms in athletes and recruits during intensive marching', *Medical and Biological Engineering and Computing*,Vol. 40, No. 3, pp. 302- 310.

Gong, S.-C. and Lee, C., 2001. 'Analysis solutions of sensitivity for pressure microsensors', *IEEE Sensors Journal* , Vol.1, No.4, pp. 340–344.

Grace, R,H., 1991. 'OEM Sensors For The'90's: An Overview Of Enabling Technologies', in *Proceedings of Electro International 1991*, pp. 648-654.

Gueuning, F. E., Varlan, M., Eugene, C. E. and Dupuis P., 1997. 'Accurate distance measurement by an autonomous ultrasonic system combining time-of-flight and phase-shift methods', *IEEE transactions on instrumentation and measurement*, vol. 46, no 6, pp. 1236-1240.

Hamel, K. A., Okita, N., Higginson, J. S., Cavanagh, P. R., 2005. 'Foot clearance during stair descent: effects of age and illumination', *Gait & Posture*, Vol. 21, No. 2, pp. 135-140.

Hsiao H, Guan J, Weatherly M., 2002. 'Accuracy and precision of two in-shoe pressure measurement systems', *Ergonomics.*, vol. 45, no. 8, pp 537-555.

Jia, G. and Madou, M.J., 2006. 'MEMS Fabrication', in: *The MEMS Handbook: MEMS Design and Fabrication*, 2nd Ed., 3, Vol. 2, ed. Gad-el-Hak, CRC Taylor and Francis, Boca Raton, Florida, USA.

Jovanov, E., Milenkovic , A., Otto , C , and de Groen , P. C, A wireless body area network of intelligent motion sensors for computer assisted physical rehabilitation, *Journal of NeuroEngineering and Rehabilitation*, vol. 2, 6.

Ko, H.S., Liu, C.W. and Gau, C., 2007. 'Micropressure sensor fabrication without problem of stiction for a wider range of measurement', *Sensors and Actuators A: Physical*, Vol. 138, No. 1, 20 July, pp. 261-267.

Kong, K. and Tomizuka, M., 2008, 'Estimation of Abnormalities in a Human Gait Using Sensor-Embedded Shoes', in *Proceedings of the 2008 IEEE/ASME Int. Conf. on Adv. Intel. Mechatronics*, July 2-5, Xian, China, pp. 1331-1336.

Kotzar, G., Freas, M., Abel, P., Fleischman, A., Roy, S., Zorman, C., Moran, J.M. and Melzak, J. 2002. 'Evaluation of MEMS materials of construction for implantable medical devices', *Biomaterials*, Vol. 23, no 13, pp.2737–2750.

Lai, D.T.H., Begg,R.K., Charry, E.,Palaniswami, M. and Hill, K., 2008. 'Measuring toe clearance using a wireless inertial sensing device', in *Proceedings of International Conference on Intelligent Sensors, Sensor Networks and Information Processing*, Sydney, Australia . December 15-18, pp. 375-380.

Lavery, L. A., Armstrong, D. G., Wunderlich, R. P., Tredwell, J. and Boulton, A. J.M., 2003. 'Predictive Value of Foot ressure Assessment as Part of a Population-Based Diabetes Disease Management Program', *Diabetes Care*, April, Vol. 26, pp.1069-1073.

Lee, N. K. S., Goonetilleke, R. S., Cheung, Y. S. and So, G. M. Y., 'A flexible encapsulated MEMS pressure sensor system for biomechanical applications', *Microsystem Technologies*, vol. 7, pp. 55-62, 2001.

Liedtke, C., Fokkenrood, S. A.W., Menger, J. T., van der Kooij, H. and Veltink, P. H., 2007, 'Evaluation of instrumented shoes for ambulatory assessment of ground reaction forces, *Gait & Posture*, Vol. 26, No. 1, June, pp. 39-47.

Ling, H., Choi, P., Zheng, Y. and Lau, K., 2007. 'Extraction of mechanical properties of foot plantar tissues using ultrasound indentation associated with genetic algorithm', *Journal of Materials Science: Materials in Medicine*, Vol. 18, No. 8, pp. 1579-1586.

Linlin, Z., Chen, X. and Guangdi, S., 2006. Analysis for load limitation of square-shaped silicon diaphragms', *Solid-State Electronics*, vol. 50, pp. 1579-1583,

Luo, Berglund & An, 1998. 'Validation of F-Scan pressure sensor system - A technical note',*Journal of Rehabilitation Research and Development*, Vol. . 35, No . 2, pp 186-191.

MacIsaac, D., and Hämäläinen, A., 2002, 'Physics and Technical Characteristics of Ultrasonic Sonar Systems', *The Physics Teacher*, vol. 40 pp. 39-46.

Mackey, J. R.,and Davis, B. L.,2006. 'Simultaneous shear and pressure sensor array for assessing pressure and shear at foot/ground interface', *Journal of Biomechanics*, Vol. 39, No. 15, pp. 2893-2897.

Magori,V. 1994. 'Ultrasonic sensors in air', in *Proceedings of IEEE Ultrasonics Symposium 1994*, pp. 471-481.

Morris, S.J., 2004, *Shoe-integrated sensor system for wireless gait analysis*, PhD Thesis, MIT, USA.

Mueller, M. J, 1999. 'Application of plantar pressure assessment in footwear and insert design', *Journal of Orthopaedics and. Sports Physical Therapy*, vol. 29, no 12, pp. 747-756.

Noble, R.A., Anthony, D., Schindel, D.W., Hutchins, D.A., Zou, L. and Sayer, M, 1995. 'The Design and Characterization of Micromachined Air-coupled Capacitance Transducer', *IEEE Transactions on Ultrasonics, Ferroelectrics, and Frequency Control*, vol. 42, no. 1, pp. 42-50.

Octavio, A., Martin, C.J., Martinez, O., Hernando, J., Gomez-Ullate, L. and Montero de Espinosa, F., 2007. 'A Linear CMUT Air-Coupled Array For NDE Based on MUMPS', in *Proceedings of IEEE Ultrasonics Symposium*, 28-31 Oct., pp. 2127-2130.

Ohya, A., Ohno,T. and Yuta, S., 1996. 'Obstacle Detectability of Ultrasonic Ranging System and Sonar Map Understanding', *Robotics and Autonomous Systems*, Vol.18, pp.251-257.

Rodgers, M.M., 1988. 'Dynamic biomechanics of the normal foot and ankle during walking and running', *Physical Therapy*, vol. 68, no 12, pp. 1822-1830.

Sabatini, A. M. and Colla, V., 1998. 'A method for sonar based recognition of walking people", Robotics and Autonomous Systems', Vol. 24, pp. 117-126, 1998.

Santarmou, E., Dozza, M., Lannocca, M., Chiari, L. and Cappello, A., 2006. 'Insole pressure sensor-based audio-biofeedback for balance improvement', *Gait & Posture*, vol. 24, pp. S30-S31.

Sieh P. and Steffen M. 2006. *Playing the E-Field: Capacitance Sensors in Action*, Sensors, viewed 11 Dec. 2006, - <http://www.sensorsmag.com/sensors/content/printContentPopup.jsp?id=369839>.

Simon, S.R., 2004. 'Quantification of human motion: gait analysis—benefits and limitations to its application to clinical problems', *Journal of Biomechanics*, Vol. 37, No. 12, pp. 1869-1880.

Simpson, R., LoPresti, E., Hayashi, S., Nourbakhsh, I. and Miller, D., 2004. 'The Smart Wheelchair Component System', *Journal of Rehabilitation Research and Development*, Vol. 41, No 3B, May/June, pp. 429 - 442.

Smith, C.V., Jr. and Schoenwald, J.S., 1984. 'A Two Tone Narrow Bandwidth Range-Rate Finding System', in *Proceedings of IEEE 1984 Ultrasonics Symposium*, pp. 465 - 468.

Song, K., Chen, C. and Huang, C. C., 2004. 'Design and experimental study of an ultrasonic sensor system for lateral collision avoidance at low speeds', in *Proceedings of 2004 IEEE Intelligent Vehicles Symposium*, 14-17 June, pp. 647 - 652.

Svilainis, L. and Dumbrava, V., 2005. 'Design of a low noise preamplifier for ultrasonic transducer', *ULTRAGARSAS*, vol. 55 no.2, , pp.28-33.

Tanwar, H., Nguyen L. and Stergiou, N., 2007. 'Force Sensitive Resistor (FSR)-based Wireless Gait Analysis Device', in *Proceedings of Telehealth - 2007*, May 31 – June 1 ,Montreal, QC, Canada.

Turner, J. D. & Austin, L., 2000. 'Review Article:Sensors for automotive telematics', *Meas. Sci. Technol.* Vol. 11 , pp. R58–R79.

Urry, S., 1999. 'Plantar pressure-measurement sensors', *Measurement Science and Technology*, vol. 10, pp. R16-R32.

van Schie, C. H. M., 2005. A Review of the Biomechanics of the Diabetic Foot., *Lower Extremity Wounds*, Vol. 4, No. 3, pp. 160-170.

Wahab, Y, Zayegh, A., and Veljanovski, R., and Begg, R.K., 2008. 'Sensitivity optimization of a foot plantar pressure micro-sensor', in *Proc. 20th IEEE International Conf. on Microelectronics 2008*. Sharjah, UAE, 14-17 Dec., pp 104-107.

Wahab, Y, Zayegh, A., Begg, R.K. and Veljanovski, R. , 2007b, 'CMUT For Human And Humanoid Locomotion Mesurement', in *Proceedings of Int. Con. on Robotics, Vision, Information and Signal Processing 2007*, Universiti Sains Malaysia, Penang, Malaysia, pp. 359-364.

Wahab, Y, Zayegh, A., Begg, R.K. and Veljanovski, R., 2007a, 'Analysis of foot to ground clearance measurement techniques for MEMS realization',in *Proceedings of the IEEE International Conference on Computer and Information Technology (ICCIT 2007*, Dhaka Bangladesh, pp. 1-5.

Wang, Z., Zhu, W., Miao, J., Zhu, H., Chao, C. and Tan, O. K., 2006, 'Micromachined thick film piezoelectric ultrasonic transducer array', *Sensors and Actuators A: Physical*, Vol. 130-131, Selected Papers from TRANSDUCERS '05 - The 13th International Conference on Solid-State Sensors, Actuators and Microsystems - Seoul, Korea, 5-9 June 2005, 14 August, pp. 485-490.

Weir, R. F. and Childress, D. S., 1997. 'A new method of characterizing gait using a Wells, L.H., 1968. 'Basic ultrasonics: 2 — The use of compression (longitudinal) waves in ultrasonic testing', *Non-Destructive Testing*, Vol. 1, No. 5, August, pp. 291-296.

Wheeler, J., Rohrer, B., Kholwadwala, D., Buerger, S., Givler, R., Neely, J., Hobart, C. and Galambos, P., 2006. 'In-Sole MEMS Pressure Sensing for a LowerExtremity Exoskeleton', *in Proceedings of The First IEEE/RAS-EMBS International Conference on Biomedical Robotics and Biomechatronics*, pp. 31-34.

Wild, S., Roglic, G., Green, R. Sicree, A. and King, H., 2004. 'Global Prevalence of Diabetes', *Diabetes Care*, Vol. 27, No 5, pp 1047-1053.

Winter, D.A., 1992. 'Foot trajectory in human gait: a precise and multi-factorial motor control task'. *Physical Therapy*, vol. 72, no 1 , pp 45-56.

Wygant, I.O., Zhuang, X., Yeh, D.T., Nikoozadeh, A., Oralkan, O., Ergun, A.S., Karaman, M. and Khuri-Yakub, B.T., 2004, 'Integrated ultrasonic imaging systems based on CMUT arrays: recent progress', in *Proceedings of the IEEE International Ultrasonics Symposium, vol. 1*, IEEE, pp. 391–394.

Yano, T., Tone, M., and Akira Fukumoto, A., 1987. 'Range Finding and Surface Characterization Using High Frequency Air Transducers', *IEEE Transactions on Ultrasonics, Ferroelectrics, and Frequency Control*, vol. UFFC 34, no. 2, pp. 232-236.

Zamali, M.S.B. and Talghader, J.J., 2006, 'Stress-mapping sensors for high-power adaptive micro-optics', *Applied Optics*, Vol. 45, No. 7, March, pp1619-1624.

14

Low-Wavelengths SOI CMOS Photosensors for Biological Applications

Olivier Bulteel, Nancy Van Overstraeten-Schlögel, Aryan Afzalian, Pascal Dupuis, Sabine Jeumont, Leonid Irenge, Jérôme Ambroise, Benoît Macq, Jean-Luc Gala and Denis Flandre
Université catholique de Louvain
Belgium

1. Introduction

Biological agents may be characterized (in terms of quantity (or concentration), purity, nature) using optical ways like spectrometry, fluorometry and real-time PCR for example. Most of these techniques are based on absorbance or fluorescence. Indeed, many biological molecules can absorb the light when excited at wavelengths close to blue and ultraviolet (UV). For example, DNA, RNA and proteins feature an absorption peak in the deep UV, more precisely around 260 and 280 nm (Karczemska & Sokolowska, 2001). This work is widely focused on those wavelengths. A biological sample concentration measurement method can be based on UV light absorbance or transmittance, as already known and realized with high-cost and large-size biomedical apparatus. But, often, the difficulties come from the limitation for measuring very small concentrations (close to a few ng/μL or lower) since the measurement of such small light intensity variations at those low wavelengths requires a precise light source, and very efficient photodetectors. Reducing the dimensions of such a characterization system further requires a small light source, a miniaturized photosensor and a processing system with high precision to reduce the measurement variations. Some light-emitting diodes (LED) performing at those UV wavelengths have recently appeared and may be used to implement the light source. Concerning the optical sensor, while accurate but high-cost photosensors in technologies such as AlGaN and SiC provide high sensitivities in UV low wavelengths thanks to their semiconductor bandgap (Yotter & Wilson, 2003), the silicon-on-insulator (SOI) layers absorb the photons in that specific range thanks to an appropriate thickness of the silicon. Adding excellent performances of low power consumption, good temperature behavior and high speed (Flandre et al., 1999; 2001), the SOI technology allows the designers for integrating a specific signal processing integrated CMOS circuit to transform the photocurrent into a digital signal for example. This opens the possibility to build a low-cost, complete and portable microsystem, including the light source, the photodetector and a recipient for the sample to characterize.

For this chapter, we start with a state-of-the-art describing the current DNA quantification methods with their advantages and disadvantages. Since we will work at low optical wavelengths, we review different ultraviolet light sources that are used in laboratories or in biomedical fields. A description of different photodetectors in various technologies, more especially in SOI, suitable for DNA quantification will then be presented. Afterwards, we detail, the SOI photodiode and the integrated circuit that were used in our experiments for characterizing DNA concentration as well as the other particular biological agents. Finally, the results of our measurements are presented and discussed.

2. Current optic-based DNA quantification methods

Nowadays the DNA concentration in liquid samples may be measured by different techniques. For example, it is possible to quantify DNA by its property to absorb light around 260 nm. However, the DNA quantities are usually too small to be detected, so the DNA concentration has to be amplified. A very-well know method to amplify DNA is the polymerase chain reaction (PCR).

2.1 PCR related methods

The polymerase chain reaction consists in a cyclic repetition of different temperature stages of a solution containing the DNA to amplify, dNTPS, primer and the DNA polymerase enzyme. A heating stage is necessary to separate the two strands of the DNA. At the lower temperature, each strand is used as a template for the synthesis by the DNA polymerase. After a consistent number of cycles, the target DNA (determined by the primer) is amplified by a factor 2^x (where x is the cycle number). The DNA concentration can next be measured by two different ways :

- the agarose gel electrophoresis. This consists in a migration of the DNA in an agarose gel under a bias voltage. The size of the double stranded DNA is revealed by a luminescent incorporation agent and estimated by comparison with a DNA ladder used as reference. The detection is visual which is inconvenient because of its dependence on the personal visual accuracy.
- the quantitative real-time PCR. This method allows the measurement of DNA concentrations during the amplification of the DNA by the addition of aspecific fluorophores. Basically, one fluorophore is initially added to the solution and engraft to the double stranded DNA along with the increase of the DNA. After each cycle, the DNA solution is illuminated and the fluorophores grafted to the DNA are emitting a light at a specific wavelength. The emitted fluorescence is thus proportional to the DNA quantity. The main problem of the real-time PCR is the relatively poor efficiency of the fluorophores and thus the light emission does not always reflect the accurate DNA concentration.

Anyway, the PCR-based methods feature the disadvantages of a long measurement time before obtaining the results. Moreover, it requires a large-sized laboratory equipment, including a specific software for analyzing the results. They also depend on the PCR amplification efficiency which is not constant with the number of cycles and thus introduce a high variance on statistical analyses.

2.2 Spectrometry

Spectrophotometers are used in molecular biology to quantify DNA and also to assess its purity. The spectrometers use a method combining optic fiber and liquid tension to illuminate a droplet of a DNA sample with a UV light. The instrument measures the DNA absorbance at 260 nm and can also perform a measurement at 280 nm to detect the presence of contaminating proteins in the sample. The spectrometers allow for quick measurement but with a poor reproducibility.

2.3 Fluorometry

Fluorescence spectroscopy is used in biological quantification techniques. It requires fluorescent dyes that can specifically bind to the DNA or RNA molecules. The fluorometry is based on a measurement 90° of a fluorescent light emitted by a dye excited by the instrument. The fluorometry features a very statistically significant (i.e. inducing a very low variance) result but implies several manipulations, and a long analysis time.

3. The UV light sources

In order to fully take advantage of the UV absorbance property of the DNA, the samples must be illuminated with a light source at appropriate wavelength and power. In laboratories, the equipments described in the previous section feature light sources that are encumbering or expensive. Hereunder is a non-extensive list of such sources :

- the large spectrum lamp. That kind of lamp is mostly used for research. For example, halogen-deuterium lamps provide a spectrum from 200 nm to 1200 nm with large emitting power. Associated with a monochromator, they allow for selecting with precision any wavelength and measurement of the spectral response of a photosensitive device. They can also be used to simulate any monochromatic light source, at present between 250 and 400 nm. But often, the whole system (including the lamp and the monochromator) is too voluminous to be integrated in a portable device.
- the flash lamp. In the spectrometers, Xenon flash lamps are used. They feature an emitting spectrum for which the high emission peak is around 260 nm. This kind of lamp provides a high power but unfortunately generates second order peaks at higher wavelengths so that a precise photosensor is required to detect only the transmitted light at 260 nm or precise filters must be integrated to cut off the parasitic wavelengths. This could lead to a sensible loss of light power.
- the laser. In the PCR apparatus for example, the light source used to excite the fluorophores has to be very powerful and narrow around the exciting wavelength. The best choice is thus a laser. But apart from these excellent optical characteristics, a laser is very expensive and not suitable for a portable application, since it requires a stabilized supply power and is not miniaturizable.
- the fluorophores. These chemical components allow the detection of a molecule. They are used in the PCR to visually follow the amplification of a target DNA during the exponential stages of the PCR. The nature of the fluorophores may be various. For example, SYBR Green fluorescent dyes bind to the double stranded DNA molecules and emit after excitation a light at a specific wavelength when the DNA is re-assembled. So the emission depends on the hybridization rate of the DNA. Another example is the Taqman probe which, contrarily to the SYBR Green, is based on the FRET principle : a probe is covalently bonded with a fluorophore and a quencher inhibits its fluorescence. Once the exonuclease activity of the polymerase degrades the probe, fluorescence is generated by the fluorochrome. But even if the nature of the fluorophore may be quite different, their common characteristic is their dependence on their affinity with their target and a relatively poor emission requiring so a long observation time (in order to integrate a sufficient photocurrent) and a very low-noise photosensor.
- the light emitting diode (LED). Finally, to combine the advantages of a high emitting light power, a controlled and narrow emitting spectrum, and a low fabrication cost, the LEDs

are an opportunistic choice. To ensure a low wavelength emission spectrum, the materials used to fabricate a UV diode are diamond (C), and Al-based materials (i.e. AlN and AlGaN) thanks to to their large bandgap, allowing a high energy photons generation when the electron-hole pairs are recombining. The UV LEDs have to be biased with relatively high forward voltage (e.g. Vd=6 V) which yields a current of about Id$\simeq$20 mA. This implies a consistent power needed to bias the diodes (compared to the power needed to supply a microelectronic integrated circuit), which also has to be very stable in time to minimize the fluctuations of the emitted light and reduce the measurements errors. However LEDs are miniaturized, portable and low-cost UV light source, making them good candidates for a complete optoelectronic microsystem aiming at biomedical applications.

4. The optical sensors for biomedical applications

In the previous laboratory equipments, optical sensors are used to measure a fluorescence phenomenon or a transmitted/absorbed light. In those equipments, the sensors are often charge coupled devices (CCD), eventually associated with a mirror network in order to select the appropriate wavelength to measure. CCDs feature the advantage of good linearity, and signal to noise ratio. But they also require a complex embedded electronic circuit to generate the clocks needed to control the charges transfers. In our case, since we target a portable, low-cost and easy-to-use system, a single device photosensor will be considered.
The most common used optical sensor to detect a signal is a photodiode. As we extensively study the UV and blue sensitive photosensors, we present a short state-of-the-art of the main available devices in each technology. A wide review of such photosensors has also been reported by Yotter & Wilson (2003). An important figure of merit for an optoelectronic sensor is the responsivity (R) :

$$R = \frac{I_{ph}}{P_{in}}[A/W] \tag{1}$$

defined as the ratio between the light induced current I_{ph}, called the photocurrent, and the incident light power at the diode surface Pin. Some papers also refer to the external quantum efficiency (QE) of the device defined as :

$$QE = \frac{\frac{I_{ph}}{q}}{\frac{P_{in}}{h\nu}}[\%] \tag{2}$$

where h is the Planck's constant and ν is the frequency related to the wavelength λ by $c = \nu \cdot \lambda$ where c is the vacuum speed of light.
Both are expressed as a function of the wavelength, so it is easy to compare devices for a given spectral range of detection, i.e, blue and UV in our case. More precisely, since DNA is absorbing at 260 nm and blue is defined from 450 to 475 nm in the electromagnetic spectrum, we can only compare the device on the specifications given in the papers. Three technology categories are studied below : bulk silicon, SOI and another regrouping some of the most common other used materials.

4.1 In bulk silicon technology

Silicon remains the lowest-cost material to fabricate a photodiode and can absorb photons whose correspond to a wavelength up to slightly more than 1100 nm thanks to its 1.1 eV bandgap (Zimmermann, 2000). Unfortunately, to realize a spectral filter, in order to only absorb photons with an associate low wavelength, a low thickness of the silicon is needed since most of the photons are absorbed in the first 5 μm of the silicon thickness. This leads to reducing as much as possible the thickness of the silicon region where the photons are absorbed and to reduce the reflections. Consequently, a high responsivity can be achieved in the appropriate wavelength by other techniques like spatial modulation of light (Chen & du Plessis, 2006) or special devices such as avalanche diode (Pauchard et al., 2000).

4.2 In SOI technology

Silicon-on-insulator is a particular silicon-based technology in which a thin silicon film is separated from a thick silicon substrate with an oxide layer (called the buried oxide, or BOX). When fabricating an integrated circuit, the electronic devices (including transistors, capacitors, resistors, ...) are realized in the top thin layer. This insulated structure features the advantage to considerably reduce the leakage currents of the transistors, reduce the parasitic capacitances of the circuits, and improve the resistance of the circuitry to the variations of temperature (at low as well as high temperature, from 100 K to 450 K (Flandre et al., 1999; 2001)).
Silicon absorbs light as a function of its thickness: the thicker the silicon, the higher the absorbed wavelengths. So, contrarily to a classical photosensor embedded in a thick silicon wafer, which absorbs most of the light from UV to near infra-red, a SOI device featuring a thin film with 100 nm of thickness allows for only absorbing light whose wavelength is under 450 nm.

4.3 Other semiconductor materials

Silicon is the most common semiconductor but other materials can be used to implement a photosensor. Thanks to their larger bandgap, materials based on Gallium Nitride (GaN) can more easily absorb photons associated to low wavelengths independently from its thickness and then achieve high responsivities below 400 nm (Chang et al., 2008; 2006; Biyikli et al., 2005; Monroy et al., 2001). Other frequently used technology is the silicon carbide (SiC) that has proven its interest by the past (Brown et al., 1998; Fang et al., 1992).

4.4 Anti reflection coatings

The advantage of depositing a dual-layer anti-reflection coating (ARC) above a photodiode has been proven (Kumer et al., 2005). It can considerably reduce the reflections of light by an accurate choice of thickness according to the index of refraction of the material and the wavelength at which the efficiency has to be improved. The most common ARCs are silicon oxide (SiO_2), silicon nitride (Si_3N_4) and alumina (Al_2O_3). Great advances have been made in the solar cell laboratory research concerning ARC. Recently, the researches are more focused on the development of texturized surfaces which are also often used to ensure a greater absorption of the light in the device with multiple reflections at the incident interface. The patterned protective layers allow an augmentation of their transmittance, leading to an increase of the quantum efficiencies of the cells (Han et al., 2009; Chu et al., 2008; Gombert et al., 2000).

4.5 Summary and comparison

The table 1 summarizes most representative results for the previously cited technologies. For classical Si photodiodes (i.e. except for avalanche diodes or else), SOI technology remains much more efficient than classical bulk silicon as can be seen on the table above.

Source	Techno	Performance
Torres-Costa et al. (2007)	Bulk Si	R=0.025@400 nm
Chen & du Plessis (2006)	Bulk Si	R=0.05@400 nm
Pauchard et al. (2000)	Bulk Si (Avalanche)	R=0.17@400 nm
Bulteel et al. (2009)	SOI	R=0.1@400 nm
Afzalian & Flandre (2005)	SOI	R=0.015@430 nm
Miura et al. (2007)	SOI	NA
Chang et al. (2008)	GaN	R=0.15@[300-400] nm
Chang et al. (2006)	GaN	R=0.18@350 nm
Biyikli et al. (2005)	AlGaN	R=0.1@250 nm
Monroy et al. (2001)	AlGaN	R=0.2@350 nm
Brown et al. (1998)	SiC	R=0.15@280 nm
Fang et al. (1992)	SiC	R=0.26@380 nm
Han et al. (2009)	Si and Patterned ARC	QE=60@400 nm

Table 1. Comparison of the photodiode characteristics among the different technologies

Comparatively, the larger bandgap materials can achieve a higher responsivity, but their fabrication cost is much higher and even if SOI technology reaches a lesser responsivity, its value remains on the same order of magnitude as the other semiconductor materials.

5. The SOI photodiode design

As previously said, a very common electronic device, but with good efficiency, used to measure the light intensity is the diode, or the PN junction. By adding an intrinsic or low-doped region between the P and N regions, we obtain a PIN diode which can reach better optical response (Zimmermann, 2000). When realizing this device in the thin film of a SOI wafer, we implement a lateral PIN diode. This device has been used in this abstract as a reference, according to the good results found in the literature and its compatible fabrication with a standard CMOS process (Afzalian & Flandre, 2005). The photocurrent, previously introduced in equation 1, can also be defined as:

$$I_{ph} = I_D - I_{Dark}[A] \tag{3}$$

where I_D is the total current flowing through the diode and I_{Dark} is the dark current of the diode, i.e. the current through the diode when subject to no illumination. Referring to equation 1, the responsivity can thus be enhanced by increasing the photocurrent, which is can be obtained by reducing the dark current and optimizing the reverse bias of the photodiode, Vd. Raising Vd indeed increases the region where the photons generate electron-hole pairs (Afzalian & Flandre, 2005), however, the generation current also increases, but so does the dark current that itself decreases the photocurrent, and thus the responsivity. It has also been demonstrated that adding an anti-reflection coating greatly improves the sensitivity of the photodiode. In our case, a silicon nitride ARC has been deposited over a silicon dioxide that came naturally with the fabrication process. The cross section of a PIN diode in a SOI technology is shown in figure 1.

For the tested technology, the dimensions according to figure 1 were T_{SUB}=800 μm, T_{BOX}=400 nm, T_{Si}=80 nm, T_{OX}=280 nm and T_{ARC}=40 nm. For the diode itself, simulations have demonstrated that an intrinsic length of Li=8 μm could reach a maximum efficiency in our detection range while the anode and cathode lengths of Ln=Lp=10 μm are fixed by the

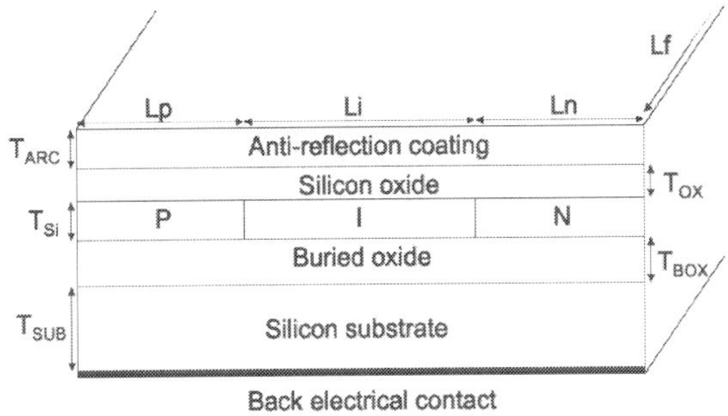

Fig. 1. Cross section of one finger of the SOI PIN photodiode

process (Flandre et al., 1999; 2001). A mathematical model has been implemented in Matlab for simulating the responsivity of our SOI device with a reflection-transmission of waves through a multi-layer device with thicknesses and refraction indexes as variables. But since the standard SOI wafer substrate and oxide are imposed by the fabrication process, while the thin Si film and the CMOS process oxide thicknesses are also constant on the wafer, the only left parametrical layer is the additional ARC. As demonstrated in (Kumer et al., 2005), we can minimize the reflected power by depositing two anti-reflecting coatings on top of a semiconductor layer. While the first ARC is the existing silicon oxide of 280 nm previously presented, the second top layer is most commonly a silicon nitride for its refraction index close to 2. Figure 2 presents the variation of responsivity at 400 nm as a function of the thickness of the silicon nitride top ARC. One can observe its periodicity as predicted in (Zimmermann, 2000; Kumer et al., 2005).

After fabrication, the photodiode responsivity has been measured by sweeping the electromagnetic spectrum in the range from 200 nm to 750 nm with a halogen-deuterium lamp and a monochromator selecting the appropriate wavelength. The comparison between the simulated and the measured responsivity is shown in figure 3.

One can observe high responsivities in the UV range while the responsivity falls down after 450 nm, which corresponds to the end of the blue range in the visible spectrum of

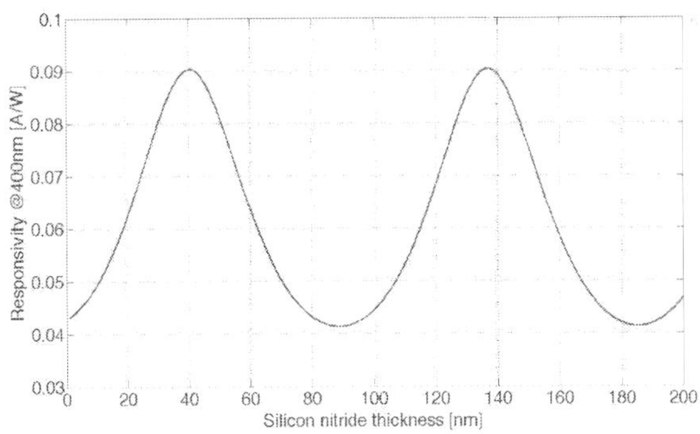

Fig. 2. Simulation of the responsivity at λ=400 nm of PIN photodiodes with a structure as in figure 1 as a function of the silicon nitride ARC.

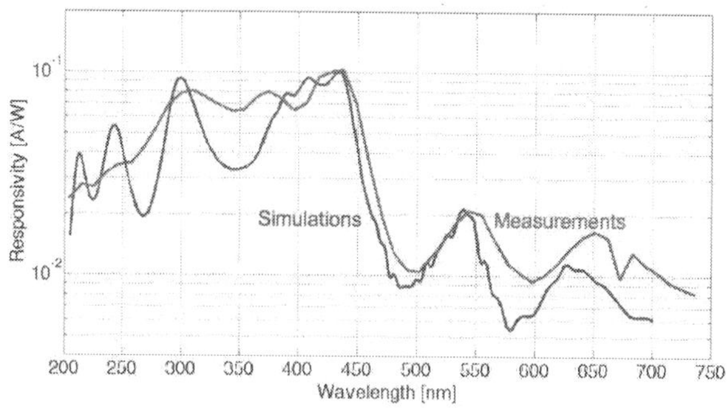

Fig. 3. Comparison between simulation and measurements of the photodiode responsivity

light. There is also a good correspondence between measurements and simulation, except for the attenuated experimental oscillations below 400 nm that can be explained by process non-uniformities. Based on the initial SOI wafer, other more accurate photodiodes can be designed according to the target light as in (Bulteel & Flandre, 2009), where it is proven that aluminum oxide ARC and silicon-on-nothing based structures may also be used to optimize such biological measurements.

6. The integrated circuit

6.1 Overview of the system

As previously mentioned, instead of directly measuring the current of the photodiode, a signal processing circuit can be fully integrated on a single chip with the photodiode, thanks to the same CMOS process and the SOI technology. An example of transimpedance circuit for measuring an analog voltage has been fully designed and measured in Afzalian & Flandre (2006). Another type of circuit can be used to transform the analog output of the photodiode into a digital signal, easy to interface with a microcontroller. An example of such a circuit is presented in figure 4.

This circuit corresponds to a current-to-frequency (I-f) converter. First, the photocurrent is processed by an integrator, and the integrated current has thus the shape of a rising voltage

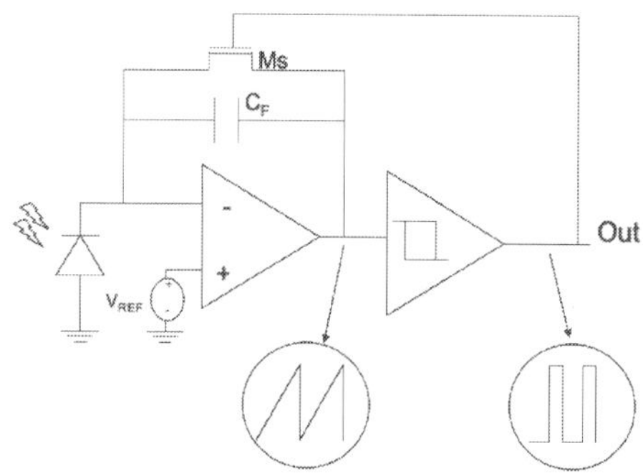

Fig. 4. Schematic of the complete photodiode and signal processing circuit

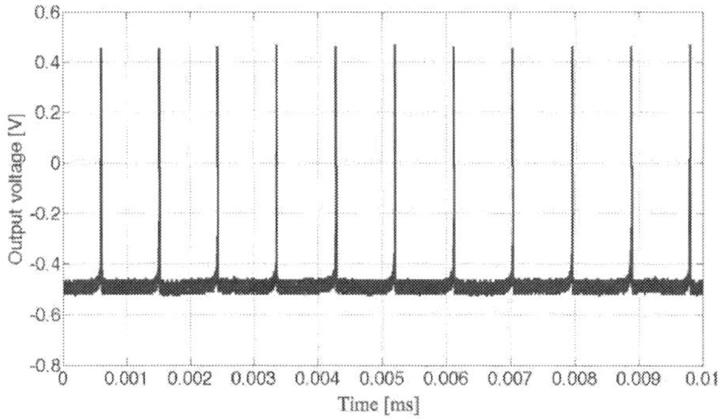

Fig. 5. Output voltage of the current to frequency circuit

whose slope directly depends on the magnitude of the photocurrent flowing through the capacitor C_F. A two-thresholds comparator (implemented in this case by a Schmitt trigger) next transforms the integrated voltage into a squared signal that resets the integrator when the output becomes high. This simple system produces a number of pulses per second proportional to the amplitude of the photocurrent. So, for a fixed time of observation, the higher the photocurrent (i.e. the higher the UV intensity), the larger the number of pulses to be measured.

6.2 Design

The system can be tuned for the application to operate. For high current, and so high pulse frequencies to measure, the bandwidth of the operational amplifier may vary, as well as its open-loop gain depending on the precision required for the integrated function. For the measured photodiode, an implementation of this circuit was designed and fabricated in our SOI technology (Flandre et al., 1999; 2001) including a Miller operational amplifier with a 60 dB open-loop gain and a 3 MHz gain-bandwidth product (GBW). A 10 pF capacitance is used as a feedback to realize the integrator function while a SOI NMOS transistor with minimal dimension and a $\frac{W}{L} = 1$ ratio was chosen to reset the integrator ensuring minimal leakage current (Luque et al., 2003). With that choice, assuming that the output dynamic of the integrator (i.e. corresponding to the difference between the two thresholds of the following trigger) is set to 1V, a 10 pA photocurrent will charge the feedback capacitance within one second. Many types of Schmitt triggers (or other comparators) can be used, also depending on the required output and the switch. A similar circuit was found in the literature (Simpson et al., 2001; Bolton et al., 2002), but featuring a single threshold comparator. In our case, due to the very low luminous intensities to measure, the currents are very small and so is the slope of the integrated signal. We thus need a larger dynamic at the integrator output implying the use of a two thresholds comparator. A standard CMOS Schmitt trigger (Filanovsky & Baltes, 1994) was used for the comparator with an input dynamic of 1V as previously said.

The circuit is powered with a 2 V voltage and consumes approximately 600 μA. The whole chip including a 0.25 mm^2 photodiode, features an area of 0.5 mm^2. Its output under illumination is shown in figure 5.

One can observe the good behavior of the circuit. The circuit has also been illuminated with lights of different powers and wavelengths, and the experiment has proved the good

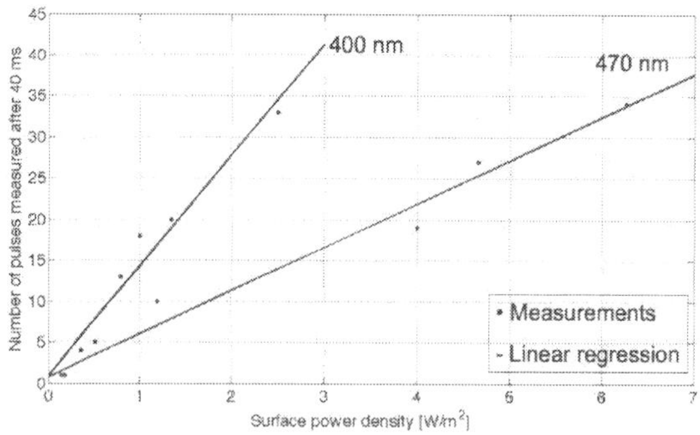

Fig. 6. Number of pulses measured in 40 ms as a function of the surface power density of light for 400 nm (black) and 470 nm (blue)

linearity of the outputs with regards to the responsivity of the photodiode (Bulteel et al., 2009) as showed in figure 6. One can observe that the slope ratios of the measurements linear regressions is of about 3 between 400nm and 470nm. When referring to the figure 3, the ratio of the responsivities at 400 nm and 470 nm is also of 3. As such, the integrated system can be used to measure environmental UV or DNA concentration.

7. Biological application of the SOI photodiodes

The current optical measurement methods (presented above in this chapter) require a lot of manipulations (e.g. pipetting, purification, etc.) and are not convenient for portable and low-cost applications. We present here an innovating system to measure DNA concentrations by optic transmittance. As previously introduced, the DNA features an absorption peak around 260 nm, so that its concentration in a liquid sample can be assessed by measuring a ray of light passing through the DNA solution. According to the Beer-Lambert law, the DNA concentration can be directly deduced from the light transmitted through the sample. Previous results demonstrated the feasibility of such a system (Bulteel et al., 2009) with a monochromator and our SOI photodiode based on measurements. The early results of the experiments were compared to spectrometry, fluorometry and quantitative real-time PCR. It was shown that the PCR featured the highest detection range but a poor precision and reproducibility. The spectrometry-based method has the lowest detection range and a poor precision. Fluorometry-based quantification presented the highest precision and a relatively good detection range, reaching the one obtained with the SOI photodiode.

7.1 The setup

Figure 7 shows a setup of the second experiment. Starting with a light source, implemented with a LED with appropriate wavelength, we can place the DNA in its container to be directly illuminated by the almost monochromatic light. Finally the sensor is positioned to receive the light that has passed through the DNA in order to measure the transmitted light.

7.2 Measurement of DNA samples in quartz containers

First of all, we wanted to confirm the literature reported results and compare them with those obtained with our system. Thus, we measured DNA samples from *Escherichia coli* in a

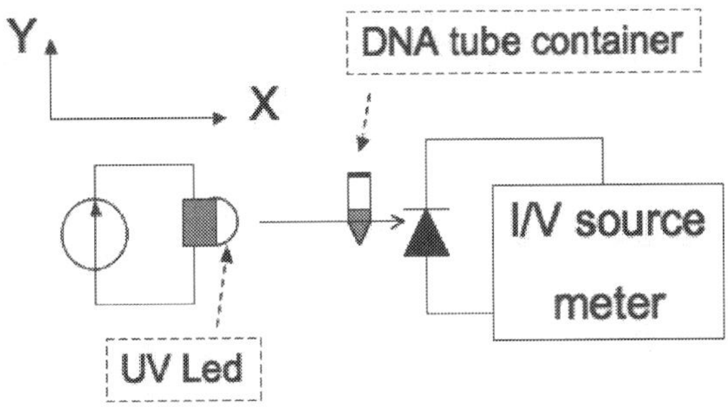

Fig. 7. Schematic of the system : a UV LED illuminates the DNA sample and the transmitted light is measured by a SOI photodiode coupled to a IV meter

reference absorption cell from Hellma. These cuvettes are 50 μL quartz containers whose good UV transmittance is a well-known property. The light is focused on a 2.5 mm diameter circular transparent window confining the DNA in a small cylinder illuminated by the light source. For the first step, the emitting wavelength of the LED was 260 nm. The LED was biased and monitored by a Keithley 236 IV source associated with a four wire connection ensuring a minimal noise floor needed for the small currents to measure (i.e. a few nA). Genomic DNA was pipetted and deposited in the quartz cuvettes with concentrations ranging from 400 ng/μL to 400 pg/μL. Three currents were measured for calibrating the system : the dark current of the photodiode, the photocurrent generated directly by the light source (denoted *Light*), and the photocurrent resulting of a blank measurement consisting of 50μL of water in the quartz cuvettes (denoted H_2O) as referred in figure 8 showing the photocurrents of the experiment. Under a Vd=-0.5 V reverse bias, a dark current average of 45 pA was measured. A monotonic relation between the photocurrent and the DNA concentration was observed. As previously demonstrated in Bulteel et al. (2009), the higher the DNA concentration, the more UV light is absorbed, and the lesser the induced photocurrent is generated in the diode. Evenly the lowest DNA concentration implied the highest photocurrent. This photocurrent

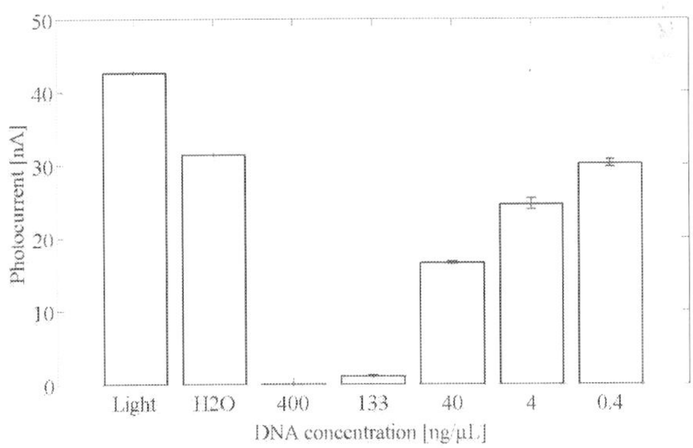

Fig. 8. Detection of different DNA concentrations (*Escherichia coli*) in the quartz cuvettes: Light and H_2O concentrations were used as references

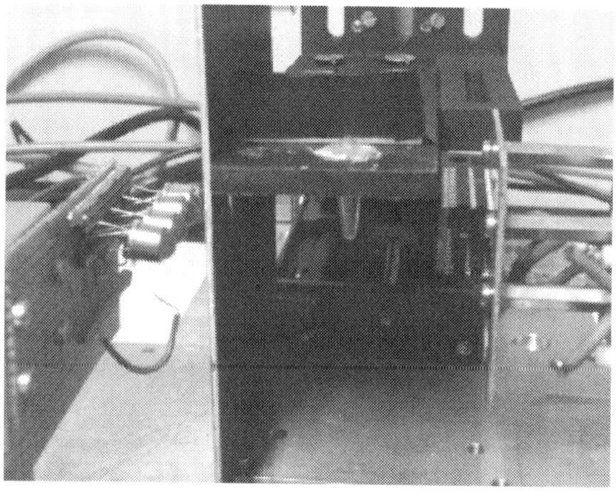

Fig. 9. Photograph of the tested system

was not significantly different from the blank sample. The error bars also shown in the figure correspond to the standard variations at each DNA concentration and pose another limit to the precision as discussed below.

8. Results of in-tube measurement with photodiode

The first step of our methodology demonstrated the principle of DNA measurements in a quartz container with a LED as light source and SOI diode as photosensor. But one condition to be fulfilled by the DNA container is to be as transparent as possible so that the light can interact with the DNA sample with as much optical power as possible. Therefore, we next practiced our experimentations on 200 μL PCR tubes, as they have already proven their usability (Bulteel et al., 2009). Another advantage is that while the quartz absorption cells require pipetting, drying and cleaning steps, the tube containers allow wasteless measurements with minimal manipulation steps and are much cheaper. A photograph of the setup is shown in figure 9.

On the left of the photograph, one can see a rack line of four LEDs emitting respectively at 260 nm, 280 nm, 295 nm and 360 nm. They are mounted on a XYZ displacer allowing for a selection of the most suitable wavelength according to the molecular nature of the biological target. The photodiode stands on the right of the picture and is encapsulated in a DIL-24 package (also mounted on a XYZ displacer for alignment) while the PCR tube is centered in the photograph on a two dimensional YZ displacer.

8.1 Detection limit and other statistical considerations

When dealing with biological samples in order to establish faithfully their concentration, it is crucial to compare the results to commonly used statistical definitions (Ripp, 1996). The most used functions are the precision limit (PL), the minimum detection limit (MDL) also called the limit of detection (LOD) for the laboratory measurements, and the limit of quantification (LOQ). Those are first linked to the blank sample measurements. So, for 20 measurements of a blank tube containing a solution without DNA (i.e. H_2O), the precision limit can be defined as :

$$PL = 3 \cdot \frac{\sigma_{Blank}}{\bar{X}_{Blank}} \tag{4}$$

Since the number of our measurements is less than 30 per sample, the results are distributed along a Student distribution, associated with its t-value. Secondly the MDL for a DNA concentration is defined with its t-value compared to the blank measurements as :

$$MDL = (t - value)_n \cdot \sigma_{Blank} = LOD \tag{5}$$

And finally, the LOQ is calculated as follow :

$$LOQ = 10 \cdot \sigma_{Blank} \tag{6}$$

The precision limit will be mainly discussed furtherly on this chapter.

8.2 Placement

The system is firstly calibrated with no assay tube. For a fixed position of the LED and the blocking mask, the photodiode is placed for obtaining a maximal value of the generated photocurrent under illumination. Then, a PCR tube containing an *europium*-diluted solution is hold on the YZ tube displacer and positioned to induce a minimal value of the photocurrent while fluorescence of the *europium* can confirm the correct alignment of the LED, the sample and the photodiode.

8.3 Description of the varying parameters

8.3.1 The light source

Since the LEDs are packaged with an hemispherical lens providing a straight illumination diagram, an aperture mask composed of a dark mask with a 2.5 mm diameter circular window is used to focus the light on the tube. The blocking mask is shown in figure 9 between the LEDs and the assay tube. The aperture mask also prevents from the diffraction of the light on the rounded boundaries of the PCR tube, which could perturb the measurements. Among the four available LEDs in the system previously presented, the two with emitting peak wavelengths of 260 nm and 280 nm were used, respectively for the DNA and proteins measurements. It is established that DNA absorbs the light at 260 nm while proteins are more sensitive to a 280 nm illumination, but both wavelengths were tested on each target, the ratios of the measurements enabling purity assessments. The LEDs have also been characterized with a spectrophotometer showing the inverse correlation between their illuminating power and the distance. Therefore a modulation of the optical power of the LED is possible when displacing it from the PCR tube.

8.3.2 The distance

As discussed above, the LED power illuminating the sample tube can be modulated by the distance between the LED and the tube. While the tubes are at 1 cm from the photodiode, and the blocking mask is also fixed (at a distance of 1.5 cm of the tube, i.e. 2.5 cm from the photodiode), the LEDs were disposed at three distances from the photodiode : 4.5 cm, 6.5 cm and 8 cm, which corresponds to a reduction of the power by respectively two and three whereas the closest distance displaying the highest power was 4.5 cm.

8.3.3 The photodiode bias

As discussed before, the choice of the photodiode bias is a trade-off between the dark and the photogenerated currents. Moreover, the measurement noise is highly related to the shot noise of the diode, defined as :

$$I^2_{Noise} = 2 \cdot q \cdot I_D [A^2/Hz] \tag{7}$$

This implies a limit for the current to fill with the MDL of the system. In the experiments, a reverse voltage sweep range from 0 V to -5 V was applied to the diode and has lead to choose a reverse bias of Vd=-0.5V to maximize the photocurrent under a constant λ=280 nm illumination. It implies a dark current I_{Dark} of about 30 pA/mm^2 for the following experiment results. The optical dynamic (OD) is the value of the current of a blank sample reported to the dark current (Bulteel et al., 2009). When PCR tubes were used, the current measured with a blank sample was of 3 nA. We then calculated that the OD was of 100, while it was of 700 with the quartz cuvettes.

8.4 Results and discussion

To validate the system, two types of samples were tested and the results are reported in this section. Firstly, pure genomic DNA (*Escherichia coli*), and secondly, spores from bacteria (*Bacillus subtilis*). Each substance was diluted into the microtubes to a volume of 50 μL (corresponding to the same volume as in the quartz cuvettes) and each tube was measured four times with the LEDs emitting at λ=260 nm and λ=280 nm. The repeated measurements are essential to take into account the tube displacements, the heterogeneity of the solution (each tube is periodically vortexed to re-homogenize the solution) and other measurement fluctuations.As discussed for the quartz calibration experiment, since the lowest concentration provides the highest photocurrent, all results are displayed as a percentage of the maximal measured current. This enables a normalization of the different tests over the optical dynamic.

8.4.1 Measurement precision

The precision of our system, as introduced above in the statistical considerations section, was calculated to be 2.16 % over 20 blank measurements and multiplied by 3 to compute the precision limit (PL) from the maximum measured current, as can been seen in the curves of figures 10-12. The intersection of the precision limit and the sample curve yields an estimate of the lowest limit of detection range.

8.4.2 The DNA

The genomic DNA was extracted from *Escherichia coli*, a Gram negative bacterium, and diluted in concentrations ranging from 400 ng/μL to 4 pg/μL. Figures 10 and 11 report the data for the DNA concentrations that have been measured for the two wavelengths (260 and 280 nm), at the three LED-to-photodiode distances.

As expected, one can observe a monotonic relation between the photocurrent and the DNA concentration in both figures and shown by the calibration data of figure 8. Nevertheless, a closer analysis of the curves can point out the influence of the parameters.

- A first observation is that the LED emitting at λ=280 nm allows a detection range down to 4 pg/μL, which is better than the detection threshold of 40 pg/μL when the LED of λ=260 nm is at a distance of 4.5 cm. Concerning the other distances, the low detection range limits appear for 4 ng/μL and 40 pg/μL at 260nm and 280 nm respectively. This observation has already been made (Bulteel et al., 2009), and the phenomenon may be explained by the fact

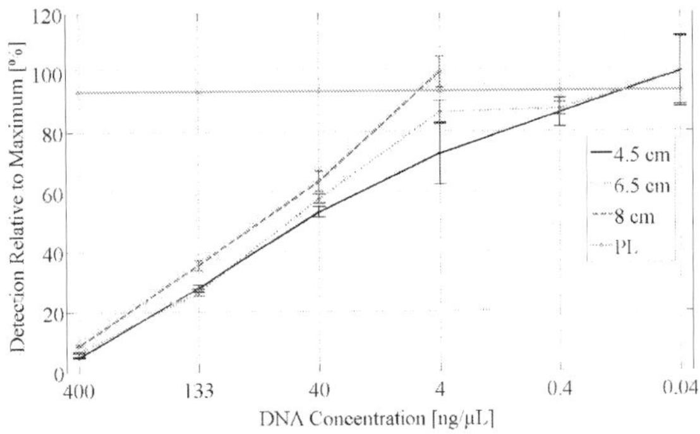

Fig. 10. Influence on the DNA concentration measurements of the distance between the LED at λ=260 nm and the photodiode : 4.5 cm (solid line), 6.5 cm (doted line), 8 cm (dashed line) and precision limit, PL (-x-)

that the peak absorption is too high at 260nm, implying a lower threshold for the detection. On the opposite, the slope of the absorption spectrum is lower at λ=280 nm (Karczemska & Sokolowska, 2001) and that would so enable more accurate measurements.

- About the LED emitting at λ=260 nm, when decreasing the power, the upper detectable concentration decreases. The upper limit of the detection seems to increase linearly with the distance. This makes sense since the measurement is made at the absorption peak wavelength. In opposition, the distance relation is less clear for λ=280 nm.
- It appears that the measurements realized at λ=280 nm are more precise with regards to standard deviation and are more reproducible than at λ=260 nm. The excessive absorption at 260 nm might disturb the level of detection, and this phenomenon may increase when if the power fits with the maximum absorption. Contrarily, the measurements carried out at 280 nm imply less variations on the results because of the lower but more reproducible

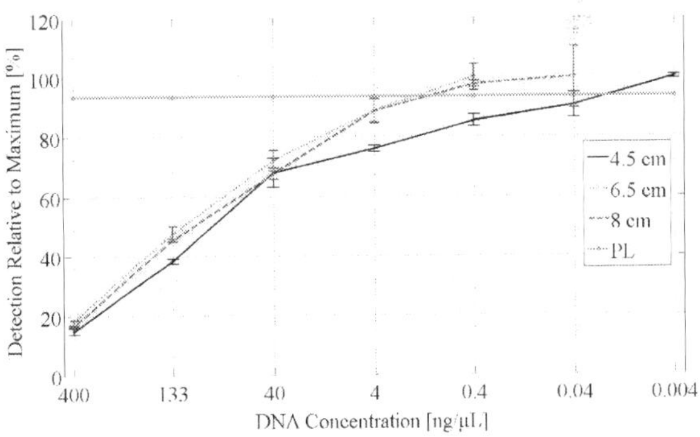

Fig. 11. Influence on the DNA concentration measurements of the distance between the LED at λ=280 nm and the photodiode : 4.5cm (solid line), 6.5cm (doted line), 8cm (dashed line) and precision limit, PL (-x-)

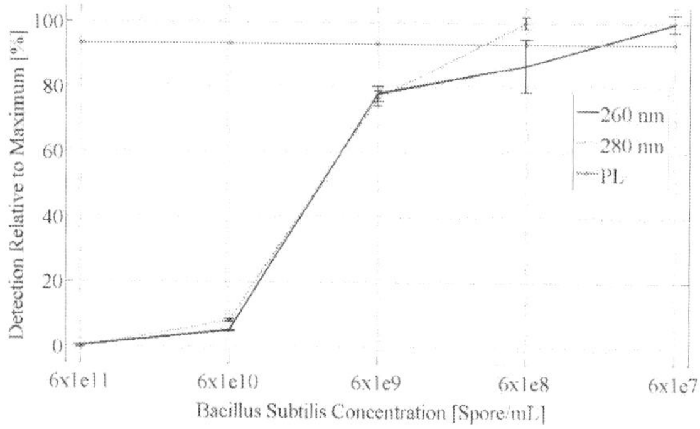

Fig. 12. *Bacillus subtilis* concentration measurements at 260 nm (solid line) and 280 nm (doted line) at a LED-to-photodiode distance of 6.5 cm. Precision limit is indicated as PL (-x-)

absorption of DNA around this wavelength.

- The standard deviation generally increases at both wavelengths, except for the shortest distance at 280 nm, with the diminution of the concentration under characterization. A usual trade-off between sensitivity and noise must hence be determined. In figure 11, the best threshold of detection then appears to be 0.02 ng/μL when the PL line crosses the measurement curve.

8.4.3 The bacteria

Lyophilized spores of a Gram positive bacterium (*Bacillus subtilis*), were resuspended in water in concentrations ranging from 6x10^{11} spores/mL to 6x10^4 spores/mL. Figure 12 presents the in-tube measurements for both wavelengths. The measurements at λ=260 nm can cover a range down to 6x10^7 spores/mL, and a decade lower for the LED at 280 nm. Nevertheless, the measurements at 280 nm are more precise in the measured range compared to those at 260 nm. Indeed the standard deviation at 260 nm for the concentration of 6x10^8 spores/mL is larger.

9. Measurements with the integrated system

As previous experiments have demonstrated that DNA concentration can be measured with a UV SOI photodiode and a UV light source, this should also be possible with the complete integrated system presented in the section 6 of this chapter. The experiment has been made by replacing the photodiode chip with a current-to-frequency converter and its associated photodiode single chip. The 260 nm LED has been used to light the DNA tubes at a distance of 4.5 cm to the tubes. It was biased with a Keithley 2400 I-V source as well as the integrated circuit. The output pulse repetition periods were measured using an Agilent MSO8104A 1-GHz real-time oscilloscope. A dark measurement gave a result of three pulses only for a 50 seconds observation period. The precision limit has been measured over 20 blank tubes as for the photodiode experiments.

In a first experiment the same DNA concentrations as used previously (i.e. from 400 ng/μL to 4 pg/μL) are measured over a time period of 10 seconds. In figure 13, the number of pulses

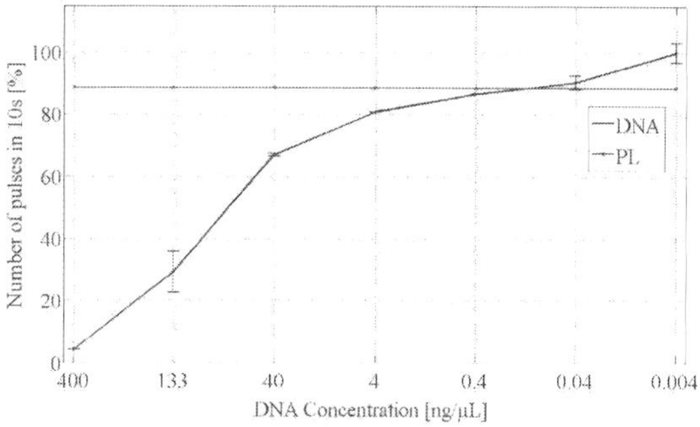

Fig. 13. DNA concentration measurement from 400 ng/μL to 4 pg/μL for 260 nm with the I-f circuit during a 10 seconds measurement period (solid line) and the precision limit (PL, -x-)

measured per sample over this period for each concentration is normalized to the maximal number of pulses associated with the lowest concentration.

One can observe in figure 13 that the circuit is able to measure DNA concentrations over the whole tested range. However, due to a 11.6 % precision limit conjugated to a small slope of the measurement curve in the low concentrations, the detection limit is of about 0.1 ng/μL. Nevertheless, for the very low DNA concentrations, a weak number of pulses are expected. It is thus important to increase the measurement time to observe a significant response. Figure 14 shows a 20 seconds measurement for the different concentrations presented above, and of two additional concentrations (i.e. from 400 pg/μL to 40 fg/μL).

On this figure, a non-ambiguous detection appears maintained down to the lowest tested DNA concentration (i.e. 40 fg/μL).

10. Improvements

One of the major limits of the system is the increase of the standard deviation of light measurements for low DNA concentrations. To reduce these variations, a first step could

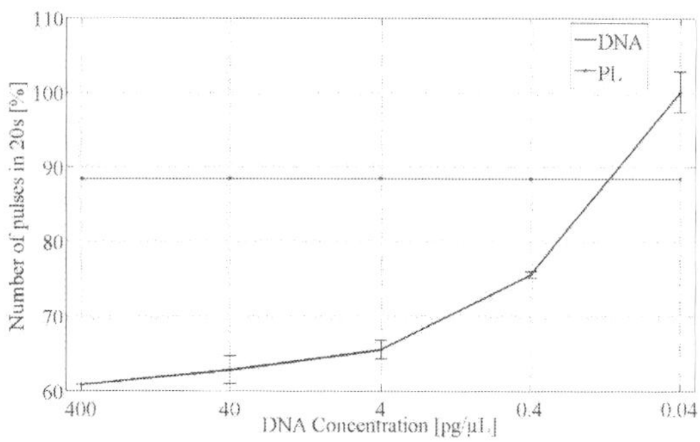

Fig. 14. DNA concentration measurement from 400 pg/μL to 40 fg/μL for 260 nm with the I-f circuit during a 20 seconds measurement period (solid line) and the precision limit (PL, -x-)

be to measure replicates and multiply the number of measurements therefore reducing the standard deviation. On the other hand, the mechanical setup may be improved. With the miniaturization of a future completely portable system, more combined measurements (e.g. concentrations, wavelengths and distances) or increasing the optical dynamic of the system (e.g. by modulating the LED power or improving the photodiode responsivity as demonstrated in Bulteel & Flandre (2009)). Regarding the integrated circuit, a digital system interface (e.g. a digital counter) can be included to automatically take measurements on a definite time period. The interface could send the data to a monitored interface by ZigBee of Wifi modulation as already made with other biological sensors (André et al., 2010). In the future the system may be adapted to measure in the air particles that respond optically to UV light. The DNA container may also be replaced by a microfluidic channel.

11. Conclusion

Our experimentations have proven the ability of new photosensors implemented in SOI technology and combined with UV LEDs to establish a monotonic relation between a DNA concentration and the resulting photocurrent after UV transmittance through assay microtubes containing the samples under test. The photodiode alone achieves a current measurement precision of 2 % and a detection range over 5 decades of concentrations, down to 4 pg/μL in optimal conditions. The threshold of quantification was estimated at 20 pg/μL. With the same PCR tubes, the photodiode is also able to establish a relation between the diode photocurrent and bacteria samples. The integrated circuit including a SOI photodiode and a CMOS current-to-frequency converter is able to measure DNA concentration down to 40 fg/μL with a precision of about 10 %. Compared to optical apparatus and laboratory equipments commonly used to quantify the concentration of biological samples, the detection limits are improved with a very high accuracy. The SOI technology next offers the possibility to integrate the measurement setup into a complete lab-on-a-chip, while the miniaturized components of the system will drive a cost reduction.

12. Acknowledgments

The authors thank Coris BioConcept for supplying the genomic DNA and the Center of Applied Molecular Technologies (CTMA) of the Université catholique de Louvain and the Defense Laboratory Department (DLD-Bio) for supplying the *Bacillus subtilis* spores.

13. References

Afzalian, A.; Flandre, A. (2005) Physical Modeling and Design of Thin-Film SOI Lateral PIN Photodiodes. *IEEE Transactions on Electron Devices*, Vol. 52, No. 6, pp. 1116-1122, June 2005, ISSN 0018-9383

Afzalian, A.; Flandre, D. (2006) Monolithically integrated 10Gbit/s photodiode and transimpedance amplifier in thin-film SOI CMOS technology. *IEE Electronics Letters*, Vol. 42, No. 24, pp. 1420-1421, ISSN 0013-5194

Andre, N.; Druart, S.; Gerard, P.; Pampin, R.; Moreno-Hagelsieb, L.; Kezai, T.; Francis, L.; Flandre, D.; Raskin, J.-P. (2010) Miniaturized Wireless Sensing System for Real-Time Breath Activity Recording. *IEEE Sensors Journal*, Vol.10, Issue 1, pp. 178 - 184, January 2010, ISSN 1530-437X

Biyikli, N.; Kimukin, I.; Tut, T.; Aytur, O.; Ozbay, E. (2005) Fabrication and characterization of solar-blind $Al_{0.6}Ga_{0.4}N$ MSM photodetectors. *Electronics Letters*, Vol. 41, No. 5, pp. 274-275, March 2005, ISSN 0013-5194

Bolton, E.; Sayler, G.; Nivens, D.; Rochelle, J.; Ripp, S.; Simpson, M. (2001) Integrated CMOS photodetectors and signal processing for very low-level chemical sensing with the bioluminescent bioreporter integrated circuit. *Sensors and actuators. B, Chemical A.*, Bol. 85, No. 1-2, pp. 179-185, June 2002, ISSN 0925-4005

Brown, D.; Downey, E.; Kretchmer, J.; Michon, G.; Shu, E.; Schneider, D. (1998) SiC Flame Sensors for Gas Turbine Control Systems. *Solid-state electronics*, Vol. 42, No. 5, pp. 755-760, ISSN 0038-1101

Bulteel, O.; Dupuis, P.; Jeumont, S.; Irenge, L.; Ambroise, J.; Macq, B.; Gala, J.-L.; Flandre,D. (2009) Low-cost miniaturized UV photosensor for direct measurement of DNA concentration within a closed tube container, *Proceedings of the fourth European congress for medical and biomedical engineering 2008*, pp. 1057-1061, ISBN 978-3-540-89207-6, Springer, Berlin

Bulteel, O.; Afzalian, A.; Flandre, D. (2009) Fully integrated blue/UV SOI CMOS photosensor for biomedical and environmental applications. *Analog Integrated Circuit Signal Processing*, Springer, October 2009, ISSN 1573-1979

Bulteel, O.; Flandre, D. (2009) Optimization of Blue/UV Sensors Using PIN Photodiodes in Thin-Film SOI Technology, *ECS Transactions of 215th ECS Meeting*, Vol. 19, Issue 4, pp. 175-180, San Francisco, CA, May 2009 , Omura, Y.; Cristoloveanu, S.; Gamiz, F.; Nguyen, B.

Chang, S.; Ko, T.; Su, Y.; Chiou, Y.; Chang, C.; Shei, S.; Sheu, J.; Lai, W.; Lin, Y.; Chen, W.; Shen, C. (2006) GaN-Based p-i-n Sensors With ITO Contacts. *IEEE Sensors Journal*, Vol. 6, No. 2, pp. 406-411, April 2006, ISSN 1530-437X

Chang, S.; Fang, Y.; Hsu, K.; Wei, T. (2008) GaN UV MSM photodetector on porous β-SiC/(111)Si substrates. *Sensors and actuators. A, Physical*, Vol. 147, No. 1, pp. 1-5, September 2008, ISSN 0924-4247

Chen, Y.; du Plessis, M. (2006) An integrated 0.35 μm CMOS optical receiver with clock and data recovery circuit. *Microelectronics Journal*, Vol. 37, Issue 9, September 2006, pp. 985-992

Chu, J.; Huang, S.; Zhu, H.; Xu, X.; Sun, Z.; Chen, Y.; Huang, H. (2008) Preparation of indium thin films without external heating for application in solar cells. *Journal of Non-Crystalline Solids*, Vol. 354, Issues 52-54, December 2008, pp. 5480-5484, ISSN 0022-3093

Fang, Y.; Hwang, S.; Chen, K.; Liu, C.; Tsai, M.; Kuo, L. (1992)An Amorphous SiC/Si Heterojunction p-i-n Diode for Low-Noise and High-Senstivity UV Detector. *IEEE Transactions on Electron Devices*, Vol. 39, No. 2, pp. 292-296, February 1992, ISSN 0018-9383

Filanovsky, I.; Baltes, H. (1994) CMOS Schmitt trigger design. *IEEE Transactions on Circuits and Systems*, Vol. 41, Issue 1, January 1994, pp. 46-49, ISSN 1057-7122

Flandre, D.; Colinge, J.-P.; Chen, J.; De Ceuster, D.; Eggermont, J.-P.; Ferreira, L.; Gentinne, B.; Jespers, P.; Viviani, A.; Gillon, R.; Raskin, J.-P.; Vander Vorst, A.; Vanhoenacker-Janvier, D.; Silveira, F. (1999) Fully-Depleted SOI CMOS Technology for Low-Voltage Low-Power Mixed Digital/Analog/Microwave Circuits. *Analog Integrated Circuits and Signal Processing*,Vol. 21, No. 3, Decembre 1999, pp. 213-228, ISSN 0925-1030

Flandre, D.; Adriaensens, S.; Akheyara, A.; Crahay, A.; Demeûs, L.; Delatte, P.; Dessard,

V.; Iniguez, B.; Nève, A.; Katschmarskyj, B.; Loumaye, P.; Laconte, J.; Martinez, I.; Picun, G.; Rauly, E.; Renaux, C.; Spôte, D.; Zitout, M.; Dehan, M.; Parvais, B.; Simon, P.; Vanhoenacker, D.; Raskin, J.-P.(2001) Fully depleted SOI CMOS technology for heterogeneous micropower, high-temperature or RF microsystems. *Solid-State Electronics*, Vol. 45, No. 4, April 2001, pp. 541-549, ISSN 0038-1101

Gombert, A.; Glaubitt, W.; Rose, K.; Dreibholz, J.; Bläsi, B.; Heinzel, A.; Sporn, D.; Döll, W.; Wittwer, V. (2000) Antireflective transparent covers for solar devices. *Solr Energy*, Vol. 68, No. 4, pp. 357-360, 2000, ISSN 0038-092X

Han, K.-S.; Lee, H.; Kim, D.; Lee, H. (2009) Fabrication of anti-reflection structure on protective layer of solar cells by hot-embossing method. *Solar Energy Materials and Solar Cells*, Vol. 93, Issue 8, August 2009, pp. 1214-1217, ISSN 0927-0248

Karczemska, A. & Sokolowska, A. (2001). Materials for DNA sequencing chip, *3rd International Conference on Novel Applications of Wide Bandgap Layers*, pp. 176, 0-7803-7136-4, Zakopane - Poland, June 2001, IEEE, Zakopane

Kumer, B.; Pandian, T.; Seekiran, E.; Narayanan, S. (2005) Benefit of dual layer silicon nitride anti-reflection coating, *Record of the Thirty-first IEEE Photovoltaic Specialists Conference 2005*, pp. 1205-1208, ISSN 0160-837, Pangalore, January 2005, pages 1205-1208, 2005

Luque, A.; Vasquez, D.; Rueda, A. (2003) Leakage current and charge injection measurement in thin-film SOI switches, *XVIII conference on Design of Circuits and Integrated Systems*, pp. 706-710

Miura, N.; Chiba, T.; Yamada, H.; Baba, S. (2007) Development of Silicon-on-Insulator (SOI) Uv Sensor IC, in *OKI Technical Review* ,Vol. 74, No. 3, Issue 221, pp.38-39, October 2007

Monroy, E.; Calle, F.; Pau, J.; Muñoz, E.; Omès, F.; Beaumont, B.; Gibart, P. (2001) AlGaN-based UV photodetectors. *Journal of crystal growth*, Vol. 230, No. 3-4, pp. 537-543, ISSN 0022-0248

Pauchard, A.; Rochas, A.; Randjelovic, Z.; Besse, P; Popovic, R. (2000) Ultraviolet Avalanche Photodiode in CMOS Technology, *Electron Devices Meeting, 2000. IEDM Technical Digest. International*, pp. 709-712, 0-7803-6438-4, San Francisco, December 2000, IEEE, San Francisco

Ripp, J. (1996) Analytical detection limit guidance & Laboratory Guide for Determining Method Detection Limits, *Wisconsin Department of Natural Resources Laboratory Certification Program*, Jeffrey Ripp, Wisconsin Department of Natural Resources, PUBL-TS-056-96, Madison (WI)

Simpson, M.; Sayler, G.; Patterson, G; Nivens, D.; Bolton, E.; Rochelle, J.; Arnott, J.; Applegate, B.; Ripp, S.; Guillorn, M. (2001) An integrated CMOS microluminometer for low-level luminescence sensing in the bioluminescent bioreporter integrated circuit. *Sensors and Actuators, B: Chemical, A.*, Vol. 72, No. 2, pp. 134-140, January 2001, ISSN 0925-4005

Torres-Costa, V.; Martín-Palma, R.; Martínez-Druart, J. (2007) All-silicon color-sensitive photodetectors in the visible. *Materials Science and Engineering : C*, Vol. 27, Issues 5-8 , September 2007, pp. 954-956, ISSN 0928-4931

Yotter, R. & Wilson, D. (2003) A Review of Photodetectors for Sensing Light-Emitting Reporters in Biological Systems. *IEEE Sensors Journal*, Vol. 3, No. 3, June 2003, pp. 288-303, ISSN 1530-437X

Zimmermann, H. (2000). *Integrated Silicon Optoelectronics*, Springer, 3540666621, Berlin.

15

LEPTS — a Radiation-Matter Interaction Model at the Molecular Level and its Use in Biomedical Applications

Martina Fuss[1], Ana G. Sanz[1], Antonio Muñoz[2], Francisco Blanco[3], Marina Téllez[4], Carlos Huerga[4] and Gustavo García[1]

[1]*Instituto de Física Fundamental, Consejo Superior de Investigaciones Científicas*
[2]*Centro de Investigaciones Energéticas, Medioambientales y Tecnológicas (CIEMAT)*
[3]*Departamento de Física Atómica, Molecular y Nuclear, Universidad Complutense de Madrid*
[4]*Hospital Universitario La Paz, Madrid*
Spain

1. Introduction

Monte Carlo-based simulations of radiation transport through biological tissues constitute an important complement to experimental dosimetry for the assessment of radiation damage in radioprotection as well as clinical applications such as diagnostics and radiotherapy. In comparison with conventional dose calculation methods that combine empirical data and deterministic algorithms, they offer significant improvements (Reynaert et al., 2007) particularly in conditions involving inhomogeneous materials or geometrically complex irradiation conditions. Therefore, various Monte Carlo (MC) codes oriented towards radiotherapeutic (Berger & Seltzer, 1973; Kawrakow, 2000; Brown, 2003; Baró et al., 1995; Agostinelli, 2003; Halbleib & Melhorn, 1984) and medical imaging (Jan, 2004; Badano & Sempau, 2006) applications have been developed in the last decades. Those programmes provide particle tracking making use of public reference databases such as Storm & Israel (1970); Cullen et al. (1997); Hubbell et al. (1975; 1985); Perkins et al. (1991b); ICRU (1984); Perkins et al. (1991a); Seltzer & Berger (1985) (for a summary, see table 1 in Verhaegen & Seuntjens (2003)) and include sophisticated elements that help reduce calculation time, e.g. condensed-history algorithms. Additionally, electrons are usually forced to instantly deposit all of their remaining energy below a certain cut-off value, further speeding up simulations. Generally, energy deposition in a given volume is assumed to be directly proportional to the number of ionization events that have been produced therein.

However, during the irradiation of biological tissues and almost irrespective of the incident radiation quality, a considerable portion of energy dose is eventually deposited in the target material by secondary electrons through multiple collisions. Only recent discoveries have shown that molecular damage (e.g., molecular dissociations or strand breaks in DNA) can be induced in biomolecules very efficiently even by sub-ionising electrons through molecular resonances (Boudaïffa et al., 2000; Huels et al., 2003) and dissociative electron attachment (Hanel et al., 2003; Abdoul-Carime et al., 2004). In view of this, an interaction model capable of giving a realistic, physically meaningful description of the effective genotoxic damage caused by the incident radiation in a biological tissue should improve on existing MC codes in the following aspects:

- The simulation has to take into account the molecular nature of the absorber medium in order to predict the physical or chemical alterations actually induced in its components. On one hand, this means that input data for a given material can no longer be computed as the sum of its atomic constituents, but needs to be supplied specifically for each molecule. On the other hand, it implies that each collision has to be simulated explicitly (event by event), without using approximations treating multiple scattering events as a single process. This approach permits to obtain particle tracks with real nanometric detail.
- All different kinds of known inelastic collisions have to be considered in the interaction model instead of restricting inelastic events exclusively to ionizations. Only by including those inelastic channels, a complete picture of the effects induced in the irradiated medium can be obtained. In particular, all relevant interaction mechanisms leading directly or indirectly to molecular dissociations need to be taken into account. These include, amongst others, neutral dissociation and dissociative electron attachment for causing chemical alterations and radical formation (which, for the particular example of biological materials, can ultimately lead to single or double breaks in RNA or DNA strands and protein malfunctions).
- Finally, low-energy electrons cannot be ignored by the interaction model by applying cut-off values. Electrons should be tracked until thermalization in order to include scattering events that occur only at low energies, even below ionization threshold. By including this amendment, also the circumstance that collectively, low-energy secondary electrons can carry away a considerable amount of energy from the primary particle's path and produce interactions in the surrounding tissue is accounted for. Consequently, interaction data has to be collected for this energy range, as well.

The global aim of a simulation fulfilling these requirements would be to predict radiation damage in biological tissues at the molecular level, ultimately by calculating how exactly specific proteins, DNA strands, or other functional elements are affected by irradiation in particular conditions (nanodosimetric approach). At present, this objective is not resolved due to the still scarce results on radiation-matter interactions for biomolecules. However, here we present the code Low-Energy Particle Track Simulation (LEPTS) which has been specifically designed by us as a tool for nanodosimetry that offers the improvements exposed above. It distinguishes fine details in the electron interaction model and gives a molecular-level description of the processes involved in radiation transport and energy degradation down to about 1 eV. Furthermore, it is a flexible programme prepared to include the results of new investigations as they become available through constant revision and maintenance of the scattering subroutines and the underlying interaction data sets. Apart from electron transport in irradiated materials of biomedical interest, also positron interactions (particularly interesting for imaging applications such as PET, positron emission tomography) can be simulated with LEPTS.

2. Programme structure

The Monte Carlo code used in our simulations (Muñoz et al., 2005; 2007a) is a general purpose code written in C++ that combines our own routines with existing MC programmes. It

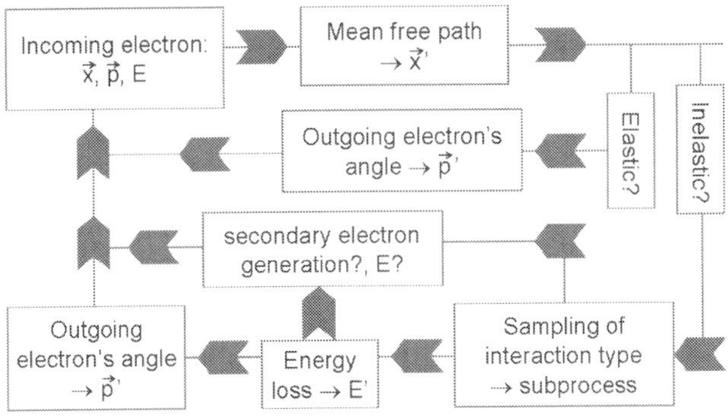

Fig. 1. Diagram depicting how LEPTS handles each collisional event.

uses geometrical and material definition facilities, sampling mechanisms, and graphical output generation from the GEANT4 toolkit (Agostinelli et al., 2003) and is also able to exchange information with PENELOPE (Baró et al., 1995). However, the programme core which provides the functions dealing with the physical interaction processes between incident particles and the target material is LEPTS, the Low-Energy Particle Track Simulation. LEPTS was developed by our group with the main purpose to improve on low-energy and secondary particle interaction models offered by other existing MC codes by providing a molecular-level description of each collisional event until thermalization using experimental input data wherever possible. Currently, electron and positron transport is calculated by LEPTS, while other radiation particles to be tracked in a target material (in particular, photons) are handed over to the corresponding routine available through GEANT-4 or PENELOPE. This combined approach offers the advantages of established radiation transport programmes for tracking many primary particles — whose main effect is to release abundant secondary particles with a certain energy range — in multiple materials on one hand. On the other hand, it provides a complex description of electrons and positrons (whether occurring as primary or secondary particles) including accurate modelling of low-energy processes on a microscopic scale. In recent years, our efforts have centered on adapting LEPTS for use in biomedical applications through the compilation of suitable input parameters and the inclusion of interaction processes that are relevant in biological tissues (e.g., neutral dissociation or electron attachment).

2.1 LEPTS

As has been explained before, the Low-Energy Particle Track Simulation is the central part of our simulation code, the actual interaction model that handles low-energy particles and especially facilitates the simulation of radiation interaction in biological materials (tissues, relevant detector materials, important organic components etc.). It is currently used for processing low-energy electron and positron interactions, typically in the energy range of 1eV up to 1keV. In order to offer a detailed description at the nanoscale, accurate physical models and the selection of input data are equally important. The methods employed in our interaction model for obtaining a realistic simulation at the molecular level are detailed below. A scheme depicting how a radiation-matter interaction event is processed is given in fig. 1. The criteria for input parameter selection will be explained in section 3.

LEPTS is a full Monte Carlo simulation, meaning that each interaction event (collision) is individually simulated starting with the position, direction and energy of the incident particle and giving as an output its new coordinates and energy as well as the possible impact it has caused in the respective molecule of the irradiated material. Unless the incident particle has been absorbed by its interaction partner (for example, via attachment to a molecule in the case of an electron or positronium formation for a positron), the radiation particle after the collision (outgoing particle) is tracked through further scattering events until its thermalization with the surrounding material, at which point it finally deposits the remaining energy. The alterations produced in the absorber, such as local energy deposition, molecular dissociations, or the generation of secondary electrons, are registered by the programme at its exact location within the volume simulated and are available for further analysis at the end of the calculation. Additionally, any secondary particles produced (e.g. through ionization) are always followed by the same means as primary particles until their absorption or thermalization. Given that for most incident radiation qualities, the final energy deposition in the medium is carried out by the multiple secondary electrons produced along the paths of primary particles, this strategy represents a very accurate mode of assessing the radiation damage inflicted.

In order to track an incoming particle, at first, the free path in the medium is sampled according to the total cross section corresponding to its momentary energy. Only once the location of the next collision is thus defined, the interaction model used by LEPTS distinguishes two classes of scattering events: elastic and inelastic scattering. Partial cross sections determine which kind of event is to take place and call the appropriate interaction routine.

For elastic collisions, since no energy is deposited in the medium, the programme samples the outgoing particle's angle according to the distribution established by the corresponding differential cross sections (DCS). In the case of inelastic collisions, different subprocesses (with their relative frequency given by the corresponding partial cross sections) are available depending on the type of incident particle, its energy, and the molecular species encountered. For electron scattering, these processes can currently include ionization (with or without Auger electron generation), vibrational and rotational excitation, electronic excitation, neutral dissociation, and dissociative attachment. In the case of positrons, also positronium formation and annihilation are simulated.

In the next step, the energy lost during the collision is determined. In the case of vibrational or rotational excitations, a fixed value is assigned which only depends on the molecule that was excited and which is calculated as the weighted mean energy of all known levels. For inelastic processes involving complete absorption of the incident particle, the total remaining energy is deposited at the interaction site. For all other inelastic channels, the energy loss is sorted from the energy loss distribution taking into account the threshold applying for a given channel. If different inelastic scattering processes can be clearly distinguished in the underlying energy loss distribution (usually an experimental energy loss spectrum), this is previously split up in order to obtain a specific distribution for each of the respective processes.

Subsequently, the outgoing particle's direction is sampled using the following approximation for the inelastic differential cross section. It has compared well to experimental inelastic DCS for materials like water (Muñoz et al., 2008b) and improves upon other common approximations such as isotropic scattering or using elastic angular distributions directly. For use with LEPTS, the elastic DCS is represented as a function of momentum transfer k to the molecular interaction partner (instead of the outgoing angle θ). Then, the inverse calculation

is done, now taking into account the inelastic nature of the collision being simulated by including an energy loss ΔE.
We thus obtain the outgoing angle after an inelastic scattering event from

$$\cos\theta = \frac{p^2 + p'^2 - k^2}{2pp'} \tag{1}$$

where p and p' are incident and final linear momenta, respectively, and the range of k is restricted by $k \in [p - p'; p + p']$.
If an ionization has taken place, a secondary electron is automatically generated and enters the simulation with the energy lost by the primary electron less the ionization energy, moving in the direction obtained when applying linear momentum conservation. Those secondary electrons are then fully tracked in the same way as primary ones until losing all of their energy or exiting the simulated volume. Finally, the interaction event has terminated and the radiation particle is ready to enter the next collision.
Since LEPTS focuses on low-energy interactions, bremsstrahlung photon production is not taken into account by the scattering subroutines currently used in our programme. This circumstance is not expected to introduce observable errors in the applications considered so far due to the relatively low particle energies. The maximum electron energy occurring in the applications presented in section 4 is approximately 3.5 MeV, where the radiation yield amounts to only 1.3 % according to data supplied by the NIST (Berger, 2000).

2.2 Information exchange with other codes

In our combination programme, a simulation is always launched using the GEANT-4 toolkit, meaning that geometrical and material settings are defined there. The initial conditions describing the incident radiation particles are however supplied by the user depending on the situation simulated. In this way, different set-ups can be considered, e.g. parallel incidence / point source / complex source shape, monoenergetic distribution / several discrete energies / continuous incident spectrum, single particle type / mixed incident species, and so on. Once an incident particle with its corresponding coordinates, direction, and energy is thus sampled, other codes can be called for tracking. Electrons and positrons are generally handed over to LEPTS, except for the purpose of comparison between different codes. PENELOPE can be used for simulating photon transport. Other kinds of particles, including photons as well, can be tracked by GEANT-4. Each code is used exclusively with their own, built-in databases.
During particle tracking, individual radiation particles are easily passed over from one programme to another. If, for example, an incident photon undergoes photoelectric effect and thus releases an electron from the absorber material, this is immediately passed over to LEPTS for simulating its further trajectory. No distinction whatsoever is made between primary and secondary particles, all of them being tracked until absorption or thermalization. Therefore, the energy released in a single interaction by any primary radiation particle (in the current example, a photon) when passing through a medium is effectively distributed among the multiple collisions along the paths of the secondary particles generated (electrons) and registered with its exact impact (type of damage induced, energy deposition) on the different absorber molecules that are affected.
Through the assignment of different kinds of particles to a certain code for track simulation, the present combined programme offers a solid base of input data and models plus punctual improvements where needed (for our intended applications, the treatment strictly event by event and the additional detail in the low-energy region). Continuous maintenance and

improvement of LEPTS and its underlying databases ensure that we obtain an up-to-date, versatile simulation model that adapts to multiple needs. Although in principle, the resulting programme is applicable to all kinds of situations, its main advantage is to offer improvements in the simulation of biological materials by accounting for recently discovered mechanisms of radiation damage of great importance at low energies.

3. Input data requirements

It is obvious that an improvement of accuracy and detail in a simulation model has to be accompanied by the corresponding revision and compilation of input parameters in order to be effective. In the present case, particularly low-energy electron and positron interaction data in materials of biomedical interest have to be collected. For each molecular component, this includes total scattering cross sections, integral and angularly differential elastic CS, partial CS for all known inelastic processes, and energy loss distributions (these may include continuous or discrete spectra depending on the collisional process(es) considered).

The interaction database for a given molecular target is compiled by critically revising and joining together published data, often completing them with our own measurements or calculations. Generally, preference is given to experimental results for considering real-life experimental conditions closer to the actual application than the rather idealized initial conditions mostly assumed in theoretical investigations. For best reliability, data are selected from sources that closely agree with other authors, if multiple results have been reported. Theoretical data are referred to when no adequate experimental ones can be encountered or as an additional orientation when different measurements are not conclusive. Mostly, they serve for extrapolating experimental values in order to extend their energy or angular range. Before a set of preferred values is definitely established for partial and total cross sections, a sum check (verifying that for each particle energy, the elastic CS plus the sum of all inelastic channels equals the total CS) is performed in order to test the congruency of the selected data. This "quality assurance" procedure on the final interaction data set helps to reveal error sources such as the inclusion of a single type of collisional event in different inelastic channels (e.g., an electronic excitation and subsequent neutral dissociation of the molecule in principle belongs equally to both partial cross sections) or the failure to discern different interaction channels due to experimental restrictions (as occurs frequently with experimental elastic cross sections that include rotational excitations because of their limited energy resolution).

For many materials, unfortunately the unavailability of sufficient data for all expected collisional processes imposes the main restriction on the accuracy (and thus, also usefulness) of a molecular-level MC simulation. While there are often extensive results on certain processes like elastic scattering or ionization, others like rotational or electronic excitation or even the total scattering cross section tend to exist only for special energy ranges (or certain outgoing angles or excited levels) due to the technical challenge of their measurement or an increased interest only in a particular state. Other channels, such as neutral dissociation, dissociative electron attachment, or positronium formation in the case of positrons, have been barely investigated for many molecules, leading to incomplete data sets that need a considerable amount of extrapolation (which introduces additional uncertainties). This means that while the simulation code can in principle model many kinds of interaction processes (and, at a given point, is easily modifiable in order to incorporate additional ones) at the molecular level, the computational detail attainable is as a matter of fact limited by the availability of suitable and self-consistent input data throughout the desired energy range. As a consequence, in the present state, LEPTS code does not distinguish the exact rotational or vibrational level after a respective excitation, and does account for the excitation of different electronic states indirectly via the corresponding energy loss distribution. Ionization is always considered to produce a single secondary electron, thus disregarding multiple ionization processes. Also, as inelastic differential CS are only rarely reported (generally, for low energies and even then only for specific conditions), the outgoing particle's angle after inelastic scattering events is approximated as described in section 2.1.

3.1 Data compilation: the example of electrons in H_2O

In the following, data collection and selection is illustrated by the example of electron interactions in water, a relatively well-studied case of electron-molecule scattering. Interaction data compiled here were used for the recent simulations of radiotherapeutic applicators presented in section 4.

3.1.1 Cross section data

The total and partial cross sections needed in order to simulate different electron scattering processes in water were obtained from experimental results whenever possible. Total electron scattering and integral ionization cross sections in water vapour were previously measured in our laboratory between 50 eV and 5 keV (Muñoz et al., 2007b) with a transmission beam technique and using synchronized electron and ion extraction pulses applied to the interaction chamber, respectively. Below 50 eV, total CS data from Čurík et al. (2006) and Szmytkowski (1987) were used. Electron-impact ionization cross sections below 50 eV were taken from Straub et al. (1996). Integral electronic excitation CS have been derived from the electron energy loss analysis carried out by Thorn and co-workers (Thorn et al., 2007a; Brunger et al., 2008; Thorn et al., 2007b) from 15 to 50 eV and have been extrapolated down to threshold and up to higher energies by assuming a double logarithmic dependence with energy. Vibrational excitation and electron attachment cross sections were taken from the recommendations made by Itikawa & Mason (2005).

For elastic collisions and neutral dissociation, integral cross sections were determined by combining experimental data and our own theoretical calculations. These were carried out with an optical potential method based on an independent atom approximation including screening corrections. Further details regarding the calculations can be found in Blanco & García (2003a;b; 2007). The model approach considers inelastic scattering as electron-electron interactions, consequently both vibrational excitation and electron attachment are excluded. Thus, when subtracting the ionization and the electronic excitation cross sections from the calculated integral inelastic cross sections, the resulting data should correspond to neutral dissociation. The good agreement with experimental results (Kedzierski et al., 1998; Harb et al., 2001) confirms this assignment. Elastic cross sections are based on experimental data from Cho et al. (2004) but include a correction for contamination with rotationally inelastic scattering. The CS values for rotational excitation are included in simulations only when considering water in the gas phase. Further details can be found in Muñoz et al. (2008b).

For high energies, the electron-molecule collision can be treated as a plane wave interaction with a sum of atoms in the framework of the first Born approximation. Integral elastic and inelastic interaction cross sections can then be represented by simple energy-dependent formulae (García & Blanco, 2000; Inokuti, 1971). For want of other data, this method was used at energies $\geq$ 10 keV. Angular distribution functions for scattered electrons were taken from our calculations, using the approximation described in section 2.1 for inelastic collisions.

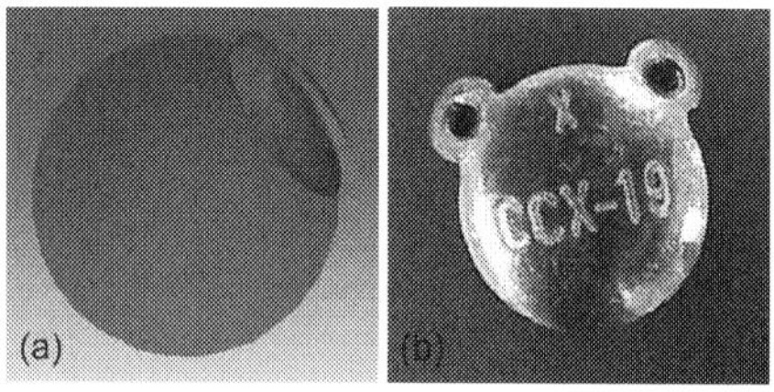

Fig. 2. Ru/Rh applicator used for the present simulation: (a) Scheme of the plaque placed around the eyeball. (b) Photo of the CCX plaque (Bebig, Germany).

3.1.2 Electron energy loss distributions

Electron energy loss distributions in H_2O were measured by us in a transmission beam set-up in order to assign the energy released in each electron-molecule interaction. After observing that the energy loss distributions did not present significant variations (uncertainty $\leq 15\%$) for incident electron energies in the range 50–5 000 eV, a unique (average) electron energy loss spectrum was used (Muñoz et al., 2008a). The mean excitation energy in water yielded by this distribution is $\leq$ 34 eV for electron energies $\leq$ 500eV and rises to about 40 eV for energies beyond the threshold for inner shell excitation/ionization.

4. Recent applications to radiotherapy

Radiotherapy of many tumours requires increased spatial precision due to the sometimes small dimensions of the treatment volume and the close proximity of organs at risk. A high accuracy energy deposition model might thus improve dose calculations (and, consequently, treatment planning and outcome). Motivated by this, the MC simulation LEPTS has been applied to determine the energy deposition in water of two radionuclides commonly used in brachytherapy, ruthenium-106 and iodine-125. The electron transport model capable of providing detailed information about secondary electron tracks, energy deposition and interaction processes at the molecular level can yield a completer picture of radiation damage in a biomedical context. In both cases, the radiation spectra emitted by the therapeutic applicators were measured by us in order to provide realistic input data and to reproduce incident radiation spectra accurately in the simulation. The localized dose deposition by both radionuclides benefits treatment outcome by sparing healthy patient tissues while delivering high doses to the clinical target volume. At the same time, these isotopes are suitable for longer-term or permanent implants, assuring the radioprotection of medical staff and third persons in close contact with patients.

The present simulations use data corresponding to a molecular medium in the gas phase without correcting for any collective effects present in liquid water. However, based on the very similar electron mass stopping powers obtained for water vapour and liquid H_2O in the keV range (Muñoz et al., 2007b), no major differences are expected when considering the liquid phase.

4.1 Ocular brachytherapy with ^{106}Ru

First, LEPTS is used to simulate brachytherapy of the eye with the beta-emitter ^{106}Ru. Uveal melanoma and other malignancies of the eye can be effectively treated by surgically implanting a concave ruthenium applicator tightly around the eyeball. As the ocular medium

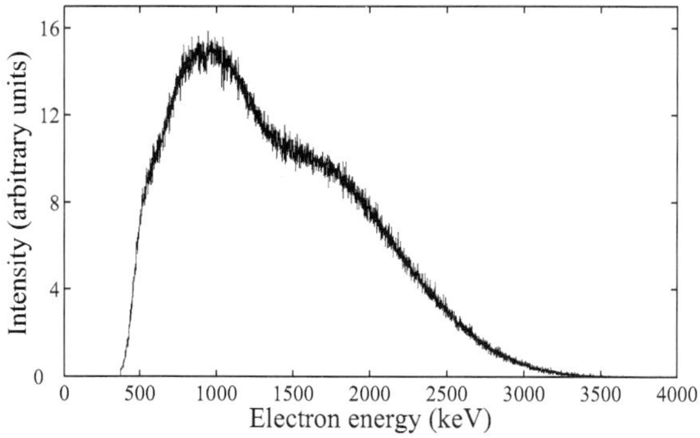

Fig. 3. Beta emission spectrum of the CCX type ophthalmic Ru-106 plaque.

can easily be mimicked by water, it constitutes an excellent system for applying the present simulation model with the interaction data set presented in section 3.1.

^{106}Ru is a β-emitter (endpoint energy 39.4 keV) that slowly ($T_{1/2}$ = 373.59 d) decays to ^{106}Rh with which it reaches secular equilibrium: it has a half-life period of 29.8 s before decaying to ^{106}Pd (stable) by different beta decays with a maximum energy of 3.541 MeV. Subsequent γ emissions from palladium have a maximum energy of 1.5623 MeV. Other probable decay energies are 2.407 MeV, 3.029 MeV and 1.979 MeV (β) and 511.86 keV, 621.93 keV and 1.050 MeV (γ) (data from the Lund Nuclear Data Service: Chu et al. (1999)). The combined electron emission spectrum of the applicator for use in the simulation was determined experimentally (Muñoz et al., 2008a) with a silicon detector and is shown in fig. 3. Note that the lowest-energy electrons emitted directly from ruthenium are absorbed within the applicator material, reducing the applicator's effective emission to the keV–MeV spectrum of its daughter nucleus rhodium.

Photon emission spectra that were measured with standard solid state spectrometers (Muñoz et al., 2008a) in order to check for a possible contamination of the source revealed gamma energies in excellent agreement with the disintegration scheme. However, in order to quantitatively relate electron and photon radiation, relative intensities of the γ emissions were taken from Chu et al. (1999).

Using a generic setup frequently found in brachytherapy of the eye with concave Ru/Rh plaques (c.f. figure 2), radiation-induced processes in the volume of interest - the eyeball approximated by liquid water - have been simulated. For this application, the incident photons were simulated using the photon interaction processes integrated in GEANT4. Once a secondary electron is generated, it is tracked using LEPTS. As the programme output, we thus obtain the exact location of each interaction event as well as the type of collision produced, the energy deposited, the change of momentum suffered by the particle, and the energy and direction of the secondary electron produced in case of ionizations.

Figure 4 shows lateral and transversal sections through the energy deposition map calculated after simulating approximately 2×10^6 primary particle histories (not taking into account those tracks that leave the volume of interest in the opposite direction, without entering the eye). (The applicator — not shown — is located to the left of the eyeball.) As expected for an efficient treatment of uveal melanoma and other tumours that are located similarly, bordering the vitreous humour, one obtains a steep dose gradient close to the applicator that becomes

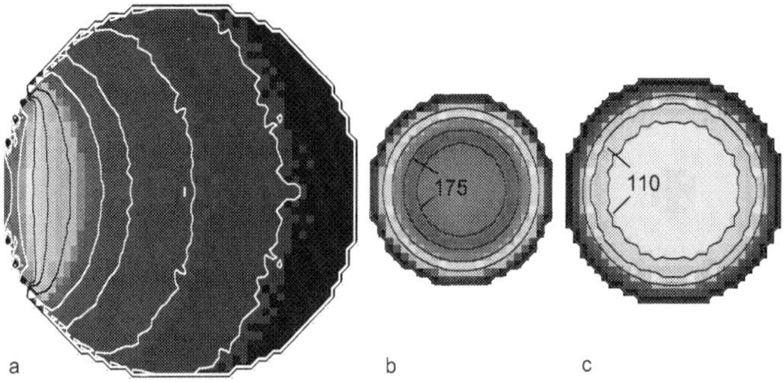

Fig. 4. Relative dose distributions produced by the ^{106}Ru plaque in the eyeball simulated as water (voxel size: $0.5 \times 0.5 \times 0.5$ mm^2). (a) Longitudinal section through the central axis of the applicator with 200%, 150%, 100%, 75%, 50%, 30%, 20%, 10% and 5% isodose lines shown. (b) Transversal section in 1 mm depth displaying 175%, 125% and 75% lines. (c) Transversal section in 2 mm depth displaying 110% and 50% lines. The same colourmap is used for all distributions.

flatter towards the centre of the eye. After normalization of dose to 100% in 2 mm depth, the relative dose absorbed in the first voxel (0-0.5mm depth) amounts to 249%, then decays to 55% in 4 mm depth (all at central axis). The relative depth dose curve along the central axis, applying the same normalization, is shown in figure 5. It can be seen that on one hand, the dose gradient is very steep within the first few mm inside the eye, but on the other hand there is still a considerable amount of energy deposited in greater depths (approximately 16% in 1 cm depth and 4% in 2 cm depth). This is due to the applicator geometry with a curved surface, the greater penetration of incident photons (compared to electrons which account for the main dose in the entrance region), and secondary electrons depositing small amounts of energy in multiple collisions while slowing down continuously. Lateral dose profiles for many different

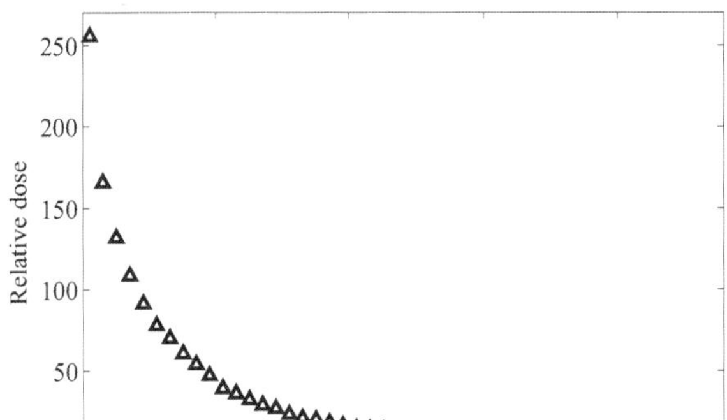

Fig. 5. Relative depth dose deposited at the central axis of the water eyeball by a CCX type Ru/Rh applicator. Normalization as in figure 4

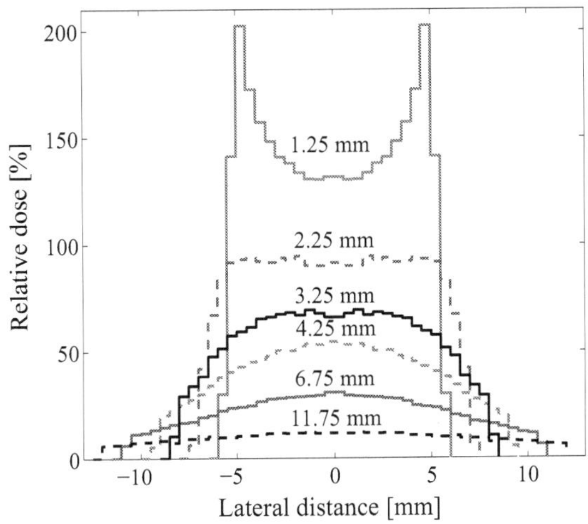

Fig. 6. Lateral dose profiles obtained for different depths in the eyeball (water sphere). Data is normalized to 100% in 2 mm depth.

depths are presented in figure 6. They exhibit two pronounced maxima in the region close to the applicator (up to 2 mm depth), reflecting its concave shape, an essentially flat central part in 2.25 mm depth, and a single, broader maximum in greater depths.

In this application, an ophthalmic brachytherapy plaque placed around the eye has been simulated by employing LEPTS for electron tracking and making use of the geometry definition facilities offered by GEANT-4, as well as its photon interaction routines. When comparing the dose distribution calculated with previous results obtained with PENELOPE on similar applicators (Sánchez-Reyes et al., 1998), they seem to be consistent within the first millimeters inside the eyeball. In depths ≥ 4 mm, the present simulation shows a shallower slope and yields larger doses at the central axis. Two possible causes are the additional dose delivered by the γ component — not accounted for in the other study — which steadily gains importance for greater depths within the medium and differences in the β spectrum used (theoretical vs. experimental spectrum). Finally, the differences in the scattering model and/or the underlying interaction data set might be responsible for the discrepancies encountered. A comparison of results obtained with PENELOPE and LEPTS in identical conditions (plaque and eye geometry, incident spectra) would be needed in order to confirm or discard the last possibility.

4.2 Brachytherapy with ^{125}I seeds

Here we show en example of how LEPTS is combined with PENELOPE in order to simulate the interaction of photon radiation with water. In particular, we investigate photon radiation with an initial energy distribution as measured for ^{125}I seeds that are used for radiotherapy of prostate cancers but can also be employed for treating lesions affecting the eye. Therefore, we do not assume any specific geometry here but center on an accurate representation of the emitted radiation and its penetration in water.

For obtaining the incident radiation spectrum in this application, a solid state Si(Li) spectrometer was used to determine the energy and intensity of the photons emitted by a

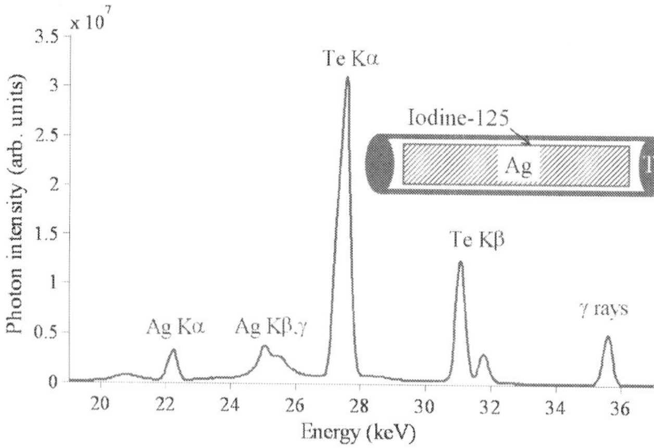

Fig. 7. Photon emission spectrum of the Amersham Health model 6711 ^{125}I seed as measured in perpendicular geometry. Gamma photons (35.49 keV) produced during ^{125}I/^{125}Te-decay as well as the most intense Kα and Kβ X-rays of Te are observed.

^{125}I brachytherapy seed (see fig. 7). ^{125}I decays to the 35.49 keV state of ^{125}Te by electron capture (half-life: 59.408 days) with 100% probability. The subsequent relaxation of nucleus and shell causes a gamma and X-ray photon emission which is considered as the primary radiation in this model. A representative spectrum shows the γ peak and various X-ray lines of tellurium in the range 27-32 keV. Additionally, X-ray lines between 22 and 26 keV with an intensity comparable to some of the photons emitted by Te were observed which are attributed to silver (present as the core of the seed onto which the radioactive iodine is adsorbed). These "contaminations" of the spectrum need to be taken into account for realistically modelling applications in brachytherapy (Rivard et al., 2004), and are thus included.
Using LEPTS in combination with PENELOPE (as explained in section 2.2), we simulated the interaction processes induced in water vapour when exposed to photon radiation according to the emission spectrum presented above. The resulting interaction map with H_2O molecules, at a density similar to that of liquid water, is shown in fig. 8. Note that up to this point, where exclusively interactions caused directly by photons are considered, only PENELOPE is used. It can be observed that in the geometry used, the photon beam remains laterally well defined, however some photon interaction events can be found even near the boundary of the simulated volume and release secondary electrons there. Photon interactions are coloured according to the type of event produced. Note that photoeffect (red dots) prevails for I-125 in water (which, for many purposes, is an acceptable approximation for human tissue), indicating that the main effect of the incident photons is to generate high-energy secondary electrons. These new electrons subsequently continue the energy deposition process by undergoing multiple scattering events until their thermalization. In this "second generation" of energy deposition events, PENELOPE is no longer involved, but electron-molecule collisions are individually simulated by LEPTS. In figure 9, one photoelectron track shown from its generation until complete thermalization, illustrates details of the energy degradation mechanism. It can be seen which different inelastic interactions with target molecules the secondary particle undergoes and how it deposits energy at many points along its track. Furthermore, additional electrons are generated by ionization events. This highlights the

Fig. 8. Simulation of 100 000 photons emitted from a 4 mm (diameter) disk according to the energy distribution measured for I-125 seeds used in brachytherapy. The simulated volume (red box) consists of $10 \times 10 \times 10$ cm^3 of water vapour at a density of 0.7320 g/cm^3. Different types of interactions are colour-coded as follows: red, photoelectric effect; green, Compton scattering; blue, Rayleigh scattering.

necessity to include accurate electron interaction data and models into simulation approaches for medical applications, as is done in the present Monte Carlo model, even if the primary radiation consists of photons as with I-125.

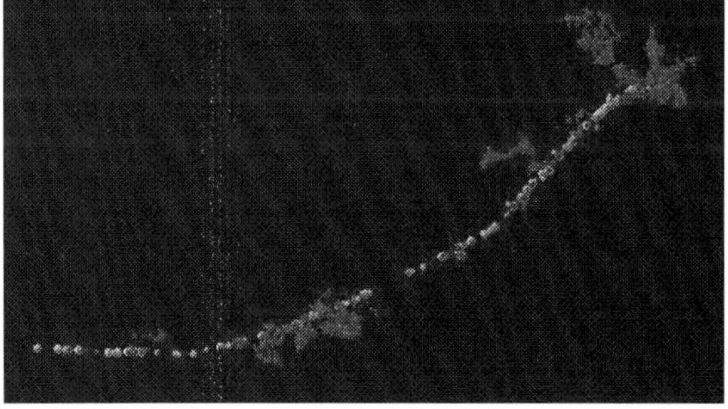

Fig. 9. Example of a photoelectron trajectory (from lower left to upper right) showing details about the electron-molecule interactions produced. Collisions are depicted using orange (ionization), yellow (neutral dissociation), green (electronic excitation), cyan (vibrational excitation), light blue (rotational excitation), and dark blue (elastic collision). For clarity, only some of the numerous elastic collisions are shown.

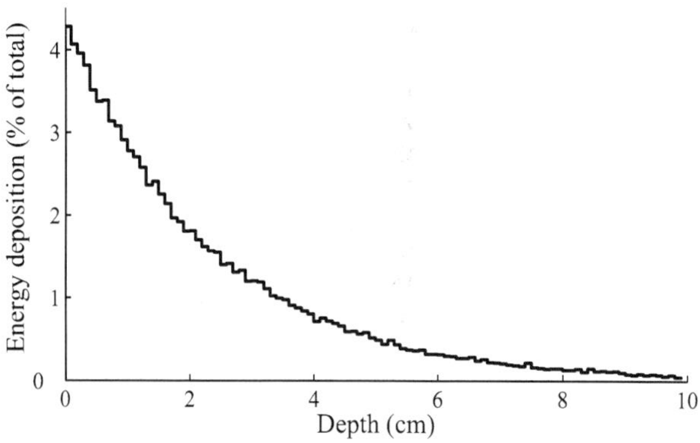

Fig. 10. Histogram showing the energy deposition by an I-125 source in water vapour at a density of 0.7320 g/cm^3 and supposing parallel photon emission. All contributions for a given depth are summed. The total energy deposited in the simulated volume ($10\times10\times10$ cm^3) is normalized to 100%.

Figure 10 depicts the energy deposition (equivalent to the relative depth dose curve) corresponding to a parallel photon beam of 4 mm diameter penetrating water at a density of 0.7320 g/cm^3. Most of the incident energy is lost immediately after entrance into the medium. 58.4% of the total energy is deposited within the first 2 cm, and 90% of the energy is deposited within 5.1 cm.

I-125 is used for radiotherapy of different tumours including ocular tumours which require a high spatial precision due to the small dimensions of the treatment volume and the close proximity of organs at risk such as the optical nerve, eye lens, lachrymal gland, etc. Simulation with a detailed energy deposition model, including an accurate representation of secondary electron interactions, thus improves dose calculations and may help to spare healthy tissues while effectively irradiating the target volume. In order to validate the present approach using LEPTS/PENELOPE for applications to radiotherapy with photon radiation, further studies will be aimed at a more realistic simulation of typical clinical cases (prostate/eye cancers), including exact geometries of radiation sources and of the relevant patient tissues.

5. Conclusions and outlook

We have presented a MC simulation code that introduces improvements in low-energy particle tracking compared to some other, currently widely used programmes (Kawrakow, 2000; Brown, 2003; Baró et al., 1995; Agostinelli, 2003). It offers a molecular-level description of the different interactions taking place between radiation particles and the traversed medium as well as a tracking model that follows electrons and positrons until thermalization. By not using any condensed-history algorithms, a series of problems that have been reported for other codes (Poon & Verhaegen, 2005; Poon et al., 2005; Bousis et al., 2008) are naturally excluded. Obviously, however, this also considerably increases the calculational resources (processing time) needed. Input data are carefully selected for each molecular material to be simulated and are updated as needed. As a result, the present simulation programme constitutes a useful tool for incorporating our knowledge on the molecular mechanisms of radiation damage into macroscopic applications and thus facilitating nanodosimetry.

Whilst the present simulation LEPTS cannot compete with the computational speed achieved by the state-of-the-art MC codes currently used for dose calculations in biomedical applications (particularly, in radiation therapy), its special treatment of low-energy particles and detailed modelling of inelastic scattering events yields a different view on radiation damage at the nanoscale by taking into account the molecular nature of the absorber medium. It could therefore give valuable clues by comparing LEPTS results with the ones obtained by other codes when considering typical "standard" situations in radiotherapy, radioprotection or medical imaging techniques (e.g., positron emission tomography). Also, a comparison of the predicted molecular-level damage due to irradiation in a tissue with the effect caused by the same irradiation at organic level will be of great interest.

Two examples of application to radiotherapy have been studied, both based on electron interaction data with water (which represents a good approximation for biological tissues for many purposes). Other data sets for use with LEPTS existing at the moment include those describing electron interactions in air (Muñoz et al., 2005), methane (CH_4, Fuss et al. (2010)) and ethylene (C_2H_4) (these two for representing simple hydrocarbons, basic building blocks in biology) and positron interactions in argon and water. A database on electron scattering by tetrahydrofuran (THF, C_4H_8O), a molecule interesting due to its strong similarity with the pentose forming part of nucleotides, is currently in preparation. With these data at our disposal, positron tracking during PET diagnostics and the simulation of electrons in THF are the next applications planned for the near future. Furthermore, particle tracking in materials composed of various different molecules will be carried out.

6. References

Abdoul-Carime, H., Gohlke, S. & Illenberger, E. (2004). Site-specific dissociation of DNA bases by slow electrons at early stages of irradiation, *Phys. Rev. Lett.* 92: 168103.

Agostinelli, S. et al. (2003). GEANT4 – a simulation toolkit, *Nucl. Instrum. Meth. A* 506: 250–303.

Badano, A. & Sempau, J. (2006). MANTIS: combined x-ray, electron and optical Monte Carlo simulations of indirect radiation imaging systems, *Phys. Med. Biol.* 51: 1545–1561.

Baró, J., Sempau, J., Fernández-Varea, J. M. & Salvat, F. (1995). PENELOPE: An algorithm for Monte Carlo simulation of the penetration and energy loss of electrons and positrons in matter, *Nucl. Instrum. Meth. B* 100: 31–46.

Berger M. J. (National Institute of Standards and Technology) (2000). Stopping-power and range tables for electrons. Available from: http://physics.nist.gov/PhysRefData/Star/Text/ESTAR.html.

Berger, M. & Seltzer, S. (1973). *ETRAN Monte Carlo code system for electron and photon transport through extended media, Radiation Shielding Information Center (RSIC) Report CCC-107,* Oak Ridge National Laboratory, (Oak Ridge, TN).

Blanco, F. & García, G. (2003a). Improvements on the quasifree absorption model for electron scattering, *Phys. Rev. A* 67: 022701.

Blanco, F. & García, G. (2003b). Screening corrections for calculation of electron scattering from polyatomic molecules, *Phys. Lett. A* 317: 458–462.

Blanco, F. & García, G. (2007). Calculated cross sections for electron elastic and inelastic scattering from DNA and RNA bases, *Phys. Lett. A* 360: 707.

Boudaïffa, B., Cloutier, P., Hunting, D., Huels, M. A. & Sanche, L. (2000). Resonant formation of DNA strand breaks by low-energy (3 to 20 eV) electrons, *Science* 287: 1658–1660.

Bousis, C., Emfietzoglou, D., Hadjidoukas, P. & Nikjoo, H. (2008). A Monte Carlo study of absorbed dose distributions in both the vapor and liquid phases of water by intermediate energy electrons based on different condensed-history transport schemes, *Phys. Med. Biol.* 53: 3739–3761.

Brown, F. B. (2003). *MCNP–A general Monte Carlo-particle transport code, version 5, Technical Report LA-UR-03*, Los Alamos National Laboratory, (Los Alamos, NM).

Brunger, M. J., Thorn, P. A., Campbell, L., Diakomichalis, N., Kato, H., Kawahara, H., Hoshino, M., Tanaka, H. & Kim, Y.-K. (2008). Excitation of the lowest lying $^3B_1$, $^1B_1$, $^3A_2$, $^1A_2$, $^3A_1$ and $^1A_1$ electronic states in water by 15 eV electrons, *Int. J. Mass Spectrom.* 271: 80–84.

Cho, H., Park, Y. S., Tanaka, H. & Buckman, S. J. (2004). Measurements of elastic electron scattering by water vapour extended to backward angles, *J. Phys. B* 37: 625–634.

Chu, S., Ekström, L. & Firestone, R. (1999). The Lund/LBNL nuclear data search, http:// nucleardata.nuclear.lu.se/ nucleardata/toi/.

Cullen, D., Hubbell, J. H. & Kissel, L. (1997). *The Evaluated Photon Data Library, '97 Version, Technical Report UCRL-LR-50400 vol 6*, Lawrence Livermore National Laboratory, (Livermore, CA). rev 5.

Čurík, R., Ziesel, J. P., Jones, N. C., Field, T. A. & Field, D. (2006). Rotational excitation of H_2O by cold electrons, *Phys. Rev. Lett.* 97: 123202.

Fuss, M., Muñoz, A., Oller, J., Blanco, F., Hubin-Franskin, M.-J., Almeida, D., Limão-Vieira, P. & García, G. (2010). Electron-methane interaction model for the energy range 0.1-10000 eV, *Chem. Phys. Lett.* 486: 110–115.

García, G. & Blanco, F. (2000). Energy dependence of the total cross section for electron scattering by chloromethanes in the energy range 0.5-10 keV, *Phys. Rev. A* 62: 044702.

Halbleib, J. A. & Melhorn, T. A. (1984). *ITS: The integrated TIGER series of coupled electron/photon Monte Carlo transport codes, Sandia Report SAND840573*, Sandia National Laboratory, (Albuquerque, NM).

Hanel, G., Gstir, B., Denifl, S., Scheier, P., Probst, M., Farizon, B., Farizon, M., Illenberger, E. & Märk, T. D. (2003). Electron attachment to uracil: Effective destruction at subexcitation energies, *Phys. Rev. Lett.* 90: 188104.

Harb, T., Kedzierski, W. & McConkey, J. W. (2001). Production of ground state OH following electron impact on H_2O, *J. Chem. Phys.* 115: 5507–5512.

Hubbell, J. H., Berger, M. J. & Seltzer, S. M. (1985). X-ray and gamma ray cross sections and attenuation coefficients, *Standard Reference Database 8*, National Institute of Standards and Technology.

Hubbell, J. H., Veigele, W. J., Briggs, E. A., Brown, R. T., Cromer, D. T. & Howerton, R. J. (1975). Atomic form factors, incoherent scattering functions and photon scattering cross sections, *J. Phys. Chem. Ref. Data* 4: 471–538.

Huels, M. A., Boudaïffa, B., Cloutier, P., Hunting, D. & Sanche, L. (2003). Single, double, and multiple double strand breaks induced in DNA by 3–100 eV electrons, *J. Am. Chem. Soc.* 125: 4467–4477.

ICRU (1984). Stopping powers for electrons and positrons, *Technical Report 37*, International Commission on Radiation Units and Measurements.

Inokuti, M. (1971). Inelastic collisions of fast charged particles with atoms and molecules—the Bethe theory revisited, *Rev. Mod. Phys.* 43: 297–347.

Itikawa, Y. & Mason, N. (2005). Cross sections for electron collisions with water molecules, *J. Phys. Chem. Ref. Data* 34: 1–22.

Jan, S. et al. (2004). GATE: a simulation toolkit for PET and SPECT, *Phys. Med. Biol.* 49: 4543–4561.

Kawrakow, I. (2000). Accurate condensed history Monte Carlo simulation of electron transport: I. EGSnrc, the new EGS4 version, *Med. Phys.* 27: 485–498.

Kedzierski, W., Derbyshire, J., Malone, C. & McConkey, J. W. (1998). Isotope effects in the electron impact break-up of water, *J. Phys. B* 31: 5361–5368.

Muñoz, A., Blanco, F., García, G., Thorn, P. A., Brunger, M. J., Sullivan, J. P. & Buckman, S. J. (2008b). Single electron tracks in water vapour for energies below 100 eV, *Int. J. Mass Spectrom.* 277: 175–179.

Muñoz, A., Blanco, F., Oller, J. C., Pérez, J. M. & García, G. (2007a). Energy deposition models at the molecular level in biological systems, *Adv. Quant. Chem.* 52: 21–57.

Muñoz, A., Oller, J. C., Blanco, F., Gorfinkiel, J. D., Limão-Vieira, P. & García, G. (2007b). Electron-scattering cross sections and stopping powers in H_2O, *Phys. Rev. A* 76: 052707.

Muñoz, A., Oller, J. C., Blanco, F., Gorfinkiel, J. D., Limão-Vieira, P., Maira-Vidal, A., Borge, M. J. G., Tengblad, O., Huerga, C., Téllez, M. & García, G. (2008a). Energy deposition model based on electron scattering cross section data from water molecules, *J. Phys. Conf. Ser.* 133: 012002.

Muñoz, A., Pérez, J. M., García, G. & Blanco, F. (2005). An approach to Monte Carlo simulation of low-energy electron and photon interactions in air, *Nucl. Instrum. Meth. A* 536: 176–188.

Perkins, S. T., Cullen, D. E., Chen, M. H., Hubbell, J. H., Rathkopf, J. & Scofield, J. (1991b). Tables and graphs of atomic subshell and relaxation data, derived from the LLNL Evaluated Atomic Data Library (EADL), Z=1100, *UCRL-50400 30*, LLNL.

Perkins, S. T., Cullen, D. E. & Seltzer, S. M. (1991a). Tables and graphs of electron-interaction cross sections from 10 ev to 100 GeV, derived from the LLNL Evaluated Electron Data Library (EEDL), *UCRL-50400 31*, LLNL.

Poon, E., Seuntjens, J. & Verhaegen, F. (2005). Consistency test of the electron transport algorithm in the GEANT4 Monte Carlo code, *Phys. Med. Biol.* 50: 681–694.

Poon, E. & Verhaegen, F. (2005). Accuracy of the photon and electron physics in GEANT4 for radiotherapy applications, *Med. Phys.* 32: 1696–1711.

Reynaert, N., van der Marck, S. C., Schaart, D. R., Van der Zee, W., Van Vliet-Vroegindeweij, C., Tomsej, M., Jansen, J., Heijmen, B., Coghe, M. & De Wagter, C. (2007). Monte Carlo treatment planning for photon and electron beams, *Rad. Phys. Chem.* 76: 643–686.

Rivard, M J and, C. B. M., DeWerd, L. A., Hanson, W. F., Huq, M. S., Ibbott, G. S., Mitch, M. G., Nath, R. & Williamson, J. F. (2004). Update of AAPM Task Group No. 43 Report: A revised AAPM protocol for brachytherapy dose calculations, *Med. Phys.* 31: 633.

Sánchez-Reyes, A., Tello, J. J., Guix, B. & Salvat, F. (1998). Monte Carlo calculation of the dose distributions of two ^{106}Ru eye applicators, *Radiother. Oncol.* 49: 191–196.

Seltzer, S. M. & Berger, M. J. (1985). Bremsstrahlung spectra from electron interactions with screened atomic nuclei and orbital electrons, *Nucl. Instrum. Meth. B* 12: 95.

Storm, E. & Israel, H. I. (1970). Photon cross sections from 1 keV to 100 MeV for elements Z=1 to Z=100, *At. Nucl. Data Tables* 7: 565–681.

Straub, H. C., Renault, P., Lindsay, B. G., Smith, K. A. & Stebbings, R. F. (1996). Absolute partial cross sections for electron-impact ionization of H_2, N_2, and O_2 from threshold to 1000 eV, *Phys. Rev. A* 54: 2146–2153.

Szmytkowski, C. (1987). Absolute total cross sections for electron-water vapour scattering, *Chem. Phys. Lett.* 163: 363–367.

Thorn, P. A., Brunger, M. J., Kato, H., Hoshino, M. & Tanaka, H. (2007b). Cross sections for the electron impact excitation of the $\tilde{a}^3b_1$, $\tilde{b}^3a_1$ and $\tilde{B}^1A_1$ dissociative electronic states of water, *J. Phys. B* 40: 697–708.

Thorn, P. A., Brunger, M. J., Teubner, P. J. O., Diakomichalis, N., Maddern, T., Bolorizadeh, M. A., Newell, W. R., Kato, H., Hoshino, M., Tanaka, H., Cho, H. & Kim, Y.-K. (2007a). Cross sections and oscillator strengths for electron-impact excitation of the $\tilde{A}^1B_1$ electronic state of water, *J. Chem. Phys.* 126: 064306.

Verhaegen, F. & Seuntjens, J. (2003). Monte Carlo modelling of external radiotherapy photon beams, *Phys. Med. Biol.* 48: R107–R164.

16

Integrated High-Resolution Multi-Channel Time-to-Digital Converters (TDCs) for PET Imaging

Wu Gao[1], Deyuan Gao[1] and Christine Hu-Guo[2], and Yann Hu[1,2]

[1]*Northwestern Polytechnical University*

[2]*Institut Pluridisciplinaire Hubert Curien (UDS, CNRS/IN2P3)*

[1]*China*

[2]*France*

1. Introduction to TDC

PET with time-of-flight (TOF) capability has been shown to provide a better reconstructed image compared to conventional positron tomography. The increase in SNR mainly depends on the size of the patient being imaged Conti (2009), the intrinsic resolution of the detector and the resolution of the TOF. In TOF-PET approach, for each detected event, the measurement of the time of flight difference between the two 511 keV photons provides an approximate value for the position of the annihilation. The approximation is directly limited to the capability of measuring the arrival time of the two photons.

In the 1980s, TOF-PET were built with an achieved timing resolution of 500 ps Moses (2007). At that time, the electronics available drastically reduced the performances of the TOF-PET. Nowadays, electronics operating in the GHz range is routine and the application-specific integrated circuits (ASIC) are commonly used Ollivier-Henry et al. (2007). The ASIC needs to include a high-precision time-to-digital converter (TDC) for each detector element to reach the required time resolution(*i.e.*, less than 100 ps)with good stability.

The objective of this chapter is to review the state-of-the-art of the TDC techniques and to select proper architecture for PET imaging systems. Both the conventional TDCs and the novel TDCs are presented. The comparison of the TDC architecture is given as well.

1.1 Conception of a TDC

A TDC is an essential electronics which quantizes small time differences between two signals (defined as "Start" and "Stop") and provides digital representations of this time interval. The funtion of a TDC is simular with an ADC. The TDC deals with the time difference rather that voltage or current differences in the ADCs, as shown in Figure 1(a). The measured time is defined as the phase difference between the positive edges of Start and Stop(Figure 1(b)). Figure 1(c) shows the transfer characteristics of a 3-bit TDC. The input is continuous time signals. The outputs are digital codes. Since the influence of the mismatches and the noise, the real transfer curve will deflect the ideal curve and generate quantization errors.

The relationship between measured time and outputs digital codes is given as

$$T_{in} = T_{LSB} \cdot \sum_{k=0}^{k=n-1} D_k \cdot 2^k \quad (1)$$

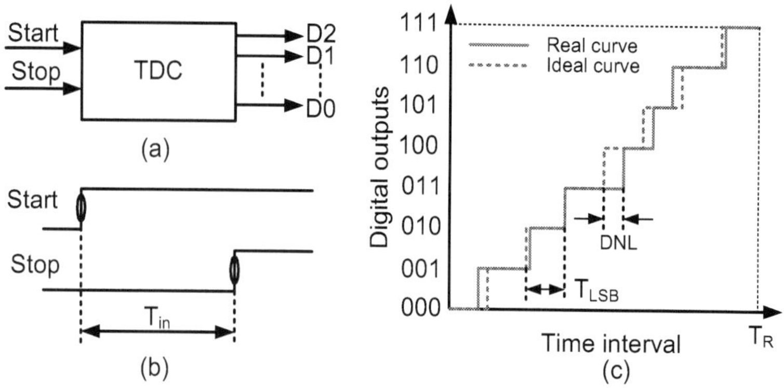

Fig. 1. Basis of time-to-digital conversion.

where T_{in} is the measured time interval between Start and Stop. T_{LSB} is the minimum unit of time measurements. n and D are the number of bits and the digital codes of the TDC outputs, respectively.

1.2 Figure of merits

The operation of a TDC is familiar with that of an ADC. So the performance merits of the ADC can be directly applied to TDC circuits. The resolution, dynamic measured range, nonlinearity and conversion speed are important characteristics to evaluate a TDC. Meanwhile, power dissipation, dead time or hit rate, and single shot precision should be considered for a TDC design.

1.2.1 Resolution

As a tool to measure time intervals, the resolution is a key parameters. The resolution of a TDC can be defined as the minimum unit of the time measurments. The dependence of the resolution is upon the circuit characteristics and noise performances.
Assuming the measured rang is T_R, the number of bits is N, the resolution is given as

$$T_{bin} = \frac{T_R}{2^N} \tag{2}$$

where T_{bin} denotes the bin size of the TDC.

1.2.2 Dynamic range

Dynamic range is the another parameter to estimate the performance of the TDC. The dynamic range is the total measured range by using the TDC. If the resolution of TDC is given, we have

$$DR = 2^N \cdot T_{LSB} \tag{3}$$

where DR refers to the dynamic range. N is the number of bits of TDC outputs.

1.2.3 Nonlinearity

The nonlinearity performances include differential nonlinearity (DNL) and integrated nonlinearity (INL). The DNL is defined as the deviation of each step from its ideal value, namely T_{LSB}. We have

$$DNL_i = T_i - T_{LSB} \tag{4}$$

where DNL_i is the ith value of the differential nonlinearity. T_i is the width of the ith step in real transfer curve.

The INL refers to a macroscopic description of the bending of a converter characteristic. It is defined as the deviation of the step position from its ideal value normalized to one T_{LSB} S.Henzler (2007). The calculation of INL is given as

$$INL_i = \sum_{n=0}^{i-1} DNL_i \tag{5}$$

1.2.4 Conversion speed

Conversion speed is a performance parameter that evaluate the speed of signal processing and device delay at each conversion time window in a TDC. This parameter is very important for high-speed applications.

1.2.5 Power dissipation

Power dissipation include both static power and dynamic power. The static power depends on the product of static consuming current and the power supply voltage.

$$P_{static} = V_{dd} \cdot I_{static} \tag{6}$$

where V_{dd} is the power supply voltage. I_{static} is the total static current. The dynamic power is determined by the switched capacitor, the power supply voltage and the clock frequency. The value is given as

$$P_{dynamic} = \alpha C \cdot V_{dd}^2 \cdot f \tag{7}$$

where α is the active factor and $0 < \alpha < 1$. C is switched capacitance. f is the clock frequency.

2. Analog TDC - the first generation

An analog TDC consists of a time-to-amplitude converter (TAC) and a high-resolution high-speed ADC, which were introduced in Tanaka et al. (1991); Bigongiari et al. (1999); Napolitano et al. (2010). The architecture of such a TDC is illustrated in Figure 2. The TAC is generally implemented by the current-integration circuit consisting of a charge-pump and a capacitor. A sample-and-hold circuit is required to provide a stable voltage signal. A high-resolution ADC digitizes this sampled voltage signal to binary codes which are the time words for the TDC.

Assuming the input time interval is T_{in}, the capacitor (C_c)is charged from zero, the amplitude of the integrated voltage is given as

$$V_{tac,amp} = \frac{1}{C_c}\int_0^{T_{in}} I_{cp}dt \approx \frac{I_{cp}}{C_c} \cdot T_{in} \tag{8}$$

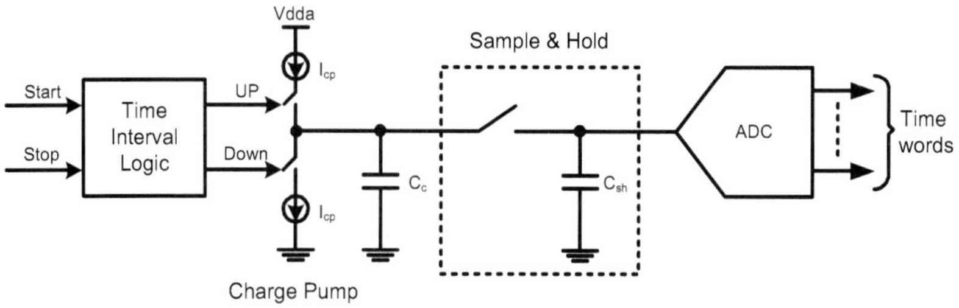

Fig. 2. Architecture of a TDC using current integration and analog-to-digital conversion.

where C_c is the charged capacitance. T_{in} is input time interval which generated from the Start and Stop signal. I_{cp} is the charging current. If I_{cp} is constant, the amplitude of the integrated voltage can be rewritten as

$$V_{tac,amp} \approx \frac{I_{cp}}{C_c} \cdot T_{in} \tag{9}$$

It illustrated that the voltage amplitude is propotional to the T_{in} with a slope of $\frac{I_{cp}}{C_c}$.
With a high-performance sample-and-hold amplifier, $V_{tac,amp}$ can be accurratly stored in C_{sh} and digitized by the ADC. Thus, we have

$$V_{tac,amp} = V_{LSB} \sum_{k=0}^{n-1} D_k \cdot 2^k + \epsilon \tag{10}$$

where V_{LSB} is the minimum resoved voltage. D_0 to D_{n-1} are the digital outputs of the ADC. ϵ is the total errors such quantization error, circuit error and noise error. From Equation 9 and 10, negalecting the errors ϵ, the relationship between the input time interval and the time words is given as

$$T_{in} \approx \frac{C_c \cdot V_{LSB}}{I_{cp}} \sum_{k=0}^{n-1} D_k \cdot 2^k \tag{11}$$

This equations means that performances of the TDC using current integration and ADC depends on both integrated precision ($\frac{C_c}{I_{cp}}$) and the resolution of ADC (V_{LSB}). Generally, with a high-resolution ADC, high-precision TDCs can be obtained.
However,the TAC and the ADC are mainly implemented by analog circuits which are not suitable for technology scaling. The design of high-performance analog and mixed-signal circuits is very complicated. Moreover, the analog circuit dissipates large static power consumption.

3. Digital TDC - the second generation

3.1 Counter-based TDC

A counter-based circuit would be the oldest and the simplest scheme. The measured time equates to the counted number multiplied by the period of the clock. The counter-based circuits have their advantages on the wide-range measurement and easier design in several technologies such as CMOS/BiCMOS process, field-programmable gate array (FPGA) Bogdan et al. (2005), and GaAs superconductive process Kirichenko et al. (2001).

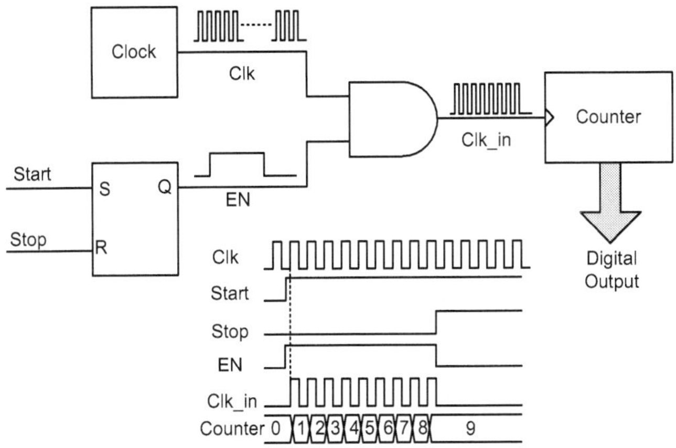

Fig. 3. The first class of the counter-based TDC Spieler (2005). The last number of the counter is the digital output which is propotional to the time difference between Start and Stop.

Two architectures of counter-based TDC have been developed. Figure 3 shows the first class of counter-based TDC. The Start and Stop signals are processed by a RS latch to generate a enable signal. This enable signal controls the width of the clock which drives the counter. The counter starts to count number when the enable signal is set to High. Thus, the last number of

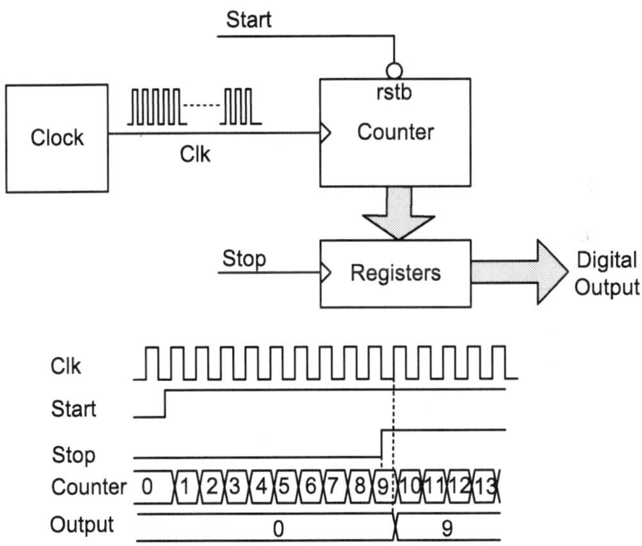

Fig. 4. The second class of the Counter-based TDC. The counter is drived by the clock and reset by the Start. The outputs of the counter is sampled by Stop. The sampled data are the digital output which is proportional to the time difference between Start and Stop.

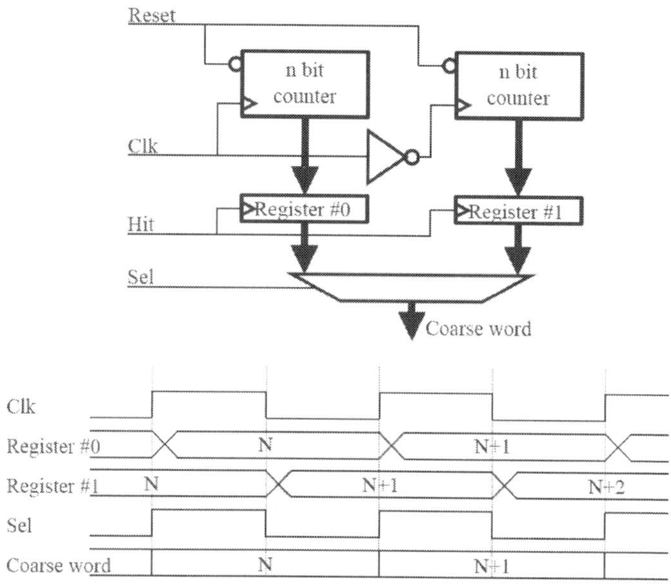

Fig. 5. The TDC using dual counters to overcome the metastability of D flip flop in the digital counters Mota (2000). Two counters operate simultaneously by using both the positive edge and the negative edge of the reference clock. Two sampled register can store the outputs of both counters. The correct data can be selected by the Sel signal.

the counter is the digital output which is proportional to the time difference bewteen Start and Stop. The counter in this architecture operates only when the Clk_in is fluctuated. Thus, low power dissipation can be achieved. However, since the RS latch and NAND gate can introduce noise on the time information from Start and Stop signals, the precision of the conversion is affected, in particular, in a high speed situation.

The second class of counter-based TDC is illustrated in Figure 4. In this architecture, the counter is drived by the clock and reset by the Start. The outputs of the counter are sampled by Stop signal. The sampled data are then stored into the registers. The stored number is proportional to the time difference between Start and Stop. This architecture can overcome the problem in the TDC shown in Figure 3. Nevertheless, the counter that operates in a continued way dissipates with large dynamic power.

Both architectures suffer from the metastability of the D filp flops in the counter. Due to the clock jitter and electronics noise, the conversion is limitted. However, the architecture shown in Figure 4 can be optimized by using Gray-code counter or dual-counter architectures. In Christiansen (1996); Mota (2000), a dual-counter was introduced of reduce the metastability. The schematic and the operational principle is depicted in Figure 5. In this architecture, two counters operate simultaneously by using both the positive edge and the negative edge of the reference clock. Two sampled register can store the outputs of both counters. The correct data can be selected by the Sel signal.

The relationship of the measured time, the converted number, the time difference and the reference clock is given by

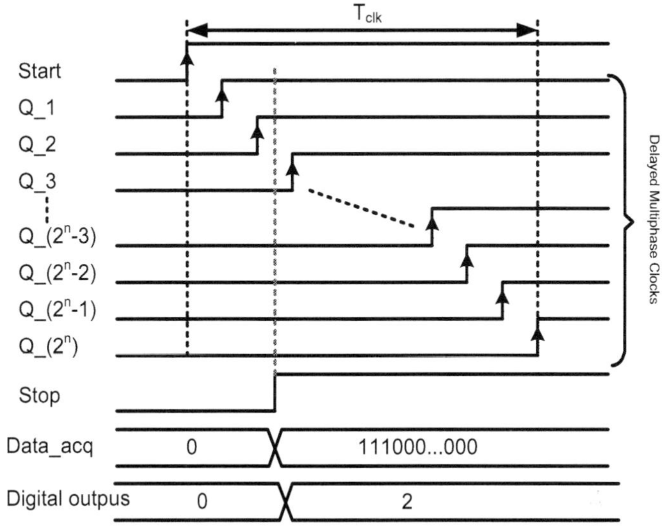

Fig. 6. The timing of the multiphase sampling.

$$T_{tdc,cnt} = T_{clk} \cdot \sum_{i=0}^{n-1} 2^{D_i} \tag{12}$$

where $T_{tdc,cnt}$ is the measured time. T_{clk} is the period of the clock. n is the number of bits for the counter. D_i is the ith digital output of the TDC. According to Equation 12, the measured range of the counter-based TDC is determined by the number of bits for the counter. Since the linearity of the conversion can not be affected by the externsion of the number of bits, the counter-based TDCs can achieve large measured range. However, the resolution is limited by the frequency of the reference clock and its conversion time depends on counted periods. These drawbacks limit its application in high-precision time interval measurement. The counter-based TDCs combined with time interpolations are usually used.

3.2 Multiphase sampling TDC

The timing of the flash sampling is shown in Figure 6. A Start signal is synchronized to the positive edge of the reference clock. The delayed clocks are generated from the Start signal with a fixed delay. The states of these delayed clocks are sampled by a common Stop signal. The acquired data are themometer codes which can be easily converted to the binary codes. The schamatic of the flash sampling is shown in Figure 7. The delay elements with the same delay are usually implemented by the stardard gate with the delay time of T_1. The resolution is determined by T_1. In this sampling method, 2^n delay clocks are required to generate n-bit binary code.

The bin size of the time measurement is given by

$$T_{bin,mps} = T_1 = \frac{T_{clk}}{2^n} \tag{13}$$

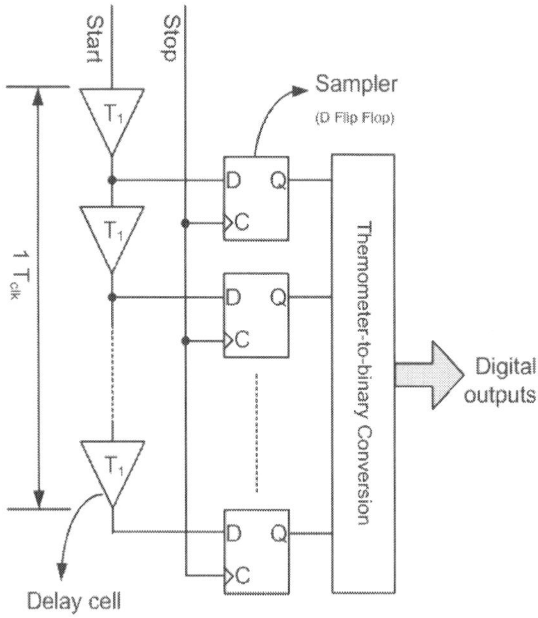

Fig. 7. The implementation of the multiphase flash sampling.

where T_1 is the delay time of each delay cell. T_{clk} is the period of the reference clock. n is the number of bits for the digital outputs. The measured time equates to the digital outputs multiplied by this bin size. Thus,

$$T_{tdc,mps} = T_{bin,mps} \cdot \sum_{i=0}^{n-1} 2^{D_i} \tag{14}$$

where $T_{tdc,mps}$ is the measured time. D_i is the ith bit of the digital outputs.

4. Sub-gate delay TDC - The third generation

The delay chain using digital gates can only deal with the resolution of gate delay which is limitted by the fabricated technology. Sub-gate delay time can be achieved by using analog delay cells built-in a delay locked loop. The multiphase sampling techniques are employed as well. However, the time interpolation such as the DLL array, the Venier delay line (VDL), and the multi-hit sampling can be used to obtain smaller time taps.

4.1 TDC based on a single DLL

The key technique of the flash sampling is to generate required delay time. The standard digital gate such as an inverter or a buffer can be employed as a delay cell. The TDCs based on gate delay were suitable for technology scaling due to its full-digital organization. However, the resolution was limited by the gate delay time. One way to get smaller time taps is to develop analog delay cells such as current-starved delay cells Swann, Blalock, Clonts, Binkley, Rochelle, Breeding & Baldwin (2004) and differential delay cells . The voltage-controlled delay

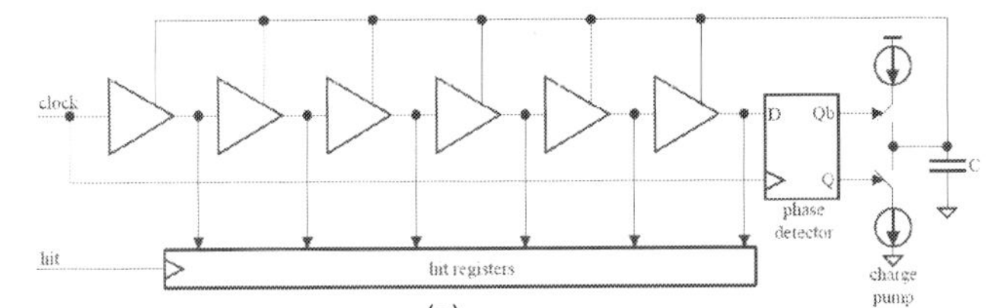

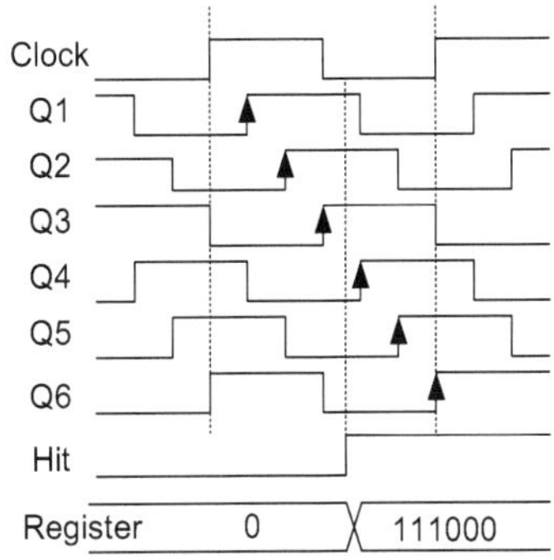

Encoding Table

Registers	TDC_out
000111	0
100011	1
110001	2
111000	3
011100	4
001110	5

(c)

Fig. 8. TDC based on a single DLL.(a)Schematic of the TDC based on a single DLL Mota (2000).(b)The timing of the flash sampling. (c)The encoding table.

line (VCDL) embedded in a delay-locked loop (DLL) can easily generate multiphase delayed clocks in one clock period Changv et al. (2002); Baronti et al. (2001). As shown in Figure 8(a), six delay cells are embedded into a charge-pump DLL. Thus, six-phase delayed clocks can be generated. A hit signal is employed as a sampling clock. When a positive edge of the hit is coming, the state of six clocks are sampled into the hit registers. The timing is illustrated in Figure 8(b). The sampled data are fake theremometer codes which should be converted to binary codes. The encoding table is shown in Figure 8(c).
The resolution of the TDC using a single DLL is given by

$$T_{bin,dll} = \frac{T_{clk}}{N} \tag{15}$$

where, $T_{bin,dll}$ denotes the bin size of the TDC. T_{clk} is the period of the clock. N is the number of delay cells in the DLL. The dependence of the resolution of the TDC based on a single DLL is upon T_{clk} and N. Since T_{clk} is limitted by the used technology, increasing N is the unique method. However, since the minimum delay time of the delay cell is limitted by the used technology as well, N has a upper limit in the practical circuits. Moreover, the mismatch of the delay cell do not allow to integrate large number of delay cells. To improve the time resolution of this architectuer, one can try to further divide the delay of the delay cells by performing phase interpolation using an array of DLLs or other time intepolation techniques.

4.2 TDC using an array of DLL

The time interpolation using an array of DLL is one of the most effective methods to improve the resolution. Two kinds of DLLs are used to construct the array. The resolution depends on

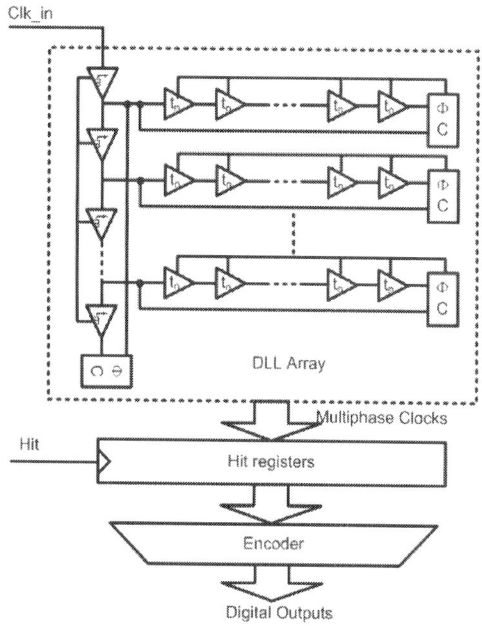

Fig. 9. TDC based on an array of DLL Christiansen (1996); Mota (2000).

the time difference of the delay cells in both DLLs. The reference clock is propogated by the array of DLLs. Smaller time taps can be obtained by using larger die area. The architecture of the TDC based on the DLL array is shown in Figure 9.
The bin size of the TDC based on the DLL array is given by

$$T_{bin,adll} = T_m - T_n = T_{clk}\left(\frac{1}{m} - \frac{1}{n}\right) = \frac{T_{clk}}{n \cdot F} \tag{16}$$

where $T_{bin,adll}$ represents the bin size of the TDC. T_m and T_n are the delay time of the delay cell in both DLLs. m and n are the number of the delay cells with the delay time of t_m and t_n. F is the number of the DLLs with the N delay cells. The bin size can be reduced by decreasing the time difference of T_m and T_n via increasing n and F. This difference can be achieved as few picoseconds. However, the jitter and the offset of the DLLs in the array limit the resolution improvement. It is very difficult to obtain the bin size of sub-picoseconds.
The principle of the time interpolation using a DLL array is, in fact, phase shift. The shift states can be illustrated in Figure 10. In this example, m, n and F are 28, 35 and 4, respectively. Thus, $T_m = 5\Delta t$ and $T_n = 4\Delta t$. Since the clock signal is continued, the positive edge of the delay clocks can be intepolated to form a time difference of Δt.
An unfortunate feature of the TDC based on the DLL array is that the array scheme is unable to produce the multiphase clocks with a number of a power of 2. This results in the digital outputs with pseudo binary codes. However, the measured result can be easily processed by off-line programming.
Since several DLLs are employed in the array, the static power dissipation is large than that in the TDC using a single DLL. Thus, low-power design should be taken into account.

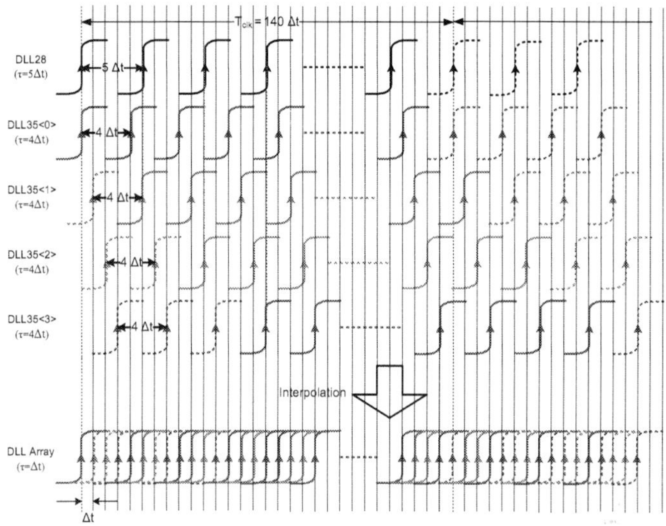

Fig. 10. Phase shift of the array of DLLs. In this example, m, n and F is 28, 35 and 4, respectively. Thus, $T_m = 5\Delta t$ and $T_n = 4\Delta t$.

4.3 TDC using a single DLL and RC delay line

Compared to the TDC using a single DLL, another method of the resolution improvement is to use multiple sampling signals delayed by the *hit* signal. The multiple sampling signals can be generated from a resistor-capacitor (RC) delay line. Since the integrated capacitor of few pF can be achieved, if the resistance is constant, the delay time, which equotes to the product of the resitance and the capacitance, can vary in the order of picoseconds as well. Thus, the bin size of the single DLL can be futher interpolated by using multiple sampling signals. The RC delay line is realized by the integrated passive elements such as Poly-resistor, Well-resistor and MOS capacitor.

Figure 11 (a) shows the architecture of the TDC based on a single DLL and a RC delay line Mota & Christiansen (1999). Assuming the number of delay cells in the DLL is N, and the number of sampling signals generated by the RC delay line is M. A register array of $N \times M$ should be arranged to store the sampled data. These sampled data are then encoded to the binary codes as the digital outputs of the TDC. The resolution of such a TDC is given by

$$T_{bin,dllrc} = \frac{T_{clk}}{N \cdot M} \tag{17}$$

where $T_{bin,dllrc}$ is the bin size of the TDC based on a single DLL and a RC delay line. T_{clk} is the period of the reference clock. If T_{clk} is constant, the bin size mainly depends on the number of delay cells in the DLL and the delayed sampling signals in the RC delay line. Theoretically, the bin size can be achieved small enough as long as the small time tap of the RC delay line can be obtained.

The implementation of the RC delay line is shown in 11 (b). Due to the parasitic resitors and capacitors, the delay of the RC delay element is basically limitted by the used technology. Since the model of the parasitic parameters for resitors and capacitors is not accurate, a digital

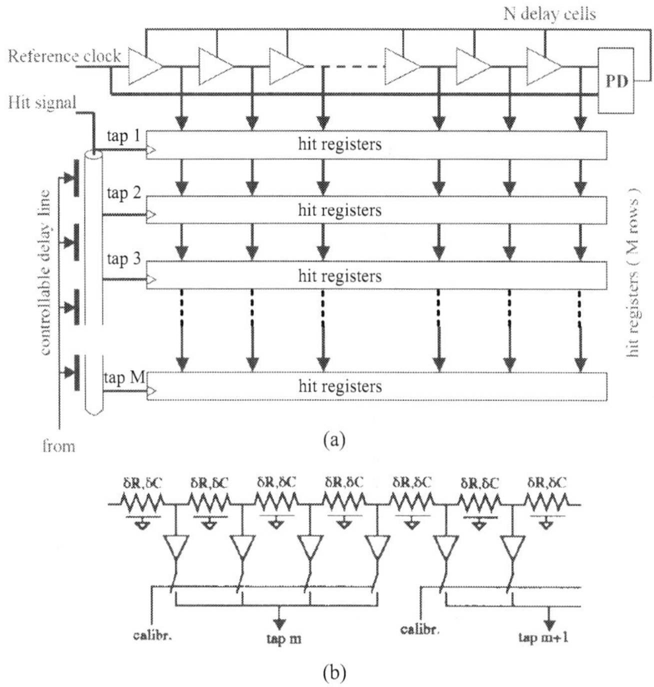

Fig. 11. TDC based on a single DLL and a RC delay line Mota & Christiansen (1999).(a) The architecture of the TDC. (b)The implementation of the RC delay line with a digital calibration circuit.

calibration circuit is required to adjust the delay time which should be compatible with the proper delay. Generally, the picoseconds-level resolution can be obtained.

4.4 TDC using Venier delay line

The Vernier sampling is shown in Figure 12. The principle of the measurements originates from the Vernier ruler. Two delay lines are required. The delay time of the delay cell in two delay lines is defferent. By using the Vernier method, the small time difference can be measured. The key point is the delay difference of the delay cell in two delay lines which should be exactly equivalent to the clock period divided by number of delay cells. In reality, the sampling process can be equivalent to the flash sampling.
The bin size of the Vernier sampling is given by

$$T_{bin,vdl} = T_1 - T_2 = \frac{T_{clk}}{2^m} \tag{18}$$

where T_1 and T_2 are the delay time of the delay cell in two delay line, respectively. m is the number of bits for digital outputs. Setting the suitable values of T_1 and T_2, the delay difference of T_1 can be interpolated by $T_{bin,vdl}$. However, the Vernier method uses multiple sampled clocks which generated from the delay line with the delay time of T_2.

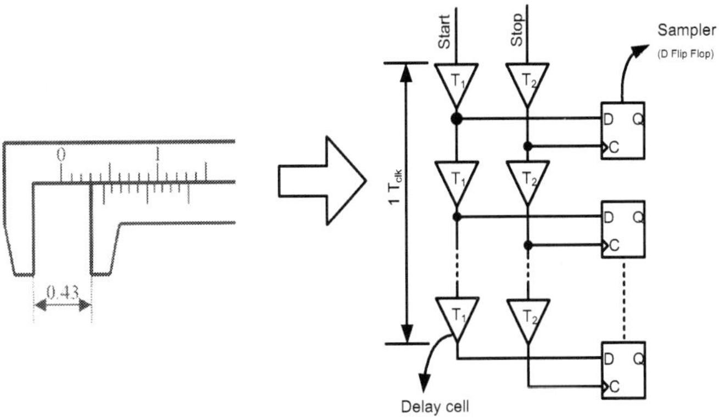

Fig. 12. Multiphase sampling using Vernier delay line Dudek et al. (2000).

To realized the TDC using vernier delay line, two DLLs should be employed. Thus, the synchronization of the multiphase clock is very important for such a circuit.

5. Sub-picosecond TDCs - the fourth generation

With the development of microelectronics and VLSI, the circuits dedictated to sub-picosecond TDC have been realized. The examples are cyclic TDCs using pulse-shrinking delay line, gated-ring-oscillator TDCs, and the TDCs using time amplifier.

5.1 Cyclic TDC using pulse-shrinking delay line

Cyclic TDC using pulse shrinking delay line Chen et al. (2000; 2005) is a low power TDC which can achieve the resolution of few picoseconds with good linearity. This TDC uses the inhomogeneity of the gates in cyclic delay line to implement the pulse shriking mechanism.
The architecture and the operational principle is shown in Figure 13. In this architecture, a Reset signal is required to ensure the T_{out} at Low level in the initial state. The input time inteval is shrinked in the delay line with a fixed width. The output of the delay line is then feedback to the input NAND gate for circular operation on the pulse shrinking until T_{out} without positive edges. A high-resolution counter is driven by T_{out} and generates digital outputs which are proportional to the measred time interval.
In the pulse-shrinking delay line, two kinds of inverters are required. One can be the standard NOT gate with the gain of one unit. The other is the inverter with the gain of β unit. Due to the difference of the input capacitance and equivalent ON resistance, the pulse will be shrinked in a fixed time interval. This shrinked delay interval depends on the dimension of the transistors, threshold voltage, power supply, temperature and other parameters. However, the influence of the temperature is an import factor for the cyclic TDC. A temperature compensation circuit is proposed in Chen et al. (2005).
Assuming the shrinked time interval is Δt, the measured time by a cyclic TDC is given by

$$T_{tdc,cyclic} = \Delta t \cdot \sum_{i=0}^{n-1} 2^{D_i} + T_{offst} \tag{19}$$

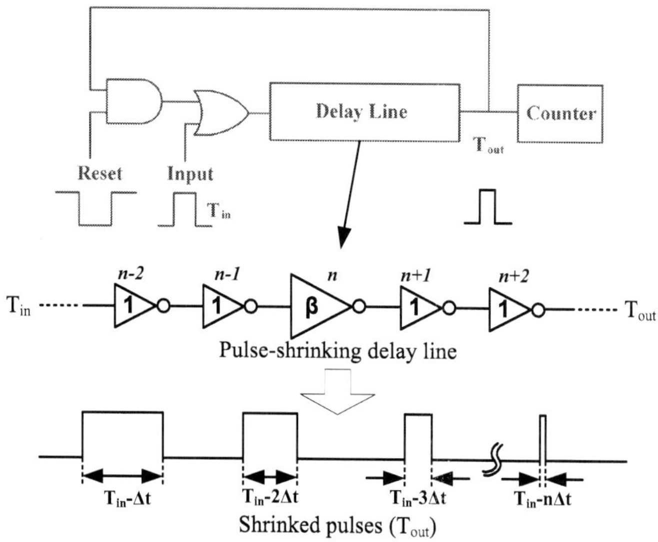

Fig. 13. Cyclic TDC using pulse-shrinking delay line Chen et al. (2000; 2005).

where $T_{tdc,cyclic}$ is the total measured time. n is the number of bits of the counter. D_i is the ith digital output of the counter. T_{offst} is the offset time interval of the TDC. This offset time interval usually exists in such a TDC. The reason is that the CMOS transistor has a cut-off frequency so that the tiny pulse can not be processed by CMOS digital circuits. The value of the offset time interval is about few picoseconds in submicron CMOS technology. Thus, the measured time of the cyclic TDC is given by both the bin size (Δt) and the offset time interval. Since it consists of pure digital circuits, the cyclic TDC finds its applications on many fields. A strong recommondation is to use a cyclic TDC as a digital phase detector Liu et al. (2008) for all-digital PLL which can be used for microprocessors, high-speed interfaces, and data recovery circuits. Moreover, the cyclic TDC can be implemented not only in standard CMOS technology but also in FPGA whose cost is lower than that of a CMOS fabrication. Futhermore, the power dissipation is low for the cyclic TDC. This is an attractive feature for some low-power portable electronics.
Cyclic TDCs using pulse shrinking can obtain a resolution of few picoseconds or several hundreds femtoseconds.

5.2 Gated-ring-oscillator TDC

For high-reslution TDCs using multiphase sampling, the resolution is mainly determined by the mismatches of delay cells. Gated-ring-oscillator (GRO) TDCs Straayer & Perrott (2009) which are a novel techique can overcome this issue and achieve sub-picoseconds level precision. The architecture and principle of the GRO TDC is depicted in Figure 14.
The GRO TDC is similar to the oscillartor-based TDC Nissinen et al. (2003) which uses the multiple outputs of the oscillator for phase measurements. However, the GRO TDC only allows the oscillator to have the phase transition during a given interval measurement. It means that the gated ring oscillator operates only when the "Enable" signal (refers to "the

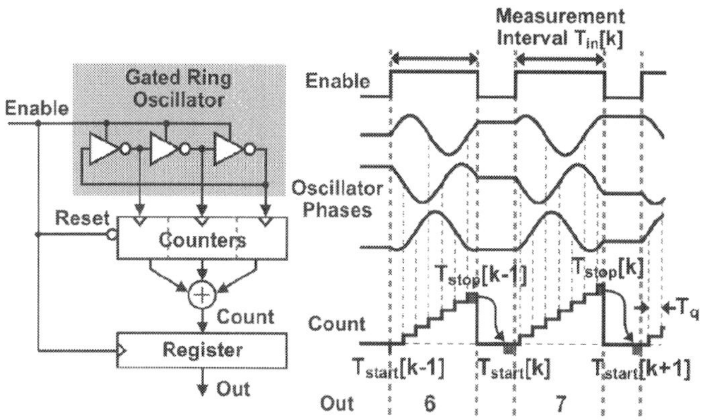

Fig. 14. Architecture and principle of gated-rign-oscillator TDCs Straayer & Perrott (2009).

measured time interval ") is high level and stops when this signal is low level. The outputs of the gated ring oscillator can be used as the clocks which drive the counter to counting numbers. One notes that the the counter is reset when the "Enable" signal is low level. Thus, the total numbers of all counters can be obtained by an binary adder. The sum of the counted number is proportional to the measured time interval.

The benefit of gating the oscillator is that the residue occurring at the end of a given measurement interval can be transferred to the next measurement interval Straayer & Perrott (2009). We have

$$T_{start}[k] = T_{stop}[k-1] \tag{20}$$

This feature can be utilized for continuous time interval measurements. Thus, the overall quatization error of the time interval measurement is given as

$$T_{error}[k] = T_{stop}[k] - T_{start}[k] = T_{stop}[k] - T_{stop}[k-1] \tag{21}$$

where T_{start} and T_{stop} are the start time interval and the stop time interval, respectively. k is the ordinal number of the measurements. This equation illuastrates that $T_{stop}[k]$ corresponds to a first-order noise shaping in the frequency domain.

Since the resolution of the GRO TDC is independent on the mismatch of the inverters, the precision can be achieved as 100 fs or less. To construct a subpicoseconds-level TDC, GRO-based architecture can be a very good choice. Moreover, GRO TDCs are realized by digital circuits which are very suitable for the technology scaling. This also introduces low static power dissipation.

However, the gated ring oscillator may suffer from non-oscillation when the time interval is enable. Thus, the design of gated ring oscillator becomes an important issue. Moreover, GRO TDCs suffer from the electronic noise and metastability as well as counter-based and delay-based TDCs.

The state-of-the-art of GRO TDCs can obtain a resolution of 100 fs.

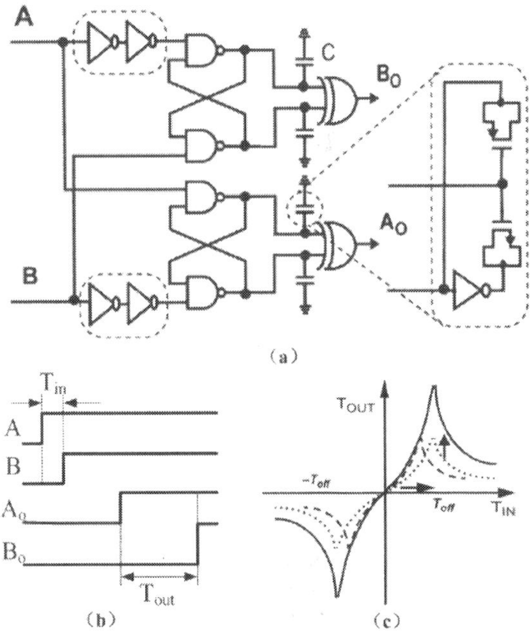

Fig. 15. Time amplifier.(a)Schematic of a time amplifier;(b)Conception of the time amplifier;(c)Characteristic of the time amplifier.

5.3 TDC based on time amplifier

It is a big challenge to measure the time interval with picoseconds-level resolution. The reason is that the performances of TDCs are mainly determined by the finite SNR and the mismatch of integrated elements. The conception of the time amplification is an effective solution for this issue. The schematic of a time amplifier (TA) which was proposed in Lee & Abidi (2007) is shown in Figure 15(a). The operation is similar with an voltage amplifer. The difference is that the TA processes a tiny time difference and outputs a larger time difference. The conception of the TA is shown in Figure 15(b). However, the circuit techniques of the TA is under developed. The state-of-the-art of the time amplifiers only can process a finite range of time interval. As shown in Figure 15(c), the transfer characteristics of the TA is not linear. Thus, the use of a TA should be based on the test results in the present age. However, the idea of time amplification gives a new research direction of TDC techniques, which needs to be optimized in the future work.

The architecture of a TA-based TDC is illustrated in Figure 16. The function of a time amplifier is simular to the preamplifier in the front-end electronics. In the neighborhood of the center point, the gain of the TA is monotone increasing, thus the behaviour of the TA is given as

$$T_{out} = K_{TA} \cdot T_{in} \tag{22}$$

where T_{in} and T_{out} are the input and output time interval, respectively. K_{TA} is the gain of the TA. Since K_{TA} is not linear, a calibration circuit is required. The TDC core could be a

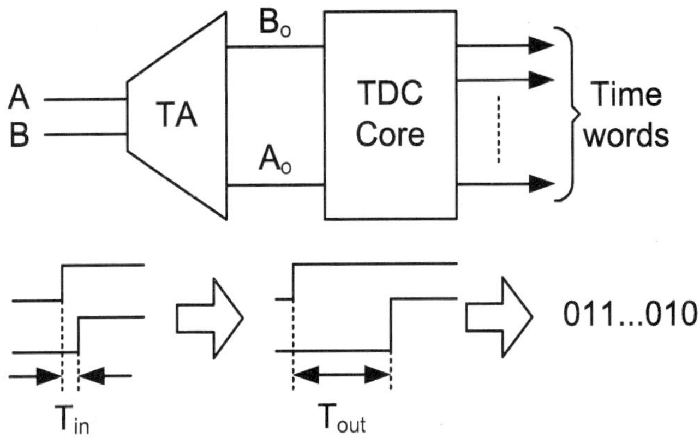

Fig. 16. Architecture of TDCs based on a time amplifier. The function of a time amplifier is simular to the preamplifier in the front-end electronics. The TDC core could be a counter-based TDC, a delay-based TDC, a GRO TDC or a TDC using a TAC and ADC.

counter-based TDC, a delay-based TDC, a GRO TDC or a TDC using a TAC and ADC. The relationship between the digital outputs of the TDC core and T_{out} is given as

$$T_{out} = T_{bin} \cdot \sum_{k=0}^{n-1} D_k 2^k \tag{23}$$

where T_{bin} is the bin size of the TDC. D_k is the digital bit. n is the number of bits for the digital outputs. From Equations 22 and 23, we have,

$$T_{in} = \frac{T_{bin}}{K_{TA}} \cdot \sum_{k=0}^{n-1} D_k 2^k \tag{24}$$

This equation means that the performances of the TA-based TDC depend on both the high-learity gain of the TA and the precision of the TDC core. With a TA, the objective of femto-second level time measurement will be realized.

The state of the art of the TA-based TDC can achieve a resolution of 1.25 ps Lee & Abidi (2007). However, the conception of time amplification can be applied to femtoseconds level time measurement.

5.4 TDCs using hybrid architecture

According to the previous disscussion, the idea of time measurement and digitizing can be categorized into three groups. First, the counter-based TDCs are used to obtain the wide measured range. Second, the TDCs using time-interpolation and multiple sampling techniques are proposed for high precision. Third, the current integration with high-resolution ADCs is introduced to profile the existed intelligent-poverty (IP) blocks (if had). However, specific applications demand custom TDC architecture with different performances. This is a motivation to develop TDCs with hybrid architecture. The mostly used hybrid architecture is counter-based TDC with time interpolation relized by a single DLL or a DLL array to persuit for both wide range and high resolution. In addition, the multiphase flash sampling together with Vernier delay line is another popular architecture for the sake of

Architecture	Counter-based	Single DLL	DLL Array	DLL+RC	VDL
Resolution	∼ns	∼100 ps	∼50 ps	∼20 ps	∼10 ps
Meas. Range	+++++	++	+++	+++	+++
Conv. speed	++	+++++	+++++	++++	++++
Power diss.	+	++	++++	++	+++
Nonlinearity	++++	++++	+++	++++	+++
Complexity	+	++	++++	+++	+++
Multi-channel	+++++	+++++	++++	+++	++++
Outputs	binary	binary	pseudo-binary	binary	binary

Table 1. Comparison of the existed TDC architectures(1)

high precision. Moreover, the time amplification can be used to these two hybrid architecture to achieve the resolution of sub-picoseconds.

6. Comparison of the TDC architectures

The performances of the existing TDC architecture are compared via the qualitative analysis. The results are listed in Table 1 and 2. The performances such as resolution, measured range, conversion speed, power dissipation, nonlinearity are considered. In addition, the design complexity, the form of digital outputs, the availible technology and the setup of multiple channels are analyzed.

From Table 1 and 2, the TDC can be divided into four groups according to the resolution. The first one is the sub-picosecond TDCs which include GRO TDC and the TDC using time amplifier. The available measured precision can be reduced 100 fs which is realized by GRO TDC. The TDC using time amplification can achieve the precision of 1 ps. The second group is picoseconds-level TDCs including the TDC using a DLL and RC delay line, VDL-based TDCs, cyclic TDC. These TDCs can achieve a resolution of about 20 picoseconds. Besides, the TDCs based on the DLL array and the TDCs using current integration and ADC techniques can be categoried to the third group which can obtain a resolution of about 50 ps ∼ 200 ps. The last is the nanoseconds and sub-nanosecond TDCs consisting of counter-based TDCs and the TDC using single DLL.

Among the existing TDCs, counter-based TDCs can achieve large meaured range. A 10-bit counter with a 100 MHz clock can operate in a dynamic range of 10.24 μs. The measured ranges of DLL-based TDCs including TDCs using a single DLl, TDCs based on a DLL array,

Architecture	GRO	Cyclic	Time Amp.	TAC+ADC	Hybrid
Resolution	∼100 fs	∼ps	∼1 ps	∼50 ps	ps ∼ ns
Meas. Range	++	+++	+	++++	++++
Conv. speed	+	++	+++	+++	+++
Power diss.	++	+	++	+++++	++++
Nonlinearity	+++++	++++	+	++	++
Complexity	+++	+++	++++	++++	+++++
Multi-channel	++	+	++++	+++	+++
Outputs	binary	binary	non-binary	binary	N/A

Table 2. Overall performances comparison of the existed TDC architectures(2)

TDC using a DLL and RC delay line, the VDL-based TDCs are determined by the clock period. The range is about several tens nanoseconds. The measured ranges of GRO TDCs, Cyclic TDCs and TDCs using current integration and ADC are larger than that of DLL-based TDCs. The value can be several picoseconds to several microseconds.

The conversion speed of TDCs depends on the measured methods. Due to flash sampling mechanisms, the counter-based TDCs and DLL-based TDC can construct flash TDCs which have high conversion speed. GRO TDCs and Cyclic TDCs require counting numbers so that the conversion time depends on the product of the counted number and the clock period. TDCs using current integration and ADC is determined by the sampling rate of the ADC.

The power dissipation of TDCs is determined by the circuit implementation of the blocks. Since the counter-based TDC and cyclic TDCs consist of counters and other digital circuits. It dissipates small static power consumption. Due to more counters required by GRO TDCs, they dissipate higher power than counter-based TDC and cyclic TDCs. DLL-based TDCs have moderate power consumption. However, since a DLL array is used, TDCs based on a DLL array consume very high power dissipation. TDCs using current integration and ADC mainly depends on the power of the used ADC.

Linearity is a very important performance parameter for TDCs. The dependence of this performance is upon both the architecture and the circuit techniques. Generally, GRO TDCs and cyclic TDCs can obtain very good performances on the linearity cause the measurement is independent on the mismatch. On the contrary, DLL-based TDCs suffer from the jitter due to the mismatch. The linearity of DLL-based TDCs is worse than that of GRO TDCs and cyclic TDCs but better than TDCs using the time amplifier and current integration. The linearity of counter-based TDCs is determined by the metastability of D flip flops. The value is better than DLL-based TDCs.

The design complexity is an issue that should be considered. Counter-based TDCs can be easily realized in modern CMOS technologies. However, the TDCs involving complex architecture and using mixed-signal circuits are difficult to be implemented. For example, the DLL-based TDCs that require low-jitter DLL techniques to generate precise multiphase clocks are typical mixed-sigal circuits. Except counter-based TDCs and TDCs using a single DLL, the design complexity of other TDCs is basically in the same level.

In the front-end electronics, the integration of multi-channel TDCs has become a trend to provide compact size, low power and high precision. Counter-based TDCs and DLL-based TDCs can be easily extended to multiple channels. However, the circuits should reused to construct multple channel architecture for GRO TDCs, cyclic TDC and TDCs using current intetration.

The specifications of hybrid TDCs can be customized according to specific applications. For example, the counter-based TDC with a DLL can obtain both high resolution and wide measured range. Thus, a hybrid TDC can obtain optimized performances via the tradeoff of resolution, speed, power, linearity and design complexity.

7. TDCs dedicated to PET imaging

In the field of PET imaging, few contributions are dedicated on the high-resolution TDC. The characteristics of these TDC are reviewed in the following items.

- A TDC that performed coincidence detection in a liquid Xenon PET prototype was introduced in Bourrion & Gallin-Martel (2006). The TDC architecture was based on dual counters and a DLL with 128 delay cells. The TDC, designed in 0.35 μm CMOS technology, was able to operate at 150 K and obtain a resolution of better than 250 ps.

- A 100-ps time-resolution CMOS TDC for PET imaging application was proposed in Swann, Blalock & et al. (2004). The TDC architecture combines an accurate digital counter and an analog time interpolation circuit to make the time interval measurement. The dynmaic range can be programmable without any timing resolution degradation by using a coarse counter. The fine conversion utilizes a time-to-amplitude converter followed by an 5-bit flash ADC. The bin size was 312.5 ps with a DNL of under ± 0.2 LSB and INL less than ± 0.3 LSB. The proposed subnanoseconds TDC was the first realization for the PET imaging applications.
- A fine resolution and process scalable CMOS time-to-digital converter (TDC) architecture was presented in Yousif & Haslett (2007). The TDC architecture uses a hierarchical delay processing structure to achieve single cycle latency and high speed of operation. The TDC had a 31 ps timing resolution and power consumption of less than 1 mW.
- A TDC based on Vernier method with 1.3ns timing resolution was realized by using only one FPGA (Kang, X., Wang, S. & et al., ?. A simple smart time-to-digital convertor based on vernier method for a high resolution lyso micropet, Vol. 4, pp. 2892 2896). The obtained resolution can meet the demand for the coincidence measurement of LYSO PET detectors with a 9 ns $\sim$ 15 ns coincidence-timing window.
- A full-custom 16-channel 625 ps TDC was proposed in Ollivier-Henry et al. (Oct. 2008) at IPHC, in 2007. The coarse conversion of the TDC was realized by dual 10-bit counter with a reference clock of 50 MHz. The dynamic range is 10 us. The fine conversion is based on the multiphase sampling techniques based on a charge-pump DLL with 32 delay cells. The TDC was designed in 0.35 μm CMOS technology.

8. Conclusions

This chapter reviews the techniques of integrated TDCs. The conception and figure of merits of a TDC is firstly given. Four generations of TDC techniques are then disscussed in detail. A comparison of these TDCs is given. At last, the TDCs dedicated to PET imaging are listed. The results show that the counter-based and time interpolation are widely used in the TDC design. Such a TDC is very suitable for the proposed PET imaging which requires a multi-channel fast TDC with a sub-nanosecond resoultion.

9. References

Baronti, F., Fanucci, L., Lunardini, D., Roncella, R. & Saletti, R. (2001). On the differential nonlinearity of time-to-digital converters based on delay-locked-loop delay lines, *Nuclear Science, IEEE Transactions on* 48(6): 2424–2431.

Bigongiari, F., Roncella, R., Saletti, R. & Terreni, P. (1999). A 250-ps time-resolution cmos multihit time-to-digital converter for nuclear physics experiments, *Nuclear Science, IEEE Transactions on* 46(2): 73–77.

Bogdan, M., Frisch, H., Heintz, M., Paramonov, A., Sanders, H., Chappa, S., DeMaat, R., Klein, R., Miao, T., Wilson, P. & Phillips, T. J. (2005). A 96-channel fpga-based time-to-digital converter (tdc) and fast trigger processor module with multi-hit capability and pipeline, *Nuclear Instruments and Methods in Physics Research Section A: Accelerators, Spectrometers, Detectors and Associated Equipment* 554(1-3): 444 – 457.

Bourrion, O. & Gallin-Martel, L. (2006). An integrated cmos time-to-digital converter for coincidence detection in a liquid xenon pet prototype, *Nuclear Instruments and Methods in Physics Research Section A: Accelerators, Spectrometers, Detectors and*

Associated Equipment 563(1): 100 – 103. Proceedings of the 7th International Workshop on Radiation Imaging Detectors - IWORID 2005.

Changv, H., J.Lin & et al., C. Y. (2002). A wide-range delay-locked loop with a fixed latency of one clock cycle, *IEEE journal of solid-state circuits* 37: 1021–1027.

Chen, C.-C., Chen, P., Hwang, C.-S. & Chang, W. (2005). A precise cyclic cmos time-to-digital converter with low thermal sensitivity, *IEEE Transactions on Nuclear Science* 52(4): 954–958.

Chen, P., Liu, S.-L. & Wu, J. (2000). A cmos pulse-shrinking delay element for time interval measurement, *Circuits and Systems II: Analog and Digital Signal Processing, IEEE Transactions on* 47(9): 954–958.

Christiansen, J. (1996). An integrated high resolution cmos timing generator based on an array of delay locked loops, *Solid-State Circuits, IEEE Journal of* 31(7): 952–957.

Conti, M. (2009). State of the art and challenges of time-of-flight pet, *Physica Medica* 25(1): 1 – 11.

Dudek, P., Szczepanski, S. & Hatfield, J. (2000). A high-resolution cmos time-to-digital converter utilizing a vernier delay line, *Solid-State Circuits, IEEE Journal of* 35(2): 240–247.

Kirichenko, A., Sarwana, S., Mukhanov, O., Vernik, I., Zhang, Y., Kang, J. & Vogt, J. (2001). Rsfq time digitizing system, *Applied Superconductivity, IEEE Transactions on* 11(1): 978–981.

Lee, M. & Abidi, A. A. (2007). A 9b 1.25 ps resolution coarse-fine time-todigital converter in 90 nm cmos that amplifies a time residue, *Proc.Symp. VLSI Circuits* pp. 168–169.

Liu, Y., Vollenbruch, U., Chen, Y., Wicpalek, C., Maurer, L., Mayer, T., Boos, Z. & Weigel, R. (2008). A 6ps resolution pulse shrinking time-to-digital converter as phase detector in multi-mode transceiver, *Radio and Wireless Symposium, 2008 IEEE*, pp. 163 –166.

Moses, W. W. (2007). Recent advances and future advances in time-of-flight pet, *Nuclear Instruments and Methods in Physics Research Section A: Accelerators, Spectrometers, Detectors and Associated Equipment* 580(2): 919 – 924. Imaging 2006 - Proceedings of the 3rd International Conference on Imaging Techniques in Subatomic Physics, Astrophysics, Medicine, Biology and Industry.

Mota, M. (2000). Design and characterization of cmos high-resolution time-to-digital converters, *PhD dissertation, UNIVERSIDADE TECNICA DE LISBOA* .

Mota, M. & Christiansen, J. (1999). A high-resolution time interpolator based on a delay locked loop and an rc delay line, *IEEE Journal of Solid-State Circuits* 34(10): 1360–1366.

Napolitano, P., Alimenti, F. & Carbone, P. (2010). A novel sample-and-hold-based time-to-digital converter architecture, *IEEE Transactions on Nuclear Science* pp. 1019–1026.

Nissinen, I., Mantyniemi, A. & Kostamovaara, J. (2003). A cmos time-todigitalconverter based on a ring oscillator for a laser radar, *ProcIEEE ESSCIRC* pp. 469–472.

Ollivier-Henry, N., Bard, P. & et al., D. B. (Oct. 2008). Imotepd: A low-jitter 16 channels time to digital converter based on delay locked loop for small animal pet imaging applications, *2008 IEEE Nuclear Science Symposium and Medical Imaging Conference* Dresden, Germany.

Ollivier-Henry, N., Berst, J., Colledani, C., Hu-Guo, C., Mbow, N., Staub, D., Guyonnet, J. & Hu, Y. (2007). A front-end readout mixed chip for high-efficiency small animal pet imaging, *Nuclear Instruments and Methods in Physics Research Section A: Accelerators, Spectrometers, Detectors and Associated Equipment* 571(1-2): 312 – 316. Proceedings of the 1st International Conference on Molecular Imaging Technology - EuroMedIm

2006.

S.Henzler (2007). Time-to-digital converter, *Springer* Springer series in advanced microelectronics.

Spieler, H. (2005). Semiconductor detector systems, *Oxford university press* .

Straayer, M. Z. & Perrott, M. H. (2009). A multi-path gated ring oscillator tdc with first-order noise shaping, *IEEE Jounal of Solid-State Circuits* 44(4): 1089–1098.

Swann, B., Blalock, B., Clonts, L., Binkley, D., Rochelle, J., Breeding, E. & Baldwin, K. (2004). A 100-ps time-resolution cmos time-to-digital converter for positron emission tomography imaging applications, *Solid-State Circuits, IEEE Journal of* 39(11): 1839–1852.

Swann, B. K., Blalock, B. J. & et al., L. G. C. (2004). A 100-ps time-resolution cmos time-to-digital converter for positron emission tomography imaging applications, *Solid-State Circuits, IEEE Journal of* 39(11): 1839–1852.

Tanaka, M., Ikeda, H., Ikeda, M. & Inaba, S. (1991). Development of monolithic time-to-amplitude converter for high precision tof measurement, *Nuclear Science, IEEE Transactions on* 38(2): 301–305.

Yousif, A. S. & Haslett, J. W. (2007). A fine resolution tdc architecture for next generation pet imaging, *IEEE Transaction on Nuclear Science* 54(5): 1574–1582.

Part 3

Imaging and Data Processing

17

Parkinson's Disease Diagnosis and Prognosis Using Diffusion Tensor Medical Imaging Features Fusion

Roxana Oana Teodorescu[1], Vladimir-Ioan Cretu[2] and Daniel Racoceanu[3]
[1,2]*"Politehnica" University of Timisoara,*
[1]*Université de Franche-Comté, Besançon*
[3]*French National Centre for Scientific Research (CNRS)*
[3]*Image and Pervasive Access Lab - IPAL UMI CNRS*
[1,2]*Romania*
[1,3]*France*
[3]*Singapore*

1. Introduction

Despite important advances in medical imaging, cognitive testing methods are still used almost exclusively nowadays for Parkinson's Disease (PD) diagnosis. These tests are evaluated and scored using predefined scales representing the disease severity like UPDRS (Unified Parkinson's Disease Rating Scale) or H&Y (Hoehn and Yahr) scale. Using the same scales, our objective is to include information extracted and fused from different medical imaging modalities, in order to obtain a quantification of the disease evolution, for diagnosis and prognosis purposes.

The dopamine, one of the main neurotransmitters, is lost when PD is installed. By the time the disease can be identified, 80-90% of the dopamine is no longer produced (Today, 2009). Medical studies concluded that the Substantia Nigra, a small anatomical region situated in the midbrain, is the producer of dopamine (Chan et al., 2007). The same anatomical region contains the motor fibres and the effect of the dopamine lost affects these fibers, as the patients lose their motor functions and start trembling once the disease starts manifesting. The importance of the motor fibers for the evolution and the early detection of the disease, represent a major medical motivation to set up a method able to extract and quantify abnormalities in the strationigral tract.

As recently a match between the dopamine level in the Substantia Nigra(SN) and the Parkinson's disease evolution has been detected (Chan et al., 2007), we are using this information further as we are studying the area where the Substantia Nigra(SN) produces the dopamine. David Vaillancourt, assistant professor at University of Illinois at Chicago has leaded a study using a scanned the part of the brain called Substantia Nigra on Parkinson's patients using DTI images and has discovered that the number of dopaminergic neurons in certain areas of this region is 50% less (Vaillancourt, 2009). His study includes 28 subjects from which half have symptoms of early Parkinson's disease and another half do not have these symptoms. This area is not well defined anatomically as there the contours are unclear. In this case, we detect the midbrain, being certain that it contains the SN. This segmented area is then studied to determine the correlation between the PD patients and the dopamine level, measured by the fractional anisotropy (Teodorescu et al., 2009b). Using a statistical evaluation, the correlation is revealed. For diagnoses purposes, we need also a value quantifying this correlation.

Another study performed to show the relationship between cerebral morphology and the expression of dopamine receptors, conducted on 45 healthy patients, reveals that on grey matter, there is a direct correlation at the SN level. This study (Woodward et al., 2009) uses T_1 weighted structural MRI images. Using Voxel-based morphometry (VBM), the authors create grey matter volumes and density images and correlate these images with Biological Parametric toolbox. Voxel-wise normalization also revealed that the grey matter volume and SN are correlated.

In order to quantify the impact of PD on the patients at the motor level, we study the motor tract to determine if there is a direct link to the loss of dopamine and the degeneration of the neural fibers of this tract. A statistical analysis of the number of fibers and their density is able to reveal if together with the loss of dopamine, the motor fibers that are inactive have a relationship with the PD severity.

1.1 Problems that we aim to solve

The main purpose of our approach is to detect PD based exclusively on the image features. We desire, based on the metrics developed at the image level, to detect PD on early stages and deduct the installation of PD - most likely cases to develop the disease. Working with medical image features, we include medical knowledge when extracting the features, based on the previous studies. The fact that the producer of dopamine is the SN area, makes it an essential volume of interest in our approach. Because this anatomical region is not well defined, we aim on extracting the midbrain, region that contains the SN.

The medical knowledge determines the area of study and the methods extracting the features required by the medical knowledge from the image level. The neural fibers affected by PD, represent the motor tract that we detect using the volume of interest. For an accurate detection, as we are using the midbrain area, where there are many neural tracts passing through, we need another volume of interest, able to select among the neural fibers starting at the midbrain level, just the motor ones. We choose the second volume as the Putamen, anatomical region where the motor tract passes also through.

These volumes of interest are detected using segmentation methods applied on medical images. The fibers are revealed using a deterministic global tractography method with the two-segmented anatomical regions as volumes of interest. The detected fibers must be evaluated and further used as a metric for PD in the diagnosis and prognosis processes. The main purpose of our work, the image based diagnosis/prognosis, determines image processing aims, as well as image analysis ones: **volumes of interest detection** achieved trough medical image segmentation, respectively **exclusive detection of the motor tract** determined by tractography.

There are other aspects that must be taken into account as well, aspects that do not derive from the medical knowledge. The **inter-patient variability** is one of these aspects and it is determined by the demographic parameters: age, sex and race of the patient. These characteristics influence the performance of the algorithms at every level. The brain structures volumes vary depending on the sex of the patient, the shape of the head differs depending on the race, and age determines brain atrophy, inducing a variation of the anatomical structures.

All these manifestations are linked to demographic parameters.
There are special limitations regarding the medical **images resolution** and specificity for the image processing algorithms. One of the main tasks is to find the appropriate slice in which to look for the volume of interest. Each slice contains different information and we rely on volumetric information when choosing the slice of interest for each of the segmentation algorithms. The **position of each patient in the image** is different, as is the size and shape of the head. This aspect determines the location of the volumes of interest of the brain (starting from the nose level or from the eyes level) or for the same number of slices, the whole brain or only a part of it (for smaller skulls the whole brain can be scanned, whereas for bigger ones, only a percentage of it, even if the scanning starts at the same level). This aspect determines an evaluation of the volume content in the image stack provided. We can place our analysis parameters, based on the center of mass of the brain.
Another aspect regarding **intra-patient variability** is the difference between the two hemispheres of the brain for the same patient. The Putamen is not symmetrically placed on the left and right side of the middle axis that separates the hemispheres, neither at the same relative position with regard to the center of mass of the brain. This is one of the challenges, together with the fact that the right side Putamen can have a different shape and size from the left side and be placed higher or lower than the other one. Tough finding the limit between the two hemispheres of the brain is another bid as it must be determined. The two hemispheres are not perfectly symmetrical and the line is not necessarily perpendicular on the horizontal axis of the image- **the intra-patient specificity**. The need to determine this axis with no connection to the specificity of the patient, determines also a need for an automatic overall detection approach.

1.2 General presentation of the methods

Using the provided images, we obtain different features from different DTI (Diffusion Tensor Imaging) modalities. By fusing the image information and using it to attach a value to the severity degree from the disease scale, we propose a new approach altogether with image processing (specific anatomical segmentation) and analysis methods. With a geometry-based automatic registration, we fuse information from different DTI image methods: FA (Fractional Anisotropy) and EPI (Echo-Planar Imaging). The specificity of the EPI resides in the tensor information, but it lacks anatomical detail, as it has a low resolution. At this point, the FA completes the informational data, as it contains the anisotropy representing the dopamine flow. As at the midbrain level, there are many fiber tracts, this area does not provide just the motor tract. The fibers from this tract cross also the Putamen. Determining the fibers that cross the two anatomical areas - midbrain and Putamen - at the same time, provides a more accurate selection using a global deterministic tractography. The midbrain can be detected and segmented on the image that contains the tensors, the EPI, but the Putamen is not detectable even on the high-resolution images like T_1 or T_2. The FA image, due to the dopamine flow, has the boundaries of the Putamen and an accurate segmentation is possible on this image.
The registration is needed as the segmented area is used for the tractography on the EPI image volume and not on the FA, where it is detected. The dopamine flow revealing the Putamen represents one type of information at the image level, different from the tensor information with anatomical detail, present on the EPI image. This is the reason for an information fusion from the two image modalities, achieved by registering the extracted Putamen map on the EPI.

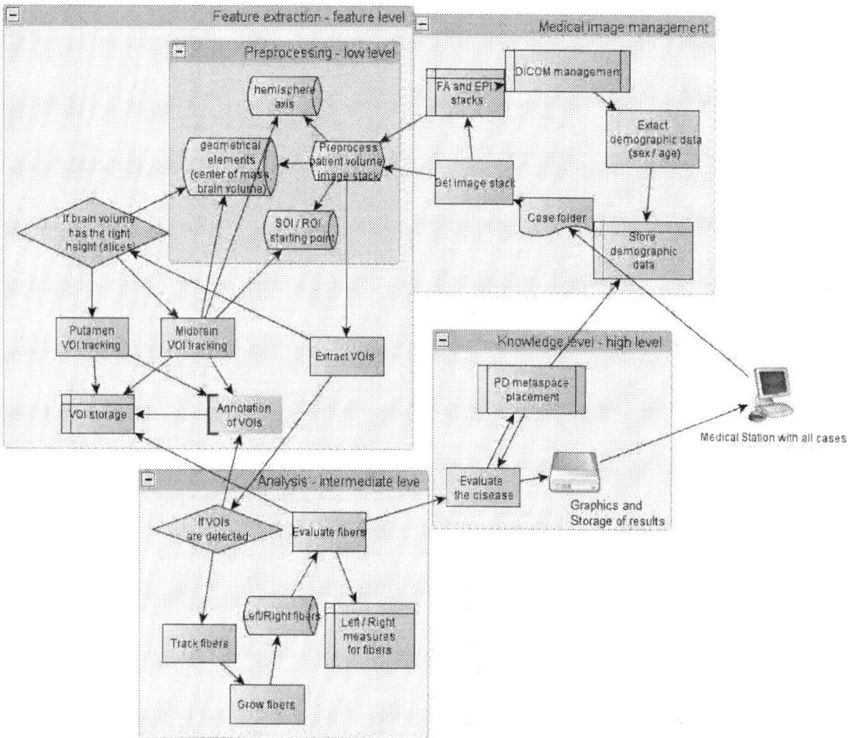

Fig. 1. PDFibAtl@s prototype integrating our methods

Once the fibers are detected, they are evaluated introducing specific metrics for the fiber density. Using a statistical method, correlation between the PD severity and the fiber values is detected. The specific fibers evaluated are analyzed. The diagnosis based on these values makes the difference between the control cases and the PD. Usually prognosis functions determine the evolution in time of a patient, but for that purpose we need a follow-up on the patients. In other cases, the prognosis function decides on the severity of a disease. For us, the prognosis is able to detect the disease severity for the PD patients.
As shown in figure 1,there are several levels where the information is manipulated:

- Image level
- Feature level
- Knowledge Level

Our prototype - PDFibAtl@s - implements the image processing and analysis methods taking the images from the medical station in DICOM format and extracting the significant features. The first level of information, the *image level,* deals with the medical image standard files and extracts the primary information from it, making the difference between the image and the protocol elements. At the *feature level,* a preprocessing step is applied to the image. The

information retrieved by feature extraction, encapsulates medical knowledge as well. The analysis part uses the tractography to determine the motor fibers. Having as input the value obtained by measuring the fibers, we develop at the *knowledge level*, the algorithms performing diagnosis and prognosis assistance.
From the clinical point of view, translational researches are necessary by next to go from the Proof of Concept (POC) to the Proof of Value (POV).
The structure of this chapter contains in the next section similar methods with the ones developed in our work and the systems that include these methods (subsec. 1.3). After presenting the protocols and characteristics of the medical images (sec. 2), we present the image processing methods (sec. 3) with the tractography approach, and the diagnosis and prognosis module performing the data analysis. These methods make the transition of information from the rough image level to the knowledge level as presented in section 4. The final conclusions together with future works and perspectives are presented in section 5.

1.3 Methods used in other approaches

We have tested several methods before designing our approach. We used our database for these tests, in order to detected the problems at the image level and define the requirements for the pre-processing stage. Different methods, provided by dedicated systems, offered a background view as well as a comparison method for evaluating our own methods.

1.3.1 Matlab based systems (SPM and VBM)

Statistical Parametric Mapping (SPM)- is a plug - in software that extends statistical processes dedicated to the functional imaging data. The software package performs analysis of brain imaging data sequences[1]. This plug-in software is designed for the Matlab environment. The SPM5 version accepts DTI images for processing and provides alignment and preprocessing using the fMRI (Functional MRI) dedicated module. Testing Statistical Parametric Mapping algorithms (Maltlab SPM toolbox), we obtain results only on the entire brain analysis and due to the image quality, the skull extraction cannot be properly performed and thus, we have interferences with the results on the anisotropy. A specific atlas, containing automatically detected anatomical volumes, represents a tool that can be applied to any type of patient.
Voxel Based Morphometry (VBM)[2] represents another module that can be integrated in Matlab with SPM, as a plug-in in SPM5. This module is able to make segmentation in WM (white matter) and GM (grey matter) based on voxel-wise comparison.
The segmentations provided by the SPM and VBM - depending on the tissue type - are not enough for our purpose, as we need specific anatomical regions as SN and the Putamen. SPM uses the atlas approach (Guillaume, 2008) for this purpose and categorizes the brain images on the race of the patients. This approach is not applicable for us, as we have a heterogeneous database. By using the atlas approach, the inter-patient variability is not considered. When performing the registration using VBM, the resulted images are "folded" and not usable for tracking.

[1]SPM site - http://www.fil.ion.ucl.ac.uk/spm/ - last accessed on May 2010
[2]Voxel based morphometry (VBM) - http://en.wikipedia.org/wiki/Voxel-based_morphometry - last accessed on May 2010

1.3.2 DTI dedicated systems

MedINRIA[3] system is designed for DTI management providing different modules for image processing and analysis procedures. In this case, the segmentation is a manual one, offering the necessary accuracy. The Fusion module of this system provides several registration methods that we are testing: the manual approach, the automatic affine registration and the diffeomorphic registration. The fact that the registration does not perform with the accuracy needed on our images to generate the correct fibers, represents the major drawback. Beside, the fact that we cannot limit, using two volumes of interest, the chosen fibers, makes us regard another option altogether for the tractography method. Even though, because of technical reasons, manual registration would be optimal for our case, we cannot use the DTI track module for the global tractography, using Log-Euclidian metrics on a deterministic approach, because it would mean choosing only one volume of interest, which cannot separate only the bundle of interest. This module provides only a local method for tractography.

Slicer 3D is another system tested with our database on the registration and tractography. The same manual segmentation approach is offered by the Slicer 3D system[4], but in this case, at the registration level, the system provides just the manual method as a valid one for our images. The tractography overcharges the memory of the computer when applying a probabilistic global approach. In some of the cases, even the registration cannot be completed by the system.

TracVis provides a probabilistic global method for tractography. This probabilistic global approach implemented in Diffusion Toolkit[5] performs the best for our database. The approach offers several methods for computing the propagation of the diffusion: FACT, second order Runge Kutta, Interpolated Streamline and Tensorline. We are testing the second order Runge Kutta, as it is the closest to our approach. Using a previous mask for the volumes of interest does not perform well on our data, but the possibility of limiting the computed fibers using a manual segmented volume of interest (VOI), or even two VOIs, provides the specific motor tract representing the bundle of interest. The drawback is the fact that this approach needs to compute all the fibers and limit them afterwards. We do not need all the fibers and this time-consuming process can be avoided with the mask volume. This possibility exists in the Diffusion Toolkit, but our mask volumes could not be read either by the Diffusion Toolkit or the TrackVis module. This aspect constrained us to perform the manual segmentation. However, even with the manually detected VOIs, the results on the fibers were either null or noisy.

1.3.3 Diagnosis and prognosis methodologies

Once the segmentation of the volumes of interest is achieved and the tractography performed, the extracted values for the fibers are analyzed for diagnosis and prognosis. We need to estimate the PD severity using the same scale as the one in the cognitive testing for estimation and comparison purpose. For the database, we are working with the provided H&Y values as a ground truth.

We have tested several classical clustering methods like KNN (K Nearest Neighbor) and KMeans but, due to the dispersions and uncertainty existent in our data, the results were not satisfactory. When deciding the way to analyze the extracted fiber values, we take into account several prognosis approaches. We need a decision-based method to analyze the features and

[3]MedINRIA - http://www-sop.inria.fr/asclepios/software/MedINRIA/ - last accessed on May 2010

[4]Slicer - http://www.slicer.org/ - last accessed on May 2010

[5]Diffuion toolkit -dtk - http://www.trackvis.org/dtk/

give an exact placement of the case on the PD scale. We can take into account rule-based systems, as they include predicates with medical knowledge. Considering fuzzy logic, we can capture the behavior of the system. Statistical methods include all possibilities for the features, but the selection of a decision threshold is very challenging and subject to sensitivity.

Working with non-probabilistic uncertainties, fuzzy sets, determines an approach based on fuzzy models. A fuzzy inference system, or fuzzy model, can adapt itself using numerical data. A fuzzy inference system has learning capability and using this aspect, the link between the fuzzy controllers and the methodologies for neural networks is possible using the Adaptive Network-Based Fuzzy Inference Systems (ANFIS). These networks have the overall input-output behavior influenced by a set of parameters. These parameters define functions that determine adaptive nodes at the network level. Applying the learning techniques from the neural networks to the fuzzy sets, allows us to determine an ANFIS structure. For us, the fuzzy sets represent the values extracted at the tractography level. These sets are defined in intervals and determine the If-Then rules. Together with these rules, the database (fuzzy sets) and a reasoning mechanism, determine a fuzzy inference system. At the reasoning part, we have to take into account the inference model (Jang & Sun, 1995).

Following an ANFIS (Bonissone, 1997), we can combine the fuzzy control offered by the medical background and statistical analysis with neural networks. The fuzzy features represent the a priori knowledge as a set of constraints - rules. One of the applications of ANFIS is presented as a mode to explain past data and predict behavior. In our approach, we use as Fuzzy Control (FC) a fuzzy set. For the FC technology we use rule inference where we make the difference between the disease stages. We adapted this approach, but as the neural networks separately did not perform well, we use adaptive interpolation functions.

1.4 Detected requirements from the tested systems

In our prototype, we use a specialized library that provides elementary image processing functions and algorithms: medical image reading and writing, basic filters and plug-ins, enables us to use algorithms already implemented and to begin our processing at a higher level of data management. Indeed *imageJ*[6] is a useful open source Java based library conceived for medical image processing and analysis that offers the possibility to develop a Java application that can be used for testing further in this library as a plug-in.

The systems that we are testing have different approach on the segmentation algorithms. MedINRIA provides a way of manually defining the regions of interest, as this is the most accurate way of segmentation.

The TrackVis module provides also the same accuracy as using the manual approach. 3D Slicer and SPM provide atlas-based approaches, but 3D Slicer does not manage to finish the computation for our images and the SPM results are blurry and not accurate. Analyzing the results obtained with these methods, we decide to adopt a geometrical-based registration with volumetric landmarks. For the segmentation method, the geometrical landmarks are used to guide specific adaptive region growing algorithms.

In our approach, we follow the ANFIS layers, from the input fiber data extracted, to the PD results, adapting the system to our needs. The ground truth is represented by the Hoehn & Yahr (H&Y) grade provided by the medical experts.

---

[6]ImageJ website -http://rsb.info.nih.gov/ij/ - last accessed on June 2010

2. Database characteristics

A number of 68 patients diagnosed clinically with PD and 75 control cases underwent DTI imaging (TR/TE 4300/90; 12 directions; 4 averages; 4/0 mm sections; 1.2 x 1.2 mm in-plane resolution) after giving informed consent. This represents, as far as we know, one of the biggest cohort of PD patients implicated in this type of study. The heterogeneity of the patients - Asians, Eurasians and Europeans - can also be used to characterize a general trend for PD prognosis. For this type of DTI images, we have 351 images that represent slices of 4 mm of brain structures taken in 13 directions at each step. In this case, we have 27 images (axial slices) that constitute a 3D brain image. The DTI images that we are using were taken with a Siemens Avanto 1.5T(B=800, 12 diffusion directions).
All the images are in DICOM format. This format is specific to the medical images, containing the header file and the image encapsulated in the "dcm" (DICOM) file.

2.1 DTI images used in our approach

From the DTI images, the **Echo Planar Images (EPI)** are among the ones with the lowest resolution. The advantage of this type of DTI is that they contain the tensor information as matrixes, giving the actual orientation of the water flow defining the brain fibers. The diffusion directions have each, as result, one volume of images.
This type of image is not appropriate for the anatomy extraction and analysis, but the tensor and anisotropy values stored represent the bottom line of fiber reconstruction, as well as the source for other images. We perform the entire image preprocessing on the EPIs, as they provide the tensor for the fibers as well. A preprocessing step for these images represents a contrast enhancement of 0.5% for a better detection of the skull and the volumes of interest.
Fractional anisotropy images result from the computation of the anisotropy level for each voxel on the EPI images. They contain not only the anisotropy values, but also the color code for it. This type of image represents the diffusion direction inside the fibers. Accordingly, the Putamen area is well defined as the motor tract reaches it and stands out as contour with high anatomical detail; therefore we use it in the automatic detection of this volume of interest.
After a registration of the volume of interest extracted from this image, we can use it together with the tensors from the EPI, in order to limit the fibers that we take into account. At this point, there is an exchange of information from one image type to another, by information fusion.

2.2 Preparing the image for processing

Due to the complex structure of the medical image-encoding manner of the DICOM format, we need to extract the useful information from the header file. During the processing and analysis steps, we only make use of the image itself, without additional information. This is the reason why we transform the image from the DICOM format to Analyze and store it as stacks of images, representing an entire brain volume for each patient and each modality.
For the axial plane, the images that we have in our database are taken in AC/PC plane - Anterior Commissure/Posterior Commissure. This axis is significant from the anatomical point of view and the radiologist uses it, because distinguishable in all the MRI images.

3. System and method presentation

Testing several systems dealing with specific treatment of DTI images, we construct our approach based on the clinical needs, as well as on the results obtained from other systems.

First, by testing other systems with our own images (subsection 1.3), we evaluate the possibilities that we have of using our images and the data flows that these images can provide.
From figure 1, we define the main processes that our information undergoes from the image level to the knowledge level. We start using EPI images, where we extract the midbrain area first. The FA images are used for automatic Putamen detection and, registering these images on the EPI, place the detected volumes at the right position on the EPI images. Once these volumes of interest are placed, the algorithm for fiber growth is applied on the EPIs and the fibers extracted are analyzed, together with the detected volumes of interest. Another part is represented by the diagnosis step followed by prognosis.

3.1 Image initialization and pre-processing

The preprocessing part has to overcome the **low resolution** of the EPI, as well as the **demographic characteristics** of the patients (age, race and sex differences). In our study, we surmount the sex differences by computing the volume of each brain, as there is a difference between female and male volume of the brain, based on smaller skull usually recorded for women.
In order to detect the elements related to the volume of interest, we consider the relative position of anatomical elements to a fixed point. We have chosen this point to be the center of mass of the brain (X_c, Y_c, Z_c). In order to determine this point, we need to consider the brain, without the skull. Another problem that we have to surmount is the intra-patient variability in the segmentation algorithms. The segmentation algorithm methods perform the detection inside the axial slices. In order to start the algorithms at the right place on the right slice, the position of this slice must be determined first. This position represents the placement of the axial plane (O_x and O_y axis inside the volume) relative to the coronal (O_x and O_z axis of the volume) and the sagittal (O_y and O_z axis of the volume) planes, on the O_z axis of the brain volume. This aspect provided us with the right placement of the algorithm at the slice level - the **placement at the volume level**. We need to find the anatomical region inside the axial image for which we need the volume definition - **placement inside the slice**, with identification of the right place for the volume detection.
From the segmentation point of view, solutions like the one proposed by SPM that performs the entire head segmentation are not applicable, as we need only our volume of interest, not a certain type of tissue. Due to the **patient variability**, we need robust VOI segmentation algorithms.
As one of the volumes is detected using an image stack (FA stack) different from the stack where we later use it (EPI stack), registration is needed. The problems with registration reside at the **landmark level** and influence the accuracy of this process. With no interference from the user, we perform a geometry based intra-patient registration with the geometrical landmarks automatically detected at the preprocessing level.
For the **bundle of interest** choice we use the two VOIs to limit the tracking starting from the midbrain area by selecting just those that reach the Putamen : deterministic global tractography. At this point, we compute measures based on the density of the fibers in the entire volume of the brain or in the volume of interest.

$$FD = \frac{F_{Nr}}{Vol_{Brain}}; \; FD_{rel} = \frac{F_{Nr}}{Vol_{VOI}} \tag{1}$$

where FD represents the fiber density computed as the number of fibers - F_{Nr} - in the volume of the entire brain - Vol_{Brain} and FD_{rel} represents the fiber density relative to the volume of interest- Vol_{VOI}. We try to overcome the age difference as well, by taking the mean age on the testing batch, as close as possible between the PD patients and the control cases. Computing the fiber volume and the brain volume, an analysis is possible to detect the geriatric effects on the brain and on the neural fibers al well.

$$FV = F_{Nr} * V_{height} * V_{width} * V_{depth} * F_{leng} \quad (2)$$

where FV represents the fiber volume computed as the product of fiber number (F_{Nr}), fiber length (F_{leng}) - constant as the fibers must pass through both regions of interest and the voxel dimensions: $V_{width}, V_{height}, V_{depth}$. According to the medical manifestation of the disease, the fiber density and volume should be diminished for the PD patients, compared with the control cases. The degradation of the fibers should also be correlated with the severity of the disease, specified by the H&Y scale.

For our system, we need several elements of image preprocessing for a good image quality, before processing. This is prevailed with morphological operators, together with segmentation algorithms and de-noises filters. Our main concerns are linked to the movement artifacts from our images that must be eliminated for a proper analysis. Due to early study and analysis, the bone tissue constituting the skull needs to be eliminated for a better further processing. At the processing level, another important matter that must be solved is preparing the parameters for our own algorithms, so that the processing algorithms can accomplish the optimal detection of the VOIs: slice detection at the volume level and adaptive anatomical detection at the image level.

3.1.1 Skull removal

As the systems considered in subsection 1.3 provided algorithms that performed the skull removal as well, we have tested these algorithms first and then developed our own, as obviously needed. The systems are tested using our own images with the characteristics specified in section 2 and we are using EPIs, as they are the ones providing the elements for the fiber growth.

Our own algorithm was applied on the EPI image and it uses KMeans classification to detect the bone tissue. This algorithm is already implemented in java and was available as a plug-in in imageJ[7]. Actually, the FA image containing the anisotropy provides the intensity for the skull voxels similar to the one representing the GM. This is the reason for the noise at the FA computation. For our purpose, we use a four-class evaluation to distinguish between the bone tissue and the GM, WM and CSF. The algorithm was not sensitive to the exterior noise, as we have applied a noise removal filter provided by the same library. In this way, all the elements outside the skull perimeter was considered as noise and eliminated.

At his point, the brain tissue represents the only information in the image. Estimation, analysis and processing on these images offer correct results on the brain tissue state.

3.1.2 Retrieving the geometrical elements

Having only the brain as information in the whole volume representation, offers us the possibility to set landmarks based on the whole volume estimation so that we can eliminate at least a part of the patient variability. This is the reason why we retrieve, using an imageJ

[7]KMeans in imageJ: http://ij-plugins.sourceforge.net/plugins/clustering /index.html - last accessed on June 2010

plug-in algorithm -object counter[8], the brain center of mass at the volume level and we are able to perform the same feature extraction at the slice level. This landmark is able to offer us an alignment for all the patients based on their volume, a central axis placement through the aligned volume. Next, we need a manner in which to find the limit the left and right side of the brain and in thus have another landmark for the patient alignment.

3.1.3 Hemisphere detection

This detection is further needed for patient alignment at the volume level to provide, together with the center of mass, a plan that passes through the center of the brain, making the distinction between the two hemispheres. For this detection, we determine the outer boundary of the brain. We analyze this boundary as a variation function determining the maximum inflexion point on the function corresponding to the occipital sinuses at the base of the occipital lobes junction.

This point, together with the center of mass of the brain, determines a sagittal plane between the two hemispheres. The same point, indicating the occipital sinuses and making the distinction between the two brain hemispheres, represents on an axial plane, together with the center of mass, an axis indicating the directionality of the head inside the image. The axis and the determined points will be used for segmentation and registration.

3.1.4 Volume management and slice detection

At the volume level, for the slice detection, we use the determined center of mass with the imageJ plug-in by Fabrice Cordelires and Jonathan Jackson called *Object Counter* [9]. This plug-in detects the 3D objects from image stacks and provides their volume, surface, the center of mass and the center of intensity. We use the volume provided for demographic parameter elimination and the center of mass for an inter-patient alignment.

Detecting the slice of interest starting from the center of mass of the brain is done by taking into account the placement of the anatomical regions that we consider as volumes of interest. For the cases with smaller brain volume, the slices could contain the entire brain, the others cannot. In order to establish the position and the content of the brain volume, we select the first and the last slice and extract the volume of the objects from these slices. We establish levels for defining the position of the midbrain relative to the determined center of mass of the brain.

$$P_{slice} = \frac{Vol_{Zslice}}{Vol_{Fslice}} * \frac{100}{ST} \tag{3}$$

where Vol_{Zslice} and Vol_{Fslice} represent the volumes of the objects in the slice with the determined center of mass, respectively the first slice on the stack; ST is the slice thickness (4 mm) and the values place the midbrain with relative to the determined center of mass with:

- Slice 0 if $P_{slice} < 60$
- Slice 1 if $60 < P_{slice} < 70$
- Slice 2 if $70 < P_{slice} < 85$
- Slice 3 if $85 < P_{slice} < 100$

[8]imageJ plug-in Object Counter: http://rsbweb.nih.gov/ij/plugins/track /objects.html - last accessed on June 2010

[9]Object Counter - http://rsbweb.nih.gov/ij/plugins/track/objects.html - last accessed on June 2010

These threshold values represent the statistical established studies with regard to the midbrain position and its placement relative to the percentage determined value. If the stack is not correct - if it does not contain the minimum slices for the midbrain and the Putamen detection - we transmit an error value for the slice of interest (-1). Once this position is determined, the Putamen algorithm starts with two slices above the midbrain-detected slice - one slice is with the midbrain, and the second one has to contain the AC/PC line. We adjust the Putamen slice if the detected volume is too small (20 pixels) or if it is placed too near to the midline. If this is the case, it means that the brain is bigger than estimated by the relative parameters and we find the Putamen one slice above the one we have placed the algorithm.

3.1.5 Finding the starting point for anatomical segmentation

Once we have the slice of interest detected for each of the volumes used on the tractography, we need algorithms that determine the placement in the image slice of the anatomical region that we are segmenting. Knowing the location of the regions based on the brain physiology, we design specific algorithms for each volume, in order to determine the stating point for the active detection algorithm.

The extraction of the volumes of interest is possible only on the images that provide a clear boundary for the anatomical regions that represent our volumes of interest. The algorithms for extraction must be placed on the right anatomical area inside the 3D image volume, for this detection to be as accurate as possible. The automatic detection is possible only after the starting point for the active volume is set. The difficulty in this case lies in finding, in the slice of interest, the right region for the active volume growth.

Detection for the starting point of the volume of interest in the **midbrain area** is done similar to the detection of the slice of interest and it is combined with the division in hemispheres of the brain. We need the hemispheres separately on account of the study of Dr. Chan (Chan et al., 2007) which states that there are different stages of development of PD in the left side and the right side of the brain. The inter-hemispherical axis detected is used when we detect the volumes of interest, as we want the algorithm to consider only the needed hemisphere. The algorithm for finding the midbrain starts from the center of mass of the volume inside the slice of interest and following the inter-hemispherical axis searches for a gray matter region placed next to this point or above it.

Detecting the starting point for the **Putamen detection algorithm** is different from the one used for the midbrain, as the Putamen is not placed on the inter-hemispherical axis and does not have a geometrically detectable point or standard distance -patient variability. We are working on the FA image as it contains the anisotropy that follows the dopamine flow and makes the Putamen more distinguishable than on the other type of images. Our algorithm is also based on the placement of the two areas relatively to the center of mass of the image as well. As this is a more complex matter there are several steps performed for achieving an adequate positioning inside the image and eliminating the inter-patient variability:

- Classification of images based on the head shape
- Segmentation on tissue type based on the voxel intensity
- Validation of the Putamen region based on the placement with reference to the center of mass

The first step represents a rough categorization of the head based on the sex variance, as well as on the subject provenance (e.g the shape of Eurasians is different of those of Europeans and Afro-Americans). We detect three main classes based on the position of the center of mass with regard to the middle of the image. The second step is meant to distinguish the anatomical areas and make easier the search for the Putamen. This segmentation is performed using the KMeans[10] plug-in based on (Jain & Dubles, 1988). We establish the number of clusters based on the tissue types the image now contains and the tolerance is left at the default value together with the randomization seed. The image containing all these clusters represents the map for the algorithm that established the volume of interest. Based on this image and the medical knowledge, our algorithm starts at the center of mass and follows the hemisphere axis. Depending on the category established at the first step, the algorithm chooses the proper level for hemisphere exploration on the left and the right side. Passing two tissue types and reaching the CSF area we then reach the Putamen. At this point, the volume-tracking algorithm can be applied.

3.2 Volume segmentation algorithms - active volume segmentation

The process of active volume determination is placed at the slice level and the stack level at the same time. At the slice level, after determining the starting point for the active tracking algorithm on the slice of interest (SOI), we move on to the growing step for the volume determination. We are thus performing a segmentation using the active contour algorithm and setting the threshold for it as voxels belonging to the other classes rather than the one we are exploring. At this point, the algorithms differ much depending on the anatomical region we want to extract, as well as on the hemisphere we are exploring. Nevertheless, after this exploration is finished, we apply this approach on the next slice and in this way, we extract volumes by making a stack of the extracted ROIs.

Regions are typically identified based on their internal homogeneity. However, the size of the shape is important when defining the homogeneity. Fractal features can provide additional information from this perspective. The region segmentation can be contour-based or region-based, depending on the restrictions applied for ending the detection process: exterior limits, respectively entropy values (Sonka & Fitzpatrick, 2009). We are using the image representing the KMeans-generated clusters as pixel intensities for the four types of classes. For the midbrain active contour, we perform a region-based detection, whereas for the Putamen, we perform a contour-based detection.

Considering a generalization on the active volume-tracking algorithm, there are several main steps to be followed:

- Seed placement inside the ROI
- Considering new points for the ROI extension
- Comparison with the voxels in the ROI and threshold elements
- Validation of the considered voxel as part of the ROI

These steps are further adapted and refined to fit our image resolution and the anatomical shapes at the same time.

In the algorithm for **detecting the volume of interest in the midbrain area**, we have two steps for detection: the definition and detection of the region of interest and the volume detection. For the region of interest, we use a snake-based algorithm applied on a segmented image with KMeans in imageJ. We segment the EPI stack in imageJ for which we intent to make the difference between the Cerebrospinal Fluid(CSF) surrounding the midbrain and the area we

[10]IJ Plugins: Clustering http://ij-plugins.sourceforge.net/plugins/clustering /index.html - last accessed on June 2010

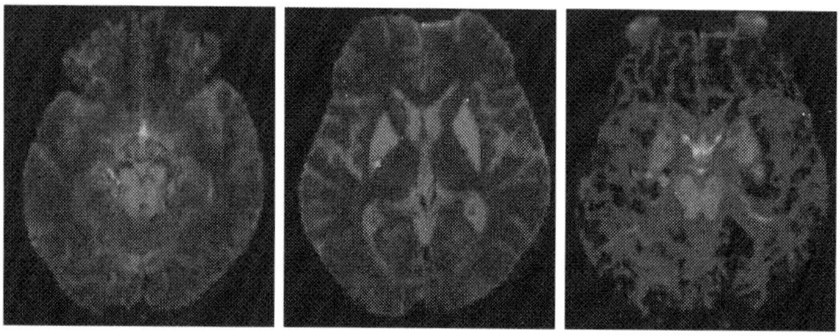

(a) (b) (c)

Fig. 2. EPI with detected VOIs: image 2(a) the midbrain on both hemispheres; image 2(b) the Putamen and image 2(c) with 3D fibers on an example

want to detect. On the gray matter class so obtained, we perform the snake-based algorithm that has the starting point determined in the preprocessing part. This exploration step ends when there is a difference between the new pixel and the previous one or we step on the midline of the brain. After finishing the algorithm on one slice we explore the slice above in similar manner. As we know from the study presented in (Starr & Mandybur, 2009), almost 80% of the SN is found in one slice (4 mm) thus, we want to make sure that in our volume of interest this anatomical region is contained and for this purpose, we take the two slices that most probably contain the midbrain.

For the Putamen volume detection, we take into account the shape of this specific anatomical region and we construct a totally different algorithm, that must overcome several obstacles: the placement of the Putamen that is not necessarily at the same level in both sides, the size of it differs very much from one hemisphere to the other, as well as its shape - intra-patient variability. In the preprocessing stage, we overcome this problem with the automatic Putamen region detection. The Putamen shape on the slice of interest - the slice above the one containing the AC/PC line- is triangular, whereas on the slice above this one is a quadrilateral shape approximation. This is the reason why, if we want a high accuracy, we have two kinds of algorithms for the Putamen tracing. One of these algorithms starts from a triangle placed at the seed place. This triangle moves its vertices only on the class of voxels belonging to the ones from the seed. It stops when reaching another class (3-5 consecutive voxels different from the ones constituting the VOI). The same manner of operating is applied for the other

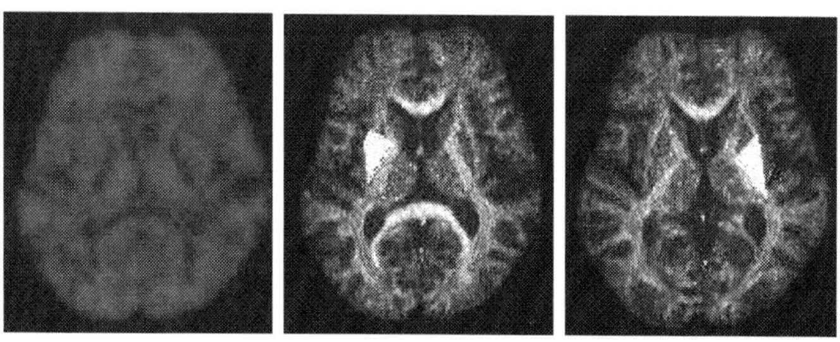

(a) (b) (c)

Fig. 3. FA image with Putamen detected (Sabau et al., 2010) starting from the KMeans clustered voxels from image 3(a) on the left side in figure 3(b), respectively the right side 3(c) approach, except the fact that it starts from a quadrilateral shape, moving at each step four vertices. We adjust the obtained shape by comparing the left and right limits and the level of the VOIs on the two hemispheres.

As shown in the flowchart from figure 4, after the positioning at the volume level in the slice of interest, the algorithm has to determine the relative position of the head inside the image in the pre-processing stage. Depending on that position, we choose the starting point for the active volume detection and move on the active volume determination. Once the starting point positioned, we choose the suitable algorithm for the shape extraction. We apply the triangular shape growing for the right side and the quadrilateral shape for the left side and the upper slices in the volume detection. These algorithms divide the starting point into three respectively four points (fig. 3). The three-point algorithm follows the triangular shape of the Putamen, which is more obvious on the slice with the AC/PC line. The choice was made by statistically determining the difference between the two algorithms and the manually segmented images that represents the ideal segmentation shape.

Both approaches consider the extension of the region of interest by taking each pixel next to the ones that represent the initial points in the clustering area. If the pixel appertains to the cluster of the initial points, it becomes one of the shape defining points - the edge of the triangle for the three points segmentation algorithm, or the edge of the quadrilateral shape for the four points segmentation algorithm. The active volume determination finishes when other clusters are encountered.

The determined area is placed with respect to the one determined on the other hemisphere. When the positioning of the two determined area is finished, the algorithm is repeated for the upper slice for the volume determination. The regions thus determined are transformed in mask images that are further transformed according to the parameters determined in the registration algorithms.

3.3 Automatic geometry-based registration

When talking about registration, we refer to matching or bringing the modalities to spatial alignment by finding the optimal geometrical transformation between corresponding image data (Teodorescu, 2010). Our approach is completely automatic as it is based on the determined geometrical landmarks used for the segmentation. These landmarks are independent of the inter-patient variability and on the imaging modality. The challenges for performing the registration reside in finding the best landmarks in both image types, finding a suitable spatial transformation and, for our type of images, preserving the tensor direction. In our case, we perform intra-subject registration, as we match images appertaining to the same subject. Our registration is a rigid one, as it contains only translations and rotations, affine transformation. As we are using homologous features, based on geometrical distances, our registration is a geometrical-based one.

For the midbrain area, we use the EPI B0 image, the one without diffusion, as it is clear enough for this purpose, even if the resolution for this type of image is poor. For the Putamen area, the contours of this anatomical region are not well detected by the algorithms on the same image modality. In this case, we use the FA image and take advantage of the anisotropy difference, represented in this type of image as a different color intensity corresponding to the dopamine flow going in different directions. This makes possible detection of the Putamen area on the FA image. However, when we use the detected Putamen, we want to do that on the EPI image and we need to know that the extracted volume is on the right place.

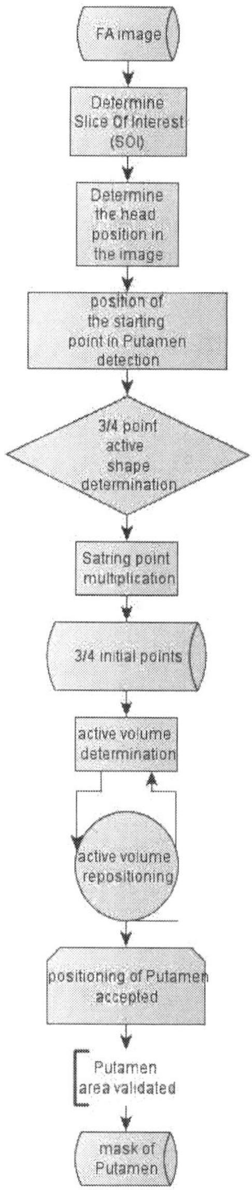

Fig. 4. Putamen detection on the FA image

3.3.1 Transformation parameters

We verify the placement of the volume of interest relative to the center of mass of the brain, as well as the external limits of this volume, relative to the same point. In order to determine the directionality of the image, we use the symmetry axis and its orientation. It gives us the angle with the horizontal and vertical image axes for the rotation and the displacement parameters. All the transformations are performed on the mask image extracted from the FA stack trough segmentation, representing the moving image in the registration process and keeping the EPI as model, representing the still image.

Analyzing the proposed technique, we can say that we perform an iconic registration (Cachier & et al., 2003) because we use on one hand the geometrical relations, as placement of the center of mass and the external limits, but on the other hand, we use the anisotropy values for defining the registered volume. As we are not using that information directly for the transformation of the image, our registration is a geometrical one (Gholinpour et al., 2007) (Maintz & Viergever, 2000). The checkpoints are the same used in our approach for the segmentation: the center of mass of the brain in both image stacks (EPI and FA) and the inter-hemispherical axis that provides the angulation parameters for the transformation. The parameters for this process are presented in 4.

$$\begin{bmatrix} x' & y' & z' & 1 \end{bmatrix} = \begin{bmatrix} cos\theta_x & sin\theta_x & 0 & d_x \\ -sin\theta_y & cos\theta_y & 0 & d_y \\ 0 & 0 & 1 & d_z \\ 0 & 0 & 0 & 1 \end{bmatrix} \begin{bmatrix} x \\ y \\ z \\ 1 \end{bmatrix} \tag{4}$$

Representing the transformation applied on the FA image in equation 4, we define the parameters for rotation, translation and skewness. The rotation angle for the transformation is computed by taking into account the symmetry axis determined for delimitation of the two brain hemispheres. The θ_x value is the angle between the axis and the O_x axis of the image and the θ_y is the angle between the same axis and the O_y of the image. We compute this angle for each image type and the difference between these angles represents the values for the transformation.

$$sin\alpha_x = \frac{SP_y}{I_1SP} \tag{5}$$

$$sin\alpha_y = \frac{SP_x}{I_2SP} \tag{6}$$

where SP is the starting point of the hemisphere axis, given by the inflexion point (occipital sinuses at the base of the Occipital Bone of the skull) placed on the lower part of the brain (posterior area of the brain) and the SP_x and SP_y are the projections of the SP point on the O_x respectively O_y axis; I_1 is the intersection between the axis and O_x; I_2 is the intersection between the axis and O_y.

We compute the α angle for the FA image and the β angle for the EPI image. The θ angle is the difference between α and β and we use it for the rotation. The translation valued from the transformation matrix from equation 4 (d_x, d_y and d_z) represents the difference between the centers of mass in the two types of images.

Another aspect of the transformation is represented by the axis orientation. The difference between the orientations of the axis determines us to flip the transformed image. This orientation is determined by the placement of the starting point (SP) and the center of mass on the image axes. Different orientation of the axis determines a flipping of the image in horizontal and/or vertical plane.

Because the FA images are generated on the AC/PC plane as well as the EPIs, there could not be any skewness problems or resizing aspects, thus we are concentrating our registration efforts on the translation and the rotation aspects. As the FA images have different orientations, we need to be sure that the volume of interest is correctly placed on the model image.

3.3.2 The feature fusion aspect

Another aspect when registering the two images information is represented by the nature of the information and the significance of the process itself. Fusing two images refers to the process of morphing them or warping them, at the image level. Both these techniques represent registration methods used and alter one of the images by incorporating the information from the other image. In this case, we are talking about fusion from another point of view, as we do not want to change the image, we put together information extracted from images with different meaning.

Putting together information from different sources enhances common characteristics and adds specific (usually complementary) elements from each source. In our case, we fuse them by putting together the displacement of the molecules and the anatomical regions, with the space displacement from the EPI respectively the FA images. The information is fused by taking the detected mask for the Putamen from the FA image and placing it with the tensor information in the EPI. We take the needed information from one image and inserting it into the other one by using registration (Maintz & Viergever, 2000)(Wirijadi, 2001). In this manner, after the images are segmented, the information from the FA image is registered to the EPI and used further for analysis and validation purposes.

3.4 Tractography

The initial method introduced by Basser (Basser et al., 2000) takes into account the diffusivity directions and the values of the tensors and Le Bihan (Le Bihan et al., 2001) takes into account the anisotropy characteristics at the tissue level for a better detection of the fibers. We choose this approach because it represents a classical approach of fiber tracking, which we can further develop and modify according to out needs. Our approach is a **global deterministic tractography** as it uses the neighbor voxels in tracking the fibers, providing the seeds as the volume of interest and using the thresholds of 0.1 for the FA value, and 0.6 for the angulation. It is a local method as it determines just a specific set of fibers, by using for selection the two-segmented volumes of interest as source and destination for the bundle of interest.

Using this approach, we are determining the fibers passing trough the midbrain area, the first volume of interest, and arriving to the Putamen volume on both sides of the brain hemispheres.

In the Basser approach, the algorithm is based on the Fernet equation for the description of the evolution of a fiber tract. This approach is specific to white matter, as the axons are the white matter. The midbrain area is gray matter. Growing fibers from the gray matter is a challenge since the number of axons in this area is much less than in the white matter and the fibers are not as well aligned as the ones in the white matter. We apply this algorithm in order to see if there are relevant fibers that we can grow between the two VOIs. Fibers too small, with anisotropy higher than 0.1, or those that do not go towards the Putamen area, whit angulation that exceeds 0.6 degrees, are not validated. The threshold values are the same as used in

(Basser et al., 2000)(Le Bihan et al., 2001)(Karagulle Kenedi et al., 2007). In this manner, with the second region of interest, taking a global tractography approach, we have an element that validates the grown fibers, without needing the SN clearly defined. The values estimated for the fibers represent the input for the diagnosis and prognosis module.

3.5 Diagnosis and prognosis

We define at this point the fiber density at 3D level on each side as presented in equation 7 where Nr_F represents the number of fibers detected on the hemisphere that we are analyzing; V represents the voxel size and Vol_{Brain} is the brain volume of the patient.

$$FD_{3D} = \frac{Nr_F * V}{Vol_{Brain}} \tag{7}$$

Once we defined, computed and then normalized the features, the learning stage for the clustering includes intervals of variation on each feature. These intervals are defined using fuzzy classes. We thus have in this case the five severity stages, the control cases class, 0 value. As we have patients for training only for PD stages 2 and 3, the other levels of PD are defined using the variation functions from the prognosis definition. After the interval definition, the rules supporting the intervals on each feature are implemented, including the medical knowledge.

We decide to use the rule-based approach, as the medical knowledge can be included, it can take into account different features at different stages of analysis and we can refine it. As presented in (Teodorescu et al., 2009a), there is a clear relation between the measured fiber values, extracted on the left hemisphere of the brain, and the severity of the disease. There are cases that do not register the fibers due to the image quality or the tracking method. In such cases, we consider the midbrain detected and the right side fibers, if detected. This approach is used also when a case can be placed in more than one class - for tangent clusters.

3.5.1 Diagnosis approach

The definition of the rules for diagnosis includes not only medical knowledge, but overcomes inter-patient variability. It takes into account the hemisphere of the brain, the density of the fibers, the volume of interest where the dopamine flow starts and the 3D density of the fibers. As presented in equation 8, after defining the clusters using the fiber density- HY_{FD}- and based on the midbrain volume- $HY_{VOI_{Vol}}$ - we evaluate the threshold and place a new case depending on these features. When conflicts appear and a decision between clusters is not obvious, an additional feature is used for diagnosis. If we do not have a positive positioning of the case on the feature axis, the VOI is not correctly determined due to image quality or insufficient slices on the volume. These conflicts generate the set of rules that we use for the expert system that determines a classification of the cases, depending on the disease severity. The fiber density (FD) values are classified on the H&Y scale. These classified FD values from the table are used next to define the rules in equation 8. When the left side fiber density does not provide a reliable value for diagnosis, the right side bundle of fibers is taken into account. If the fibers are not determined, the volumes of interest are taken as measures for diagnosis. By testing the rules in equation 8 we obtain the variation function of the FD according to the severity of PD.

$$\begin{aligned}
&If(HY_{FD} = HY_{VOI_{Vol}} \wedge HY_{FD} \neq -1)\ then\ HY = HY_{FD}\\
&If(HY_{FD} = -1 \wedge HY_{VOI_{Vol}} \neq -1)\ then\ HY = HY_{VOI_{Vol}}\\
&If(HY_{FD} \neq -1 \wedge HY_{VOI_{Vol}} = -1)\ then\ HY = HY_{FD}\\
&If(HY_{FD} \neq -1 \wedge HY_{VOI_{Vol}} \neq -1) \wedge (HY_{FD} \neq HY_{VOI_{Vol}}))\ then\\
&If(FD_{3D} \neq 0)\ then\ HY = 2\\
&else\ HY = 0\\
&If(HY_{FD} = -1 \wedge HY_{VOI_{Vol}} = -1) then\ The\ image\ is\ invalid!
\end{aligned} \tag{8}$$

For the moment, at this level, only the difference between the control and the PD cases is possible using this rule-based algorithm. At the PD level, only cases rated stage 2 and 3 can be classified, as these are the cases used for training. For new cases, as well as for variation study on the features, we consider the clusters and determine their variation.
In ANFIS architecture, the next step is represented by the rule strengths definition. We define a set of rules based on the detected clusters and include the medical knowledge as well.
Based on the intervals determined on the H&Y scale, each variable has a set of data, part of a rule: the FD variable determines the first rule from equation 8 and delivers the HY_{FD} scale value. The $FD_{3D}L$ metric determines the $HY_{3D}L$ from the set of rules. For determining the $HY_{VOI_{Vol}}$ value we are using values from $R1_{vol}$. The volume obtained for the midbrain, expressed as Vol_{avg} is correlated with H&Y as well and is used on the set of rule equations.
From diagnosis to prognosis, there is apparently only one step. While the diagnosis based on the rules is matching the patients into the classes that it was trained to recognize, the prognosis can place patients at levels that are not learned by the system. The diagnosis makes a classification of the patient by placing it in one of the disease stages or the control case. The prognosis offers the value of the correlation between the disease and the affected features and by extrapolation is able to find the evolution stage of the features for early cases of the disease.

3.5.2 From diagnosis to prognosis

Prognosis systems learn from the formerly acquired data and by analyzing and studying it, a pattern is revealed and used for new cases. Prediction systems using artificial intelligence can be based on neural networks, on fuzzy logic, on genetic algorithms or on expert systems. The interference among different PD levels at the feature level does not provide a clear boundary for classification using neural networks. We tested the KMeans and KNN approaches and they did not offer satisfactory results on our data. The interference among different feature groups at the class level represents a fuzzy dispersion on the features space. The rule-based expert system, using the fuzzy feature classes identifies the known stages of PD, but it does not offer the possibility for prognosis.
At this stage, the learning and classes are already defined and we intend to find a function by using interpolation among the existing points, representing the patient features on the disease severity. The ANFIS architecture at this stage has already defined the functions for determining the consequence parameters that provide the final decisional value. In our case we define the interpolation functions for this purpose. The intervals with their limitations can be considered as weights in defining the interpolation functions for the ANFIS approach. Like the RBFN (Radial Basis Function Network) model, in this case the weights represent the medical constraints, encapsulated in the intervals, and the variation functions are in our case the interpolation functions. The function found in this manner should be used for extrapolation onto disease areas that are not detectable at this moment. The function describes

the disease variation based on features and for any new patient, a correct placing of the case on the PD scale.
The interpolation methods are based on the shape of the mesh function, which can be: linear, polynomial or spline. Analyzing our data set, a linear approach is not possible due to the dispersed points on the plot. A polynomial approach is challenging at the parameter level and at the degree level as well. The cubic spline interpolation method has weights attached to each flat surface to guide the bending of the variation function, but the challenge at this point is to find the correct variations among the weights.
Looking at the polynomial approach, the Lagrange function that determines the parameters and can be adapted easily is a good choice for our data. This is a good choice also because each time we have a new input, the basis polynomials are recalculated and thus we improve our prediction each step of the way. With the help of weights we can improve the polynomial functions and define the spline as Lagrange functions. For a definition of a polynomial using the Lagrange approach we need the coefficients determined using equation 9. In this function, the points (x_i,y_j) represent the features extracted at the image level.

$$L(x) = \sum_{i=0}^{n} y_i * \prod_{j=0,j\neq i}^{n} \frac{x - x_j}{x_i - x_j} \tag{9}$$

Using the data from the training set we determine a forty degree polynomial that computes the coefficients using equation 9. This kind of function is hard to handle, as it becomes very complicated and in the case of new points in the data evaluation takes a lot of time and is not accurate. At this point, we divide the feature points in the H&Y space into sets and define a variation function for each set of points. A two point set definition determines a linear function and we already know that the variation is nonlinear; therefore we start from three set points. A five-degree polynomial function becomes too complicated so the highest degree of polynomial representation on an interval is a four-degree polynomial function.

3.5.2.1 Specific prognosis adaptive methods

When we provide a new case for analysis, we extract the fiber features and we try to place it on an interval, determining the left and right closest values. Defining the interval where the new value needs to be placed, we determine the H&Y values corresponding to the interval and the middle value of the same interval. The three H&Y values provide the data for the rule-based diagnosis system. This system provides the final value for the new case.
When a new point is to be evaluated and its H&Y value determined, we have several steps to perform. We perform this estimation using the "ideal" set of points. The position of the new point (X) among the others is determined by finding the next point higher (X_M) and lower (X_m) - figure 5 - and recurrently determining polynomial functions(LF) for evaluating the new value(X).
This algorithm describes an Independent Adaptive Polynomial Evaluation (IAPE) method as it is applied both on PD and controls determining the most likely polynomial that can be applied on these data. This method is a hybrid ANFIS approach as it uses as back-propagation the difference between polynomials at each stage but it works like the RBF using the Lagrange polynomials.
An extension of this approach, adapted for PD cases, is called PD Adaptive Polynomial Evaluation method (PD-APE). The estimation function is used basically for the PD patients, adding the condition that if HY_1 or HY_2 have as result 0, the other value is taken as result. This condition does not affect the results of the overall performance. The variation function

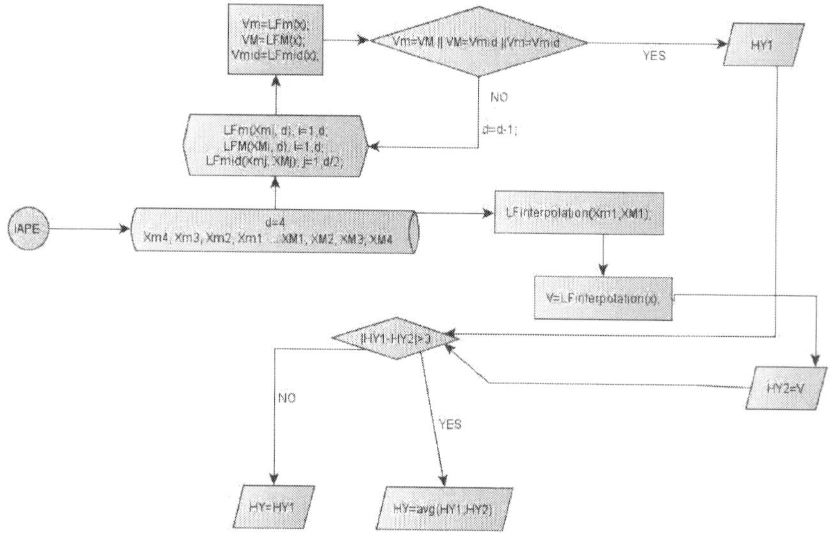

Fig. 5. Independent Adaptive Polynomial Evaluation (IAPE)- When evaluating a new feature X, starting from fort degree polynomials (d=5) computed for neighbor values, we obtain HY1, a first evaluation of the PD severity. A second evaluation using an interpolation on the two closest values is determined as well: HY2. Using these estimations, the final HY value representing the severity is determined.

with this condition performs the best on the accuracy level. From the ANFIS point of view this method takes into the second layer the firing strength given by the PD appurtenance. Determining the control and the PD cases first and then applying the function that provides the best interpolation for the set of points represents a fuzzy adaptive method for prognosis. This variation function uses for the control cases the second-degree polynomial method and for the patient cases the PD adaptive polynomial evaluation method.

4. Testing and results

There are several stages of evaluation in our system. At the image processing level, the preprocessing stage provides the automatic landmarks for the segmentation and the registration methods. At the image processing level, the neurologist validates the midbrain detection. The Putamen segmentation is evaluated against the manual one, performed by a specialist. By comparing the detected fibers obtained after the tractography with the ones determined using the manual detected Putamen directly on the EPI, we evaluate the registration. The registration method is a fully automatic geometric registration. This method was visually validated as well, in collaboration with the radiologists.

4.1 Test sets and requirements

Testing procedures must assure that they are sensitive to our parameters, and robust to other exterior factors. Thus, we construct several testing batches by varying parameters that we need our system to be robust to. We apply this procedure for the demographical parameters. The whole database contains 66 patients and 66 control cases that managed successfully to generate the segmented areas. We dispose of 68 patients and 75 control cases, but due to the image stacks unable to provide the entire volume between the midbrain and the Putamen, several were eliminated from the test, as they did not have valid images. We use this database to evaluate the methods developed using a test batch (42 patients: 21 PD cases and 21 controls - on which we have the manual Putamen segmented) .

At the image processing level, we have as input data the images and we test the automatic detection against the manual one. At the feature level, we have as input data the extracted values for the neural fibers on the left and the right side, the detected volumes on both sides and/or the new computed parameters: FD, FD_{3D}, FD_{rel}, FV.

For the diagnosis and prognosis, the ground truth is represented by the H&Y value given by the medical doctors using the cognitive tests. The neurologist also performs the validation of the fibers, so that we can be sure of detecting the right bundle of fibers for further study.

4.2 Evaluation of the segmentation algorithms

There are several characteristics when analyzing the result of a region-based segmentation. Comparing an image segmentation result to ground truth segmentation - the manual detected one from the specialist- represents one way of evaluating the automatic segmentation. Another way would be to estimate the overlap between the ground truth image and the segmented one. There can be over-segmentation or under-segmentation when the two images overlap, but one of them is bigger than the other one. When there is a ground truth region that the segmentation does not contain, we are dealing with a missed region. A noise region manifests as a region identified in the segmented image, but not contained in the noise region.

Midbrain automatic detection is preformed on the EPI stack with no diffusion direction. The algorithm providing the segmentation presented is applied on the test set and our specialist studies the results. Validating the algorithm actually means verifying if it managed to segment the whole midbrain and just this part, without taking part of the surrounding tissue or the CSF (see fig. 2(a)). This is the criterion followed by the neurologist in validating the algorithm.

For the **Putamen detection** the evaluation is performed by comparing the manually segmented images with the automatically detected ones. Performing a logical AND operation at the image level between the two Putamen slices at the pixel level, we are using the imageJ Image Calculator on the segmented volumes. The error rate estimated the difference area on our segmentation algorithm compared with the manual one.

Also, a validation done by the neurologist is necessary for this step. For the registration performed on the detected volume, we use medical knowledge for validation and visual evaluation.

When using just the triangular segmentation of the Putamen, we detect an error rate of 34.66% on the left side and 35.75% on the right side of the brain. When evaluating the alignment algorithm based on the center of mass, the relative error rate is 37.16% on the left side and 39.6% on the right side.

The results show a smaller error rate for the left Putamen area, which has more clear boundaries than the right Putamen area. This is consistent with the medical approach as PD patients usually are more affected on the left side of the brain by this disease.

As the Putamen correct placement determines the validation for the strationigral fibers, its placement together with the correct detection of the volume, determine the number of fibers and directly affect the analysis results.

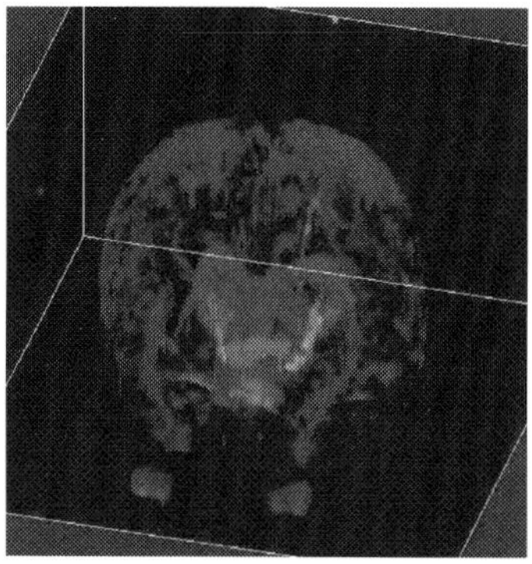

Fig. 6. 3D View of the grown fibers from PDFibAtl@s: the detected midbrain in pink; the two Putamen volumes on each side in red and the fibres in green.

4.3 Evaluation of the registration method

In our approach, the registration process with the acquired parameters determined is fully automatic. It uses the EPI stack with no diffusion and the FA one. The results can be visually verified as we are applying the transformation on the Putamen mask and we transpose the image on the EPI. Thus, we verify the correct anatomical position.

For fiber evaluation, the number of fibers identified for each patient represents the measure of a correct or incorrect segmentation. The tracking algorithm does not change, but it is sensitive to the Putamen area. This is the reason why values above 20 fibers, represent a misplacement of the Putamen area or an incorrect detection - this happens when our algorithm detects more than just the strationigral tract. Based on these elements, we define the metrics for the sensitivity, specificity and accuracy.

With these classes, the overall performance of the algorithms on the existing data, corresponds to 63% of specificity, 81% of sensitivity and 78.5% of accuracy.

4.4 Tractography evaluation

The motor tract is automatically detected in our case by growing the fibers between the two volumes of interest: midbrain area and the Putamen. This is consistent with a global tractography method. After computing the FD and FV on each side of the brain, we study the effects of PD in each bundle of interest. For this purpose, we perform the T-Test making the correlation between FD/FV and H&Y scale. As the FD is dependent on the FV, the two parameters have the same variation. For the medical relevance on correlating the H&Y parameter with the fibers, we test the obtained values using WinSPC (Statistical Process control Software).

We first evaluate the PD-APE prognosis function on a test batch, representing the manually processed Putamen detection (37 PD patients and 52 control cases that provided valid features after the fiber extraction). Together with the manual Putamen data, in the training function, we include five PD patients from the initial valid 42. With an accuracy rate of 32.43% on the patients and 46.15% on the control data, the overall system provides an accuracy of 40.44% .

When updating the Putamen detection, we perform a reevaluation of the diagnosis and prognosis module on the entire automatic methods applied on the database (68 patients and 66 controls).

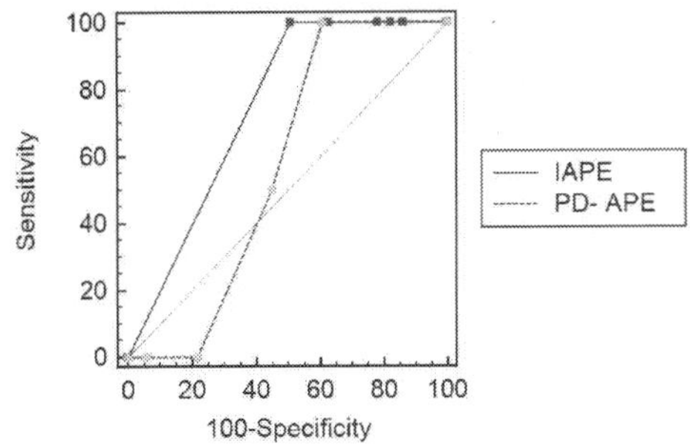

Fig. 7. The two ROC curves for IAPE and PD-APE methods applied on the database (143 cases: 68 patients and 75 controls). The AUC values for IAPE and PD-APE are 0.745, respectively 0.569. By evaluating the ROC difference between the two tested methods, the AUC indicates a difference of 0.176.

The patients are characterized by the value of the sensitivity - maximum value for the Independent Adaptive Polynomial Evaluation (IAPE) approach with 62.16%. On the control cases, the specificity represents the evaluation value that characterizes it - maximal value for the second degree polynomial approach is 43.9%. The accuracy represents the overall performance of the algorithms that performs the best on PD Adaptive Polynomial Evaluation (PD-APE) method, generating a value of 44.87%.

The overall performance of the prognosis module is provided by the ROC curve. We compute this metric using the SPSS 17.0 (Statistical Package for the Social Sciences) for the patient estimation. By evaluating the IAPE method for this case, we obtain an area under the curve (AUC) of 0.705, whereas for the PD-APE, we obtain 0.959. This indicates a much better performance on the patients' data for the second method.

We evaluate the prognosis performances on the control and patients' data, to estimate the overall capacity of the proposed methods at this level. We compare the ROC curves for different methods and for this purpose, we use the MedCalc[11] software. This software provides two approaches for the ROC curve estimation: De Long and Hanley & McNiel. Using the database results on IAPE, the AUC values for these two ROC estimation approaches were the same. We further use the De Long approach when evaluating the ROC, as the error rate provided on the same test is slightly lower compared with the McNiel approach (0.1%). For the PD-APE method of prognosis, we obtain a value of 0.569 for AUC and for IAPE, the same metric has a value of 0.745. Comparing the two curves, the difference between the areas is 0.176 - figure 7.

4.5 Computational speed and requirements

We use Java for all the systems with imageJ toolbox and bio-medical imaging plug-ins [12]. The initialization of the preprocessing part is done by enhancing the contrast for the EPI images and by removing the noise. For the 3D visualization, we are using the Volume Viewer from imageJ [13].

[11] MedCalc 11.3.3.0 - www.medcalc.be

[12] Bio-medical image - http://webscreen.ophth.uiowa.edu/bij/ - last accessed on May 2010

[13] Volume Viewer 3D - http://rsbweb.nih.gov/ij/plugins/volume-viewer.html - last accessed on March 2010

The algorithm is tested on Intel core Quad CPU Q660 (2.4GHz; 4.0G RAM) and the average time for each patient is 4.68 min with the automatic detection and the fiber growth algorithm. If with DTI tracker from MedINRIA took us 3 min just to have the fibers, without segmentation or other preliminary preparation, but with our prototype it takes us an average of 2 min. A similar time (1.2 min) is provided using a probabilistic global method with the Diffusion Tracking module (TrackVis) for image selection and the tractography, without segmentation and computation for the fiber metrics.

5. Conclusion and Future work

Proposing a fully automatic way for estimating the severity of the PD, based on the information provided by the image, represents altogether a new demarche. The prognosis represents another scientific act, based on measurable functionality and specific features, to determine at a higher scale, the diseases severity, even on early cases. These scientific aims are reached by studying the images and the possibility to extract and use the information specific to the disease from these images. This research corresponds to the learning and understanding part on the image modality study and specific elements. The methods developed for preparing the images and volume-based analysis are created for sustaining the more complex systems corresponding to the volume segmentation algorithms. The tractography method, using the extracted volumes of interest, offers not only a much better time on processing but also the selectivity needed by the diagnosis and prognosis model.

Our approach is important from the clinical point of view, offering a new method for the neurologists in PD and a mean to verify/confirm their diagnosis and prognosis. From the technical standpoint, the fusion is novel, as it combines the tensor based information and the anatomical details. This system provides data for H&Y estimation and PD prognosis.

Analyzing the results obtained by each new method, we have to take into account the fact that the image quality together with patient variability influences the algorithms.

The main breakthrough initiated by this study is represented by the method able to predict PD by offering a view on the early cases as well, not only on those starting from the second stage of the disease. This evaluation method based on the image attributes, on the anatomical and neurological aspects of the patient, offers a measurable value of the severity of the disease. As the H&Y test is based on the cognitive facet, our method is complementary to the test, but is placed on the same scale.

PDFibAtl@s is a new system, able to automatically detect the volumes of interest for PD diagnosis using the DTI images and a geometrical approach. The algorithms included in this platform are original and are based not only on the brain geometry, but also including medical knowledge by taking into account the position of different anatomical structures at the brain level, hence the atlas dimension. Concerning the fusion contribution of our work, it brings together the FA clarity at the Putamen level with the tensors matrix for the fiber tracking algorithms. Our algorithm automatically detects the elements that until now were obtained by user interaction: detection of the slice of interest, detection of volumes of interest, automatic detection of the registration parameters. Introducing parameters for fiber evaluation and eliminating the demographic factors at the atlas level, as well as at the volume level represents another important contribution.

Our new prototype represents a first attempt to provide not only image-based analysis and features for PD diagnosis, but also an automatic system specialized for this task. There is place for improvements, like in any new system, but the results obtained so far are encouraging.

The accuracy of the system can be augmented, especially at the prognosis level by applying a specially designed function.

6. Acknowledgements

This study has been performed in collaboration with Dr. Ling-Ling CHAN (MD) from the Singapore General Hospital[14]; the support of the French National Centre for Scientific Research (CNRS)[15] and the Romanian Research Ministry (TD internship 64/2008). Help was also provided by Nicolas Smit (ISEN)[16] and from "Politehnica" University of Timisoara[17] Anda Sabau, Cristina Pataca and Claudiu Filip.

7. References

Basser, P. J., Pajevic, S., Pierpaoli, C., Duda, J. & Aldroubi, A. (2000). In vivo fiber tractography using dt-mri data, *Magnetic Resonance in Medicine* 44: 625–632.

Bonissone, P. P. (1997). Adaptive neural fuzzy inference systems (anfis): Analysis and applications, GE CRD Schenectady, NY USA.

Cachier, P. & et al. (2003). Iconic feature based non-rigid registration: the pasha algorithm, *Computer Vision and Image understanding* 89: 272–298.

Chan, L.-L., Rumperl, H. & Yap, K. (2007). Case control study of diffusion tensor imaging in parkinson's disease, *J. Neurol. Neurosurg. Psychiatry* 78: 1383–1386.

Gholinpour, A., Khetanarvaz, N. & et al. (2007). Brain functional localization: a survey of image registration techniques, *IEEE Transactions on Medical Imaging* 26: 1–20.

Guillaume (2008). Spm documentation, pdf technical report. Trust Center for Neuroimaging. http://www.fil.ion.ucl.ac.uk/spm/doc/ - last accessed on May 2010.
URL: *http://www.fil.ion.ucl.ac.uk/spm/doc/*

Jain, A. K. & Dubles, R. C. (1988). *Algorithms for Clustering Data*, Prentice Hall Advanced Reference Series, Prentice Hall.

Jang, J.-S. R. & Sun, C.-T. (1995). Nuero-fuzzy modeling and control, *The Proceesings of IEEE* 83: 387–406.

Karagulle Kenedi, A., Lehericy, S. & Luciana, M. (2007). Altered diffusion in the frontal lobe in parkinson disease, *AJNR Am J Neuradiol Brain - Original Research* 29: 501–05.

Le Bihan, D., Mangin, J.-F., Pupon, C. & Clark, C. A. (2001). Diffusion tensor imaging : concepts and application, *Journal of Magnetic Resonance Imaging* 13: 534–546.

Maintz, A. J. & Viergever, M. A. (2000). A survey of medical image registration, *Medical Image Analysis* 1 and 2: 1–32.

Sabau, A., Teodorescu, R. & Cretu, V. (2010). Automatic putamen detection on dti images. application to prakinson's disease, *ICCC-CONTI* 1: 1–6.

Sonka, M. & Fitzpatrick, J. M. (eds) (2009). *Handbook of Medical Imaging*, Vol. 2 Medical Image Processing and Analysis of *Diagnostic Imaging - Handbooks.*, 3 edn, SPIE Press, P.O. box 10 Bellingham, Washington 98227-0010 USA. ISBN 0-8194-3621-6.
URL: *http://link.aip.org/link/doi/10.1117/3.831079*

Starr, C. & Mandybur, G. (2009). Grant to improve targeting in parkinsons surgery, University of Cincinnati neuroscience institute. Mayfield Clinic.

[14]SGH - http://www.sgh.com.sg/Pages/default.aspx
[15]CNRS - Centre National de la Recherche Scientifique www.cnrs.fr
[16]INSEN-Institut Supérieur de l'Electronique et du Numérique, Lille, France
[17]PUT - www.cs.upt.ro

Teodorescu, R. O. (2010). *Parkinson's Disease Prognosis using Diffusion Tensor Imaging Features Fusion (Pronostic de la Maladie de Parkinson basé sur la fusion des caractristiques d'Images par Résonance Magnétique de Diffusion)*, PhD thesis, "Politehnica University of Timisoara, Romania Université de Franche-Comté, Besançon, France.

Teodorescu, R. O., Racoceanu, D. & Chan, L.-L. (2009a). Hy compliant for pd detection using epi and fa analysis, Presentation Number: NIH09-NIH01-88. Natcher Auditorium, National Institutes of Health in Bethesda, MD USA.

Teodorescu, R., Racoceanu, D. & Chan, L. e. a. (2009b). Parkinsons disease detection using 3d brain mri fa map histograms correlated with tract directions, *RSNA* 8015681: 1. Chacago, IL USA.

Today, M. N. (2009). Brain bank appeal aims to double number of brain donors, www.medicalnewstoday.com. Parkinsons awareness week 2009, 20-26 April. URL: *http://www.medicalnewstoday.com*

Vaillancourt, D. e. a. (2009). Imaging technology may trace development of parkinsons disease, *University of Illinois at Chicago, Rush University* 1: 3. URL: *http://www.medicalnewstoday.com/articles/143566.php*

Wirijadi, O. (2001). Survey of 3d image segmentation methods, *Fraunhoffer technical report* 1: 1.

Woodward, N., Zald, D. & Ding, Z. e. a. (2009). Cerebral morphology and dopamine d2/d3 receptor distribution in humans: a combined [18f] fallypride and voxel-based morphometry study, *NeuroImage* 46: 31–38.

18

Non-Invasive Foetal Monitoring with Combined ECG - PCG System

Mariano Ruffo[2,3], Mario Cesarelli[2], Craig Jin[1], Gaetano Gargiulo[1,2,3], Alistair McEwan[1], Colin Sullivan[4], Paolo Bifulco[2], Maria Romano[2], Richard W. Shephard[3], and André van Schaik[1]

[1]*School of Electrical and Information Engineering (EIE), The University of Sydney*
[2]*Dept. of Biomedical, Electronic and Telecommunications Engineering, "Federico II" University of Naples*
[3]*HEARD Systems, Sydney*
[4]*David Read Laboratory, Dept. of Medicine, The University of Sydney*
[1,3,4]*Australia*
[2]*Italy*

1. Introduction

Although modern ultrasound provides remarkable images and biophysical measures, the technology is expensive and the observations are only available over a short time. Longer term monitoring is achieved in a clinical setting using ultrasonic Doppler cardiotocography (CTG) but this has a number of limitations. Some pathologies and some anomalies of cardiac functioning are not detectable with CTG. Moreover, although frequent and/or long-term foetal heart rate (FHR) monitoring is recommended, mainly in high risk pregnancies, there is a lack of established evidence for safe ultrasound irradiation exposure to the foetus for extended periods (Ang et al., 2006). Finally, high quality ultrasound devices are too expensive and not approved for home care use. In fact, there is a remarkable mismatch between ability to examine a foetus in a clinical setting, and the almost complete absence of technology that permits longer term monitoring of a foetus at home. Therefore, in the last years, many efforts (Hany et al., 1989; Jimenez et al., 1999; Kovacs et al., 2000; Mittra et al., 2008; Moghavvemi et al., 2003; Nagal, 1986; Ruffo et al., 2010; Talbert et al., 1986; Varady et al., 2003) have been attempted by the scientific community to find a suitable alternative.

The development of new electronic systems and sensors now offers the potential of effective monitoring of the foetus using foetal phonocardiography (FPCG) and foetal electrocardiography (FECG) with passive, fully non-invasive low cost digital recording systems that could be suitable for home monitoring. These advances provide the opportunity of extending the recordings of the current commonly used CTG from relative short to long term, and provide new previously unavailable measures of cardiac function.

In this chapter, we present highlights of our research into non-invasive foetal monitoring. We introduce the use of FECG, FPCG and their combination in order to detect the foetal heart rate (FHR) and potential functional anomalies. We present signal processing methodologies, suitable for longer-term assessment, to detect heart beat events, such as first and second heart sounds and QRS waves, which provide reliable measures of heart rate, and offer the potential of new information about measurement of the systolic time intervals and foetus circulatory impedance.

2. Foetal monitoring

The most important aim of foetal surveillance is to avoid intrauterine death or permanent damage to the foetus. So, in industrialized countries, all pregnant women periodically take pregnancy and foetal well-being checks, which include measuring the pattern of foetal growth and maturation, oxygen availability and cardiac functions.
The foetal heart rate (FHR) is currently monitored for routine ante partum surveillance in clinical practise (Babbitt, 1996) and it is thought to be an indicator of a correctly functioning nervous system (Baser et al. 1992). FHR analysis as a means of monitoring foetal status has become widely accepted and continuous FHR monitoring should be recommended, particularly for high-risk pregnancies (Kovacs et al, 2000; Moghavvemi et al., 2003; Varady et al., 2003).
There are two situations for which FHR provides important information about the condition of the foetus. It is known that FHR monitoring is able to distinguish between the so called *reactive* foetus and the so called *non-reactive* foetus (Bailey et al., 1980). A foetus is considered *reactive* if the FHR will temporarily accelerate in response to stimulation (e.g. during a uterine contraction). Alternatively a foetus is considered *non-reactive* if no accelerations were observed or they did not meet the criteria for a reactive test (Rabinowitz et al., 1983). The above mentioned classification is considered a reasonably reliable indicator of foetal development and well-being (Babbitt, 1996). It is also known that a normal reactive foetus is less likely to suffer foetal distress during labour (Janjarasjitt, 2006).
FHR can be monitored by means of different techniques: CTG, magnetocardiography, electrocardiography (ECG) and phonocardiography (PCG). We describe these techniques in the following sections.

2.1 Ultrasonic Doppler cardiotocography (CTG)

CTG is one of the most commonly used, non-invasive pre-natal diagnostic techniques in clinical practice, both during ante partum and labour (Romano et al., 2006). In some countries, the CTG is considered a medical report with legal value (Williams and Arulkumaran, 2004). Since its introduction in the 1960s, electronic foetal monitoring has considerably reduced the rate of perinatal morbidity and mortality (Shy et al., 1987). It can be used from the 24th week of gestation onwards even if, in clinical routine, it is generally used in the last weeks of gestation only (from the 35th week). During CTG diagnostic monitoring, FHR and uterine contractions (UC) are simultaneously recorded by means of an ultrasound Doppler probe and a pressure transducer (Cesarelli et al., 2009), respectively.
In order to record a FHR signal an ultrasonic beam is aimed at the foetal heart. The ultrasound reflected from the beating heart walls and/or moving valves is slightly Doppler shifted as a result of the movement. After demodulation the Doppler shift signal is used to detect the heart beats in order to extract the FHR. The ultrasonic frequencies used are generally within the range of 1-2 MHz (Karlsson et al., 1996).
The advantage of the Doppler ultrasound technique is that one can be virtually assured that a recording of FHR will be obtained. The disadvantages of such systems are that they require intermittent repositioning of the transducer and are only suitable for use by highly

trained operators. Because the procedure involves aiming a directional beam of a 2 MHz ultrasound at the small target a foetal heart presents, the use of Doppler ultrasound is not suitable for long periods of FHR monitoring. Moreover, as previously mentioned, although frequent and/or long-term FHR monitoring is recommend, mainly in risky pregnancies, it has not been proven that long applications of ultrasound irradiation are absolutely harmless for the foetus (Kieler et al., 2002).

The major limitation of the Doppler ultrasound technique is its sensitivity to maternal movements that result in Doppler-shifted reflected waves, which could be stronger than the foetal cardiac signal (Hasan et al., 2009). Thus the CTG technique is inappropriate for long-term monitoring of FHR, as it requires the subject to remain immobile. Moreover, the detection of the heart beats relies upon a secondary effect (the mechanical movement of the heart and/or the cardiac valves) and it is therefore not as accurate for FHR analysis as detection of the QRS complex from FECG. In addition, FHR is the only parameter obtained by CTG and some pathologies and anomalies of cardiac functionality are not detectable from the FHR alone. Research has shown that a global assessment of morphological and temporal parameters of the FECG or FPCG during gestation can provide further information about the well-being of the foetus (Martenset al, 2007; Varady et al., 2003; Kovacs et al., 2000; Hany & Dripps, 1989).

2.2 Foetal magnetocardiography

Foetal magnetocardiography (FMCG) consists of the measurement of the magnetic fields produced by the electrical activity of the foetal heart muscle (Janjarasjitt, 2006). The recording uses the SQUID (Superconducting Quantum Interference Device) biomagnetometry technique. The FMCG is morphologically and temporally similar to the FECG since the electrical field and the magnetic field are generated in conjunction by the activity of the heart.

Because of the disadvantages of the FMCG such as size, cost, complexity of the required instrumentation, and again the need to minimise subject movement (Wakai, 2004; Zhuravlev et al., 2002; Mantini et al., 2005), FMCG is currently mainly a research tool and little used in clinical practice. However, a considerable advantage over FECG is that FMCG can be recorded reliably from the 20th week onwards, unaffected by the insulating effects of the vernix caseosa, and with virtually no interference from the maternal ECG. Hence, the FMCG result can help to classify arrhythmias, such as heart blocks and atria flutter, and to diagnose a prolonged QT-syndrome (Mantini et al., 2005; Wakay, 2004; Zhuravlev et al., 2002).

2.3 Foetal phonocardiography

The preliminary results obtained by Baskaran and Sivalingam (Tan & Moghavvemi, 2000) have shown that there are significant differences in the characteristics of FPCG signals between intrauterine retarded and normal growth during pregnancy. This preliminary study has further inspired investigations into the possibility to employ FPCG to identify foetuses at risk. This could be a significant contribution to the pressing clinical problem faced by some abortions and preterm babies. FPCG records foetal heart sounds using a passive, non-invasive and low cost acoustic sensor (Varady et al., 2003; Kovacs et al., 2000; Hany & Dripps, 1989). This signal can be captured by placing a small acoustic sensor on mother's abdomen and, if appropriately recorded, is very useful in providing clinical indication. Uterine Contractions (UCs) may be simultaneously recorded by means of a pressure transducer.

Even though the heart it is not fully developed in a foetus, it is still divided into two pairs of chambers and has four valves. During the foetal cardiac cycle, when the ventricles begin to contract, the blood attempts to flow back into the atrial chambers where the pressure is lower: this reverse flow is arrested by the closing of the valves (mitral and tricuspid), which produces the first heart sound (S1). After, the pressure in the ventricular chambers increases until the pulmonary valves open and the pressurized blood is rapidly ejected into the arteries. The pressure of the remaining blood in the ventricles decreases with respect to that in the arteries and this pressure gradient causes the arterial blood to flow back into the ventricles. The closing of the pulmonary valves arrest this reverse flow and this gives rise to the second heart sound (S2) (McDonnell, 1990).

A disadvantage of FPCG is that it is not possible to fully automate the signal processing for detecting the hear sounds because the signal characteristics depend on the relative positioning of the foetus with respect to the sensor. This results in a variable signal intensity and spectrum. Moreover, recordings are heavily affected by a number of acoustic noise sources, such as foetal movements, maternal digestive and breathing movements, maternal heart activity and external noise (Mittra et al., 2008; Ruffo et al., 2010).

Despite the disadvantages mentioned above, FPCG provides valuable information about the physical state of the foetus during pregnancy and has the potential for detection of cardiac functionality anomalies, such as murmur, split effect, extra systole, bigeminal/trigeminal atrial. Such phenomena are not obtainable with the traditional CTG monitoring or other methods (Chen et al, 1997; Moghavvemi & Tan, 2003; Mittra et al., 2008).

2.4 Foetal electrocardiography

FECG (Echeverria et al., 1998; Pieri et al., 2001) has also been extensively studied, but it is difficult to obtain high quality recordings, mainly because of the very poor signal to noise ratio (SNR). Moreover, the automated analysis of FECG is less accurate than that of CTG (Varady et al., 2003).

ECG is a recording of the electrical potentials generated by heart muscle activity. Aristotle first noted electrical phenomena associated with living tissues and Einthoven was the first one demonstrating the measurement of this electrical activity at the surface of the body, which resulted in the birth of electrocardiography (Janjarasjitt, 2006).

Electronic foetal monitoring for acquiring the FECG can be external to the mother, internal, or both. The internal monitoring method is invasive because of the placement of a small plastic device through the cervix. A foetal scalp electrode (a spiral wire) is placed just beneath the skin of the foetal scalp. This electrode then transmits direct FECG signal through a wire to the foetal monitor in order to extract the FHR. Because the internal foetal monitor is attached directly to the scalp of the foetus, the FECG signal is usually much clearer and more consistent than the signal recorded by an external monitoring device. However, the most important problem is a risk of infection which increases significantly in long term recordings (Murray, 2007). Hence, a foetal scalp electrode cannot be used ante partum period (Hasan, 2009). In contrast, external methods utilizing abdominal FECG have a greater prospect for long-term monitoring of FHR (e.g., 24 h) and foetal well-being. We have shown that the FECG can be obtained non-invasively by applying multi-channel electrodes placed on the abdomen of a pregnant woman (Gargiulo et al., 2010).

The detection of FECG signals by means of advanced signal processing methodologies is becoming a very essential requisite for clinical diagnosis. The FECG signal is potentially precious to assist clinicians during labour for more appropriate and timely decisions, but disadvantages such as low SNR, due to the different noise sources (Hasan et al., 2009), and the necessity of elaborate signal processing have impeded the widespread use of long-term external FECG recordings.

3. Processing of the FPCG Signal

In an adult, the heart (a sound generator) is closer to the transducer than in a foetus, where it may be separated from the probe by a distance of up to ten times the foetal heart diameter (Talbert, 1986). In addition, the foetal heart is a much weaker sound generator than the adult heart. Generally, the foetal heart sounds can be heard in only a small area of the mother's abdomen of usually no more than 3 cm in radius, although sometimes this range can extend to a 12 cm radius (Zuckerwar et al., 1993).

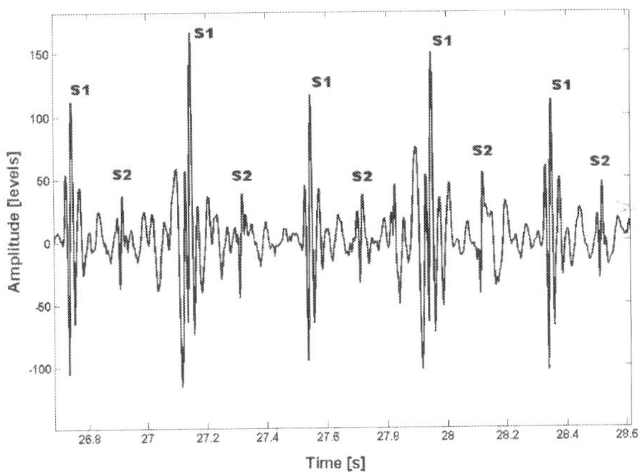

Fig. 1. Example of a FPCG signal (37th gestational week) recorded by a portable phonocardiograph and digitized with a sampling frequency of 333 Hz and 8-bits ADC.

In figure 1 examples of S1 and S2 events are shown. S1 contains a series of low frequency vibrations, and it is usually the longest and loudest heart sound; S2 typically has higher frequency components than S1, and its duration is shorter. In adults a third sound (S3) characterized by low frequency may be heard in correspondence with the beginning of the diastole, during the rapid filling of the ventricles and also a fourth heart sound (S4) in correspondence with the end of the diastole, during atrial contraction (Reed et al, 2004). In FPCG recordings, S3 and S4 sounds are practically undetectable (Mittra et al., 2008) and the power spectral densities and relative intensities of S1 and S2 are a function of foetal gestation age (Nagal, 1986). Whenever the closing of the cardiac valves creates a sound, the acoustic waves travel through a complex system of different tissue layers up to the maternal abdominal surface: amniotic fluid, the muscular wall of the uterus, layers of fat and possibly bony and cartilaginous material. Each layer attenuates the acoustic wave's amplitude due to absorption and reflection arising from the impedance mismatch that occurs at the boundary of two different layers. The result is attenuation of signals and a poor SNR (Jimenez et al., 1999; Mittra et al. 2008).

Recorded FPCG signals are heavily affected by other noise sources (Varady et al., 2003; Bassil & Dripps, 2000; Mitra et al., 2008; zhang et al., 1998), such as:

- acoustic noise produced by foetal movements;
- maternal digestive sounds;
- maternal heart activity sounds (MHAS);
- maternal respiratory sounds;
- movement of measuring sensor during recording - shear noise;
- external noise originating from the environment - ambient noise.

The above interference signals are non-stationary and have to be removed from another non-stationary signal: the foetal heart sound (FHS). Thus, a crucial issue is the correct recognition of FHS associated with each foetal heart beat and the subsequent reconstruction of the FHR signal (Varady et al., 2003; Bassil & Dripps, 2000; Kovacs et al., 2000; Moghavvemi et al., 2003; Mittra et al., 2007).

Most of the early effort in the area of FPCG monitoring was focused on sensor development. More recent studies focused on FHR estimation and different signal processing algorithms have been developed to perform foetal heart beat identification, such as: matched filtering (a technique commonly used to detect recurring time signals corrupted by noise); non-linear operators designed to enhance localised moments of high energy, such as the Teager energy operator proposed by James F. Kaiser (Kaiser, 1990); autocorrelation techniques in order to emphasize the periodic components in the foetal heart signal while reducing the non-periodic components; quadratic energy detectors that incorporate frequency filtering with energy detection (Atlas et al., 1992); neural networks; and linear prediction.

Except for some studies, the proposed methods have mainly aimed at detecting heart sound occurrences, but not their precise location in time. Moreover, no detailed quantitative results assessing the reliability of the proposed methods have been published.

In (Ruffo et al., 2010) we presented a new algorithm for FHR estimation from acoustic FPCG signals. The performance of the algorithm was compared with that of CTG, which is currently considered the gold standard in FHR estimation. The results obtained showed that the algorithm was able to obtain obtains the FHR signal reliably. An example of the comparison is shown in Figure 2.

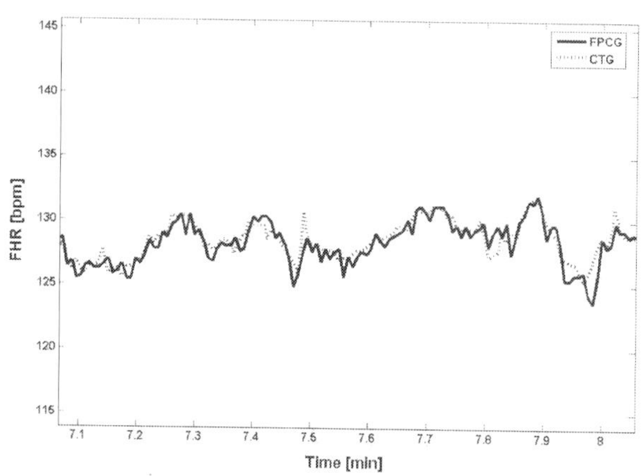

Fig. 2. Comparison between a FHR estimated from FPCG signal and FHR simultaneously recorded by means of CTG

3.1 FHR extraction from FPCG

In FHS extraction, S1 is often considered as a good time marker for the heart beat, because of its high energy with respect to the other portions of the FPCG signal, and its lower morphologic variability (Pieri et al., 2001; Ahlstrom et al., 2008). Thus, once each S1 is detected, the correspondent FHR series can be easily estimated measuring the time between each S1.

A possible algorithm for FHR extraction based on S1 enhancement and detection was presented by Ruffo et al. (Ruffo et al., 2010). A block diagram of this algorithm is shown in figure 3. In addition to the extraction of the FHR, the detected S1 sequence it is also used to identify the fainter S2.

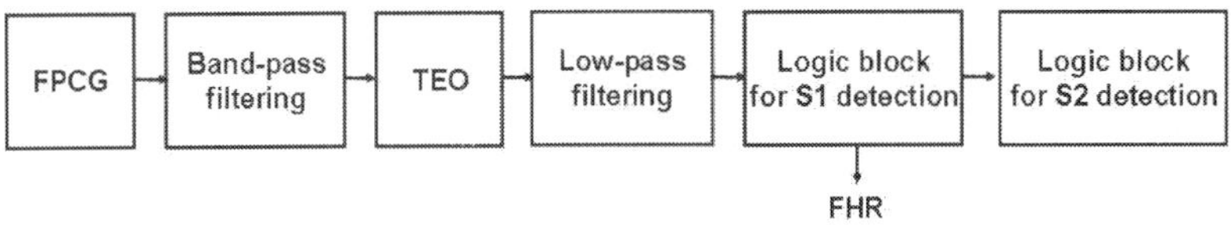

Fig. 3. Block diagram of the FHR from FPCG algorithm

Before entering into the detailed explanation of each block, it is worthwhile to recall that interference in FPCG recording is usually below 20 Hz (mostly internal noise, such as MHAS and digestive sounds) and above 70 Hz (externals noise) (Varady et al., 2003; Bassil & Dripps, 2000; Kovacs et al., 2000; Mittra et al. 2008). Moreover, the frequency content of S1 and S2 partially overlap, so that it may be difficult to distinguish them in the frequency domain. However, in the time domain they are separable since the time correlation between them is known (Varady et al., 2003; Kovacs et al., 2000; Jimenez et al., 1999; Mittra et al. 2008). Thus, the algorithm described in figure 3 has been designed accordingly. Particularly the first filtering block, the band-pass filter, is designed to cut out most of the interference. It is a 100th order digital band-pass filter having 3 dB band equal to 34-54 [Hz] centred at 44 Hz. (Ruffo et al., 2010).

The output of the filter is fed to the Teager Energy Operator (TEO) block (Kaiser, 1990). This non-linear time operator is implemented here for S1 enhancement. It is able to identify signal tracts characterized by local high energy (Kaiser, 1990). The resulting signal will have a further enhanced S1.

Because of the residual noise, the TEO output needs further digital filtering (Kaiser, 1993). In the presented algorithm such a filter is implemented with a 30 Hz cut-off frequency 5th order low-pass filter (Ruffo et al., 2010). The result of the filtering will be an enhancement of the lobes corresponding to the possible locations of S1.

Finally, the signal is sufficiently pre-processed to perform the S1 extraction. Such extraction is performed using a peak by peak analysis with a strategy very close to that reported in (Varady et al., 2003; Bassil & Dripps, 2000; Kovacs et al., 2000; Ahlstrom et al., 2008). After an initial training, peaks within a fixed time interval (based on inter-distance consistency of the previous eight identified beats) are classified as candidate beats. Among them, the peaks with amplitude greater than a fixed threshold (based on the amplitude regularity of the previous eight identified beats) are classified as probable heart beats.

The time interval considered for a candidate beat is set to be equal to T_0 + 0.65*MEAN, T_0 + 1.35*MEAN, where T_0 is the position of the last detected S1 and MEAN is the mean of the time distance between two consecutive detected S1 events on the previous eight beats. The coefficients 0.65 and 1.35 were heuristically chosen in order to take in consideration acceptable variations of FHR and to reject, at the same time, extreme outliers. The amplitude threshold is half of the mean value of the previous eight detected S1 amplitudes. In the case of detection of multiple peaks with an amplitude higher than the threshold in the same time interval, the algorithm chooses the peak which has position P_i that minimizes the distance $||T_0-P_i| - MEAN|$. To illustrate how the logic block for S1 detection works, its flow chart is depicted in figure 4.

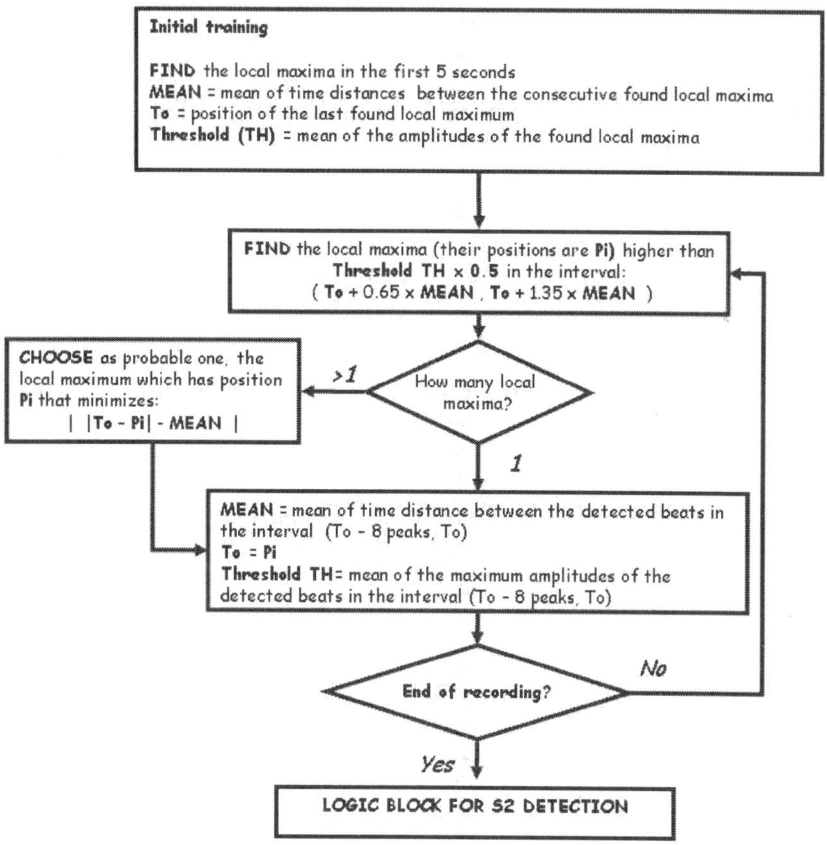

Fig. 4. The logic block for S1 detection

Finally, for each of the detected S1, the timing of the event occurrence is established following an approach similar to the ones used in ECG processing for QRS detection (Kohler et al., 2002; Bailon et al., 2002; Rozentryt et al., 1999): for each identified S1 event, the algorithm chooses the time occurrences of the maximum amplitude of the peak as time markers.

In addition, the algorithm generates a reliability index for each detected S1 event. The value assigned to the reliability index from the algorithm is a function of the local SNR and number of candidates that the logic block has found for the corresponding beat; the index can assume three different values (high, medium, low) in a similar way to some CTG devices used in clinical practise (Ruffo et al., 2010).
Once the S1 detection is complete, the search for S2 events is executed by the next logic block. As for the previous logic block, in order to identify an S2 event, remaining large signal amplitudes are analyzed with regard to the consistency of their distance from the corresponding S1 events and their amplitude regularity. According to Kovacs et al., the time interval between S1 and S2 (SSID) in milliseconds is a function of the corresponding FHR value (Kovacs et al., 2000): SSID = 210 - 0.5 * FHR. If Tn represents the position in milliseconds of the last detected peak S1, the algorithm searches for S2 candidate peaks with a position in a fixed time interval T equal to Tn + SSID - 50 , Tn + SSID + 50. The algorithm deals with multiple peak detection with a strategy similar to the one for multiple S1 detection described above. The flow chart for this logic block is depicted in figure 5, an example of results of the entire algorithm on an excerpt of data is shown in figure 6.

4. Processing of the FECG signal

The FECG can be recorded from the maternal abdominal region using a multi-lead system that covers the entire area. The raw recorded waveform is similar to the maternal one (often recorded with an additional chest lead. However, if the signals are correctly processed it will be possible to recognize three important features that are helpful indicators for foetal well being assessment and diagnosis such as (Peddaneni, 2004):

- Foetal heart rate
- Waveforms amplitudes
- Waveforms duration.

Unfortunately there is a lack of meaningful abdominal FECG recordings mainly because of the very low SNR due to the various interference sources (Hasan et al., 2009). Some of the issues are:
Base-line wander: respiration and body movements can cause electrode-skin impedance changes generating a baseline drift (Janjarasjitt, 2006). The baseline drift due to the respiration presents itself as a large amplitude sinusoidal component at low frequency and can cause amplifier saturation and signal clipping;
Power line interference: induced by the main electrical power source (60 or 50 Hz);
Maternal ECG (mECG): this is likely the main interferer. Since the maternal ECG amplitude is considerably higher than the FECG (in an abdominal recordings, the amplitude of the maternal QRS is typically around 1 mV while the foetal QRS amplitude is around 60 μV), the larger signal may obscure the smaller one. Moreover, the spectra of maternal and foetal signals overlap, so that it is not possible to separate them through conventional selective filtering (Janjarasjitt, 2006);
EMG: generated by muscle contraction and generally associated with movements and uncomfortable positions for the patient. EMG can generate artefacts that are characterized by a relatively large high-frequency content (Janjarasjitt, 2006). The situation is far worse during uterine contractions which add to the FECG some peculiar artefacts due to the uterine EMG (electrohysterogram); however, it is useful to monitor FECG during uterine contractions because the FHR in response to the contractions is an important indicator of the foetal health (Peddaneni, 2004).

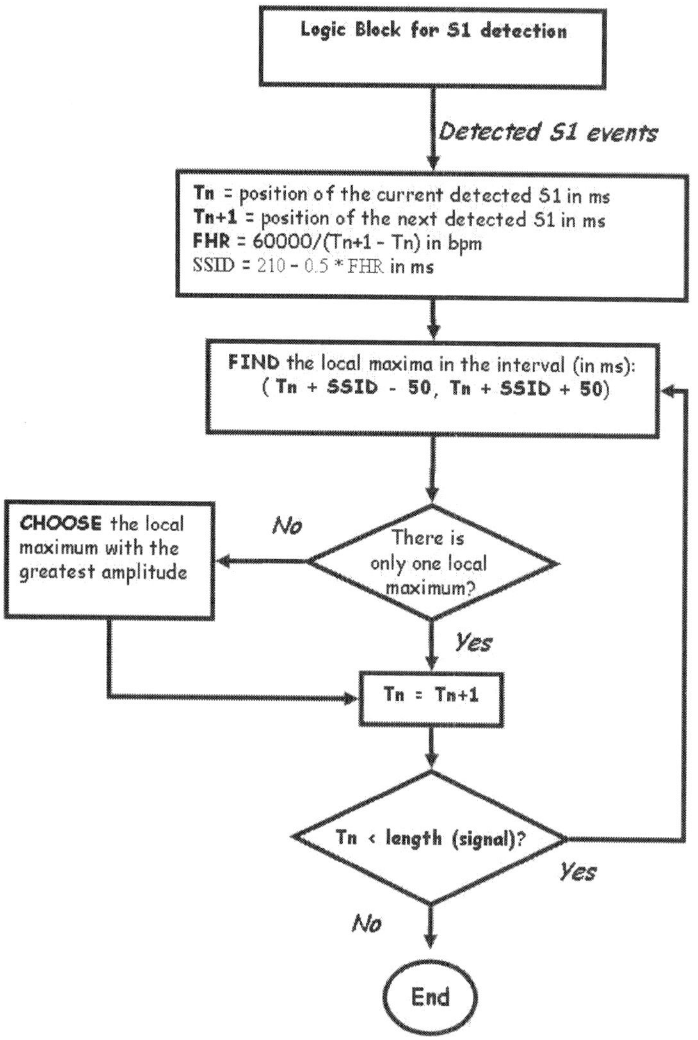

Fig. 5. Flow chart of the logic block for S2 detection

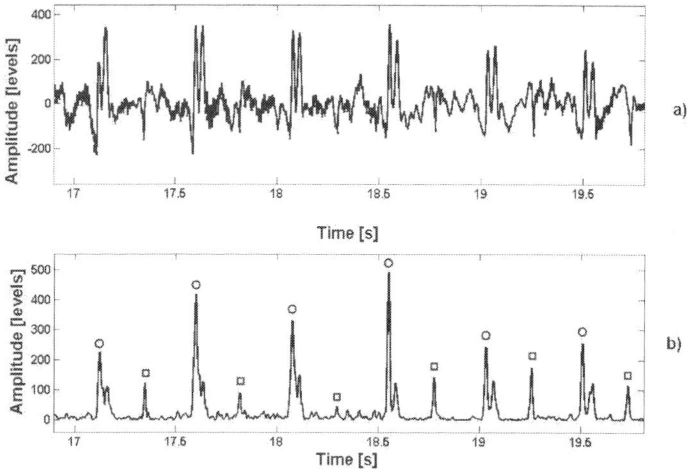

Fig. 6. Examples of detected S1 events (circles) and detected S2 events (squares): a) FPCG signal; b) Low-pass filtering block output

Inherent noise in electronic equipment: all electronic equipment generates noise. This noise cannot be eliminated - even the use of high-quality electronic components can only minimize it.

In addition to all the issues described above, there is an inter- and intra-subject variability related to the gestational age and the position of the electrodes during the acquisition of the signal. Finally, another issue that has to be considered in FECG recording, is the attenuation of the FECG signal due to the electrically insulating properties of the vernix caseosa, which develops around the 28th to 32nd weeks of gestation (Janjarasjitt, 2006). Despite all the above mentioned issues, the FECG is a unique tool to assess foetal well being.

Cardiac events in an ECG are associated with alphabetical labels as shown in figure 7. One cycle of a normal heart beat consists of waves, complexes, intervals, and segments representing as follows:

- P wave: the firing of the sinoatrial node and atrial depolarization;
- PR interval: the atrial depolarization and atrioventricular delay;
- QRS complex: the ventricular depolarization;
- Q wave: the initial negative deflection due to ventricular depolarization;
- R wave: the first positive deflection due to ventricular depolarization;
- RR interval: the time interval between consecutive R waves;
- S wave: a second negative deflection of ventricular depolarization;
- ST segment: a part of the ventricular depolarization process;
- T wave: the ventricular repolarization;
- QT interval: the time interval which ventricular depolarization and repolarization take.

The analysis of FECG permits the evaluation of cardiac parameters in order to identify eventual cardiac pathologies (Symonds et al., 2001), such as acidosis (Janjarasjitt, 2006). It can also give other information about premature ventricular contractions, activity of the autonomic nervous system, cardiac arrhythmia, uterine contraction, etc. It is important to monitor the ST interval since it reflects the function of the foetal heart muscle during stress tests. Rosen and Kjellmer (Rosen & Kjellmer, 1975) observed progressive changes in the ST interval prior to the bradycardia in the FECG tracings in experimental hypoxia and it is known that oxygen deficiency causes neurological damage. The ST waveform can be assessed qualitatively by its shape but also quantitatively, by the height of the T wave in relation to the amplitude of QRS wave (T/QRS ratio). Greene et al. (Greene et al., 1982) found a correlation between high values of the T/QRS ratio with persistently elevated ST waveforms and anaerobic metabolism in chronically instrumented lambs. In addition, in adults, ST depression with T wave elevation is also seen in myocardial ischemia and may represent an index of myocardial ischemic hypoxia when the myocardium action potential change is not uniform. Finally, it is know that ST waveform monitoring is used to identify myocardial infarction or coronary insufficiency (Braunwald et al., 1976).

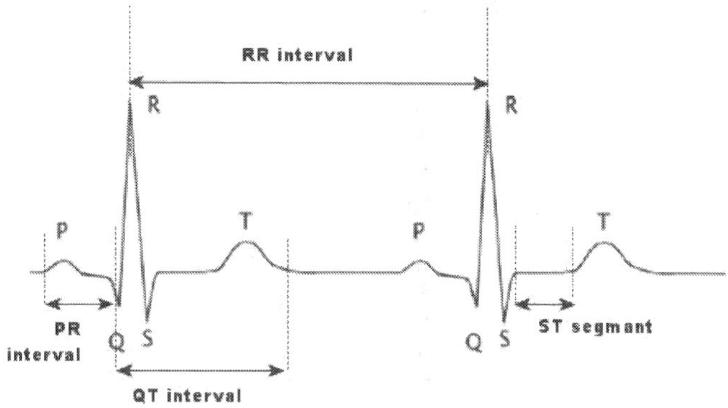

Fig. 7. An example of ECG signal and its components

4.1 FHR extraction from FECG

The extraction of the FHR from FECG is not a trivial signal processing issue. In the literature it is possible to find different techniques to extract FHR from abdominal ECG recordings: Neural Networks (Camps et al., 2001; Kezi et al., 2006), Dynamic Neural Network (Camps et al., 2001; camps et al. 2004), Least Mean Square (Camps et al., 2004; Roberts & Mullis, 1987), Orthogonal Basis Function (Longini et al., 1977), Subtraction of an Average Pattern (Bundin & Abboud, 1994), Wavelet Transform (Hasan, 2009; Mochimaru et al., 2004; Mallat & Hwang, 1992), State Space Projection (Ritcher et al., 1998; Schreiber et al., 1998), Temporal structure (Kardec & Cichocki, 2001; Zhi-Lin & Zhang, 2006), Polynomial networks (Assaleh & Al-Nashash, 2005), and Independent Component Analysis (Stone, 2002; Hyvarinen & Oja, 2000). However, there is no agreement about which one is the best technique. Our method is based on Independent Component Analysis (ICA). ICA is essentially a method for extracting individual signals from mixtures of signals under the physically realistic assumption that different physical processes generate unrelated signals. The simple and generic nature of this assumption ensures that ICA is being successfully applied in a diverse range of research fields (Stone, 2002). In our case it is possible to assume that the foetal and maternal signals are the independent components.

A number of different methods for implementing ICA have been published. Aapo Hyvärinen in 1997 introduced a family of algorithms that are grouped under the epithet fixed-point or FastICA algorithms (Hyvarinen, 1997). In principle, all the FastICA algorithms find independent components by separately maximising the negentropy (negative entropy) of each mixture (Yan et al., 2000). It is also known from the literature that FastICA algorithms usually offer fast and efficient approach for the pre-processing of FECG with multiple signals of interest, in particular when the SNR is low. Moreover, no specific a priori knowledge is required in order to identify components generated from different sources. However, the main disadvantage of this technique is that it requires different ECG leads (Stone, 2002; Hyvarinen & Oja, 2000). These additional leads mean a larger number of electrodes is then required. In addition, because the foetus moves, it is clear that a standard location for the sensors does not exist. Enough electrodes must be used to ensure a good informative content for the foetal extraction, but the number of electrodes should not be excessive because this could be uncomfortable for the mother. As a compromise, we used four electrodes placed on the maternal abdomen and an additional electrode placed on the right leg as the reference.

One of the known limitations of ICA is that the number of the output channels cannot be larger than the number of input signals. However, since the number of independent sources in the recorded signals could be greater than the number of the abdominal leads employed, it is important to reduce, as much as possible, the known sources of noise (such as maternal ECG, baseline wander, power-line interference, and motion artifacts) prior to ICA.

In our case, a bank of sharp notch filters (with Q-factor equal to 30) at 50 Hz and its higher harmonic components (100, 150 and 200 Hz) is used to suppress the power line interference. Next, a 10th order band-pass filter with a bandwidth range of 3 - 40 [Hz] is used because the frequencies of interest for the QRS extraction lie mainly inside this frequency range. This filter reduces high frequency noises coming from motion artefacts and also reduces low frequency baseline wander.

The maternal ECG needs to be reduced as well. In our case, the maternal QRS waves are detected and erased by means of a threshold detection (proportional to the local root mean square value of the signal), and for each detected maternal QRS, the average wave, computed on the previous detected five QRS waves, is then subtracted.

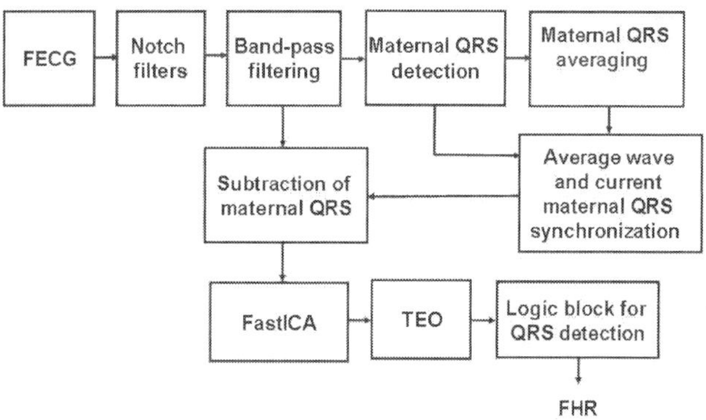

Fig. 8. Flow chart of the algorithm for FHR extraction

The FastICA algorithm described is summarized in the block diagram depicted in figure 8. The independent component that best represented the FECG was chosen manually.
In order to extract FHR, the foetal QRS waves were detected using the same strategy used for the FPCG. Foetal QRS waves were enhanced by means of TEO and then detected using a similar process employed for S1 events detection (Kohler et al., 2002; Bailon et al., 2002; Rozentryt et al., 1999). An excerpt of data showing QRS detection is depicted in figure 9.

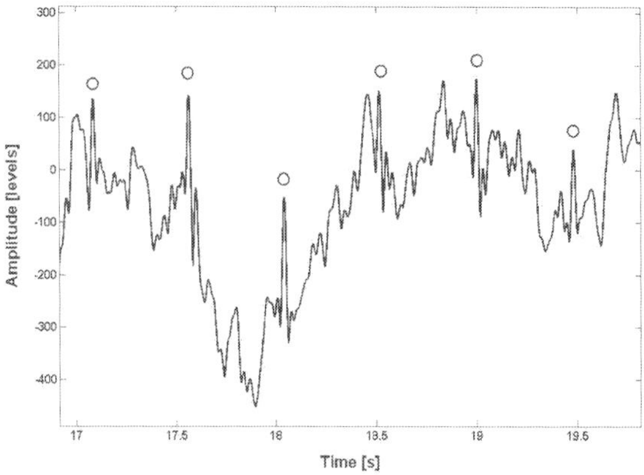

Fig. 9. Examples of detected QRS events (circles)

5. Combined FECG-FPCG monitoring and future development

A longer-term non-invasive assessment to evaluate foetal distress could be achieved by means of the measurement of the systolic time intervals (FSTI) of the foetal heart (Fleming et al., 1986). In the literature, the most satisfactory available technique for FSTI measurement consists of recording simultaneously FECG and valve movements by means of a Doppler ultrasound device (De Vore et al., 1981; Giolardino et al., 1986; Adam et al., 1979; Robinson et al., 1978). However in order to identify foetal cardiac valve movements, FPCG could be a possible alternative to the Doppler ultrasound system (Fleming et al., 1986). This would overcome the problem caused by the directionality of the ultrasound beam and, in addition, it would avoid long term exposure to ultrasound waves.
In order to estimate FSTI from FPCG and FECG signals it is necessary to extract different heart beat events. In particular, from FPCG, it is necessary to detect the vibrations which identify the mitral valve closure, aortic valve closure, aortic valve opening (a lower-frequency component resulting from the ejection recoil) at the commencement of systole. Instead to estimate the FSTI from the FECG, it is necessary to extract the QRS complex, because the pre-ejection period (PEP), can be defined as the time interval from the onset of the Q-wave to the aortic valve opening) (Fleming et al., 1986).
The proposed algorithms provide all the required information; the occurrence of PEP can be estimated by means of the QRS wave detection while the timing of the other events can be estimated by the detection of S1 and S2. In both S1 and S2, the main part of the complex consists of large vibrations, due to the movements of the valves (Luisada et al., 1949). Therefore, division of each S1 and S2 into different phases which correspond to different

valvular events (mitral valve closure and opening and aortic valve closure) is relatively easy (Fleming et al., 1986).

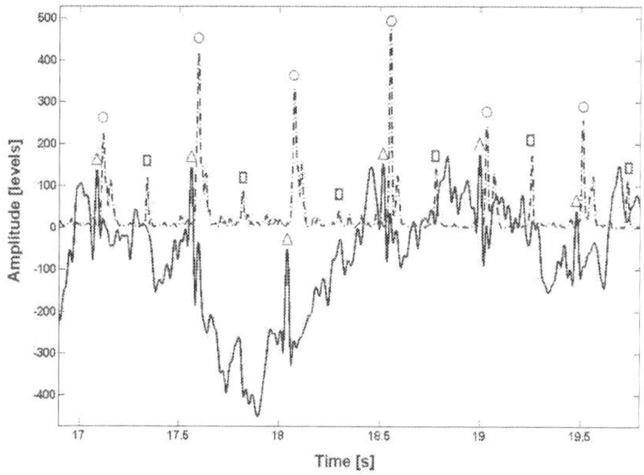

Fig. 10. Examples of detected QRS events (triangles), S1 events (circles) and S2 events (squares) in a combined recording; solid line represents FECG, dashed line represents FPCG (low-pass filtering block output)

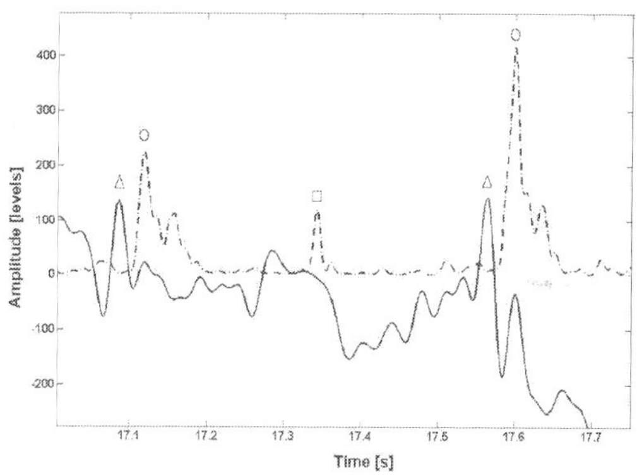

Fig. 11. Magnified section from figure 10

CTG monitoring is limited to the clinical recording duration (typically only 20-30 minutes) and it does not provide information about the foetal circulatory impedance on a continuous basis or over longer periods. Our results will encourage the further development of processing strategies to obtain further information about the foetal circulatory impedance. By monitoring of the time difference between occurrence of particular events on the FECG signal (such as P waves) and the corresponding foetal heart sounds, it is possible to provide information about the circulatory impedance. For example, in the case of placental insufficiency, the placental resistance rises and a larger pressure is generated in the foetal ventricles; this causes a lengthening of the time interval between the P wave and the occurrence of S1. In this way, it would be possible to monitor any increase of this time interval over a long period of time to identify a foetus at risk.

Further information to assess the foetus well-being can be estimated from the FECG and FPCG signals separately. FECG processing allows ST interval analysis. Synchronized averaged FECG can improve the SNR. R-peaks can be detected and aligned in a given time window (e.g. 30 seconds or more). Then all the recognized FECG can be averaged, with the expected improvement in SNR proportional to the square root of the number of FECG considered in the averaging operation. In this way it is possible to reduce the noise and analyze the ST interval which reflects the condition of the heart muscle under load. This could be useful for clinicians when deciding on obstetric interventions (Ross et al., 2004).
Future developments will aim to detect from the FCPG signal cardiac functioning anomalies (such as murmur, split effect, extrasystole, bigeminal/trigeminal atria contraction; phenomena which cannot be studied with the traditional CTG technique).

6. References

Adam A.H., Doig J.R., Fleming J.E.E., Smith M.C., Houston A., Adam K. & Aitchison T. (1979). Fetal Heart Electromechanical Intervals. *Recent Advances in Ultrasonic Diagnosis*, Vol. 12, Ed. Kurjak A.

Ahlstrom C., Lanne T., Ask P. & Johansson A. (2008). A method for accurate localization of the first heart sound and possible applications. *Physiol. Meas.* Vol. 29, pp. 417-428

Ang E. S. B. C., Gluncic V., Duque A., Schafer M. E. & Rakic P. (2006). Prenatal exposure to ultrasound waves impacts neuronal migration in mice. *Proceedings of the National Academy of Sciences,* Vol. 103, pp. 12903-12910

Assaleh K. & Al-Nashash H. (2005). A novel technique for the extraction of fetal ECG using polynomial networks. *Biomedical Engineering, IEEE Transactions,* Vol. 52, no. 6, pp. 1148-1152

Atlas, L. & Fang, J. (1992). Quadratic Detectors for General Nonlinear Analysis of Speech. *IEEE Proc. ICASSP'92, San Francisco, CA,* March 23-26, 1992, pp. II-9-II-12,

Babbitt N. E. Antepartum fetal surveillance. (1996). Nonstress test, contraction stress test, and biophysical profile. *S D J Med.* Vol 49 (11), pp. 403–408

Bailey D., Flynn A.M., Kelly J. & O'Conor M. (1980). Antepartum fetal heart rate monitoring in multiple pregnancy. *Br J Obstet Gynaecol.* Vol. 87 (7), pp. 561-564

Bailon R., Olmos S., Serrano P., Garcıa J. & Laguna P. (2002). Robust Measure of ST/HR Hysteresis in Stress Test ECG Recordings. *Computers in Cardiology,* Vol. 29, pp. 329–332

Baser I., Johnson T.R. & Paine L.L. (1992). Coupling of fetal movement and fetal heart rate accelerations as an indicator of fetal health. *Obstet Gynecol.* 1992 Jul; 80(1), pp. 62-6

Bassil H. E. & Dripps J. H. (1989). Real time processing and analysis of fetal phonocardiographic signals. *Clin. Phys. Physiol. Meas.,* Vol. 10, Suppl. B, 67-74. Printed in UK

Braunwald E. & Maroko P.R. (1976). ST-segment mapping. Realistic and unrealistic expectations. *Circulation* 54 (4), pp. 529- 532

Budin N. & Abboud S. (1994). Real Time Multichannel Abdominal Fetal ECG Monitor Using Digital Signal CoProcessor. *Computers in Biology and Medicine,* Vol. 24 (6). pp. 451-462

Campbell S. & Trickey N, Whittle MJ. (1984). Report of the Royal College of Obstetricians and Gynaecologists Working Party on routine ultrasound examination in pregnancy. R Co11, *Obstet Gynecol*

Camps G., Martinez M. & Soria E. (2001). Fetal ECG extraction using an FIR neural network. *Computers in Cardiology*, pp. 249-252

Camps-Valls G., Martínez-Sober M., Soria-Olivas E., Guerrero-Martínez J. & Calpe-Maravilla J. (2004) Foetal ECG recovery using dynamic neural networks. *Artificial Intelligence in Medicine*, Vol. 31(3), pp. 197-209

Cesarelli M., Romano M. & Bifulco P. (2009). Comparison of short term variability indexes in cardiotocographic foetal monitoring. *Computers in Biology and Medicine* vol. 39 issue 2, pp. 106-118

Chen D., Durand L.G. & Lee H. C. (1997). Time-frequency analysis of the first heart sound. Part 1: Simulation and analysis. *Med. Biol. Eng. Compu.* , 35, pp. 306-310

DeVore G.R., Donnerstein R.L., Klcinman C.S. & Hobbins J.C. (1981) Real-time-directed M-mode echocardiography: A new technique for accurate and rapid quantitation of the fetal preejection period and ventricular ejection time of the right and left ventricles. *Am J Obstet Gynecol*; 141, pp. 470-471

Echeverria J.C., Ortiz R., Ramirez N., Medina V. & Gonzalez R. (1998). A reliable method for abdominal ECG signal processing. *IEEE - Computers in Cardiology* Vol 25

Gargiulo G., McEwan A., Nasehi Tehrani J., Jin C., Van Schaik A., Bifulco P., Maria R., Ruffo M., Shephard R., Cesarelli M., Mohamed A. & Calvo R. (2010). Dry Electrode Bio-potential recordings. *IEEE/EMBS* Aug. 31 to Sep. 4

Giorlandino C., Gentili P., Vizzone A., Rizzo G. & Arduini D. (1986). A new method for the measurement of pre-ejection period in the human fetus. *Br J Obstet Gynecol*; Vol. 93, pp. 307-309

Goddard B. A. (1996) A Clinical Foetal Electrocardiograph, *Med. Biol. Engineering* 4, pp. 159–167

Greene K.R., Dawes G.S., Lilja H., & Rosen K.G. (1982). Changes in the ST waveform of the fetal lamb electrocardiogram with hypoxemia. *Am J Obstet Gynecol* Vol. 144(8), pp. 950–958

Hasan M. A., Reaz M. B. I., Ibrahimy M. I., Hussain M. S. & Uddin J. (2009). Detection and Processing Techniques of FECG Signal for Fetal Monitoring. *Biological Procedures Online*, Publisher Springer New York, Vol. 11, no 1, pp. 263-295, 27 March 2009

Hyvarinen A. (1997). A family of fixed-point algorithms for independent component analysis, Acoustics. *Speech and Signal Processing*, 1997 ICASSP-97, IEEE International Conference on, vol.5, vol. 5, pp. 3917-3920

Hyvärinen A. & Oja E. (2000). Independent component analysis: algorithms and applications. *Neural Networks* Volume 13, Issues 4-5, pp. 411-430

Janjarasjitt S. (2006). A new QRS detection and ECG signal extraction technique for fetal monitoring, Department of Electrical Engineering and Computer Science Case Western Reserve University

Jimenez A., Ortiz M.R., Pena M.A., Charleston S., Aljama A.T. & Gonzalez, R. (1999). The use of wavelet packets to improve the detection of cardiac sounds from the fetal phonocardiogram. *Computers in Cardiology* , 26-29 Sept. 1999, pp. 463 - 466

Kaiser J.F. (1990). On a simple algorithm to calculate the 'energy of a signal. *ICASSP-Albuquerque, New Mexico Vol 90*, pp. 381-384,

Kaiser J.F. (1993). Some useful properties of teager's energy operators. *IEEE International Conference ICASSP-93* Acoustics, Speech, and Signal Processing, Vol 3, pp. 149-152

Kardec Barros A. & Cichocki A. (2001). Extraction of Specific Signals with Temporal Structure. *Neural Computation*, September 2001, Vol. 13, Issue 9

Karlsson B., Pourcelot D., Pourcelot L. & Berson M. (1996). Miniature sensor for Doppler ultrasound Fetal Heart Rate monitoring. Increased patient comfort and ergonomy in use. *IEEE Instrumentation and Measurement Technology Conference Brussels*, Belgium, June 4-6.

Kezi S. V. C., Kanagasabapathy P. & Johnson S. (2006). Fetal ECG Extraction using Softcomputing Technique. **Journal of Applied Sciences**, Vol.6, No.2, pp. 251-256

Kieler H., Cnattingiust S., Haglund B., Palmgren J. & Axelsson O. (2002). Ultrasound and adverse effects. *Ultrasound in Obstetrics and Gynecology*. Vol. 20, Issue 1, pp. 102-103

Köhler B. U., Hennig C. & Orglmeister R. (2002). The Principles of Software QRS Detection. *IEEE Engineering In Medicine And Biology* January/February, 2002

Kovacs F., Torok M., Habermajer I. (2002). A rule-based phonocardiographic method for long-term fetal heart rate monitoring. *IEEE Trans. on Biomed. Eng.*, vol. 47, no 1, January 2000

Longini R. L., Reichert T. A., Man Cho Yu J. & Crowley J. S. (1977) Near-Orthogonal Basis Functions: A Real Time Fetal ECG Technique. *Biomedical Engineering, IEEE Transactions on*, vol. BME-24, no.1, pp. 39-43, Jan. 1977

Luisada A. A., Mendoza F. & Alimurung M. M. (1949). The duration of normal heart sounds. *British Heart Journal*. 1949 January; 11(1), pp. 41–47

Mallat S. & Hwang W.L. (1992). Singularity detection and processing with wavelets, Information Theory. *IEEE Transactions on*, vol.38, no.2, pp. 617-643, Mar. 1992

Mantini D., Comani S., Alleva G. & Romani G.L. (2005). Fetal cardiac time intervals: validation of an automatic tool for beat-to-beat detection on fetal magnetocardiograms. *IJBEM*. Vol. 7, No. 1

Martens S. M. M., Rabotti C., Mischi M. & Sluijter R. J. (2007). A robust fetal ECG detection method for abdominal recordings. *IOP Publishing Physiological Measurement*, 7 March 2007

McDonnell, J.T.E. (1990). Knowledge-based interpretation of foetal phonocardiographic signals. *IEE Proceedings*, Vol. 137, No. 5, pp. 311-318

Mittra A.K., Shukla A. & Zadgaonkar A.S. (2007). System simulation and comparative analysis of foetal heart sound de-noising techniques for advanced phonocardiography. Int. *J. Biomedical Engineering and Technology*, Vol. 1, No. 1

Mittra A.K., Choudhary N.K. & Zadgaonkar A.S. (2008). Development of an artificial womb for acoustical simulation of mother's abdomen. *Int. J. Biomedical Engineering and Technology*, Vol. 1, No. 3

Mochimaru F., Fujimoto Y. & Ishikawa Y. (2004). The Fetal Electrocardiogram by Independent Component Analysis and Wavelets. *Japanese Journal of Physiology*, Vol.54, pp. 457-463

Moghavvemi, M., Tan, B.H. & Tan, S.Y. (2003). A non-invasive PC based measurement of fetal phonocardiography. *Journal of Sensors and Actuators*, Vol. A 107, pp. 96–103

Murray M. L. (2007). Antepartal and intrapartal fetal monitoring. Springer Publishing Co.

Nagal J. (1986). New diagnostic and technical aspects of fetal phonocardiography. *European Journal of Obstetrics and Gynecology and Reproductive Biology*, Vol. 23, pp. 295–303

Peddaneni H. (2004). Comparison of algorithms for fetal ECG extraction, University of Florida

Pieri J.F., Crowe J.A., Hayes-Gill B.R., Spencer C.J. & Bhogal K. (2001). Compact long-term recorder for the transabdominal foetal and maternal electrocardiogram. *Med. Biol. Eng. Comput.*, Vol. 39, pp. 118-125

Rabinowitz R., Persitz E. & Sadovsky E. (1983). The relation between fetal heart rate accelerations and fetal movements. *Obstet Gynecol.* 1983 Jan;61(1), pp. 16-8

Reed T.R., Reed N.E. & Peter F. (2004). Heart sound analysis for symptom detection and computer aided diagnosis. *Journal of Simulation Modeling Practices and Theory*, Vol. 12, pp. 129–146

Richter M., Schreiber T. & Kaplan D.T. (1998). Fetal ECG extraction with nonlinear state-space projections. *Biomedical Engineering, IEEE Transactions on*, vol. 45, no.1, pp. 133-137, Jan 1998

Roberts R.A. & Mullis C.T. (1987). Digital signal processing, Adison-Wesley, Reading, Mass

Robinson H.P., Adam A.H., Fleming J.E.E., Houston A. & Clark D.M. (1978). Fetal electromechanical intervals in labour. *Br J Obstet Gynecol;* 3, pp. 172-177

Romano M., Bracale M., Cesarelli M., Campanile M., Bifulco P., De Falco M., Sansone M. & Di Lieto A. (2005). Antepartum cardiotocography: a study of fetal reactivity in frequency domain. *Comput Biol Med.* 2006 Jun;36(6), pp. 619-33. Epub 2005 Jul 11

Rosen K.G. & Kjellmer I (1975). Changes in the fetal heart rate and ECG during hypoxia. *Acta Physiol Scand,* Vol. 93(1), pp. 59–66

Ross G. , Devoe L. D. & Rosen K. G. (2004). St-Segment Analysis Of The Fetal Electrocardiogram Improves Fetal Heart Rate Tracing Interpretation And Clinical Decision Making. *J Matern Fetal Neonatal Med.* 2004 Mar; Vol. 15 (3), pp. 181-5

Rozentryt P., Leski J., Sroczynski J. & Czogala E. (1999). A new beat-by-beat spectrotemporal analysis of variability in ECG morphology. *Med Sci Monit;* Vol 5(4), pp. 777-785

Ruffo M., Cesarelli M., Romano M., Bifulco P., & Fratini A. (2010). An algorithm for FHR estimation from foetal phonocardiographic signals, *Biomedical Signal Processing and Control* 5, pp. 131-141

Schreiber T., Richter M. (1998). Nonlinear projective filtering in a data stream. *Wuppertal preprint WUB* -98-8

Shy K.K., Larson E.B. & Luthy DA. (2002). Evaluating a new technology: the effectiveness of electronic fetal heart rate monitoring. *Annu Rev Public Health.* 1987; Vol. 8, pp. 165-90

Stone J. V., Independent component analysis: an introduction. *TRENDS in Cognitive Sciences,* Vol.6 No.2, pp. 59-64, February 2002

Symonds E.M., Sahota D. & Chang A. (2001). Fetal electrocardiography. *Imperial College Press, London*

Talbert D.G., Davies W.L., Johnson F., Abraham N.G., Colley N. & Southall D.P. (1986). Wide bandwidth fetal phonography using a sensor matched to the compliance of the mother's abdominal wall. *IEEE Trans Biomed Eng* 1986; Vol. 33, pp. 175-181

Tan B.H. & Moghavvemi M. (2000). Real time analysis of fetal phonocardiography. *Proceedings of IEEE TENCON* 2000

Varady P., Wildt L., ´N Benyo´ Z. & Hein A.. An advanced method in fetal phonocardiography. (2003). *Computer Methods and Programs in Biomedicine,* Vol. 71, pp. 283-296

Wakai R.T. (2004). Assessment of fetal neurodevelopment via fetal magnetocardiography. *Experimantal Neurology, Vol.* 190, pp. S65-S71

Williams B. & Arulkumaran S. (2004). Cardiotocography and medicolegal issues. *Best Pract Res Clin Obstet Gynaecol*. Jun; Vol 18(3), pp. 457-66

Yan Li, Powers D. & Peach J. (2000) Comparison of Blind Source Separation Algorithms. *Advances in Neural Networks and Applications*, WSES, pp.18-21

Zhang, X., Durand, L., Senhadji, L., Lee, H. & Coatrieux, J. (1998). Time-frequency scaling transformation of the phonocardiogram based of the matching pursuit method. *IEEE Transactions on Biomedical Engineering*, Vol. 45, No. 8, pp. 972–979

Zhi-Lin Zhang & Zhang Yi. (2006). Robust extraction of specific signals with temporal structure, Neurocomputing, *New Issues in Neurocomputing: 13th European Symposium on Artificial Neural Networks*, Vol. 69, Issues 7-9, pp. 888-893

Zhuravlev Y.E., Rassi D., Mishin A.A. & Emery S.J. (2002). Dynamic analysis of beat-to-beat fetal heart rate variability recorded by squid magnetometer: quantification of sympatho-vagal balance. *Early Human development*, Vol. 66, pp. 1-10

Zuckerwar A.J., Pretlow R.A., Stoughton J.W.& Baker D.A. (1993). Development of a piezopolymer pressure sensor for a portable fetal heart rate monitor. *IEEE Trans Biomed Eng*, Vol. 40(9), pp. 963-9

19

Parametric Modelling of EEG Data for the Identification of Mental Tasks

Simon G. Fabri, Kenneth P. Camilleri and Tracey Cassar
Department of Systems and Control Engineering, University of Malta
Malta

1. Introduction

Electroencephalographic (EEG) data is widely used as a biosignal for the identification of different mental states in the human brain. EEG signals can be captured by relatively inexpensive equipment and acquisition procedures are non-invasive and not overly complicated. On the negative side, EEG signals are characterized by low signal-to-noise ratio and non-stationary characteristics, which makes the processing of such signals for the extraction of useful information a challenging task.

When a person performs specific events, such as cued imagery tasks, left-hand or right-hand movements, imagined motor tasks and auditory tasks, corresponding variations in the characteristics of the person's EEG signal take place. These are typically identified by so-called event-related potentials (ERP). For example, event-related potentials associated with real and imagined motor tasks exhibit frequency-specific characteristics: a decrease in EEG band power occurs on the contra-lateral side, a phenomenon known as Event-Related Desynchronization (ERD), followed some time later by an increase in band power on the ipsi-lateral side, known as Event -Related Synchronization (ERS). Hence the detection and identification of ERD and ERS phenomena would enable the classification of mental activity. Such techniques can find useful application in *brain-computer interface* (BCI) systems where EEG data is measured from the brain and processed by a computer so as to, for example, detect and classify real or imagined left and right-hand movements for the execution of useful tasks such as wheelchair navigation (Pfurtscheller *et al.*, 2006). Several signal processing techniques have been proposed to classify left and right-hand movement from the EEG signal either by detecting ERD and ERS phenomena directly, or by the application of appropriate signal analysis techniques which are characterised by the ERD/ERS phenomena. These include the inter-trial variance approach, the Short-time Fourier Transform, Wavelet Transform methods and Source Localization methods (Pfurtscheller & Lopes da Silva, 1999; Qin *et al.*, 2004).

A different approach, on which this chapter will focus, aims to capture the dynamics of the EEG signal by means of auto-regressive (AR) or auto-regressive moving average (ARMA) parametric models (Pardey *et al.*, 1996). This chapter will specifically address the use of such models for the identification and classification of imagined left and right-hand movements. It will start with a literature review on the use of AR and ARMA parametric models for EEG signals and their practical applications. It then proceeds to report, in a unified manner, a number of novel contributions proposed and published by the authors as summarized below.

The first contribution proposes a novel three-mode classifier which uses the parameters of the AR model as a feature for distinguishing between no hand movement and left-hand or right-hand movement (Cassar *et al.*, 2010b). The quality of the classifier depends on the optimal estimation of the AR model parameters. The Kalman filter presents itself as a versatile tool for on-line estimation of model coefficients. However, the performance of the Kalman filter depends critically on its initialisation and the correct setting of the Kalman filter parameters, which are generally unknown. (Khan & Dutt, 2007) showed that the Expectation Maximization (EM) algorithm could be used to estimate the Kalman filter parameters and hence obtain AR coefficient estimates which improve the identification of ERD. Following the same approach, this chapter shows that the EM algorithm for Kalman filter initialization, together with the proposed three-mode classifier, yields better scores than two-mode classifiers typically proposed in the literature for brain computer interface applications.

Additionally, it is shown that a potentially richer interpretation of the AR parameters can be obtained through their relation with the poles of the model. It is argued that these poles provide explicit dominant frequency information which may be useful to describe, represent and identify ERD/ERS phenomena taking place over time. Such dominant frequencies can be individually tracked, showing that poles in the alpha band represent ERD phenomena which are related to hand movement.

The final contribution focuses on the selection of the AR or ARMA model order; an important aspect of parametric techniques. Several approaches have been proposed for the estimation of model order from the data, each having its own advantages and disadvantages. In order to obtain a more robust model order estimation, this chapter reviews an improved criterion developed by the authors in (Cassar *et al.*, 2010a) which leads to a lower probability of error for model order estimation in the case of multivariate systems. The performance of this criterion is tested by extensive Monte Carlo analysis and it is also used to fit an ARMA model to real EEG data.

2. Literature review

Parametric modelling has long been recognized as a versatile tool for the analysis of EEG data (Bohlin, 1973; Isaksson *et al.*, 1981). Nevertheless, this is still an active area of research and several open problems need to be addressed in order to successfully deploy these techniques for practical applications such as EEG driven, brain-computer interface systems. Linear parametric models have been widely used to fit EEG data. The auto-regressive moving average (ARMA) model structure, or variations based upon this structure, are commonly employed. The tutorial paper by (Pardey *et al.*, 1996) provides good explanations on the use of parametric modelling techniques for time series analysis, with emphasis on EEG data and autoregressive models. The concept of signal stationarity is addressed and the use of adaptive and non-adaptive models is discussed, together with the issues of model complexity and stability.

EEG data is generally considered to be non-stationary because its statistical characteristics change with time, depending upon the mental states that are active at any given time instant. In order to handle this feature, one approach is to assume that over short time intervals the signal remains stationary. A batch processing algorithm is then applied to estimate the optimal parameters which best fit the measurements taken over each of these short time intervals. This approach leads to non-adaptive models, where AR or ARMA structures are normally used. The Burg algorithm or the Levinson-Durbin algorithm are used to estimate the parameters of the model. Alternatively the model's parameter estimates are updated recursively at every time instant with the arrival of new data samples, typically by means of the Kalman filter algorithm. This approach leads to so-called adaptive models because the model parameters adapt themselves recursively to the characteristics of the data measurements taken along the course of time (Pardey *et al.*, 1996; Isaksson *et al.*, 1981). The term "time varying auto-regressive" (TVAR) is also used to refer to this technique when AR model structures are applied.

Several papers on different aspects of adaptive modelling for EEG signal analysis and applications have been published. For example, (Shloegl *et al.*, 1997) used the Adaptive Autoregressive Method (AAR) together with a linear discriminant classifier to investigate EEG data from two subjects executing imagined left-hand and right-hand movements. The AAR parameters were estimated by a Recursive Least Squares (or Kalman filter) algorithm. The parameters at a specific classification time instant were applied for linear discriminant analysis and an error rate calculated. By repeating this at different classification time instants, the dependence of error rate upon time was determined. It was concluded that left-hand and right-hand movements could be discriminated on the basis of the estimated AAR parameters instead of the more traditional method based upon the analysis of signal energy in specific frequency bands. In order to analyze non-stationary EEG data, TVAR models were used in (Krystal *et al.*, 1999) where the evolution of the models was represented by latent components having a time-varying frequency leading to a representation made up of: damped sinusoid components with amplitude, phase and frequency characteristics that vary temporally; and high-frequency sinusoid components. In this paper, these latent components were plotted and tracked to provide insights into the EEG variation in time. The work of (Li, 2007) investigated how a time varying AR model can be used to estimate the complexity and synchronization of an EEG signal in order to identify epileptic seizures. The onset of a seizure is detected by a change in complexity of the AR model, where complexity is measured by the model order that is required to adequately represent the EEG signal. In (Tarvainen *et al.*, 2001) the Kalman smoother is adopted instead of the more common LMS or RLS algorithms for adaptive ARMA modelling of non-stationary EEG. An ARMA(6,2) model was used to track alpha band characteristics of a subject having eyes opening and closing. The study suggests that the Kalman smoother method gives more reliable tracking compared to the other algorithms. The problem of model order estimation was also pointed out in this paper, indicating methods that could be used to handle this problem. However an order of (6,2) was arbitrarily selected and deemed to be suitable for all the experiments in this work.

Three different model order estimation techniques for fitting an AR model to EEG data were studied by (Palaniappan *et al.*, 2000). The model order selection criteria considered in this work are the Final Prediction Error, Akaike's Information Criterion and Reflection Coefficient. The parameters of the resulting AR models were used to generate the Power Spectral Density which was applied as an input to a neural network classifier. Out of the three criteria, the Reflection Coefficient criterion resulted in models which gave the best classification performance and lower optimum order.

When a combination of signals from multiple EEG channels is used for analysis, a multivariate (vector) model is often used to fit this data. The advantages of multivariate modelling techniques for biomedical signals are explained in (Rezek, 2006), where an example of multivariate AR (MVAR) modelling for sleep EEG is demonstrated. The work of (Anderson *et al.*, 1998) introduced the use of multivariate AR models for mental state classification. The performance of classification of two mental tasks – relaxed state and mental multiplication –

using features derived from univariate (scalar) AR and 6-channel MVAR models was studied. The results showed that the MVAR features have a slightly better classification performance and better consistency. Adaptive on-line MVAR was explored in (Arnold *et al.*, 1998), adapting the use of the Kalman filter from the univariate case to the multivariate model. A trivariate AR model of order 22 was used, from which spectral parameters were extracted yielding relevant information regarding neural communication processes. A multivariate adaptive autoregressive model is proposed in (Ding *et al.*, 2000) for the analysis of non-stationary, multichannel event-related potentials originating from the cerebral cortex. The model parameters, captured over successive time windows, are used to derive spectral quantities by means of which the cortical dynamics can be illustrated. In (Pei & Zheng, 2004) a multivariate AR model is fitted to EEG signals from two channels recorded from a subject performing left-hand and right-hand movements. They show that the parameters of the multivariate AR model can be used to form a feature vector for discriminant analysis based upon the Mahalanobis distance, and that the performance of the multivariate approach surpasses that of a univariate AR model. In (Schloegl & Supp, 2006), multivariate AR models are applied to event-related EEG data for the analysis of multichannel spectral properties of EEG.

Some research studies have investigated whether nonlinear models are more suitable than linear models for fitting EEG data. In (Popivanov *et al.*, 1998), linear (AR) and a non-linear analysis (point-wise dimension, Kolmogorov entropy, largest Lyapunov exponent and non-linear prediction) of EEG data arising from voluntary movement were compared. The study concluded that linear and non-linear components in the EEG of voluntary movement co-exist and that both the linear and the non-linear methods detected EEG transitions prior to the movement. The results of the study also indicate that the two classes of methods do not have temporally coincident measures and were thus supposed to detect different dynamics of the EEG signal. The paper by (Inoue *et al.*, 2004) addresses the issue of nonlinearity by proposing the use of a Quasi-AR model for EEG data during motor tasks. This model has a linear structure, similar to AR, but nonlinear parameters and hence it could capture the nonlinear dynamics of the EEG signal. The model parameters were estimated by a recursive prediction error method. The features obtained from the spectrum of the Quasi-AR model were used for discrimination between left and right-hand movement tasks. This approach showed superior performance when compared with conventional AR models. Two linear and two nonlinear models were compared by (Jain & Deshpande, 2004). Their analysis shows that the Bilinear model structure gives better results for EEG than AR, ARMA and Polynomial AR models. Unfortunately it is also the most computationally demanding of all four. The Bilinear AR model has also been studied by (Poulos *et al.*, 2010) in the context of person identification from EEG. The results of this study also show that the Bilinear model gives superior results than an AR model, indicating the presence of information bearing nonlinearities in the EEG signal, and the capability of the Bilinear model to extract these nonlinear components.

(Atry *et al.*, 2005) address the problem of noise. They propose an EEG signal purification technique on specific channels using the fitted parametric models prior to classification, so as to mitigate the effects of noise and improve classification results by up to 15%. They consider univariate AR, multivariate AR and Box-Jenkins models. (Kelly *et al.*, 2002) investigate the use of an autoregressive model with exogenous input (ARX) to model event-related potentials from the EEG of a subject executing left-hand and right-hand tasks. Classification results derived from the use of features from this model and features from other approaches are compared. It is concluded that the ARX model leads to the best results in the feature extraction stage. This analysis and results are developed further in (Burek *et al.*, 2005). AR modelling has also been applied to the inverse problem of EEG source localisation or current distribution estimation. In (Galka *et al.*, 2004) a new interpretation of the dynamic inverse problem for estimating local current vectors in the brain was proposed by breaking away from the classical constrained least squares formulation and reformulating the problem as a spatiotemporal AR model.

Several other relevant publications can be found in the literature. However, due to space limitations, the rest of the chapter will review in some detail the authors' own contributions to EEG data analysis covering parameter estimation and its effect on classification results, the relation between model poles and EEG characteristics, and the problem of model order estimation. However, due to space limitations, the rest of the chapter will review in some detail the authors' own contributions to EEG data analysis (Cassar *et al.*, 2010a; Cassar *et al.*, 2010b). These concern the parameter estimation problem and its effect on classification results, the relation between model poles and EEG characteristics, and the problem of model order estimation.

3. Classification of imagined hand movements and their effect on AR pole variations

One popular technique for brain-computer interfacing involves the acquisition of EEG signals from a person who interacts with a computer by imagining the movement of his/her left-hand or right-hand. This method opens up the possibility of a communication channel between a person who is subject to serious motor impairments and a computer. The execution of such imagined actions gives rise to a pattern of specific variations in particular frequency bands of the person`s EEG (Penny *et al.*, 1998). Just prior to the imagined event, a decrease in power is typically detected in the alpha band (8-12Hz) of EEG signals captured from the controlateral side of the imagined hand movement. This is called Event Related Desynchronization (ERD) (Pfurtscheller & Lopes da Silva, 1999). When the imagined movement is stopped, an increase in power is typically exhibited in the beta (13-30Hz) band of the EEG signals captured from the ipsilateral side of the relevant hand movement. This is called Event Related Synchronization (ERS). Therefore, if ERD and ERS phenomena are identified from EEG signals, there exists a potential for the classification of the imagined action *i.e.* whether the person imagined a left-hand or a right-hand movement.

Towards this end, one approach is to model the EEG signals by means of an auto-regressive (AR) parametric model (Pardey *et al.*, 1996). The parameters of the model are typically estimated from the EEG signals by using the Yule-Walker equations or a Kalman filter/smoother. These parameters, which are sometimes assumed to be constant and sometimes time-varying, can then be used as a feature vector to classify the underlying event related potential (Huan & Palaniappan, 2005; Anderson *et al.*, 1998). This process is typically cast as a 2-mode classifier, one mode for each of the two possible actions, namely imagined left or right-hand movement. This chapter proposes to identify also the background periods, where no imagined actions are taking place, as a third class that is distinct from the two classes representing left-hand or right-hand movement. It will be shown that this approach, together with a Kalman Smoother algorithm for parameter estimation that is initialized by the Expectation Maximization algorithm, will lead to improved classification results.

It is assumed that the EEG signal is modelled by a linear AR model of order p, characterized by the following difference equation in the discrete-time domain:

$$y_t = -\sum_{k=1}^{p} a_t^{(k)} y_{t-k} + \upsilon_t \quad (1)$$

where y_t represents the EEG signal recorded at time t, $a_t^{(k)}$ is the kth time-varying AR model parameter and υ_t is a random Gaussian process of zero mean and covariance R. The AR model is fitted to EEG data measurements by estimation of parameters $a_t^{(k)}$. In this work, the Kalman Smoother (Maybeck, 1979) is used to find the optimal value of the parameters which fit the data in the least square error sense. Equation (1) is first re-written in state space form:

$$x_t = \Phi x_{t-1} + \omega_t \quad (2)$$

$$y_t = H_t x_t + \upsilon_t \quad (3)$$

where x_t is the vector of AR parameters $[a_t^{(1)} a_t^{(2)} ... a_t^{(p)}]^T$ which requires estimation by the Kalman Smoother. H_t is the vector of past EEG measurements $[y_{t-1} y_{t-2} ... y_{t-p}]$ and ω_t is a random Gaussian process of zero mean and covariance Q which allows a random walk of the parameter vector x_t. Although state matrix Φ is sometimes set to be the identity matrix, this could be detrimental to the estimation of the AR parameters. (Khan & Dutt, 2007) show that the accuracy of the Kalman Smoother algorithm is very much dependent on the values assigned to Φ, the noise covariances Q and R, and the initial conditions of the parameter vector and its covariance. They show that if these are estimated by the Expectation-Maximization algorithm, rather than set randomly to some reasonable values, the Kalman Smoother algorithm yields AR parameter estimates which capture better the dynamics and spectra of event related potentials.

The Kalman Smoother algorithm consists of a set of forward recursion Equations (4) to (8), also known as the Kalman filter equations, followed by the set of backward recursion Equations (9) to (11) as shown here:

$$x_t^{t-1} = \Phi x_{t-1}^{t-1} \quad (4)$$

$$P_t^{t-1} = \Phi P_{t-1}^{t-1} \Phi' + Q \quad (5)$$

$$K_t = P_t^{t-1} H_t' \left(H_t P_t^{t-1} H_t' + R \right)^{-1} \quad (6)$$

$$x_t^t = x_t^{t-1} + K_t \left(y_t - H_t x_t^{t-1} \right) \quad (7)$$

$$P_t^t = P_t^{t-1} - K_t H_t P_t^{t-1} \quad (8)$$

$$J_{t-1} = P_{t-1}^{t-1} \Phi' \left(P_{t-1}^{t-1} \right)^{-1} \quad (9)$$

$$x_{t-1}^n = x_{t-1}^{t-1} + J_{t-1} \left(x_t^n - \Phi x_{t-1}^{t-1} \right) \quad (10)$$

$$P_{t-1}^{n} = P_{t-1}^{t-1} + J_{t-1}\left(P_t^n - P_t^{t-1}\right)J_{t-1}^{'} \tag{11}$$

where the initial conditions x_0^0 and P_0^0 are estimated together with Φ, Q and R by the Expectation-Maximization algorithm as detailed in (Khan & Dutt, 2007; Cassar *et al.*, 2010b).
The following comparative analysis will utilize the above algorithms to analyze EEG data from a subject performing imagined left and right-hand movements. It is shown that the classification results based upon a 3-mode classifier with the Kalman Smoother initial conditions estimated by Expectation-Maximization, are superior to both the 2-mode classifier and to a Kalman Smoother that is initialized with arbitrary values.

The EEG data utilized for this analysis was recorded by Dr. Allen Osman from the University of Pennsylvania which was made available for the Neural Information Processing Systems (NIPS 2001) Brain-Computer Interface Workshop (Sajda *et al.*, 2003). This data consists of 59 channels of EEG signals sampled at 100Hz. The experimental protocol starts off with a blank screen for 2 seconds. This is followed by a fixation point for 500ms indicating the start of the trial. A letter 'E' or 'I', is then displayed for 250ms to indicate whether the subject is requested to perform an explicit or an imaginary movement. The fixation cross is shown again for 1s and in the next 250ms the subject is told whether to act with the left-hand, right-hand, both hands or not at all through the letters 'L', 'R', 'B', 'N' displayed on the screen. After another fixation cross presented for 1s, an 'X' appears for 50ms acting as the synchronization cue to perform the requested response. The trial ends with the fixation cross being displayed for the next 950ms. This analysis will utilize the EEG from channels C3 and C4 (10/20 electrode placement system) arising from the imagined left or right-hand movements of Subject 2, for which 90 left and 90 right-hand trials are available. In order to enhance spatial activity of the EEG, the Hjorth derivation is applied to the signals (Pfurtscheller & Lopes da Silva, 1999).

The Kalman Smoother algorithm is applied on this data so as to estimate the parameters of a 7th order AR model. For the purpose of comparative analysis, the initial conditions Φ, Q, R, x_0^0 and P_0^0 are set in two different ways:

a. an arbitrary initialization, with Φ set to be an identity matrix I, Q = 0.001xI, R = 1, $x_0^0 = 0$ and $P_0^0 = 10\text{x}I$,
b. using the Expectation-Maximization (EM) code provided by (Khan, 2007). This estimation starts off by using the Kalman Smoother. The EM algorithm is then used to estimate the initial conditions. Rather than working on each individual trial, the EM initialized parameters are found from all trials in the training set and an average is calculated. This allows for smoother estimates of the AR parameters. Once the EM initialized system parameters are obtained, they are fed to the Kalman Smoother to estimate the AR parameters of each trial in the data set.

3.1 A three-mode classification approach

The novel approach presented here is to consider that the process is characterized by three possible modes:

a. Background Mode; effective during the time period prior to 3.75s where the subject is told the type of movement to perform. At 3.75s, the subject is aware of the required task and hence the EEG characteristics are expected to change.

b. Left Movement Mode; effective from 3.75s up to 6s and characterized by ERD activity on the controlateral channel (C4) and no ERD activity on the ipsilateral channel (C3).
c. Right Movement Mode; effective from 3.75s up to 6s and characterized by ERD activity on the controlateral channel (C3) and no ERD activity on the ipsilateral channel (C4).

AR parameters are estimated for the whole 6s time period of each signal from channels C3 and C4, for both cases of left-hand and right-hand movement. For the case of arbitrary setting of initial conditions, these are kept fixed throughout the whole length of data irrespective of whether the EEG signal is in a background or a movement state. For classification purposes, a feature vector is generated by concatenating the AR parameters estimated from signals recorded at C3 and C4 respectively, leading to a 14-element feature vector. To train the classifier, the parameters at each time instant up to 3.75s are considered as Background Mode, whereas the parameters at C3 and C4 for each time instant between 3.75s and 6s for a left task are considered for the Left Movement Mode. Similarly, the parameters at C3 and C4 for each time instant between 3.75s and 6s for a right task are considered for the Right Movement Mode.

For the EM initialization approach, different initial conditions are estimated for each of the 3 modes of operation. Taking the EEG signal on channel C4 during a left task as an example, two sets of AR parameters are estimated; one obtained by using the initial conditions from the Background Mode and another obtained by using the initial conditions from the Left Movement Mode. Similarly for channel C3 during a right task, one set of AR parameters is estimated assuming Background Mode initial conditions and another set assuming Right Movement Mode initial conditions. These AR parameters are concatenated, leading to a 28-element feature vector in this case. The time periods used to train this classifier are the same as those for the arbitrary initialization.

The available 90-trial data was split into two: the first 45 trials were used for training and the rest for testing, for both imagined left and right-hand movements respectively. For comparative purposes, the classification results using both arbitrary initialization as well as initial conditions estimated by the EM algorithm will be shown next. For Background Mode classification results, the number of trials at each time instant between 0 and 3.75s which were classified as correct have been considered. For Left Movement and Right Movement Mode classification, the total number of correctly classified movement tasks at each time instant between 3.75s and 6s were considered. Figure 1 shows the percentage of correctly classified results for the case of arbitrary initialization. It is clear that for the Background Mode there occur frequent misclassifications as either a left or a right-hand movement. Classifications results improve to just below 80% at around 5s when the imagined movement is actually performed.

A significant improvement is obtained when the initial conditions are estimated with the Expectation-Maximization algorithm, as shown in the classification results of Figure 2. There is a significant improvement in the classification of the Background Mode because the estimated parameters are very smooth and differ from those during the movement periods. Classification is close to 100% during the first 2s but it reduces as the movement period approaches. At around 5s, when the movement is performed, the classification score approaches 90%, as opposed to 80% for the arbitrary initialization case.

Additional insight can be obtained by the construction of a confusion matrix. Table 1 and Table 2 show the confusion matrices for the two different initialization approaches. The arbitrarily initialized case leads to around 64% and 65% correct classification for left and right movement respectively and it performs very poorly when classifying the background period. Many of these time instances are classified as an imagined right-hand movement instead. The EM initialized case gives superior performance with background periods being identified with a score of 89%, a significant improvement on the 39% score of the previous case. There is also improvement in the classification of right and left-hand movement, where scores of 68% and 80% respectively, are obtained. As in the previous case, a number of left modes (around 22%) are incorrectly classified as right modes. These classification results compare well with the 76% overall classification obtained by Dornhege *et. al.* in the NIPS 2001 workshop, where a 2-mode classifier was used (Sajda *et al.*, 2003).

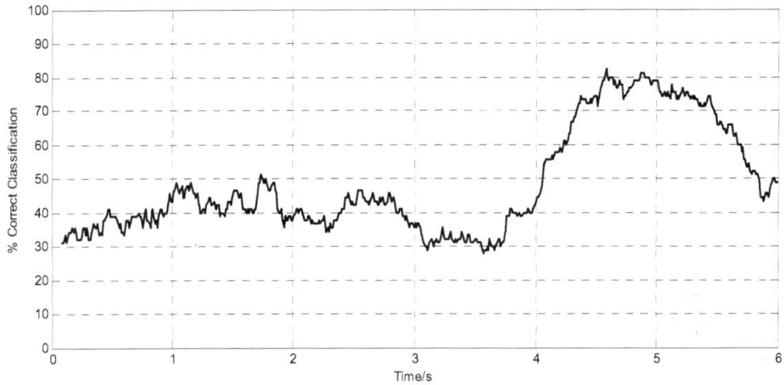

Fig. 1. Percentage correct classification for arbitrary initialization

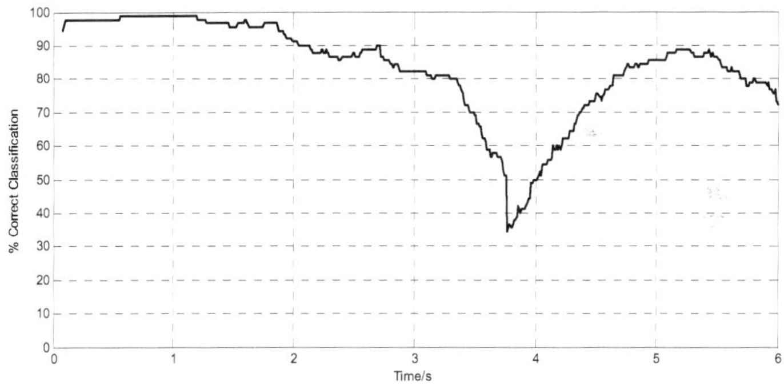

Fig. 2. Percentage correct classification for EM-based initialization

		Actual Mode		
		Background	Left	Right
Predicted Mode	Background	38.68%	14.52%	22.35%
	Left	24.11%	63.87%	12.76%
	Right	37.20%	21.51%	64.89%

Table 1. Confusion matrix for arbitrary initialization

		Actual Mode		
		Background	Left	Right
Predicted Mode	Background	89.32%	9.59%	8.96%
	Left	3.50%	68.12%	11.50%
	Right	7.19%	22.29%	79.89%

Table 2. Confusion matrix for EM-based initialization

3.2 Interpretation in terms of AR pole variation

Another contribution of this work centres on the analysis of the variation of the AR parameter estimates with time, together with the corresponding poles of the model, during the 6s time interval of the trial. The transfer function of the AR model in the z-domain is:

$$G(z) = \frac{1}{1 + \sum_{k=1}^{p} a_t^{(k)} z^{-k}} \tag{12}$$

The poles of the model are given by the roots of the denominator of Equation (12). These poles can therefore be calculated at every time instant from the AR parameter estimates $a_t^{(k)}$ and marked on a pole-zero plot whose x-axis represents the real part of the pole and the y-axis represents the imaginary part. The frequency associated with a given pole is proportional to the angle it subtends with the positive x-axis on the pole-zero plot.

The resulting poles obtained at each time instant for imagined left-hand trials are plotted in Figure 3 and 4, which show both the pole-zero plot and the variation of the magnitude of the poles with time. Note that the latter displays four plots instead of seven because 3 pairs of poles are complex conjugates and their magnitudes are equal. These poles are computed from the average of the AR parameters over the 90 available trails.

Figure 3(a) shows the poles obtained from the model fitted to data from channel C3 when the Kalman Smoother is initialized arbitrarily. Figure 3(b) follows the same pattern, but for channel C4. Figures 4(a) and 4(b) show the corresponding plots for the case of EM-based initialization.

An analysis of the pole variations gives some interesting insights on the EEG data which are otherwise not directly apparent from the AR parameter estimates. In all cases, the angle of the obtained poles indicates that there is concentrated activity at around 12Hz (alpha band), 24Hz (beta band) and 40Hz (gamma band). Activity in the alpha and beta bands is synonymous with this type of data (Pfurtscheller & Lopes da Silva, 1999). All plots also show that on the ipsilateral side (C3 for the case of left-hand trials) the poles do not vary much with time and that their magnitude remains fairly constant. This contrasts with the activity on the contralateral side (C4 for the case of left-hand trials) where, during the imagined hand movement, a significant decrease in the magnitude of the alpha and beta poles occurs. This indicates that on the contralateral side there is a significant change in pole magnitude between background and movement periods, which corresponds to ERD. This characteristic is correspondingly reflected in the trajectories of the poles shown in the pole-zero plots, which are more spread out on the contalateral side (C4) than the pole trajectories on the ipsilateral (C3) side.

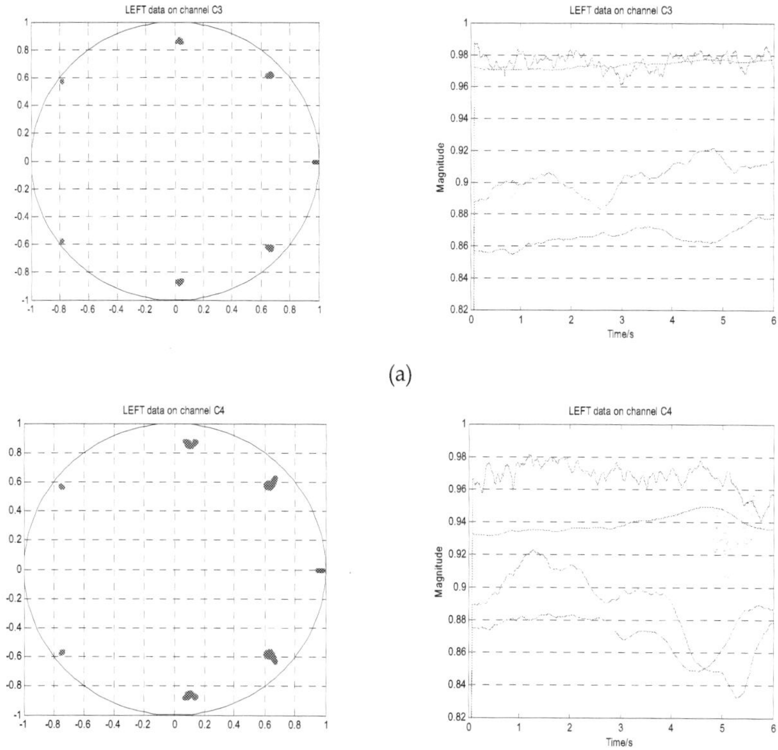

(a)

(b)

Fig. 3. Pole trajectories and magnitudes for imagined left-hand movement arising from arbitrary initialization. (a) corresponds to C3 and (b) corresponds to C4

4. Model order estimation

In system identification, the effectiveness of the model that is used to fit a data set depends critically on the determination of a suitable model order. There exist various techniques for the estimation of model order. These can be categorized into three main groups. One group is based on the prior estimation of model parameters using a set of candidate models of different order. Information criteria such as the Akaike Information Criterion or Minimum Description Length are then used to find the best compromise between model complexity and best fit within the candidate models of this set. These methods incur computational complexity due to the consideration of multiple candidate models.

Another group of methods, which do not require prior estimation of model parameters, use eigendecomposition of the input/output data covariance matrix to estimate the model order. This approach, based on the Minimum Description Length criterion, was applied to univariate ARMA and ARX models by Liang et al. (1993). The method was shown to be able

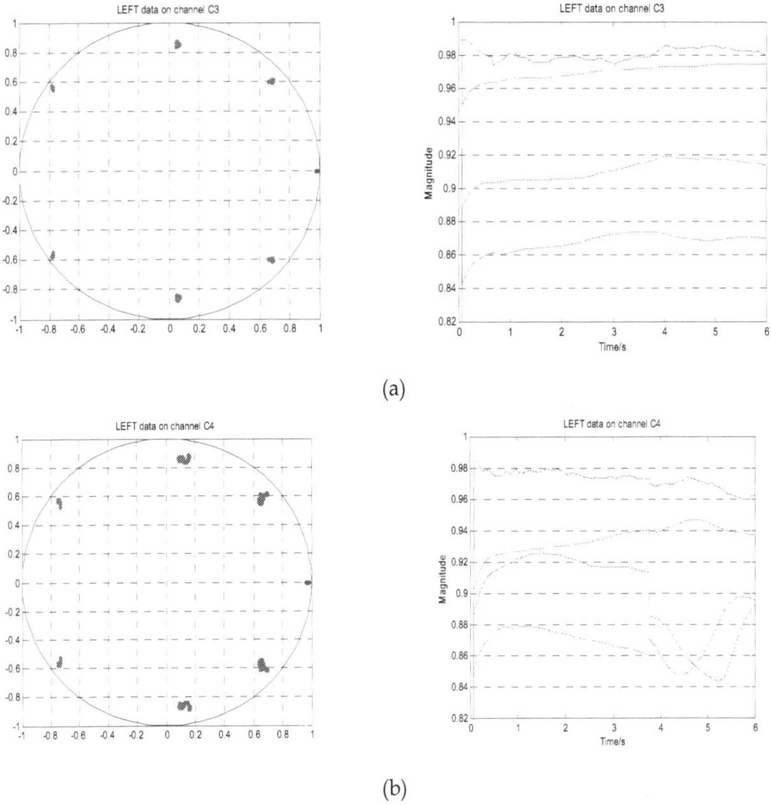

Fig. 4. Pole trajectories and magnitudes for imagined left-hand movement arising from EM-based initialization. (a) corresponds to C3 and (b) corresponds to C4

to estimate the correct model order even in the presence of limited noise conditions. These methods are more computationally efficient than the previous group. The third group of methods estimate the model order and model parameters simultaneously. They utilize a Bayesian approach and are normally very demanding computationally.

The work presented in this section, which is based on the second group of methods, proposes a modified criterion to that of (Liang *et al.*, 1993) which leads to a lower probability of error for model order estimation. As in (Lardies & Larbi, 2001), which extended Liang's method to multivariate AR models, this work will not be restricted to univariate models. However in (Lardies & Larbi, 2001), the effects of different model order, model parameters and data lengths are not investigated. In this work, an extensive Monte Carlo analysis will be applied in order to evaluate such effects. Finally the approach is applied to real EEG data recorded from a subject performing motor imagery tasks.

A multivariate ARMA model is given by the difference equation

$$y_t = -A_1 y_{t-1} - \ldots - A_p y_{t-p} + B_1 e_{t-1} + \ldots + B_q e_{t-q} + e_t + \upsilon_t \tag{13}$$

where $y_t \in R^n$ represents the output data on n channels measured at time t, A_i and $B_i \in R^{n \times n}$, represent the AR and MA parameter matrices respectively, p and q represent the AR and MA orders, $e_t \in R^n$ represents the input to the model which is a white Gaussian noise process having zero mean and covariance C, and $\upsilon_t \in R^n$, which represents observation or modeling error, is also a random white noise process having covariance Q_υ.
Extending the approach of (Liang *et al.*, 1993) to the multivariate case, assuming that N time samples of the output data are available, Equation (13) can be written as follows:

$$D_{p,q}\theta_{p,q} = \upsilon \tag{14}$$

where $D_{p,q}, \theta_{p,q}, \upsilon$ are defined as follows:

$$D_{p,q} = \begin{pmatrix} y_1^T & 0 & \cdots & 0 & e_1^T & 0 & \cdots & 0 \\ \vdots & y_1^T & \cdots & 0 & \vdots & e_1^T & & 0 \\ \vdots & \vdots & \cdots & & \vdots & \vdots & \cdots & \\ y_N^T & y_{N-1}^T & \cdots & y_{N-p}^T & e_N^T & e_{N-1}^T & \cdots & e_{N-q}^T \end{pmatrix} \tag{15}$$

$$\theta_{p,q} = \begin{pmatrix} A_0^T & \cdots & A_p^T & -B_0^T & \cdots & -B_q^T \end{pmatrix}^T \tag{16}$$

$$\upsilon = \begin{pmatrix} \upsilon_1^T & \cdots & \upsilon_N^T \end{pmatrix}^T \tag{17}$$

with A_0 and B_0 assumed to be identity matrices.
In order to compose the input/output matrix $D_{p,q}$, the unknown input signal e_t needs to be estimated. This could be done by preliminarily fitting a high order AR model to the output data y_t using a least squares approach to estimate the corresponding AR parameters. As explained in (Cassar *et al.*, 2010a), these AR parameters are next used to generate an estimate for e_t which, together with the output data, is used to compose $D_{p,q}$ as defined in Equation (15). This matrix is then used to generate the covariance data matrix $R_{p,q}$ defined as:

$$R_{p,q} = D_{p,q}^T D_{p,q} \tag{18}$$

The relevance of this matrix becomes evident when the Minimum Description Length criterion is used for the estimation of model order. This criterion strikes a compromise between model complexity and the maximum likelihood estimator of the parameters, by minimizing the following cost function:

$$J_{MDL}(p,q) = -\log f(\upsilon_1, \cdots, \upsilon_N) + 0.5n^2(p+q+1)\log N \tag{19}$$

where $f(\upsilon_1, \cdots, \upsilon_N)$ is the probability density function of noise υ. For a multivariate Gaussian model, this density function is given by the normal distribution equation:

$$f(\upsilon_1, \cdots, \upsilon_N) = \frac{1}{(2\pi)^{N/2}|Q_\upsilon|^{N/2}} \exp\left(-\frac{1}{2|Q_\upsilon|}\theta^T R_{p,q}\theta\right) \tag{20}$$

which, after substitution in (20), yields

$$J_{MDL}(p,q,\theta) = \frac{N}{2}\log 2\pi + \frac{N}{2}\log\left|Q_{\upsilon}\right| + \frac{1}{2Q_{\upsilon}}\theta^T R_{p,q}\theta + \frac{1}{2}n^2(p+q+1)\log N \tag{21}$$

Given a fixed model order (p,q), the covariance matrix Q_{υ} which minimizes Equation (21) is $Q_{\upsilon} = \theta^T R_{p,q}\theta$. As shown by (Lardis & Larbi, 2001), the minimum value of the determinant of Q_{υ} is obtained from an eigendecomposition of the covariance data matrix $R_{p,q}$ as follows:

$$R_{p,q} = \begin{bmatrix} V_L & V_S \end{bmatrix} \begin{bmatrix} \lambda_L & 0 \\ 0 & \lambda_S \end{bmatrix} \begin{bmatrix} V_L^T \\ V_S^T \end{bmatrix} \tag{22}$$

where λ_L is a diagonal matrix whose terms consist of the first $(p+q)n$ largest eigenvalues of $R_{p,q}$, the columns of V_L contain the corresponding eigenvectors, λ_S is a diagonal matrix whose terms are the $2n$ smallest eigenvalues and the columns of V_S contain the corresponding eigenvectors of $R_{p,q}$.

If an orthogonality constraint is imposed on θ, then the value of θ which minimizes (21) is the matrix of eigenvectors V_S which correspond to the smallest eigenvalues of $R_{p,q}$ (Lardis & Larbi, 2001). Due to the orthonormality of the eigenvectors, it turns out that $Q_{\upsilon} = \lambda_s$ and $\left|Q_{\upsilon}\right| = \prod_{i=1}^{n}\lambda_S(i)$. Following substitution in (21) and some manipulation, the following result is obtained

$$\frac{2}{N}J_{MDL}(p,q) = \log\left(\prod_{i=1}^{n}\lambda_S(i)\right)N^{n^2(p+q)/N} \tag{23}$$

An analysis of matrix J_{MDL} shows that the eigenvalues of $R_{p,q}$ are large for model orders less than the true order. By contrast, they decrease significantly for orders which are greater than the true order (Liang *et al.*, 1993). Hence if $J_{MDL}(p,q)$ is organized such that the AR order p increases along the columns and the MA order q increases along the rows, as shown in Figure 5, it will be possible to identify a 'corner' which corresponds to the true order of the multivariate model.

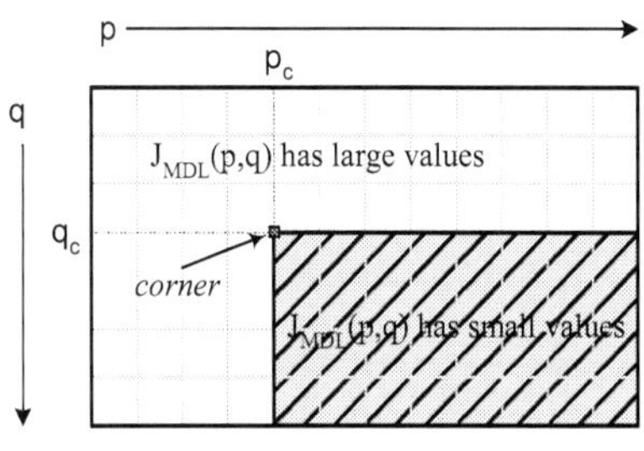

Fig. 5. The values of J_{MDL} for a range of p and q values. The corner gives the model order

For the univariate case, (Liang *et al.*, 1993) generate a column ratio (CR) and a row ratio (RR) table to identify the transition between the two regions shown in Figure 5. The CR entry at (p,q) is constructed by dividing $J_{MDL}(p-1,q)$ by $J_{MDL}(p,q)$. Similarly, the RR table is determined by dividing $J_{MDL}(p,q-1)$ by $J_{MDL}(p,q)$. The optimal model order is then chosen by taking the value of the p column which corresponds to the largest value in the CR table, and the value of q row which corresponds to the largest value in the RR table.

In the multivariate ARMA case, the situation becomes complicated because additional spurious peaks tend to appear in the CR and RR tables, thereby making it difficult to select the peak which actually corresponds to the corner that identifies the true model order. This phenomenon often gives rise to incorrect estimation of the model order. In order to address this problem, a modified criterion is proposed to enhance the value of the corner, as described next.

The CR and RR tables are constructed as described previously, but then an element-by-element product of these two tables is performed so as to generate a product matrix P_M. This has the tendency of enhancing the value of the true peak in matrix P_M, because it is reinforced by peaks appearing in the same location within both the CR and RR tables. On the other hand, the contribution of incorrect peaks is diminished because their location will not be consistent between the two tables. Nevertheless, experimental analysis has shown that there may be situations where the product matrix P_M exhibits a number of comparable peaks in close proximity, with the maximum peak not necessarily corresponding to the correct corner. Given that a significant change in value is expected between the point corresponding to the correct corner and its neighbours, the modified criterion also checks whether neighbouring locations exhibit a value that is relatively much smaller than the peak being analyzed. A relative difference corresponding to a factor of 5 was found to be suitable from Monte Carlo analysis. Hence the modified criterion can be described by the following algorithm:

1. Form the CR and RR tables by computing $J_{MDL}(p-1,q)/J_{MDL}(p,q)$ and $J_{MDL}(p,q-1)/J_{MDL}(p,q)$ respectively.
2. Perform an element by element product of CR and RR to generate the product matrix P_M.
3. Find the largest value in P_M and check whether its neighbours, corresponding to a one step increase in p and q satisfy the following conditions:
   a. $P_M(p,q) \geq 5P_M(p,q+1)$
   b. $P_M(p,q) \geq 5P_M(p+1,q)$
4. If the conditions in step 3 are satisfied, (p, q) are taken to be the model order. If the conditions in step 3 are not satisfied, recursively go through the other values of P_M in descending order until a (p, q) pair that satisfies both conditions (a) and (b) is found. This is chosen as the optimal model order.
5. If none of the values in P_M satisfy the above, recursively reduce the factor of 5 appearing on the right-hand side of the equations in conditions (a) and (b) above, until the correct corner, and hence optimal model order, is identified.

4.1 Performance analysis

Probability arguments were applied in (Cassar *et al.*, 2010a) to show that the modified criterion proposed in the previous section has less chance of model order estimation error than the criterion proposed by (Liang *et al.*, 1993). Cassar *et al.* showed that if Liang's criterion estimates q correctly and the proposed criterion does not, then Liang's criterion would always estimate p incorrectly except for one specific exceptional condition. Similarly, if Liang's criterion estimates p correctly and the proposed criterion does not, then Liang's criterion would always estimate q incorrectly except for a second, very specific exceptional condition. Extensive Monte Carlo trials demonstrated that the probability of occurrence of the above-mentioned two exceptional conditions is close to zero *i.e.* there were no cases during the Monte Carlo trials where the proposed criterion gave an error while Liang's criterion did not. This led to the conclusion that the probability of error of the proposed criterion is bounded above by the probability of error of Liang's criterion (Cassar *et al.*, 2010a).

In order to evaluate the proposed order estimation technique, Monte Carlo analysis was performed. One hundred different two-channel, minimum phase ARMA models with p = 2 and q = 2 were generated. The magnitude of the poles and zeros of these models was randomly chosen within the range of 0.6 to 0.99, and their phase between 1 degree and 180 degrees. Each of these models was subjected to different random realizations of e_t, υ_t. The Monte Carlo trials were conducted with different signal-to-noise ratios (SNR). 2000 samples were considered for each model. The order of the preliminary AR model used to estimate the input signal e_t was set to 10. The proposed modified criterion and Liang's criterion were applied and, in both cases, the percentage amount of correctly estimated model orders was noted.

The results are shown in Table 3. Note the improvement in performance obtained by using the proposed criterion, where the percentage of correct hits always exceeds Liang's criterion, even with low SNR. For every model, the mean square error between the true and estimated model order was calculated across the 2000 samples. The mean and standard deviation of these errors across the 100 different models were then calculated and are shown in the last two columns of Table 3. Once again, note the improved performance of the modified criterion with order estimation error being consistently lower on average, than that of Liang's criterion. The difference between the errors obtained from the two criteria was tested for statistical significance by means of a *t*-Test. With a significance level of 0.05, the results from the no noise case up to the case with SNR of 10dB, indicate that the difference between the errors of the two criteria is indeed statistically significant.

SNR/dB	**Percentage of Correct Hits**		**Mean Error ± Std. Dev.**	
	Liang's Criterion	Modified Criterion	Liang's Criterion	Modified Criterion
no noise	32	97	0.50± 0.35	0.03± 0.17
25	44	94	0.43± 0.39	0.06± 0.24
20	39	90	0.49± 0.41	0.09± 0.29
15	38	83	0.55± 0.45	0.16± 0.35
10	28	59	0.69± 0.44	0.39± 0.48
5	15	29	0.83± 0.36	0.81± 0.76

Table 3. Results of Monte Carlo analysis utilizing 100 models

4.2 Results with EEG data

The proposed technique was applied on a real EEG measurements obtained from data set 3a of the BCI Competition III where a subject performed a cued motor imagery task while EEG

was recorded from 60 channels at a sampling frequency of 250Hz. The data was bandpass filtered between 1 and 50Hz by a notch filter. The subject, facing a computer screen, was asked to perform one of four possible imaginary movements: left-hand, right-hand, foot or tongue. For this analysis, only the trials for left-hand and right-hand movement were considered. 36 left-hand and 36 right-hand artifact-free trials were averaged over the 4s period during which movement is performed, utilizing data from channels C3 and C4.
A multivariate ARMA model was set up to capture the dynamics of this data. The proposed modified criterion was then applied, which estimated a model order of $p = 2$ and $q = 1$. The product matrix P_M which gave rise to this model order is shown in Figure 6, exhibiting a distinctive peak at the location corresponding to the recommended model order. For comparison purposes, the classical Akaike Information Criterion was also applied to estimate the model order for this data. The Akaike criterion estimated the same model order as the proposed criterion ($p = 2$ and $q = 1$). However, the computational efficiency of the proposed criterion is superior to that of the Akaike criterion. The former took 0.6 seconds of processing time to generate the model order result, whereas the latter required approximately 4 seconds (both tests performed on an Intel Core 2 Duo PC having a 2GHz processor and 2 GB RAM).

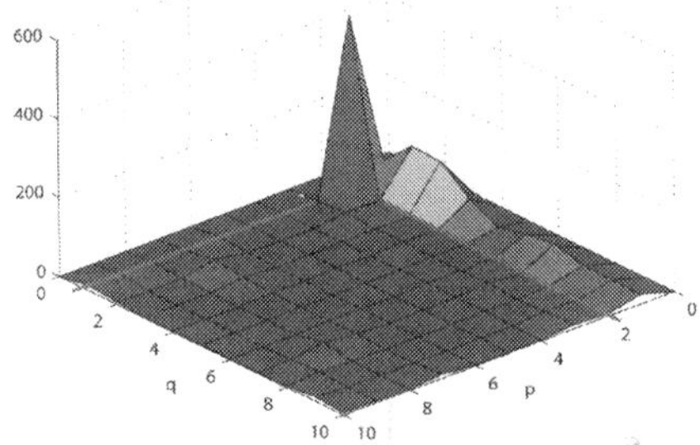

Fig. 6. The product matrix P_M for the EEG data obtained from the modified criterion

Using this recommended model order, the parameters of the ARMA model were then estimated using a Kalman filter initialized by the EM algorithm. This model was used to reconstruct the data within a frequency range of 0 to 45Hz. Auto and cross spectra of the original data and the reconstructed data were then calculated for model evaluation purposes. These are shown in Figure 7, indicating clearly that the recommended model order captures well the dynamics of the EEG data.

5. Conclusion

This chapter has investigated the use of parametric models for the identification of mental tasks from EEG data, with specific emphasis on linear modelling techniques. Following a brief review of relevant papers which appear in the literature, it was shown how improved classification results can be obtained from EEG data recorded during imagined hand movement trials. This improvement is the result of a 3-mode classifier which makes use of AR parameters estimated during periods of left movement, right movement and inactivity, together with a Kalman Smoother initiated by the Expectation-Maximization algorithm.

In addition it was shown how the trajectories of the poles of the AR model relate with ERD phenomena pertaining to imagined hand movements, in a more direct way than the model parameters. Finally a new model order selection criterion was proposed for the multivariate ARMA case, which is more accurate than alternative criteria developed for univariate ARMA. The efficacy of the proposed criterion was exhibited with extensive Monte Carlo analysis under different conditions of signal-to-noise ratio.

The use of EEG data for the identification of mental tasks carries with it several interesting possibilities for future applications. From these possibilities, brain-computer interfacing is one of the leading and most challenging ones. One hopes that the improvements documented in this chapter, together with other techniques which are continuously being developed by the research community, would contribute to the advancement of brain-computer interface technology so as to make it more practical, robust and realistic.

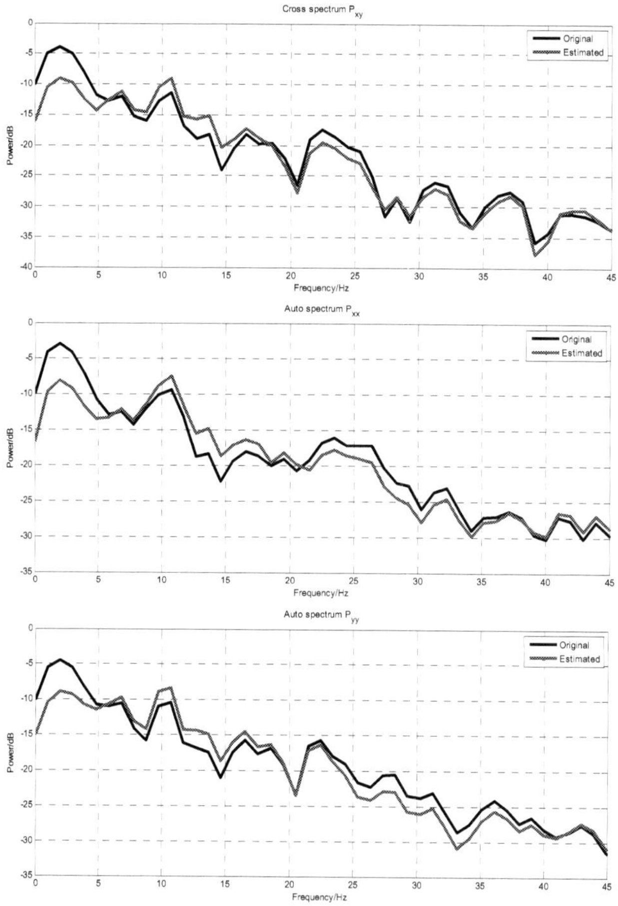

Fig. 7. Cross and auto spectra of the original EEG averaged data and the reconstructed data from the estimated model

6. References

Anderson, C. W.; Stolz, E. A. & Shamsunder, S. (1998). Multivariate Autoregressive Models for Classification of Spontaneous Electroencephalogram During Mental Tasks, *IEEE Transactions on Biomedical Engineering*, 45(3), 277-286.

Arnold, M.; Miltner, W. H. R.; Witte, H.; Bauer, R. & Braun, C. (1998). Adaptive AR Modeling of Nonstationary Time Series by Means of Kalman Filtering, *IEEE Transactions on Biomedical Engineering*, 45(5), 553-562.

Atry, F.; Omidvarnia, A.H. & Kamaledin Setarehdan, S. (2005). Model Based EEG Signal Purification to Improve the Accuracy of the BCI Systems, *Proceedings of the 13th European Signal Processing Conference EUSIPCO*, Antalya, Turkey.

Bohlin, T. (1973). Comparison of Two Methods of Modeling Stationary EEG Signals, *IBM J. Res. Dev.*, 17(3), 194-205.

Burke, D.P.; Kelly, S.P.; de Chazal P.; Reilly, R.B. and Finucane, C. (2005). A Parametric Feature Extraction and Classification Strategy for Brain-computer Interfacing, *IEEE Transactions on Neural Systems and Rehabilitation Engineering*, 13(1), 12-17.

Cassar, T.; Camilleri, K. P. & Fabri, S. G. (2010a). Order Estimation of Multivariate ARMA Models, *IEEE Journal of Selected Topics in Signal Processing*, 4(3), 494-503.

Cassar, T.; Camilleri, K. P. & Fabri, S. G. (2010b), Three-mode Classification and Study of AR Pole Variations of Imaginary Left and Right Hand Movements, *Proceedings of the Biomed 2010 Conference*, Austria.

Galka, A.; Yamashita, O.; Ozaki, T.; Biscay, R. & Valdes-Sosa, P. (2004). A solution to the dynamical inverse problem of EEG generation using spatiotemporal Kalman filtering, *NeuroImage*, 23, 435-453.

Huan, N.J. & Palaniappan, R. (2005). Classification of Mental Tasks Using Fixed and Adaptive Autoregressive Models of EEG Signals, *Proceedings of the 2nd International IEEE EMBS Conference on Neural Engineering*, Arlington, Virginia, 633-636.

Inoue, K.; Kajikawa, R.; Nakamura, T.; Pfurthscheller, G. & Kumamaru, K. (2004). EEG Signal Analysis Based on Quasi-AR Model - Application to EEG Signals during Right and Left Motor Imagery, *Proceedings of the SICE Annual Conference*, Japan, 2197-2201.

Isaksson, A.; Wennberg, A. & Zetterberg L.H. (1981). Computer Analyis of EEG Signals with Parametric Models, *Proceedings of the IEEE*, 69(4), 451-461.

Jain, S. & Deshpande, G. (2004). Parametric Modeling of Brain Signals, *Biotechnology and Bioinformatics, 2004. Proceedings. Technology for Life: North Carolina Symposium on , 85- 91.*

Kelley, S.; Burke, D.; de Chazal, P. & Reilly R. (2002). Parametric Models and Spectral Analysis for Classification in Bran-computer Interfaces, *Proceedings of the 14th International Conference on Digital Signal Processing*, Greece.

Khan, M.E. (2007). http://people.cs.ubc.ca/~emtiyaz/software.html [last visited Sep 2010].

Khan, M. E. & Dutt, D. N. (2007). An Expectation-Maximization Algorithm Based Kalman Smoother Approach for Event-Related Desynchronization (ERD) Estimation from EEG, *IEEE Transactions on Biomedical Engineering*, 54(7), 1191-1198.

Krystal, A. D.; Prado, R. & West. M. (1999). New Methods of Time Series Analysis of Non-Stationary EEG Data: Eigenstructure Decompositions of Time Varying Autoregressions, *Clinical Neurophysiology*, 110(12), 2197-2206.

Lardies, J. & Larbi, N. (2001). A new method for model order selection and modal parameter estimation in time domain, *Journal of Sound and Vibration*, 245(2), 187-203.

Li, X. (2007). Complexity and Synchronization Measures of EEG with a Time Varying Parametric Model, *Life Science Data Mining (Wong, S. & Li, C-S. Eds.)*, World Scientific Press, Chapter 5.

Liang, G; Wilkes, D. M. & Cadzow, J. A. (1993). ARMA Model Order Estimation Based on the Eigenvalues of the Covariance Matrix, *IEEE Transactions on Signal Processing*, Vol. 41, No. 10, 3003-3009.

Maybeck, P.S. (1979). *Stochastic Models, Estimation and Control*, Academic Press, San Diego.

Palaniappan, R.; Raveendran, P.; Nishida, S. & Saiwaki, N. (2000). Autoregressive Spectral Analysis and Model Order Selection Criteria for EEG Signals, *TENCON 2000 Proceedings, vol.2, 126-129.*

Pardey, J.; Roberts, S. & Tarassenko, L. (1996). A Review of Parametric Modelling Techniques for EEG Analysis, *Med. Eng. Phys.*, 18, 2-11.

Pei, X-M. & Zheng C-X. (2004). Feature Extraction and Classification of Brain Motor Imagery Task Based on MVAR Model, *Proceedings of the Third International Conference on Machine Learning and Cybernetics*, Shanghai, 3726-3730.

Penny, W.D.; Roberts S.J. & Stokes M.J. (1998). Imagined hand movements identified from the EEG mu-rhythm, *Technical Report TR-98-1.*

Pfurtscheller, G. & Lopes da Silva, F. H. (1999). *Handbook of Electroencephalography and Clinical Neurophysiology: Event Related Desynchronization*, Elsevier, 044482999 7 (volume), 0444 80125 1 (series).

Pfurtscheller, G.; Graimann, B. & Neuper, C. (2006). EEG-Based Brain-Computer Interface System, *Wiley Encyclopedia of Biomedical Engineering (Akay, M. Ed.)*, Wiley, 978 0471 740360.

Popivanov, D.; Mineva, A. & Dushanova, A. (1998). Tracking EEG Signal Dynamics During Mental Tasks, *IEEE Engineering in Medicine and Biology*, 17(2), 89-94.

Poulos, M.; Rangoussi, M.; Alexandris, N. & Evangelou A. (2010). Person Identification from the EEG using Nonlinear Signal Classification, *Methods of Information in Medicine*, Issue 4, 64-75.

Qin, L.; Deng, J.; Ding, L. & He, B. (2004). Motor Imagery Classification by Means of Source Analysis Methods, *Proceedings of the 26th Annual International Conference of the IEEE Engineering in Medicine and Biology Society*, Vol.2, 4356-4358.

Rezek, I. (2006). Multivariate Biomedical Signal Processing, *Wiley Encyclopedia of Biomedical Engineering (Akay, M. Ed.)*, Wiley, 978 0471 249672.

Sajda, P.; Gerson A.; Mueller K. R.; Blankertz B. & Parra L. (2003). A data analysis competition to evaluate machine learning algorithms for use in brain computer interfaces, *IEEE Trans Neural Syst. Rehabil. Eng.*, 11(2), 184-185.

Shloegl, A.; Neuper, C & Pfurtscheller G. (1997). Subject Specific EEG Patterns During Motor Imaginary, *Engineering in Medicine and Biology Society, 1997. Proceedings of the 19th Annual International Conference of the IEEE , vol.4, pp.1530-1532.*

Shloegl, A. & Supp, G. (2006). Analyzing Event-related EEG Data With Multivariate Autoregressive Parameters, *Progress in Brain Research*, Vol. 159, Elsevier, 0079-6123, 135-147.

Tarvainen, M. P.; Ranta-aho, P. O.; Karjalainen, P. A. (2001). Time-Varying ARMA modelling of Nonstationary EEG using Kalman Smoother Algorithm, *Proceedings of the 2001 Finnish Signal Processing* Symposium, FinSig01, 28-31.

20

Automatic Detection of Paroxysms in EEG Signals using Morphological Descriptors and Artificial Neural Networks

Christine F. Boos, Fernando M. de Azevedo
Geovani R. Scolaro and Maria do Carmo V. Pereira
University Federal of Santa Catarina
Brazil

1. Introduction

The first recordings of brain activity in the form of electrical signals, through the use of a galvanometer and insertion of two electrodes on the scalp of an individual, were conducted in 1875 by British scientist Richard Caton. Since then, the electroencephalogram (EEG) has been used to denote the neural electrical activity of the brain (Sanei & Chambers, 2007).
The EEG signal acquisition can be performed by introducing electrodes inside the brain tissue (depth EEG), the placement of electrodes directly into the exposed surface of the cerebral cortex (electrocorticogram - ECoG) or the positioning of electrodes in a non-invasive, on the surface of the scalp (scalp EEG - sEEG).
The human scalp EEG, in relation to its physical characteristics, occupies a frequency band of 0Hz to 100 Hz and an amplitude range of 2μV to 200μV, however, in general, the signal is concentrated between 0,5Hz and 60Hz with an average amplitude of 50μV (Coimbra, 1994).
These frequency and amplitude value of the EEG signal are influenced by a series of characteristics, such as: location in the cerebral cortex from where recording was acquired, age of the subject, physical (sleep, wake, coma, etc.) and behavioral (depression, excitement, euphoria, stress, etc.) state of the subject. Furthermore, the signal can also be distorted by artifacts interference from many sources, for example, extra cerebral electrical potentials from the patient, the electrodes, the signal acquisition system and external electromagnetic interferences. This means that the recordings may have variability among patients under identical circumstances and in the same patient over time. The presence of this variability contributes to the great difficulty presented in attempts to mathematically model the electrographic patterns commonly present in the EEG signal. Nevertheless these patterns have a relative regularity in frequency, morphology and amplitude - whichever they are - i.e. the frequency spectrum of the EEG is usually divided into frequency bands that may be related to different physical states and behavior (Sanei & Chambers, 2007):

- alpha band - 8 to 13 Hz - common rhythm in normal patients and more easily observable while the subject is awake, relaxed and with its eyes closed;
- beta band - 13 to 22 Hz - common rhythm in normal adult patients during wakefulness. Dominant in the pre-central region of the brain but also occurs in other brain regions. Subdivided into: beta I, 13 to 17 Hz - present during intense

activation of central nervous system (CNS) - and beta II, 18 to 22 Hz - decreases during intense activation of the CNS;

- theta band – 4 to 8 Hz – rhythm frequent in children, in central and temporal region of the brain. Typical of early stages of sleep. Some transient components of this rhythm have been found in normal adult patients;
- delta band – 0,5 to 4 Hz – common rhythm in children, especially infants, in a state of deep sleep. The presence of this wave in adults under a state of alert may indicate abnormalities.

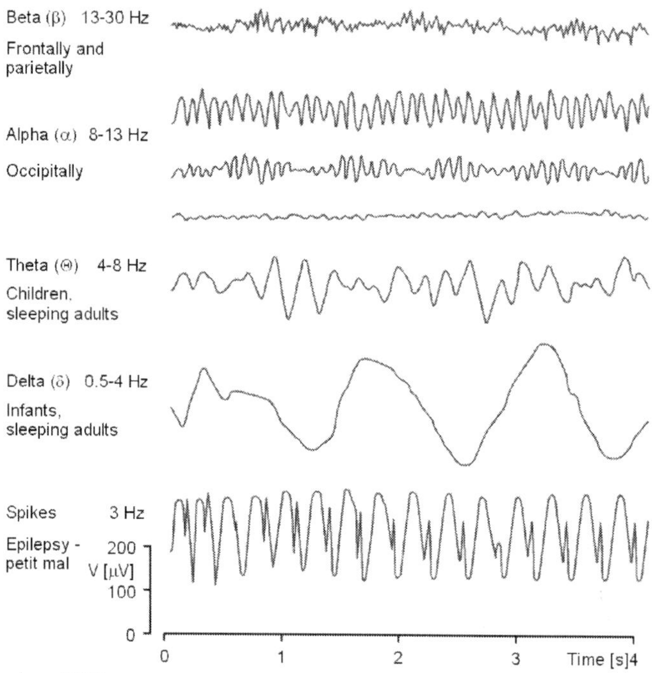

(Sanei & Chambers, 2007)

Fig. 1. Examples of common electrographic patterns present in the EEG signal

The EEG recording has applicability on, among others: monitoring alertness, coma and brain death; locating damaged areas after head injury, stroke and tumor; testing afferent pathways; monitoring anesthesia depth; researching physiology and sleep disorders; researching epilepsy and localizing the seizure focus (Sanei & Chambers, 2007).

Epilepsy is a disorder of the brain characterized by an enduring predisposition to generate epileptic seizures and by the neurobiological, cognitive, psychological and social consequences of this condition. The definition of epilepsy requires the occurrence of at least one epileptic seizure, which is a transient occurrence of signs and/or symptoms due to abnormal excessive or synchronous neuronal activity in the brain (Fisher et al., 2005).

Neurologists can make a diagnosis of epilepsy simply through anamneses however EEG signal analysis is a commonly used and important tool to: clinical diagnosis, support in

defining the type of epilepsy syndrome, provide information for planning drug therapy and also help in deciding the feasibility of surgical intervention.
The occurrence of certain electrographic events, called epileptiform events, in EEG signal is a strong indicator of this pathology presence. An expert in reading these records (EEGer) spends a considerable amount of time reviewing each record, especially when they are acquired for long term monitoring (more than 24 hours) and with many channels - between 24 and 128 leads (Pillay & Sperling, 2006).
In attempt to facilitate the analysis of EEG recordings by neurologists (or other experts) many studies have proposed automated systems for this analysis. Unfortunately few of them are actually being used worldwide mainly because the available systems for automatic detection of epileptiform events have a relative high number of false identifications (false positives), resulting in little or no effective time save for the process (Wilson & Emerson, 2002). This means that the low specificity of the systems still discourages EEGers to delegate the task of thorough analysis of the thousands of EEG screens (each with up to 128 continuous signals) in the search for events whose maximum length is 200ms and the amplitude values are in the range of microvolts (μV).

2. Automatic detection of paroxysms

The Biomedical Engineering Institute (IEB-UFSC) of the Federal University of Santa Catarina (UFSC) has as one of their areas of expertise and interest the acquisition, analysis and processing of bioelectrical signals, with emphasis in electroencephalogram (EEG), electrocardiogram (ECG), electromyogram (EMG) and electrooculogram (EOG) signals. Currently within this area there are two research lines, both using neural networks, for automatic detection of epileptiform events: one applies methodologies based on Wavelet Transform and the other one uses a parameterization[1] of the EEG signal.

2.1 Approaches based on wavelet transform

The Wavelet Transform is a tool that allows you to make a more comprehensive analysis of the signal due to the fact that it is possible to obtain information in both time and frequency domains simultaneously. This Transform is a powerful tool for the analysis of non-stationary signals (Wilson et al., 2004) making it ideal for EEG signal analysis. Its basic principle of operation is extract approximation and detail coefficients of the signal at each decomposition carried out, i.e., get high and low frequencies features of the signal for each level of decomposition. Wavelet Transform can be used for the parameterization, filtering and/or feature extraction of the EEG signals and also be very involved in the construction of hybrid intelligent systems for the automatic detection of epileptiform events, providing relatively good results when applied as a preprocessor for Artificial Neural Networks (Kalayci & Özdamar, 1995; Hoffmann et al., 1996; Oweiss & Anderson, 2001; Quiroga et al . 2001; Adeli et al., 2003; Khan & Gotman, 2003; Argoud et al., 2006, Pang et al., 2003, Liu et al., 2006; Argoud et al., 2006; Mohamed et al., 2006; Subasi, 2007; Indiradevi et al., 2008; Ocak, 2008; Abibullaev et al., 2009th, 2009b; Ocak, 2009; Scolaro & Azevedo, 2010).

---

[1] In this study, the term parameterization refers to the representation of an EEG signal by means of parameters related to morphological characteristics of this signal and these parameters will be called morphological descriptors.

2.2 Approaches based on parameterization of the signal

A comparative study of various algorithms used in automatic detection methods, conducted by Wilson and Emerson in 2002, showed that the methods use some form of parameterization of the EEG signal usually get good results.

The first studies involving the parameterization as a tool for the detection of epileptiform events in EEG recording were published by Gotman and Gloor (Gotman, 1976; Gotman & Gloor, 1982) followed by the research of Webber (1994), Walckzak & Nowack (2001), Litt (2001) and Tzallas et al. (2006) among others that have obtained promising results.

However with the advances in mathematical methods and the increasing capacity of computer processing the investigations were directed to other approaches (Halford, 2009), for example, the Wavelet Transform, entropy, statistical methods and/or a combination of these and other methods (Kaneko et al. 1999; Diambra, 1999, Liu et al., 2002; Saab & Gotman, 2005; Tzallas et al., 2006; Übeyli, 2009; Kumar, 2010). Nevertheless we did not abandon the parameterization approach (Guedes et al., 2002, Pereira 2003, Pereira et al., 2003; Sovierzoski, 2009, Boos et al., 2010a, 2010b).

According to the literature, so far one of the most used and successful methods applied in systems for automatic detection of paroxysms is Gotman's (Hoef et al., 2010). This method performs spike modeling through parameters, that in this work will be called morphological descriptors[2], before detection. Gotman's method deals with the EEG signal by dividing it into segments and sequences, both ascending and descending, which are categorized by duration, absolute amplitude and length variation coefficient (which gives information on the cadency of the EEG). In this system, the detection of a paroxysm occurs when the descriptors' values for each epoch exceeds a pre-determined threshold.

Although the literature allows access to various studies that use morphological descriptors to characterize the EEG signal, it is necessary a detailed analysis of the applicability, relevance and effectiveness of each descriptor that will be used.

Therefore our objective is to discuss a methodology for the preparation and evaluation of a set of descriptors for modeling paroxysms through the use of descriptors that are already available in the literature as well as others proposed by us in attempt to improve the differentiation between epileptiform events and other electrographic manifestations that occur in the signal.

3. Methodology

This section will present the recordings and methodologies used for both the development of the descriptors' ensemble and the experiments used as an evaluation tool for the proposed set.

3.1 EEG recordings

All of the EEG signals used in this study belong to a database with nine records acquired from seven adult patients with confirmed diagnosis of epilepsy. They have a sampling frequency of 100Hz and were acquired through 24 (1 record) and 32 channels (8 records).

A bipolar montage (Fig. 2.) type zygomatic-temporal (Zygo-Db-Temp) was used, with 25 electrodes in positions Zy1, Zy2, Fp1, Fp2, F3, F4, F7, F8, F9, F10, CZ, C3, C4, T3, T4, T5, T6,

---

[2] The use of the term morphological descriptor is because we believe that this term is more appropriate within the context of parameters referring to morphological characteristics of a signal.

T9, T10, P3, P4, P9, P10, O1, O2 of the 10/20 system and two electrodes positioned for acquisition of electrooculogram (EOG).

For the acquisition process the signals went through analog filtering to isolate the range of 0,5 to 40Hz. We also observed the need to perform additional filtering to remove the baseline wandering effect (DC frequency - 0Hz) and eliminate noise caused by power line interference (60Hz), and it was necessary to perform interpolation of the signal to a sampling frequency of 200Hz.

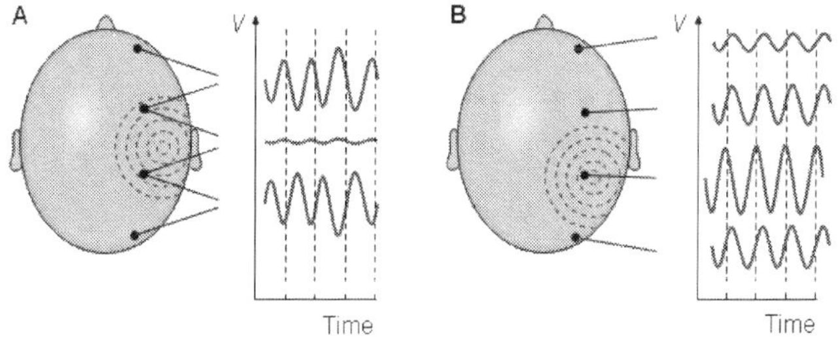

(Malmivuo & Plonsey, 1995)

Fig. 2. EEG signal differences presented when a bipolar (A) and unipolar or referential (B) montage is used. In the bipolar montage the signal is a result of potential difference between pairs of electrodes while for the unipolar montage the signal is obtained by the difference in potential between an electrode and a reference point (equal for the whole montage)

3.2 Morphological descriptors

The literature on the automatic detection of epileptiform events contains a considerable amount of morphological descriptors used in different methodologies and/or developed systems. For our experiments we selected the descriptors most reported in literature: the maximum amplitude of the event, event duration, the length variation coefficient, crest factor and entropy.

The maximum amplitude and duration of the event are self-explanatory. The length variation coefficient - used to measure the regularity of the signal - is the ratio of standard deviation and the mean value of the signal. The crest factor is the difference between the maximum and minimum amplitudes, divided by the standard deviation (Webber et al., 1994). The entropy, reported in several studies - e.g. Quiroga (1998), Esteller (2000), Srinivasan et al. (2007) and Naghsh-Nilchi & Aghashahi (2010) - provides a value for the complexity of the signal under analysis.

These descriptors are widely used, however they may not guarantee the complete differentiation between the events presented by the recordings and also because of this the existing systems for automatic detection have only a moderate performance. Thus, through a detailed analysis of the EEG signals that are being used, new descriptors based on the physical and/or morphological signal can be developed in attempt to improve the performance of the automatic detection process.

The main focus for the development of new descriptors was to find characteristics in the EEG signals that further highlighted the epileptiform events from other types of events. The latter are called non-epileptiform events (Fig. 3.) and for our database they are represented by:

a. normal background EEG activity;
b. alpha waves;
c. blinks;
d. artifacts originated from EMG (muscle activity), external electromagnetic interference, among others.

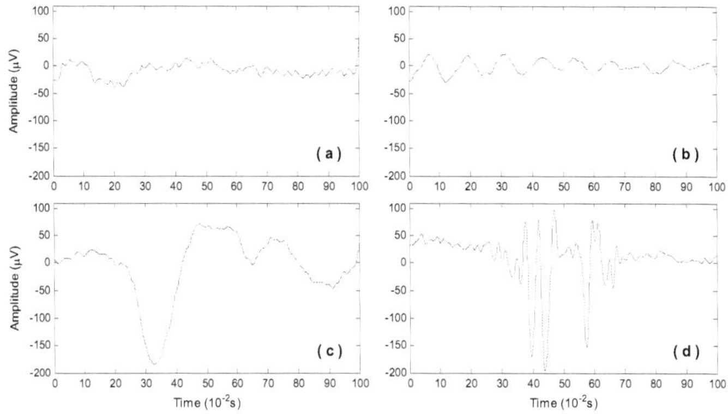

Fig. 3. Morphology of the main non-epileptiform events found in our EEG signals database

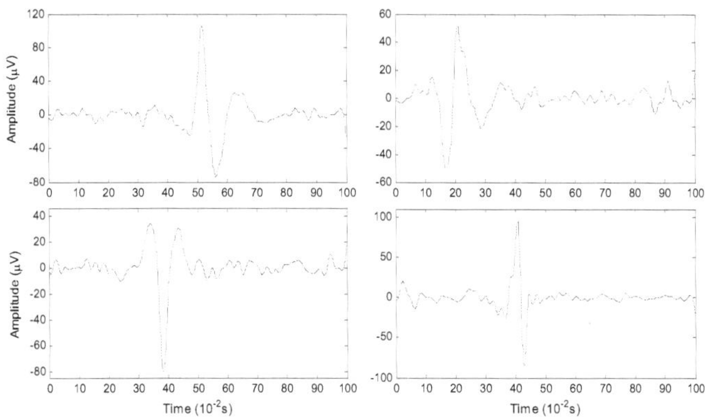

Fig. 4. Morphology presented by the epileptiform events in the recordings under analysis

Looking at the obtained records we realized that due to the use of a bipolar montage (Fig.2) the epileptiform events can appear in four different ways (Fig. 4.). In other words, because of the type of montage the spikes and sharp waves may appear with both electronegative and electropositives amplitude peaks, however to be considered a paroxysm they still have to be followed by a slow wave.

The basic morphological characteristics of an epileptic event are related to their amplitude and duration. The spikes have duration of 20 to 70ms, while a sharp wave has duration of 70 to 200ms. Since both events can be a paroxysm and making a distinction between them makes little sense from a clinical point of view, we can consider that the duration epileptiform events varies from 20 to 200ms. The amplitudes values of both spikes and sharp waves are also varied but when considering them epileptiform events the amplitude (module value) usually lies between 20μV and 200μV (Niedermeyer, 2005). Examples of morphological descriptors related to the amplitude and duration of a typical epileptiform event are (Fig. 5.):

- maximum amplitude (Amax);
- minimum amplitude (Bmin);
- difference between the points of occurrence of extreme amplitude (Tdif);
- difference between the maximum and minimum amplitudes (DifAB).

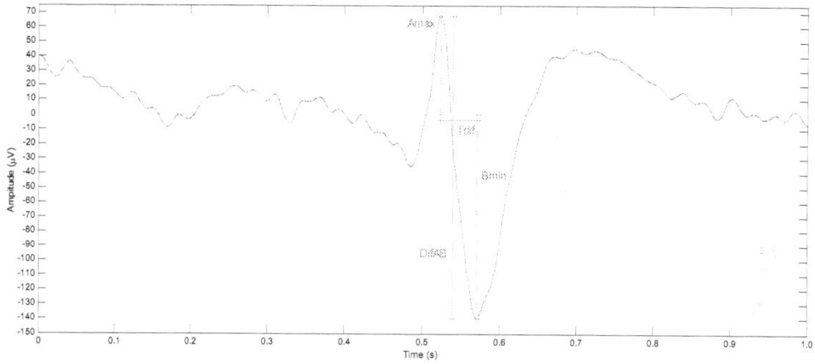

Fig. 5. Morphological descriptors related to the amplitude and duration of paroxysms

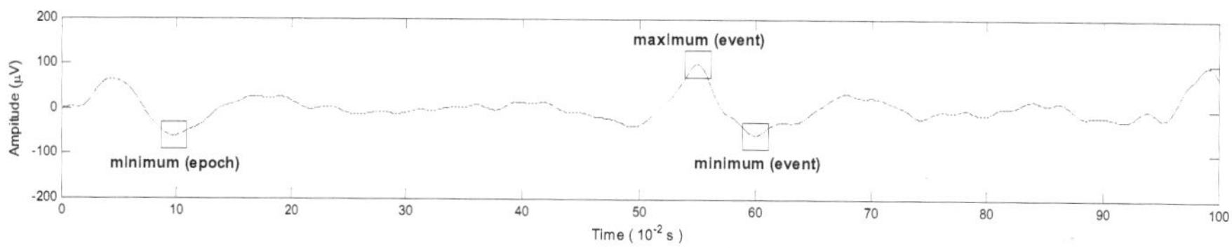

Fig. 6. EEG signal presenting maximum amplitude corresponding to an epileptiform event and minimum amplitude corresponding to another (different) event

Also regarding the amplitudes within the epoch under review (in this case 1 second of the signal) the points of maximum and minimum amplitude may not belong to the same event (Fig. 6.). Analyzing this fact, we could see that to be a paroxysm (event we want to correctly identify) the event should have a time difference between maximum and minimum amplitudes in the range of 35 to 100ms (half duration the slowest event). For this, as illustrated in Fig 7, we determined a 300ms segment centered at the event appearing in the epoch under review and within this segment we calculated the following descriptors: maximum amplitude (Amax_pts); minimum amplitude (Bmin_pts); distance between extreme amplitudes (DifAB_pts) and time difference (Tdif_pts) between the maximum and minimum amplitudes.

Another feature that can be observed is that an epileptiform event, particularly the spike, has more acute peaks when compared to the obtuse peaks of alpha waves or blinks (Fif. 3b and Fig. 3c). This fact allows another opportunity to discriminate between events since the

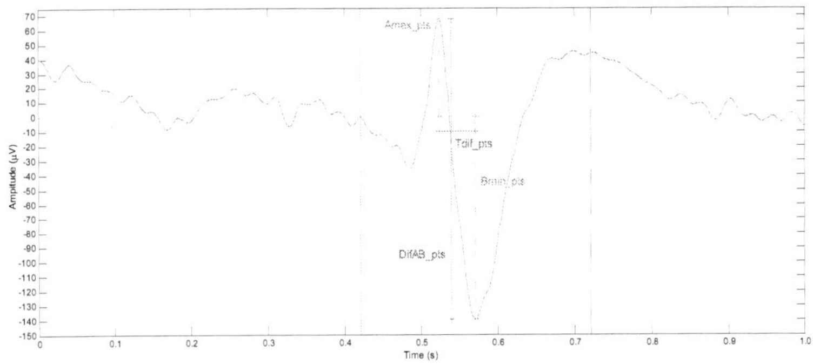

Fig. 7. Maximum amplitude (Amax_pts), minimum amplitude (Bmin_pts), distance between extreme amplitudes (Tdif_pts) and time difference between amplitudes (DifAB_pts), all within the 300ms segment centered on the event under analysis

process of automatic detection can confused them, which is a detrimental factor to the system performance. Based on these observations we analyzed the vertex angle of the peaks through the extreme amplitudes and zero crossing points adjacent to the beginning and the end of the event.

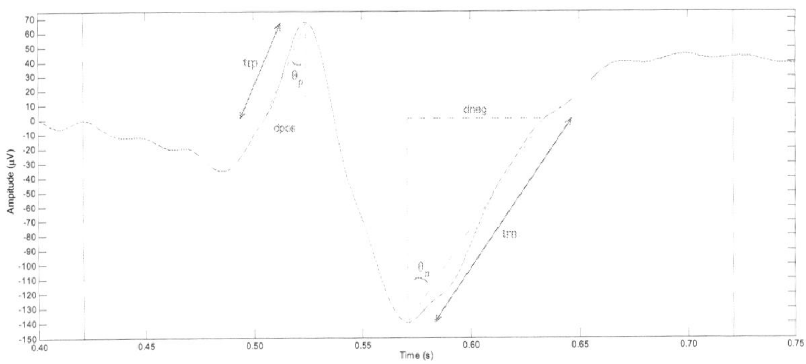

Fig. 8. Vertex angle of positive and negative epileptiform event, calculated from the maximum and minimum amplitude, respectively

The calculated angles (Fig. 8.), taking an epileptiform event as example, refer to the angle influenced by the peak's initial inclination and the angle that suffers influence of beginning slope of the slow wave. Based on the calculation of these angles (θp and θn) we determined other descriptors:

- base of the peaks directly adjacent to the beginning and the end of the event (dpos and dneg, depending in order of appearance of the peaks);
- angle of the analyzed event apex (θ);
- tangents of the angles of peak apex (tgp and tgn);
- tilt of the slopes directly adjacent to the beginning and the end of the event (trp and trn);
- event basis (dbase).

The morphology of a paroxysm can also often be confused with the morphology of artifacts (from various sources) present in the EEG signal. However, as can be seen in Fig. 9. the typical waveforms of these noises usually have a relative high frequency. This means that the high amplitudes appear with minimum time differences between them, which are the opposite of paroxysms that usually have more widely spaced peaks because they are always followed by a slow wave.

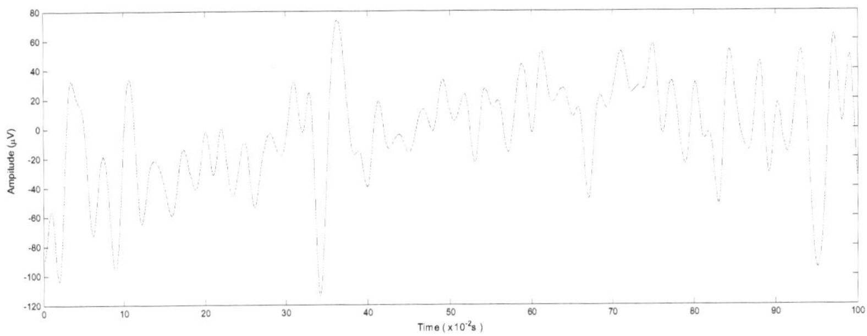

Fig. 9. Example of typical morphology of an artifact (noise) present in the EEG signal

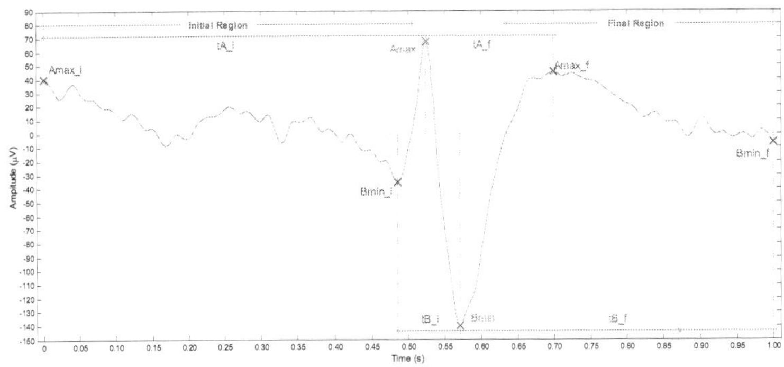

Fig. 10. Descriptors for the differentiation between epileptiform events and artifacts, considering distances (time) between the points of maximum and minimum amplitude

The descriptors proposed to make the distinction between noise and epileptiform events can be based on relations of time and amplitude differences in the epoch when dividing it in two regions (initial and final) adjacent to the event. Experiments were performed and from them we projected the following descriptors:

- amplitude and time difference between maximum amplitudes of the event (Amax), initial (Amax_i) and final regions (Amax_f): DifA_i, tA_i, DifA_f and tA_f;
- amplitude and time difference between minimum amplitudes of the event (Bmin), initial (Bmin_i) and final regions (Bmin_f): DifB_i, tB_i, DifB_f, tB_f.

Further analysis of the morphology and other characteristics of events that occur in the EEG recordings can be performed. In this research it is proposed only the addition of descriptors based on the classical statistical indices of average, standard deviation and variance. These descriptors, were calculated for both the epoch under analysis (one second) and the 300ms segment. Thus, considering the descriptors selected from the literature and those we developed after a review of the recordings, we obtained a final set of 45 morphological descriptors (Table 1).

Origin if the descriptors	Descriptors identifications
Amplitude	Amax, Bmin, DifAB, Amax_pts, Bmin_pts, DifAB_pts
Duration	Tdif, Tdif_pts, T
Vertex angle of the peaks	θ, θp, θn, dbase, dpos, dneg, trp, trn, tgp, tgn
Initial region of the epoch	Amax_i, Bmin_i, DifA_i, tA_i, DifB_i, tB_i
Final region of the epoch	Amax_f, Bmin_f, DifA_f, tA_f, DifB_f, tB_f
Statistical indexes[1]	desvio, media, var, coef, CF, desvioC, mediaC, varC, coefC, CFC
Entropy[1,2]	entrop_log, entrop_norm, entrop_logC, entrop_normC

[1] The letter 'C' at the end of the identification means that the descriptor was calculated for the segment of 300ms.

[2] We calculated two types of entropy: normalized (norm) and logarithm of "energy".

Table 1. Summary of the elements that compose the final set of 45 morphological descriptors selected and developed for this research

3.3 Morphological descriptors evaluation

In the previous item (3.2) 45 morphological descriptors were presented. Some of them were chosen among those universally used and others were defined in our previous work.

After the creation of the descriptors' set it is necessary to analyze this ensemble in order to verify the significance of each element of the group in the differentiation of events. For this research we chose to use correlation analysis and application of Hotelling's T^2 test (Härdle & Simar, 2007) for individual assessment and Artificial Neural Networks (Eberhart & Dobbins, 1990; Zurada, 1992; Haykin, 1994) to verify the complete set performance.

The correlation analysis was made evaluating the correlation matrices of descriptors for pairs of events. We examined the correlation between morphological descriptors calculated from epochs containing paroxysm and epochs with non-epileptiform (blinks, artifacts, alpha waves and background EEG activity). The criterion for possible exclusion of any element (descriptor) of the designed set was the existence of high correlation values (above 50%) for all pairs of events considered.

The Hotelling's T^2 test consisted in calculating the difference between the values of each descriptor in epochs with epileptiform transients and epochs with non-epileptiform events. The assessment of this test was made comparing the results of these differences with a predetermined T^2 critical value (a threshold). Based on this test a descriptor is considered relevant when its T^2 result is greater than the pre-determined critical value.

Some descriptors such as the tangents of the positive (θp) and negative (θn) angles, length variation coefficient (coef) and crest factor (CF) had T^2 test result relatively close to the critical value and thus these elements could have been removed from the set. However as the correlation value achieved by these same descriptors was not high and their exclusion did not affect significantly the sensitivity and specificity of the neural networks implemented in this study. We chose to not exclude them from the final set.

For the verification that the descriptors can indeed provide sufficient information so a classifier can make the discrimination between events the set was arranged at the input of several Artificial Neural Networks.

The networks used are all Feedforward Multilayer Perceptron with Backpropagation algorithm and supervised learning. The basic architecture of each network was of an input layer with 45 neurons and output layer with only one neuron. The number of neurons in the hidden layer and the application of input stimuli normalization[3] were varied in each of the networks so we could find the best configuration and analyze the effect of this normalization. Some other features of neural networks implemented are:

- activation function of output and hidden layers: hyperbolic tangent;
- number of neurons in the hidden layer (N): 7 to 11 neurons;
- batch update of the synaptic weights (after every training epoch);
- learning rate and momentum were respectively: 0,01 and 0,9.

Finally, the training and test of networks were made with two different compositions of files (Table. 2.): a set of files classified only by the presence or absence of paroxysms and another set where the files were classified by type of event (sharp waves, spikes, blinks, normal background EEG activity, alpha waves and artifacts).

Composition	Process	Signal classification used		No. of files
Composition I	Training	Epileptiform event		47
		Non-epileptiform event		73
	Test	Epileptiform event		30
		Non-epileptiform event		23
Composition II	Training and test[a]	Epileptiform event	Sharp wave	10
			Spike	10
		Non-epileptiform event	EEG background activity	5
			Alpha waves	10
			Artifacts	5
			Blinks	5

Table 2. Composition of files according to different classifications of EEG signals events, used for training and tests of the neural networks created

4. Results

Several networks with the same basic architecture and features showed in the previous section were trained and tested using both types of file composition (Table 2.). The normalization of input stimuli was tested in all implemented networks.

The set of descriptors (computed for each file) were attributed directly to the networks' input and the stopping criteria for training, used in our experiments, was the minimum error (1%) and the maximum number of iterations allowed (100.000 epochs).

[3] The term normalization refers to the operation of correcting the amplitude of EEG recordings in which the maximum amplitude is greater than the one of a paroxysm (± 200µV). The applied correction is the ratio between the signal and its mean value.

The best results obtained after the simulations with all these networks are presented in Table 3, where the following statistical indices can be observed:

- Success rate (SR);
- True positive (TP), true negative (TN), false positive (FP) and false negative (FN);
- Sensibility (SE) e specificity (SP);
- Positive predictive value (PPV) and negative predictive value (NPV).

ANN specifications	SR	TP	TN	FP	FN	SE	SP	PPV	NPV
8N hidden / 10^5 epochs[a]	81%	27	19	4	3	0,90	0,83	0,87	0,86
9N hidden / 10^5 epochs[a]	79%	27	20	3	3	0,90	0,87	0,90	0,87
8N hidden / 10^5 epochs[a,c]	79%	27	16	7	3	0,90	0,70	0,79	0,84
8N hidden / 10^5 epochs[b]	80%	18	24	1	2	0,90	0,96	0,95	0,92
9N hidden / 11863 epochs[b]	89%	17	24	1	3	0,85	0,96	0,94	0,89
9N hidden / 12026 epochs[b,c]	68%	19	19	6	1	0,95	0,76	0,76	0,95

a Training and test with files from composition I.
b Training and test with files from composition II.
c The input stimuli was normalized.

Table 3. Best results achieved with the Artificial Neural Networks created

According to results presented in Table 3 the use of files with signals classified by the occurrence of paroxysms showed success rate (the correct identification of test signals) of 79% whereas with the files of the composition II this rate was around 90%. The best network implementations for each type of files showed sensitivity of 90% and 85% and specificity of 87% and 96%.

The effect of normalizing the network's input stimuli that we observed during the simulations was a reduction in the specificity values due to the number of false positives generated (for example, for the network with nine hidden neurons the false positives increased from one to six).

5. Conclusions

The use and determination of morphological descriptors seems to be simple because it is a direct data collection with relatively basic calculations such as, for example, calculating the dimensions of amplitude and duration of the event. However, this process requires *a priori* knowledge of information about the system or entity which characteristics will be cataloged. In other words, for the case of automatic detection of epileptiform events in EEG recordings is necessary to carry out preliminary studies about the morphology of the signals to be analyzed.

Another significant aspect when using morphological descriptors is the assessment of the selected descriptors as input of the classifier used. It is important to perform an evaluation to demonstrate the contribution of each descriptor for the capability of the ensemble in making the distinction between events of interest. In this study we used correlation analysis and Hotelling's T^2 test to identify which descriptors could be excluded from the created set in order to provide a performance improvement of the automatic detection process. The methods applied for this assessment did not result in significantly high improvements in the automatic detection, but this does not invalidate its use because the classifier (neural network) used on the experiments showed promising results.

Thus, it becomes necessary to study other advanced and robust analysis tools that can within a tolerance (error) threshold, provide more consistent results. Therefore we are using multivariate analysis (Principal Component Analysis, Independent Component Analysis) alone or in combination with other statistical techniques for assessing the relevance of the descriptors in attempt to optimize the size of the set needed to perform automatic detection through neural networks (or other classifier) without causing significant performance loss for the system in which the descriptors are inserted.

6. References

Abibullaev B.; Seo H. D. & Kang W. (2009a) A Wavelet Based Method for Detecting and Localizing Epileptic Neural Spikes in EEG. *Proceedings of the 2nd International Conference on Interaction Sciences: Information Technology, Culture and Human.* pp. 702-707, 9781605587103, Seoul, Korea, November 2009, ACM, New York.

Abibullaev B.; Kim M. S. & Seo H. D. (2009b) Seizure Detection in Temporal Lobe Epileptic EEGs Using the Best Basis Wavelet Functions. *Jornal of Medical Systems.* Vol.34, No.4, May 2009, pp. 755-765, 0148-5598.

Adeli, H.; Zhou, Z. & Dadmehr, N. (2003). Analysis of EEG records in an epileptic patient using wavelet transform. *Jornal of Neuroscience Methods.* Vol.123, February 2003, pp. 69-87, 0165-0270.

Argoud, F.I.M.; De Azevedo, F.M.; Marino Neto, J. & Grillo, E. (2006). SADE3: an effective system for automated detection of epileptiform events in long-term EEG based on context information. *Medical & Biological Engineering & Computing.* Vol.44, No.6, June 2006, Springer, pp. 459–470, 0140-0118.

Boos, C. F.; Pereira, M. C. V.; Argoud, F. I. M.; Azevedo, F. M.. (2010a). Analysis and definition of morphological descriptors for automatic detection of epileptiform events in EEG signals with artificial neural networks. *Proceedings of the 3rd IEEE International Conference on Computer Science and Information Technology.* Vol.5, pp. 349-353, 978-1-4244-5537-9, Chengdu, Sichuan, China, July 2010, IEEE Press.

Boos, C. F.; Pereira, M. C. V.; Argoud, F. I. M.; Azevedo, F. M.. (2010b). Morphological descriptors for automatic detection of epileptiform events. *Proceedings of the 32nd Annual International Conference of the IEEE Engineering in Medicine and Biology Society.* pp. 2435-2438, 978-1-4244-4124-2, Buenos Aires, Argentina, August-September 2010, IEEE Press.

Coimbra, A. J. F.; Marino J.; Freitas, C. G.; Azevedo, F. M., Barreto, J. M. (1994). Automatic Detection of Sleep-Waking States Using Kohonen Neural Networks. *Proceedings of the I Congresso Brasileiro de Redes Neurais,* Itajubá, Brazil, October 1994, pp. 327-331.

Diambra, L.; Fiqueiredo, J.C.B.; Malta,C.P. (1999). Epileptic Activity Recognition in EEG Recording, *Physica A,* Vol.273, No.3, November 1999, Elsevier, pp.495-505, 0378-4371.

Eberhart, R & Dobbins, R. (1990). *Neural Network PC Tools: A Practical Guide.* Academic Press, 0122286405, San Diego, California.

Esteller, R. (2000). Detection of Seizure Onset in Epileptic Patients from Intracranial EEG Signal. PhD. Thesis, School of Electrical and Computer Engineering Georgia Institute of Technology, 2000.

Fisher, R.S.; Boas, W.E.; Blume,W., Elger, C.; Genton, P.; Lee, P.; Engel Jr, J. (2005) Epileptic Siezures and Epilepsy: Definitions Proposed by the International League Against

Epilepsy (ILAE) and International Bureau for Epilepsy (IBE). *Epilepsia*, Vol.46, No.4, March 2005, p.470-472, 1528-1167.

Gotman, J. (1982). Automatic recognition of epileptic seizures in the EEG, *Electroencephalography and Clinical Neurophysiology*, Vol.54, No.5, November 1982, pp. 530-540, 0013-4694.

Gotman, J.; Gloor, P. (1976). Automatic recognition and quantification of interictal epileptic activity in the human scalp EEG, *Electroencephalography and Clinical Neurophysiology*, V.41, No.5, November 1976, pp. 513-529, 0013-4694.

Guedes, J. R. ; Pereira, M. C. ; Azevedo, F. M. ou de Azevedo, F.M. (2002). Parameterization of the EEG Signal Applied to the Detection of Epileptiform Events. *Proceedings of the 2nd European Medical and Biological Engineering Conference*, Vol.3(1), pp. 444-445, Vienna, Austria, December 2002, IFMBE.

Halford, J. J. (2009). Computerized epileptiform transient detection in the scalp electroencephalogram: Obstacles to progress and the example of computerized ECG interpretation. *Clinical Neurophysiology*, Vol.120, No.11, November 2009, pp. 1909–1915, 1388-2457.

Haykin, S. (1994) *Neural Networks: A Comprehensive Foundation*, Macmilliam College Publishing Company, 0-13-226556-7, Englewood Cliffs.

Hoef, L.; Elgavish, R.; Knowlton, R. C. (2010). Effect of Detection Parameters on Automated Electroencephalography Spike Detection Sensitivity and False-Positive Rate. *Journal of Clinical Neurophysiology*, Vol.27, No.1, February 2010, pp. 12-16, 0736-0258

Hoffmann, K.; Feucht, M.; Witte, H.; Benninger, F & Bolten, J. (1996). Analysis and classification of interictal spikes discharges in Benign Partial Epilepsy of Childhood on the basis of the Hilbert transform, *Neuroscience Letters*, Vol. 211, No.3, June 1996, pp. 195-198, 0304-3940.

Indiradevi, K.P.; Elias, E.; Sathidevi, P.S.; Nayak, S.D. & Radhakrishnan, K. (2008). A multi-level wavelet approach for automatic detection of epileptic spikes in the electroencephalogram, *Computers in Biology and Medicine*, V.38, No.7, July 2008, pp. 805-816, 0010-4825.

Kalayci, T. & Özdamar, O. (1995). Wavelet preprocessing for automated neural network detection of EEG spikes, *IEEE Engineering in Medicine and Biology Magazine*, Vol.14, No.2, March 1995, pp. 160-166, 0739-5175.

Kaneko, H.; Suzuki, S. S.; Akamatsu, M. (1999). Multineuronal Spike Classification Based on Multisite Electrode Recording, Whole-Waveform Analysis, and Hierarchical Clustering. *IEEE Transactions on Biomedical Engineering*, Vol.46, No.3, March 1999, pp. 280-290, 0018-9294.

Khan, Y.U. & Gotman, J. (2003). Wavelet based automatic seizure detection in intracerebral electroencephalogram, *Clinical Neurophysiology*, Vol.114, No.5, May 2003, pp. 898-908, 1388-2457.

Kim, K. H.; Kim, S. J. (2000). Neural Spike Sorting Under Nearly 0-dB Signal-to-Noise Ratio Using Nonlinear Energy Operator and Artificial Neural-Network Classifier. *IEEE Transactions on Biomedical Engineering*, Vol.47, No.10, October 2000, pp. 1406-1411, 1406-1411.

Kumar, S. P.; Sriraam, N.; Benakop, P.G.; Jinaga, B.C. (2010). Entropies based detection of epileptic seizures with artificial neural network classifiers, *Expert Systems with Applications*, Vol.37, No.4, April 2010, pp. 3284-3291, 0957-4174.

Litt, B.; Esteller, R; Echauz, J; D'Alessandro, M.; Shor, R.; Henry, T.; Pennell, P.; Epstein, C.; Bakay, R.; Dichter, M. & Vachtsevanos, G. (2001). Epileptic Seizures May Begin Hours in Advance of Clinical Onset: A Report of Five Patients, *Neuron*, Vol.30, No.1, April 2001, pp. 51-64, 0896-6273.

Liu, H.S.; Zhang, T. & Yang, F.S. (2002). A multistage, multimethod approach for automatic detection and classification of epileptiform EEG, *IEEE Transactions on Biomedical Engineering*, Vol. 49, No.12, December 2002, pp. 1557-1566, 0018-9294.

Malmivuo, J.; Plonsey, R. (1995). *Bioelectromagnetism: Principles and Applications of Bioelectric and Biomagnetic Fields*, Oxford University Press, 0-19-50-5823-2, New York.

Mohamed, N.; Rubin, D.M. & Marwala, T. (2006). Detection of epileptiform activity in human EEG signals using Bayesian neural networks, *Neural Information Processing – Letters and Reviews*, Vol.10, No.1, January 2006, pp. 231–237, 1738-2572.

Naghsh-Nilchi, A.R. & Aghashahi, M. (2010). Epilepsy seizure detection using eigen-system spectral estimation and Multiple Layer Perceptron neural network, *Biomedical Signal Processing and Control*, Vol.5, No.2, April 2010, pp. 147-157, 1746-8094.

Niedermeyer, E. & Silva F. L. (1993). *Electroencephalography: Basic Principles, Clinical Applications, and Related Fields*. Williams & Wilkins, 0-683-06511-4, Philadelphia.

Ocak, H. (2008). Automatic detection of epileptic seizures in EEG using discrete wavelet transform and approximate entropy, *Expert Systems with Applications*, Vol.36, No.2, Part 1, March 2009, pp. 2027-2036, 0957-4174.

Ocak, H. (2008). Optimal classification of epileptic seizures in EEG using wavelet analysis and genetic algorithm, *Signal Processing*, Vol.88, No.7, July 2008, pp. 1858-1867, 0165-1684.

Oweiss, K.G. & Anderson, D.J. (2001). Noise reduction in multichannel neural recordings using a new array wavelet denoising algorithm, *Neurocomputing*,Vol.38-40, June 2001, pp. 1687-1693, 0925-2312.

Pang, C.C.C.; Upton, A.R.M.; Shine, G. & Kamath, M.V. (2003). A Comparison of Algorithms for Detection of Spikes in the Electroencephalogram, *IEEE Transactions on Biomedical Engineering*, Vol.50, No.4, April 2003. pp. 521-526, 0018-9294.

Pereira, M. C. V. (2003). *Avaliação de técnicas de pré-processamento de sinais do EEG para detecção de eventos epileptogênicos utilizando redes neurais artificais*. Thesis (PhD), Biomedical Engineering Institute, University Federal of Santa Catarina, 2003.

Pereira, M. C. V.; Azevedo, F.M. & Argoud, F. I. M. (2003). Investigation About Pre-Processing in the Input of an Artificial Neural Network for Analysis of Epileptogenic Events in EEG Signals. *Proceedings of the World Congress on Medical Physics and Biomedical Engineering*, pp.103-103, Sydney, Australia, IFMBE.

Pillay, J. & Spearling, M. R. (2006). Interictal EEG and the Diagnosis of Epilepsy, *Epilepsia*, Vol.47, No.1, October 2006, pp. 14-22, 1528-1167.

Quiroga, R. Q. (1998). *Quantitative Analysis of EEG Signals: Time-Frequency Methods and Chaos Theory*. Thesis (PhD), Institute of Physiology, Medical University Lübeck and Institute of Signal Processing, Medical University Lübeck, 1998

Quiroga, R.Q.; Sakowitz, O.W.; Basar, E. & Schürmann, M. (2001). Wavelet Transform in the analysis of the frequency composition of evoked potentials, *Brain Research Protocols*, Vol.8, No.1, August 2001, pp. 16-24, 1385-299X.

Saab. M. E. & Gotman, J. (2005). A system to detect the onset of epileptic seizures in scalp EEG, *Clinical Neurophysiology*, Vol.116, No.2, February 2005, pp. 427-442, 1388-2457.

Sanei, S. & Chambers, J.A. (2007). *EEG Signal Processing*, John Wiley & Sons, 978-0-470-02581-9, West Sussex.

Scolaro, G.R. & Azevedo, F.M. (2010). Classification of Epileptiform Events in Raw EEG Signals using Neural Classifier, *Proceedings of the 3rd IEEE International Conference on Computer Science and Information Technology*. Vol.5, pp. 368-372, 978-1-4244-5537-9, Chengdu, Sichuan, China, July 2010, IEEE Press.

Sovierzoski, M. A. (2009). *Avaliação de descritores morfológicos na identificação de eventos epileptiformes*. Thesis (PhD), Biomedical Engineering Institute, University Federal of Santa Catarina, 2009.

Srinivasan, V.; Eswaran, C. & Sriraam, N. (2007). Approximate Entropy-Based Epileptic EEG Detection Using Artificial Neural Networks, *IEEE Transactions on Information Technology in Biomedicine*, Vol.11, No.3, May 2007, pp.288-295, 1089-7771.

Subasi, A. (2007). Application of adaptive neuro-fuzzy inference system for epileptic seizure detection using wavelet feature extraction, *Computers in Biology and Medicine*, Vol.37, No.2, February 2007, pp. 227-244, 0010-4825.

Tzallas, A.T.; Karvelis, P. S.; Katsis, C. D.; Fotiadis, D.I., Giannopoulus, S. & Konitsiotis, S. (2006). A Method for Classification of Transient Events in EEG Recordings: Application to Epilepsy Diagnosis, *Methods of Information in Medicine*, Vol.45, No.6, March 2006, pp. 610-621, 0026-1270.

Übeyli, E. D. (2009). Statistics over features: EEG signals analysis, *Computers in Biology and Medicine*, Vol.39, No.8, August 2009, pp. 733-741, 0010-4825.

Walczak, S. & Nowack, W. J. (2001) An Artificial Neural Network Approach to Diagnosing Epilepsy Using Lateralized Bursts of Theta EEGs, *Journal of Medical Systems*, Vol.25, No.1, February 2001, pp. 1-22, 0148-5598.

Webber, W. R. S.; Litt, B.; Wilson, K. & Lesser, R. P. (1994). Practical Detection of Epileptiform Discharges (EDs) in the EEG Using an Artificial Neural Network: a Comparison of Raw and Parameterized EEG Data, *Electroencephalography and Clinical Neurophysiology*, Vol.91, No.3, September 1994, pp. 194-204, 0013-4694.

Wilson, S. B.; Emerson, R. (2002). Spike Detection: a Review and Comparison of Algorithms, *Clinical Neurophysiology*, Vol.113, No.12, December 2002, pp. 1873-1881, 1388-2457.

Wilson, S.B.; Scheuerb, M.L.; Emerson R.G. & Gabor, A.J. (2004). Seizure detection: evaluation of the Reveal algorithm, *Clinical Neurophysiology*, Vol.115, No.10, October 2004, pp. 2280-2291, 1388-2457.

Zurada, J. M. (1992). *Introduction to Artificial Neural Systems*, West Publishing Company, 0-314-93391-3, St. Paul.

21

Multivariate Frequency Domain Analysis of Causal Interactions in Physiological Time Series

Luca Faes and Giandomenico Nollo
Department of Physics and BIOtech Center
University of Trento
Italy

1. Introduction

A common way of obtaining information about a physiological system is to measure one or more signals from the system, consider their temporal evolution in the form of numerical time series, and obtain quantitative indexes through the application of time series analysis techniques. While historical approaches to time series analysis were addressed to the study of single signals, recent advances have made it possible to study collectively the behavior of several signals measured simultaneously from the considered system. In fact, multivariate (MV) time series analysis is nowadays extensively used to characterize interdependencies among multiple signals collected from dynamical physiological systems. Applications of this approach are ubiquitous, for instance, in neurophysiology and cardiovascular physiology (see, e.g., (Pereda et al., 2005) and (Porta et al., 2009) and references therein). In neurophysiology, the time series to be analyzed are obtained, for example, sampling electroencephalographic (EEG) or magnetoencephalographic (MEG) signals which measure the temporal dynamics of the electro-magnetic fields of the brain as reflected at different locations of the scalp. In cardiovascular physiology, the time series are commonly constructed measuring at each cardiac beat cardiovascular and cardiorespiratory variables such as the heart period, the systolic/diastolic arterial pressure, and the respiratory flow. It is well recognized that the application of MV analysis to these physiological time series may provide unique information about the coupling mechanisms underlying brain dynamics and cardiovascular control, and may also lead to the definition of quantitative indexes useful in medical settings to assess the degree of mechanism impairment in pathological conditions.

MV time series analysis is not only important to detect *coupling*, i.e., the presence or absence of interactions, between the considered time series, but also to identify driver-response relationships between them. This problem is a special case of the general question of assessing *causality*, or cause-effect relations, between (sub)systems, processes or phenomena. The assessment of coupling and causality in MV processes is often performed by linear time series analysis approaches, i.e. approaches in which a linear model is supposed to underlie the generation of temporal dynamics and interactions of the considered signals (Kay, 1988; Gourevitch et al., 2006). While non-linear methods are continuously under development

(Pereda et al., 2005; Faes et al., 2008), the traditional linear approach remains of great interest for the study of physiological signals, mainly because it has the important advantage to be strictly connected to the frequency-domain representation of multichannel data. Indeed, physiological signals such as the brain and cardiovascular ones are rich of oscillatory content and thus lend themselves to spectral representation. Typical examples of physiological rhythms are the EEG dynamics, typically observed within the well-bounded frequency bands from delta to gamma (Nunez, 1995), and the cardiovascular oscillations, characterized by spectral peaks within the so-called low frequency (LF, ~0.1 Hz) and high frequency (HF, synchronous with respiratory activity) bands (Akselrod et al., 1981). As a consequence, the linear frequency-domain evaluation of coupling and causality constitutes an eligible approach to characterize the interdependence among specific oscillations manifested within the same frequency band in two or more physiological signals.

While an unique and universally accepted definition of causality does not exist, in time series analysis inference about cause-effect relationships is commonly based on the notion introduced by Nobel Prize winning Clive Granger (Granger, 1969). Granger causality was mathematically formalized within a linear time-domain framework widely applied in economy and finance but rapidly spread to other fields including the analysis of physiological time series. This notion of causality is defined in terms of predictability and exploits the direction of the flow of time to achieve a causal ordering of dependent processes. The definition may be contextualized in a different way for bivariate (based on two signals only) and MV (based on more than two signals) analysis; in the MV formulation, a distinction between direct causality from one series to another and indirect causality (i.e., causality between two series mediated by other series) is achieved (Faes et al., 2010b). Moreover, while the most intuitive definition of causality accounts for lagged effects only (i.e., effects of the past of a time series on the present of another), the concept of instantaneous causality, describing influences which occur within the same lag, is crucial for the evaluation of causal relationships among processes (Lutkepohl, 1993). Finally, the different facets of the concept of causality may be related to the concept of coupling between two processes, according to which the presence or absence of an interaction is detected and measured, but the directionality of such interaction is not elicited.

The notions of causality and coupling are commonly formalized in the context of a MV autoregressive (MVAR) representation of the available time series, which allows to derive time- and frequency-domain pictures of these concepts respectively through the model coefficients and through their spectral representation. Accordingly, several frequency domain measures of causality and coupling have been introduced and applied in recent years. Coupling is traditionally investigated by means of the coherence (Coh) and the partial coherence (PCoh), classically known, e.g., from Kay (1988) or (Bendat & Piersol, 1986). Measures able to quantify causality in the frequency domain have been proposed more recently: the most used are the directed transfer function (DTF) (Kaminski & Blinowska, 1991), the directed coherence (DC) (Baccala et al., 1998), and the partial directed coherence (PDC) (Baccala & Sameshima, 2001). All these measures have been used extensively for the analysis of physiological time series, and applications showing their usefulness for the interpretation of interaction mechanisms among, e.g., EEG rhythms or cardiovascular oscillations, are plentiful in the literature (see, for instance, (Porta et al., 2002; Schlogl & Supp, 2006; Astolfi et al., 2007; Faes & Nollo, 2010a)). Despite this, several issues have to be taken into account for their correct utilization. While the relationships existing among these indices are generally understood, and most of the properties linking these measures to the different concepts of causality and coupling are known, an organic joint description and contextualization in relation to the underlying time domain concepts is lacking. Also for this reason, the interpretation of frequency-domain coupling and causality measures is not always straightforward, and this may lead to an erroneous description of connectivity and related mechanisms. Examples of ambiguities emerged in the interpretation of these measures are the debates about the ability of PCoh to measure some forms of causality (Albo et al., 2004; Baccala & Sameshima, 2006), and about the specific kind of causality which is reflected by the DTF and DC measures (Kaminski et al., 2001; Baccala & Sameshima, 2001; Eichler, 2006). An aspect which is perhaps more problematic regards the structure of the model used to represent the data prior to computation of the frequency domain measures, which commonly accounts for lagged but not for instantaneous effects among the series. Despite this, the significance of instantaneous correlations among the series is almost never tested in practical applications, and the possible effects on coupling and causality measures of forsaking such correlations have not been investigated thoroughly. Very recent studies have suggested that neglecting instantaneous interactions in the model representation may lead to heavily modified connectivity patterns (Hyvarinen et al., 2008; Faes & Nollo, 2010b).

The mission of this chapter is to enhance the theoretical interpretability of the available frequency domain measures of coupling and causality derived from the MVAR representation of multiple time series. To this end, a common framework for the definition of Coh, PCoh, DC/DTF, and PDC is provided on the basis of the frequency domain MVAR representation, and is exploited to relate the various measures to each other as well as to the specific coupling or causality definitions which they underlie. The chapter is structured as follows: Sect. 2 presents a comprehensive definition of the various forms of causality and coupling that can be observed in MV processes; Sect. 3 particularizes these definitions for standard MVAR processes, derives the corresponding frequency domain measures of coupling and causality, and discusses their interpretation; Sect. 4 proposes an extended MVAR representation to be used in the presence of significant instantaneous correlations in the observed process, whereby novel frequency domain causality measures are defined and compared to the existing ones; Sect. 5 briefly discuss the practical application of the measures on physiological time series; and Sect. 6 concludes the chapter.

2. Causality and coupling in multivariate processes

Let us consider M stationary stochastic processes y_m, m=1,...,M. Without loss of generality we assume that the processes are real-valued, defined at discrete time ($y_m=\{y_m(n)\}$; e.g., are sampled versions of the continuous time processes $y_m(t)$, taken at the times $t_n=nT$, with T the sampling period) and have zero mean (E[$y_m(n)$]=0, where E[$\cdot$] is the statistical expectation operator). A MV closed loop process is defined as:

$$y_m(n)=f_m(Y_m,\acute{Y}_l \,|\, l\neq m)+w_m(n)\,, \quad l,m=1,\ldots,M, \tag{1}$$

where f_m is the function linking the set of the p past values of the m-th process, collected in $Y_m=\{y_m(n-1),\ldots,y_m(n-p)\}$, as well as the sets of the present and the p past values of all other processes, collected in $\acute{Y}_l=\{y_l(n),Y_l\}=\{y_l(n),y_l(n-1),\ldots,y_l(n-p)\}$, $l\neq m$, to the present value $y_m(n)$, and w_m is a white noise process describing the error in the representation. Given two processes y_i and y_j, i,j=1,...,M, different definitions of causality and coupling between the processes may be defined as discussed in the following, and summarized in Table 1.

		Strictly causal MVAR representation	Extended MVAR representation
DIRECT			
a) direct causality	$y_j \to y_i$	PDC, $\pi_{ij}(f)$	PDC, $\tilde{\pi}_{ij}(f)$
b) extended direct causality	$y_j \overset{\cdot}{\to} y_i$	-	ePDC, $\chi_{ij}(f)$
c) direct coupling	$y_i \leftrightarrow y_j$	PCoh, $\Pi_{ij}(f)$	
DIRECT+INDIRECT			
a) causality	$y_j \Rightarrow y_i$	DC, $\gamma_{ij}(f)$	DC, $\tilde{\gamma}_{ij}(f)$
b) extended causality	$y_j \overset{\cdot}{\Rightarrow} y_i$	-	eDC, $\xi_{ij}(f)$
c) coupling	$y_i \Leftrightarrow y_j$	Coh, $\Gamma_{ij}(f)$	

Table 1. Frequency domain measures of causality and coupling between two processes y_i and y_j of a multivariate closed loop process. Note that causality and direct causality measure lagged effects only, while extended causality and extended direct causality measure combined instantaneous and lagged effects.

Denoting as $Z_j=\{Y_l \,|\, l=1,...,M, l\neq j\}$ the set of the past values of all processes except y_j, *direct causality* from y_j to y_i, $y_j \to y_i$, exists if the prediction of $y_i(n)$ based on Z_j and Y_j is better than the prediction of $y_i(n)$ solely based on Z_j. *Causality* from y_j to y_i, $y_j \Rightarrow y_i$, exists if a cascade of direct causality relations $y_j \to y_m \cdots \to y_i$ occurs for at least one value m in the set $(1,\ldots,M)$; if $m=i$ or $m=j$ causality reduces to direct causality. This last case is obvious for a bivariate closed loop process (M=2), where only one definition exists and agrees with the notion of Granger causality (Granger, 1969) involving only the relations between two processes. For multivariate processes ($M\geq3$) the definition of direct causality agrees with the notion of *prima facie* cause introduced in (Granger, 1980); the definition of causality is a generalization including also causal indirect effects between two processes, i.e., effects mediated by one or more other processes in the MV closed loop.

While the definitions provided above are based on the exclusive consideration of lagged effects from one series to another, the interactions modeled in (1) consider also the possible instantaneous effects, i.e. effects which occur within the same lag. If we consider the directed interaction from y_j to y_i, lagged causality (with lag $k\geq1$) occurs if $y_j(n-k)$ is useful to predict $y_i(n)$, while instantaneous causality (with lag k=0) occurs if $y_j(n)$ is useful to predict $y_i(n)$. These two concepts may be combined together to provide extended causality definitions as follows. Denoting as $Z_{ij}=\{Y_i, \acute{Y}_l \,|\, l=1,...,M, l\neq j, l\neq i\}$ the set of the past values of y_i and the present and past values of all other processes except y_j, *extended direct causality* from y_j to y_i, $y_j \overset{\cdot}{\to} y_i$, exists if the prediction of $y_i(n)$ based on Z_{ij} and $\acute{Y}_j$ is better than the prediction of $y_i(n)$ solely based on Z_{ij}. *Extended causality* from y_j to y_i, $y_j \overset{\cdot}{\Rightarrow} y_i$, exists if a cascade of extended direct causality relations $y_j \overset{\cdot}{\to} y_m \cdots \overset{\cdot}{\to} y_i$ occurs for at least one value m in the set $(1,\ldots,M)$; again, if $m=i$ or $m=j$ extended causality reduces to extended direct causality.

Definitions of coupling between two processes are derived from the causality definitions as follows. *Direct coupling* between y_i and y_j, $y_i \leftrightarrow y_j$, exists if $y_i \overset{\cdot}{\to} y_m$ and $y_j \overset{\cdot}{\to} y_m$; while the most obvious case is when $m=i$ or $m=j$, two processes are considered as directly coupled also when they both directly cause a third common process ($m\neq i$, $m\neq j$). *Coupling* between y_i and

y_j, $y_i \Leftrightarrow y_j$, exists if $y_m \dot{\Rightarrow} y_i$ and $y_m \dot{\Rightarrow} y_j$; again, coupling may arise when the of the two processes causes the other ($m=i$ or $m=j$), or when both processes are caused by other common processes ($m \neq i$, $m \neq j$). Thus, the coupling definitions generalize the concept of causality accounting for both forward and backward interactions between two processes.
An illustrative example of the described causality and coupling relations is reported in Fig. 1. In the diagrams, the set of interactions is represented with a network where nodes correspond to processes and connecting arrows depict direct causality relations.

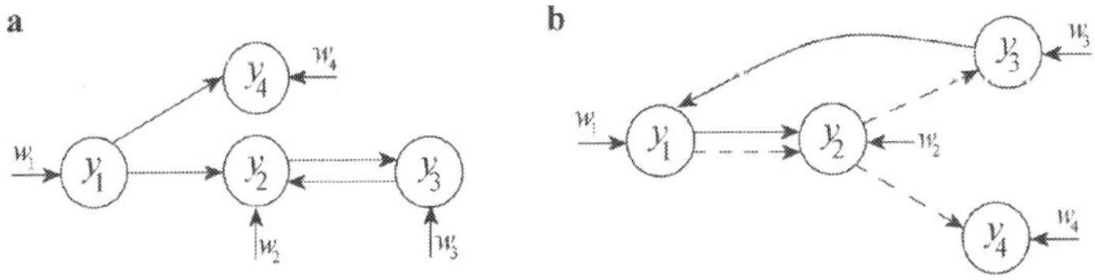

Fig. 1. Examples of networks of interacting processes exhibiting only lagged interactions (**a**) and combined instantaneous and lagged interactions (**b**). Lagged and instantaneous effects are depicted with solid and dashed arrows, respectively.

Fig. 1a shows a network of M=4 interacting processes in which only lagged effects from one process to another are present. In this situation, extended causality reduces to causality due to the absence of instantaneous effects. The direct causality relations imposed in the net are $y_1 \rightarrow y_2$, $y_2 \rightarrow y_3$, $y_3 \rightarrow y_2$, and $y_1 \rightarrow y_4$. Since direct causality is a condition sufficient for causality, we observe also $y_1 \Rightarrow y_2$, $y_2 \Rightarrow y_3$, $y_3 \Rightarrow y_2$, and $y_1 \Rightarrow y_4$; moreover, the cascade $y_1 \rightarrow y_2 \rightarrow y_3$ determines an indirect effect such that causality $y_1 \Rightarrow y_3$ exists. Direct coupling follows from direct causality, so that $y_1 \leftrightarrow y_2$, $y_2 \leftrightarrow y_3$, and $y_1 \leftrightarrow y_4$, but is also caused by the common driving exerted by y_1 and y_3 on y_2, so that $y_1 \leftrightarrow y_3$. Finally, coupling is present between each pair of processes: $y_1 \Leftrightarrow y_2$, $y_2 \Leftrightarrow y_3$, $y_1 \Leftrightarrow y_4$, and $y_1 \Leftrightarrow y_3$ result from the causality relations, while $y_2 \Leftrightarrow y_4$ and $y_3 \Leftrightarrow y_4$ result from the common driving exerted by y_1 respectively on y_2 and y_4, and on y_3 and y_4. In Fig. 1b, instantaneous effects are considered together with lagged ones. In this case, direct causality occurs only when lagged effects are present, i.e., over the directions $y_1 \rightarrow y_2$, $y_3 \rightarrow y_1$. Extended direct causality follows from lagged and/or instantaneous direct causality, so that we have $y_1 \dot{\rightarrow} y_2$, $y_2 \dot{\rightarrow} y_3$, $y_2 \dot{\rightarrow} y_4$, and $y_3 \dot{\rightarrow} y_1$. As no indirect lagged causality is present, causality follows exclusively from direct causality, i.e. $y_1 \Rightarrow y_2$, $y_3 \Rightarrow y_1$. On the contrary, extended causality is observed very often because of the existence of several cascades of instantaneous and/or lagged effects: we observe indeed $y_1 \dot{\Rightarrow} y_2$, $y_1 \dot{\Rightarrow} y_3$, $y_1 \dot{\Rightarrow} y_4$, $y_2 \dot{\Rightarrow} y_1$, $y_2 \dot{\Rightarrow} y_3$, $y_2 \dot{\Rightarrow} y_4$, $y_3 \dot{\Rightarrow} y_1$, $y_3 \dot{\Rightarrow} y_2$, $y_3 \dot{\Rightarrow} y_4$. Direct coupling follows from extended direct causality: $y_1 \leftrightarrow y_2$, $y_2 \leftrightarrow y_3$, $y_2 \leftrightarrow y_4$, $y_3 \leftrightarrow y_1$ (no common driving of two processes on a third one is observed). Finally, coupling is detected between all pairs of processes as the network is fully connected (i.e., there are no isolated groups of processes).
While causality definitions cannot be explored by means of conventional statistical operators, the concepts of coupling and direct coupling may be quantified through standard analysis of the correlation structure of the observed processes. Specifically, defining as $\mathbf{Y}(n)=[y_1(n) \cdots y_M(n)]^T$ the observed M×1 vector process, as $\mathbf{R}(k)=E[\mathbf{Y}(n)\mathbf{Y}^T(n-k)]$ its M×M correlation matrix evaluated at lag k, and as $\mathbf{P}(k)=\mathbf{R}(k)^{-1}$ the inverse correlation matrix, coupling $y_i \Leftrightarrow y_j$ and direct coupling $y_i \leftrightarrow y_j$ are quantified at the time lag k respectively by the correlation coefficient and the partial correlation coefficient (Whittaker, 1990):

$$\rho_{ij}(k)=\frac{r_{ij}(k)}{\sqrt{r_{ii}(k)r_{jj}(k)}}, \quad \eta_{ij}(k)=-\frac{p_{ij}(k)}{\sqrt{p_{ii}(k)p_{jj}(k)}}, \tag{2}$$

where $r_{ij}(k)$ and $p_{ij}(k)$ are the i-j elements of $\mathbf{R}(k)$ and $\mathbf{P}(k)$. The correlation and partial correlation coefficients are normalized measures of the linear interdependence existing between $y_i(n)$ and $y_j(n-k)$, and of the linear interdependence between $y_i(n)$ and $y_j(n-k)$ after removing the effects of all remaining processes. As such, ρ_{ij} and η_{ij} quantify the correlation and the "direct correlation" (i.e., the correlation that cannot be accounted for by the influence of any other process) between y_i and y_j. To identify the frequency-domain analogous of these two coefficients, we consider the spectral representation of the vector process $\mathbf{Y}(n)$, which is provided by the $M\times M$ spectral density matrix $\mathbf{S}(f)$, defined as the Fourier transform (FT) of the correlation matrix $\mathbf{R}(k)$. The spectral matrix contains the spectrum of $y_i(n)$, $S_{ii}(f)$, and the cross-spectrum between $y_i(n)$ and $y_j(n)$, $S_{ij}(f)$, as diagonal and off-diagonal terms, respectively (i,j=1,...,M). In analogy with the time domain definitions, the spectral matrix and its inverse, $\mathbf{P}(f)=\mathbf{S}(f)^{-1}$, are exploited to provide frequency-domain measures of coupling and direct coupling, respectively through the *coherence* (Coh) and the *partial coherence* (PCoh) functions (Bendat & Piersol, 1986):

$$\Gamma_{ij}(f)=\frac{S_{ij}(f)}{\sqrt{S_{ii}(f)S_{jj}(f)}}, \quad \Pi_{ij}(f)=\frac{P_{ij}(f)}{\sqrt{P_{ii}(f)P_{jj}(f)}}, \tag{3}$$

As the functions in (3) are complex-valued, their squared modulus is commonly used to measure the strength of coupling and direct coupling in the frequency domain. Specifically, the magnitude-squared Coh $|\Gamma_{ij}(f)|^2$ measures the strength of the linear, non-directed interactions between the processes y_i and y_j as a function of frequency, being 0 in case of uncoupling and 1 in case of full coupling. The squared PCoh $|\Pi_{ij}(f)|^2$ measures the strength of the direct, non-directed interaction between y_i and y_j, i.e. the strength of the interaction remaining after subtracting the effect of the remaining processes. We stress that, due to the symmetrical nature of these measures, they cannot provide information about causality; such an information may be extracted, as explained in the following, from the coefficients of a parametric representation of the time series.

3. Causality and coupling in MVAR processes

3.1 Time domain definitions

The joint multivariate process $\mathbf{Y}(n)$ can be represented as the output of a MV linear shift-invariant filter (Kay, 1988):

$$\mathbf{Y}(n)=\sum_{k=-\infty}^{\infty}\mathbf{H}(k)\mathbf{U}(n-k), \tag{4}$$

where $\mathbf{U}(n)=[u_1(n)\cdots u_M(n)]^T$ is a vector of M zero-mean input processes and $\mathbf{H}(k)$ is the $M\times M$ filter impulse response matrix. A particular case of the general model in (4), extensively used in time series analysis, is the MV autoregressive (MVAR) model (Kay, 1988):

$$\mathbf{Y}(n)=\sum_{k=1}^{p}\mathbf{A}(k)\mathbf{Y}(n-k)+\mathbf{U}(n), \tag{5}$$

where p is the model order, defining the maximum lag used to quantify interactions. The input process $\mathbf{U}(n)$, also called innovation process, is assumed to be composed of white and uncorrelated noises; this means that the correlation matrix of $\mathbf{U}(n)$, $\mathbf{R}_U(k)$=E[$\mathbf{U}(n)\mathbf{U}^T(n-k)$], is zero for each lag k>0, while it is equal to the covariance matrix Σ=cov($\mathbf{U}(n)$) for k=0. One major benefit of the representation in (5) is that it allows to interpret properties of the joint description of the processes $y_m(n)$ —like coupling or causality— in terms of the estimated coefficients $\mathbf{A}(k)$. In fact, the i-j element of $\mathbf{A}(k)$, $a_{ij}(k)$, quantifies the causal linear interaction effect occurring at lag k from y_j to y_i. As a consequence, the definitions of causality and coupling provided above for a general closed-loop MV process can be specified for a MVAR process in terms of the off-diagonal elements of $\mathbf{A}(k)$ as follows: $y_j \rightarrow y_i$ if $a_{ij}(k)\neq 0$ for at least one k=1,…,p; $y_j \Rightarrow y_i$ if $a_{m_s m_{s-1}}(k_s)\neq 0$ for at least a set of $L\geq 2$ values for m_s (with $m_0=j$, $m_{L-1}=i$) and a set of lags $k_0,\dots,k_{L-1}$ with values in (1,…,p); $y_i \leftrightarrow y_j$ if $a_{mi}(k_1)\neq 0$ for at least one k_1 or $a_{mj}(k_2)\neq 0$ for at least one k_2; $y_i \Leftrightarrow y_j$ if $a_{m_s m_{s-1}}(k_s)\neq 0$ for at least a set of $L\geq 2$ values for m_s (either with $m_0=m$, $m_{L-1}=i$ or with $m_0=m$, $m_{L-1}=j$) and a set of lags $k_0,\dots,k_{L-1}$. Thus, causality and coupling relations are found when the pathway relevant to the interaction is active, i.e., is described by nonzero coefficients in $\mathbf{A}$. Note that the extended definitions of causality and direct causality cannot be tested from the coefficients of the MVAR model (5), as the model does not describe instantaneous interactions. We refer to Sect. 3.3 to see how the MVAR coefficients may be related to causality and coupling effects in an illustrative example.

3.2 Frequency domain definitions

The spectral representation of a MVAR process is derived considering the FT of the representations in (4) and (5), which yield respectively the equations $\mathbf{Y}(f)=\mathbf{H}(f)\mathbf{U}(f)$ and $\mathbf{Y}(f)=\mathbf{A}(f)\mathbf{Y}(f)+\mathbf{U}(f)$, where $\mathbf{Y}(f)$ and $\mathbf{U}(f)$ are the FTs of $\mathbf{Y}(n)$ and $\mathbf{U}(n)$, and the $M\times M$ transfer matrix and coefficient matrix are defined in the frequency domain as:

$$\mathbf{H}(f)=\sum_{k=-\infty}^{\infty}\mathbf{H}(k)e^{-j2\pi fkT},\quad \mathbf{A}(f)=\sum_{k=1}^{p}\mathbf{A}(k)e^{-j2\pi fkT}. \tag{6}$$

Comparing the two spectral representations, it is easy to show that the coefficient and transfer matrices are linked by: $\mathbf{H}(f)=[\mathbf{I}-\mathbf{A}(f)]^{-1}=\bar{\mathbf{A}}(f)^{-1}$. This relation is useful to draw the connection between the cross-spectral density matrix $\mathbf{S}(f)$ and its inverse $\mathbf{P}(f)$, as well as to derive frequency domain estimates of coupling and causality in terms of the MVAR representation. Indeed, the following factorizations hold for a MVAR process (Kay, 1988):

$$\mathbf{S}(f)=\mathbf{H}(f)\Sigma\mathbf{H}^H(f),\quad \mathbf{P}(f)=\bar{\mathbf{A}}^H(f)\Sigma^{-1}\bar{\mathbf{A}}(f), \tag{7}$$

where the superscript ^{H} stands for the Hermitian transpose. The (i-j)th elements of $\mathbf{S}(f)$ and $\mathbf{P}(f)$ can be represented in the compact form:

$$S_{ij}(f)=\mathbf{h}_i(f)\Sigma\mathbf{h}_j^H(f),\quad P_{ij}(f)=\bar{\mathbf{a}}_i^H(f)\Sigma^{-1}\bar{\mathbf{a}}_j(f), \tag{8}$$

where $\mathbf{h}_i(f)$ is the i-th row of the transfer matrix ($\mathbf{H}(f)=[\mathbf{h}_1(f)\cdots\mathbf{h}_M(f)]^T$) and $\bar{\mathbf{a}}_i(f)$ is the i-th column of the coefficient matrix ($\bar{\mathbf{A}}(f)=[\bar{\mathbf{a}}_1(f)\cdots\bar{\mathbf{a}}_M(f)]$). Under the assumption that the input white noises are uncorrelated even at lag zero, their covariance cov($\mathbf{U}(n)$) reduces to the diagonal matrix Σ=diag(σ^2_i), and its inverse to the matrix Σ^{-1}=diag($1/\sigma^2_i$) which is diagonal as well (σ^2_i is the variance of u_i). In this specific case, (8) factorize into:

$$S_{ij}(f)=\sum_{m=1}^{M}\sigma_m^2 H_{im}(f)H_{jm}^*(f),\ P_{ij}(f)=\sum_{m=1}^{M}\frac{1}{\sigma_m^2}\overline{\mathbf{A}}_{mi}^*(f)\overline{\mathbf{A}}_{mj}(f) \tag{9}$$

The usefulness of the factorizations in (9) is in the fact that they allow to decompose the frequency domain measures of coupling and direct coupling previously defined into terms eliciting the directional information from one process to another. Substituting (8) and (9) into (3), the Coh between y_i and y_j can be factored as:

$$\Gamma_{ij}(f)=\frac{\mathbf{h}_i(f)\boldsymbol{\Sigma}\mathbf{h}_j^{\mathrm{H}}(f)}{\sqrt{\mathbf{h}_i(f)\boldsymbol{\Sigma}\mathbf{h}_i^{\mathrm{H}}(f)}\sqrt{\mathbf{h}_j(f)\boldsymbol{\Sigma}\mathbf{h}_j^{\mathrm{H}}(f)}}=\sum_{m=1}^{M}\frac{\sigma_m H_{im}(f)}{\sqrt{S_{ii}(f)}}\frac{\sigma_m H_{jm}^*(f)}{\sqrt{S_{jj}(f)}}=\sum_{m=1}^{M}\gamma_{im}(f)\gamma_{jm}^*(f), \tag{10}$$

where the last term contains the so-called *directed coherence* (DC). Thus, the DC from y_j to y_i is defined as (Baccala et al., 1998):

$$\gamma_{ij}(f)=\frac{\sigma_j H_{ij}(f)}{\sqrt{\sum_{m=1}^{M}\sigma_m^2\left|H_{im}(f)\right|^2}}. \tag{11}$$

Note that the directed transfer function (DTF) defined in (Kaminski & Blinowska, 1991) is a particularization of the DC in which all input variances are all equal ($\sigma^2_1=\sigma^2_2=\cdots=\sigma^2_M$) so that they cancel each other in (11). The factorization in (10) justifies the term DC, as $\gamma_{ij}(f)$ can be interpreted as a measure of the influence of y_j onto y_i, as opposed to $\gamma_{ji}(f)$ which measures the interaction occurring over the opposite direction from y_i to y_j. Further interpretation of the DC in terms of coupling strength is achieved considering its normalization properties:

$$0\le\left|\gamma_{ij}(f)\right|^2\le 1\ ,\ \sum_{m=1}^{M}\left|\gamma_{im}(f)\right|^2=1\,. \tag{12}$$

The inequality in (12) indicates that the squared DC $|\gamma_{ij}(f)|^2$ measures a normalized coupling strength, being 0 in the absence of directed coupling from y_j to y_i at the frequency f, and 1 in the presence of full coupling. The equality indicates that $|\gamma_{ij}(f)|^2$ measures the coupling strength from y_j to y_i as the normalized proportion of $S_{ii}(f)$ which is due to y_j, i.e. is transferred from u_j via the transfer function $H_{ij}(f)$. Indeed, combining (9) and (12) it is easy to show that the spectrum of the process y_i may be decomposed as:

$$S_{ii}(f)=\sum_{m=1}^{M}S_{i|m}(f)\ ,\ S_{i|m}(f)=\left|\gamma_{im}(f)\right|^2 S_{ii}(f). \tag{13}$$

where $S_{i|m}(f)$ is the part of $S_{ii}(f)$ due to y_m; $S_{i|i}(f)$ measures the part of $S_{ii}(f)$ due to none of the other processes, which is quantified in normalized units by the squared DC $|\gamma_{ii}(f)|^2$. Note that the useful decomposition in (13) does not hold for the DTF, unless all input variances are equal to each other so that the DC reduces to the DTF. For this reason, in the following we will consider the DC only, as it provides a similar, but more general and interpretable in terms of power content, measure of frequency domain causality.

In a similar way to that followed to decompose the Coh, the PCoh defined in (3) can be factored, using (8) and (9), as:

$$\Pi_{ij}(f)=\frac{\bar{\mathbf{a}}_i^{\mathrm{H}}(f)\mathbf{\Sigma}^{-1}\bar{\mathbf{a}}_j(f)}{\sqrt{\bar{\mathbf{a}}_i^{\mathrm{H}}(f)\mathbf{\Sigma}^{-1}\bar{\mathbf{a}}_i(f)}\sqrt{\bar{\mathbf{a}}_j^{\mathrm{H}}(f)\mathbf{\Sigma}^{-1}\bar{\mathbf{a}}_j(f)}}=\sum_{m=1}^{M}\frac{\frac{1}{\sigma_m}\bar{A}_{mj}(f)}{\sqrt{P_{jj}(f)}}\frac{\frac{1}{\sigma_m}\bar{A}_{mi}^*(f)}{\sqrt{P_{ii}(f)}}=\sum_{m=1}^{M}\pi_{mj}(f)\pi_{mi}^*(f), \quad (14)$$

where the last term contains the *partial directed coherence* (PDC) functions. The PDC from y_j to y_i is thus defined as (Baccala et al., 2007):

$$\pi_{ij}(f)=\frac{\frac{1}{\sigma_i}\bar{A}_{ij}(f)}{\sqrt{\sum_{m=1}^{M}\frac{1}{\sigma_m^2}\left|\bar{A}_{mj}(f)\right|^2}}. \quad (15)$$

As suggested by the factorization in (14), the PDC extracts the directional information from the PCoh, and is thus a measure of the direct directed interaction occurring from y_j to y_i at the frequency f. The normalization properties for the squared modulus of the PDC are:

$$0\leq\left|\pi_{ij}(f)\right|^2\leq 1\ ,\ \sum_{m=1}^{M}\left|\pi_{mj}(f)\right|^2=1, \quad (16)$$

suggesting that $|\pi_{ij}(f)|^2$ quantifies the interaction from y_j to y_i as the normalized proportion of $P_{jj}(f)$ which is which is sent to y_i, via the coefficients $\bar{A}_{ji}(f)$. Indeed, we have that:

$$P_{jj}(f)=\sum_{m=1}^{M}P_{j\to m}(f)\ ,\ P_{j\to m}(f)=\left|\pi_{mj}(f)\right|^2 P_{jj}(f), \quad (17)$$

where $P_{j\to m}(f)$ is the part of $P_{jj}(f)$ sent to y_m; in particular, $P_{j\to j}(f)$ measures the part of $P_{jj}(f)$ which is not sent to the other processes, and is expressed in normalized terms by the squared PDC $|\pi_{jj}(f)|^2$. The quantity which we denote as PDC was named "generalized PDC" in (Baccala et al., 2007), while the original version of the PDC (Baccala & Sameshima, 2001) was not including inner normalization by the input noise variances. Our definition (15) follows directly from the decomposition in (14); besides, this definition shares with the Coh, PCoh and DC functions the desirable property of scale-invariance, contrary to the original PDC that may be affected by different amplitudes for the considered signals.

Although both DC and PDC may be regarded as frequency domain descriptors of causality, there are important differences between these two estimators. First, as the DC and the PDC are factors in the decomposition of Coh and PCoh, respectively, they measure causality and direct causality in the frequency domain. In fact, the PDC $\pi_{ij}(f)$ is nonzero if and only if direct causality $y_j\to y_i$ exists, because the numerator of (15) contains, with $i\neq j$, the term $\bar{A}_{ij}(f)$, which is nonzero only when $a_{ij}(k)\neq 0$ for some k and is uniformly zero when $a_{ij}(k)=0$ for each k. As to the DC, one can show that, expanding $\mathbf{H}(f)=\bar{\mathbf{A}}(f)^{-1}$ as a geometric series, the transfer function $H_{ij}(f)$ contains a sum of terms each one related to one of the (direct or indirect) transfer paths connecting y_j to y_i (Eichler, 2006). Hence, the DC $\gamma_{ij}(f)$ is nonzero whenever any path connecting y_j to y_i is significant, i.e., when causality $y_j\Rightarrow y_i$ occurs. Another important difference between DC and PDC is in the normalization: as seen in (12) and in (16), $\gamma_{ij}(f)$ is normalized with respect to the structure that receives the signal, while $\pi_{ij}(f)$ is normalized with respect to the structure that sends the signal. Summarizing, we can state that the DC measures causality as the amount of information flowing from y_j to y_i through all (direct and indirect) transfer pathways, relative to the total inflow entering the structure at which y_i is measured; the PDC measures direct causality as the amount of information flowing from y_j to y_i through the direct transfer pathway only, relative to the total outflow leaving the structure at which y_j is measured. We note that this dual interpretation highlights advantages and disadvantages of both measures. The DC has a meaningful physical interpretation as it measures causality as the amount of signal power transferred from one process to another, but cannot distinguish between direct and indirect causal effects measured in the frequency domain. Conversely, the PDC reflects clearly the underlying interaction structure as it provides a one-to-one representation of direct causality, but is hardly useful as a quantitative measure because its magnitude quantifies the information flow through the inverse spectral matrix elements (which do not find easy interpretation in terms of power spectral density).

3.3 Theoretical example

To discuss the properties and compare the behavior of the frequency domain measures of causality and coupling summarized in Table 1, we consider the MVAR vector process of order p=2, composed by M=4 processes, generated by the equations:

$$\begin{cases} y_1(n) = 2\rho\cos(2\pi f_1)y_1(n-1) - \rho^2 y_1(n-2) + u_1(n) \\ y_2(n) = y_1(n-1) + 0.5y_3(n-1) + u_2(n) \\ y_3(n) = 2\rho\cos(2\pi f_3)y_3(n-1) - \rho^2 y_3(n-2) + 0.5y_2(n-1) + 0.5y_2(n-2) + u_3(n) \\ y_4(n) = y_1(n-2) + u_4(n) \end{cases}, \tag{18}$$

with ρ=0.9, f_1=0.1 and f_3=0.3, where the inputs $u_i(n)$, i=1,2,3, are fully uncorrelated and with variance σ^2_i. The process (18) is one of the possible MVAR realizations of the diagram of Fig. 1a. The coupling and causality relations emerging from the diagram, discussed in Sect. 2, can be interpreted here in terms of the MVAR coefficients set in (18). In fact, the nonzero off-diagonal values of the coefficient matrix ($a_{21}(1)$=1, $a_{23}(1)$=0.5, $a_{32}(1)$=0.5, $a_{32}(2)$=0.5, $a_{41}(2)$=1) determine direct causality and causality among the processes —and consequently direct coupling and coupling— in agreement with the definitions particularized at the end of Sect. 3.1. For instance, $a_{21}(1)$ and $a_{32}(2)$=0.5 determine direct causality $y_1 \rightarrow y_2$ and $y_2 \rightarrow y_3$ as well as causality $y_1 \Rightarrow y_2$, $y_2 \Rightarrow y_3$ (direct interaction) and $y_1 \Rightarrow y_3$ (indirect interaction). The diagonal values of the coefficient matrix determine autonomous oscillations in the processes. Indeed, the values set for $a_{ii}(k)$, $a_{ii}(1)=2\rho\cos(2\pi f_i)$, $a_{ii}(2)=-\rho^2$, generate complex-conjugate poles with modulus ρ and phases $\pm 2\pi f_i$ for the process y_i (the sampling period is implicitly assumed to be T=1). In this case, narrow-band oscillations at 0.1 Hz and 0.2 Hz are set for y_1 and y_3.
The trends of spectral and cross-spectral density functions are reported in Fig. 2.
The spectra of the four processes, reported as diagonal plots in Fig. 2a (black), exhibit clear peaks at the frequency of the two imposed oscillations: the peaks at ~0.1 Hz and ~0.3 Hz are dominant for y_1 and y_3, respectively, and appear also in the spectra of the remaining processes according to the imposed causal information transfer. The inverse spectra, computed as the diagonal elements of the inverse spectral matrix $\mathbf{P}(f)$, are also reported as diagonal plots in Fig. 2b (black). Off diagonal plots of Fig. 2a and Fig. 2b depict respectively the trends of the squared magnitudes of Coh and PCoh; note the symmetry of the two

functions ($\Gamma_{ij}(f)=\Gamma^*_{ji}(f)$, $\Pi_{ij}(f)=\Pi^*_{ji}(f)$), reflecting the fact that they measure coupling and direct coupling but cannot account for directionality of the considered interaction. As expected, Coh is nonzero for each pair of processes, thus measuring the full connectivity of the considered network. PCoh is clearly nonzero whenever a direct coupling relation exists ($y_1 \leftrightarrow y_2$, $y_2 \leftrightarrow y_3$, $y_1 \leftrightarrow y_4$, $y_1 \leftrightarrow y_3$), and is uniformly zero between y_2 and y_4 and between y_3 and y_4 where no direct coupling is present.

Figs. 3 and 4 depict the decomposition of spectra and inverse spectra, as well as the trends of DC and PDC functions resulting from these decompositions.

Fig. 3a provides a graphical representation of (13), showing how the spectrum of each process can be decomposed into power contributions related to all processes; normalizing these contributions one gets the squared modulus of the DC, as depicted in Fig. 3b. In the example, the spectrum of y_1 is decomposed in one part only, deriving from the same process. This indicates that none part of the power of y_1 is due to the other processes. The absence of external contributions is reflected by the null profiles of the DC from y_1 to y_2, to y_3 and to y_4 seen in Fig. 3b; as a result, the squared DC $|\gamma_{11}(f)|^2$ has a flat unitary profile. On the contrary, the decompositions of y_i, with i=2,3,4, results in contributions from the other processes, so that the squared DC $|\gamma_{ij}(f)|^2$ is nonzero for some $j \neq i$, and the squared DC $|\gamma_{ii}(f)|^2$ is not uniformly equal to 1 as a result of the normalization condition. In particular, we observe that the power of the peak at f_1=0.1 Hz is entirely due to y_1 for all processes, determining very high values of the squared DC in the first column of the matrix plot in Fig. 3b, i.e., $|\gamma_{i1}(f_1)|^2$=1; this behavior represents in the frequency domain the causality relations imposed from y_1 to all other processes. The remaining two causality relations, relevant to the bidirectional interaction between y_2 and y_3, concern the oscillation at f_2=0.3 Hz, which is

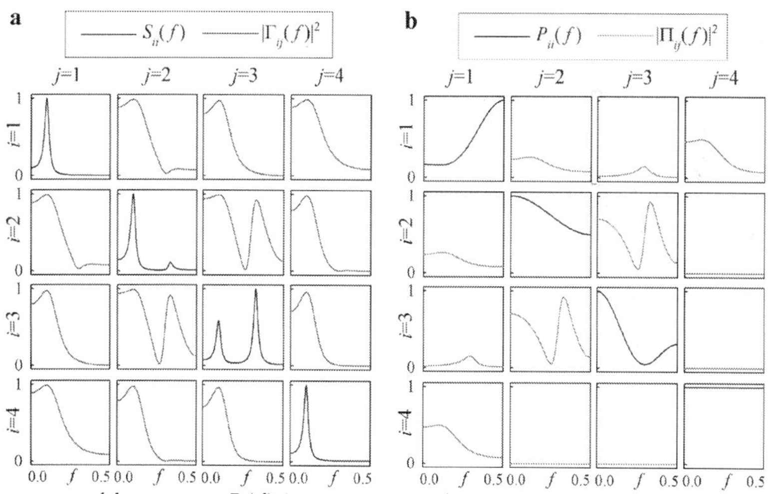

$S_{ii}(f)$: spectrum of the process y_i; $P_{ii}(f)$: inverse spectrum of y_i; $\Gamma_{ij}(f)$: coherence between y_j and y_i; $\Pi_{ij}(f)$: partial coherence between y_j and y_i.

Fig. 2. Spectral functions and frequency domain coupling measures for the theoretical example (18).

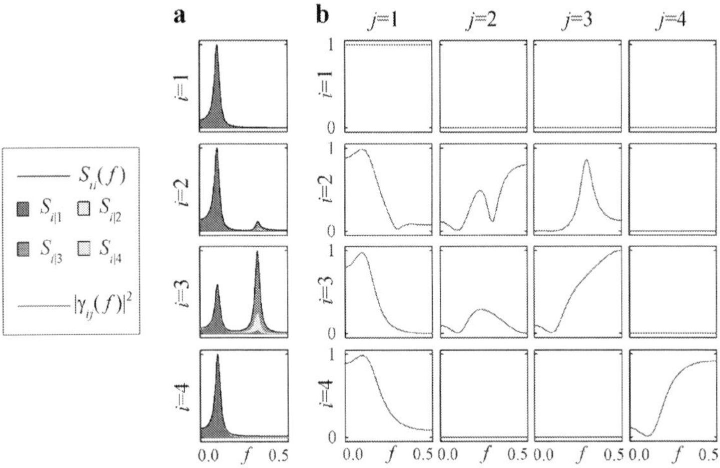

Fig. 3. Decomposition of the power spectrum of each process y_i in (18), $S_{ii}(f)$, into contributions from each process y_j ($S_{i|j}$, shaded areas in each plot) (**a**), and corresponding DC from y_j to y_i, $\gamma_{ij}(f)$ (**b**) depicted for each i,j=1,...,M.

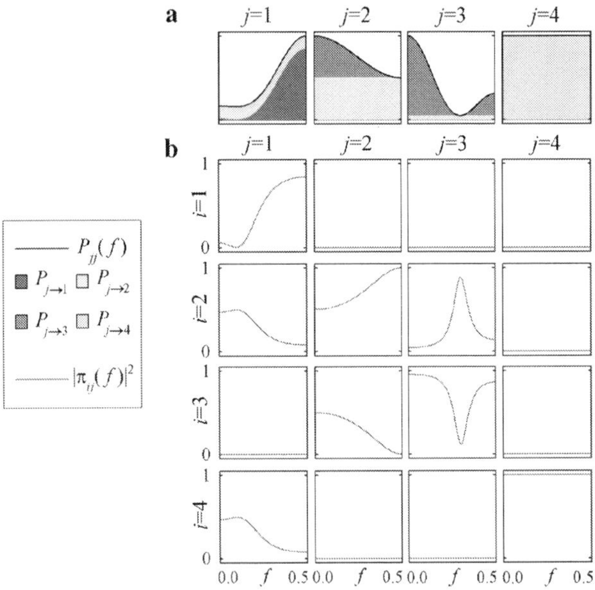

Fig. 4. Decomposition of the inverse power spectrum of each process y_j in (18), $P_{jj}(f)$, into contributions towards each process y_i ($P_{j\to i}$, shaded areas in each plot) (**a**), and corresponding PDC from y_j to y_i, $\pi_{ij}(f)$ (**b**) depicted for each i,j=1,...,M.

generated in y_3 and then transmitted forward and backward to y_2. This behavior is reflected by the spectral decomposition of the peak at ~0.3 Hz of the spectra of y_2 and y_3, which shows contributions from both processes, and then in the nonzero profiles of the DCs $|\gamma_{23}(f)|^2$ and $|\gamma_{32}(f)|^2$ (with peaks at ~0.3 Hz). To complete the frequency domain picture of causality, we observe that the DC is uniformly zero along all directions over which no causality is imposed in the time domain (e.g., compare Fig. 3b with Fig. 1a).

A specular interpretation to the one given above holds for the decomposition of the inverse spectra into absolute and normalized contributions sent to all processes, which are depicted for the considered example in the area plot of Fig. 4a and in the matrix PDC plot of Fig. 4b, respectively. The difference is that now contributions are measured as outflows instead as inflows, are normalized to the structure sending the signal instead to that receiving the signal, and reflect the concept of direct causality instead that of causality. With reference to the proposed example, we see that the inverse spectrum of y_1 is decomposed into contributions flowing out towards y_2 and y_4 (yellow and cyan areas underlying $P_{11}(f)$ in Fig. 4a), which are expressed in normalized units by the squared PDCs $|\pi_{21}(f)|^2$ and $|\pi_{41}(f)|^2$. While y_2 and y_3 affect each other (absolute units: $P_{2\to3}\neq0$, $P_{3\to2}\neq0$; normalized units: $|\pi_{32}|^2\neq0$ and $|\pi_{23}|^2\neq0$) without being affected by the other processes ($|\pi_{i2}|^2=0$, $|\pi_{i3}|^2=0$, i=1,4), y_4 does not send information to any process ($P_{4\to i}=0$, $|\pi_{i4}|^2=0$, i=1,2,3). As can be easily seen comparing Fig. 4 with Fig. 1a, the profiles of $P_{j\to i}$ and $|\pi_{ij}|^2$ provide a frequency domain description, respectively in absolute and normalized terms, of the imposed pattern of direct causality. We note also that all inverse spectra contain a contribution coming from the same process, which describes the part of $P_{jj}(f)$ which is not sent to any of the other processes ($P_{j\to j}$ in Fig. 4a). After normalization, this contribution is quantified by the PDC $|\pi_{jj}|^2$, as depicted by the diagonal plots of Fig. 4b.

4. Causality and coupling in the presence of instantaneous interactions

4.1 MVAR processes with instantaneous effects

The MVAR model defined in (5) is a strictly causal model, in the sense that it accounts only for lagged effects, i.e. the effects of the past of a time series on another series, while instantaneous effects (i.e., effects of $y_j(n)$ on $y_i(n)$) are not described by any model coefficient. The problem with this model representation is that any zero-lag correlation among the observed series y_i, when present, cannot be described by the model because $\mathbf{A}(k)$ is defined only for positive lags (k=0 is not considered in (5)). Neglecting instantaneous effects in the MVAR representation of multiple processes implies that any zero-lag correlation among the processes is translated into a correlation among the model inputs (Lutkepohl, 1993). As a result, the input covariance matrix Σ=cov($\mathbf{U}(n)$) is not diagonal. We will see in the next subsections that, since non-diagonality of Σ contradicts the assumptions of spectral factorization, the presence of significant instantaneous interactions may be detrimental for the estimation of causality and direct causality through the DC and PDC estimators.

As an alternative to using the strictly causal model (5), the multivariate process $\mathbf{Y}(n)$ can be described including instantaneous effects into the interactions allowed by the model. This is achieved considering the extended MVAR process (Faes & Nollo, 2010b):

$$\mathbf{Y}(n)=\sum_{k=0}^{p}\mathbf{B}(k)\mathbf{Y}(n-k)+\mathbf{W}(n), \qquad (19)$$

where $\mathbf{W}(n)=[w_1(n),...,w_M(n)]^T$ is a vector of zero-mean uncorrelated white noise processes with diagonal covariance matrix $\Lambda=\text{diag}(\lambda^2_i)$. The difference with respect to strictly causal MVAR modelling as in (5) is that now the lag variable k takes the value 0 as well, which brings instantaneous effects from $y_j(n)$ to $y_i(n)$ into the model in the form of the coefficients $b_{ij}(0)$ of the matrix $\mathbf{B}(0)$. In the extended MVAR model, absence of correlation among the noise inputs w_i, i.e. diagonality of $\Lambda=\text{cov}(\mathbf{W}(n))$, is guaranteed by the presence of the instantaneous effects. Thus, the assumption that the input is a white noise vector process is always fulfilled by the extended representation.
The relation between the strictly causal representation and the extended representation can be established moving the term $\mathbf{B}(0)\mathbf{Y}(n)$ from the right to the left side of (19) and then left-multiplying both sides by by the matrix $\mathbf{L}^{-1}=[\mathbf{I}-\mathbf{B}(0)]$. The comparison with (5) yields:

$$\mathbf{A}(k)=\mathbf{L}\mathbf{B}(k)=[\mathbf{I}-\mathbf{B}(0)]^{-1}\mathbf{B}(k), \tag{20}$$

$$\mathbf{U}(n)=\mathbf{L}\mathbf{W}(n), \quad \Sigma=\mathbf{L}\Lambda\mathbf{L}^T . \tag{21}$$

These relationships indicate that the two representations coincide in the absence of instantaneous effects, and that the assumption of uncorrelated inputs is not satisfied in the presence of instantaneous effects. In fact, in the model (5) the input noise covariance Σ is not diagonal whenever $\mathbf{B}(0)\neq 0$ (and $\mathbf{L}\neq\mathbf{I}$). If the matrix $\mathbf{B}(0)$ has all zero entries we have $\mathbf{L}=\mathbf{I}$ and the model (19) reduces to (5) ($\mathbf{A}(k)=\mathbf{B}(k)$, $\mathbf{U}(n)=\mathbf{W}(n)$, $\Sigma=\Lambda$). By contrast, the existence of $\mathbf{B}(0)\neq 0$ makes coefficients $\mathbf{B}(k)$ differ from $\mathbf{A}(k)$ at each lag k. This property is crucial as it says that different patterns of causality may be found depending on whether instantaneous effects are included or not in the MVAR model used to represent the available data set.
Contrary to the strictly causal MVAR model which may describe only lagged interactions, the extended MVAR representation allows to detect any type of interaction defined in Sect. 2 and Table 1 from the elements $b_{ij}(k)$ of the matrix coefficients $\mathbf{B}(k)$. Specifically, direct causality $y_j\rightarrow y_i$ and extended direct causality $y_j \dot{\rightarrow} y_i$ are detected if $b_{ij}(k)\neq 0$ for at least one $k=1,\ldots,p$, and for at least one $k=0,1,\ldots,p$, respectively. Causality $y_j \Rightarrow y_i$ and extended causality $y_j \dot{\Rightarrow} y_i$ are detected if $b_{m_s m_{s-1}}(k_s)\neq 0$ for a set of lags $k_0,\ldots,k_{L-1}$ with values in $(1,\ldots,p)$ and with values in $(0,1,\ldots,p)$, respectively. Direct coupling $y_i\leftrightarrow y_j$ is detected if $b_{ji}(k)\neq 0$ and/or $b_{ij}(k)\neq 0$ for at least one $k=0,1,\ldots,p$. Coupling $y_i \Leftrightarrow y_j$ is detected if $b_{m_s m_{s-1}}(k_s)\neq 0$ for a set of $L\geq 2$ values for m_s (either with $m_0=j$, $m_{L-1}=i$ or with $m_0=i$, $m_{L-1}=j$) and a set of lags $k_0,\ldots,k_{L-1}$.

4.2 Frequency domain analysis of extended MVAR processes

The spectral representation of an extended MVAR process is obtained taking the FT of (19) to yield $\mathbf{Y}(f)=\mathbf{B}(f)\mathbf{Y}(f)+\mathbf{W}(f)$, where

$$\mathbf{B}(f)=\mathbf{B}(0)+\sum_{k=1}^{p}\mathbf{B}(k)e^{-j2\pi fkT} \tag{22}$$

is the frequency domain coefficient matrix. The representation evidencing input-output relations is $\mathbf{Y}(f)=\mathbf{G}(f)\mathbf{W}(f)$, where the transfer matrix is given by $\mathbf{G}(f)=[\mathbf{I}-\mathbf{B}(f)]^{-1}=\overline{\mathbf{B}}(f)^{-1}$. Given these representations, the spectral matrix $\mathbf{S}(f)$ and its inverse $\mathbf{P}(f)$ are expressed for the extended MVAR model as:

$$\mathbf{S}(f)=\mathbf{G}(f)\Lambda\mathbf{G}^{\mathrm{H}}(f),\ \mathbf{P}(f)=\overline{\mathbf{B}}^{\mathrm{H}}(f)\Lambda^{-1}\overline{\mathbf{B}}(f), \tag{23}$$

By means of some matrix algebra involving the spectral representations of (5) and (19), as well as (21), it is easy to show that the spectral matrix (and its inverse as well) resulting in (23) are exactly the same as those obtained in (7). This demonstrates the equivalence of the spectral representation for strictly causal MVAR processes and extended MVAR processes. Consequently, also the concepts of coupling and direct coupling are equivalent for the two process representation, since Coh and PCoh estimated as in (3) depend exclusively on the elements of $\mathbf{S}(f)$ and $\mathbf{P}(f)$. For this reason, a single estimator for Coh and PCoh is indicated in Table 1. A substantial difference between the conditions without and with instantaneous effects arises when coupling relations are decomposed to infer causality. We remark that the original formulation of DC and PDC holds fully only under the assumption of uncorrelation of the input processes, leading to diagonality of Σ and Σ^{-1}. When such an assumption is not fulfilled, the spectral factorizations in (9) do not hold anymore and the DC and PDC may become unable to identify causality and direct causality in the frequency domain. On the contrary, since the extended MVAR representation leads to diagonal input covariance matrices Λ and Λ^{-1} by construction, the factorizations in (9) are valid (using $\mathbf{B}(f)$ and $\mathbf{G}(f)$ as coefficient and transfer matrices in place of $\mathbf{A}(f)$ and $\mathbf{H}(f)$) still in the presence of instantaneous interactions among the observed processes. In particular, the following factorizations hold for the Coh:

$$\Gamma_{ij}(f)=\frac{\mathbf{g}_i(f)\Lambda\mathbf{g}_j^{\mathrm{H}}(f)}{\sqrt{\mathbf{g}_i(f)\Lambda\mathbf{g}_i^{\mathrm{H}}(f)}\sqrt{\mathbf{g}_j(f)\Lambda\mathbf{g}_j^{\mathrm{H}}(f)}}=\sum_{m=1}^{M}\frac{\lambda_m G_{im}(f)}{\sqrt{S_{ii}(f)}}\frac{\lambda_m G_{jm}^{*}(f)}{\sqrt{S_{jj}(f)}}=\sum_{m=1}^{M}\xi_{im}(f)\xi_{jm}^{*}(f) \quad (24)$$

and the PCoh:

$$\Pi_{ij}(f)=\frac{\bar{\mathbf{b}}_i^{\mathrm{H}}(f)\Lambda^{-1}\bar{\mathbf{b}}_j(f)}{\sqrt{\bar{\mathbf{b}}_i^{\mathrm{H}}(f)\Lambda^{-1}\bar{\mathbf{b}}_i(f)}\sqrt{\bar{\mathbf{b}}_j^{\mathrm{H}}(f)\Lambda^{-1}\bar{\mathbf{b}}_j(f)}}=\sum_{m=1}^{M}\frac{\frac{1}{\lambda_m}\bar{B}_{mj}(f)}{\sqrt{P_{jj}(f)}}\frac{\frac{1}{\lambda_m}\bar{B}_{mi}^{*}(f)}{\sqrt{P_{ii}(f)}}=\sum_{m=1}^{M}\chi_{mj}(f)\chi_{mi}^{*}(f), \quad (25)$$

where $\mathbf{g}_i(f)$ is the i-th row of $\mathbf{H}(f)$ and $\bar{\mathbf{b}}_i(f)$ is the i-th column of $\bar{\mathbf{B}}(f)$. The last terms of (24) and (25) contain the so-called *extended DC* (eDC) and *extended PDC* (ePDC), which are defined, for the extended MVAR model including instantaneous effects, respectively as:

$$\xi_{ij}(f)=\frac{\lambda_j G_{ij}(f)}{\sqrt{S_{ii}(f)}}=\frac{\lambda_j G_{ij}(f)}{\sqrt{\sum_{m=1}^{M}\lambda_m^2|G_{im}(f)|^2}}, \quad (26)$$

and as (Faes & Nollo, 2010b):

$$\chi_{ij}(f)=\frac{\frac{1}{\lambda_i}\bar{B}_{ij}(f)}{\sqrt{P_{jj}(f)}}=\frac{\frac{1}{\lambda_i}\bar{B}_{ij}(f)}{\sqrt{\sum_{m=1}^{M}\frac{1}{\lambda_m^2}|\bar{B}_{mj}(f)|^2}}. \quad (27)$$

The normalization conditions in (12) and (16) keep holding for the eDC and the ePDC defined in (26) and in (27). Hence, the squared eDC and ePDC $|\xi_{ij}(f)|^2$ and $|\chi_{ij}(f)|^2$ maintain their meaning of normalized proportion of $S_{ii}(f)$ which comes from y_j, and normalized proportion of $P_{jj}(f)$ which is sent to y_i, respectively, even in the presence of significant zero-lag interactions among the observed processes. In other words, we have that the meaningful decompositions in (13) and (17) are always valid for the eDC and the ePDC, respectively. On the contrary, these decompositions hold for the DC and the PDC only if instantaneous effects are negligible; when they are not, DC and PDC can still be computed through (11) and (15) but, since the factorizations in (9) are not valid when Σ is not diagonal, their numerator is no more a factor in the decomposition of Coh and PCoh, and their denominator is no more equal to $S_{ii}(f)$ or $P_{jj}(f)$. As we will see in a theoretical example in the next subsection, these limitations may lead to erroneous interpretations of causality and direct causality in the frequency domain.

When we use the extended measures in (26) and (27), the information which flows from y_i to y_j is both lagged (k>0) and instantaneous (k=0), because it is measured in the frequency domain by the function $\mathbf{B}(f)$ which incorporates both $\mathbf{B}(0)$ and $\mathbf{B}(k)$ with k>0. Therefore, eDC and ePDC measure in the frequency domain the concepts of extended causality and extended direct causality, respectively (see Table 1). If we want to explore lagged causality in the presence of zero-lag interactions, we have to exclude the coefficients related to the instantaneous effects from the desired spectral causality measure. Hence, we set:

$$\tilde{\mathbf{B}}(f)=\overline{\mathbf{B}}(f)+\mathbf{B}(0)=\mathbf{I}-\sum_{k=1}^{p}\mathbf{B}(k)e^{-j2\pi fkT} \quad , \quad \tilde{\mathbf{G}}(f)=\tilde{\mathbf{B}}(f)^{-1} \tag{28}$$

and then we define the following DC and PDC functions:

$$\tilde{\gamma}_{ij}(f)=\frac{\lambda_j\tilde{G}_{ij}(f)}{\sqrt{\sum_{m=1}^{M}\lambda_m^2\left|\tilde{G}_{im}(f)\right|^2}} \quad , \quad \tilde{\pi}_{ij}(f)=\frac{\frac{1}{\lambda_i}\tilde{B}_{ij}(f)}{\sqrt{\sum_{m=1}^{M}\frac{1}{\lambda_m^2}\left|\tilde{B}_{mj}(f)\right|^2}} . \tag{29}$$

Since they are derived exclusively from time domain matrices of lagged effects, $\tilde{\gamma}_{ij}(f)$ and $\tilde{\pi}_{ij}(f)$ measure respectively causality and direct causality in the frequency domain (see Table 1). We stress that, even though measuring the same kind of causality, the DC and PDC given in (29) are different from the corresponding functions given in (11) and (15), because the presence of instantaneous effects leads to different estimates of the coefficient matrix, or of the transfer matrix, using strictly causal or extended MVAR models. Only in the absence of instantaneous effects ($\mathbf{B}(0)$=0) DC and PDC estimated by the two models are the same, and are also equivalent to eDC and ePDC.

4.3 Theoretical example

In this section we compare the behavior of the different measures of frequency domain causality in a MVAR processes with imposed connectivity patterns including instantaneous interactions. The process is defined according to the interaction diagram of Fig. 1b, and is generated by the equations:

$$\begin{cases} y_1(n)=2\rho_1\cos(2\pi f_1)y_1(n-1)-\rho_1^2 y_1(n-2)-0.4y_3(n-1)+w_1(n) \\ y_2(n)=y_1(n)+0.2y_1(n-1)-\rho_2^2 y_2(n-2)+w_2(n) \\ y_3(n)=0.8y_2(n)+w_3(n) \\ y_4(n)=0.6y_2(n)+w_4(n) \end{cases} , \tag{30}$$

with ρ_1=0.95, f_1=0.125, ρ_2=0.8, and where the inputs $w_i(n)$, i=1,…,4 are fully uncorrelated white noise processes with variance equal to 1 for w_1 and w_4, equal to 2 for w_2, and equal to 8 for w_3. The diagonal values of the coefficient matrix are set to generate autonomous oscillations at ~0.125 Hz and ~0.25 Hz for y_1 and y_2, respectively. The nonzero off-diagonal coefficients set the direct directed interactions, which are exclusively instantaneous from y_2 to y_3 and from y_2 to y_4, exclusively lagged from y_3 to y_1, and mixed instantaneous and lagged from y_1 to y_2. The coupling and causality relations resulting from this scheme are described in detail in Sect. 2.1, with reference to Fig. 1b.
The MVAR process (30) is suitably described by the MVAR model with instantaneous effects of Fig. 5a, in which the use of coefficients describing both instantaneous and lagged effects allows to reproduce identically both the set of interactions imposed in (30) and the connectivity pattern of Fig. 1b. On the contrary, when a strictly causal MVAR process in the form of (5) is used to describe the same network, the resulting model is that of Fig. 5b. The strictly causal structure in Fig. 5b results from the application of (20) and (21) to the extended structure, leading to different values for the coefficients. As seen in Fig. 5, the result is an overestimation of the number of active direct pathways, and a general different estimation of the causality patterns. For instance, while in the original formulation (30) and in the extended MVAR representation of Fig. 5a direct causality is present only from y_1 to y_2 and from y_3 to y_1, a much higher number of direct causality relations is erroneously represented in Fig. 5b: in some cases instantaneous effects are misinterpreted as lagged (e.g., from y_2 to y_3 and from y_2 to y_4), in some other spurious connections appear (e.g., from y_1 to y_3 and from y_1 to y_4). The misleading connectivity pattern of Fig. 5b is the result of the impossibility for the model (5) to describe instantaneous effects. In the strictly causal representation, these effects are translated into the input covariance matrix (according to (20)): indeed, not only the input variances are different, but also cross-correlations between the input processes arise; in this case, we have σ^2_{12}=1, σ^2_{13}=0.8, σ^2_{14}=0.6, σ^2_{23}=2.4, σ^2_{24}=1.8, σ^2_{34}=1.44, whereas λ^2_{ij}=0 for each i≠j.

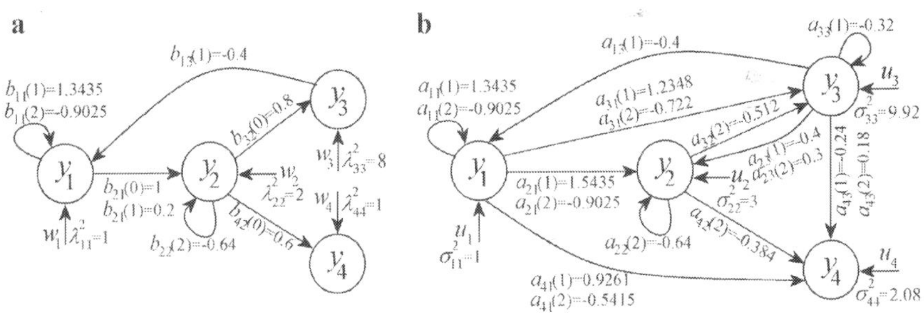

Fig. 5. Extended MVAR representation (**a**) and strictly causal MVAR representation (**b**) of the MVAR process generated by the equations in (30).

Fig. 6 reports the spectral and cross-spectral functions of the MVAR process (30). We remark that, due to the equivalence of eqs. (7) and (22), the profiles of spectra and inverse spectra, as well as of Coh and PCoh, perfectly overlap when calculated either from the strictly causal or from the extended MVAR representation. Despite this, these profiles are readily interpretable from the definitions of coupling and direct coupling only when the extended representation is used, while they do not describe the strictly causal representation. For instance, the PCohs reported in Fig. 6b have a one-to-one correspondence with the extended MVAR diagram of Fig. 5a, as a nonzero PCoh is shown in Fig. 6b exactly when a direct coupling is described by the coefficients in Fig. 5a (i.e., between y_1 and y_2, y_2 and y_3, y_2 and y_4, and y_1 and y_3). On the contrary, the PCoh profiles do not explain the direct coupling interactions which may be inferred from the strictly causal model in Fig. 5b: e.g., the nonzero coefficients $a_{41}(1)$ and $a_{41}(2)$ suggest the existence of direct coupling $y_1 \leftrightarrow y_4$,while such a coupling is not reflected by nonzero values of the PCoh $\Pi_{14}(f)$.

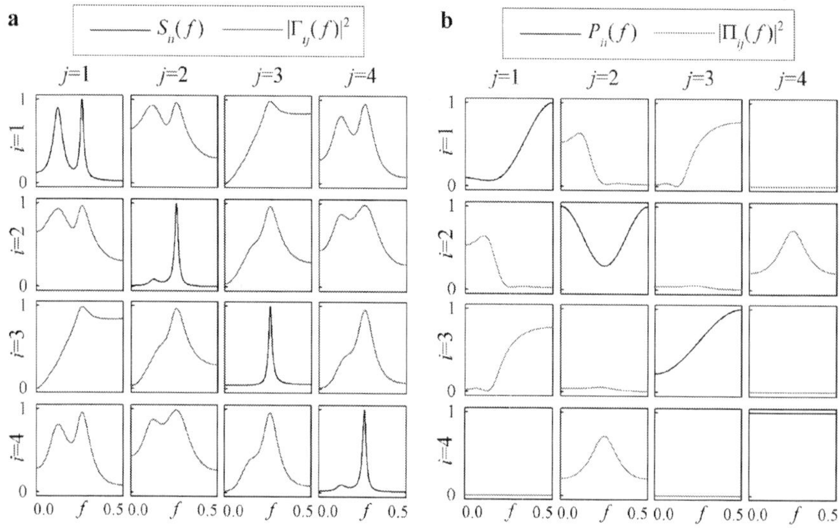

$S_{ii}(f)$: spectrum of the process y_i; $P_{ii}(f)$: inverse spectrum of y_i; $\Gamma_{ij}(f)$: coherence between y_j and y_i; $\Pi_{ij}(f)$: partial coherence between y_j and y_i.

Fig. 6. Spectral functions and frequency domain coupling measures for the theoretical example (30).

The problems of using the strictly causal MVAR representation in the presence of instantaneous effects become even more severe when one aims at disentangling the coupling relations to measure causality in the frequency domain. In this case, the spectral representations closely reflect the time domain diagrams, but —quite for this reason— only the extended spectral profiles are correct while the strictly causal one may be strongly misleading. This is demonstrated in Figs. 7 and 8, depicting respectively the frequency domain evaluation of causality and direct causality for the considered theoretical example.

As shown in Fig. 7, the extended MVAR representation of the considered process yields a frequency-domain connectivity pattern which is able to describe all and only the imposed direct connections: the PDC correctly portrays (lagged) direct causality from y_1 to y_2 and from y_3 to y_1, being zero over all other directions (black dashed curves in Fig. 7a); the ePDC portrays all extended causality relations, being nonzero only from y_1 to y_2 (mixed instantaneous and lagged effect), from y_3 to y_1 (lagged effect), as well as from y_2 to y_3 and from y_2 to y_4

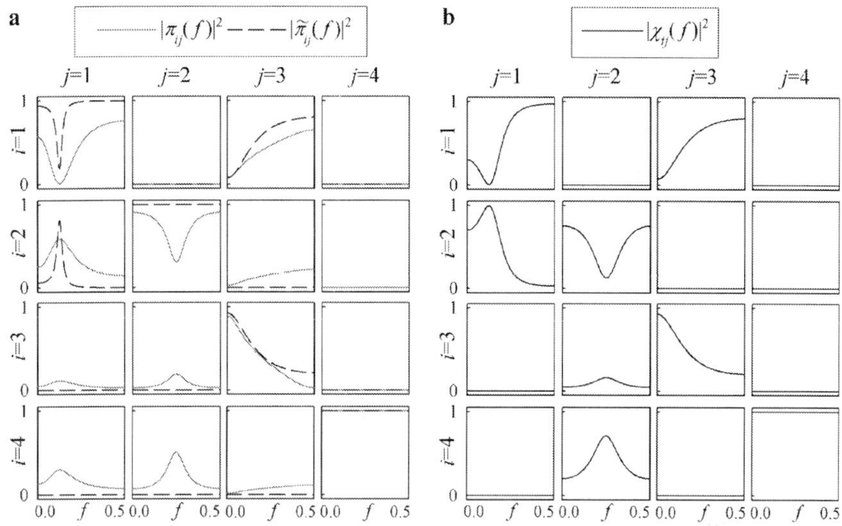

Fig. 7. Diagrams of squared PDC for the strictly causal MVAR representation ($|\pi_{ij}(f)|^2$) and the extended representation ($|\tilde{\pi}_{ij}(f)|^2$) (**a**), and of squared ePDC ($|\chi_{ij}(f)|^2$, **b**), for the theoretical example (30).

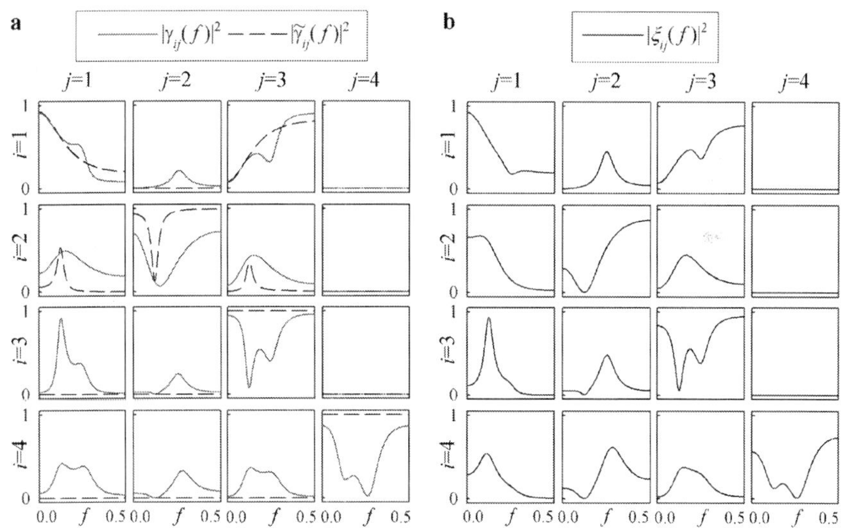

Fig. 8. Diagrams of squared DC for the strictly causal MVAR representation ($|\gamma_{ij}(f)|^2$) and the extended representation ($|\tilde{\gamma}_{ij}(f)|^2$) (**a**), and of squared eDC ($|\xi_{ij}(f)|^2$, **b**), for the theoretical example (30).

(instantaneous effect) (Fig. 7b). On the contrary, utilization of the strictly causal MVAR representation leads to erroneous interpretation of lagged direct causality. Indeed, as seen in Fig. 7a (red solid curves), the PDC interprets as lagged the instantaneous connections from y_2 to y_3 and from y_2 to y_4. Moreover, spurious causality effects are measured, as the PDC is nonzero from y_1 to y_3, from y_1 to y_4 and from y_3 to y_4, albeit no direct effects (neither lagged nor instantaneous) are imposed in (30) over these directions.

A similar situation occurs when causality and extended causality are studied in the frequency domain through DC-based functions. Fig. 8a shows that the pattern of causality relations imposed in (30) (i.e., $y_1 \Rightarrow y_2$, $y_3 \Rightarrow y_1$, and $y_3 \Rightarrow y_2$) is not reflected by the DC measured from the strictly causal model through eq. (11). The DC profile (blue solid curves) describes indeed many other causal effects besides the two correct ones; precisely, all (direct or indirect) causality relations emerging from the diagram of Fig. 5b are measured with nonzero values of the DC and thus interpreted as lagged causal effects. These effects are actually due to instantaneous interactions, and thus should not be represented by the DC as it is a measure of lagged causality only. The correct representation is given using the DC measured from the extended MVAR model through eq. (29): in this case, the only nonzero squared DCs are those measured over the three directions with imposed causality, while the squared DC is zero over all other directions (black dashed curves in Fig. 8a). The relations of causality emerging thanks to the instantaneous effects are detected by the eDC computed through (29) and plotted in Fig. 8b, which is able to measure also instantaneous effects in addition to the lagged ones. Thus, we see that a correct frequency domain representation of causality and extended causality is given by the DC and eDC functions derived from the extended MVAR representation of the considered process.

5. Practical analysis

5.1 Model identification

The practical application of the theoretical concepts described in the previous sections is based on considering the available set of time series measured from the physiological system under analysis, $\{y_m(n), m=1,\ldots,M; n=1,\ldots N\}$, as a finite-length realization of the vector stochastic process describing the evolution of the system over time. Hence, the descriptive equations of the MVAR processes (5) and (19) are seen as a model of how the observed data have been generated. To obtain the various frequency domain functions measuring causality and coupling, estimation algorithms have to be applied to the observed time series for providing estimates of the model coefficients, which are then used in the generating equations in place of the true unknown coefficient values. Obviously, the estimates will never be the exact coefficients, and consequently the frequency domain measures estimated from the real data will always be an approximation of the true functions. The goodness of the approximation depends on practical factors such as the data length, and on the type and parameters of the procedure adopted for the identification of the model coefficients. In the following, we describe some of the possible approaches to identify and validate the MVAR models in (5) and (19) from experimental data.

Identification of the strictly causal MVAR model (5) can be performed with relative ease by means of classic regression methods. The several existing MVAR estimators (see, e.g., (Kay, 1988) or (Lutkepohl, 1993) for detailed descriptions) are all based on the principle of minimizing the prediction error, i.e. the difference between actual and predicted data. A simple, consistent and asymptotically efficient estimator is the MV least squares method. It is based first on representing (5) through the compact representation **Y=AZ+U**, where **A**=[**A**(1)$\cdots$**A**(p)] is the $M\times pM$ matrix of the unknown coefficients, **Y**=[**Y**(p+1)$\cdots$**Y**(N)] and **U**=[**U**(p+1)$\cdots$**U**(N)] are $M\times(N-p)$ matrices, and **Z**=[$\mathbf{Z}_1\cdots\mathbf{Z}_p$] is a $pM\times(N-p)$ matrix having $\mathbf{Z}_i$=[**Y**(i)$\cdots$**Y**(N-p+i-1)] as i-th row block of (i=1,...M). Given this representation, the method estimates the coefficient matrices through the well known least squares formula: $\hat{\mathbf{A}}=\mathbf{YZ}^T[\mathbf{ZZ}^T]^{-1}$, and the input process as the residual time series: $\hat{\mathbf{U}}=\hat{\mathbf{A}}\mathbf{Z}-\mathbf{Y}$. As to model order selection, one common approach is to set the order p at the value for which the Akaike figure of merit (Akaike, 1974), defined as $AIC(p)=N \log \det\Sigma+M^2p$, reaches a minimum within a predefined range of orders (typically from 1 to 30). While the presented model identification and order selection methods have good statistical properties, more accurate approaches exist; e.g., we refer the reader to (Schlogl, 2006) for a comparison of different MVAR estimators, and to (Erla et al., 2009) for an identification approach combining MVAR coefficient estimation and order selection.

The identification of the extended MVAR model (19) is much less straightforward, because the estimation of instantaneous causality is hard to extract from the covariance information (which is, *per se*, non-directional). In principle, availing of an estimate of the instantaneous effects, described by the matrix **B**(0) in the representation (19), identification of the extended MVAR model would follow from that of the strictly causal model describing the same data. Indeed, we recall from (20) and (21) that lagged coefficients and residuals may be estimated for the extended model as $\hat{\mathbf{B}}(k)=[\mathbf{I}-\mathbf{B}(0)]\hat{\mathbf{A}}(k)$ and $\hat{\mathbf{W}}(n)=[\mathbf{I}-\mathbf{B}(0)]\hat{\mathbf{U}}(n)$. Hence, the key for extended MVAR identification is to find the matrix **B**(0) which satisfies the instantaneous model $\mathbf{U}(n)=\mathbf{LW}(n)=[\mathbf{I}-\mathbf{B}(0)]^{-1}\mathbf{W}(n)$, and then to use it together with estimates of **A**(k) and **U**(n) to estimate **W**(n) and **B**(k) for each $k\geq1$.

The basic problem with the instantaneous model is that it is strictly related to the zero-lag covariance structure of the observed data and, as such, it suffers from lack of identifiability. In other words, there may be several combinations of **L** (or, equivalently, **B**(0)) and **W**(n) which result in the same **U**(n), and thus describe the observed data **Y**(n) equally well. The easiest way to solve this ambiguity is to impose *a priori* the structure of instantaneous causation, i.e. to set the direction (though not the strength) of the instantaneous transfer paths. Mathematically, this can be achieved determining the mixing matrix **L** and the diagonal input covariance of the extended model, Λ=cov(**W**(n)), by application of the Cholesky decomposition to the estimate of input covariance of the strictly causal model, Σ=cov(**U**(n)) (Faes & Nollo, 2010b). While this decomposition agrees with (21), the resulting **L** is is a lower triangular matrix, and **B**(0) is also lower triangular with null diagonal. To fulfill this constraint in practical applications, the observed time series have to be ordered in a way such that, for each $j<i$, instantaneous effects are allowed from $y_j(n)$ to $y_i(n)$ ($b_{ij}(0)\neq0$) but not from $y_i(n)$ to $y_j(n)$ ($b_{ji}(0)=0$). This can be done in some applications by means of physical considerations, e.g., based on the temporal order of the events of interest for each measured variable. Following this approach, frequency domain causality was assessed between heart period, arterial pressure and respiration variability in a recent study (Faes & Nollo, 2010a). Nevertheless, if similar prior knowledge is not available, as happens e.g., in the analysis of EEG data, other ways have to be followed to overcome problem of identifiability of the extended model. The most promising one seems that based on exploiting non-Gaussianity in the identification. Indeed, (Shimizu et al., 2006) demonstrated that, if the input process **W**(n) has a non-Gaussian distribution, no prior knowledge on the network structure is needed to identify the instantaneous model. The proposed algorithm

estimates $\mathbf{B}(0)$ in two steps (see (Shimizu et al., 2006) for details): first, independent component analysis (ICA) is performed on the estimated residuals $\mathbf{U}(n)$, finding a mixing matrix $\mathbf{M}$ which represents an unordered and non-normalized version of $\mathbf{L}$; second, an appropriate row-permutation followed by normalization is applied to $\mathbf{M}^{-1}$ to get an estimate of $\mathbf{L}^{-1}$, and thus of $\mathbf{B}(0)=\mathbf{I}-\mathbf{L}^{-1}$. This algorithm has been exploited to demonstrate identifiability of the extended MVAR model in (Hyvarinen et al., 2008). More recently, the full algorithm has been proposed to estimate frequency domain causality, and used to assess patterns of directional cortical connectivity from multichannel EEG (Faes et al., 2010a).

5.2 Validation

Although model identification allows to find the estimates of coefficients and input covariances which easily lead to the desired frequency-domain measures of coupling and causality, validation steps need to be performed to guarantee a correct interpretation of the obtained results. In fact, proper checking has to be performed, in both time and frequency domains, in order to confirm the suitability of the estimated model for describing the observed data and to assess the significance of the estimated coupling strengths.

Model validation refers to the use of a range of diagnostic tools which are available for checking the adequacy of the estimated structure. While validation tests are rarely used in the practical application of tools like the DC or the PDC, they constitute actually fundamental safeguards against drawing erroneous inferences consequently to model misspecification. A striking example is the undervaluation of the impact of instantaneous effects in the assessment of frequency domain causality, which we demonstrated in this chapter and might be avoided by proper checking of the significance of instantaneous correlations in experimental multichannel data. While a thorough description of the statistical tools for model validation is beyond the scope of this work, here we remark the model assumptions that must be verified prior to frequency domain analysis. The identification of strictly causal MVAR models should result in temporally uncorrelated and mutually independent residuals $\hat{\mathbf{U}}(n)$. These assumptions may be checked, e.g., using the Ljung-Box portmanteau test for whiteness and the Kendall's τ test for independence. Independence of the residuals has to be checked particularly at zero lag; when this assumption is violated, one should allow instantaneous effects to be modeled moving from the strictly causal to the extended MVAR representation. If performed without incorporating prior assumptions in the model formulation, the extended MVAR identification should result also in non-Gaussian residuals $\hat{\mathbf{W}}(n)$; non-Gaussianity may be tested, e.g., by the Jarque-Bera test for non-normal distribution. All the diagnostic tests mentioned here are excellently reviewed in (Lutkepohl, 1993).

Another issue of great practical importance is the assessment of the significance of any frequency domain index of coupling or causal coupling. Due to practical estimation problems, nonzero values are indeed likely to occur at some frequencies even in the case of absence of a true interaction between the two considered processes. This problem is commonly faced by means of statistical hypothesis testing procedures based on setting a threshold for significance at the upper limit of the confidence interval of the considered index, where confidence intervals are based on the sampling distribution of the index computed under the null hypothesis of absence of interaction. Comparing at each specific frequency the estimated index with the threshold allows rejection or acceptance of the null hypothesis, and thus detection or denial of coupling or causality, according to the predetermined level of significance. The sampling distribution in the absence of coupling or causality may be derived theoretically or empirically: theoretical approaches are elegant and computationally more efficient, empirical ones are more general and free of approximations. For a detailed description of the two approaches we refer to (Koopmans, 1974; Schelter et al., 2006; Eichler, 2006), where the statistical properties of Coh, DC/DTF, and PDC are studied and corresponding analytical threshold for significance are derived, and to (Faes et al., 2004; Faes et al., 2010b), where empirical significance levels are estimated for the same functions on the basis of surrogate data generation procedure devised specifically for each function.

6. Conclusion

In this chapter we have discussed the theoretical interpretation of the most common frequency-domain measures of coupling (Coh, PCoh) and causality (DC, PDC) in MV time series. We have shown that: (i) each of these measures reflects a specific time-domain definition of coupling or causality (see Table 1); (ii) while Coh and PCoh are symmetric measures, they can be decomposed into factors eliciting directionality, these factors being exactly the DC and the PDC; (iii) the squared modulus of the DC and the PDC measure respectively the fraction of power of the output signal which is received from the input signal, normalized to all incoming contributions, and of inverse power of the input signal which is sent to the output signal, normalized to all outgoing contributions. The picture emerging from these results suggests that both DC and PDC should be computed for the complete inference of frequency-domain causality in MV time series: DC measures causality in meaningful physical terms as power contributions, but cannot separate direct effects from indirect ones; PDC determines the correct interaction structure in terms of direct causal effects, but its absolute values lack of straightforward interpretability.

In addition, we emphasized the necessity extending the MVAR modeling approach traditionally used to assess frequency-domain causality whenever the time resolution of the measurements is lower than the time scale of the lagged influences occurring in the observed MV process. In such a case, the interpretation of the lagged effects may change considerably if instantaneous effects are not included in the model. We showed how the traditional DC and PDC computed from the strictly causal model may lead to misleading connectivity patterns, while the correct interpretation is obtained defining the two functions from the coefficients of the extended model. Moreover, we introduced novel frequency-domain measures of causality and direct causality (eDC and ePDC) which were shown to reflect extended causality definitions combining both lagged and instantaneous causality from one signal to another.

7. References

Akaike, H. (1974). A new look at the statistical model identification. *IEEE Transactions on Automation and Control*, Vol. 19, pp. 716-723

Akselrod, S.; Gordon, D.; Ubel, F. A.; Shannon, D. C.; Berger, A. C. & Cohen, R. J. (1981). Power spectrum analysis of heart rate fluctuation: a quantitative probe of beat-to-beat cardiovascular control. *Science*, Vol. 213, pp. 220-222

Albo, Z.; Di Prisco, G. V.; Chen, Y.; Rangarajan, G.; Truccolo, W.; Feng, J.; Vertes, R. P. & Ding, M. (2004). Is partial coherence a viable technique for identifying generators of neural oscillations? *Biological Cybernetics*, Vol. 90, No. 5, pp. 318-326

Astolfi, L.; Cincotti, F.; Mattia, D.; Marciani, M. G.; Baccala, L. A.; De Vico, F. F.; Salinari, S.; Ursino, M.; Zavaglia, M.; Ding, L.; Edgar, J. C.; Miller, G. A.; He, B. & Babiloni, F. (2007). Comparison of different cortical connectivity estimators for high-resolution EEG recordings. *Human Brain Mapping*, Vol. 28, No. 2, pp. 143-157

Baccala, L.; Sameshima, K. & Takahashi, D. Y. (2007). Generalized partial directed coherence, *Proceedings of the 2007 15th International Conference on Digital Signal Processing*, pp. 163-166, Cardiff, UK

Baccala, L. A. & Sameshima, K. (2001). Partial directed coherence: a new concept in neural structure determination. *Biological Cybernetics*, Vol. 84, No. 6, pp. 463-474

Baccala, L. A. & Sameshima, K. (2006). Comments on 'Is partial coherence a viable technique for identifying generators of neural oscillations?': Why the term 'Gersch Causality' is inappropriate: common neural structure inference pitfalls. *Biological Cybernetics*, Vol. 95, No. 2, pp. 135-141

Baccala, L. A.; Sameshima, K.; Ballester, G.; Valle, A. C. & Timo-Iaria, C. (1998). Studying the interaction between brain structures via directed coherence and Granger causality. *Applied Signal Processing*, Vol. 5, pp. 40-48

Bendat, J. S. & Piersol, A. G. (1986). *Random data: analysis and measurement procedures*, John Wiley & Sons, New York

Eichler, M. (2006). On the evaluation of information flow in multivariate systems by the directed transfer function. *Biological Cybernetics*, Vol. 94, No. 6, pp. 469-482

Erla, S.; Faes, L. & Nollo, G. (2009). Robust estimation of partial directed coherence by the vector optimal parameter search algorithm, *Proceeding of the 4-th IEEE-EMBS Conference on Neural Engineering*, pp. 6280-6283, Antalya, Turkey

Faes, L.; Erla, S.; Tranquillini, E.; Orrico, D. & Nollo, G. (2010a). An identifiable model to assess frequency-domain Granger causality in the presence of significant instantaneous interactions, *Proceedings of the 32th Annual International Conference of the IEEE-EMBS*, pp. 1699-1702, Buenos Aires, Argentina

Faes, L. & Nollo, G. (2010a). A method to assess frequency domain causality in the presence of instantaneous effects and its application to short term cardiovascular variability. *Methods of Information in Medicine*, Vol. 49, No. 5, doi: 10.3414/ME09-02-0030

Faes, L. & Nollo, G. (2010b). Extended causal modelling to assess partial directed coherence in multiple time series with significant instantaneous interactions. *Biological Cybernetics*, in press; doi: .1007/s00422-010-0406-6.

Faes, L.; Nollo, G. & Chon, K. H. (2008). Assessment of Granger causality by nonlinear model identification: application to short-term cardiovascular variability. *Annals of Biomedical Engineering*, Vol. 36, No. 3, pp. 381-395

Faes, L.; Pinna, G. D.; Porta, A.; Maestri, R. & Nollo, G. (2004). Surrogate data analysis for assessing the significance of the coherence function. *IEEE Transactions on Biomedical Engineering*, Vol. 51, No. 7, pp. 1156-1166

Faes, L.; Porta, A. & Nollo, G. (2010b). Testing Frequency Domain Causality in Multivariate Time Series. *IEEE Transactions on Biomedical Engineering*, Vol. 57, No. 8, pp. 1897-1906

Faes, L. & Nollo, G. (2010a). Assessing frequency domain causality in cardiovascular time series with instantaneous interactions. *Methods of Information in Medicine*, Vol. 49, pp. 453-457

Faes, L. & Nollo, G. (2010b). Extended causal modelling to assess partial directed coherence in multiple time series with significant instantaneous interactions. *Biological Cybernetics*, Vol. 103, No. 5, pp. 387-400

Gourevitch, B.; Bouquin-Jeannes, R. L. & Faucon, G. (2006). Linear and nonlinear causality between signals: methods, examples and neurophysiological applications. *Biological Cybernetics*, Vol. 95, No. 4, pp. 349-369

Granger, C. W. J. (1969). Investigating causal relations by econometric models and cross-spectral methods. *Econometrica*, Vol. 37, pp. 424-438

Granger, C. W. J. (1980). Testing for causality: a personal viewpoint. *J. Econom. Dynam. Control*, Vol. 2, pp. 329-352

Hyvarinen, A.; Shimizu, S. & Hoyer, P. O. (2008). Causal modelling combining instantaneous and lagged effects: an identifiable model based on non-Gaussianity, *Proceedings of the 25th International Conference on Machine Learning*, pp. 1-8, Helsinki

Kaminski, M.; Ding, M.; Truccolo, W. A. & Bressler, S. L. (2001). Evaluating causal relations in neural systems: granger causality, directed transfer function and statistical assessment of significance. *Biological Cybernetics*, Vol. 85, No. 2, pp. 145-157

Kaminski, M. J. & Blinowska, K. J. (1991). A new method of the description of the information flow in the brain structures. *Biological Cybernetics*, Vol. 65, No. 3, pp. 203-210

Kay, S. M. (1988). *Modern spectral estimation. Theory & application*, Prentice Hall, Englewood Cliffs, New Jersey

Koopmans, L. H. (1974). *The spectral analysis of time series*, Academic Press, New York

Lutkepohl, H. (1993). *Introduction to multiple time series analysis*, Springer, Berlin Heidelberg New York

Nunez, P. L. (1995). *Neocortical dynamics and human EEG rhythms*, Oxford University Press, USA

Pereda, E.; Quiroga, R. Q. & Bhattacharya, J. (2005). Nonlinear multivariate analysis of neurophysiological signals. *Progress in Neurobiology*, Vol. 77, No. 1-2, pp. 1-37

Porta, A.; Aletti, F.; Vallais, F. & Baselli, G. (2009). Multimodal signal processing for the analysis of cardiovascular variability. *Philosophical Transactions of the Royal Society of London Series A-Mathematical Physical and Engineering Sciences*, Vol. 367, No. 1887, pp. 391-409

Porta, A.; Furlan, R.; Rimoldi, O.; Pagani, M.; Malliani, A. & van de Borne, P. (2002). Quantifying the strength of the linear causal coupling in closed loop interacting cardiovascular variability signals. *Biological Cybernetics*, Vol. 86, No. 3, pp. 241-251

Schelter, B.; Winterhalder, M.; Eichler, M.; Peifer, M.; Hellwig, B.; Guschlbauer, B.; Lucking, C. H.; Dahlhaus, R. & Timmer, J. (2006). Testing for directed influences among neural signals using partial directed coherence. *Journal of Neuroscience Methods*, Vol. 152, No. 1-2, pp. 210-219

Schlogl, A. (2006). A comparison of multivariate autoregressive estimators. *Signal Processing*, Vol. 86, pp. 2426-2429

Schlogl, A. & Supp, G. (2006). Analyzing event-related EEG data with multivariate autoregressive parameters. *Progress in Brain Research*, Vol. 159, pp. 135-147

Shimizu, S.; Hoyer, P. O.; Hyvarinen, A. & Kerminen, A. (2006). A linear non-Gaussian acyclic model for causal discovery. *Journal of Machine Learning Research*, Vol. 7, pp. 2003-2030

Whittaker, J. (1990). *Graphical models in applied multivariate statistics*, Wiley, Chichester

22

Biomedical Image Segmentation Based on Multiple Image Features

Jinhua Yu[1,2], Jinglu Tan[1] and Yuanyuan Wang[2]
[1]*University of Missouri*
[2]*Fudan University*
[1]*USA*
[2]*China*

1. Introduction

Image segmentation is a procedure that partitions an image into disjointing segments with each segment sharing similar properties such as intensity, color, boundary and texture. In general, three main types of image features are used to guide image segmentation, which are intensity or color, edge, and texture. In other words, image segmentation methods generally fall into three main categories: intensity-based (or color-based), edge-based, and texture-based segmentations.

Intensity-based segmentation assumes that an image is composed of several objects with constant intensity. This kind of methods usually depends on intensity similarity comparisons to separate different objects. Histogram thresholding (Otsu, 1979; Sahoo et al., 1988), clustering (Bezdek, 1981; Pappas, 1992), and split-and-merge (Tyagi & Bayoumi, 1992; Wu, 1993) are examples of intensity-based segmentation methods.

Edge-based segmentation has a strong relationship with intensity-based segmentation, since edges usually indicate discontinuities in image intensity. Edge-based segmentation uses different methods to describe the salient edges in images. Then, the boundaries of objects are detected by edge grouping or edge-driven active contour construction. Widely-used methods in edge-based segmentation include Canny (Canny 1986), watershed (Vincent & Soille, 1991) and snake (Kass et al., 1998; Xu & Prince, 1998).

Texture is another important characteristic used to segment objects in an image. Most texture-based segmentation algorithms map an image into a texture feature space, then statistical classification methods (Randen & Husoy, 1999) are usually used to differentiate texture features. Co-occurrence matrix (Zucker & Terzopoulos, 1980), directional gray-level energy (Hsiao & Sawchuk, 1989), Gabor filters (Jain & Farrokhnia, 1991), and fractal dimension (Mandelbrot, 1976; Pentland 1984) are frequently used methods to obtain texture features.

Biomedical images usually suffer from certain imaging artifacts stemming from different imaging modalities. Because of imperfect illumination, signal attenuation or signal superposition in biomedical images, intensity-based segmentation methods are often ineffective in differentiating neighboring tissues with similar intensity features. Further, because of noises in biomedical images, detected tissue edges are often discontinuous, obstructed, or obscure. It remains a problem in edge-based segmentation to interpret and connect discontinuous edges. As a high-level image characteristic, texture reflects the spatial arrangement of intensity, color or shape. Texture features could be easily spoiled by imperfect imaging conditions mentioned above. As a result, a single image feature is usually not sufficient to produce satisfactory segmentation for biomedical images. Multiple image features can be combined to enhance segmentation. This chapter provides three applications illustrating how multiple image features are integrated for segmentation of images generated from different modalities.

2. Fetal abdominal contour measurement in ultrasound images

Because of its noninvasiveness, ultrasound imaging is the most prevalent diagnostic technique used in obstetrics. Fetal abdominal circumference (AC), an indicator of fetal growth, is one of the standardized measurements in antepartum ultrasound monitoring. In the first application, a method that makes effective use of the intensity and edge information is provided to outline and measure the fetal abdominal circumference from ultrasound images (Yu et al., 2008a; Yu et al., 2008b).

2.1 Algorithm overview

Fig. 1 summarizes the segmentation algorithm for abdomen measurement.

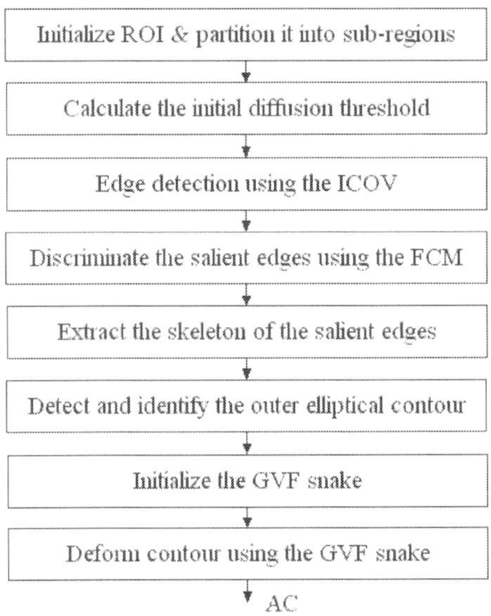

Fig. 1. Flowchart of segmentation algorithm for abdomen measurement.

In the first step, a rectangle enclosing the contour of the target object, is given by the operator (as shown in Fig. 2(a)), then a region of interest (ROI) is defined in the form of an elliptical ring within the manually defined rectangle. The outer ellipse of the ring inscribes the rectangle. The inner ellipse is 30% smaller than the outer ellipse. To accommodate edge strength variations, the ROI is equally partitioned into eight sub-regions. In the second step, the initial diffusion threshold is calculated for each sub-region. Instantaneous coefficient of variation (ICOV) is used to detect the edges of the abdominal contour in the third step. The detected edges are shown in Fig. 2(b). The fuzzy C-Means (FCM) clustering algorithm is then used to distinguish between salient edges of the abdominal contour and weak edges resulting from other textures. Salient edges are then thinned to serve as the input to the next step. As shown in Fig. 2 (c), bright pixels are the salient edges, and dark lines within the bright pixels are the skeleton of the edges. In the sixth step, randomized Hough transforms (RHT) is used to detect and locate the outer contour of AC. The detected ellipse for AC is shown in Fig. 2 (d). To improve AC contour extraction in the seventh and eighth steps, a GVF snake is employed to adapt the detected ellipse to the real edges of the abdominal contour. The final segmentation by the GVF snake is shown in Fig. 2(e). For comparison, the original ROI image and the manual AC contour are shown in Fig. 2(f) and 2(g), respectively.

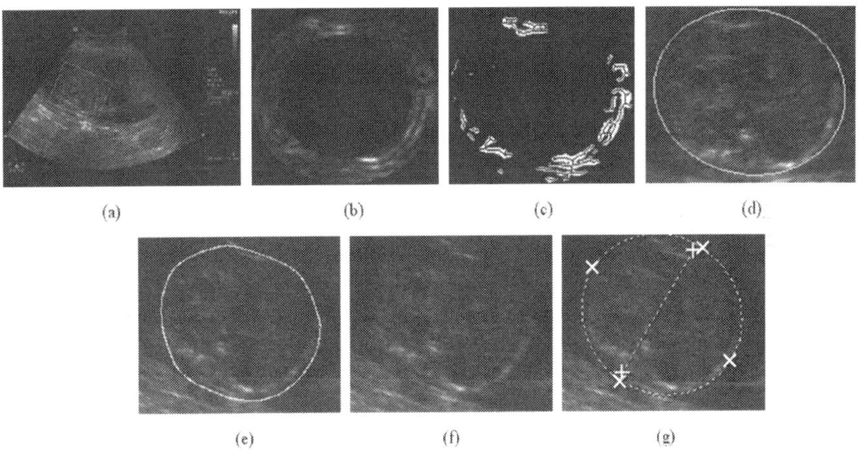

Fig. 2. Segmentation and measurement of fetal abdomen. (a) ROI definition, (b) Edge map detected by ICOV, (c) Salient edges with skeleton, (d) Initial contour obtained by RHT, (e) Final abdominal contour, (f) Original image, (g) Manually extracted abdominal contour.

2.2 Edge detection of the abdominal contour

For images that contain strong artifacts, it is difficult to detect boundaries of different tissues without being affected by noise. A regular edge detector such as Canny operator (Canny, 1986), Haralick operator (Haralick 1982) or Laplacian - of - Gaussian operator (FjØrtoft et al., 1998) can not provide satisfactory results. The instantaneous coefficient of variation (ICOV) (Yu & Acton, 2004) provides improvement in edge-detection over traditional edge detectors. The ICOV edge-detection algorithm combines a partial differential equation-based speckle-reducing filter (Yu & Acton, 2002) and an edge strength measurement in filtered images. With the image intensity at the pixel position (x,y) denoted as I, the strength of the detected edge at time t, denoted as $q(x,y;t)$, is given by

$$q(x,y;t)=\sqrt{\frac{\left|\left(\frac{1}{2}\right)\|\nabla I\|^2-\left(\frac{1}{16}\right)\left(\nabla^2 I\right)^2\right|}{\left(I+\left(\frac{1}{4}\right)\nabla^2 I\right)^2}} \tag{1}$$

where ∇, ∇^2, $\| \ \|$, and $| \ |$ are the gradient, Laplacian, gradient magnitude, and absolute value, respectively. The speckle reduction is achieved via a diffusion process, which is determined by a diffusion coefficient defined as

$$c(q) = \frac{1}{1 + [q^2(x,y;t) - q_0^2(t)] / [q_0^2(t)(1 + q_0^2(t))]} \tag{2}$$

where $q_0(t)$ is the diffusion threshold to determine whether to encourage or inhibit the diffusion process. The selection of an appropriate $q_0(t)$ has paramount effects on the performance of speckle reduction hence the performance of edge detection. To be adaptive to edge strength variation, the ROI is equally partitioned into eight sub-regions. The initial diffusion threshold q_0 for each sub-region is formulated as

$$q_0 = \frac{\sqrt{\mathrm{var}[SR]}}{\overline{SR}} \tag{3}$$

where var[SR] and $\overline{SR}$ are the intensity variance and mean of each sub-region SR. $q_0(t)$ is approximated by $q_0(t) = q_0 \exp[-t/6]$, where t represents the discrete diffusion time step.

2.3 Edge map simplification

In order to distinguish between salient edges of the abdominal contour and weak edges from other textures, the fuzzy C-Means (FCM) clustering algorithm (Bezdek, 1980) is employed. Let $X=\{I_1, I_2, \ldots, I_n\}$ be a set of n data points, and c be the total number of clusters or classes. The objective function for partitioning X into c clusters is given by

$$J_{FCM} = \sum_{j=1}^{c} \sum_{i=1}^{n} \mu_{ij}^2 \left\| I_i - m_j \right\|^2 \tag{4}$$

where m_j, $j=1,2,\ldots,c$ represent the cluster prototypes and μ_{ij} gives the membership of pixel I_i in the jth cluster m_j. The fuzzy partition matrix satisfies

$$U = \left\{ \mu_{ij} \in [0,1] \;\middle|\; \sum_{j=1}^{c} \mu_{ij} = 1 \quad \forall i \quad and \quad 0 < \sum_{i=1}^{N} \mu_{ij} < N \quad \forall j \right\} \tag{5}$$

Under the constraint of (5), setting the first derivatives of (4) with respect to μ_{ij} and m_j to zero yields the necessary conditions for (4) to be minimized. Based on the edge strength, each pixel in the edge map is classified into one of three clusters: salient edges, weak edges, and the background. Then salient edges (bright pixels in Fig. 2(c)) are thinned (dark curves in Fig. 2(c)) to serve as the input to the next step.

2.4 Initial abdominal contour estimation & contour deformation

Randomized Hough transform (RHT) depends on random sampling and many-to-one mapping from the image space to the parameter space in order to achieve effective object detection. An iterative randomized Hough transform (IRHT) (Lu et al., 2005), which applies the RHT to an adaptive ROI iteratively, is used to detect and locate the outer contour of AC. A parametric representation of ellipse is:

$$a_1x^2 + a_2xy + a_3y^2 + a_4x + a_5y + 1 = 0 \tag{6}$$

At the end of each round of the RHT, the skeleton image is updated by discarding the pixels within an ellipse which is 5% smaller than the detected ellipse. At the end of IRHT iterations, edges located on the outer boundary remain; and the detected ellipse converges to the outer contour of the abdomen.

The active contour model, or snake method as commonly known, is employed to find the best fit between the final contour and the actual shape of the AC. A snake is an energy-minimizing spline guided by external constraint forces computed from the image data and influenced by image forces coming from the curve itself (Kass et al., 1988). To overcome problems associated with initialization and poor convergence to boundary concavities of a classical snake, an new external force field called gradient vector flow (GVF) is introduced (Xu & Prince, 1998). The GVF field is defined as the vector field $v(x, y)$ that minimizes the following energy functional

$$E = \iint \mu |\nabla \mathbf{v}|^2 + |\nabla f|^2 |\mathbf{v} - \nabla f|^2 \, dxdy \tag{7}$$

where μ is a parameter governing the tradeoff between the first term and the second term in the integrand, ∇ is the gradient operator which is applied to each component of v separately, and f represents the edge map. Fig. 2(e) shows the final segmentation by the GVF snake with the skeleton image as the object and the detected ellipse (Fig. 2(d)) as the initial contour.

2.5 Algorithm performance

Fig. 3 gives results of automatic abdominal contour estimation and manual delineation on four clinical ultrasound images. The four images represent some typical conditions that often occur in daily ultrasound measurements. The first row is for a relatively ideal ultrasound image of abdominal contour. There is plenty of amniotic fluid around the fetal body to give good contrast between the abdominal contour and other tissues. The second row represents a circumstance, in which one of fetal limbs superposed on the top left of the abdominal contour. The next row shows a case where the part of contour is absent as a result of shadow. Other circumstances may cause partial contour absence, such as signal dropout, improper detector positioning, or signal attenuation. The last row shows a case of contour deformation because of the pressure on the placenta. The first column to the third column show the original images, delineations by physicians, and the final contour by the GVF snake, respectively.

The method takes advantage of several image segmentation techniques. Experiments on clinical ultrasound images show that the accurate and consistent measurements can be obtained by using the method. The method also provides a useful framework for ultrasound object segmentation with a priori knowledge of the shape. Beside the fetal head, the vessel wall in the intravascular ultrasound, and the rectal wall in the endorectal ultrasound are other potential applications of the method.

3. Cell segmentation in pathological images

Pathological diagnosis often depends on visual assessment of a specimen under a microscope. Isolating the cells of interest is a crucial step for cytological analysis. For instance, separation of red and white pulps is important for evaluating the severity of tissue infections. Since lymphocyte nuclei are densely distributed in the white pulps, the nucleus

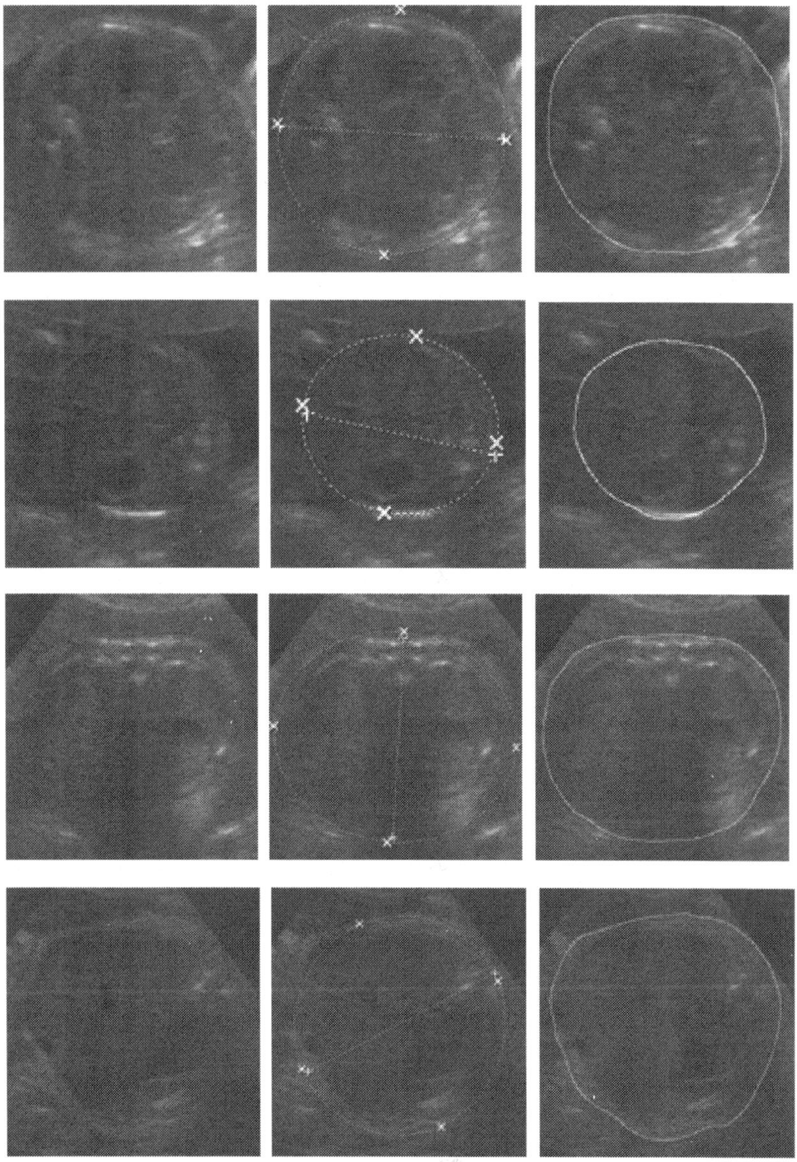

Fig. 3. Abdominal contour estimation on four clinical images. First column, from top to bottom: images represent relatively good, superposition interference, contour absence, and contour deformation, respectively. Second column: delineations by physicians. Third column: detected ellipses by the IRHT. Fourth column: final contours obtained by the GVF snake.

density serves as a segmentation criterion between red and white pulps. The second application demonstrates a cell segmentation method which incorporates intensity-based, edge-based and texture-based segmentation techniques (Yu & Tan, 2009).

3.1 Algorithm overview

Fig. 4 gives the flowchart of the cell segmentation algorithm. The algorithm first uses histogram adjustment and morphological operations to enhance a microscopic image, reduce noise and detect edges. Then FCM clustering is utilized to extract the layer of interest (LOI) from the image. Following preprocessing, conditional morphological erosion is used to mark individual objects. The marker-controlled watershed technique is subsequently employed to identify individual cells from the background. The main tasks of this stage are marker extraction and density estimation. The segmented cells are the starting point for the final stage, which then characterizes the cell distribution by textural energy. A textural energy-driven active contour algorithm is designed to outline the regions of desired object density. In the final stage, two important parameters are determined by the result of object segmentation, which are the window size for fractal dimension computation and the termination condition for the active contour algorithm.

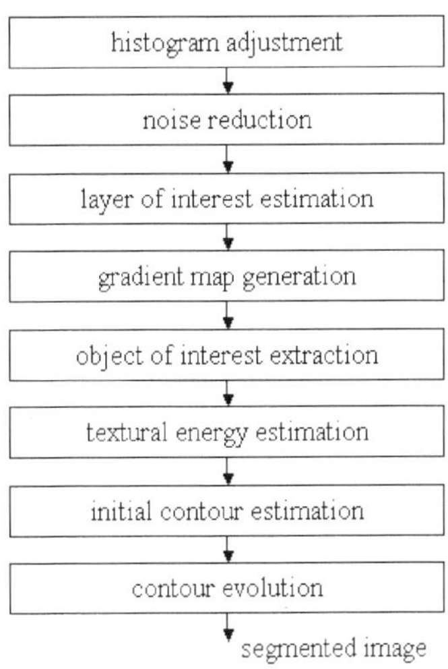

Fig. 4. Flowchart of the cell segmentation algorithm

3.2 Image preprocessing

The preprocessing stage consists of several subtasks including image enhancement, noise reduction, gradient magnitude estimation and preliminary LOI extraction. Fig. 5(a) shows an image of rat spleen tissue. The tissue section was stained with haematoxylin and eosin (H&E) for visual differentiation of cellular components. Under a microscope, nuclei are usually dark blue, red blood cells orange/red, and muscle fibers deep pink/red. The density of the lymphocytes is a key feature to differentiate red and white pulps. The white pulp has lymphocytes and macrophages surrounding central arterioles. The density of the lymphocytes in the red pulp is much lower than that in the white pulp. Evaluating the severity of infection requires identifying the infected regions or the white pulp. To simplify the subsequent processing procedure, color images are transformed into gray level images. Histogram adjustment (Larson *et al.*, 1997) is used to widen the dynamic range of the image and increase the image contrast. Following image enhancement, grayscale morphological reconstruction (Vincent, 1993) is used to reduce noise and simplify image construction. Although morphological reconstruction can smooth slow intensity variations effectively, it is sensitive to sharp intensity variations, such as impulsive noise. Since median filtering can remove transient spikes easily and preserve image edges at the same time, it is applied to the image obtained from morphological reconstruction. Fig. 5(b) shows the output image after histogram adjustment, morphological reconstruction and median filtering. FCM is used to classify each pixel according to its intensity into c categories. Then the category with the high intensity is defined as LOI. Fig. 5(c) shows the LOI obtained from FCM clustering. A gradient magnitude image (Fig. 5(d)) is computed for subsequent use by a watershed algorithm.

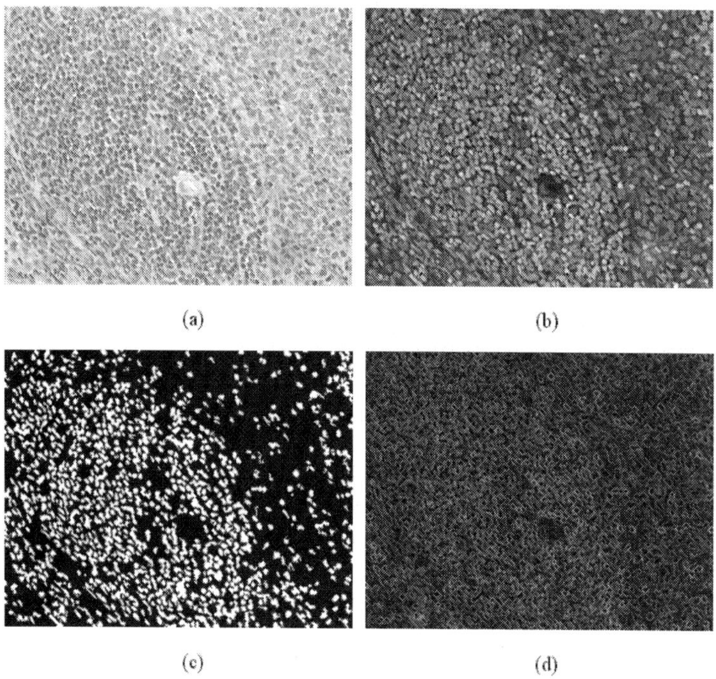

Fig. 5. Preprocessing of microscopic image. (a) Original image. (b) Image after histogram adjustment, morphological reconstruction and median filtering. (c) LOI obtained from FCM clustering. (d) Morphological gradient map.

3.3 Object segmentation

After the preprocessing stage, objects are extracted from the background. From Fig. 5(c), we can see that touching objects can not be separated by using FCM clustering, which will lead to errors in density estimation. Watershed (Vincent & Soille, 1991; Yang & Zhou, 2006) is known to be an effective tool to deal with such a problem. Simulation of an immersion process is an efficient algorithm to compute the watershed line. The gradient magnitude image is used for watershed computation. The gradient is treated as a topographical map with the height of each point directly related to its gradient magnitude. The topography defined by the image gradient is flooded through holes pierced at the bottom of valley. The flooding progresses at constant rate from each hole upwards and the catchment basins containing the holes are flooded. At the point where waters would mix, a dam is built to avoid mixing waters coming from different catchment basins. Since each minimum of the gradient leads to a basin, the watershed algorithm usually produces too many image segments.

Several techniques (Yang & Zhou, 2006; Hairs *et al.*, 1998 ; Jackway, 1996) have been proposed to alleviate this problem. Marker-controlled watershed is the most commonly used one, in which a marker image is used to indicate the desired minima of the image, thus predetermining the number and location of objects. A marker is a set of pixels within an object used to identify the object. The simplest markers can be obtained by extracting the regional minima of the gradient image. The number of regional minima could, however, be large because of the intensity fluctuations caused by noise or texture. Here, conditional erosion (Yang & Zhou, 2006) is used to extract markers. Fine and coarse erosion structures are conditionally chosen for erosion operations according to the shape of objects, and the erosions are only done when the size of the object is larger than a predefined threshold. The coarse and fine erosion structures utilized in this work are shown in Fig 6. Fig. 7(a) shows the marker map obtained and Fig. 7(b) gives segmented objects.

0	0	1	0	0
0	1	1	1	0
1	1	1	1	1
0	1	1	1	0
0	0	1	0	0

(a)

0	1	0
1	1	1
0	1	0

(b)

Fig. 6. Structuring element (SE). (a) Coarse SE. (b) Fine SE.

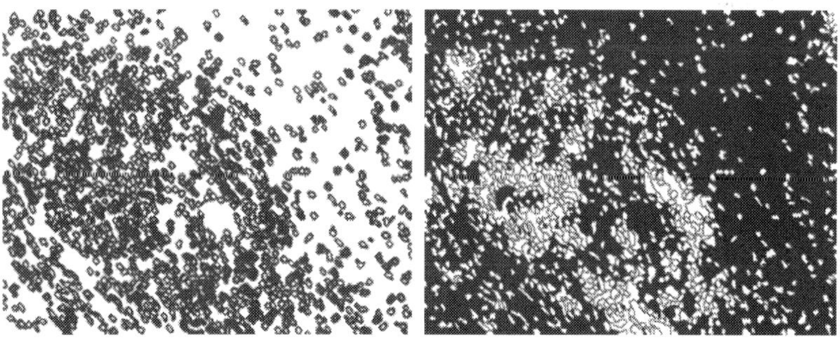

(a) (b)

Fig. 7. Object segmentation. (a) Marker map. (b) OI segmentation by marker-controlled watershed.

3.4 Final segmentation

Many image features can be used to characterize the spatial density of objects. An object image may be characterized as an image texture. It has been long recognized that the fractal model of three-dimensional surfaces can be used to obtain shape information and to distinguish between smooth and rough textured regions (Pentland, 1984). In this application, fractal dimension is used to extract textural information from images. Several methods have been reported to measure the fractal dimension (FD). Among these methods, differential box-counting (DBC) (Chaudhuri & Sarkar, 1995) is an effective and commonly used approach to estimating fractal dimension of images.

Assume that an $M \times M$ image has been partitioned into grids of size $m \times m$, where $M/2 \geq m > 1$ and m is an integer. Then the scale ratio r equals to m/M. Consider the image as a three-dimensional (3D) surface, with (x, y) denoting 2D position and the third coordinate (z) denoting the gray level of the corresponding pixel. Each grid contains $m \times m$ pixels in the x-y plane. From a 3D point of view, each grid can be represented as a column of boxes of size $m \times m \times m'$. If the total number of gray levels is G, then $m' = [r \times G]$. $[\cdot]$ means rounding the value to the nearest integers greater than or equal to that value. Suppose that the grids are indexed by (i, j) in the x-y plane, and the minimum and maximum gray levels of the image in the (i, j)th grid fall in the kth and the lth boxes in the z direction, respectively, then

$$n_{r(i,j)} = l - k + 1 \tag{8}$$

is the contribution of the (i, j)th grid to N_r, which is defined as:

$$N_r = \sum_{i,j} n_i(i,j) \tag{9}$$

N_r is counted for different values of r (i.e., different values of m). Then, the fractal dimension can be estimated as:

$$D = \frac{\log(N_r)}{\log(1/r)} \tag{10}$$

The FD map of an image is generated by calculating the FD value for each pixel. A local window, which is centered at each pixel, is used to compute the FD value for the pixel. Fig. 8(a) shows the textural energy map generated from fractal dimension analysis.

An active contour model is used to isolate the ROI based on the texture features. Active contour model-based algorithms, which progressively deform a contour toward the ROI boundary according to an objective function, are commonly-used and intensively-researched techniques for image segmentation. Active contour without edges is a different model for image segmentation based on curve evolution techniques (Chan & Vese, 2001). For the convenience of description, we refer to this model as the energy-driven active contour (EDAC) model for the fact that the textural energy will be used to control the contour deformation. The energy functional of the EDAC model is defined by

$$\begin{aligned} F(c_1, c_2, C) = {} & \mu \cdot Length(C) + \nu \cdot Area(inside(C)) \\ & + \lambda_1 \int_{inside(C)} \left| I_0(x,y) - c_1 \right|^2 dxdy \\ & + \lambda_2 \int_{outside(C)} \left| I_0(x,y) - c_2 \right|^2 dxdy \end{aligned} \tag{11}$$

where $I_0(x, y)$ is the textural energy image, C is a variable contour, and c_1 and c_2 are the averages of I_0 inside and outside C, respectively. $\mu \geq 0$, $\nu \geq 0$, λ_1, $\lambda_2 > 0$ are weighting parameters.

To apply the EDAC model, an initial contour must be chosen. From the previous step, the FD-based texture feature map represents the textural energy distribution of OIs. FCM clustering is utilized to estimate the initial contour for EDAC. The active contour evolution starts from the region with the highest object intensity, which corresponds to the region with the highest textural energy. FCM is used to classify textural energy into c clusters, and the region corresponding to the cluster with the highest textural energy is chosen as the initial contour. Fig. 8(b) shows the final contour obtained from EDAC.

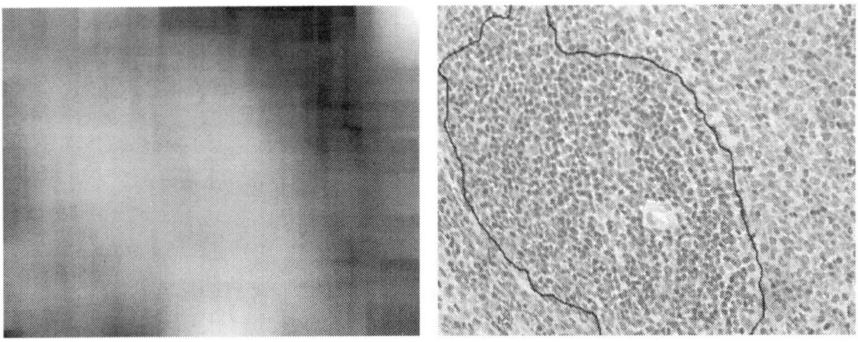

(a) (b)

Fig. 8. Final segmentation. (a) Textural energy generated from fractal dimension analysis. (b) Initial contour. (c) Final segmentation obtained from EDAC.

3.5 Algorithm performance

Fig. 9(a) shows another microscopic spleen tissue image. Fig. 9(b) to (e) show the results of preprocessing, object segmentation, textural energy map computation, and final segmentation. From Fig. 9(b), it is clear that the noise is reduced and the intensity variation is suppressed, which will benefit LOI extraction based on FCM. In Fig. 9(c), touching nuclei are effectively separated by the marker-controlled watershed algorithm. From the textural feature image shown in Fig. 9(d), the high- and low-density regions produce different textural energy levels. Accurate classification of the regions, however, may not result if it is only based on the textural feature. The energy-driven active contour with an appropriate stopping criterion gives satisfactory segmentation. From the results obtained with microscopic images, it can be seen that the image segmentation algorithm is effective and useful in this kind of applications.

The algorithm is a hybrid segmentation system which integrates intensity-based, edge-based and texture-based segmentation techniques. The method provides not only a closed contour corresponding to a certain object density but also density-related information in this contour. The experiment results show the effectiveness of the methodology in analysis of microscopic images.

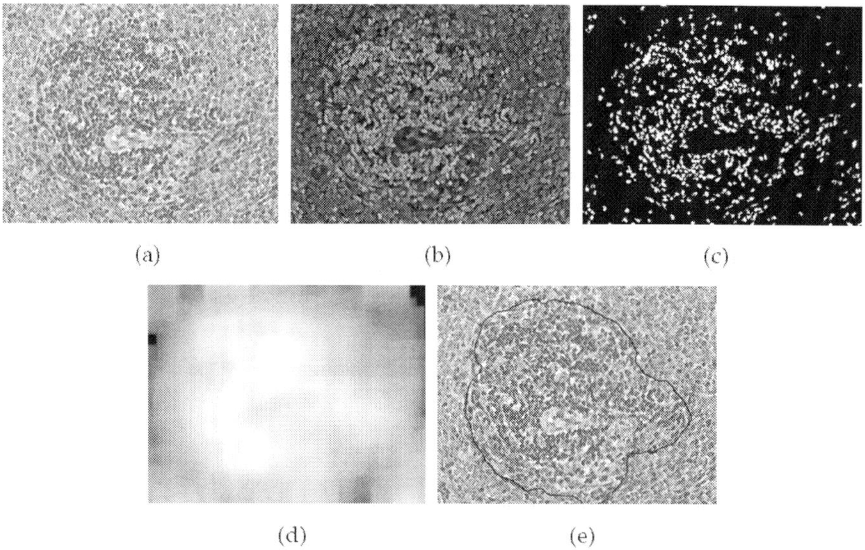

Fig. 9. Microscopic image segmentation. (a) Original image. (b) Image after preprocessing. (c) Object segmentation. (d) Textural energy map. (e) Final segmentation.

4. Molecular image segmentation

The final application is about molecular marker identification in molecular images. Molecular imaging allows clinicians to visualize molecular markers and their interactions in vivo, which represents a step beyond imaging at the anatomical and functional levels. Owing to their great potential in disease diagnosis and treatment, molecular imaging techniques have undergone explosive growth over the past few decades. A method that integrates intensity and texture information under a fuzzy logic framework is developed for molecular marker segmentation (Yu & Wang, 2007).

4.1 Algorithm overview

A two-dimensional fuzzy C-means (2DFCM) algorithm is used for molecular image segmentation. The most important feature of the FCM is that it allows a pixel to belong to multiple clusters according to its degree of membership in each cluster, which makes FCM-based clustering methods able to retain more information from the original image as compared to the case of crisp segmentation. FCM works well on images with low levels of noise, but has two disadvantages used in segmentation of noise-corrupted images. One is that the FCM does not incorporate the spatial information of pixels, which makes it sensitive to noise and other imaging artifacts. The other is that cluster assignment is based solely on distribution of pixel intensity, which makes it sensitive to intensity variations resulting from illumination or object geometry (Ahmed et al., 2002; Chen & Zhang, 2004; Liew et al., 2005).
To improve the robustness of conventional FCM, two steps are considered in the design of the algorithm. Because the SNR of molecular images is low, image denoising is carried out

prior to segmentation. A denoising method which combines a Gaussian noise filter with an anisotropic diffusion (AD) technique is used to reduce noise in molecular images. Since the Gabor wavelet transform of molecular images is relatively robust to intensity variations, a texture characterization method based on the Gabor filter bank is used to extract texture information from images. Spatial constraints provided by denoising and texture information provided by the Gabor wavelet are embedded in the objective function of a two-dimensional fuzzy clustering (2DFCM) algorithm.

4.2 Molecular image denoising

Ling and Bovik (Ling & Bovik, 2002) proposed a method to smooth molecular images by assuming an additive Gaussian model for noise. As a result, molecular images may be assumed to contain a zero-mean Gaussian white noise.

The FIR filter is well known for its ability to remove Gaussian noise from signals but it does not work very well in image processing since it blurs edges in an image. The Gaussian noise filter (GNF) (Russo, 2003) combining a nonlinear algorithm and a technique for automatic parameter tuning, is a good method for estimation and filtering of Gaussian noise. The GNF can be summarized as follows. Let $X=\{x_1, x_2,\ldots, x_n\}$ be a set of n data points in a noisy image. The output $Y=\{y_1, y_2,\ldots, y_n\}$ is defined as

$$y_i = x_i + \frac{1}{N_R}\sum_{x_r \in N_i} \varsigma(x_r, x_i), \quad i = 1,\cdots,n \tag{12}$$

$$\zeta(x_i, x_j) = \begin{cases} x_i - x_j & |x_i - x_j| \le p \\ \left(\dfrac{3p - |x_i - x_j|}{2}\right)\operatorname{sgn}(x_i - x_j) & p < |x_i - x_j| \le 3p \\ 0 & |x_i - x_j| > 3p \end{cases} \tag{13}$$

where N_i stands for the neighborhood configuration with respect to a center pixel x_i, N_R is the cardinality of N_i. The automatic tuning of parameter p is a key step in GNF. Let $MSE(k)$ denote the mean square error between the noisy image filtered with $p=k$ and the same image filtered with $p=k$-1. A heuristic estimate of the optimal parameter value is

$$\hat{p} = 2(k_m - 2) \tag{14}$$

where

$$MSE(k_m) = MAX\{MSE(k)\} \tag{15}$$

The GNF can remove intensity spikes due to the Gaussian noise, but, it has limited effect on suppressing minor intensity variations caused by the neighbourhood smoothing. Since the conventional FCM is a method based on the statistic feature of the image intensity, a piecewise-smooth intensity distribution will be greatly beneficial. More desirable denoising would result if the GNF is followed with a SRAD filter, which was introduced in Section 2.2. Suppose that the output of the SARD is represented by $X^*=\{x_1^*, x_2^*,\ldots, x^{n*}\}$. Fig. 10 shows the denoising results of GNF and SRAD.

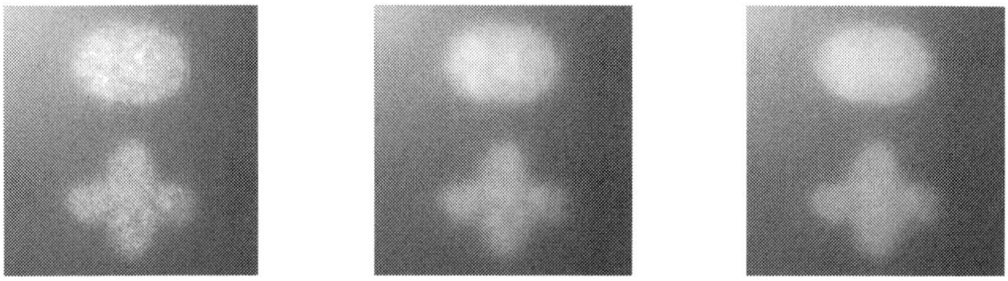

(a) (b) (c)

Fig. 10. Denoising by GNF and SRAD. (a) Original image. (b) After GNF filtering. (c) After GNF and SRAD filtering.

4.3 Texture characterization

A molecular image reveals the distribution of a certain molecule (Ling & Bovik, 2002). Since photons have different transport characteristics in different turbid tissues, a molecular image can be divided into several separate regions with each region having similar intensity (implying similar molecular concentration) and certain kind of textural pattern. Because photon distribution in a turbid tissue is usually not uniform, intensity within a region usually changes gradually. This intensity variation can cause errors when one attempts to segment images using intensity-based classification methods. Intuitively, if a feature insensitive to the slowly-varying intensity can be introduced into the classification, the image segmentation could be improved. Here a texture characterization method based on the Gabor wavelet is utilized to obtain this desirable feature.

A Gabor function in the spatial domain is a sinusoidal-modulated Gaussian function. The impulse response of the Gabor filter is given by

$$h(x,y;\mu,\theta)=\exp\left\{-\frac{1}{2}\left[\frac{x^2}{\sigma_x^2}+\frac{x^2}{\sigma_y^2}\right]\right\}\cdot\cos(2\pi\mu x) \tag{16}$$

where $x=x'\cos\theta+y'\sin\theta$, $y=-x'\sin\theta+y'\cos\theta$, (x, y) represent rotated spatial-domain rectilinear coordinates, u is the frequency of the sinusoidal wave along the direction θ from the x-axis, σ_x and σ_y define the size of the Gaussian envelope along x and y axes respectively, which determine the bandwidth of the Gabor filter. The frequency response of the filter is given by

$$H(U,V)=2\pi\sigma_x\sigma_y\left(\exp\left\{-\frac{1}{2}\left[\frac{(U-u)^2}{\sigma_u^2}+\frac{V^2}{\sigma_v^2}\right]\right\}+\exp\left\{-\frac{1}{2}\left[\frac{(U+u)^2}{\sigma_u^2}+\frac{V^2}{\sigma_v^2}\right]\right\}\right) \tag{17}$$

where $\sigma_u=1/2\pi\sigma_x$, $\sigma_v=1/2\pi\sigma_y$. By tuning u and θ, multiple filters that cover the spatial frequency domain can be obtained. Gabor wavelets with four different scales, μ $\{\frac{\pi}{4\sqrt{2}},\frac{\pi}{4},\frac{\pi}{2\sqrt{2}},\frac{\pi}{2}\}$, and eight orientations, θ $\{\frac{0\pi}{8},\frac{1\pi}{8},\cdots,\frac{7\pi}{8}\}$ are used. Let $X(x, y)$ be the intensity level of an image, the Gabor wavelet representation is the convolution of $X(x, y)$ with a family of Gabor kernels; i. e.,

$$G_{\mu,\theta}(x,y)=X(x,y)*h(x,y;\mu,\theta) \tag{18}$$

where * denotes the convolution operator, $G_{u,\theta}$ is the convolution result corresponding to the Gabor kernel at scale μ and orientation θ. The next step is to compute the textural energy in $G_{u,\theta}$. The textural energy is a measure widely used to characterize image texture. The energy that corresponds to a square window of image $G_{u,\theta}$ centered at x and y is defined as

$$E_{\mu,\theta}(x,y)=\frac{1}{M^2}\sum_{(i,j)\in W_{xy}}\left|F(G_{\mu,\theta}(i,j))\right| \tag{19}$$

where M^2 is the total number of pixels in the window, and F(.) is a non-linear, sigmoid function of the form

$$F(t)=\tanh(\alpha t)=\frac{1-e^{-2\alpha t}}{1+e^{-2\alpha t}} \tag{20}$$

where a equals to 0.25. The texture feature image is finally given by

$$T(x,y)=\frac{1}{32}\sum_{\mu,\theta}E_{\mu,\theta}(x,y) \tag{21}$$

As an example, Fig. 11(a) shows a synthetic image with intensity inhomogeneity. Fig. 11(b) shows the texture feature image. From this example, it is seen that the texture feature characterization using the Gabor wavelet is insensitive to intensity inhomogeneity.

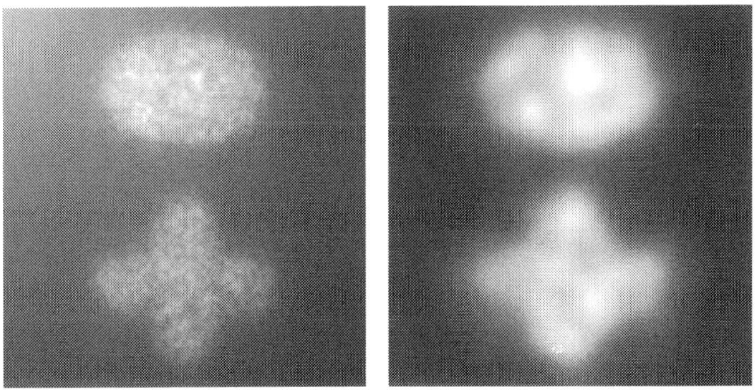

(a) (b)

Fig. 11. Texture feature characterization. (a) Original image with intensity inhomogeneity. (b) Texture energy images for different u and θ. (c) Texture feature image.

4.4 2DFCM

The two-dimensional fuzzy C-Means (2DFCM) algorithm is constructed by integrating both the intensity and the texture information. Suppose that the denoised molecular image is $X^*=\{x_1^*, x_2^*,\ldots, x_n^*\}$ and the texture feature image is $T=\{t_1, t_2,\ldots, t_n\}$, the objective function of 2DFCM can be expressed as

$$J_{2DFCM}=\sum_{j=1}^{c}\sum_{i=1}^{n}\mu_{ij}^b\left\|x_i-m_j\right\|^2+\alpha\sum_{j=1}^{c}\sum_{i=1}^{n}\mu_{ij}^b\left\|x_i^*-m_j\right\|^2+\beta_i\sum_{j=1}^{c}\sum_{i=1}^{n}\mu_{ij}^b\left\|t_i-v_j\right\|^2 \tag{22}$$

where α controls the effect of denoising on clustering, m_j represents the prototype of intensity image. The influence of texture characterization on the clustering procedure can be controlled by a constant vector β_i, $(i=1,\ldots,n)$, and the prototype of texture image is represented by v_j, $(j=1,\ldots,c)$. The choice of β_i is based on the following principle. If t_i is large, implying dominant textural energy, β_i should be large; if t_i is small, β_i should be also small. β_i is determined by $\beta_i=(Bt_i)/\max(T)$. Both α and B are determined by trial-and-error.

The optimization problem under constraint U in (5) can be solved by using a Lagrange multiplier λ in the following functional,

$$F=\sum_{j=1}^{c}\sum_{i=1}^{n}\mu_{ij}^{b}\left\|x_i-m_j\right\|^2+\alpha\sum_{j=1}^{c}\sum_{i=1}^{n}\mu_{ij}^{b}\left\|x_i^*-m_j\right\|^2+\beta_i\sum_{j=1}^{c}\sum_{i=1}^{n}\mu_{ij}^{b}\left\|t_i-v_j\right\|^2+\lambda\left(1-\sum_{j=1}^{c}\mu_{ij}\right) \quad (23)$$

Taking the derivative of F with respect to μ_{ij} and setting the result to zero, we can obtain an equation for μ_{ij} with λ unknown

$$\mu_{ij}=\left\{\frac{\lambda}{b[(x_i-m_j)^2+\alpha(x_i^*-m_j)^2+\beta_i(t_i-v_j)^2]}\right\}^{\frac{1}{(b-1)}} \quad (24)$$

Utilize constraint U, λ can be solved as

$$\lambda=\left\{\sum_{k=1}^{c}\left\{b[(x_i-m_j)^2+\alpha(x_i^*-m_j)^2+\beta_i(t_i-v_j)^2]\right\}^{\frac{1}{(b-1)}}\right\}^{b-1} \quad (25)$$

By substituting (25) into (24), a necessary condition for (22) to be at a local minimum will be obtained as

$$\mu_{ij}=\frac{\left[(x_i-m_j)^2+\alpha(x_i^*-m_j)^2+\beta_i(t_i-v_j)^2\right]^{-\frac{1}{(b-1)}}}{\sum_{k=1}^{c}\left[(x_i-m_k)^2+\alpha(x_i^*-m_k)^2+\beta_i(t_i-v_k)^2\right]^{-\frac{1}{(b-1)}}} \quad (26)$$

Similarly, by zeroing the derivatives of F with respect to m_j and v_j, we have

$$m_j=\frac{\sum_{i=1}^{n}\mu_{ij}{}^{b}(x_i+\alpha x_i^*)}{(1+\alpha)\sum_{i=1}^{n}\mu_{ij}{}^{b}},\quad v_j=\frac{\sum_{i=1}^{n}\mu_{ij}{}^{b}t_i}{\sum_{i=1}^{n}\mu_{ij}{}^{b}} \quad (27)$$

The procedure of 2DFCM can be summarized in the following steps:

1. Filter the image by GNF followed by SRAD to generate the denoised image X^*;
2. Filter the image by Gabor wavelet band and compute the texture feature image T;
3. Formulate the 2D histogram with the denoised image X^* and the texture feature image T; Estimate the number of clusters (c) and initial prototypes (M), and
4. Repeat following steps until the centroid variation is less than 0.001:

a. Update the membership function matrix with (26).
b. Update the centroids with (27).
c. Calculate the centroid variation and before and after updating.

4.5 Algorithm performance

The performance of the 2DFCM is first tested with simulated molecular images, from which the ground truth is available. Simulated molecular images are obtained by using MOSE (Monte Carlo optical simulation environment) (Li et al., 2004; Li et al., 2005) developed by the Bioluminescence Tomography Lab, Departments of Radiology & Departments of Biomedical Engineering, University of Iowa (http://radiology.uiowa.edu/). MOSE is based on the Monte Carlo method to simulate bioluminescent phenomena in the mouse imaging and to predict bioluminescent signals around the mouse.

The optimized α and B in the 2DFCM should be obtained by trial-and-error. α=3.5 and B=36 are used. The computation time of the algorithm for an image of 128×128 is approximately 12 seconds on a personal computer. About two-thirds of the time is consumed in texture characterization based on Gabor wavelet. The first example is for applying the algorithm to a synthetic cellular image and comparing the 2DFCM with FCM. The synthetic image is shown in Fig. 12(a). The segmentation results by 2DFCM and FCM are presented in Figs. 12(b) and (c), respectively.

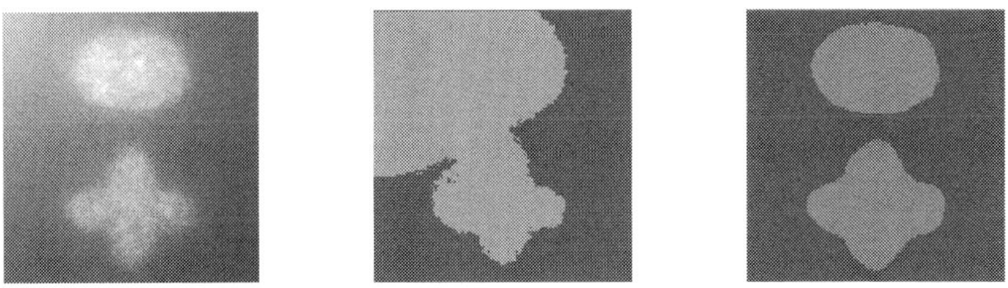

(a) (b) (c)

Fig. 12. Segmentation results on the first synthetic image. (a) The synthetic image generated by MOSE. (b) Segmentation by FCM. (c) Segmentation by 2DFCM.

In the second example, the algorithm is applied to a real molecular image (256×256) (as shown in Fig. 13(a)). Figs. 13(b) and (c) show the denoising result by the GNF plus SRAD, and the texture feature image obtained by the Gabor wavelet bank, respectively. Figs. 13(d) and (f) show the segmentation results of by FCM and 2DFCM, respectively. In order to illustrate the segmentation results clearly, the contours of the region of interest in the classification image are extracted and superimposed on the original image. Figs. 13(e) and (g) give the contour comparisons.

From the experimental results, we can see that denoising by GNF plus SRAD are satisfactory. The Gabor wavelet bank can represent the texture information in the molecular image without disturbance by intensity variation. Intensity inhomogeneity degenerates segmentation by the FCM. Since the 2DFCM utilizes both the intensity and texture information simultaneously, it produces more satisfactory results than the FCM.

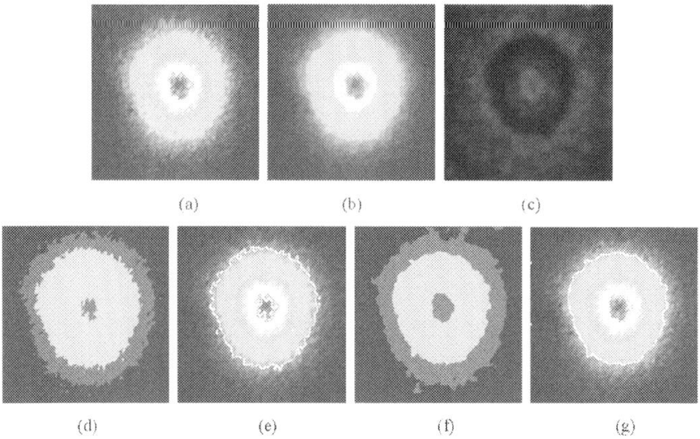

Fig. 13. Segmentation results for a real molecular image. (a) Original image. (b) Denoising result by GNF plus SRAD. (c) Texture feature image. (d) Segmentation result by FCM. (e) Contour obtained from (d) superimposed on the original image. (f) Segmentation result by 2DFCM. (g) Contour obtained from (f) superimposed on the original image.

5. Conclusion

In this chapter, segmentation of three different kinds of biomedical images is discussed. Biomedical images obtained from different modalities suffer from different imaging noises. Image segmentation techniques based on only one image feature usually fail to produce satisfactory segmentation results for biomedical images. Three methodologies are presented for the segmentation of ultrasound images, microscopic images and molecular images, respectively. All these segmentation methodologies integrate image features generated from image intensity, edges and texture to reduce the effect of noises on image segmentation. It can be concluded that a successful medical image segmentation method needs to make a use of varied image features and information in an image.

6. References

Ahmed, M.N.; Yamany, S.M.; Mohamed, N.; Farag, A.A. & Moriarty, T. (2002). A modified fuzzy c-means algorithm for bias field estimation and segmentation of MRI data. *IEEE Trans. Med Imag.*, Vol. 21, No. 3, (March 2002) (193-199), ISSN: 0278-0062

Bezdek, J.C. (1981). A convergence theorem for the fuzzy ISODATA clustering algorithm. *IEEE Trans. Pattern Anal. Mach. Intell.*, Vol. 2, No. 1, (January 1980) (1-8), ISSN: 0162-8828

Bezdek, J.C. (1981). *Pattern Recognition with Fuzzy Objective Function Algorithms*, Kluwer Academic Publishers, ISBN: 0306406713, Norwell, MA, USA

Canny, J.F. (1986). A computational approach to edge detection. *IEEE Trans. Pattern Anal. Mach. Intell.*, Vol. 8, No. 6, (November 1986) (679-698), ISSN: 0162-8828

Chan, T.F. & Vese, L.A. (2001). Active contours without edges, *IEEE Trans. Image Process.*, Vol. 10, No. 2, (February 2001) (266-277), ISSN: 1057-7149

Chaudhuri, B.B. & Sarkar, N. (1995). Texture segmentation using fractal dimension. *IEEE Trans. Pattern Anal. Mach. Intell.*, Vol. 17, No. 1, (January 1995) (72-76), ISSN: 0162-8828

Chen, S. & Zhang, D. (2004). Robust image segmentation using FCM with spatial constraints based on new kernel-induced distance measure. *IEEE Trans. Syst., Man, Cybern.*, Vol. 34, No.4, (April 2004) (1907-1916), ISSN: 0018-9472

FjØrtoft R., Lopés A., Marthon P. & Cubero-Castan E. (1998). An optimal multiedge detector for SAR image segmentation. *IEEE Trans Geosci Remote Sensing*, Vol. 36, No. 3, (May 1998) (793-802), ISSN: 0196-2892

Haris, K.; Efstratiadis, S.N.; Maglaveras, N. & Katsaggelos, A.K. (1998). Hybrid image segmentation using watersheds and fast region merging. *IEEE Trans. Image Process.*, Vol. 7, No. 12, (December 1998) (1684-1699), ISSN: 1057-7149

Haralick R. (1982). Zero crossing of second directional derivative edge operator. *Proceedings of SPIE Symp Robot Vision*, pp. 91-99, Washington, DC, May 1982.

Hsiao, J.Y. & Sawchuk, A.A. (1989). Supervised texture image segmentation using feature smoothing and probabilistic relaxation techniques. *IEEE Trans. Pattern Anal. Mach. Intell.*, Vol. 11, No. 12, (December 1989) (1279-1292), ISSN: 0162-8828

Jackway, P. (1996). Gradient watersheds in morphological scale-space. *IEEE Trans. Image Process.*, Vol. 5, No. 6, (June 1996) (913-921), ISSN: 1057-7149

Jain, A.K. & Farrokhnia, F. (1991). Unsupervised texture segmentation using Gabor filters. *Pattern Recognition*, Vol. 24, No. 12 (December 1991) (1167-1186), ISSN: 0031-3203

Li, H.; Tian, J.; Cong, W.X.; Wang, L.V.; Hoffman, E.A. & Wang G. (2004). A mouse optical simulation environment (MOSE) to investigate bioluminescent phenomena in the living mouse with Monte Carlo method. *Academic Radiology*, vol. 11, no. 9, (September 2004) (1029-1038), ISSN: 1076-6332

Li, H.; Tian, J.; Luo, J.; Wang, G. & Cong, W.X. (2005). Interactive graphic editing tools in bioluminescent imaging simulation. *BioOptics of SPIE 2005*, pp. 22-24, San Diego, Jan. 2005. California USA.

Liew, A.W.C.; Yan, H. & Law, N.F. (2005). Image segmentation based on adaptive cluster prototype estimation. *IEEE Trans. Fuzzy Syst.*, Vol. 13, No. 4, (August 2005) (444-453), ISSN: 1063-6706

Ling, J. & Bovik, A.C. (2002). Smoothing low-SNR molecular images via anisotropic medina-diffusion. *IEEE Trans. Med Imag.*, Vol. 21, No. 4, (April 2002) (377-384), ISSN: 0278-0062

Kass, M.; Witkin, A. & Terzopoulos, D. (1988). Snakes: active contour models. *Int. J. Comput. Vis.*, Vo. 1, No. 4, (January 1998) (321-331), ISSN: 0920-5691

Larson, G.W.; Rushmeier, H. & Piatko, C. (1997). A visibility matching tone reproduction operator for high dynamic range scenes. *IEEE Trans. Vis. Comput. Gr.*, Vol. 3, No. 4, (October-December 1997) (291-306), ISSN: 1077-2626

Lu, W.; Tan, J. & Floyd, R. (2005). Automated fetal head detection and measurement in ultrasound images by iterative randomized Hough transform. *Ultrasound Med Biol.*, Vol. 31, No. 7, (July 2005) (929-936), ISSN: 0301-5629

Mandelbrot, B.B. (1976). How long is the coast of Britain? Statistical self-similarity and fractal dimension. *Science*, Vol. 156, No. 37, (May 1967) (636-638), ISSN: 0036-8075

Otsu, N. (1979). A threshold selection method from gray-level histograms. *IEEE Trans. Syst., Man, Cybern.*, Vol. 9, No. 1, (January 1979) (62-66), ISSN: 0018-9472

Pappas, T.N. (1992). An adaptive clustering algorithm for image segmentation, *IEEE Trans. Signal Process.*, Vol. 40, No. 4, (April 1992) (901-914), ISSN: 1053-587X

Pentland, A.P. (1984). Fractal based description of natural scenes, *IEEE Trans. Pattern Anal. Mach. Intell.*, Vol. 6, No. 6, (November 1984) (661-674), ISSN: 0162-8828

Randen, T. & Husoy, J.H. (1999). Filtering for texture classification: a comparative study. *IEEE Trans. Pattern Anal. Mach. Intell.*, Vol. 21, No. 4, (April 1999) (291-310), ISSN: 0162-8828

Russo, F. (2003). A method for estimation and filtering of Gaussian noise in images. *IEEE Trans. Instrum. & Meas.*, Vol. 52, No. 4, (August 2003) (1148-1154), ISSN: 0018-9456

Sahoo, P.K.; Soltani, S.; Wong, A.K.C. & Chen, Y.C. (1988). A survey of thresholding techniques. *Comput. Vis. Graph. Image Process.*, Vol. 41, No. 2, (February 1988) (233-260), ISSN: 0734-189X

Tyagi, A. & Bayoumi, M.A. (1992). Image segmentation on a 2-D array by a directed split and merge procedure. *IEEE Trans. Signal Process.*, Vol. 40, No. 11, (November 1992) (2804-2813), ISSN: 1053-587X

Vincent, L. (1993). Morphological grayscale reconstruction in image analysis: application and efficient algorithm. *IEEE Trans. Image Process.*, Vol. 2, No. 2, (April 1993) (176-201), ISSN: 1057-7149

Vincent, L. & Soille, P. (1991). Watersheds in digital spaces: an efficient algorithm based on immersion simulations, *IEEE Trans. Pattern Anal. Mach. Intell.*, Vol. 13, No. 6, (June 1991) (583-598), ISSN: 0162-8828

Wu, X. (1993). Adaptive split-and-merge segmentation based on piecewise least-square approximation. *IEEE Trans. Pattern Anal. Mach. Intell.*, Vol. 15, No. 8, (August 1993) (808-815), ISSN: 0162-8828

Xu, C. & Prince, J.L. (1998). Snakes, shapes, and gradient vector flow, *IEEE Trans. Image Process.*, Vol. 7, No. 3, (March 1998) (359-369), ISSN: 1057-7149

Yang, X.; Li, H. & Zhou, X. (2006). Nuclei segmentation using marker-controlled watershed, tacking using mean-shift, and Kalman filter in time-lapse microscopy. *IEEE Trans. Circuits and Systems*, Vol. 53, No.11, (November 2006) (2405-2414), ISSN: 1057-7122

Yu, J. & Wang, Y. (2007). Molecular image segmentation based on improved fuzzy clustering. *Int. J. Bio. Imag.*, Vol. 2007, (July 2007) (1-9), ISSN: 1687-4188

Yu, J.; Wang, Y.; Chen, P. & Shen, Y. (2008a). Fetal abdominal contour extraction and measurement in ultrasound images. *Ultrasound Med Biol.*, Vol. 34, No. 2, (February 2008) (169-182), ISSN: 0301-5629

Yu, J.; Wang, Y. & Chen, P. (2008b). Fetal ultrasound image segmentation system and its use in fetal weight estimation. *Med. Biol. Eng. Comput.*, Vol. 46, No. 12, (December 2008) (1227-1237), ISSN: 0140-0118

Yu, J. & Tan, J. (2009). Object density-based image segmentation and its applications in biomedical image analysis. *Comput. Meth. Prog. Bio.*, Vol. 96, No. 3, (December 2009) (193-204), ISSN: 0169-2607

Yu Y. & Acton S.T. (2002). Speckle reducing anisotropic diffusion. *IEEE Trans Image Process*, Vol. 11, No. 11, (November 2002) (1260-1270), ISSN: 1057-7149

Yu Y. & Acton S.T. (2004). Edge detection in ultrasound imagery using the instantaneous coefficient of variation. *IEEE Trans Image Process*, Vol. 13, No. 12, (December 2004) (1640-1655), ISSN: 1057-7149

Zucker, S. & Terzopoulos, D. (1980). Finding structure in co-occurrence matrices for texture analysis. Comput, *Graph. Image Process.*, Vol. 12, No. 3, (March 1980) (286-308), ISSN: 0146-664X

23

A General Framework for Computation of Biomedical Image Moments

G.A. Papakostas, D.E. Koulouriotis, E.G. Karakasis and V.D. Tourassis
Democritus University of Thrace, Department of Production Engineering and Management
Greece

1. Introduction

Image moments have been successfully used as images' content descriptors for several decades. Their ability to fully describe an image by encoding its contents in a compact way makes them suitable in many disciplines of the engineering life, such as image analysis (Sim et al., 2004), image watermarking (Papakostas et al., 2010a) and pattern recognition (Papakostas et al., 2005, 2007, 2009a, 2010b). Apart from the *geometric moments*, which are firstly introduced, several moment types have been presented due time (Flusser et al., 2009). Orthogonal moments are the most popular moments widely used in many applications owing to their orthogonality property that permits the reconstruction of the image by a finite set of its moments with minimum reconstruction error. This orthogonality property comes from the nature of the polynomials used as kernel functions, which they constitute an orthogonal base. As a result the orthogonal moments have minimum information redundancy meaning that different moment orders describe different image parts of the image. The most well known orthogonal moment families are: Zernike, Pseudo-Zernike, Legendre, Fourier-Mellin, Tchebichef, Krawtchouk, dual Hahn moments, with the last three ones belonging to the discrete type moments since they are defined directly to the image coordinate space, while the first ones are defined in the continue space.

Recently, there is an increased interest on applying image moments in biomedical imaging, with the reconstruction of medical images (Dai et al., 2010; Papakostas et al., 2009b; Shu et al., 2007; Wang & Sze, 2001) and the description of image's parts with particular properties (Bharathi & Ganesan, 2008; Iscan et al., 2010; Li & Meng, 2009; Liyun et al., 2009) by distinguishing diseased areas from the healthy ones, being the most active research directions the scientists work with.

Therefore, a method that computes fast and accurate the orthogonal moments of a biomedical image is of great importance. Although many algorithms and strategies (Papakostas et al., 2010c) have been proposed in the past, these methodologies handle the biomedical images as "every-day" images, meaning that they are not making use of specific properties of the image in process.

The authors have made a first attempt to compute the Krawtchouk moments of biomedical images by taking advantage of the inherent property of the biomedical image to have limited number of different intensity values (Papakostas et al., 2009c). Based on this observation and by applying the ISR method (Papakostas et al., 2008a) an image is decomposed to a set of image slices consisting of pixels with the same intensity value, an image representation that enables the fast computation of the image moments (Papakostas et al., 2009d).

This first approach has shown very promising results, by giving more space to apply it to more moment families and biomedical datasets under a general framework, which is presented in this chapter.

2. Image moments

A general formulation of the $(n+m)^{th}$ order image moment of a NxN image with intensity function $f(x,y)$ is given as follows:

$$M_{nm} = NF \times \sum_{x=1}^{N}\sum_{y=1}^{N} Poly_n(x)Poly_m(y)f(x,y) \tag{1}$$

where NF is a normalization factor and $Poly_n(x)$ is the nth order polynomial value of the pixel point with coordinate x, used as a moment kernel. According to the type of the polynomial kernel used in (1), the type of the moments is determined such as Geometric, Zernike, Pseudo-Zernike, Fourier-Mellin, Legendre, Tchebichef, Krawtchouk and dual Hahn.

For example, in the case of Tchebichef moments (Papakostas et al., 2009d, 2010c) the used polynomial has the form of the normalized Tchebichef polynomial defined as follows:

$$Poly_n(x) = \tilde{t}_n(x) = \frac{t_n(x)}{\beta(n,N)} \tag{2}$$

where

$$t_n(x) = (1-N)_n\, {}_3F_2(-n,-x,1+n;1,1-N;1) = \sum_{k=0}^{n}(-1)^{n-k}\binom{N-1-k}{n-k}\binom{n+k}{n}\binom{x}{k} \tag{3}$$

is the nth order Tchebichef polynomial, ${}_3F_2$, the generalized hypergeometric function, $n,x = 0,1,2,\ldots,N-1$, N the image size and $\beta(n,N)$ a suitable constant independent of x that serves as scaling factor, such as N^n.

Moreover the normalization factor NF has the following form:

$$NF = \frac{1}{\tilde{\rho}(p,N)\tilde{\rho}(q,N)} \tag{4}$$

where $\tilde{\rho}(n,N)$ is the normalized norm of the polynomials

$$\tilde{\rho}(n,N) = \frac{\rho(n,N)}{\beta(n,N)^2} \tag{5}$$

with

$$\rho(n,N) = (2n)!\binom{N+n}{2n+1}, \quad n = 0,1,\ldots,N-1 \tag{6}$$

Based on the above assumptions, the final computational form of the $(n+m)^{th}$ order Tchebichef moments of a NxN image having $f(x,y)$ intensity function takes the following form:

$$T_{nm} = \frac{1}{\tilde{\rho}(n,N)\tilde{\rho}(m,N)} \sum_{x=0}^{N-1} \sum_{y=0}^{N-1} \tilde{t}_n(x)\tilde{t}_m(y) f(x,y) \tag{7}$$

Working in the same way, the computational formulas of Geometric, Zernike, Pseudo-Zernike, Legendre, Krawtchouk and dual Hahn moments can be derived (Papakostas et al., 2009d, 2010c) based on the general form of (1).

3. A general computation strategy

Generally, there are four main computation strategies (Papakostas et al., 2010c) that have been applied to accelerate the moments' computation speed: 1) the *Direct Strategy (DS)*, which firstly used, since it is based on the definition formulas of each moment family, 2) the *Recursive Strategy (RS)*, which is characterized by the mechanism of recursive computation of the kernel's polynomials, 3) the *Partitioning Strategy (PS)*, according to which the image is partitioned into several smaller sub-images in order to reduce the maximum order need to computed and finally 4) the *Slice-Block Strategy (SBS)*, which decomposes a gray-scale image to intensity slices and rectangular blocks, developed by the authors (Papakostas et al., 2008a, 2009d).

Among the four above strategies the last one has the advantage to collaborate with the RS and PS strategies (Papakostas et al., 2010c), by resulting to more efficient computation schemes. Moreover, the SBS strategy can be applied to any moment family defined in the cartesian coordinate system (for the case of the polar coordinate system, appropriate transformation to the cartesian system is needed) in a common way, establishing it a general computation framework.

After the presentation of the main principles of the SBS methodology, this method will be applied to compute the moments of several families, for the case of biomedical images, which they constitute a special case of images where the benefits of the SBS strategy are significantly increased.

The principal mechanisms used by the SBS strategy are the *ISR (Image Slice Representation)* and *IBR (Image Block Representation)* methodologies, which decompose an image into intensity slices and a slice into rectangular blocks, respectively.

The main idea behind the ISR method is that we can consider a gray-scale image as the resultant of non-overlapped image slices, whose pixels have specific intensities. Based on this representation, we can decompose the original image into several slices, from which we can then reconstruct it, by applying fundamental mathematical operations.

Based on the above image decomposition, the following definition can be derived:

Definition 1: *Slice* of a gray-scale image, of a certain intensity f_i, is the image with the same size and the same pixels of intensity f_i as in the original one, while the rest of the pixels are considered to be black.

As a result of Definition 1, we derive the following Lemma 1 and 2:

Lemma 1: Any 8-bit gray-scale image can be decomposed into a maximum of 255 slices, where each slice has pixels of one intensity value and black.

Lemma 2: The binary image as a special case of a gray-scale image consists of only one slice, the binary slice, where only the intensities of 255 and 0 are included.

Based on the ISR representation, the intensity function $f(x,y)$ of a gray-scale image can be defined as an expansion of the intensity functions of the slices:

$$f(x,y) = \sum_{i=1}^{s} f_i(x,y) \tag{8}$$

where s is the number of slices (equal to the number of different intensity values) and $f_i(x,y)$ is the intensity function of the ith slice. In the case of a binary image s is 1 and thus $f(x,y)=f_1(x,y)$.

In the general case of gray-scale images, each of the extracted slices can be considered as a two-level image and thus the IBR algorithm (Papakostas et al., 2008a, 2009d) can be applied directly, in order to decompose each slice into a number of non-overlapped blocks.

By using the ISR representation scheme, the computation of the $(n+m)^{th}$ order orthogonal moment (1) of a gray-scale image $f(x,y)$, can be performed according to the equations

$$\begin{aligned} M_{nm} &= NF \times \sum_x \sum_y Poly_n(x) Poly_m(y) f(x,y) \\ &= NF \times \sum_x \sum_y Poly_n(x) Poly_m(y) \left(\sum_{i=1}^{s} f_i(x,y) \right) \\ &= NF \times \sum_x \sum_y Poly_n(x) Poly_m(y) \left(f_1(x,y) + f_2(x,y) + \ldots + f_s(x,y) \right) \Leftrightarrow \end{aligned} \tag{9}$$

$$\begin{aligned} M_{nm} &= NF \times \sum_x \sum_y Poly_n(x) Poly_m(y) f_1(x,y) + \\ &+ NF \times \sum_x \sum_y Poly_n(x) Poly_m(y) f_2(x,y) + \ldots \\ &+ NF \times \sum_x \sum_y Poly_n(x) Poly_m(y) f_s(x,y) \\ &= f_1 \left[NF \times \sum_{x_1} \sum_{y_1} Poly_n^1(x_1) Poly_m^1(y_1) \right] + \\ &+ f_2 \left[NF \times \sum_{x_2} \sum_{y_2} Poly_n^2(x_2) Poly_m^2(y_2) \right] + \ldots \\ &+ f_s \left[\sum_{x_s} \sum_{y_s} Poly_n^s(x_n) Poly_m^s(y_n) \right] \\ &= f_1 M_{nm}^1 + f_2 M_{nm}^2 + \ldots + f_s M_{nm}^s \end{aligned} \tag{10}$$

where f_i and M_{nm}^i, $i=1,2,\ldots,s$ are the intensity functions of the slices and the corresponding $(n+m)^{th}$ order moments of the ith binary slice, respectively.

The corresponding moment of a binary slice M_{nm}^i is the moment computed by considering a block representation of the image (Papakostas et al., 2008a, 2009d), as follows:

$$M_{nm}^{i}=\sum_{j=0}^{k-1}M_{nm}\left(b_j\right)=\sum_{j=0}^{k-1}\sum_{x=x_{1,b_j}}^{x_{2,b_j}}\sum_{y=y_{1,b_j}}^{y_{2,b_j}}Poly_n\left(x\right)Poly_m\left(y\right)$$
$$=\sum_{j=0}^{k-1}\left(\sum_{x=x_{1,b_j}}^{x_{2,b_j}}Poly_n\left(x\right)\right)\left(\sum_{y=y_{1,b_j}}^{y_{2,b_j}}Poly_m\left(y\right)\right) \tag{11}$$

where x_{1,b_j},x_{2,b_j} and y_{1,b_j},y_{2,b_j} are the coordinates of the block b_j, with respect to the horizontal and vertical axes, respectively.
A result of the above analysis (10) is the following Proposition 1:
Proposition 1: The $(n+m)^{th}$ order discrete orthogonal moment of a gray-scale image is equal to the "intensity-weighted" sum of the same order discrete orthogonal moments of a number of binary slices.
The SBS strategy has been applied successfully in computing the geometric moments (Papakostas et al., 2008a), the orthogonal moments (Papakostas et al., 2009d) and the DCT (Papakostas et al., 2008b, 2009e), by converging to high computation speeds in all the cases.
The performance of the SBS methodology is expected to be higher for the case of the biomedical images, since the limited number of different intensities of these images, enables the construction of less intensity slices and therefore bigger homogenous rectangular blocks are extracted.

4. Biomedical images – A special case

As it has already been mentioned in the previous sections, the application of the SBS strategy can significantly increases the moments' computation rate for the case of biomedical images, as compared with the "every-day" images. This is due to the fact that the biomedical images are "intensity limited" since the pixels' intensities are concentrated mostly in a few intensity values. For example, let see the two "every-day" images Lena and Barbara as illustrated in the following Fig. 1, along with their corresponding histograms.
These images having a content of general interest, present a more normally distributed pixel's intensities into the intensity range [0-255].
On the contrary, in the case of biomedical images the intensities are concentrated in a narrower region of the intensity range. Figure 2, shows four sample images from three different kinds of biomedical images BRAINX, KNIX (MRI images), INCISIX (CT images) retrieved from (DICOM) and MIAS (X-ray images) (Suckling et al., 1994). All the images have 256x256 pixels size, while each dataset consists of 232 (BRAINIX), 135 (KNIX), 126 (INCISIX), 322 (MIAS) gray-scale images.
It is noted that in the above histograms the score of the 0 intensity is omitted for representation purposes, since a lot of pixels have this intensity value, causing the covering of all the other intensity distributions.
A careful study of the above histograms can lead to the deduction that the most pixels' intensities are limited to a small fraction of the overall intensity range [0-255]. This means that the images' content is concentrated in a few intensity slices. This fact seems to be relative to the images' nature and constitutes an inherent property of their morphology. From (10) and (11) it is obvious that the performance of the SBS method is highly dependent on the image's intensity distribution, meaning that images with less intensities and big

blocks enable the achievement of high moments' computation rates, conditions that are satisfied by the biomedical images.

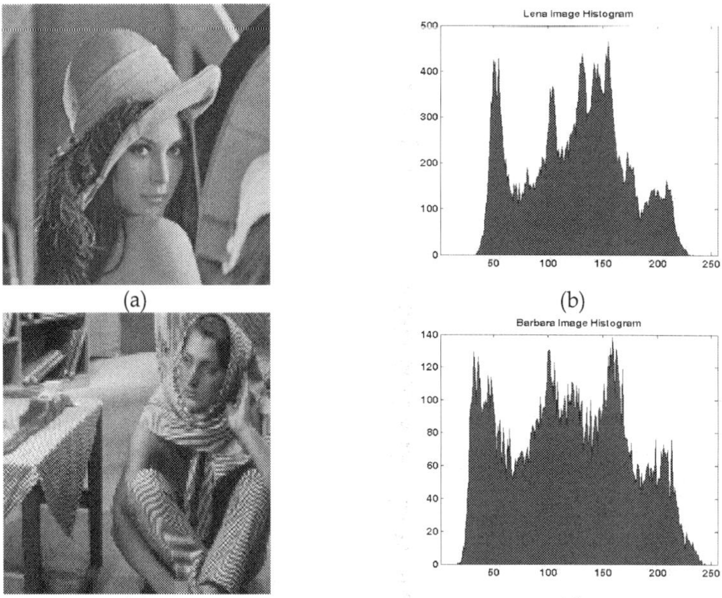

(a) (b) (c) (d)

Fig. 1. "Every-day" images and their histograms: (a)-(b)Lena image and its histogram, (c)-(d) Barbara image and its histogram.

5. Experimental study

In order to investigate the performance of the SBS strategy in computing the biomedical image moments, a set of experiments have been arranged. For this reason five representative moment families the *Geometric Moments (GMs), Legendre Moments (LMs), Tchebichef Moments (TMs), Krawtchouk Moments (KMs)* and *dual Hahn Moments (DHMs)*, are computed to the entire four datasets of Fig.2, up to a maximum order from 0 to 50 with step 5. The variance (σ) and mean (μ) values of the SBS strategy results are summarized in the following Table 1.

	BRAINIX	KNIX	INCISIX	MIAS
Block Extraction Time(msecs)	0.0234/1.1117	0.1189/1.8363	0.0874/1.9470	0.0442/0.9915
Num. of Blocks	1.7477E+07/28325	4.6382E+07/48291	2.3089E+06/56265	3.7785E+07/22053
Num. of Intensity Slices	740.1785/213.7845	305.7875/231.5407	136.3860/241.7169	220.6238/237.5280

Table 1. Performance statistics (σ/μ) of applying SBS to the datasets.

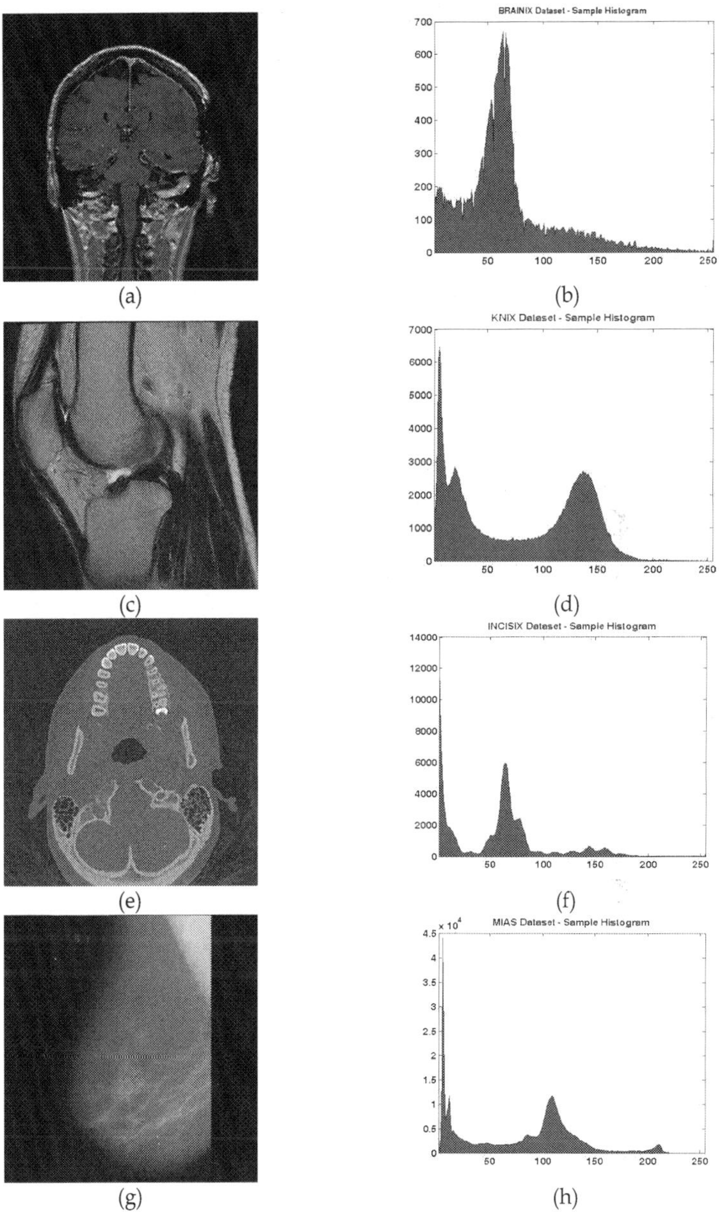

Fig. 2. Biomedical images and their histograms: (a)-(b) BRAINIX sample image and its histogram, (c)-(d) KNIX sample image and its histogram, (e)-(f) INCISIX sample image and its histogram, (g)-(h) MIAS sample image and its histogram.

From the above results, it can be realized that the extraction of the homogenous block does not add a significant overhead to the entire computation procedure (small mean values with low variability), since it needs a little time to be executed. On the other hand, the high variance on the number of blocks and intensity slices, reveal a complicated dependency of the computation time on these two main factors, as far as the size of the blocks and the distribution of the blocks on the intensity slices are concerned.

In order to study the timing performance of the SBS strategy, a comparison of its behaviour with that of the DS methodology, for the case of the four biomedical datasets has been taken place. Since, the SBS strategy can effectively be collaborated with other fast strategies (RS and PS) (Papakostas et al., 2010c), only a comparison with the DS methodology is needed to highlight its advantages. The mean values of the computation time in each case are illustrated in the following Table 2, 3 and 4. From these results it is obvious that the proposed method needs less time to compute the moments of any order, as compared to the DS one. This outperformance varies by the moment family, since each family needs a different time to compute its moments.

Order	Moment Families (BRAINIX Dataset)									
	GMs		LMs		TMs		KMs		DHMs	
	DS	*SBS*	*DS*	*SBS*	*DS*	*SBS*	*DS*	*SBS*	*DS*	*SBS*
0	15	9	4	2	23	14	198	125	11775	7207
5	554	349	3452	2110	2352	1455	7663	4864	713050	436919
10	1877	1185	14611	8929	15087	9348	28091	17814	2617380	1601577
15	3955	2493	36663	22446	47139	29211	64455	40764	5716791	3497941
20	6808	4289	72640	44454	108589	67167	119837	75595	10037777	6142626
25	10441	6573	125502	76874	208647	128912	196699	123978	15590386	9541093
30	14844	9339	200755	122885	355676	219857	298193	187821	22386172	13700734
35	19980	12567	298700	183023	556002	343423	426135	268199	30487995	18667254
40	25843	16266	423570	259605	825554	509665	584561	367523	39895856	24423207
45	32487	20465	577570	354053	1168458	720985	774426	486405	50549799	30948566
50	39909	25147	767700	470815	1598002	988073	1000782	627991	62496927	38267424

Table 2. Timing performance (msecs) for the case of BRAINIX dataset.

Order	Moment Families (KNIX Dataset)									
	GMs		LMs		TMs		KMs		DHMs	
	DS	*SBS*	*DS*	*SBS*	*DS*	*SBS*	*DS*	*SBS*	*DS*	*SBS*
0	13	11	4	3	25	21	200	171	11762	9975
5	508	443	3261	2746	2455	2082	7820	6697	708705	601321
10	1720	1501	14204	11950	15517	13143	28786	24624	2598280	2204667
15	3824	3346	36354	30605	48075	40717	65699	56164	5693130	4831323
20	6623	5799	72407	60926	110151	93218	121549	103819	9999761	8486341
25	10108	8851	125500	105649	209637	177333	199574	170328	15565313	13211695
30	14233	12461	200015	168363	355661	300744	302023	257620	22380144	18996004
35	19047	16675	296031	249264	555787	469906	431928	368258	30466446	25858760
40	24590	21519	420693	354320	823488	696162	592365	504798	39823488	33801678
45	30806	26959	574196	483628	1170698	989141	783864	667674	50473687	42842306
50	37735	33021	759956	640210	1605292	1355880	1012044	861656	62430595	52992467

Table 3. Timing performance (msecs) for the case of KNIX dataset.

Order	Moment Families (INCISIX Dataset)									
	GMs		LMs		TMs		KMs		DHMs	
	DS	*SBS*	*DS*	*SBS*	*DS*	*SBS*	*DS*	*SBS*	*DS*	*SBS*
0	13	12	4	4	32	30	201	188	11922	11145
5	496	475	3578	3338	3272	3050	7783	7275	722863	675832
10	1685	1614	15295	14254	20771	19302	28372	26505	2660991	2487824
15	3572	3422	38163	35545	67594	62776	70776	66143	5864036	5482582
20	6188	5929	75896	70658	153916	143171	138969	129886	10284282	9615163
25	9475	9078	131719	122599	266591	247966	235428	220038	15971863	14932422
30	13464	12904	208231	193770	425457	395679	359150	335315	22919177	21427273
35	18187	17431	322708	300266	671490	624761	522587	487417	31164529	29135577
40	23591	22614	504327	469081	983175	914848	706469	658649	40724145	38072365
45	29692	28472	726877	675879	1346551	1252703	913268	851339	51649763	48285960
50	36558	35077	932814	867355	1816793	1690125	1156850	1078288	63889158	59727774

Table 4. Timing performance (msecs) for the case of INCISIX dataset.

Order	Moment Families (MIAS Dataset)									
	GMs		LMs		TMs		KMs		DHMs	
	DS	*SBS*	*DS*	*SBS*	*DS*	*SBS*	*DS*	*SBS*	*DS*	*SBS*
0	13	6	4	2	24	11	197	89	11835	4809
5	509	240	3333	1522	2398	1099	7856	3571	710597	290989
10	1714	809	14452	6593	15442	7091	28732	13070	2609070	1067752
15	3623	1712	36858	16863	48365	22174	65639	29875	5710608	2337811
20	6272	2964	73305	33510	110365	50572	121797	55539	10042048	4113727
25	9628	4550	127805	58579	209384	96111	199562	90988	15602271	6392757
30	13653	6456	202445	92886	355803	163355	301687	137453	22409641	9184141
35	18387	8697	300303	137786	557843	256311	431414	196660	30481570	1249575
40	23830	1274	425532	195223	824113	378585	590462	269338	39851184	1634314
45	29986	4187	581006	266380	1162588	534107	783667	357651	50506603	2072049
50	36819	7432	770337	353421	1584871	728010	1012265	461968	62485283	2564557

Table 5. Timing performance (msecs) for the case of MIAS dataset.

A more descriptive way to present the performance of the SBS methodology is by computing the *Computation Time Reduction (CTR)*, defined in the following equation (12) and depicted in Fig.3 for the case of all moment families and biomedical image datasets.

$$CTR-\% = \frac{Time^{DS} - Time^{SBS}}{Time^{DS}} \times 100 \tag{12}$$

The above diagrams clearly show that the reduction of the computation time by using the SBS strategy is significant for all the cases. More precisely, this reduction varies between 37%-50%, 12%-25%,0%-7.5% and 50%-95% for the BRAINX, KNIX, INCISIX and MIAS datasets respectively. This diversity of the reduction owing to the different intensity distribution each image dataset presents, forming different number of blocks as shown in Table 1.

Another important outcome from the above plots is that all the moment families give near the same reduction for the same dataset and moreover this reduction is quite stable as the moment order increases (DHMs constitutes an exception for the case of MIAs dataset, where the reduction is significant higher (95%), for the high moment orders, as compared with the rest moment families (58%)).

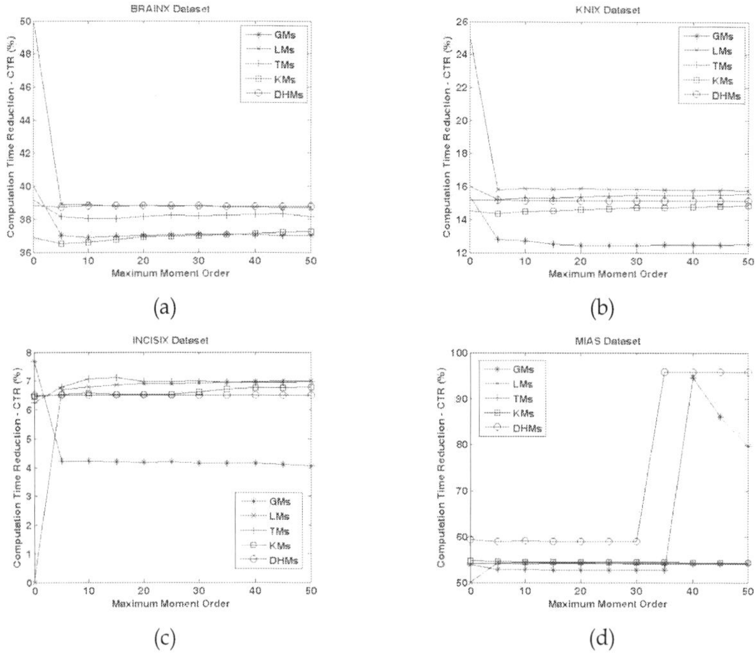

Fig. 3. Computation time reduction for the case of (a) BRAINIX, (b) KNIX, (c) INCISIX and (d) MIAS, datasets.

6. Conclusion

A morphology-driven methodology that improves the computation rates of the biomedical image moments was presented and analyzed in the previous sections. The usage of the introduced methodology can reduce the computation overhead by a significant factor depending on the image intensity morphology. This improvement is mainly achieved due to the biomedical images' nature dealing with their intensities distribution, which boosts the performance of the proposed computation scheme.

7. References

Bharathi, V.S. & Ganesan, L. (2008). Orthogonal moments based texture analysis of CT liver images. *Pattern Recognition Letters*, Vol. 29, No. 13, pp. 1868-1872.

Dai, X.B.; Shu, H.Z.; Luo, L.M.; Han, G.N. & Coatrieux, J.L. (2010). Reconstruction of tomographic images from limited range projections using discrete Radon transform and Tchebichef moments. *Pattern Recognition*, Vol. 43, No. 3, pp. 1152-1164.

DICOM, Retreived 16/08/2010 from http://pubimage.hcuge.ch:8080/.

Flusser, J.; Suk, T. & Zitova, B. (2009). *Moments and Moment Invariants in Pattern Recognition*. Wiley. Chichester.

Iscan, Z.; Dokur, Z. & Ölmez, T. (2010). Tumor detection by using Zernike moments on segmented magnetic resonance brain images. *Expert Systems with Applications*, Vol. 37, No. 3, pp.2540-2549.

Suckling, J et al (1994) "The Mammographic Image analysis society digital mammogram database. *Exerpta Medica. International Congress Series* 1069, pp. 375-378.

Li, B. & Meng, M.Q.-H. (2009). Computer-based detection of bleeding and ulcer in wireless capsule endoscopy images by chromaticity moments. *Computers in Biology and Medicine*, Vol. 39, No. 2, pp. 141-147.

Liyun, W.; Hefei, L.; Fuhao, Z.; Zhengding, L. & Zhendi, W. (2009). Spermatogonium image recognition using Zernike moments. *Computer Methods and Programs in Biomedicine*, Vol. 95, No. 1, pp. 10-22.

Papakostas, G.A.; Karras, D.A.; Mertzios, B.G. & Boutalis, Y.S. (2005). An efficient feature extraction methodology for computer vision applications using wavelet compressed Zernike moments", *ICGST International Journal on Graphics, Vision and Image Processing, Special Issue: Wavelets and Their Applications*, Vol. SI1, pp. 5-15.

Papakostas, G.A.; Boutalis, Y.S.; Karras, D.A. & Mertzios, B.G. (2007). "A new class of Zernike moments for computer vision applications. *Information Sciences*, Vol. 177, No.13, pp. 2802-2819.

Papakostas, G.A.; Karakasis, E.G. & Koulouriotis, D.E. (2008). Efficient and accurate computation of geometric moments on gray-scale images. *Pattern Recognition*, Vol. 41, No. 6, pp. 1895-1904.

Papakostas, G.A.; Karakasis, E.G. & Koulouriotis, D.E. (2008b). On accelerating the computation of 2-D discrete cosine transform in image processing. *International Conference on Signals and Electronic Systems (ICSES'08), (IEEE Xplore)*, pp. 7-10, Krakow - Poland.

Papakostas, G.A.; Boutalis, Y.S.; Karras, D.A. & Mertzios, B.G. (2009a). Pattern classification by using improved wavelet compressed Zernike moments. *Applied Mathematics and Computation*, Vol. 212, No. 1, pp. 162-176.

Papakostas, G.A.; Karras, D.A. & Mertzios, B.G. (2009b). Performance of the orthogonal moments in reconstructing biomedical images. *Proceedings of 16th International Workshop on Systems, Signals and Image Processing (IWSSIP'09), (IEEE Xplore)*, pp. 1-4, Chalkida - Greece.

Papakostas, G.A.; Karakasis, E.G. & Koulouriotis, D.E. (2009c). Computing orthogonal moments in biomedical imaging. *Proceedings of 16th International Workshop on Systems, Signals and Image Processing (IWSSIP'09), (IEEE Xplore)*, pp. 1-4, Chalkida - Greece.

Papakostas, G.A.; Koulouriotis, D.E. & Karakasis, E.G. (2009d). A unified methodology for efficient computation of discrete orthogonal image moments. *Information Sciences*, Vol. 179, No. 20, pp. 3619-3633.

Papakostas, G.A.; Koulouriotis, D.E. & Karakasis, E.G. (2009e). Efficient 2-D DCT computation from an image representation point of view", pp. 21-34, *Image Processing*, InTech.

Papakostas, G.A.; Tsougenis, E.D. & Koulouriotis, D.E. (2010a). Near optimum local image watermarking using Krawtchouk moments", *IEEE International Workshop on Imaging Systems and Techniques (IST'10)*, pp. 459-462, Thessaloniki - Greece.

Papakostas, G.A.; Karakasis, E.G. & Koulouriotis, D.E. (2010b). Novel moment invariants for improved classification performance in computer vision applications. *Pattern Recognition*, Vol. 43, No. 1, pp. 58-68.

Papakostas, G.A.; Koulouriotis, D.E. & Karakasis, E.G. (2010c). Computation strategies of orthogonal image moments: a comparative study. *Applied Mathematics and Computation*, Vol. 216, No. 1, pp. 1-17.

Shu, H.Z.; Zhou, J.; Han, G.N.; Luo, L.M. & Coatrieux, J.L. (2007). Image reconstruction from limited range projections using orthogonal moments. *Pattern Recognition*, Vol. 40, No. 2, pp. 670-680.

Sim, D.G.; Kim, H.K. & Park, R.H. (2004). Invariant texture retrieval using modified Zernike moments. *Image and Vision Computing*, Vol. 22, No. 4, pp. 331-342.

Wang, T.J. & Sze, T.W. (2001). The image moment method for the limited range CT image reconstruction and pattern recognition. *Pattern Recognition*, Vol. 34, No. 11, pp. 2145-2154

24

Modern Trends in Biomedical Image Analysis System Design

Oleh Berezsky, Grygoriy Melnyk and Yuriy Batko
Ternopil National Economic University
Ukraine

1. Introduction

1.1 Automated microscopy systems

Nowadays the combination of progressive information technologies, modern methods and algorithms of processing, analysis and synthesis of images together with medicine has resulted in the emergence of a new branch or field, called telemedicine. Telemedicine is distant diagnostics based on image analysis and processing of human organs cells. There are the following directions in this field: medical-biological research automation (that is computer systems design, which provides input, processing and analysis of images); development and application of algorithms of biomedical images pre-processing, which improves quality of images; image analysis (feature extraction, classifiers development, etc.) and data transfer network technologies. This problem has been studied by many scientists.

Today the analysis of medical-biological specimens (cytological and histological smears) in diagnostic laboratories is conducted by visual inspection. This process is routine and labour intensive. That's why the automated microscopy systems (AMSs) - software-hardware complexes appeared for the digital processing of microscopic images. AMS includes motorized controlled microscope, video camera, optical adapters, computer, and specialized software modules. In general the medical complexes for automated microscopy are made to provide higher productivity of medical work; improve analysis accuracy, availability of intensive labour-consuming and rare analyses, quality control, telemedicine; to collect and archive specimen image; and better learning, service and certification. AMS provides the following levels of microscopic analyses automations:

1. Visual analysis, documenting and telemedicine;
2. Analysis of images in order to determine the specimen characteristics;
3. Automation of movements and inspection of specimen.

Morphometry of cells is only the one of the automated methods in AMS. Basic steps of cytological and histological analysis are the following: selection of an object of investigation, preparation for microscope inspection, microscopy techniques application, qualitative and quantitative analysis of images. Type, structure and functions of the system are dictated by actual task, objects class of research and financial ability of user.

Problem definition. The actual tasks are projecting of AMS hardware and software structures based on the hardware components existing in the market and development of the own software for histological and cytological image analysis.

1.2 Components of automated microscopy systems

In general, AMSs are divided into research-based and specialized (Egorova 2005, Egorova 2006). Research AMS is used for development of new methods of diagnostics. Specialized AMS provides implementation of a standardized clinical research. The key feature of research-based AMS is the use of multifunctional microscopes and cameras with increased sensitiveness and resolution. The research method is not preset, but formed by a user.

For microbiology investigations the world market offers AMSs or their components from different manufacturers, such as Carl Zeiss, Leica, Olympus, Nikon, Micromed (Russia), Motic (China), Konus (Italy).

Let's shortly describe the process of research with the help of AMS (Egorova, 2005). At the beginning, specimen is set on the microscope stage. The selected image area is displayed on the screen. All the necessary adjustment and image acquisition is derived in real-time. The image can be processed with filters, and it can be followed with text comments and calibrating marker. AMS allows selecting micro-objects on image in the automatic, semi-automatic or manual modes. The selected micro-objects are measured automatically and the results of measuring are displayed in a tabular form (Medovyi, 2006). Micro-objects can be classified according to any of the measured parameters. The results of analysis can be printed and saved in a database.

1.2.1 Software overview

The basic advantage of the use of software tools is a transition from subjective and qualitative analysis to objective and quantitative analysis. The basic disadvantage here is complication of adjustment and occurrence of errors of measurement.

AMS allows acquiring image by a photo camera, video camera, and scanner or from a file. The results of researches are displayed on a screen in a table form, or charts. Measuring accuracy is provided by calibration of camera with calibrating slide. Software complexes give a user a wide spectrum of tools for processing and analysis of biomedical images (BMI) and video stream (Richardson, 2005), in particular, in genetic, cytological, histological researches etc. The characteristic features of the modern systems are a high level of automation, possibility of remote work and decreasing of dependence on specialised video recording devices.

For the construction of the generalized structure of AMS, design and functions of existent software tools were investigated (table 1). In particular, comparison was based on the followings parameters:

- method of information acquisition: an image is acquired from real-time source (support of technology of MCI/TWAIN) or loading from a disk;
- modes of segmentation algorithms operation: manual (the operator in the manual mode selects micro-objects), automated (the operator learns the algorithm) or automatic (the parameters of algorithm are set automatically);
- previous processing of image: noise reduction, correction of brightness, contrast, filtration, selection to the area of interest, etc;
- calculation of numerical features of micro-objects: perimeter, area, nucleocytoplasmic relationship, diameter, corner between two segments, etc;
- calculation of statistical features: mathematical expectation, standard deviation, maximal (minimum) value, etc;
- presentation of results in a form of diagrams, histograms, or charts;

№	Software	Support of additional formats of files	Converting of file to other format	Editing of image	Converting to other colour space	A selection of micro-objects in manual / automated / automatic modes	Calculation of characteristic features	Determination of co-ordinates of convex rectangle	Use of plugging	Use of scenarios	Forming of reports	Communication with third-party software	Printing	Tuning of parameters	Calibration of camera	Presence of the help system
1	Image Tool v.2.00	+	+	+	+	+/-/-	+	-	-	+	+	-	+	+	-	+
2	Image Warp	-	+	+	-	+/-/-	+	-	+	+	+	-	+	+	-	+
3	"Imager-CG"	-	+	+	-	+/-/-	+	-	-	-	+	-	+	+	-	+
4	VideoTest-Morpho 3.2	+	+	+	+	+/+/-	+	-	+	+	+	-	+	+	-	+
5	Vido-Test Morphology 5.0	+	+	+	+	+/+/+	+	-	+	+	+	+	+	+	+	+
6	Micromed Images	+	+	+	-	+/-/-	+	-	-	+	+	-	+	+	-	+
7	Screen Meter	-	-	-	-	+/-/-	+	-	-	-	+	-	-	+	-	+
8	Image Expert Pro 3	-	+	+	+	+/+/-	+	-	+	+	+	-	+	+	-	+
9	Image Expert™ Gauge	-	+	+	+	+/+/-	+	-	+	+	+	-	+	+	-	+
10	AnalySIS Five	-	+	+	+	+/+/-	+	-	+	+	+	-	+	+	-	+
11	Bio Vision	-	+	+	+	+/+/-	+	-	+	+	+	-	+	+	-	+
12	QCapture PRO 6.0	-	+	+	+	+/+/-	+	-	+	+	+	-	+	+	-	+
13	Motic Images Advanced 3.2	+	+	+	+	+/+/+	+	+	+	+	+	+	+	+	-	+
14	MCID™ Core	-	+	+	+	+/+/-	+	-	+	+	+	-	+	+	-	+
15	Image-Pro Plus 6.2	+	+	+	+	+/+/-	+	-	+	+	+	-	+	+	-	+
16	MetaMorph 7.5	-	+	+	+	+/+/-	+	-	+	+	+	-	+	+	-	+
17	ImageJ (NIH, USA)	-	+	+	+	+/-/-	+	-	+	+	+	-	+	+	-	+
18	Pixels	-	-	+	-	+/-/-	+	-	-	-	+	-	+	+	-	+
19	NIH Image	-	+	+	+	+/+/+	+	+	+	+	+	+	+	+	-	+
20	Xite v3.45	-	-	+	-	+/-/-	+	-	-	-	+	-	+	+	-	+
21	DiaMorph	-	+	+	+	+/+/+	+	+	+	+	+	+	+	+	-	+

Table 1. Comparison of software

- co-operating with third-party software: MS Word, MS Excel, MS Access, FoxPro, etc;
- the use of scripts and presence of built-in language for the batch processing;
- presence of the detailed technical documentation.

1.2.2 Hardware components overview

The typical structure of hardware consists of microscope, video camera or photo camera, computer, printer and monitor (Egorova, 2005). The subsystem of image acquisition (Berezsky, 2008, b) consists of light microscope, camera, photo adapter, objective changing device, focusing device, stage moving device, specimen supplying device and illumination device (figure 1).

Minimum requirements for the computer is processor with 1 GHz frequency, amount of main memory is not less than 1 GB and USB or IEEE interfaces for incorporation with a digital camera (Egorova, 2005).

The transmitted light microscope consists of a stand, to which all units are fastened: illumination device, specimen stage, systems of imaging and visualization. The basic characteristics of microscope is its class, magnification ratio, optical resolution, size of the linear field view on object and degree of optical aberration correction (Egorova 2005). For cytology and histology AMSs use the biological direct microscopes of work, laboratory and research classes.

Biological microscopes have the following methods of research: light field, phase contrast, polarization and luminescence. Microscope includes three basic functional parts (Egorova, 2006): illumination system, imaging system, and visualization system.

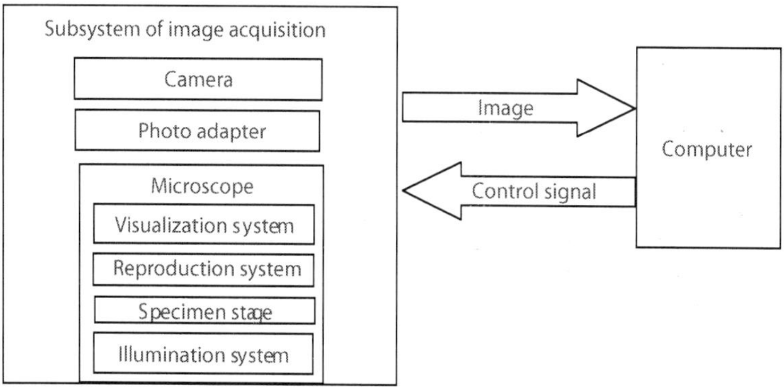

Fig. 1. Structure of AMS hardware

The illumination system of light microscope is intended for creation of uniform luminous flux and consists of light source and optical-mechanical system (field stop, collector, and condenser). The imaging system provides the first degree of magnification and includes objective fastening unit, objective, optical filters changing device and focusing device. The visualization system is intended to acquire the real image of micro-object on the retina of eye, film, and screen monitor with an additional magnification. Visualizing part is located between the image plane of objective and eyes of observer (or camera).

To capture image with a microscope the following cameras are used: digital single-lens reflex camera, digital non reflex photo camera, and digital video camera (Wu, 2008). The general device of input in microscopy is digital video camera. Firms, engaged in development and trade of the special video cameras for a microscopy are: Carl Zeiss (Germany), Axiovision, Motic (China), Tucsen (China), Lumenera Corp. (Canada), SPOT Imaging Solutions (USA). For digital photo- and video cameras basic characteristics are the following: a dynamic range of sensor, signal-noise ratio, resolution, and fastening compatibility with a microscope. For mechanical connection of camera and video port of microscope the special photo adapter is used. It provides an image transfer without distortions with the certain coefficient of magnification on the photosensitive matrix of camera. Let's summarize the basic parameters of devices, on which AMS are synthesized, in a table 2.

For planning of the system it is necessary to define the area of its application, magnification degree for specific medical research, sizes of micro-objects and level of automation. The choice of specific components of the system is based on heuristic rules. The basic tasks of AMS designing are: selection of optical elements of microscope, choice of digital camera and proper photo adapter, optical connection of system devices, and electric connection of devices.

The minimal requirements to the microscope during the histological researches with the use of AMS are the following: class not lower than laboratory, objectives magnification 10, 40; eyepieces with field of 20 mm or 18 mm, and mounted powerful illumination device. For histology application the use of differential- interference contrast allows to attain better results.

One of the basic parameters of microscope is resolution, which determines quality of the obtained image (Egorova, 2006). Resolution depends on the numerical aperture of objective and condenser, and also on the wave-length of light.

The level of AMS automation depends on its setting and desired speed of specimen analysis. For automation the device of focusing motorization, moving of specimen stage, changes of current objective and changes of filter are set on a microscope.

Camera is chosen according to the problem specifications: type of the investigated specimen, system of illumination, size of necessary increase, geometrical sizes of the least micro-object. Therefore, the main characteristics of camera are the following: type of sensor (monochrome, colour), resolution of sensor, and type of fastening of camera objective (Rietdorf, 2005). For histological specimen research, the coloured camera with a resolution not less than 1280x1024 points, the interface of USB connecting, mounting of objective of C-mount, CCD by sensor and relation of signal/noise not less than 65 dB are recommended (Egorova, 2005).

Optical connection of camera and microscope. It is possible to select three methods to acquire microscopic image by means of a digital camera (Murphy, 2001). Usually light rays quit the eyepiece of microscope in form parallel rays, but with the help of focusing it is possible to get a consilient bunch. The first method consists in that the objective of camera is placed as near as possible to the eyepiece of microscope. The system is used for editing of digital video camera or digital camera. However, such system requires setting up the special adapter that would firmly fasten the lens of camera on the ocular tube of microscope.

The second method consists in the direct projecting of image from objective on sensor of camera. For this purpose, when fastening to the ocular tube, eyepiece and lens of camera are removed, and the proper adapter is set (without optical elements). When fastening to the special video port on a microscope, the proper adapter, which is included in the complete set of microscope, is set.

Device	Basic parameters
Microscope	Type: light microscope System: monocular, binocular Manufacturer: Carl Zeiss, Nikon, Olympus, Leica, Motic Class: educational, laboratory (mechanical), work (motorized), research (digital) Photo adaptation: without video port, with video port Amount of objectives: 4 pieces, ×4, ×10, ×40, ×100 Type of objectives: dry, immersion Class of objectives: without correction of aberration, semi plan, achromatic, achromatic - aplanatic Numerical aperture of objective. Research methods: light field, dark field, phase contrast, polarized light, fluorescence Condenser: regular, achromatic, achromatic - aplanatic Illumination: halogen lamp, light-emitting diode Specimen stage: mechanical, motorized Accessories: photo adapter, digital camera
Video camera	Manufacturer: CarlZeiss, Nikon, Webbers, Olympus, Qimaging, MicroCam, CARTON, ScopeTek, KONUS, Motic Type of sensor: monochrome, colour Type of sensor: CCD, CMOS Resolution: 1, 2, 3, 5, 8 MPixel Sensor sensitivity: 0,8v/lux.sec with 550 nm (colour CMOS) Signal-noise ratio: larger than 45 dB Dynamic range larger than 60 dB (colour CMOS) Matrix size: 1/3", 1/2", 2/3" Frame rate during video capturing in maximal resolution Interface: IEEE 1394, video composite, USB Type of objective mounting: C-mount, T-mount
Computer	Processor with 2 GHz clock frequency Memory: not less then 1 GB Video card with 256 NB video RAM Hard drive with capacity not less than 250 GB
Monitor	Size: minimum 17", advisable 19"
Printer	For the reports - laser printer For the pictures of specimens - colour inkjet printer

Table 2. Basic parameters of AMS hardware devices

The third method consists in adapter, set up between a camera and video port, which has the own optical system, so-called reverse objective. Its purpose is to reproduce correctly an image on-the-spot of sensor, namely to decrease the size of image from objective, so that it covers a sensor area fully. Relation of linear sizes of sensors toward eyepiece field of view is described in fig. 3.

Some reverse lenses are in a position to change an image, that is, they work as a transfocator. Digital cameras, developed specially for a microscopy, are assembled by means of the first and third methods.

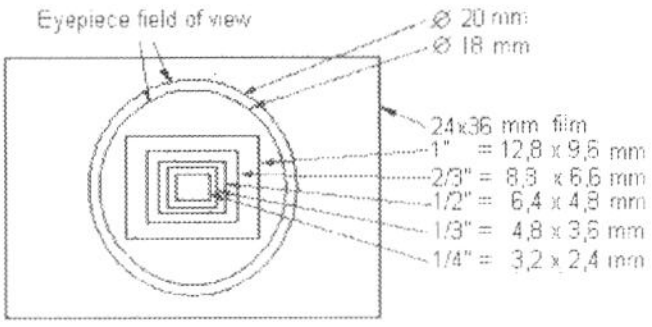

Fig. 3. Correlation of sizes of digital camera matrix and main image of microscope

The digital scale is calculated according to the expression:

$$m = d_{YFO}{}^{*}k_M \,/\, w$$

in which m is a linear digital scale, micrometer/pixel;
d_{YFO} - a diameter of field of view on the object, micrometer;
k_M - a coefficient of the overlap of field of view by the matrix (Fig. 3); and
w - number of pixels on the horizontal row of sensor.

2. Automated microscopy system design

2.1 Design of AND-OR tree for AMS hardware

The tasks of systems structures synthesis are hard to formalize on the whole (Berezsky, 2009, a). Input information for structural synthesis consists of description of designed object demands, its operating condition and limited elements composition. Output is the information about composition of the system and methods of elements connection. Formally, decision support task for structural synthesis is possible to present in such way:

$$DSS = \langle \mathbf{A}, \mathbf{K}, M, RS \rangle$$

where $\mathbf{A} = \langle A_1, A_2, ..., A_n \rangle$ is a set of alternatives, $\mathbf{K} = \langle K_1, K_2, ..., K_n \rangle$ is a set of criteria, M:$\mathbf{A} \to \mathbf{K}$ is a model, which allows to find the criteria vector for every alternative, RS - a decision rule, which provides the choice of optimum alternative. For every alternative there is an ordered set of attributes $\mathbf{X} = \langle X_1, X_2, ..., X_p \rangle$. If mathematical model $\mathbf{X} \to \mathbf{K}$ is unknown, an approach of expert system is used. In most cases the tasks of structural synthesis are solved with the help of heuristic methods. The set of alternatives **A** can be presented as $\mathbf{A} = \langle \mathbf{P}, \mathbf{E} \rangle$, where **P** is a set of rules, **E** is a set of system elements. Morphological tables and AND-OR tree for **P** and **E** are used for description.

Morphological tables represent alternatives as $\mathbf{M} = \langle \mathbf{X}, \mathbf{R} \rangle$, where **X** is a set of object characteristics (functions), **R** is a set of methods of functions implementation. The disadvantage of morphological tables is ignoring forbidden elements combination in structures and mutual independence of realizations set R_i. These disadvantages are absent in AND-OR tree, which is an aggregate of morphological tables. In AND-OR tree the "AND" node corresponds to a partial morphological table M_j, each "OR" node that is incidental to M_j table, corresponds to the set of variants of realization of i- function.

AND-OR tree based synthesis anticipates the existence of decision rules in every "OR" node. These rules are based on and related to the demands of requirement specification. During their creation it is necessary to use such production rules as:

IF condition 1, condition 2, condition n, THEN action 1, action 2, action m.

On the basis of AMS classification and analysis of its structure we can build the AND-OR tree for system structure according to the set of its functions and characteristics (Fig. 4) (ribs which are connected to "And" nodes are marked with arcs). For system design it is necessary to define the application field, magnification degree of actual medical research, micro-objects sizes and level of automation. IIS can be built on the basis of digital or Photo Adapted Microscopes and camera. Selecting of actual system components is based on their characteristics using heuristic rules. The level of AMS automation depends on its purpose and desired speed of specimen analysis. For automation purpose microscopes can include devices of focusing motorization, moving of specimen table, objective and filter changing.

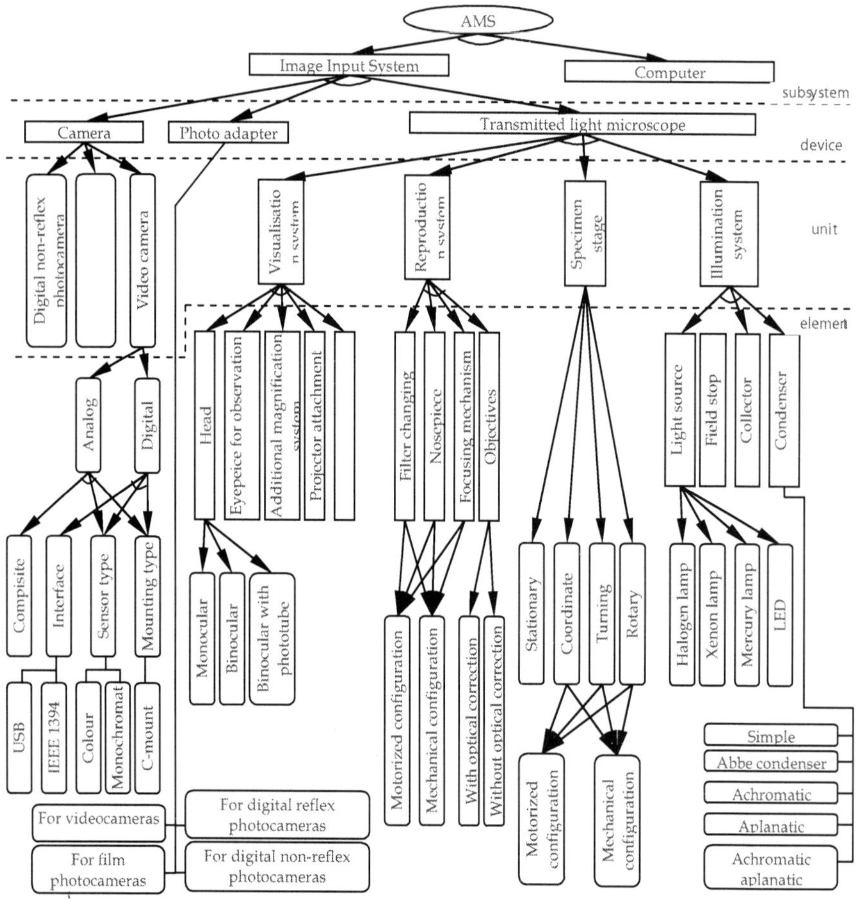

Fig. 4. AND-OR tree of hardware part of AMS

AMS consists of the image input system (IIS) and computer. Typical IIS consists of camera, photo adapter and light microscope. The IIS components are based on optical compatibility properties and connected with the special photo adapter, which can be put in the phototube of trinocular head, in the eyepiece tube of binocular head or in the special adapter on the microscope stage.

Let us define parameters, which can help to choose alternative variants of system arrangement:

1. Medical field: cytology, histology, haematology, chromosome analysis, and telemedicine;
2. Research types: morphometry, cytophotometry, and densitometry;
3. Research methods: bright field microscopy: phase contrast, differential interference contrast, dark field;
4. Magnification ratio: 80 - 1000;
5. Micro-object size: micrometer;
6. Digital scale: micrometer/pixel;
7. Level of automation.

On the basis of AND-OR tree for the choice of separate components of the system we will bring fragment of product rules, which form the alternative variants of configuration of the system.

If medical field is histology,
  then AMS consists of IIS and computer.
If medical field is histology **and** research method is light microscopy,
  then IIS consists of a camera, photo adapter and transmitted light microscope.

The product rules allow us to generate the set of variants of structural arrangement of the system, which satisfies a requirement specification. Parametric optimization is conducted on the set of possible solutions.

2.2 Design of software ASM part AND-OR tree

We will build the AND-OR tree for the synthesis of alternative variants of creation of programming constituent, which is based on the conducted analysis systems of morphometric analysis (Berezsky, 2009, b). The basic criteria, which influence on the choice of the systems, are (Berezsky, 2009, c): quality of input images, type of micro-objects, types of numerical descriptions of micro-objects, and their statistical descriptions (Fig. 5).

We will build alternative decision AND-OR tree, using the parameters:

1. medical area: cytology, histology, haematology, analysis of chromosomes, telemedicine;
2. source data type: local, global;
3. quality of entrance images: with noise, without noise;
4. level of automation;
5. type selection of objects;
6. necessary characteristics;
7. types of research objects : separate objects, groups of objects;
8. the way of results delivery: internal or external software.

We will show fragment rules of how to choose the product structures of the programming system for morphometric analysis.

If medical area is histology **and** class of the system is specialized
  then system is automated.
If medical area is histology
  then the system consists of the module of input information, module of previous processing, module of selection of objects and module of determination of informative descriptions.

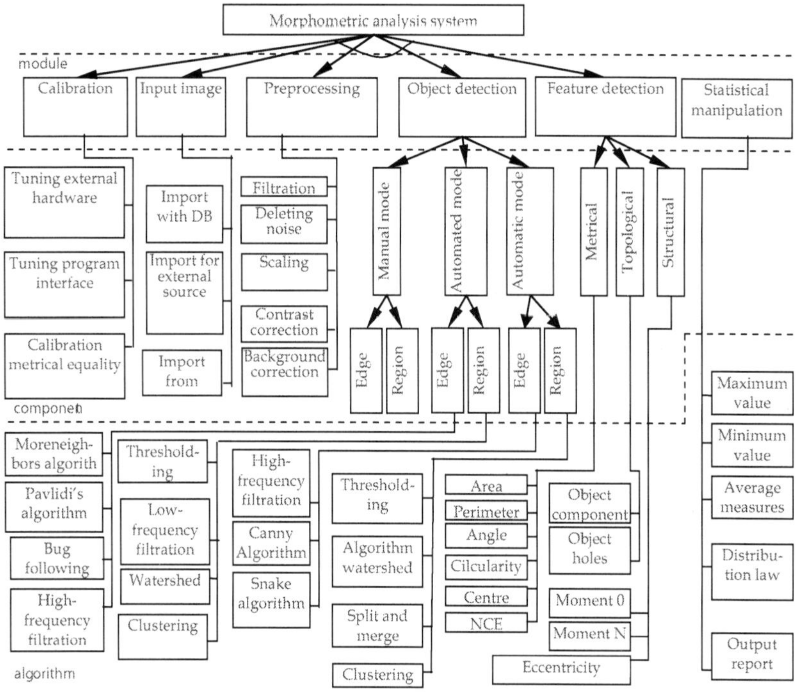

Fig. 5. AND-OR tree for software part of AMS

2.3 Examples of logical production rules for specialized AMS

Karyotyping

The basic method of chromosomal violation diagnostics in reproductive medicine is a cytogenetic research - karyotyping. Rules for AMS constructions are the following:

Hardware

If karyotyping, **then** microscope (class (work), objective (10x, 100x).

If karyotyping with Q-painting, **then** microscope (method (fluorescence)).

If karyotyping, **then** camera (type (digital), sensor (monochrome, CCD), resolution (1280x1024).

If karyotyping, **then** computer (processor (2,4 GHz), RAM (1 GB), HDD (250 GB), video adapter (256 MB)).

Software

If karyotyping, **then** software includes such modules: image pre-processing, editing, storage is to DB, print of results.

DNA Research

CGH Method. The kernel of every cell has chromosomes, in which there are genes that consist of segments of desoxyribonucleic acid (DNA), where genetic information is accumulated and saved. In order to expose quantitative violations in a genome it is possible to apply the method of comparative hybridization (Comparative Genome Hybridization - CGH). Investigated and normal donor DNA is marked by means of fluorophors of different colour. After leading through FISH, metaphases are analysed on a fluorescent microscope, and with the help of the specialized program of computer analysis of images, intensity of fluorescence of two fluorophors on all length of every chromosome is determined. AMS construction rules are the following:

If method CGH, **then** microscope (class (work), method (fluorescence), block for colour filters mounting, objective (magnification (10x, 100x)).

If method CGH, **then** camera (digital) and camera (black and white) and sensor (type CCD, resolution (1280x1024), charge accumulation mode)

Computer

If method CGH, **then** computer (processor (Pentium IV 2,4 GHz)), computer (RAM (512MB)), computer (HDD (250GB)), computer (video card (256MB RAM)).

Software

If method CGH, **then** software includes such modules: image pre-processing, editing, storage is in DB, print of results, specialized functions.

Spermatology is medical-biological branch, which is engaged in research of sperm of man and animal.

Interest to the analysis of human sperm is closely related to the needs of genesial medicine, which solves the problems of birth of children, birth control and planning of family.

The systems of computer analysis, based on technologies of digital processing of video images, allow with the less waste of time estimate the parameters of sperm more objectively and avoid subjectivity of interpretation of results, which happens in standard spermogram. Moreover, determination of additional indexes of mobility appeared, such as, curvilinear speed and linearness of motion. The use of the similar systems for automation of analysis of sperm underlay direction in andrology - CASA. AMS construction rules are the following:

If CASA, **then** microscope (class (work), objective (magnification 20x)).

If CASA, **then** video camera (digital, coloured, sensor (type (CCD), resolution (above 640x480), frame rate(50 fps))).

Computer

If CASA, **then** computer (processor (Pentium IV 2,4 GHz)), computer (RAM (512MB)), computer (HDD (250GB)), computer (video card (256MB RAM)).

Software

If CASA, **then** software includes such modules: image pre-processing, editing, storage is in DB, printing of results, specialized functions.

Hematology

Hematology is the section of medicine that investigates structure and functions of blood system (blood, organs of blood formation), reasons and mechanisms of development of blood illnesses, and develops the methods of their recognition, treatment and prophylaxis.

AMS construction rules are:

Microscope

If hematology, **then** microscope (class work), objective (magnification 10x, 100x), specimen table (motorized)).

Camera

If hematology, **then** camera (digital, coloured, sensor (type (CCD), resolution (1280*1024), adjustability on colours)).

Computer

If hematology, **then** computer (processor (Pentium IV 2,4 GHz), RAM (512MB), HDD (160GB), video adapter (512MB RAM)).

Software

If hematology, **then** software includes such modules: image pre-processing, editing, storage in DB, printing of results, blood cells atlas, specialized functions.

2.4 Functions of microscopic image processing and their realization

Let us consider the components of the typical AMS(s) software and algorithms of their realization.

3.1 Micro-objects segmentation task

We will make the table of the use of the proper methods of segmentation according to the type of investigated micro-objects (Table 3).

All the process of analysis can be divided into such stages: image acquisition (loading, sight selection, etc.) (Pratt, 2007), pre-processing (noise reduction, recoding, etc.) (Duda, 2000), (Shapiro, 2001), analysis (segmentation) of image (*Gonzalez, 2008)* (Duda, 2000) (Wismullera, 2004) and description (extraction of characteristic features) (Avtandilov, 1990) (Jahne, 2005) of micro-objects.

Amount of types micro-objects	Type of objects	Clearness of border	Algorithm
Single objects	Objects one to the type	clear border	threshold segmentation, high-frequency filtration
		not clear border	watershed, clusterization
	Objects of different types	clear border	threshold segmentation, clusterization, region growing
		not clear border	watershed, clusterization
Groups of objects	Objects one to the type	clear border	clusterization, high-frequency filtration
		not clear border	threshold segmentation, clusterization
	Objects of different types	clear border	clusterization, region growing, watershed
		not clear border	watershed, clusterization

Table 3. Criteria of choice of algorithms of image segmentation

One of the important stages of automation of analysis process of biomedical preparations is a selection of micro-objects (Avtandilov, 1990). This task is solved by means of images digital analysis (Pratt, 2007). Principal reason of complication of histology research automation is high variability and low contrast of the most histological structures.

One of the most widely used segmentation BMI approaches is the selection of micro-objects borders. It is predefined by clear borders of micro-objects. This group includes the following algorithms: threshold segmentation, active contours algorithm, high-frequency filtration,

etc. As a rule, algorithms of this group are used in the morphological operations (Al-Jarrahb, 2008) of dilatation and erosion (Batko, 2009). The choice of segmentation thresholds is based on a priori information about micro-objects and analysis of histograms of brightness distribution (Furman, 2003).
Advantages of these algorithms are high speed action and realization simplicity. And disadvantages are low efficiency of work with poorly contrasting images, work with imposition of micro-objects, and work with uneven backgrounds.
Another approach for solving micro-objects detection problems is a selection micro-object form on the template. The main task is to find that part of image (the micro-object contour) that better coincides with the form of standard micro-object. Advantage ot this approach is possibility of work with images with well-known set of templates. Among the disadvantages of this approach we determine the result dependence on template accuracy and exactness, high complication and, as a result, low speed action.
The third approach is based on determination of areas, which are identical to micro-objects. Among the algorithms of this group there are: clusterization of image (Forsyth, 2004), sectional segmentation, increase of areas, images marking and others. The selection of areas has found its wide application in morphometric researches, because often a structure of fabric is a background, and it does not give it possible to select a cell, because its elements have brightness and different levels of brightness, which coincide with the brightness of background. Difficulties at the choice of starting points of segmentation (by chance, or on the basis of a priori information) are the main disadvantages of algorithms of this group.

4. AMS design and testing example in the area of histology and cytology

We describe the examples of AMS design for histology and cytology purpose and determine the rules for AMS design (Berezsky, 2009, a).
Rules for hardware are the following:
If medical field is histology **and** medical field is cytology, **then** AMSs consist of IIS and computer.
If medical field is histology, **and** medical field is cytology, **and** research method is light microscopy, **then** IIS consists of camera, photo adapter and transmitted light microscope.
If medical field is histology, **or** cytology, **and** research method is light microscopy, **then** IIS consists of camera, photo adapter and transmitted light microscope.
Rules for software are the following:
If class of the system is research, **then** system is manual.
If medical area is histology **and** medical field is cytology, **then** the system consists of: module of manual selection of objects, module of input information, module of pre-processing, and module of determination of informing descriptions.
Structure of AMS software
The structure of the projected AMS software is presented in fig. 6. For the acquisition images the module of information input was implemented. The module information input allows working with loaded and captured in real-time images. The module of pre-processing is provided for improvement of images quality, emphasis of characteristic features of micro-objects and choice of areas of interest. For the selection of micro-objects there is a module of segmentation. It provides three algorithms of selection: pixel-wise (manual), block and automated (based on key points). To acquire the characteristic features of objects, the

contour and texture analyses are used. By means of the algorithms of contour analysis the followings characteristic features are calculated: perimeter, length, angle of slope of micro-object, and others. For the statistical analysis of data the module of statistical processing, which provides the calculation of maximum, minimum and medium values of elements selection, is implemented. The important stage of work of the system is presenting of findings both in electronic and printing variants. The module of reports formation is implemented for this purpose.

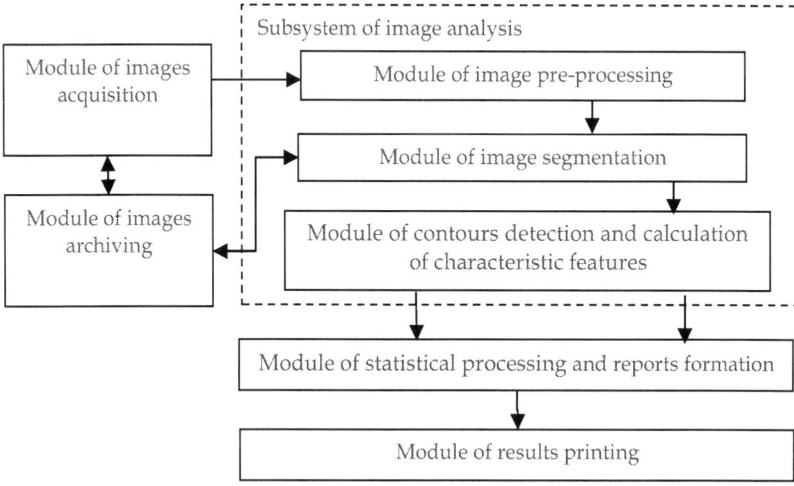

Fig. 6. Flow diagram of AMS software

Software is developed in Delphi IDE for Windows of the based work stations. The use of technology of TWAIN allowed organizing co-operation with majority of modern hardware tools, including video cameras. TWAIN is the industrial standard of interface of software tool for the transmission of images from different hardware tools in OS Windows and Macintosh (scanner, web-camera, video camera etc). Important advantage of the developed system is possibility of large size images processing. We will consider the algorithms of realization of the modules of software consistently.

Module of images acquisition. Input images can be loaded from a disk or captured from a video recording hardware. The system allows capturing an image from a video recording hardware in real-time mode. Video information, which is captured from a video recording hardware, is displayed in the working window of the system. To transfer an image into the working area of the program, double click of the left button mouse is used. After that the program stops displaying of video stream and transfers captured image to module of pre-processing.

Module of image pre-processing. In order to remove artefacts, improve quality and perform additional processing, functions of image pre-processing are used. Among accessible functions there are:

- selection of image part;
- down-scaling of image;
- transformation from one colour base to another;

- correction of image brightness;
- correction of colour gamut.

Module of image segmentation. According to the tasks and necessary selection of objects a user is able to choose three variants of selection (Berezsky, 2010):

- pixel-wise selection of objects;
- block selection of objects;
- selection of objects on the basis of characteristic points.

These algorithms can be compared according to the followings criteria: exactness, speed of selection and level of process automation. Exactness is defined as relationship of the correctly selected points (that belong to the object and amount of the ignored points that do not belong to the object) and the points selected by mistake (points that were selected, but do not belong to the object and the ignored points that belong to the object). Speed of selection is determined as time necessary for the selection of micro-objects in the selected area. Level of automation is a relationship of amount of the selected points, necessary for the selection of all objects in the selected area that the system selects to the amount of points selected by the operator.

During the implementation of manual pixel-wise selection exactness is maximum, however, process automation is not present. As result, there is more investigation time (Hea, 2008). During the implementation of block processing exactness of selection is sufficient. The result of such selection sometimes needs partial correction. The level of automation and speed is high.

During the implementation of processing on the basis of characteristic points exactness of selection is sufficient. The result of such selection sometimes needs partial correction. The level of automation is the greatest among the algorithms offered in the system. The results of comparison of algorithms of selection of micro-objects are presented in a table 4.

№	Algorithm	Exactness	Speed of selection	Level of automation
1	Pixel wise selection	>99%	>30c	0
2	Block selection	97%	10-15c	92%
3	Selection on the basis of characteristic points	95%	3-5c	99%

Table 4. Comparison of algorithms of selection of objects

Module of contours detection and calculation of characteristic features. For the calculation of contour features, the additional processing of received data is foreseen in the system (Berezsky, 2009, f). This additional analysis is provided by means of functions:

- passing a contour;
- selection of major axis;
- selection of characteristic points;
- contour approximation.

Except visual information, the program presents the results of its work in a tabular format. During statistical analysis the system calculates the following morphometric characteristics:

- area of nuclei;
- area of cytoplasm;
- area of cell;
- nucleocytoplasmic relationship (NCR);

- medium selective;
- minimum value of selection;
- maximum value of selection.

The calculation of additional informative characteristics is also foreseen in the program, in particular:

- measuring of distance between two points;
- relationship between lengths of two segments;
- corner between two unparallel segments.

The use of this module allows conducting the previous statistical processing of the received data. The received results allow the expert to conduct the preliminary estimation of findings.

Module of statistical processing and reports formation. In order to increase functional possibilities in the software system, the functions of co-operating with other external software tools are foreseen, in particular, with tabular editor MS Excel (Berezsky, 2009, e). An information transfer takes place with the help of OLE functions, which realize the interface of co-operation between a software tool and tabular editor. The use of MS Excel allowed decreasing of loading on the system and substantial increasing of statistical processing possibilities, and presenting the findings in a diagram format.

Module of results printing. The standard dialog box of information output is implemented on a print. An information transfer is carried out by built-in to MACAW functions, which realize the interface of co-operation between a software tool and printing unit. A user is able to choose a necessary device for a print, amount of copies, amount of pages on a sheet etc.

Module of images archiving. There is a set of procedures and functions for work with the base of information (Berezsky, 2008, a). Basic functions are: search of image in the base of information and formation of reports.

4.1 Testing of the module of image segmentation

The computer system is used for analysis and research of cytological images of multi-layered images of epithelium for the different types of dysplasia of epithelium of uterus neck of women of reproductive age (Berezsky, 2009, d). The results of work of segmentation algorithms are described on the example of images of cells of uterus neck. In Fig. 7.

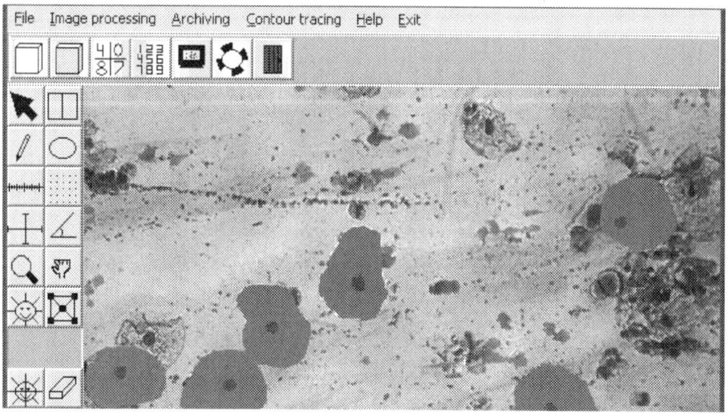

Fig. 7. The example of selection of micro-objects during pixel segmentation

After completion of segmentation procedure, the program forms a report, which indicated descriptions of the selected objects. The example of report is presented in the table 5.

Number of cell	Area of nuclei	Area of cell	Area of cytoplasm	NCR
1	369	18475	18106	0,02038
2	365	19379	19014	0,0191964
3	628	18006	17378	0,0361376
4	467	20712	20245	0,0230674
5	360	16509	16149	0,0222924
6	324	15271	14947	0,0216766
7	463	18085	17622	0,026274
Medium values	425,1428571	18062,42857	17637,28571	0,0241463
Minimum values	324	15271	14947	0,0191964
Maximum values	628	20712	20245	0,0361376
Medium square deviation	104,5457293	1785,717023	1752,86924	0,0057403

Table 5. Descriptions of micro-objects are during a pixel selection

4.3 Approbation of the module of image archiving

Test DB of images contains about 500 full-colour cytological and histological images of tumour cells. Storage of the following information is foreseen in DB of BMI:

- Image of sample. This information is saved in a graphic file. The name of file is encoded on the basis of date, when the sample was received, and identification code of a patient in the medical establishment.
- Quantitative results of the sample, processed by the program. This information is saved in a tabular form. The name of file is identical to the name of file with digital sample image. In this file the saved information is about the kernel area, cell, cytoplasm area, and nucleocytoplasmic relationship of the selected cells. Besides, some statistical information is saved: areas of maximum, medium, and minimum of kernel, cell, cytoplasm and NCR.
- Annotation of sample image. This information is saved in a text format. The name of file is identical to the name of file with digital image. In this file the saved information is about the date of material reception, type of material, diagnosis, method of treatment and so on.

The developed system additionally checks process of treatment, analyses the results of inspections of group of people, etc. Two functions of work with data base are implemented for this purpose: search of image and forming of summarizing report about the group of images. General view of window of information search in a database is possible to see in fig. 8.

The result of search in DB is the description of image. In the case of absence of the proper files the system informs about an error message. If the file with a text representation is absent, the user is able to fill the proper fields. If the file with quantitative results is absent, the user must do additional testing of image.

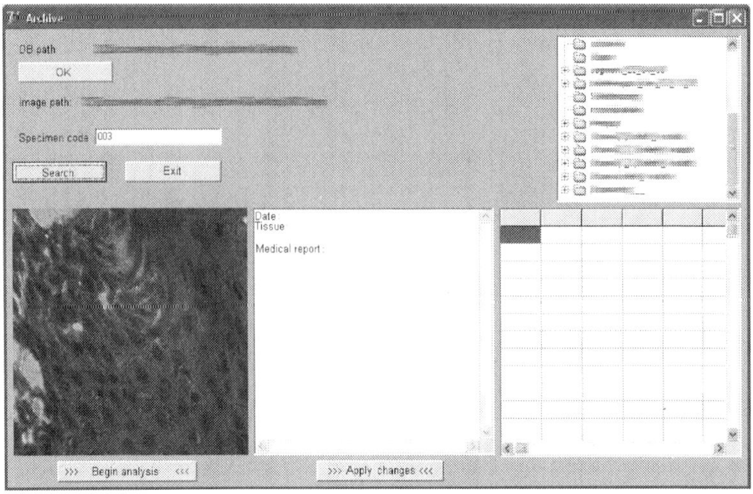

Fig. 8. The result of image search of image based on its description

5. Conclusion

The performed researches proved that at the present time in the modern market there is a wide spectrum of software and hardware tools for AMS design. Modern AMSs have different hardware and software specification, which is reflected on their cost. But even the universal AMS can not completely satisfy the demands of clinical practice and, moreover, scientific researches. Therefore, researches in the area of AMS design are important, especially those that are oriented on the specialized use. This article is devoted to this significant problem.

In this work the following results are achieved:

- Review and classification of AMS are provided: hardware and software. AND-OR tree for the generation of set of alternatives of structure and rules of products are developed. AND-OR tree allows to decrease power of set of alternative decisions restricted by requirement specification;
- The example of development of the software system, which is intended for acquisition, processing, analysis and storage of biomedical images, is shown;
- The use of modular design and object-oriented technique of programming resulted in easy modification and flexibility of the software system adjustment.

6. Acknowledgment

This work was supported by project IOSU-10-2008-"B" "Information-analytical system for research and diagnosis of tumour (cancer) cells based on their images analysis".

7. Reference

Al-Jarrahb, M.A.; Al-Omarib, F.A.; Matalkaa, I.; Kanaan F.M. & Obeidatc, F.N. (2008) Image-based discriminating morphological features for gastric atrophy assessment: A step to go further. *Pathology – Research and Practice*, Vol. 204, pp. 235–240, ISSN 0344-0338

Avtandilov G.G. (1990) Medicine morphometry. Handbook. (1990), Meditsina, Moscow

Batko, Yu. & Berezsky, O (2009), Object contour tracing algorithm with backward movement, *Artificial intelligence*, Vol.3, 2009, pp.516-523, ISSN 1561-5359

a. Berezsky O.M.; Melnyk G.M. & Batko Yu.M (2008) Biomedical Image Search and Retrieval Algorithms, *Computing*, Vol. 7, pp.108–114., ISSN 1727-6209

b. Berezsky, O.M.; Batko, Yu.M. & Melnyk, G.M. (2008) Information-analytical system for research and diagnosis of tumour cells based on their images analysis. *Herald of the Khmelnitsky National University*, Vol.1, No. 3, pp. 120–130

a. Berezsky O.M.; Batko, Yu.M.; Berezska K.M. & Melnyk G.M. (2009) Design of computer systems for biomedical image analysis *Proceedings of the X-th International Conference "The Experience of Designing and Application of CAD Systems in Microelectronics"*, pp.186–192, Lviv-Polyana, 24-28 February 2009, Lviv-Polyana

b. Berezsky O.M.; Batko Yu.M.; Berezska, K.M. & Melnyk G.M. (2009) Alternative decision synthesis under structural design of automated microscopy systems. *Herald of National University "Lvivska politechnika". Computer science and information technologies*, No. 638, pp. 64–72.

c. Berezsky O.M.; Batko, Yu.M. & Melnyk G.M. (2009) Computer system of biomedical system analysis. *Herald of National University "Lvivska politechnika". Computer science and information technologies*, No. 650, pp. 11–18.

d. Berezsky, O.M.; Batko, Yu.M.; Datsko, T.V.; Melnyk, G.M.; Bodnar, J.J.; Datsko I.A. & Voloshyn V.D. (2009) Morphometrical analysis of duct epithelium of mammary gland under unproliferative mastopathy with cytological analysis. *Proceedings of international conferense "Morphological condition of tissue and organs of organism systems under norm and pathology"*, pp.47-48, June 2009 p., Ternopil.

e. Berezsky, O.M.; Berezska, K.M. & Melnyk G.M. (2009) Algorithms of statistical processing of biomedical images. *Proceedings of international conference "Intellectual Systems of Decision Making and The Problems of Computational Intelligence (ISDMCI'2009"*, pp. 23–29, Kherson, May 2009.

f. Berezsky, O.M. & Grytsyk, V.V. (2009) Methods and algorithms of analysis and synthesis of complex images on the basis of theoretical-group approach, *Reports of the National Academy of Sciences of Ukraine*, Vol. 11, 2009, pp. 64–79, ISSN 1025-6415

Berezsky, O.M.; Batko, Yu.M. & Melnyk, G.M. (2010), Biomedical image segmenattion method, *Herald of the Khmelnitsky National University*, Vol. 1, pp.188-196.

Duda, R. O.; Hart, P. E. & Stork, D. G. (2000), *Pattern Classification (2nd Edition)*, Wiley-Interscience, ISBN 0471056693

Egorova, O.; Klykova, E. & Panteleev, V. (2005). *Computer microscopy*, Tehnosfera, ISBN 5-94836-025-3, Moscow

Egorova, O. (2006), *Familiar on microscope. The step in XXI century. Light microscopes for biology and medicine*, "Reporttsentr M", ISBN 5-949-939-060-1, Moscow

Forsyth, D. & Ponce, J. (2004) *Computer Vision. A modern approach*, Williams, Moscow

Furman J.A.; Krevetsky, A.V; Peredreev, A.K.; Rozhentsov, A.A.; Hafizov, R.G.; Eroshina, I.L. & Leuhin A.N. (2003). *Contour analysis introduction; application in image and signal processing. 2-nd ed.*, Fizmatlit, Moscow

Gonzalez, R. & Woods, R. (2008) *Digital Image Processing (3rd Edition)*, Prentice-Hall, Inc.

Hea, L.; Peng, Z.; Everding, B.; Wang, X.; Han, C. Y.; Weiss, K. L. & Wee W. G. (2008) A comparative study of deformable contour methods on medical image segmentation. *Image and Vision Computing*, Vol. 26, pp. 141–163

Jahne B. (2005) *Digital Image Processing*, Springer, ISBN 3540627243, Berlin

Medovyi, V.S.; Parpara A.A., Pyatnitskii A.M., Sokilinskii, B.Z. & Dem'yanov V.L. (2006) An automated microscopy system MECOS-C2 and its trials, *Biomedical Engineering*, No 4, pp. 197-202, Plenum Publishing Corp.

Murphy, D. B. (2001). *Fundamentals of light microscopy and electronic imaging*, Wiley-Liss, Inc., ISBN 047125391X, Canada

Pratt W.K. (2007). *Digital Image Processing: PIKS Inside, 4-th Edition*, John Wiley and Sons, Inc., ISBN 0471767778, New York.

Rietdorf, J. (2005). *Microscopy Techniques. Advances in Biochemical Engineering/Biotechnology*, Springer, ISBN 3540236988, Berlin

Richardson J. (2005). *Videocoding. H.264 and MPEG-4 - Next Generation standards*, Tehnosfera, ISBN 5-94836-041-5, Moscow

Shapiro, L.G. and Stockman, G.C. (2001) *Computer Vision*, Prentice Hall., ISBN 013-0307963.

Wismullera A.; Vietzea, F.; Behrendsa J., Meyer-Baeseb A., Reisera M., Helge Ritter (2004). Fully automated biomedical image segmentation by self-organized model adaptation. *Neural Networks*, Vol. 17, pp. 1327–1344

Wu, Q.; Merchant, F. A. & Castleman, K. R. (2008), *Microscope Image Processing*, Elsevier, USA, ISBN 978-0-12-372578-3,Boston.

25

A New Tool for Nonstationary and Nonlinear Signals: The Hilbert-Huang Transform in Biomedical Applications

Rui Fonseca-Pinto
School of Technology and Management
Polytechnic Institute of Leiria
Portugal

1. Introduction

Time-frequency techniques constitutes a major improvement in signal analysis, namely at the field of biomedical signals in which the interdisciplinary nature of the proposed questions implies the development of new strategies to answer to specific problems. Time-frequency analysis using Wavelets, Wigner-Ville transform and more recently the Hilbert-Huang Transform (HHT) constitutes the core of these tools with applications in biomedical signals in last years.

The non-linearity and non-stationarity nature of these signals puts HHT as a powerful tool to process signals with those properties, avoiding artefacts related to the use of linear and stationary assumptions.

Classical spectral analysis using Fourier Transform still the most commonly used method when one wants to measure the global power-frequency distribution (power spectrum) of a given signal.

In all areas of knowledge, Fourier-based analysis of time-series data faces constraining limitations. In biomedical signals, the critical constraining factors are the shortness of total data span, the non-stationarity of the data and the nonlinearity of the underlying physiological process.

Methods using Short Time Fourier Transform (STFT) are able to extract the spectral information by defining short time windows and locally computing the Fourier transform, thereby coping with non-stationary phenomena. The frequency resolution is inversely proportional to the window length, and changes in time resolution (window length) compromise the frequency resolution. Even with optimized joint time-frequency localization, the trade-off between time and frequency resolution is unavoidable.

In spite of these limitations, classical Fourier spectral analysis is still widely used to process biomedical data, for lack of alternatives. The uncritical use of Fourier spectral analysis and the careless adoption of the stationary and linear assumptions may give misleading results.

Wavelet theory developed in the 90's of last century was a significant contribution to tackle the problem of non-stationarity in time-series analysis. In common with Fourier-based analysis such as STFT, wavelet analysis yields a time-frequency representation, the main difference being that the decomposition is not based on sinusoidal functions, but rather using a so-called "mother function", from which "daughter" wavelets are obtained by means of scaling procedures.

Nonetheless, wavelet theory is also limited by the fundamental uncertainty principle, according to which time and frequency cannot simultaneously be resolved with the same precision. The issue of non-linearity remains problematic. Besides, wavelet analysis entails the choice of the wavelet mother, and that choice may not be optimal for the time-series being studied.

The Hilbert-Huang Transform is a time-frequency technique whose philosophy is different from others, as the core of the technique consists in a signal decomposition *a posteriori*, enabling the extraction of the inner scales of each signal.

This chapter is meant to illustrate the potential of this technique by showing is performance in two applications in signal/image processing using medical data. The first example is about inner body regulation by autonomic nervous system. This is a classical topic in internal medicine, in which classical spectral techniques mostly had been used. For those interested in explore new techniques in these area, this chapter contains a state of the art in this subject and presents a new approach to this problem. The other application is an image feature extraction of lesion borders and artefact removal, based on 1D signal processing technique.

We start by reviewing some basic ideas of signal processing techniques, avoid as possible, strong mathematical notation.

2. Classical spectral analysis and new time-frequency methods

Spectral analysis using Fourier Transform (FT) is the most commonly used method when one wants to measure the global power-frequency distribution (power spectrum) of a given signal, forming a bridge between two spaces (time and frequency). This relationship is regulated by the Fourier Transform (FT) of a signal s defined by

$$S(f) = F\{s(t)\} = \int_{-\infty}^{+\infty} s(t)e^{-i\omega t}dt, \text{ where } \quad \omega = 2\pi f \tag{1}$$

and by Inverse Fourier Transform (IFT)

$$s(t) = F^{-1}\{S(f)\} = \int_{-\infty}^{+\infty} S(f)e^{-i\omega t}df \tag{2}$$

Equation (2) states that signal s can be expressed as the sum of complex exponentials of different frequencies, whose amplitudes are the complex quantities $S(f)$ defined by (1). In practice the frequency content is usually represented as the magnitude squared of (1); $|S(f)|^2$.

In all areas of knowledge, Fourier-based analysis of time-series data faces constraining limitations. In biomedical signals, the critical constraining factors are the shortness of total data span, the non-stationarity of the data and the nonlinearity of the underlying physiological process.

Methods using Short Time Fourier Transform (STFT) are able to extract the spectral information by defining short time windows and locally computing the Fourier transform, thereby coping with non-stationary phenomena.

The frequency resolution is inversely proportional to the window length, and changes in time resolution (window length) compromise the frequency resolution. Even with optimized joint time-frequency localization, the trade-off between time and frequency resolution is unavoidable (Gabor D, 1993).

In spite of these limitations, classical Fourier spectral analysis is still widely used to process biomedical data, for lack of alternatives. The uncritical use of Fourier spectral analysis and the careless adoption of the stationary and linear assumptions may give misleading results (Huang N et al., 1998).

Wavelet theory developed in the 90's of last century (Daubechies I, 1988; Daubechies I, 1992; Meyer Y, 1993) was a significant contribution to tackle the problem of non-stationarity in time-series analysis. In common with Fourier-based analysis such as STFT, wavelet analysis yields a time-frequency representation, the main difference being that the decomposition is not based on sinusoidal functions, but rather using a so-called "mother function", from which "daughter" wavelets are obtained by means of scaling procedures.

Nonetheless, wavelet theory is also limited by the fundamental uncertainty principle, according to which time and frequency cannot simultaneously be resolved with the same precision. The issue of non-linearity remains problematic. Besides, wavelet analysis entails the choice of the wavelet mother, and that choice may not be optimal for the time-series being studied.

Recently Huang and its co-workers developed a method in which the issue of non-linearity is treated, by using a procedure to decompose the signal according to its own scale properties. This method enables to obtain for each signal a set of orthogonal functions, i.e. a set of a basis functions. It is a data driven and *a posteriori* method, contrasting with other class of decompositions, whose basis functions are established *a priori* (trigonometric functions, and wavelets) and in the former case with constant amplitude and frequency (sinusoidal functions). This method proposed by Huang in 1998 (Huang N.E et al 1998) is known by Hilbert-Huang Transform (HHT) comprise two parts, the EMD - Empirical Mode Decomposition, and the Hilbert Spectral Analysis (HSA).

2.1 Short Time Fourier Transform – STFT

The strength of classical Fourier analysis is that it allows the decomposition of a signal into its individual frequency components and establishes the relative intensity of each frequency component. Due to the infinite durations of these basis functions, any time-local information is spread over the whole frequency spectrum.

To overcome the time localization issue, Gabor introduced a sliding window to well localize variations in time domain. This procedure is known by Short Time Fourier Transform - STFT. When the applied window follows a Gaussian shape, this STFT is also called Gabor Transform.

Similar to the FFT case, the magnitude squared of STFT is used in practice (the spectrogram), giving now information as a function of time and frequency, and is define by

$$S(t,f)=\left|\int_{-\infty}^{+\infty} s(\tau)h(t-\tau)e^{-i\omega\tau}d\tau\right|^2 \tag{3}$$

The major advantage of STFT is that if a signal has most of its energy in the interval $[-T,T]$ and in the frequency range $[-\omega,\omega]$, then its STFT will be localized in the region

$[-T,T]\times[-\omega,\omega]$ in the time-frequency plane. The uncertainty principle prevents de possibility of having arbitrary high resolution in both time and frequency domains, since it lowers-bounds the time bandwidth product of any basis function by $\Delta T \Delta\omega \geq 1/4\pi$, where $(\Delta T)^2$ and $(\Delta\omega)^2$ are the variances of time function and its Fourier Transform respectively.

2.2 Wavelet Transform – WT

Wavelet Transform (WT) mitigates the limitations of FT and STFT by having a basis function which can be both shifted and dilated or contracted. By decomposing the time-scale plane, WT enhances time and frequency domains representation of signals, as is the first proposed method comprises an adaptative nature.

WT[1] of a signal s is expressed as

$$C(a,b) = \int s(t)\overline{\varphi}_{a,b}(t)dt \tag{4}$$

Where $\overline{\varphi}_{a,b}(t)$ is defined as,

$$\overline{\varphi}_{a,b}(t) = \frac{1}{\sqrt{a}}\overline{\varphi}\left(\frac{t-b}{a}\right) \tag{5}$$

In (4) $C(a,b)$ are the wavelet coefficients. $\overline{\varphi}(.)$ is known as the mother wavelet, and $\overline{\varphi}_{a,b}(.)$ is its stretched and translated version with a and b as its scale and translation parameters.

For a detailed explanation about WT is possible to find several references, in particular Daubechies, 1992 and Addison P, 2002, among other good books.

2.3. Hilbert-Huang Transform - HHT

The Hilbert-Huang transform is a time-frequency technique consisting of two parts. In the first part, EMD the signal is decomposed into Implicit Mode Functions -IMF's, putting forward the scale characteristics imbedded in the signal. In the second part, the Hilbert transform is applied to the IMF's, yielding a time-frequency representation (Hilbert spectrum) for each IMF.

HHT has been applied to different fields of science since is first application to fluid dynamics in water waves and ocean engineering (Ding et al., 2007; Rao & Hsu, 2008), financial applications (Huang N et al., 2003), system identification (Xun & Yan, 2008; Quek T et al, 2003) medical signals (Tang J. et al., 2007; Salisbury & Sun, 2007; Caseiro P. et al., 2010). By it's owns characteristics biomedical signals are indicated to HHT analysis.

An IMF is a function that satisfies two conditions:

1. in the whole data set, the number of extrema and the number of zero crossings must either be equal or differ at most by one;
2. at any point, the mean value of the envelope defined by the local maxima and the envelope defined by the local minima is zero.

Unfortunately, most time-series do not meet these criteria. At any given time, the data may involve more than one oscillatory mode. This is the reason why the simple Hilbert Transform cannot provide the full description of the frequency content in general data

---

1 In fact, CWT for, Continuous Wavelet Transform.

(Cohen L, 1995). Thus, it is necessary to extract the oscillatory modes (IMF's) from the data, by means of the EMD procedure, which is implemented by an algorithm comprising the following steps:

1. Identify all extrema of $x(t)$;
2. Interpolate between minima to obtain the lower envelope $x_L(t)$, and between maxima to obtain the upper envelope $x_U(t)$;
3. Calculate the average envelope $e(t) = \dfrac{x_L(t) + x_U(t)}{2}$;
4. Extract the intrinsic oscillatory mode $d(t) = x(t) - e(t)$;
5. Iterate on the residual $e(t)$.

In practice, the above procedure has to be refined by first iterating steps 1 to 4 upon the detail signal $d(t)$, until the latter can be considered as a zero-mean signal according to some stopping criterion (Huang et al, 1998). In Figure 1 at left, is possible to verify that after first iteration of this shifting procedure, the signal do not achieve the two conditions for IMF. After a set of iterations (varying within different signals) the zero mean is reached and the first mode of oscillation is them achieved, as is possible, as is possible to observe in Figure 1 at right.

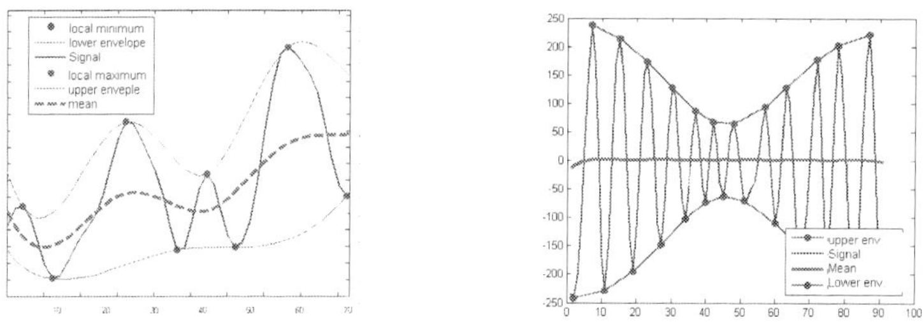

Fig. 1. Left - first iteration of shifting. Right - first IMF after several iterations

Interpolation in step 2 is made using cubic splines; however other interpolation techniques may be applied (Long SR et al, 1995). The aim of this repeated operation is to eliminate the riding waves and to achieve more symmetrical wave-profile by smoothing the uneven amplitudes. Once this is achieved, the detail is considered as the effective IMF, the corresponding residual is computed and step 5 follows. An example of a EMD decomposition is presented in Figure 2, were the signal is in the first row, giving in this case 5 oscillatory intrinsic modes (or scales) of oscillation.

Having obtained the IMF's components, it is possible to apply the Hilbert Transform (HT) to each component, to get instantaneous frequency.

The HT of a real signal $x(t)$ is defined as

$$H[x(t)] = x * \frac{1}{\pi t} = y, \tag{6}$$

or using the convolution definition,

$$y(t) = \frac{1}{\pi} P \int_{-\infty}^{\infty} \frac{x(\tau)}{t - \tau} d\tau \tag{7}$$

where P indicates the Cauchy principal value. From $y(t)$ it is possible to define the analytical signal $z(t) = x(t) + iy(t)$ or, in polar form, $z(t) = a(t)e^{i\theta(t)}$, in which

$$a(t) = \sqrt{x^2(t) + y^2(t)}\,, \quad \theta(t) = \arctan\left(\frac{y(t)}{x(t)}\right). \tag{8}$$

Instantaneous frequency is defined using the instantaneous variation of phase,

$$\omega = \frac{d\theta(t)}{dt} \tag{9}$$

This is the second part of the HHT (Hilbert spectral analysis, HSA), and it entails writing the signal in the form

$$x(t) = \sum_{j=1}^{n} a_j(t) e^{i\int \omega_j(t)dt}. \tag{10}$$

We can thus obtain the amplitude and the instantaneous frequency as a function of time $H(\omega,t)$. This time-frequency representation is called the Hilbert Spectrum (HS). This spectral representation offers a totally different interpretation when compared to the classical Fourier representation. In Fourier terms, the existence of energy at some frequency implies the existence of a component of a sine or a cosine wave throughout the whole time-series or a significant part of it. A time-frequency technique allows for the extraction of the frequency content at each time point. The HS of the signal whose decomposition is in Figure (2) is presented in Figure (3)

To obtain a measure of the total amplitude (or energy) contribution from each frequency value, we can compute the Marginal spectrum defined by

$$h(\omega) = \int_0^T H(\omega,t)dt. \tag{11}$$

Similarly it is possible to achieve a measure of the energy of the signal with respect to time, if we compute the Instantaneous Energy Density Level, IE defined by

$$IE(t) = \int_\omega H(\omega,t)^2 d\omega. \tag{12}$$

As already reported elsewhere in the text, the uncritical use of Fourier derived techniques may lead to the extraction of ambiguous information from the data, and in other cases, may lead to failure to extract properties and characteristics of the signal. The use of HHT allows for a decomposition of the signal that resorts to an adaptative set of basis functions. It is therefore possible to use HHT without a predefined choice of parameters.

3. Time-frequency analysis in biomedical signals: applications

In this chapter two examples of HHT applications are shown. The first in the field of Sympathovagal balance (SVB) and the other uses digital images of the surface of the skin (dermoscopic images).

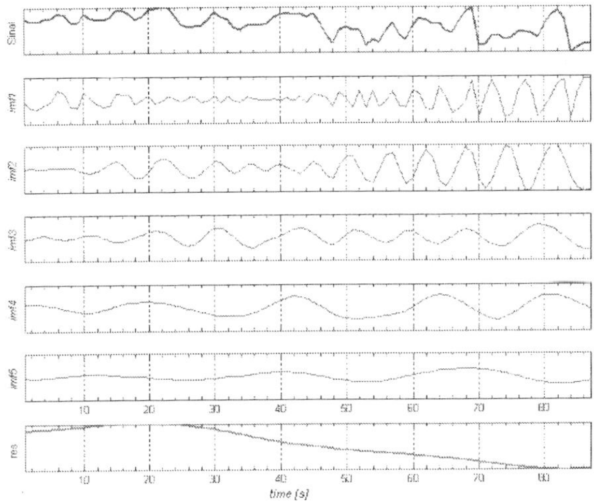

Fig. 2. Signal (first row) and EMD decomposition plus trend or residue (in last row)

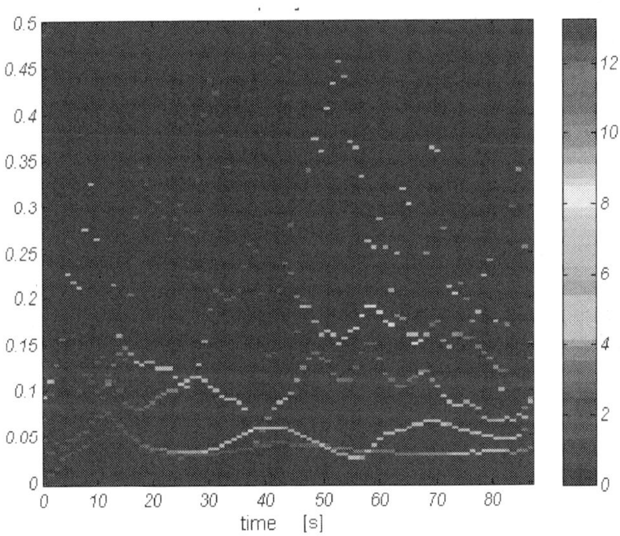

Fig. 3. Hilbert Spectrum of the signal whose decomposition is in Figure 2

3.1 Sympathovagal Balance – SVB

The Nervous System (NS) is one of the human body systems enrolling more complexity, whose interactions among others systems are yet partially unknown. Discovering how it behaves, and is complex relationships within the whole body, is still a major challenge for those who are interested in understanding how the human body really works.

The Autonomic Nervous System (ANS) is a breach of the Peripheral Nervous System (PNS). The ANS is a neural network suitable to regulate cardiovascular function and work at a subconscious level by regulating visceral functions. The main function of the ANS is control cardiac output and blood supply at central and peripheral levels. Cardiac output is controlled by ANS and is modulated by its main components: Sympathetic Nervous System (SNS) and Vagal System[2] (VS).

The variation in Heart Rate (HR) is defined as the variability of the time-series of heart beats, and is called Heart Rate Variability (HRV). Epidemiological Studies showed that a decrease in HRV is one of the best predictors of arrhythmic events and sudden death after myocardial infraction.

One way to study cardiovascular neuronal regulation is to perform a spectral analysis of heart rate variability and blood pressure signals. Usually, spectral procedures are designed to separate the full spectrum of the signal into two main frequency bands associated with vagal and sympathetic subdivisions of the autonomous nervous system.

Regulation of blood pressure is a continuous phenomenon. Short term adaptation is mainly dependent on sympathetic outflow to arterial muscle, and largely controlled by baroreflexes. Changing from supine to upright position leads to gravitational dependent pooling of blood in dependent parts, namely legs, distal portion of arms and venous abdominal plexes, thereby reducing ventricular feeling, cardiac output and blood pressure. Blood pressure lowering is sensed by baroreceptors in carotid bodies, giving rise to a reflex mediated by sympathetic activation, which determines arterial vasoconstriction and cardiac acceleration (Joyner M & Shepherd J, 1997; Shepherd R & Shepherd J, 1988).

Provocative manoeuvres can be used to evaluate autonomic vagal and/or sympathetic outflows indirectly. With these approaches, autonomic behaviour is inferred from measurements of cardiovascular variables. The analysis of heart rate and blood pressure variability applying Fast Fourier Transform (FFT) and autoregressive (AR) spectral analysis to these signals has made a very important contribution to autonomic evaluation (Ducla-Soares JL et al, 2007).

Heart rate varies during inspiration and expiration[3]. The most evident fluctuations of HR are related to respiration and manifest as increased HR during inspiration and decreases HR during expiration (Hales, 1735). It has been clearly shown that a linear relationship exists between heart frequency and vagal activity. The influence of the ANS has been recognized in HR short-term variability and is mediated by vagal system. Experimental data has clearly shown that vagal activation slows heart rate and inversely, vagal block determines heart rate increases (Freeman R, 1997).

The direct quantification of vagal activity in humans is difficult as recording directly from the nerve is highly invasive. The degree of RSA provides a quantitative measure of the vagal outflow to the myocardium, since RSA is generated by cardiac vagal nerve traffic. Spectral analysis techniques have been applied to HRV in order to estimate the frequency component centred about the respiratory frequency, termed high frequency band (HF) of the spectrum (0.15 Hz - 0.4Hz). In studies whose experimental conditions may vary the respiratory frequency, the value of this central frequency constitutes crucial information. For

---

[2] Also known by Parasympathetic Nervous System (PaNS).

[3] The influence of respiration in HR has been known for more than one century and is called Respiratory Sinus Arrhythmia (RSA).

instance, breathing at slow frequency, as is the case during deep breathing manoeuvre[4] at 6 cycles per minute, heart frequency oscillations fall in the low frequency (LF) part of the power spectrum. In HRV data is also possible to find a lower frequency component centred around 0.1 Hz, related to the Meyer Waves[5] and baroreceptors.

Spectral analysis of HRV data also shows a Low Frequency band (0.04 Hz-0.15Hz), which physiological significance is more difficult to establish, as the pharmacological blockage in vagal activity also produce reduction in LF power. Some researchers have being settled that LF variability may have a vagal and sympathetical component and therefore they state that LF is not a pure measure of sympathetic activity (Akselrod et al, 1985; Malliani et al, 1991; Eckberg, 1997). Other studies indicate that LF[6] represents the primary sympathetic modulation of heart rate. The ratio LF/HF is defined as the Sympathovagal balance (SVB) (Pagani et al, 1986; Malliani et al, 1991).

Behind the two above mentioned LF and HF frequency bands, RR interval power spectrum can present also two more bands, the Very Low frequency band (VLF) and the ultra low frequency band (ULF) whose spectral densities can be reliably analysed from long-term recordings (more then 18 hours).

3.1.1 Review of classical spectral methods to obtain SVB: a physiological and technical challenge

HRV time-series (RR intervals) is obtained form ECG data using algorithms designed to detect the QRS complexes, and time between R waves. Before trying to detect the R waves, the ECG signals are detrended using a locally weighted robust regression algorithm. Usually a vertical and horizontal threshold are established (the former to define a level that R wave must exceed, and the later to prevent detecting an R wave for a period of time after one was detected).

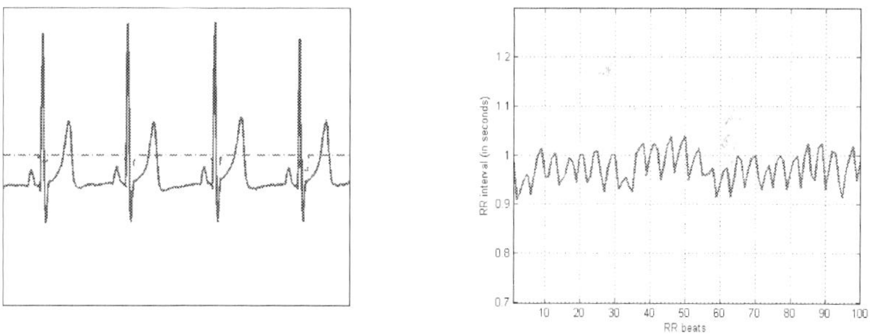

Fig. 4. Left - ECG and QRS detection. Difference in time between R waves plotted as a function of the RR beats is the tachogram, presented at right

---

[4] This is a autonomic test in which the subject is instructed to breath deeply at a rate of 6 breaths per minute, paced by a metronome (deep metronomic breathing). This and head-up-tilt test are the most commonly used strategies to standardize respiratory changes and their relation to heart rate, hence to vagal activity.

[5] Slow waves at one cycle in 10 seconds associated with sympathetic activation.

[6] In particular the ratio LF/(LF+HF), which is the normalized LF power.

After R waves identification, the HRV is calculated as the difference in time between RR waves (see Figure 4 at right). This information in time units, plotted as a function of the RR beats is known in the literature by tachogram.

The simplest form to extract information from a time-series is the inspection in time domain. By using time domain methods, is possible to calculate HR in any point, or intervals between successive normal ECG complexes, as well other statistic measures (NN intervals[7], RMSSD[8]) obtained from direct measures of HR or by differences between NN intervals. In time domain is possible to use also geometric models. More details about time-domain methods can be fund in (Malik, 1996).

RR signal represents de heart period at discrete points, but this representation is no suitable for FFT analysis as these points are not equally spaced. In order to produce RR data suitable for classical spectral analysis, the RR signal must be interpolated and re-sampled at higher uniform rate, usually at 2 or 4 Hz (Carvalho J et al., 2003).

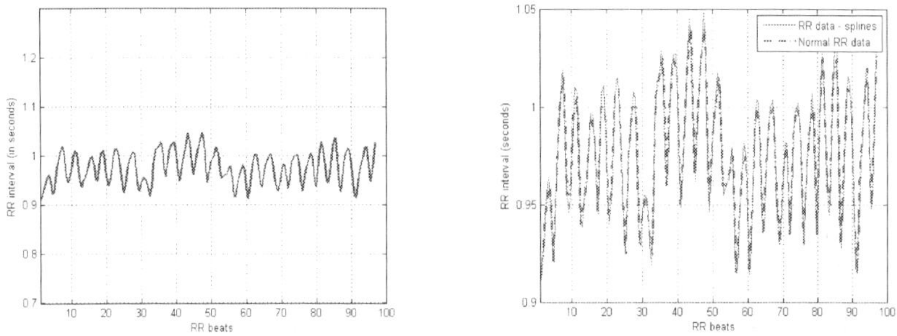

Fig. 5. Left - RR time-series after interpolation by cubic splines. In the right both signals are presented (before and after interpolation)

Parametric autoregressive modelling (AR[9], ARMA[10]) and nonparametric Fourier Transform methods (e.g. DFT[11]) provide classical frequency-domain methods to analyse HRV from RR interpolated signal.

Parametric methods by AR models uses linear prediction defined as

$$\hat{s}(k) = \sum_{i=0}^{p} b_i w(k-i) - \sum_{i=1}^{p} a_i s(k-i) \tag{13}$$

where s is the signal, a and b are prediction parameters and $w(k)$ white noise.

Non parametric spectral methods using DFT are usually implemented by an algorithm for fast computation of the DFT, which uses a recursive algorithm known by Fast Fourier Transform - FFT. The spectrum visualization in AR models is usually smoother then Fourier based ones (see Figure 6). In order to approximate results obtained form AR models from those obtained by FFT, the order of the AR model must increase. To get a good spectral

[7] Intervals between adjacent QRS complexes.

[8] Squared root of the mean squared differences of successive NN intervals.

[9] Autoregressive Model.

[10] Autoregressive Moving Average.

[11] Discrete Fourier Transform

estimation we must use order 12 in AR model for a sampling rate of 2Hz, and order 15 for a sampling rate of 4Hz (Carvalho J et al, 2003).

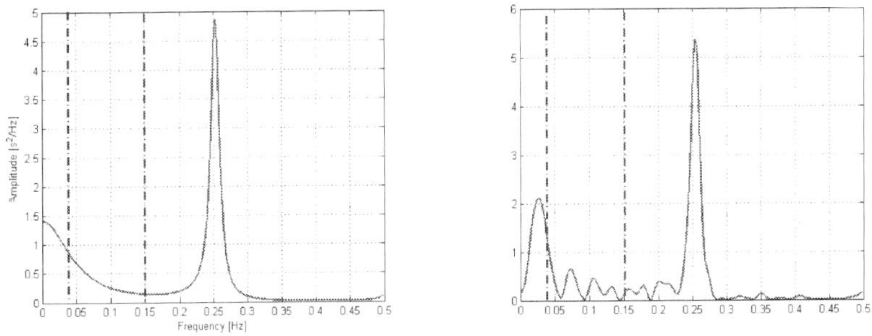

Fig. 6. Spectral analysis of RR signal in figure 2. Left: using AR model order 12. At right is present the spectrum of the same signal using FFT with an Hamming window

Using the HRV data from Figure 5 and spectral analysis in Figure 6, is possible to see a bigger energy input from high frequency band (0.15 Hz - 0.4 Hz), whose main frequency is 0.25Hz showing the RSA enrolment in HF band, representing the contribution of the Vagal System during this period of 100 heart beats.

The classical spectral analysis presented above, were designed for whole signal, abolishing time information. Form Figure 6 we just know that a wave of frequency around 0.25 Hz persist in all signal, lacking the time information. This required information of frequency in time is not possible using the classical frequency definition. Instead, an instantaneous frequency definition is required, being this one of the main characteristics of time-frequency analysis.

Behind the non-consensual physiological interpretation of LF frequency band, classical methods possesses these constrains related with lack of time guidance.

3.1.2 Access to SVB by HHT

The access to Sympathovagal Balance is an interdisciplinary problem, and in last years had been treated within research groups with Mathematicians, Engineers, Doctors and Medical Staff, see as an example the Guidelines of Task Force of The European Society of Cardiology and The North American Society of Pacing and Electrophysiology. Nevertheless the interdisciplinary nature of the panel, those guidelines was stated in 1996, lacking time-frequency techniques.

Today powerful techniques of time-frequency analysis were used by engineers to process data from all knowledge areas, as is the case of medical signal processing. Instantaneous frequency is defined mainly using the Hilbert Transformation (HT), and time-frequency techniques from different classes (atomics and energy) are today completely established. From STFT, WT and Wigner- Ville Transform (WVT) is possible to use numerous variants. HHT - Hilbert-Huang transform presents good skills to process these kind of data, diverging from the previous time-frequency techniques by lacking for an yet complete analytical formulation. This was the case regarding WT in the 80's of the last century, when a French mathematician *Ingid Daubechies* completed the Wavelet theory.

Using those recent time-frequency representations, new approaches had been proposed to process RR data in spectral domain, by using points sampled synchronously with each heartbeat. By this way, frequencies are expressed in 1/heartbeat units. Working with frequencies (in Hz) is possible, but it would require re-sampling and interpolation procedures that may be problematic in high variability signals such as these (Fonseca-Pinto et al, 2010).

As we presented before, the algorithm enrolled the first part of the HHT (Empirical Mode Decomposition) behaves like a filter bank (Flandrin P, 2004), and this allows the separation of the spectrum in two main frequency bands (high frequency band, HF, and low frequency band, LF) without a predefined cut-off frequency. In order to study the modulation of the sympathetic nervous system activity, signals of Diastolic Blood Pressure (DBP) and Heart Rate Variability (HRV) were obtained following a protocol to extract values of DBP and HRV at each heartbeat (RR interval). These signals were obtained during the head-up tilt test and deep breathing manoeuvre, following the same procedures as in (Ducla-Soares J L et al 2007). In the former test, distinct postural positions are studied, including a 60-degree tilt of the bed where the subject is resting. In the latter test, the subject is instructed to breath deeply at a rate of 6 breaths per minute, paced by a metronome (deep metronomic breathing). This is one of the most commonly used strategies to standardize respiratory changes and their relation to heart rate, hence to vagal activity.

In the method presented next, DBP signals were used to access the Sympathetic modulation of SVB, and the HR signal is used to follow vagal output. By this formulation the SVB is constructed based in two signals (main indirect measures to access SVB), allowing a more realistic picture of the complex interactions performed to obtain homeostasis. DBP also reflects the vasoconstriction and is more sensitive to pressure changes.

Methods

The first step to achieve the separation in two frequency bands is to normalize[12] the HRV and DBP signals and to submit them to the EMD procedure. As stated before, in the present study we presented a new formulation by assigning the highest frequency modulation to the IMF1 of the heart rate signal, and the lowest frequency modulation to the sum of IMF2 and IMF3 obtained from the diastolic blood pressure signal as

$$x_{HF} = IMF_1(HR) \ , \ \ x_{LF} = IMF_2(DBP) + IMF_3(DBP). \tag{14}$$

As the number of IMF's is not a constant within different signals, in those cases with only two IMF's, the lower frequency content is obtained just considering the IMF2 from DBP.

This reconstruction in modes leads to a spectrum separation in two frequency bands. By this way it is possible to reproduce the two main frequency bands (LF and HF) related respectively with sympathetical system and vagal system used in studies with FFT and Wavelets (Parati G et al., 1995; Ducla-Soares J L et al., 2007). In the case of deep breathing, the highest frequency content is obtained from the IMF2 of the heart rate, considering the shift in heart rate towards the LF band, already mentioned and reported in (Sleight & Casadei, 1995).

The next step is the computation of the Hilbert spectrum associated with the high frequencies $H_{HF}(\omega,t)$, and the low frequencies $H_{LF}(\omega,t)$. For each case, a two-dimensional representation of the energy fluctuation with time is obtained (see equation (15)):

[12] Signals are divided by the maximum value of each one.

$$PS_{HF} = \int_{\omega} H_{HF}(\omega,t)^2 d\omega \,; \qquad PS_{LF} = \int_{\omega} H_{LF}(\omega,t)^2 d\omega \qquad (15)$$

By considering a time range that is adequate from the point of view of the experiment (e.g. 5 heartbeats before and after the tilt), it is possible to calculate the energy contribution in function of time, related to the LF band and to the HF band, by computing IHF, ILF and Index defined by

$$IHF = \int_0^T PS_{HF}dt; \quad ILF = \int_0^T PS_{LF}dt; \quad Index = \frac{ILF}{IHF}. \qquad (16)$$

Studies to evaluate the Sympathovagal balance involve postural manoeuvres, and it is critical to pinpoint fluctuations that happen synchronously with postural changes, or shortly before or after them. If the above time range is small when compared with the duration of the test, a better sensitivity to energy variations can be achieved.

Related to the issue of critical data length, simulation studies were carried out in order to understand the influence of the signal length in the number of IMF's produced by EMD. These recent studies were made using was made using fGn (fractional Gaussian noise) signals, and allowed to define a measure to establish the minimum data length needed to obtain a predetermined number of IMF's. In this proposed methodology, it is crucial that the number of IMF's are at least three (or two in some cases) in order to obtain the meaningful separation of frequency content, as explained above. According to previous simulation studies (Fonseca-Pinto R et al, 2009), to obtain 2 or 3 IMF's, the average number of signal samples required is 36 (RR beats).

The Hilbert-Huang Spectrum was obtained following Matlab™ routines adapted from (Rilling G, 2003). These routines contain functions of the TFTB (time-frequency) toolbox (Auger F, 2009).

Results

As a first example of the access to SVB using this HHT formulation we present in Figure 7 the HR and DBP signals from a period of 42 heart beats. In this registration is possible to observe a slow variation in DBP at the beginning (between 10th and 20th heart beat), and a more effective variation in HR increasing is variation mainly at the end of the record. In the same figure at right, we can track in time the energy fluctuation of the two frequency bands. Figure 8 at right show a prominent contribution of vagal system mainly after the 33rd heart beat period were HR decreases. In the period between 10th and 20th heart beat, HR increases and is possible to observe a decrease in vagal output and an bigger sympathetic input by improve PS_{DBP}.

In fact, this time-frequency derived technique by HHT, when compared with the classical representation presents greater advantages. To compare both spectra we present the classical spectral representation in Figure 6.

In fact, using Figure 8, all above local interpretations were impossible. We just are able to say that HF spectrum and LF spectrum present similar contribution, as the area above the curve for the two main frequencies roughly is similar. In fact the LF/HF ratio is in this case bigger than one. It is also important here to register that in the HHT based method the LF spectrum is obtained for a different signal (DBP) and by this way is impossible fully compare both spectra.

Another example is showed in Figure 9. In this sketch is possible to observe at right both signals of HR and DBP during 50 heart beats.

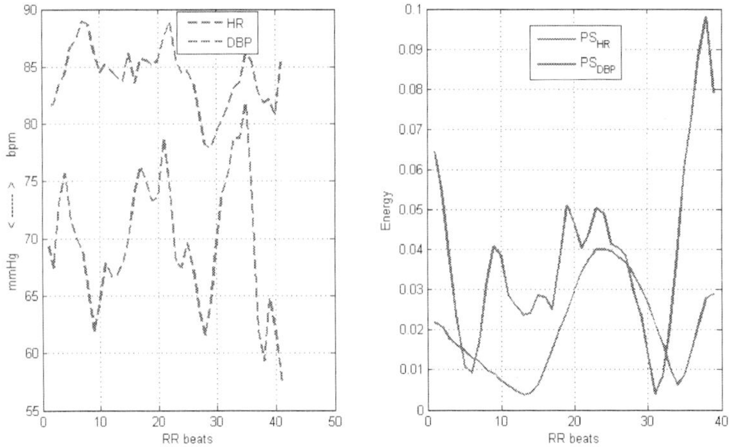

Fig. 7. SVB by HHT- left: HR and DBP signals -Right: Instantaneous Energy fluctuation of Vagal and Sympathetic systems

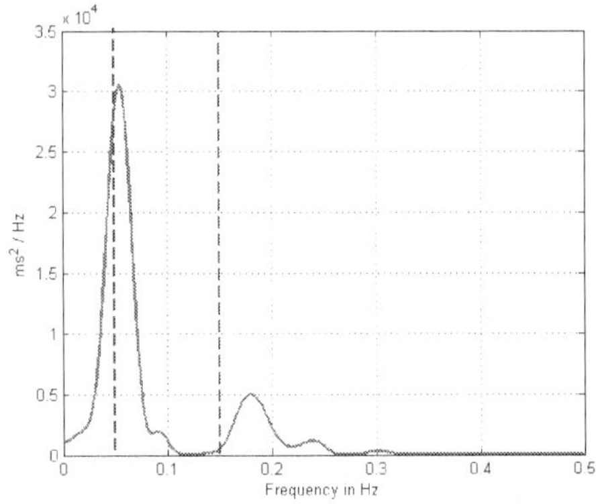

Fig. 8. Classical Spectrum of HR signal in figure 5. Vertical dashed lines mark LF (0.04Hz-0.15Hz) range

During the firsts 20th heart beats we assist at an increase in HR and a decrease in DBP. In fact, during almost all record, DBP possesses a descendent behaviour. This initial deed of HR is elucidated in the figure at right by an SVB (LF/HF) bigger than unity. Actually in this period the vagal system varies slowly. At the end (between 40th and 50th heart beat) DBP increases and HR decrease and once more SVB is bigger than one. In fact we assist variability in DBP conducted by an Sympathetical inflow. This is enhanced by the fact that HR continues is descending path, hence vagal system contribution in insufficient to balance LF component.

As we do previously the classical spectrum is also presented in Figure 11. In this case we also use other time-frequency method to be able to compare two time-frequency methods.

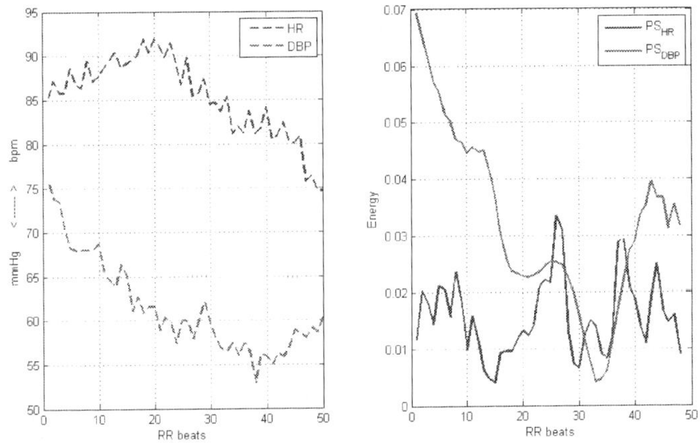

Fig. 9. SVB by HHT- left: HR and DBP signals -Right: Instantaneous Energy fluctuation of Vagal and Sympathetic systems

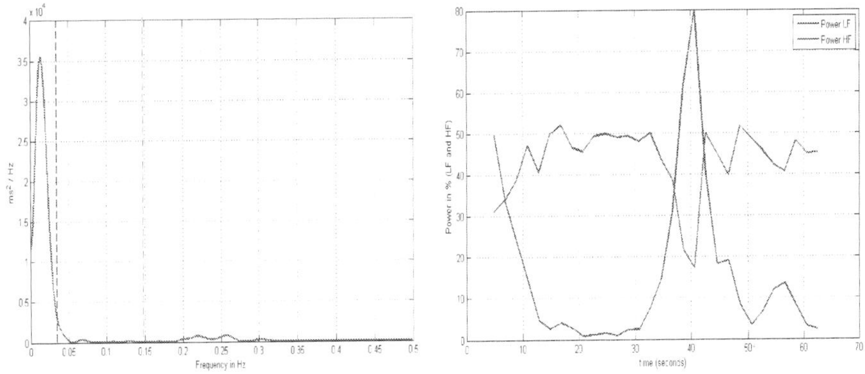

Fig. 10. Left - Classical Spectrum of HR signal in Figure 7. Right - Power spectrum in % of HF an LF bands by STFT

The low energy values in Figure 9 are also presented in the classical spectrum in Figure 10 at left, and once more only global interpretations are allowed. At right in Figure 10 we present the STFT power of the LF and HF bands in percentage. This plot when compared to the HHT energy variation presents a global similar shape, but by construction (STFT uses a sliding window) only reflects variation between adjacent windows, being this the reason for few irregularities.

The last example of this chapter is obtained using the *101511*[13] criterion as presented in (Fonseca-Pinto et al, 2009; Fonseca-Pinto et al., 2010b)) for the Head-Up-Tilt test. HR and DBP signals plotted are in Figure 11.

---

[13] This was established for HUT test wit HHT and used 10 heart beats before the tilt manoeuvre and 26 after (in mean 15 during tilt and the rest after).

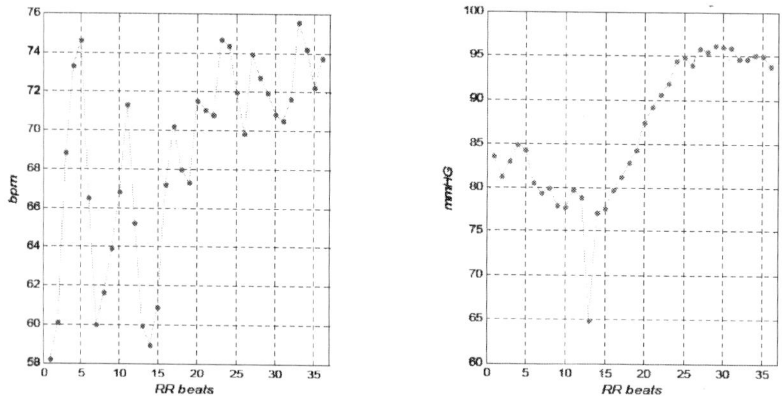

Fig. 11. HR and DBP during 36 heart beats including HUT test

In Figure 12 is possible to observe the instantaneous energy variation obtained by HHT. The increase in DBP after 15th heart beat is conditioned by and sympathetic inflow, and the big variability in HR until 15th heart beat, is captured by the Instantaneous energy representation in Figure 13. In all this period, in which we assist to a contention in HRV (by increasing vagal flow) and then in a preeminent DBP increase (by increase the sympathetic contribution) SVB can be calculated at each heart beat. In fact, this is one of the main differences in using or not interpolation, and by this way, losing time information.

When we assist to a postural change, blood goes to inferior members and to distal parts of superior members. As a result compensatory mechanisms act by increasing sympathetical activity, whose action can be immediate (at the order of seconds) or during hours. When this compensatory mechanisms acts immediately, such regulation must by inferred in beat-to-beat fluctuation, being this the natural scale for getting autonomic regulatory information.

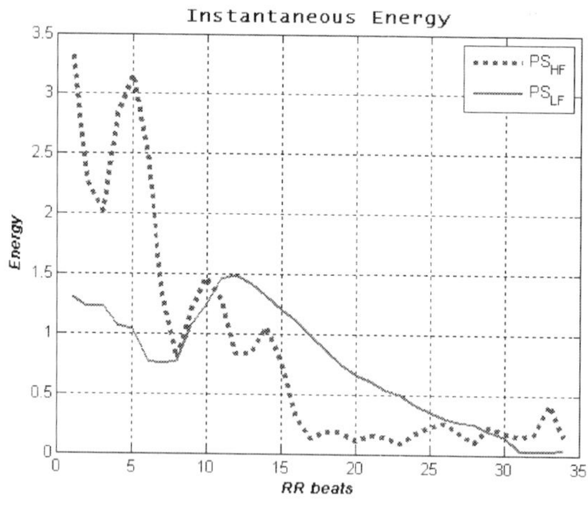

Fig. 12. Instantaneous Energy fluctuation of HF and LF spectrum by HHT

3.2 Lesion border detection and artefact removal in dermoscopic images

Skin cancer is one of the cancer types with most rapidly increasing prevalence and is also one of the most common form of malignancy in humans (Celebi et al., 2007). It is expected that its impact in public health will increase significantly in the coming decades in the absence of effective intervention today (Boyle et al., 2007).

Early detection of skin lesions is critical to prevent this kind of malignancies. Dermatologists use epiluminescence microscopy, or dermatoscopy as is usually called, to perform early diagnosis of melanocytic lesions and to track the progression thereof.

Dermatoscopy uses a polarized light source and a magnifying lens. A fluid is usually spread on the skin surface to minimize light scattering, and thus increase the performance of this technique. The use of this fluid and the presence of hairs, give rise to conspicuous artefacts in dermatoscopic images.

The classification of some melanocytic lesions is sometimes difficult, even for experienced specialists. The lesion border is especially relevant for diagnosis since it allows to gather information about the shape of the lesion, growth path, and growth rate.

The early detention of lesions is crucial to prevent malignancies. Early detection requires periodic monitoring of suspected lesions. Currently dermatologists often resort to digital dermoscopes and computer storage of the information. Computers can also be used to perform automatic lesion border detection. The presence of artefacts may induce artificial borders, thereby jeopardizing the efficiency of automatic detection algorithms (Fonseca-Pinto et al., 2010a)). Artefact removal is a required pre-processing step to improve the quality of detection.

3.2.1 IEMD and image processing

EMD was developed for one-dimensional signals but is possible to extend this procedure to two dimensional arrays. In this work, a 2D extension of EMD is presented, called Image Empirical Mode Decomposition (IEMD). The obtained modes are called 2dIMF's.

An image is an array of pixels that can be treated as a matrix. Each row of this matrix stands for the energy of this set of pixels, and therefore is possible to plot this information. By this way we obtain a one-dimensional signal and it is possible to apply EMD to this one-dimensional signal.

Performing EMD in succession to all rows leads to a set of IMF's for each row, and the set of all IMF's of the same order constitutes a set of 2dIMF's.

Dermoscopic images used in this work are obtained in RGB format and therefore they need to be pre-processed to before application of IEMD. Each image in RGB format corresponds to an array with dimensions $(m, n, 3)$ allowing the extraction of components R, G and B to be individually treated as described above. The final set of 2dIMF's is obtained after each individual matrix processing, by summing up the results. An example of 2dIMF extraction by IEMD from a dermoscopic image is presented in Figure 14.

Dermoscopic images involve some artefacts directly related to this kind of images, i.e. hairs and air bubbles. The correct outline of lesion borders is critical for diagnosis, and the efficiency of automatic lesion border detection is hampered by artefacts.

Artefact removal comprises two steps: 1) detection of corrupted pixels, and 2) assignment of new intensity value associated to those pixels, while trying to minimize changes in the relevant image features.

The above presented IEMD decomposition is used in this work to detect artefacts. Figure 14 suggests that 2dIMF's capture the main visible artefacts.

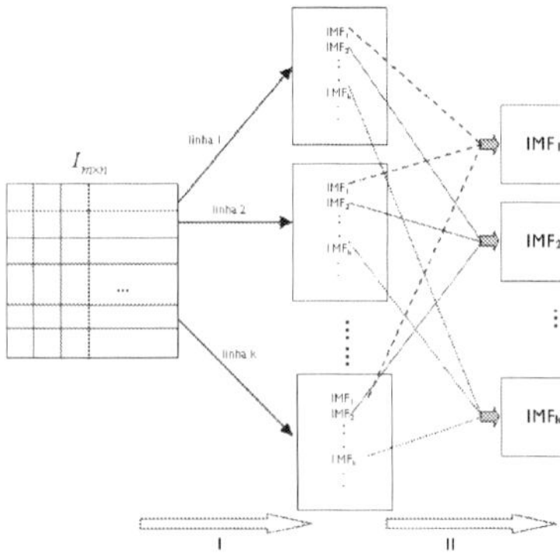

Fig. 13. IEMD extraction from the original matrix

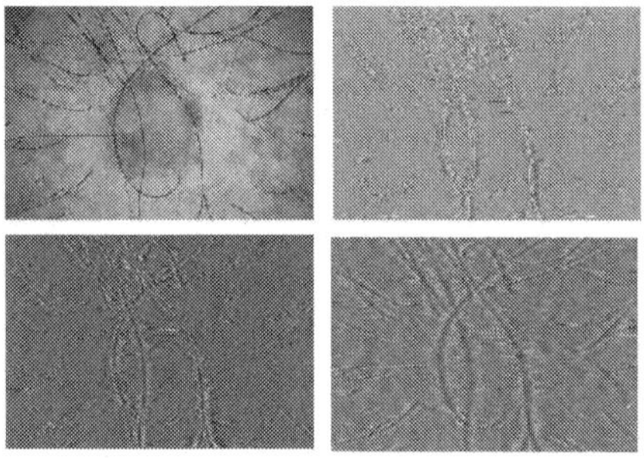

Fig. 14. Dermoscopic image (top left), 2dIMF1 (top right), 2dIMF2 and 3 (bottom images)

3.2.2 Artefact removal by IEMD

Air bubbles and hairs represent bursts of high frequency oscillation that are efficiently captured by the firsts 2dIMF's. These high variation regions are enhanced by applying the following algorithm to 2dIMF1 presented in Figure 16.

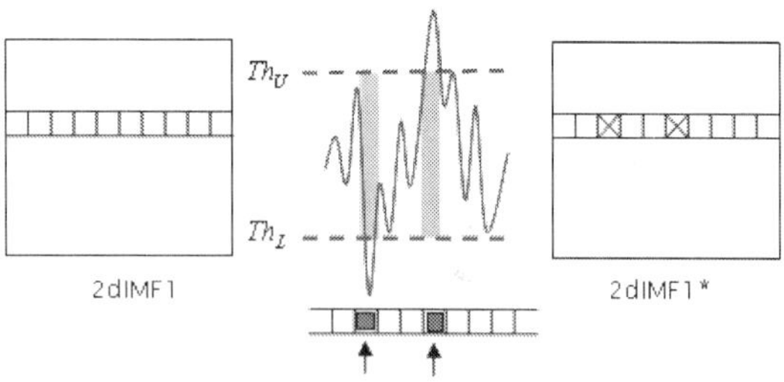

Fig. 15. Detection of anomalous pixels in 2dIMF1

After IEMD we get the first component (2dIMF1, with dimensions $r \times c$) and the maximum (M) and minimum (m) energy value is calculated

$$M = \max_{\substack{i=1,\dots,r \\ j=1,\dots,c}} \{2dIMF1(i,j)\}; \quad m = \min_{\substack{i=1,\dots,r \\ j=1,\dots,c}} \{2dIMF1(i,j)\} \tag{17}$$

and the inner variation is calculated by $R = M + |m|$.

Using this inner variation above defined we set an empirically chosen threshold range. This threshold range is symmetric and the Th of Figure 15 is calculated by $Th = R \times h$, resulting in a percentage of the inner variation characterized by the h value as defined by the user for each image component.

After this step the reassignment of anomalous pixels can be made using several strategies. In this work we chose a simple approach that consists of averaging the values of neighbouring, non-artefact pixels.

This IEMD procedure amounts in fact to filtering. However, contrary to common filter procedures, this technique targets only those pixels where artefacts exist, leaving the remaining image unchanged. It is not a blind procedure, but rather an adaptative and oriented strategy to remove artefacts in dermoscopic images.

As stated in the beginning, automatic border detection is important to improve early diagnosis and the presence of artefacts decreases the efficiency of lesion border detection (specifically, the presence of hairs induces artificial lesion borders). Common filters (in this case low pass filters) applied to these images tend to mask those artefacts, and have the disadvantage of decreasing image resolution. Besides, they tend to blur important diagnosis features such as pigmented networks and blue-white zones.

Dermoscopic images used as examples were obtained from the database of the skin cancer society of Australia in *www.dermoscopyatlas.com* . Low pass filtering used as a comparative model was created with *imfilter.m* function from Matlab using symmetric boundary options.

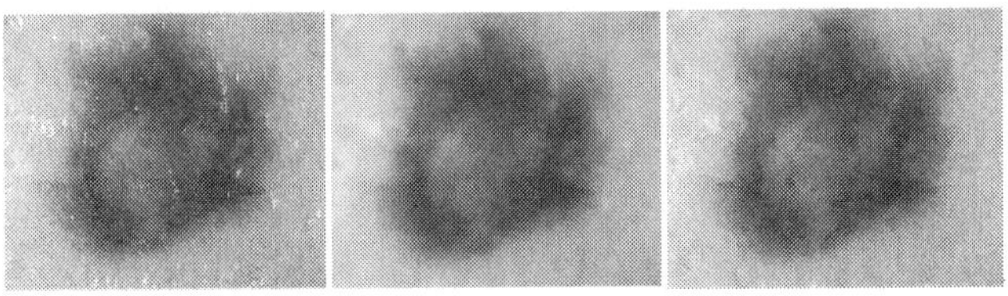

Fig. 16. Dermoscopic image with air bubbles (left), image after classical low pass filtering (middle) and image after IEMD filtering

The performance of IEMD artifact removal is illustrated in Figure 16 in which a dermoscopic image of a melanoma is presented. In this case it is possible to detect several air bubbles due to fluid application on the skin. The image after classical low pass filtering (in the middle) presents poor resolution. The image after IEMD artifact removal (right) indicates a clearly better performance in terms of image resolution preservation.

3.2.3 IEMD as a filter in automatic border lesion detection

After the IEMD artefact removal, we use *bwtraceboundary.m* from the Matlab™ signal processing toolbox to detect border lesions. In the present work we compare the performance of this routine applied to the original dermoscopic image (original), to the image filtered by a classical low pass filter (classical filter) and to the image after being submitted to IEMD (IEMD filter).

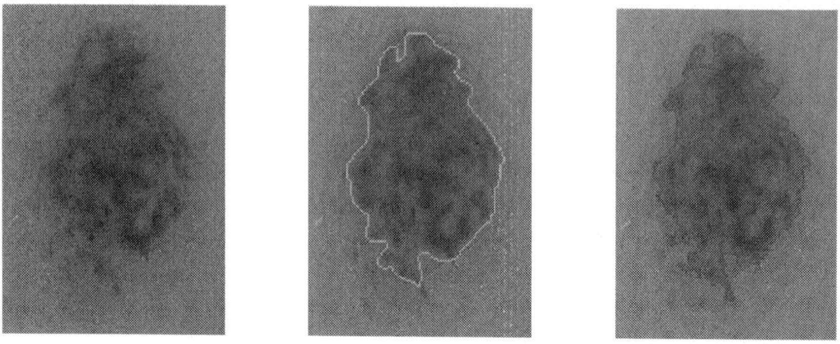

Fig. 17. Automatic border detection without filtering (left), with classical filter (middle) and with IEMD filter (right)

The first example presented in Figure 17 is an *acral melanocytic naevus*. In this case air bubbles are presented and as expected they corrupt the efficiency of automatic border detection, as can be seen in Figure 17 on the left. The two filtering schemes (classical and IEMD) are presented at the same figure at the centre and right. Selective filtering, in this case, resulted in improved border detection (notice the small lesion area at the bottom, missed by classical filtering approach and detected by IEMD).

In the second example, presented in Figure 18, both main artefact sources (air bubbles and hairs) are present, resulting in a tough challenge for the artefact removal algorithm.

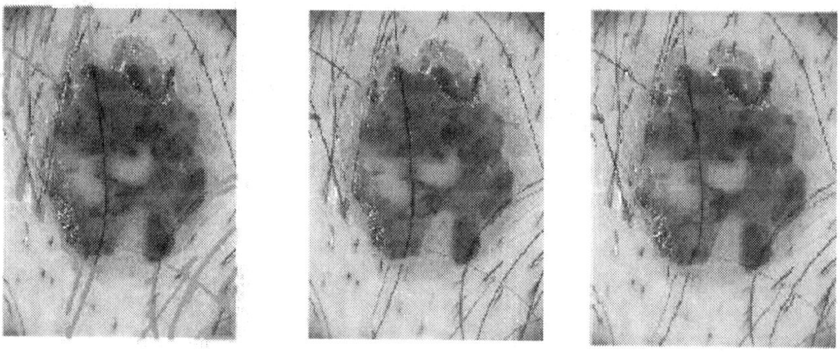

Fig. 18. Automatic border detection without filtering (left), with classical filter (middle) and with IEMD filter (right)

As expected, the automatic border detection of this image without any kind of filtering leads to nonsense results and produces artificial borders in the lesion like those presented in Figure 18 at left. After filtering, it is possible to see that both filtering schemes produce much more reasonably looking borders. Classical filtering leads to soft borders, as opposed to IEMD, where the lesion outline seems to be more realistic.

We present in Figure 19 another example of automatic border detection. This is a melanocytic lesion melanoma *acral lentiginous* and in this case only air bubbles are present. After lesion border automatic detection it is possible to see that, again, IEMD leads to a more detailed outline of the border, as opposed to the softer border yielded by classical filtering, due to the filter-induced blurring.

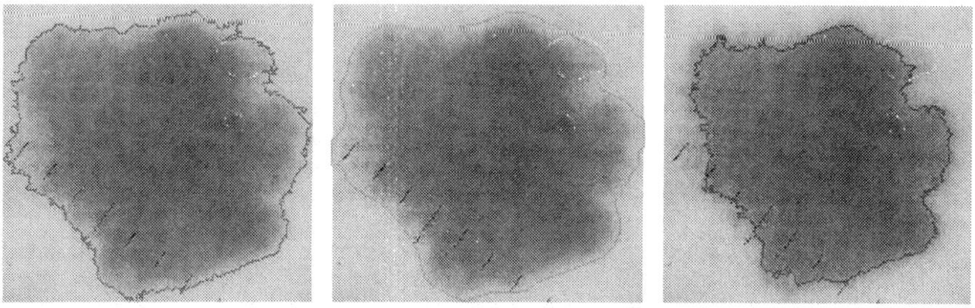

Fig. 19. Automatic border detection without filtering (left), with classical filter (middle) and with IEMD filter (right)

4. Conclusion

The way we have to access to information from systems is, sometimes enrolled in complicated schemes and finally what we get is more a function of the process and less a function of the true phenomenon. In fact, a truly data processing technique must be designed in order to let the data talk! As we have seen, hinders related with stationarity and linearity may cause constrains, when they are overlooked.

To find solutions to old problems, new strategies must be used, as is the case in the EMD decomposition, scratching with traditional an *a priori* basis assumption. In this specific case, as long as whole methodology were empirical and without an analytical formulation, we have to face results with some prudence, filtered by a stable theoretical knowledge in signal processing, allowing to use those results with tranquillity.

People who work with this technique always sited Heaviside, an English Mathematician how said in other context

"Shall I refuse my dinner because I do not fully understand the process of digestion?"

5. Acknowledgements

This Chapter reflects part of the work done during my PhD in the Institute of Biophysics and Biomedical Engineering (IBEB) at the Faculty of Sciences in Lisbon, hence I whish to thank my supervisor Professor Alexandre Andrade.

Data for testing the methodology to access to SVB was obtained in the Laboratory of Autonomic Nervous System at the Hospital de Santa Maria em Lisbon. I want to thank for the data and also for all support from Professor José Luis Ducla-Soares and is team.

6. References

Addison P (2002), *The Ilustrated Wavelet Transform Handbook*, Institute of Physics, ISBN 0750306920.

Auger F, Flandrin P, Gonçalvès P, Lemoine O. *Time frequency toolbox for Matlab*, Freeware at URL (http://tftb.nongnu.org). Accessed 24 May 2009.

Akselrod S, Gordon D, Madwed JB, Snidman NC, Shannon DC, Cohen RJ(1985), Hemodynamic regulation: Investigation by spectral analysis, *Am. J. Physiol.* 18, H867-H875

Boashash B (1992), Estimate and interpreting the instantaneous frequency of a signal: I - Fundamentals, *Proc IEEE* 80, 520-538.

Carvalho JLA, Rocha A, Junqueira L, Souza Neto J, Santos I, Nascimento F (2003); A tool for Time-frequency analysis of heart rate variability, *Proceedings of the 25th annual International Conference of the IEEE EMBC*, 2574-2577.

Caseiro P, Fonseca-Pinto R, Andrade A, Screening of Obstructive Sleep Apnea using Hilbert-Huang Decomposition of Oronasal Airway Pressure recordings, *Medical Engineering and Physics*, 2010.

Cohen L (1995), *Time-Frequency Analysis*. Prentice-Hall,. Englewood Clis, NJ, 1995

Daubechies I (1992), *Discrete Wavelet Transform: Frames*, Chap III of X Lectures on Wavelets. Capital City Press, pp 53-106.

Daubechies I. (1988). Orthonormal Bases of Compactly Supported Wavelets, *Comm. Pure Applied Math.*, Vol 41, pp. 906-966.

Ding H, Huang Z, Song Z, Yan Y (2007) Hilbert–Huang transform based signal analysis for the characterization of gas–liquid two phase flow; *Flow measurement and instrumentation*:18, 37-46.

Ducla-Soares J L, Santos-Bento M, Laranjo S, Andrade, A, Ducla-Soares E, Boto J P, Silva-Carvalho L, Rocha I. (2007). Wavelet analysis of autonomic outflow of normal subjects on head-up tilt, cold press test, valsalva manoeuvre and deep breathing, *Journal of Experimental Physiology*, 92, 677-687.

Eckberg DL. (1997). Sympathovagal balance: a critical appraisal. *Circulation 96*, 3224-3232.

Flandrin P, Gonçalvès P, Rilling G. (2004), Empirical Mode Decomposition as a filter bank, *IEEE Signal Processing Letters*, Vol XI .

Fonseca-Pinto R, Ducla-Soares J. L, Araújo F, Aguiar P, Andrade A (2009), On the influence of time-series length in EMD to extract frequency content: Simulations and models in biomedical signals, *Medical Engineering & Physics* 31 713–719.

Fonseca-Pinto R, Caseiro P, A. Andrade (2010a)), Bi-dimensional Empirical Mode Decomposition (BEMD) in dermoscopic images: artefact removal and border lesion detection; *Proceedings of the 7th IASTED international Conference Signal Processing, Pattern recognition and Applications*; 341-345

Fonseca-Pinto R , Andrade A , Araújo F, Aguiar P, Ducla-Soares J.L (2010b)), Access to Sympathovagal Balance (SVB) using Hilbert-Huang Transform (HHT), *Proceedings of the Matemathical Methods in Engineering conference 2010, MME2010.*

Freeman R. (1997). *Non invasive evaluation of heart rate variation. The time domain. Clinical Autonomic Disorders* (2nd edition) Philadelphia, Lippincott-Raven Publishers : 297-307.

Gabor D, Theory of communication, (1993) *IEEE J. Comm. Eng.* 93: 429-457.

Huang N.E, Shen Z, Long SR, Wu MC, Shih HH, Zheng Q, Yen N-C, Tung CC, Liu HH (1998), The Empirical mode decomposition and the Hilbert spectrum for nonlinear and nonstationary time-series analysis. *Proc R Soc Lond A* 454: 903-995.

Huang N, Wu M, Qu W, Long S, Shen S. (2003), Applications of Hilbert-Huang transform to non-stationary financial time series analysis; *Applied stochastic models in business and industry* - Vol 19, 245-268.

Joyner M, Shepherd J. (1997). *Autonomic regulation of circulation: Clinical Autonomic Disorders* (2nd edition) Philadelphia, Lippincott-Raven Publishers : 61-71.

Long S R, Huang N E, Tung C C, Wu M L, Lin R Q, Mollo-Christensen, E &Yuan Y. (1995), The Hilbert techniques: an alternate approach for non-steady time series analysis. *IEEE Geoscience Remote Sensing Soc.* Lett. 3, 6-11.

Malik M. (1996), Heart rate variability: Standards of measurement, physiological interpretation, and clinical use, Task Force of The European Society of Cardiology and The North American Society of Pacing and Electrophysiology, *European Heart Journal* 17, 354-381.

Malliani A, Pagani M, Lombardi F, Cerutti D. (1991). Cardiovascular neural regulation explored in the frequency domain, *Circulation,* 84, 482 - 492.

Meyer Y. (1993). Wavelets: Algorithms and Applications, *Society for Industrial and Applied Mathematics,* Philadelphia, pp. 13-31, 101-105.

Parati G, Saul J.P, Di Rienzo M, Mancia G. (1995). Spectral analysis of blood pressure and heart rate variability in evaluating cardiovascular - A critical appraisal, *Hypertension,* 25, pp 1276-1286.

Quek T, Tua S, Wang Q. (2003), Detecting anomalies in beams and plate based on the Hilbert-Huang transform of real signals; *Smart materials and structures*- vol12 , 447-460.

Rao R, Hsu E-C (2008) Hilbert-Huang Transform Analysis Of Hydrological And Environmental Time Series; *Water Science and Technology Library*-vol 60.

Rilling G., Flandrin P., Gonçalves P. (2003), On Empirical Mode Decomposition and its Algorithms, *IEEE-EURASIP Workshop on Nonlinear Signal and Image Processing NSIP-03,* Grado (Italy). URL code in:
http://perso.ens-lyon.fr/patrick.flandrin/emd.html.

Salisbury J, Sun Y(2007). Rapid screening test for sleep apnea using a nonlinear and nonstationary signal processing technique; *Medical Engineering & Physics,* 29(3):336-43.

Shepherd R, Shepherd J. (1988). *Control of blood pressure and the circulation in man, Autonomic Failure: A textbook of clinical disorders of the autonomic nervous system* (2nd edition) ,Oxford, Oxford University Press,:80-96.

Sleight P, Casadei B. (1995). *Relationships between heart rate, respiration and blood pressure variabilities, Hear rate variability*. Armonk, NY. Futura Publishing Company : 311-327.

Tang J, Zou Q. Tang Y, Liu B, Zhang Xiao-kai (2007) Hilbert-Huang Transform for ECG De-Noising; *Bioinformatics and Biomedical Engineering*, 664-667.

Xun J, Yan S (2008). A revised Hilbert–Huang transformation based on the neural networks and its application in vibration signal analysis of a deployable structure; *Mechanical Systems and signal processing*-Vol 22, 1705-1723.

Part 4

Computation and Information Management

26

Periodic-MAC: Improving MAC Protocols for Biomedical Sensor Networks Through Implicit Synchronization

Stig Støa[1,2,3] and Ilangko Balasingham[1,2,4]
[1]The Intervention Centre, Oslo University Hospital,
[2]Institute of Clinical Medicine, University of Oslo,
[3]Novelda AS,
[4]Dept. Electronics and Telecommunications,
Norwegian University of Science and Technology,
Norway

1. Introduction

Wired biomedical sensors have facilitated increasingly advanced clinical decisions support systems in specialized medical settings over the last decades. Reliable hemodynamic monitoring of cardiac and pulmonary function is mandatory for individual tailoring of treatment of critically ill patients. Sensors provide the hemodynamic parameters that reveal impending clinical problems, and initiate caregiver intervention. Biomedical sensor technologies include invasive or non-invasive sensors for intermittent or continuous monitoring of vital physiological parameters used in hemodynamic treatment at point-of-care. A hemodynamic sensor portfolio thus involves multiple sensors either attached to the patient, or embedded in biomedical devices used for treatment. The criticality of such systems is evident, as they are used for direct life support in a setting where quality, stability and continuity of real-time data is vital (Øyri et al., 2010). For the last few decades, biomedical sensors and patient monitors used in hemodynamic monitoring have been based on wired solutions. However, a digital revolution is now taking place in healthcare. Medical profiles for wireless standards, such as Bluetooth or ZigBee standards, have currently been developed and adopted by the Continua Health Alliance (Caroll et al., 2007). In the standardization bodies IEEE, ISO and CEN TC 251, improvement of care by reuse of medical device data has been addressed for many years; In particular the IEEE 1073 Standard for Medical Device Connection. A consortium of Scandinavian research institutions, technology startup companies, sensor producers, and a hospital based test facility collaborated to develop a portfolio of multiple experimental wireless sensor prototypes for a platform compliant with the X73 PoC-MDC (ISO11073/IEEE1073)(Galarraga et al., 2006) medical device communication outline (Øyri et al., 2010). Other research groups have evaluated implementations of wireless clinical alerts from pager systems (Major et al., 2002 and Reddy et al., 2005). Yao and Warren investigated how to apply the ISO/IEEE 11073 Standards to wearable home health monitoring systems (Yao & Warren., 2005). There is a demand for a point of care clinical decision support systems providing real time processing of biomedical sensor data displayed as continuous waveform streams. This may be based on a wireless biomedical sensor network which will pave the way for a range of new applications within clinical decision support for healthcare professionals. Wireless connections can transfer digitalized data which, along with other digital data, may enable novel clinical and logistics applications. The wireless systems may also eliminate some of the adverse events typically associated with wires, and enhance the mobility of the patient in the recovery period. The use of wireless sensors would enable greater flexibility for both the patient and medical staff, as the same sensors could follow the patient during the cycle of treatment.

In-hospital deployment of wireless sensor networks defies many of the common assumptions related to medium access control (MAC) protocols. Wireless sensor networks are most often assumed to react on events. This might not be true for clinical decision support systems where the main flows of data are continuous waveform streams. These data streams vary greatly in bandwidth requirements, but the requirements for bandwidth are typically higher than for traditional sensor networks. In such systems we can assume that there are short routes between the source and destination, and the importance of previously sampled data rapidly decreases as time passes, since the main objective is real-time decision support. Failure to access the channel within a short period of time will, in many cases, render the data useless.

Loss of data over a wireless medium is strongly dependent on the channel state of the wireless medium. Data may be lost due to noise interference from other systems like WI-FI and Bluetooth, or path loss variations, a fading effect known as shadowing. Our own investigations show that the main cause of data loss in said networks are due to packet collisions that can be avoided by improving packet scheduling on the MAC layer. We utilize the property that sensors, especially sensors in biomedical sensor networks, transmit at fixed intervals, which is a direct result of the time required to continuously sample each data packet. Knowing that the channel access can be approximated as a periodic instance, we can predict the channel availability with a given probabilistic model, and reduce the channel occupation rate. Thereby reducing the number of retransmissions and enabling operation closer to saturation.

Energy conservation is another important challenge to meet in order to guarantee a minimum operational time of the sensors. Since the power consumption of a transceiver is markedly high during channel listening, the best way to achieve energy conservation is to turn off the radio electronics on every network node for as long as possible. Considering the above, periodic operation is the key factor for energy efficiency and robust communication.

This paper explores how the periodic operation of sensors can be utilized when scheduling transmissions through a wireless interface. Often, the transmission of data packets will be a natural periodic operation, because the sensors themselves sample periodically, with a fixed sample frequency. As a result, the period between each transmission, determined by the time that is required to fill a data packet, will also be fixed. TDMA-based protocols are naturally energy conserving because they have a built-in duty cycle, and do not suffer from collisions. However, maintaining a TDMA schedule in an ad-hoc network is not an easy task and requires much node complexity. TDMA-based protocols usually require the nodes to form communication clusters. Thus, when the number of nodes within a cluster changes, due to the addition or removal of sensor nodes, it is not easy for them to dynamically change their frame length and time slot assignment. Therefore, the scalability is not as efficient as that of a contention-based protocol. In a contention-based MAC algorithm, e.g. CSMA, the key element in optimizing the energy consumption is to minimize the duration of a receiver's on time before the actual data exchange takes place. In addition to data transmission and reception, this time interval may also include signaling, handshaking, collision avoidance mechanisms, plus the necessary transmit/receive turnaround and calibration time. To combine the strengths of these two protocols we suggest using a CSMA/TDMA hybrid protocol that can take advantage of the property of periodicity, and in a decentralized manner predict the channel availability with a given probabilistic model. By storing, in a local TDMA table, the time(s) where CSMA results in a successful transmission, and reusing these time slots in future transmission periods, the operation gradually becomes similar to TDMA scheduling. The decentralization in itself does not necessarily prevent the use of centralized control, but rather reduces the risk of a single point of failure, since the protocol may operate with or without a network coordinator. Therefore, the hybrid protocol can improve the performance and safety of both coordinated and uncoordinated networks.

Since the introduction of computer networks, a great number of data scheduling protocols have been proposed. Typically, these protocols are based on the OSI model (ITU-T X.200), where conceptually similar functions are performed in what is described as a layer. Each layer provides services to the layers above, and receives services from the layer below. Many of these protocols have later been adapted to wireless sensor networks (WSN). Because of the strict requirement of power conservation, and the low bandwidth in WSNs, the interconnection of nodes in a network has taken a new approach by moving toward cross layer protocols. By sharing information between the transmission layers, network nodes can adapt their transmission schedules based on the wireless channel state information they receive from the lower layers that monitor the physical transmission medium. With this approach, a number of scheduling protocols for wireless networks have been proposed to optimize energy conservation, routing, and transmission scheduling. In recent years some protocols have also been developed to combine the strengths of TDMA and CSMA. S-MAC (Ye et al. 2002) auto-synchronizes its sleep schedules, where the node powers down to conserve energy, by forming virtual clusters. Thus, the sleep schedule becomes a periodic operation. TRAMA (Rajendran et al., 2003) is another approach that is closer to TDMA scheduling. TRAMA avoids assigning time slots to nodes with no traffic, and scheduling is adapted based on traffic. Rhee et al. developed Z-MAC (Rhee et al., 2005), which reserves time slots for priority data, but allows nodes that do not necessarily have priority over a given slot to "steal" the time slot when the owner does not have data to send. This enables Z-MAC to switch between CSMA and TDMA depending on the level of contention. Hence, Z-MAC acts like CSMA under low contention but acts like TDMA while under high contention. However, the S-MAC, TRAMA, and Z-MAC protocols require control messages in the form of schedule exchange or central coordination, adding additional protocol overhead. Sticky CSMA-CA (Singh et al., 2007) utilizes implicit synchronization by recording periodic transmissions from neighboring nodes. Sticky CSMA-CA is based on the assumption that all the real-time flows in the network are either naturally periodic or have been shaped by the higher layers as periodic streams with the same period. The periodic nodes access the medium using CSMA-CA and stick to a periodic schedule upon successful transmission. Independently, our own research led to the development of Periodic-MAC protocol (Støa & Balasingham, 2008). Some of the features that separate this protocol from the above protocols is how it introduces memory into the CSMA-CA mechanism, and the fact that no network coordinator is required. For instance, Sticky CSMA-CA maintains a log of the channel transmissions by monitoring the channel over a given time duration, whilst the Periodic MAC maintains a table containing the positions in time, relative to the completion time of the last data packet, that had previously resulted in a successful transmission. In this way, no monitoring of the channel

is needed, and the node can power down for longer periods. Periodic MAC does not utilize RTS/CTS, and does not require any communication other than the data delivery followed by an acknowledgment from the receiver. Periodic-MAC protocol is devised on the assumption that some wireless sensor networks are either naturally, or shaped periodic, however Periodic MAC only requires the transmitters to share a common harmonic of their transmission period. That is, Periodic-MAC should be able to handle multirate as well as homogeneous network traffic. An evaluation of Periodic MAC (Støa & Balasingham, 2009) shows that the protocol also performs very well when there is interference by hidden terminals or random noise.
This paper contributes to understanding and solving several important scheduling problems associated with hybrid protocols based on the assumption of periodic operation. If we assume the nodes in these networks are multi-rate and inhomogeneous, close to optimal scheduling can be determined as a dynamic process by considering a limited number of transmission periods. In Section 2 we describe the Periodic-MAC algorithm, which utilizes this property by iteratively running through a set of solutions that have previously resulted in successful transmissions. However, to simplify the analysis of a network with periodic operation, in Section 3, we will assume that the nodes can only store one such solution. In Section four we look at possible improvements of the algorithm. We conclude in Section 5.

2. Periodic-MAC protocol description

The Periodic-MAC protocol was devised for one hop star topology networks that we would expect to find in hospital environments, such as the operating theater. This network carries data packets containing waveform data intended for real time monitoring of the intensive care unit, or for use during surgery. Since the wave form data appears on the monitor for only a short period, Periodic-MAC relies on the assumption that a data packet is only valid for a limited period of time. Because of this, there is no queuing of packets on the sensor nodes. This reduces the overhead of retransmitting data when the data is no longer useful, and enables normal operation closer to network capacity. When the network is in saturation, the full capacity of the wireless medium is utilized by the sensor nodes. Retransmission of corrupted packages would then start to fill the queues, further adding additional traffic load, resulting in decreased network throughput. Since the protocol assumes that the individual sensors operate periodically, it does not consider nodes that are event driven. Events that would cause alarms should therefore be triggered by the monitoring device.
Crucial for the efficiency of a wireless sensor network protocol is its contention resolution mechanism. When more than one node attempts to transmit a frame at the same time, a collision occurs, and subsequently all frames become corrupted. The standard mechanism for contention resolution in computer networks is the carrier sense multiple access. The Periodic-MAC protocol uses the CSMA-CA algorithm of the IEEE 802.15.4 Standard. This standard has been specifically devised to support wireless sensor networks, and specifies the medium access control and physical layers. For the physical layer, 27 communication channels in three different frequency ranges are defined in the industrial, scientific and medical (ISM) bands; 16 channels in the 2.4 GHz band, 10 channels at 915 MHz and 1 channel at 868 MHz. We consider IEEE 802.15.4 operating in the 2.4 GHz band with 250 kbps data rate. An IEEE 802.15.4 network operates either in a beacon enabled or non-beacon enabled mode. In beacon enabled mode the network uses a slotted CSMA-CA mechanism to access the channel, and in the non-beacon mode it uses more conventional CSMA-CA. Thus far only non-beacon mode has been considered for Periodic-MAC. Although the proposed algorithm has similarities to slotted CSMA-CA, the nodes do not depend on any coordinator as in the

beacon enabled network.

2.1 CSMA/CA algorithm

The basic time unit of the IEEE 802.15.4 MAC protocol is the *aUnitBackoffPeriod*, which is the length of 20 symbol periods or 320 μs. Two variables are maintained by the nodes: BE and NB. BE is the backoff exponent that determines the number of *aUnitBackoffPeriods* a node should delay prior to performing clear channel assessment (CCA), and NB is the number of times a node has been denied channel access due to channel unavailability. The delay period is referred to as the binary exponential backoff (BEB). BE and NB are incremented for each new delay. After reaching a predefined number, *aMaxBE*, BE will not change until it has been reset. When NB reaches its maximum value given by the parameter *macMaxCSMABackoffs*, the packet is either discarded, or the algorithm starts over with initial parameters until the maximum number of retransmissions *aMaxFrameRetries* is reached.

2.2 Implicit synchronization and packet lifespan

Since Periodic-MAC does not queue any data packets, the packets are dropped as soon as a new packet is ready for transmission. This period is dependent on the sampling rate of the sensor and the number of samples a packet can contain. These two variables thus define the packet lifespan. Implicit synchronization can then be achieved if the packet lifespan of each node is aligned. If the lifespan of each packet is perfectly aligned, TDMA may be applied. However, Periodic-MAC only requires that the lifespan of each packet are aligned relative to each other. One way to achieve alignment is to choose a packet lifespan for each node that can be factorized by an integer number. For example, consider three nodes with packet lifespans of 200 ms, 400 ms and 800 ms, respectively. If all nodes have a packet ready at a given time, then all nodes will have a second packet ready 800 ms later. In this case the network traffic will have *global* periodic operation with a period that can be determined by the least common multiple of the individual packet lifespans. In order for the nodes to synchronize their schedules in a decentralized manner, without exchanging transmission schedules among the nodes, the nodes use feedback, in the form of receiver acknowledgments or clear channel assessments (CCA), to learn when other nodes are using the channel. If CCA fails, or no receiver acknowledgment is returned, the node will try to avoid this particular time in the future. The *global* periodic operation of the network thereby sets the minimum time it takes for the nodes to obtain the complete behavior of the network. Figure 1 illustrates how the degree of periodicity, given by the least common multiple of the transmission periods, effects the algorithm's learning process. Considering different constellations of 3 individual transmission periods (packet life spans) equally distributed among 30 nodes, the fraction of packets colliding during one second intervals is recorded by Periodic-MAC computer simulation, with the results shown in Figure 1(a). Similarly, the number of transmissions that timed out due to the CSMA-CA algorithm reaching *macMaxCSMABackoffs* is also shown in Figure 1(b). Finally, Figure 1(c) shows the total delivery ratio after 20 seconds of operation as a function of network traffic load. Traffic is increased by adding groups of three nodes with different transmission periods. It is clear that when there is a high degree of periodicity in the network, the algorithm converges faster toward TDMA scheduling, and the performance of the network increases.

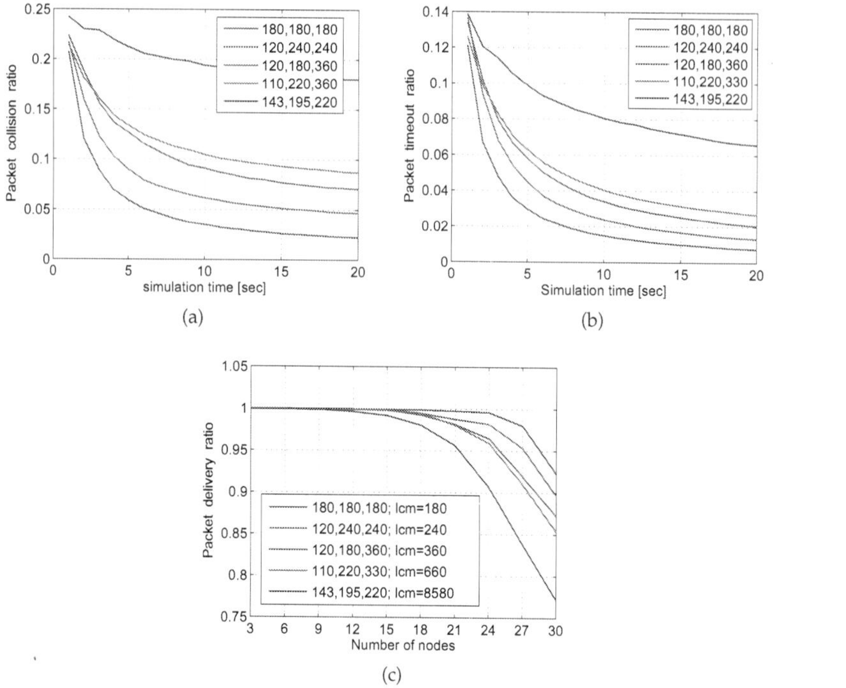

Fig. 1. Effect on the algorithm learning based on the degree of periodicity. Legend show the packet lifespan in milliseconds. The least common multiple is shown in the legend. Figure (a); second per second recording of the fraction of packets colliding. Figure (b); failures due to the algorithm reaching *macMaxCSMABackoffs*. Figure (c); total delivery ratio after 20 seconds of operation.

2.3 Periodic-MAC algorithm

The algorithm utilizes the CSMA-CA algorithm as described in Section 2.1, with the exception that the BEB periods are stored for future transmission attempts. Each node is required to maintain a table where it stores the BEB values. The BEB values are always relative to the start of the packet life cycle. If the node updates BEB more than once before successfully transmitting its data, the sum of all BEB, in addition to the time spent on failed transmission attempts, is stored. If the transmission does not complete successfully, no value is stored. When the node schedules a new transmission, it will always check if there are any entries in the table. If entries exists, the node schedules its transmission with a delay according to the table entry, without using the CSMA-CA algorithm. Otherwise, the regular CSMA-CA algorithm is used. If a transmission fails after selecting a delayed timeslot from the table, and *aMaxFrameRetries* is not reached, the node continues using the CSMA-CA algorithm. If this second attempt using CSMA-CA succeeds, a second entry is added to the table. In this way the nodes build up a table based on feedback from earlier transmission attempts. As this learning process continues, the scheduling gradually becomes like TDMA. In order for the

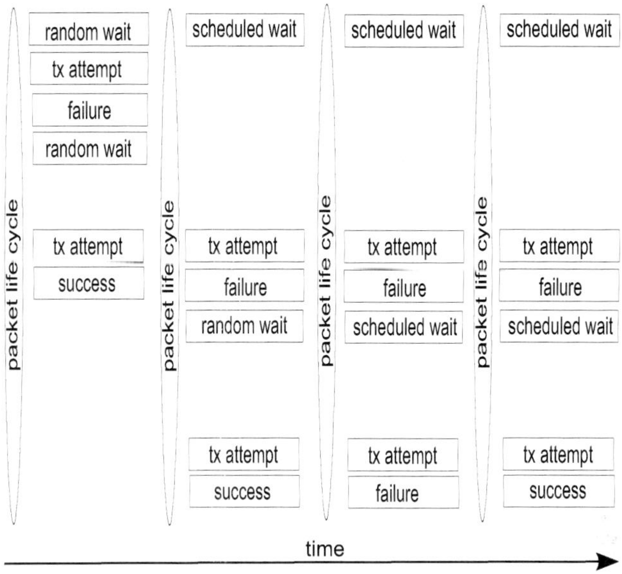

Fig. 2. Illustration of Periodic-MAC algorithm and the packet life cycle.

nodes to dynamically adapt to changes in the traffic flow of the network, the table size must have a finite length. If a transmission ends in failure after attempting all table entries, the table is either partially or completely reset. A typical scenario of the algorithm is illustrated by Figure 2. In the illustration, two entries are stored in the table (scheduled wait) after performing CSMA-CA (random wait). Three packets are successfully transmitted and one packet is dropped.

3. Analysis of the periodic channel access using one table entry

For simplicity, we analyze the periodic channel access of a network with only one table entry per node. These networks are illustrated by Figures 3 and 4. While Figure 3 illustrates a network where all the nodes have the same transmission period, Figure 4 shows a scenario where the nodes access the channel with different periods. We consider the two scenarios as a homogeneous and inhomogeneous network, respectively. We will also explore how the algorithm can work without the use of binary backoff, by simply randomly choosing one of the time slot that are within the nodes packet lifespan. The number of time slots to choose from and their duration will therefore depend on the packet lifespan and is carefully chosen so that each packet lifespan contains an integer number of time slots.

3.1 Homogeneous network

Consider the scenario illustrated by Figure 3, where there are N number of channels competing for channel access in one of M time slots available at the beginning of every period. In this example, the total number of ways the nodes can randomly choose a specific slot, is given as $M^N = 3^3 = 27$ ways. Let $\mathbf{s}_l$ be a vector containing the probabilities of $\mathbf{x} \in \{1,2,..,N\}$ transmissions succeeding in state l. The state is defined by the number of nodes that have

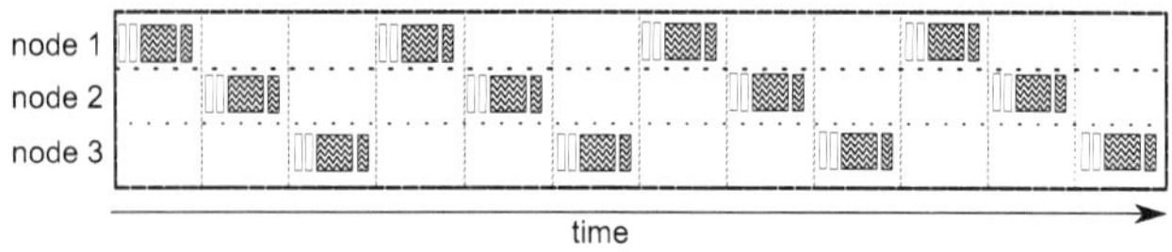

Fig. 3. Homogeneous network with optimal channel alignment.

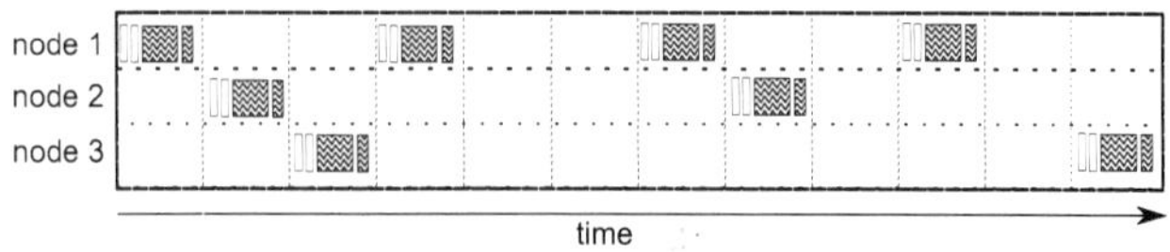

Fig. 4. Inhomogeneous network with optimal channel alignment.

locked on to one of the time slots, indicating that a successful transmission has occurred in this slot. Thus, $l \in \{0, 1, .., N\}$. Once a node acquires a lock, its transmission schedule is fixed for all future periods. Let $\lambda(k)_l$ be a state probability vector containing the probabilities of reaching any state, given the current state l, after k transmission periods.

3.1.1 Estimating the probability of successful transmission and lock probability

In the current example, the probabilities of successful transmission, $\mathbf{s}_l$, will only depend on the lock state. We can therefore define a single matrix S containing $\mathbf{s}$ for all states. We solve S for the current example by identifying, for all states, how many of the possible combinations will result in $\mathbf{x}$ number of successful transmissions. Note that $S_{l,(N-1)}$ will always be zero since at least two packets have to be involved in a collision.

$$S = \begin{pmatrix} \frac{3}{3} * \frac{1}{3} * \frac{1}{3} & \frac{3}{3} * \frac{3}{3} * \frac{2}{3} & 0 & \frac{3}{3} * \frac{2}{3} * \frac{1}{3} \\ \frac{1}{3} * \frac{1}{3} & \frac{3}{3} * \frac{2}{3} & 0 & \frac{2}{3} * \frac{1}{3} \\ 0 & \frac{2}{3} & 0 & \frac{1}{3} \\ 0 & 0 & 0 & 1 \end{pmatrix} = \begin{pmatrix} \frac{1}{9} & \frac{6}{9} & 0 & \frac{2}{9} \\ \frac{1}{9} & \frac{6}{9} & 0 & \frac{2}{9} \\ 0 & \frac{2}{3} & 0 & \frac{1}{3} \\ 0 & 0 & 0 & 1 \end{pmatrix}$$

When nodes lock on a slot and consider using only this time slot for later transmissions, the number of ways to arrange the schedule in the next period decreases exponentially. Once all nodes have a lock, there will only be one way to arrange the transmission schedule, and the probability of successful transmission is guaranteed for the remaining periods. If the number of nodes becomes large, it is impractical to calculate the probabilities using combinatorics. In this case the probabilities can easily be found empirically by assigning locked nodes different numbers between 1 and M, and having a computer select a random number in the same range for the remaining nodes. The duplicates indicate collisions. Then, an approximation of S can be found by averaging over a large number of selections.

Assuming the initial state is 0, and none of the nodes have a lock, it is apparent that the probability of having zero, one or three locks in the next period is equal to $\mathbf{s}_0$. Given a period where we have one lock and one successful transmission, $S_{1,1}$, there is a $\frac{N-1}{N} = \frac{2}{3}$ probability of a new lock, since one of the nodes already has a lock. In any case, the number of locks cannot decrease.

Define the state transition probability matrix L. Then the single step probability matrix $L = (\lambda_{li})$ is the probability that the next state will be i given that the current state is l.

$$L = \begin{pmatrix} S_{0,0} & S_{0,1} & S_{0,2} & S_{0,3} \\ 0 & S_{1,1} * \frac{1}{3} & S_{1,1} * \frac{2}{3} & S_{1,3} \\ 0 & 0 & S_{2,1} & S_{2,3} \\ 0 & 0 & 0 & S_{3,3} \end{pmatrix} = \begin{pmatrix} \frac{1}{9} & \frac{6}{9} & 0 & \frac{2}{9} \\ 0 & \frac{3}{9} & \frac{4}{9} & \frac{2}{9} \\ 0 & 0 & \frac{2}{3} & \frac{1}{3} \\ 0 & 0 & 0 & 1 \end{pmatrix}$$

Since the initial state $\lambda(0)_0$ is known, we can express the state probabilities after k periods as

$$\lambda(k) = \lambda(0)L^k, \tag{1}$$

where k is also used as the exponent of L. In order to analyze the evolution of the lock probability, define $\Lambda(k)$ to be the expected number of locks after k periods.

$$\Lambda(k) = \lambda(k)\mathbf{x}^T, \tag{2}$$

where T symbolizes the transposed of vector $\{\mathbf{x}\} = [0, 1, 2.., N]$.

3.1.2 Estimating the effective throughput

After identifying the probabilities of S, the probability of successful transmissions during the k'th period is only dependent on the current state. The success probability in period k can therefore be calculated by

$$\mathbf{s}(k) = \lambda(k)S. \tag{3}$$

Let $\hat{\mathbf{s}}_k$ be the expected number of successful transmissions, during period k, and let the effective throughput, Θ, be the fraction of nodes that successfully transmit their data packet during this period. Θ is thus defined as

$$\Theta = \hat{\mathbf{s}}_k / N. \tag{4}$$

Similar to Equation (2), the expected number of successful transmissions during the k'th period can be calculated as follows

$$\hat{\mathbf{s}}_k = \mathbf{s}(k)\mathbf{x}^T. \tag{5}$$

Following the above example, where we consider three transmissions scheduled for each period, the average effective packet throughput after the first period is $\frac{\hat{\mathbf{s}}_1}{3} = \frac{4}{9}$. Note that Θ would remain constant for all periods when using regular CSMA without locking.
Figure 5 shows the effective throughput, Θ, and the lock probability, Λ, as a function of time (periods) for different traffic load. Notice that although the two are clearly correlated, Θ will converge at a slower rate because the transmission schedules of nodes without a lock might still collide with those that are locked. Here N varies while M is 18.

3.2 Inhomogeneous network

Many sensor networks consist of sensors with very different sampling rates, which in turn lead to different transmission intervals. However, the behavior of the network may be simplified so that the method for calculating the probability of successful transmission, and lock probability, is similar to that of a homogeneous network. Assuming that all transmission periods are individually periodic, they will share a common harmonic. The network will then behave in a periodic manner with a global period, T^{gbl}, equal to the least common multiple of the individual transmission periods. Since some nodes only transmit once within a global period, we first consider one T^{gbl} when calculating probabilities of successful transmission.

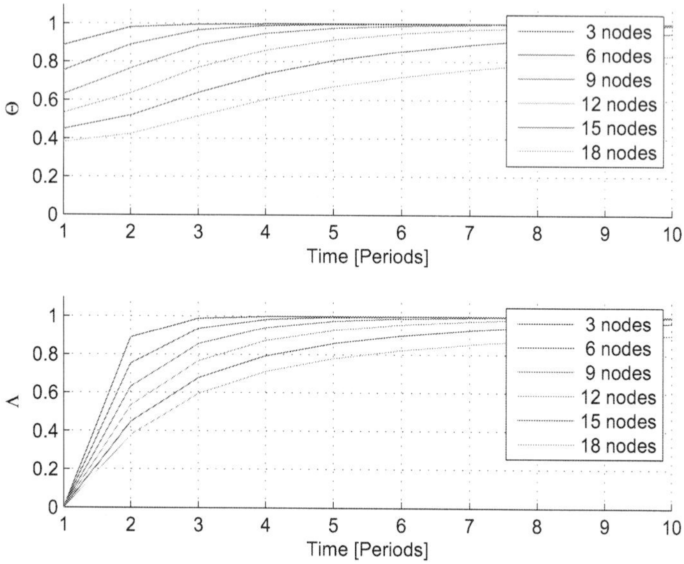

Fig. 5. Effective throughput, Θ, and lock probability, Λ, with M=18

Let T_i^{loc} $i \in \{1,2,..,N\}$, be a subset of T^{gbl}, with a duration equal to the shortest local period. N number of subsets then sum up to the duration of one T^{gbl}. By realizing that no matter how we shift our schedules, since they are periodic, the fraction of T_i^{loc}, in T^{gbl}, with a given number of scheduled nodes will be constant. We can therefore calculate the average success probability matrix $\bar{S}^{loc}$. Define $[S^{loc}]_i$ as a single matrix for each of the N subsets and identify the probabilities of having successful transmissions in each of them. $[S^{loc}]_i = (S_{lj})_i$ is the probability of j successful transmissions given that the current state is l,

$$\bar{S}^{loc} = \frac{1}{N}\sum_{i=1}^{N}[S^{loc}]_i\,. \tag{6}$$

Now, $\bar{S}^{loc}$ can be used to calculate the lock state probabilities in the same manner as for the homogeneous network, and we can use Equation (1) and (3) to calculate the success probability in a given local period. Because some nodes might transmit only once during T^{gbl}, it makes sense to calculate the effective throughput for T^{gbl}, which is N times that of T^{loc}. The effective throughput is then

$$\hat{s}_k = N * \bar{S}^{loc} * \mathbf{x}^T. \tag{7}$$

3.3 Deciding the time slot duration

When deciding the duration of a time slot, several factors need consideration. In order to ensure that all slots are utilized, the slot should have a duration that is at least that of a data package transmission. Note that this is not an assumption in most CSMA systems. If the network is not fully synchronized, longer slots should be considered, but regardless, a given number of slots should sum up to exactly one *global period*, T^{glb}. If the number of slots does not sum up to exactly one global period, the alignment of the slots will continually shift relative to each other. The optimal duration of a slot when the network is fully synchronized can easily be found by dividing T^{glb} by the maximum time required to successfully transmit a data packet. This will assure that the slot will have room for an entire packet, and minimizes the time between transmissions where the channel is left idle. Assuming two nodes, A and B, are within range, and that the network is not fully synchronized, node A's slots may overlap with two of node B's slots. As a result only half of the slots can be utilized. Because of this, slot duration in the case of unsynchronized transmissions should be twice that of synchronized transmissions, in order to apply the same method of calculating throughput and lock probability for both synchronized and unsynchronized transmissions.

In order to decide on a suitable slot duration, considering that we are using the IEEE 802.15.4 physical layer for transmission, we analyze the packet length, and transmission period, of the nodes in the network. The maximum channel occupation time required per transmission attempt with the IEEE 802.15.4 protocol is

$$2(CCA + aTurnaroudTime) + TX + aMaxAckWaitDuration = 40 + 266 + 54 \quad symbolperiods,$$

which sums up to 360 symbol durations. As previously mentioned, the transmission periods can be shaped in a way such that they all become periodic with a common harmonic frequency. In order to allow for a maximum number of different transmission periods, while still keeping the global period as short as possible, the slot duration should have a length that maximizes the number of factors in T^{glb}. For instance, 360 can also be expressed as n!/2, and would therefore be a good choice if we were deciding a duration for T^{glb}, since any product of the numbers between 1 and 6 can be used as a divisor to create local periods. However, we will consider that the sampling rates are already decided, and instead search for a suitable T^{loc}. With channel capacity of 250 kbps and 4 bits per symbol, there are 62500 symbols per second, which gives the minimum slot time 360/62500=5.8 ms. This slot duration may further be adjusted to fit the sensor sampling frequency by adding a small number of symbol durations while keeping a balance between T^{glb} and T^{loc}. This implies that if $\hat{T^{loc}} = T^{loc} + \mathbb{N}$ then $T^{gbl} * \frac{\hat{T^{loc}}}{T^{loc}}$ is still a integer factor of T^{loc}.

Considering we have three sensors sampling at frequencies 100Hz, 200Hz, and 300Hz, respectively. The local periods for each node can be expressed as

$$[T^{loc}]_x = \mathbb{A}_x * \frac{360 + c}{62500} \qquad , \ seconds. \tag{8}$$

Here $\mathbb{A}$ is an integer satisfying

$$\mathbb{A}_x = \frac{62500\mathbb{P}_x}{(360 + c)R_x} \qquad , \ \mathbb{A}_x \in \mathbb{N}\,, \tag{9}$$

where c is a constant used to extend the slot duration as needed, R is the sampling rate in Hz and $\mathbb{P}$ is the integer number of samples in each data packet. For all x, $[T^{loc}]_x$ satisfies

$$\frac{[T^{loc}]_x}{min\{[T^{loc}]_x\}} = \mathbb{N}. \tag{10}$$

If the payload cannot be adjusted to make T^{loc} exactly a factor of 5.8 ms, the slot size is lengthened such that it becomes equal to an integer number of *sample* periods on all of the nodes. In the current example, we choose c such that (360+c)/62500 = $1/gcd(R)$ $\rightarrow c = 265$. gcd is the greatest common divisor of R. The slot duration is then 10 ms, and T^{gbl} is consequently lengthened by a factor of (360+c)/360. Also, Equation (10) and (9) can be satisfied to make the network either homogeneous or inhomogeneous. By choosing $\mathbb{P}_x = [16,32,48]$, $x \in [1,2,3]$, given that we have the sample rates $\{R\} \in [100,200,300]$, $[T^{loc}]_x$ becomes constant for all x and the network becomes homogeneous with T^{gbl} equal to $lcm(\{T^{loc}\})$=160 ms. To minimize the overhead due to header data in the data packet, larger packets are preferable. Assuming a data packet can contain 48 samples and maximum packet length is chosen, $\mathbb{P}_x$=[48,48,48], the network become inhomogeneous with $\{T^{loc}\} = [480,240,160]$ ms and T^{gbl} equal to $lcm(\{T^{loc}\})$=480 ms.

3.4 Performance of Simplified Protocol

Simulations of the two networks consisting of groups of sensors with the transmission periods described above was performed, and the delivery ratio for different number of nodes is shown in Figure 6(c). Let scenario A be the scenario with transmission periods of 160 ms, and scenario B the scenario with transmission periods of 120 ms, 240 ms, and 480 ms. The different transmission periods are equally distributed among the nodes. The delivery ratios for each of the two scenarios, as a function of time, are shown in Figures 6(a) and 6(b). Since scenario A consists of sensors with the same transmission period, the global network period is short, and the network algorithm adapts quickly. Scenario B has a global network period that is 3 times that of scenario A, resulting in a slightly longer learning period. However, in order to make the network in scenario A homogeneous, the number of packets to be transmitted was increased since they now carry fewer data samples. Also, more channel capacity is wasted on the idle period needed to align the time slots. This causes a lower throughput in scenario A when the number of nodes is high. Figure 6(c) shows a rapid decrease in performance for scenario A, indicating that all the time slots are occupied with 15 nodes in the network, and the network cannot be scaled any further. Note also that the performance of scenario B starts to decrease sooner than for scenario A. When the network is homogeneous, all transmission periods are orthogonal which ensures that two or more nodes will not lock onto the same slot. However, in scenario B, if a node with a long packet lifetime locks onto a slot before the nodes with shorter packet lifespans has fixed their schedules, the latter may find a lock between transmissions of the first node, resulting in future collisions. In scenarios such as scenario B, the node should only lock temporarily until it has successfully transmitted its entire data packet for a minimum duration of one global period.

3.5 Hidden terminals

One of the strengths of Periodic-MAC is its resilience to influence from the well known *hidden terminal problem*. With the presence of hidden terminals, selected nodes in the network do not operate within reach of each other, and are therefore unable to detect each others transmissions. The hidden terminal problem arises when the receiver of a message is within range of two nodes that are hidden from each other. Let node A and node B be the hidden nodes, and node C the node within reach of both A and B. When node A transmits a data packet to node C, node B might be transmitting at the same time, rendering node C unable to receive the message from A. The scenario is illustrated in Figure 7. Periodic-MAC is more resilient to this problem because the scheduling is done based on the feedback, or the lack

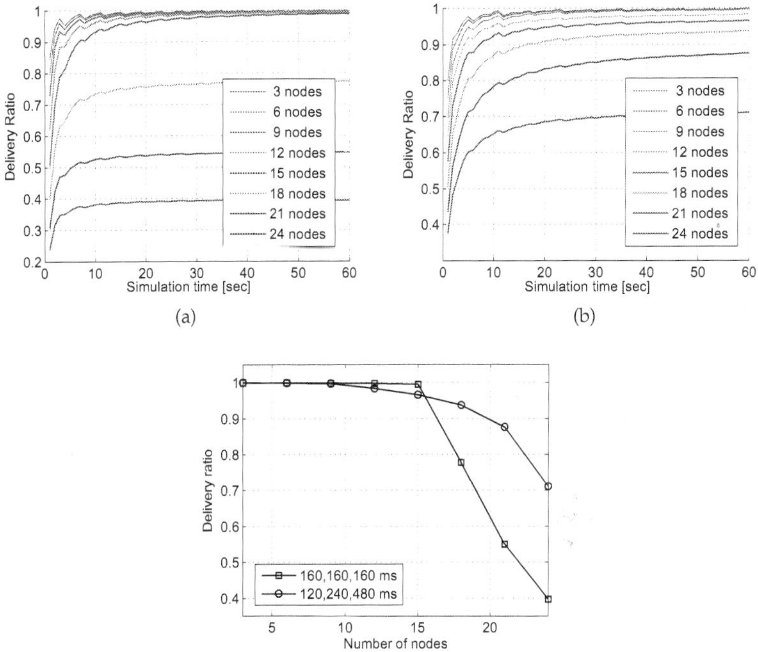

(c)

Fig. 6. Past second delivery ratio for nodes with transmission periods 160 ms versus time(a), and with transmission periods 120 ms, 240 ms, and 480 ms (b). (c) shows the delivery ratio of the two scenarios for a different number of nodes.

of such, from the receiver. If the receiver cannot receive a transmission because of a hidden terminal, no feedback is given, and the nodes therefore indirectly receive information about the transmission schedule of nodes that are hidden.

In the case of slotted Periodic-MAC with one table entry, the algorithm learning process is indifferent to the hidden terminal altogether. This is because the nodes will only lock onto a time slot if the receiver acknowledges that the transmission was successfully received. Hence, performance of the network scenario illustrated by Figure 7 will be equal to a scenario where

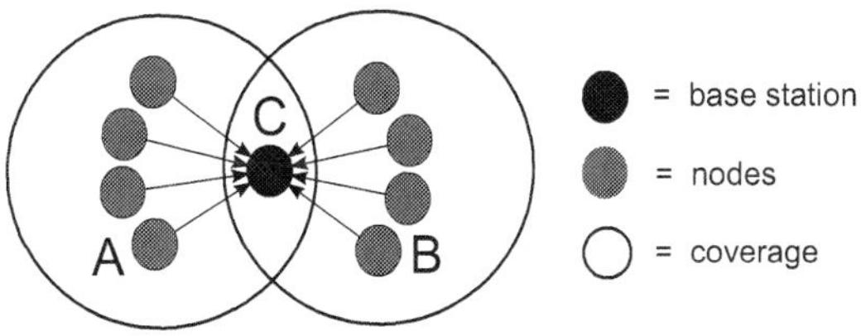

Fig. 7. Illustration of a hidden terminal scenario. A and B are hidden from each other while communicating with C.

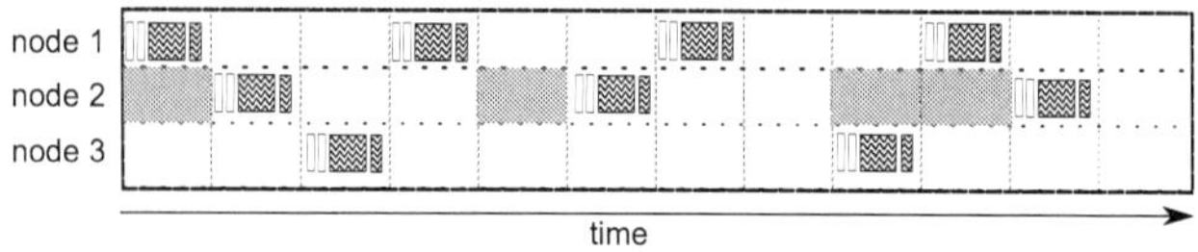

Fig. 8. Inhomogeneous network with dynamic channel alignment.

all the nodes are within reach of each other. Note that this only applies when the intended receiver is a node within reach of all nodes. This scenario illustrates an important property. Since base stations and access points usually do not share the same restriction on power conservation as the sensor nodes, they operate with higher transmission power to increase coverage.

4. Discussion

4.1 Periodic channel access using multiple table entries

As was explained in Section 3.4, two inhomogeneous nodes may lock onto the same slot if no counter measures are applied. In contrast to the simplified protocol described in the previous section, the original Periodic-MAC utilizes multiple table entries to enable dynamic shifting of the scheduling. Consider Figure 8, where node 2 shifts its transmission schedule by one slot for the first two transmissions, and then by two slots for every third transmission. In this example optimal scheduling is achieved when node 2 shifts its schedule by one or two slots depending on the modulo of the life cycle. This dynamic shifting of the schedule is achieved by iteratively traversing the table entries which are all solutions that had previously resulted in successful transmissions. This is, however, a suboptimal solution since the node will have to power up and do a clear channel assessment for every table entry. Another possible scenario, as a result of this sub optimality, occurs when two packets collide on a transmission attempt using the fixed schedule. This indicates that the two nodes have packet life cycles that are closely aligned and perform CCA at the same time. In this case, unless the remaining transmission attempts fail and the scheduling table is reset on one of the nodes, a collision will occur every time the two schedules overlap. To prevent this scenario, the algorithm needs a way to delete table entries that frequently result in collision. An improvement of the protocol is therefore possible by counting the number of successful transmissions between every failure. This number can then be used to determine when to skip a table entry.

4.2 Nodes entering the network

Sensors are usually not switched on at exactly the same time, which causes changes in the network topology when new sensors are switched on. As new nodes enter the network, the existing nodes may already have adapted to a TDMA schedule. Additional nodes will then likely influence these schedules, and a new learning process will begin. If several nodes have to start the learning period from zero, this might create a cascade effect, causing all nodes to reset their schedules. This would have a dramatic effect on the algorithm. However, the new nodes accessing the network will perform CCA until they find the channel to be idle. The network is most vulnerable to cascade effects when it operates close to saturation. In this case it will take some time for the new nodes to access the channel. Once they find the channel to be idle, the nodes will occupy the channel for a period of time, which may overlap with the current schedule of another node, or at a later time due to non-orthogonal transmission periods. Since the existing nodes have built up a table with several possible scheduling

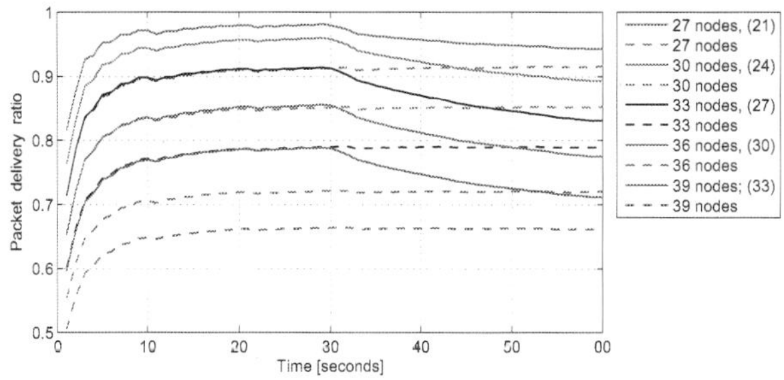

Fig. 9. Delivery ratio as a function of time. Additional nodes entering the network after 30 seconds.

options, it might still be possible for them to transmit using another table entry. With the introduction of new nodes, the scheduling will therefore gradually adapt. A simulation of nodes entering the network was performed using the simulator described in (Støa & Balasingham, 2008). Figure 9 shows the delivery ratio, during the past second, for a different number of nodes over a period of 60 seconds. The graphs with dashed lines are groups of nodes all starting simultaneously, and graphs with solid lines are groups where 6 of the nodes start with a delay. The same color indicates that the total number of nodes are equal. After 30 seconds, most of the nodes have operated with TDMA scheduling, and the 6 additional nodes enter the network. The figure shows that the added nodes do not have an immediate impact, but rather gradually converge toward the delivery ratio that is obtained for the nodes that started simultaneously.

5. Conclusion

In this paper the properties of sensor networks with periodic operation have been scrutinized. An analysis of the hybrid protocol Periodic-MAC, and how the degree of network periodicity influences the protocol has been performed. Because of the number of variables involved, and the fact that the channel state probabilities change over time, a simplified version of Periodic-MAC was presented in order to highlight some of the most important properties of hybrid scheduling protocols that are based on the assumption of periodic operation. Even though Periodic-MAC was devised as a decentralized protocol, the simplified protocol operating using CSMA-CA with a fixed contention window similar to slotted CSMA-CA, indicates that the protocol can be used in combination with centralized networks. By combining the two, the risk of a single point of failure is reduced. By utilizing the property that sensors, especially in biomedical sensor networks, transmit at fixed intervals, close to full channel efficiency can be achieved by reusing previously successful transmission times. Periodic-MAC has shown that it can efficiently distribute the transmission schedules, in a dynamic and decentralized way, where the performance is close to TDMA scheduling.

6. References

Øyri, K.; Støa, S. & Fosse, E. (2010). A Biomedical Wireless Sensor Network for Hemodynamic Monitoring, *Proceedings of The Fifth International Conference on Body Area Networks*, Corfu, Greece, September 2010, IEEE press, to appear.

Støa, S. & Balasingham, I. (2008). A decentralized MAC layer protocol with periodic channel access for biomedical sensor networks. *First International Symposium on Applied Sciences on Biomedical and Communication Technologies (ISABEL '08)*, pp. 1-5, ISBN 978-1-4244-2647-8. IEEE conference proceedings, Aalborg, Denmark, October 2008.

Støa, S. & Balasingham, I. (2009). A decentalized MAC layer protocol with periodic channel access evaluated with presence of interference. *Second International Symposium on Applied Sciences in Biomedical and Communication Technologies*, pp. 1-6, ISBN 978-1-4244-4641-4, IEEE conference proceedings, Bratislava, Slovak Republic, November 2009.

Caroll, R.; Cnossen, R.; Schnell, M. & Simons, D. (2007). Continnua: An Interoperative Personal Healthcare Ecosystem. *Pervasive Computing*, Vol. 6, No. 4, (October 2007), 90-94.

Galarraga, M.;Serrano, L.; Martinez, I. & Toledo, P. (2005). Standards for medical device communication: X73 PoC-MDC, *Medical and Care Compunetics 3*, Bos, L.; Roa, L.; Yogesan, K; O'Connel, B.; Marsh, A & Blobel, B., (Ed.), pp. 242-256, IOS Press - Studies in Health Technology and Informatics, ISBN: 1-58603-620-3, Netherlands.

Major, K.; Shabot M. M. & Cunnen, S. (2002). Wireless clinical alerts and patient outcomes in the surgical intensive care unit, *Am. Surg.*, Vol. 68, No. 12, (December 2002), 1057-1060.

Reddy, M.C.; McDonald, D. W.; Pratt, W. & Shabot, M. M. (2005). Technology, work, and information flows: lessons from the implementation of a wireless pager system, *J. Biomed. Inform.*, Vol. 38, No. 3 (June 2005), 229-238.

Yao, J. & Warren, S. (2005). Applying the ISO/IEEE 11073 standards to wearable home health monitoring systems, *J. Clin. Monit. Comput.*, Vol. 19, No. 6 (December 2005), 427-436.

Rajendran, V.; Obraczka, K. & Garcia, J. J. (2003). Energy efficient, collision-free medium access control for wireless sensor networks. *Proceedings of the 1st. ACM Conf. on Embedded Networked Sensor Systems*, pp. 181-192, ISBN, Los Angeles, CA, USA, November 2003, IEEE.

Rhee, I.; Warrier, A.; Aia, M.; Min, J. & Sichitiu, M.L. (2008). Z-MAC: a Hybrid MAC for Wireless Sensor Networks, *IEEE/ACM Transactions on Networking*, Vol. 16, No. 3 (June 2008), 511-524, ISSN:1063-6692.

Singh, S.; Acharaya, P. A. K.; Madhow, U. & Belding-Royer, E. M. (2007). Sticky CSMA/CA: Implicit synchronization and real-time QoS in mesh networks, *Ad Hoc Networks*, Vol. 5, No. 6 (August 2007), 744-768, ISSN:1570-8705.

27

Biomedical Electronic Systems to Improve the Healthcare Quality and Efficiency

Roberto Marani and Anna Gina Perri
Laboratorio di Dispositivi Elettronici
Politecnico di Bari, Dipartimento di Elettrotecnica ed Elettronica
Bari,
Italy

1. Introduction

The most recent developments of electronics, informatics and telecommunications let imagine applications in the biomedical engineering field to improve the healthcare quality (She et al., 2007). In particular a number of systems has been developed in the telemedicine and home care sectors which could guarantee an efficient and reliable home assistance allowing a highly better quality of life in terms of prophylaxis, treatment and reduction of discomfort connected to periodic out-patient controls and/or hospitalization for the patients afflicted by pathologies (such as cardiac decompensation or obstructive chronic bronchopathy), and allowing considerable savings on sanitary expenses.

In this chapter we present a review of our principal projects in biomedical electronic field, developed at the Electronic Device Laboratory of Polytechnic of Bari, Italy.

Firstly we propose a medical electronic-computerized platform for diagnostic use, which allows the doctor to carry out a complete cardio-respiratory control on remote patients in real time. The system has been patented and has been designed to be employed also to real-time rescue in case of emergency without the necessity for data to be constantly monitored by a medical centre, leaving patients free to move. For this purpose the system has been equipped with highly developed firmware which enables automated functioning and complex decision-making. In fact, when an emergency sign is detected through the real-time diagnosing system, it sends a warning message to people able to arrange for his/her rescue. A Global Positioning System (GPS) also provides the patient coordinates. All this occurs automatically without any intervention by the user. The system might be useful also to sportsmen. Thanks to its characteristics it can help to reduce hospitalization rates and length of stays thereby improving health costs and quality of life. Moreover the system, in its version for diagnostic use, has been verified by the heart specialists of the Institute of Cardiology in the General Hospital (Polyclinic) of the University of Bari.

We also propose a low-cost, electronic medical device, designed for the non-invasive continuous real-time monitoring of breathing functions. It diagnoses respiratory pathologies by the electronic three dimensional (3-D) auscultation of lung sounds, performing a correlation between lung sounds and diseases.

Moreover we present a new system for acquiring simultaneously some health parameters which are strongly correlated: breathing rate and kinetic activity. The system is based on a couple of sensors, which are very light, absolutely non- invasive and compatible with every day life.

For breathing sensing we use an already known method involving a belt to sense the thorax dilatation, but we apply a new kind of dilatation sensor on the belt based on a conductive rubber, which is new in breathing detection, quite cheap and sensitive.

Breathing rate observation is quite useless when no information is available on patient activity that could cause breathing rate change. Therefore we present also a kinetic activity sensor based on commercial accelerometer. Signals from these sensors are amplified filtered and elaborated and feed to the ADC of a micro-controller. Experimental results have shown a clear correlation between these signals, inducing us to stress the importance of coupling breathing and kinetic activity monitoring, particularly in patients with lung and heart diseases.

At last we present a new system for cardioholter applications, characterized by the possibility to send an ElectroCardioGram (ECG) by Bluetooth to 6 or 12 leads. Moreover it is also equipped with GPS module for the patient location in real time. Particularly it proves useful indefinite places such as nursing homes and rest homes for elderly people. However by using a mobile phone the system also allows transmission within a long range by GPRS/GSM.

All designed systems, prototyped and tested, are characterized by originality, by plainness of use, as they planned with a very high level of automation (so called "intelligent" devices).

2. Heart and lung auscultation system for diagnostic use on remote patients

Although there are already available instruments for the remote monitoring of ECG (Prolux et al., 2006), the contemporary Cardiac and Pulmonary tele-Auscultation (ACP) is not carried out yet for the lack of adequate instruments and clinical validation of the methods.

However the known tele-electrocardiographs are able to transfer the electrocardiograms only after the acquisition, not in real time and are mostly and strongly orientated towards the sanitary emergencies. In fact they are typically installed on ambulances and need a skilled staff for the utilization (Woolard et al., 2005) (Kyriacou et al., 2002).

On the other hand it is essential to observe the electrocardiogram is not the only source of information useful to evaluate the patient health.

It is obvious, therefore, that there is a rather limited offer of the current market with regard to the requirements which a health service should meet, if it is in the lead with regard to the effective potentialities offered by the present technology.

Particularly we recognize deficiency or total absence of reliable and valid telemedicine platforms which allow the follow up of patients and the execution of all the main vital parameters, such as electrocardiograms, spirometry, oximetry, cardiac tones, lung sounds, with a doctor in a different place regard to the patient.

In this paragraph we describe (Convertino et al., 2009) a medical electronic-computerized platform for diagnostic use, which allows the doctor to carry out a complete cardio-respiratory control on remote patients in real time. The system has been patented (Italian patent n.0001354840, 2009) and has been designed to be employed also to real-time rescue in case of emergency without the necessity for data to be constantly monitored by a medical centre, leaving patients free to move.

As if the doctor is present personally near the patient, the system allows him to receive in real time the following data:

1. auscultation of cardiac tones and broncho-pulmonary sounds
2. electrocardiogram
3. arterial blood pressure
4. oximetry
5. respiration frequency
6. phonocardiography
7. spirometry
8. image and audio of the patient with high quality.

The system consists of two parts: a patient station and a doctor position, both compact and light easily transportable, both are composed of committed laptop, hardware and software. The patient unit is equipped with miniaturized diagnostic instruments and is suitable also for paediatrics use. Many patient stations can correspond to one doctor position.

The system is modular and allows to select and to install some of the suitable diagnostic instruments, even though it is prearranged for the plug and play installation of the others (for example only the electrocardiograph can be installed and then also the phonendoscope, etc.).

The electrocardiogram could record up to 12 derivations and the software is able to interpret the data and to automatically carry out the reading and the diagnosis of the trace which should be confirmed by the doctor. It is possible to carry out monitoring without time limits and always in real time. This makes possible the capture of uneven heartbeats or also intermittent ones of other nature. The acquire trace is registered and filed.

The tele-phonendoscope is of electronic kind and obtains biological sounds in the [20 Hz, 1 kHz] frequency range and can be used in three modes in order to improve the cardiac and pulmonary auscultation: membrane, bell and extensive modality. Moreover, it allows the 75% suppression of the external noise.

It is equipped with software for the real time spectrum analysis and it starts automatically at the beginning of the auscultation procedure. The positioning of the phonendoscope is led by a remote doctor thanks to the full time audio/video communication and the biological sounds can be simultaneously heard either by the patient (or by an operator helping the patient in the examination) or by the doctor in remote.

The biological sounds are also registered during the acquisition with significant advantages for diagnosis accuracy and for possibility of carrying out diagnostic comparisons with previous records.

The tele-spirometer allows to carry out the FVC, VC, MVV tests and to determine the respiratory frequency and it is autodiagnostic.

The finger (optic) tele-saturimeter allows to carry out the monitoring (check without time limit) of the SpO_2 value as it is equipped with plug-in which permits the tracing of the saturation values curve that will be presented in real time to the doctor.

The filing of the data concerning the carried out examination occurs in a dynamic database both on the patient position and on the doctor position; the data will be filed by ordering them for each patient.

Thus to each patient a clinical record will be associated containing all his data. This kind of filing is very useful to carry out diagnostic comparisons on the evolution of a disease or on the outcome of a therapy, and it eases him of the burden of having the record documentation regarding him personally. In the patient database there is also a filed schedule containing the personal details of the patient, the case history in addition to various notes, values of blood tests, the outcome of other diagnostic tests, treatments undertaken during the time, therapy in course, etc.

This system also makes possible to transmit echograms, X-rays radiograms and other tests in digital form to the doctor and also their filing in the patient data base.
The doctor can also prescribe other subsequent clinical tests advised and/or treatments to undertake.
The system does not present connectivity limits of any kind find and requires a 320 Kb/s minimum band or a UMTS Mobile telephone.
The system has a user friendly software interface very easy to be used, which implements the one touch philosophy, and requires extremely reduced operating costs.
The patient can ask for a medical examination and the doctor can accept or refuse to examine him if busy. As a result of the doctor's availability, the medical examination can start and the doctor can ask for the necessary tests through a simple "click".
This system has been planned/designed in the observance of the current regulations for medical devices, informatic safety and privacy.
The system, therefore, is marked by three distinct and basic fundamental characteristics:

1. the real time data transmission by assuring the remote doctor the simultaneous control of the data during their acquisition;
2. the possibility to carry out a complete telematic medical examination, including the tele-auscultation, all the operations the doctor performs when he examines the patient directly at home or at the surgery and even more, since the system is equipped with typically diagnostic instruments not available at the family doctor but at hospital units;
3. the possibility to establish a continuous audio/video communication during the examination, in order that the same doctor can interact with the patient, verifying the correct positioning of the sensors and having also a very high quality image of the patient, which can be useful for diagnostic aims.

Among the most evident and important applications we can indicate the following ones:

1. home tele-assistance of cardiac patients in decompensation or of chronic patients with pathologies attributed to the cardio-circulatory or respiratory apparatus;
2. mass prophylaxis with complete cardio-respiratory control, frequently and at low cost;
3. tele-consultation;
4. follow-up of patients discharged early (precociously) and in need of tele-protection;
5. closed-circuit monitoring of the health of patients waiting for hospitalization.

The reduction of hospitalization time, using home tele-protection, and the avoided hospitalization of patients in decompensation monitored at home imply large economic saving. The shorter patient presence in hospitals reduce the waiting lists in a remarkable way.
Moreover there is today a growing need for inexpensive and reliable health monitoring devices (Jovanov et al., 2003). able to record data, to analyze them in real time and, if possible, to transmit them to a receiving unit by exploiting wireless technology, but the market still does not seem to offer any reliable GPRS or Bluetooth-based, effective and low-cost health-monitoring telemetric systems.
Although telemetric systems are already used in hospitals, they do not seem to fully exploit all the potential of modern technology and seem to suffer from some important limitations. In fact, many devices are specifically intended for emergencies (Pavlopoulos et al., 1998) and can transmit ECG results, as well as those from the monitoring of some other parameters. Such systems are inadequate for continuous health monitoring, not easy to use and have to be managed only by qualified operators, which makes them unsuited for personal use and domestic applications. Moreover one of the limitations of existing devices lies in the fact that they are not wearable and allow only to monitor ECG, saturation and some other

parameters separately, otherwise extraordinary bandwidth would be needed in order to transfer all data, especially via GSM (at the limited speed of 9200 kbit/s). GPRS and UMTS technologies result from the development of GSM transmission of packet data.

The combination of the latest suitable telecommunication solutions (GPRS and Bluetooth) with new algorithms and solutions for automatic real-time diagnosis, cost-effectiveness (both in terms of purchase expenses and data transmission/analysis) and simplicity of use (the patient will be able to wear it) can give the designed system useful for remote health monitoring, allowing real-time rescue operations in case of emergency without the necessity for data to be constantly monitored.

For this purpose the proposed system has been equipped with highly developed firmware which enables automated functioning and complex decision-making. It is indeed able to prevent lethal risks thanks to an automatic warning system. All this occurs automatically without any intervention by the user.

Each monitored patient is given a case sheet on a Personal Computer (PC) functioning as a server (online doctor). Data can also be downloaded by any other PC, palmtop or smartphone equipped with a browser. The system reliability rests on the use of a distributed server environment, which allows its functions not to depend on a single PC and gives more online doctors the chance to use them simultaneously.

The whole system consists of three hardware units and a management software properly developed. The units are:

- Elastic band: the sensors for the measurement of health parameters are embedded in an elastic band to be fastened round the patient's chest.
- Portable Unit (PU), which is wearable and wireless (GPRS/Bluetooth). This PU allows, by an Internet connection, the transmission, continuous or sampled or on demand, of the health parameters and allows the GPS satellite localization and the automatic alarm service, on board memory. Moreover PU has an USB port for data transfer and a rechargeable battery.
- Relocable Unit (RU): GPRS/Bluetooth Dongle (on PC server, i.e. online doctor).
- Management Software: GPS mapping, address and telephone number of nearest hospital, simultaneous monitoring of more than one patient, remote (computerized) medical visits and consultation service, creation and direct access to electronic case sheets (login and password)

Fig. 1 shows a picture of the PU. The very small dimensions are remarkable, even if it is only a prototype, realized at the Electronic Devices Laboratory of Polytechnic of Bari, and more reduction in dimensions is still possible.

The system, in particular the PU, collects data continuously. These are stored in an on-board flash memory and then analyzed real-time by an on-board automatic diagnosis software. Data can be sent to the local receiver, directly to the PC server (online doctor), or to an internet server, which allows anyone to download them once identified with his/her own login and password.

Data can be transmitted as follows:

1. real time continuously
2. at programmable intervals (for 30 seconds every hour, for example)
3. automatically, when a danger is identified by the alarm system
4. on demand, whenever required by the monitoring centre
5. offline (not real-time), downloading previously recorded (over 24 hours, for example) data to a PC.

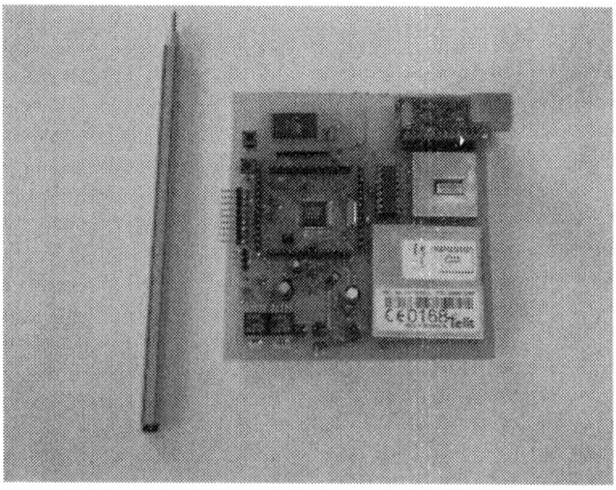

Fig. 1. A picture of the Portable Unit.

In all cases patients do not need to do anything but simply switching on.

When an emergency sign is detected through the real time diagnosing system, the PU automatically sends a warning message, indicating also the diagnosis, to one person (or even more) who is able to verify the patient health status and arrange for his/her rescue. In order to make rescue operations as prompt as possible, the PU provides the patient's coordinates using the GPS unit and the Management Software provides in real time a map indicating the position of the patient, as shown in Fig. 2.

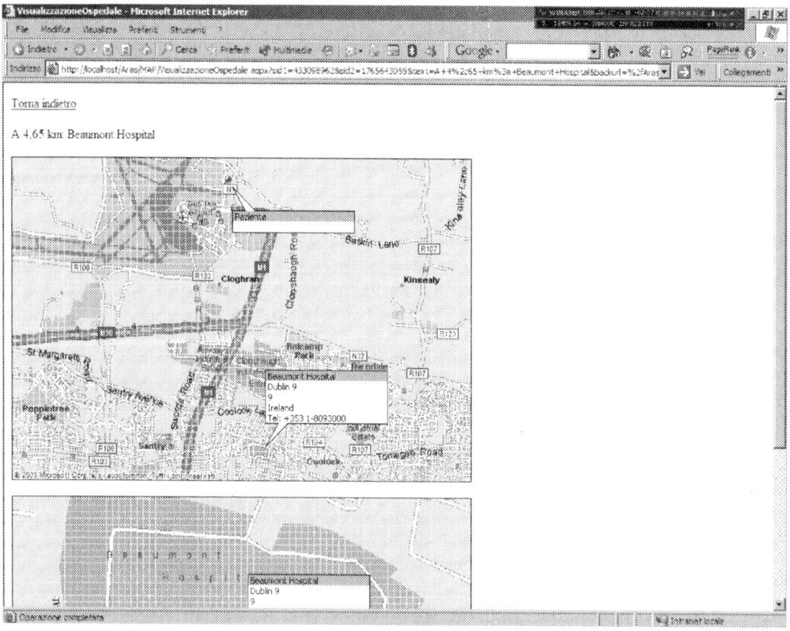

Fig. 2. GPS mapping with address and telephone number of nearest hospital.

Fig. 3 shows a picture of an electrocardiogram transmitted by Bluetooth and plotted on a Personal Computer by the proper developed management software.

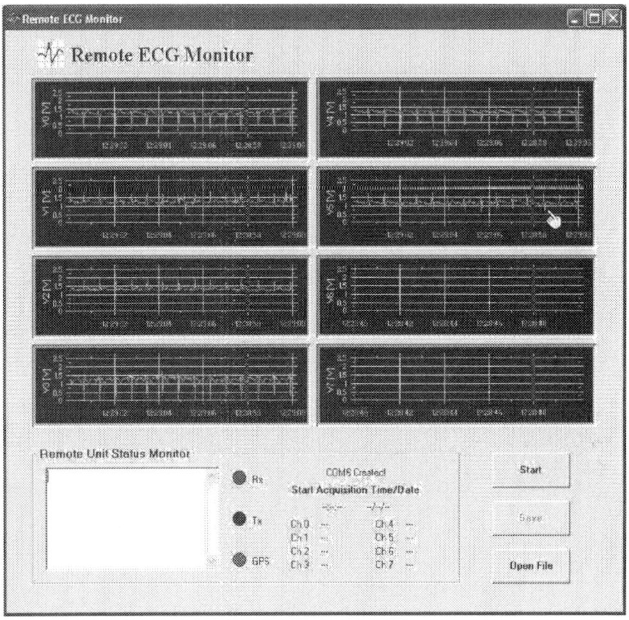

Fig. 3. Example of acquisition by Bluetooth of an electrocardiogram.

The system, in its version for diagnostic use, has been used in a routine clinical context in order to evaluate the feasibility and accuracy of the ACP carried out via Internet compared with the traditional auscultation (T).

At the Cardiac Decompensation Unit of Bari Polyclinic 21 patients (16 males, 5 females, in stable clinical conditions) have been examined. Each patient has been examined by two experienced heart specialists (Obs1 and Obs2) in two successive phases (I-ACP and T-ACP). The I-ACP check-up has been carried out by the instrumentation which the system is equipped with. The audio signal of high quality obtained from the cardio-pulmonary auscultation has been transmitted on internet through a standard ADSL connection from a patient position to a remote doctor position. The observer was able to listen and simultaneously record an audio file (WAV Format) of the ACP. A trained nurse placed the membrane on two auscultations spots under the visual guide of the doctor by means of a properly positioned webcam. The T-ACP check-up has been carried out with a traditional sound phonendoscope. The listened reports were recorded in a data file with preclassified reports. The obtained data have been analysed in terms of uniformity and examined with fisher's exact test ($p < 0,05$) and the kappa-test (where applicable).

In Tab. 1 the data of the ACP carried out both via internet and in a traditional way have been shown for the observer 1 and for the observer 2 (intra-observer analysis).

Moreover, the data registered by the two observers according to the two different ways of check-up (intra-observer analysis) have been compared.

Cardio pulmunary auscultation
Acoustic vs web
Intra-observer / inter-observer analysis

	Obs 1	Obs 2	Web	Acoustic
Total	217/231 (93.9%)	214/231 (92.6%)	224/231 (97.0%)	219/231 (94.8%)
Cardiac	81/84 (96.4%)	79/84 (94.0%)	79/84 (94.0%)	83/84 (98.8%)
Pulmonary	60/63 (95.2%)	59/63 (93.7%)	59/63 (93.7%)	62/63 (98.4%)
Cronology of systolic murmurs	19/21 (90.5%) k=0.82	18/21 (85.7%)	17/21 (81.0%)	19/21 (90.5%) k=0.82
Inspiratory crepitations	20/21 (95,2%) k=0.64	19/21 (90.5%)	20/21 (95.2%)	21/21 (100%) k=0.47

Table 1. Data of the ACP carried out both via internet and in a traditional way.

The intra-observer concordance of I-Vs IACP (number of concordant reports, (%)) for the observer 1 and the observer 2 have been respectively:

- 217/231 (93.9%) and 214/231 (92.6%) (ns) for the total reports,
- 81/84 (96.4%) and 79/84 (94.0%) (ns) for the cardiac reports,
- 60/63 (95.2%) and 59/63 (93.7%) (ns) for the pulmonary reports.

The intra-observer concordance of observer 1 has been 19/21 (90.5%, kappa = 0,82) for the chronology of the systolic murmurs and 20/21 (95.2%, kappa = 0,64) for teleinspiratory crepitations.

The inter-observer concordances for I-Vs T-ACP have been respectively:

- 224/231(97.0%) versus 219/231(94.8%) (ns) for the total reports,
- 79/84(94.0%) versus 83/84 (98.8%)(ns) for the cardiac reports,
- 59/63(93.7%) versus 62/63(98.4%) (ns) for the pulmonary reports.

The detailed analysis of each specific typology of report has been carried out.

The cardiac and pulmonary auscultation, evaluated in our series of cases through concordance analysis, has shown a high concordance of pulmonary and cardiac listener reports both for the traditional approach and for the telemedicine one via Internet.

The intra-observer and inter-observer concordances have not been significantly different for the two observers in the two operational contexts, showing that the cardiopulmonary auscultation with our system is an innovative diagnostic method able to improve the present procedures of telemonitoring.

3. Multichannel system for electronic auscultation of the pulmonary sounds

In this paragraph we describe a low-cost, electronic medical device for the non-invasive continuous real-time monitoring of breathing functions, designed by us within a research program on the remote and non-invasive monitoring of the health, which has been developed at the Electronic Devices Laboratory of the first Faculty of Engineering at Bari Polytechnic, with the support of national university medical centres (Marani et al., 2010).

The system diagnoses respiratory pathologies by the electronic three dimensional (3-D) auscultation of lung sounds (Sovijärvi et al., 2000) (Earis et al., 2000), performing a correlation between lung sounds and diseases.
A block diagram of the designed device is shown in Fig. 4.

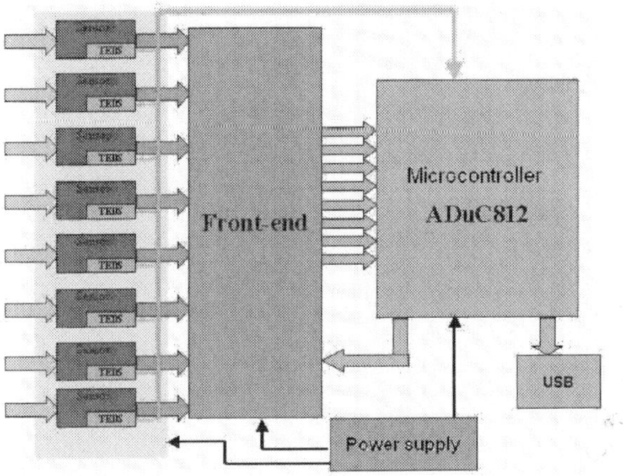

Fig. 4. Block diagram of the designed device.

The signals, coming from analog sensors, are suitably processed by the front-end and sampled at 1 KHz frequency and, then, converted into digital format with 12-bit resolution, therefore guaranteeing high noise immunity.
The Front-End processes the signal to adapt the voltage values coming from the sensors to the input dynamic range (between 0 V and 2.5 V) of the Analog-Digital Converter (ADC) included into the microcontroller.
Sensors can be unipolar (i.e. output voltages can be only positive or negative) or bipolar, where both positive and negative voltages are present. In both cases, the output signal amplitude can be greater than 2.5 V, if each sensor includes an integrated amplifier.
The Front-End must diminish or amplifier the signal coming from each sensors, depending on its level and the input dynamic range of the ADC. If the signal is bipolar, a level shift is required to obtain a new signal greater than zero.
Since the signal processing depends on the sensor features, several shift-voltage values, each time determined by the microcontroller, have to be simultaneously produced (Kirianaki, 2002).
Moreover, the gain of the amplifier has to be dynamically changed.
We have used only two programmable integrated circuits, controlled by a low-cost and high reliability (with particular reference to thermal drift phenomena) microcontroller, by implementing a device self-configuration procedure of the device to avoid any further maintenance work (such as calibration, front-end setting) by the user.
Microcontroller is required to program the Front-end functions, depending on sensor type, recognized by means of the implemented plug and play. The *Three Wire Serial Interface* Connections protocol has been used to establish a dialog between the Front-End and the microcontroller.

We have used the ADuC812 Microcontroller, produced and distributed by *Analog Devices*, a low-cost device, which is very suitable to the design specifications.
A block diagram of the ADuC812 is shown in Fig. 5.

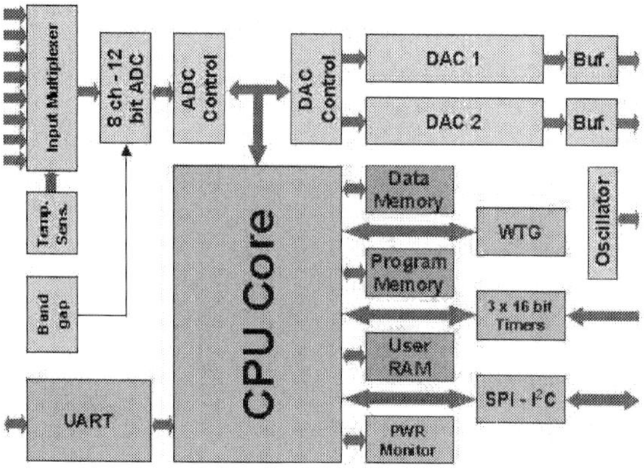

Fig. 5. Block diagram of the ADuC812 Microcontroller.

The Microcontroller allows the data acquisition from 8 multiplexed channels, at a sample frequency up to 200 KHz, and can address up to 16 MB of external data memory. The core is a 8052 compatible CPU, asynchronous output peripherals (UART) and synchronous serial SPI and I²C.
The Sensor Plug and Play has been realized through implementation of IEEE standard P1451.4, with *1-wire system* Communication Protocol.
Each sensor includes a transducer electronic data-sheet (TEDS), which stores the most significant informations relevant to the sensor type (manufacturer, offset, output range, etc). Based on the stored data, microcontroller identifies the sensor and sets the Front-End device to suitably process the signal and perform the Analog-Digital conversion in very accurate manner. Each TEDS is a serial type Electrically-Erasable-Programmable Read Only Memory (EEPROM), connected to the microcontroller by only two wires.
The realized prototype is shown Fig. 6.

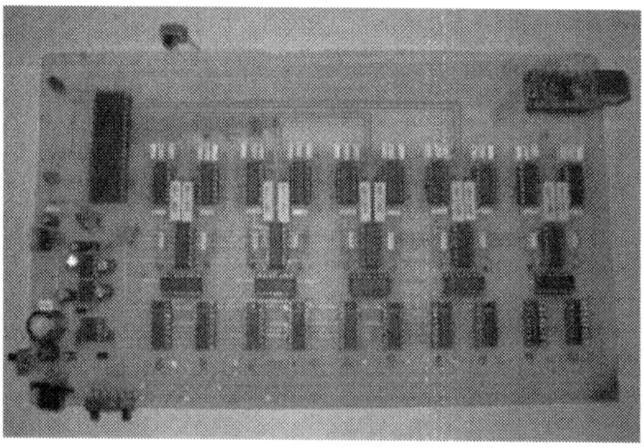

Fig. 6. The prototype: a double-sided printed circuit board.

The device, characterized by compactness and small-size, performs self-configuration, data-acquisition and conversion, data transfer to a Personal Computer and post-processing (such as ventilator setting). All the data can be processed in real time, but an external memory support can be used to realize a data-bank accessible from any PC.
Fig. 7 shows the graph of a signal both while recording it (real time) and after saving it.

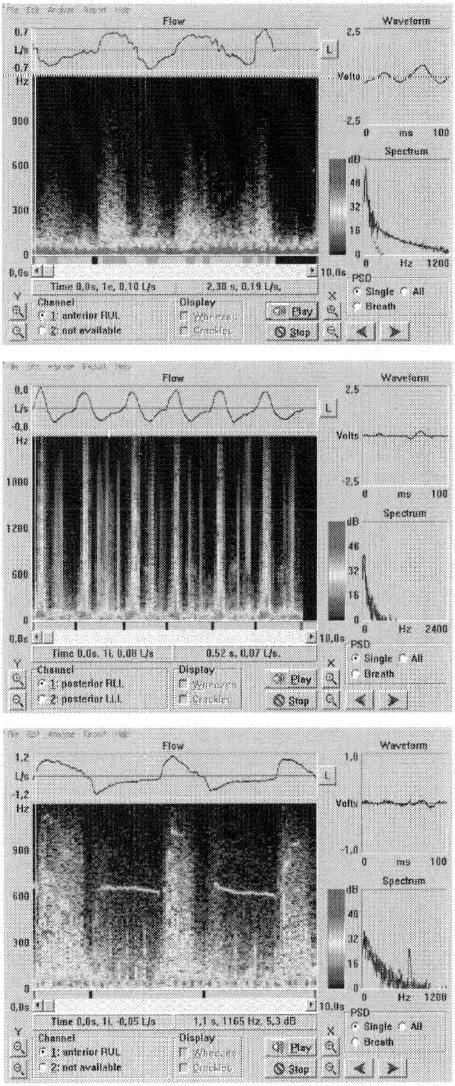

Fig. 7. Graphs of some lung sounds (respectively *Normal, Crackle, Wheeze*).

A research (Grasso et al., 2000) has pointed out the effectiveness of the frequency analysis of lung sounds for the diagnosis of pathologies.
The experiment illustrated below shows that computerized tomography (CT) results perfectly match those of a simple frequency analysis of previously recorded lung sounds.
Some studies (Vena et al., 2002) have been carried out on the frequency analysis of lung sounds and researchers have set the threshold for the detection of pulmonary pathologies at 500 Hz (see Fig. 8).

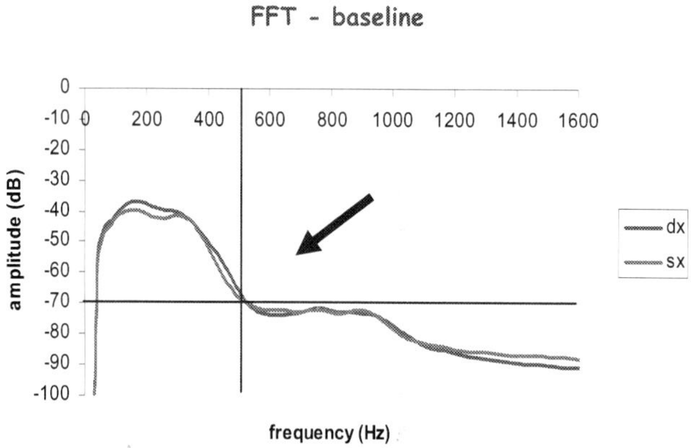

Fig. 8. FFT – spectrum of a lung sound in a patient with no pulmonary pathologies.

Spectrum components over that threshold (500 Hz) may be indicative of pulmonary disease.
It is widely known that in patients treated with mechanical ventilation a gradual PEEP increase (PEEP = positive end-expiratory pressure) results in a progressive re-expanding of alveoli which were previously collapsed due to a pathology.
The obtained experimental results, reported in Fig. 9, show that a gradual PEEP increase – from 5 to 20 – has effected a gradual reduction in lung damage, thereby leading to improvement in the patient's respiratory health.
The CT results, shown in the first column, perfectly match those of the frequency analysis on the right.
Moreover, there are also research projects about pulmonary acoustic imaging for the diagnosis of respiratory diseases. In fact, the respiratory sounds contain mechanical and clinical pulmonary information. Many efforts have been devoted during the past decades to analysing, processing and visualising them (Kompis et al., 2001).
We can now evaluate deterministic interpolating functions to generate surface respiratory acoustic thoracic images (Charleston-Villalobos et al., 2004) (Marani et al., 2010).
Moreover the following options are available:

- temporal graph of a breathing sound
- frequency graph of a breathing sound
- spectrogram of a breathing sound
- temporal graph of the airflow
- measurement of both airflow and inspiratory/expiratory volume.

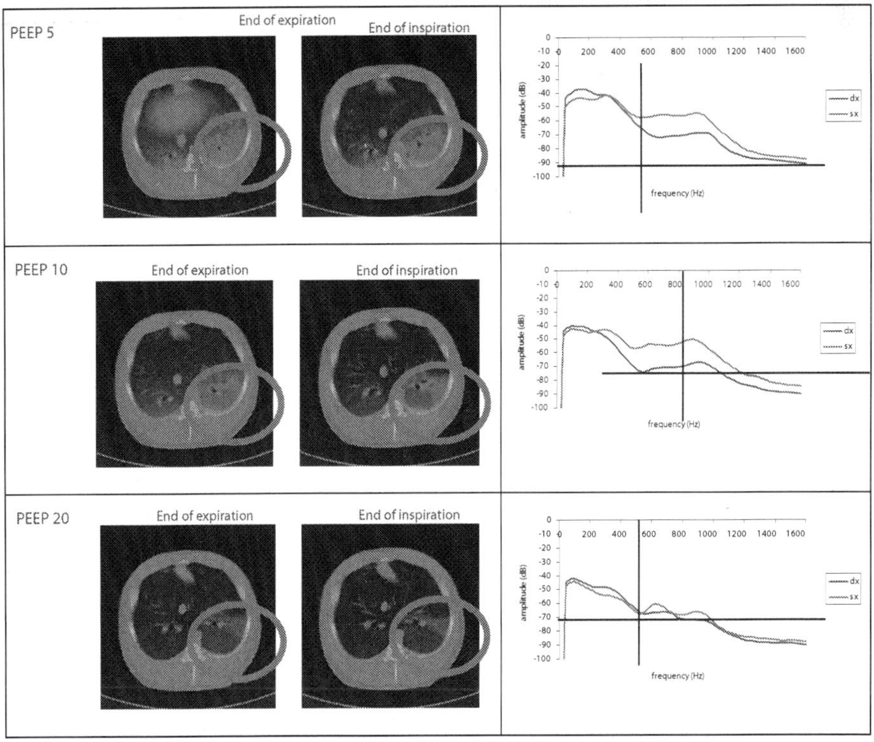

Fig. 9. Correlation between CT results and spectrum analysis of lung sounds.

4. A system for continuous monitoring of breathing and kinetic activity

In physical activity monitoring often only one parameter at a time is detected (Welkowitz et al., 1976) since otherwise patient movement capabilities would be compromised. This is unsatisfactory since correlation among parameters is necessary to reject parameters alteration due to everyday life, but also it is necessary to detect correlated parameter alteration due to medical causes. Let's think about how everyday activities could modify heart rhythm, breathing rate and body temperature.

Moreover the employed sensors have to be very light, non-invasive and absolutely compatible with the ordinary day activities.

In this paragraph we present a new system for acquiring simultaneously some health parameters which are strongly correlated: breathing rate and kinetic activity.

The system is based on a couple of sensors, which are very light, absolutely non- invasive, and compatible with everyday life.

For breathing sensing we use the already known method, the plethysmography (Konno et al., 1967) involving a belt to sense the thorax dilatation, but, in order to eliminate the practical inconveniences due to the presence of metal coils on the thorax, we apply a new kind of dilatation sensor on the belt based on a conductive rubber, which is new in breathing detection, quite cheap and sensitive.

Breathing rate observation is quite useless when no information is available on patient activity that could cause breathing rate change. Therefore we present also a kinetic activity sensor based on commercial accelerometer.
Signals from these sensors are amplified, filtered and elaborated and feed to the ADC of a micro-controller.
Experimental results, as we will illustrate later, have shown a clear correlation between these signals. The evaluation of correlation between breathing rate and kinetic activity requires a complex mathematical procedure, which is currently under development. Actually we can assert that the breathing and kinetic activity monitoring allows in particular to better understand the origin of tachypnea events whether they come from physical activities or not. Furthermore, in patients with lung and heart diseases, it is very useful for the doctor to understand when tachypnea begins during physical activities, and how long it persists after the subject stops.

4.a Breathing monitoring

In past years two main methods for breathing monitoring have been developed (Webster, 1998) (Moore et al., 2004) (Tarassenko et al., 2002). In the first method, the air flow is sensed while in the second one the breast dilatation is sensed.
Air flow monitoring is accurate but is very uncomfortable, since it requires tubing or placing sensors both in mouth and in nose (Lay-Ekuakille et al., 2010) (Wei et al., 2010). This would rule out 24 hours logging. For our project we are so forced toward the breast dilatation monitoring, which may be quite less accurate and very sensitive to arms movements but is much more comfortable.
For breast dilatation monitoring, piezoelectric strain gauge sensors are quite problematic (Bonato, 2003) since the charge generated at typical breathing frequencies (0.25 Hz) can be difficultly amplified. Moreover the temperature effect and the ageing on these sensors may produce a drift of the direct component of the signal. This problem could be solve by the introduction of a low-frequency filter, having a cut-off frequency less than breathing one.
Accelerometers are not suitable, because the tiny breathing acceleration available (about 0.02 g) is much smaller than the gravity acceleration g and body movement acceleration.
Breast dilatation monitoring is well accomplished using a breast elastic belt (Kim et al., 2006) so sensing the belt stress makes sense breathing possible.
Aside from several stress sensors we have designed a new, very interesting conductive rubber sensor, being it also quite cheap and easy tailored. Conductive rubbers are made by mixing carbon or iron powder in the chemical reactants used to produce rubbers. They have been applied as flexible conductors and as pressure sensors, but we did not found application as dilatation sensors. Indeed conductivity of these rubbers are sensitive to stress, but among the large kinds of conductive rubbers available, not all are suited for this application.

4.a.1 The conductive rubber selection

We look for conductive rubber satisfying these specifications:

- high sensitivity to the stress
- rubber should stand the stress applied to the breast belt, about 10 N
- moderate resistivity, between 0.1 Ω·m and 10 Ω·m.

This value range of resistivity depends on measurement problems, as the sensor is supplied at constant current. In fact, for low values of resistivity, either we would have a low voltage to the sensor and therefore an amplifier would be necessary, or higher currents would be required with consequent higher battery consumption not suited for an apparatus to wear for 24 hours. On the other hand, for high values of resistivity, we could have some reliability problems regards to the rubber contacts (Fig. 10), which would have an higher area.

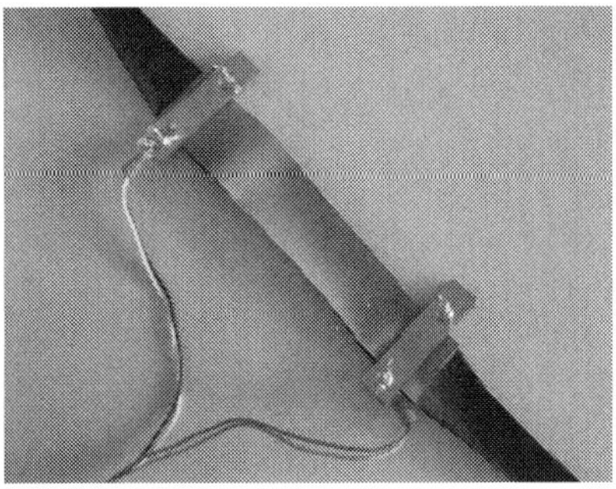

Fig. 10. Rubber contacts.

We have used a sample of conductive rubber, from Xilor, whose resistivity was only $7{\cdot}10^{-5}$ $\Omega{\cdot}m$, constituted by an aggregate of small conductive spheroids, about 20 μm wide, as shown in Fig. 11, in which it is clear the structure composed of microspheres of rubber.

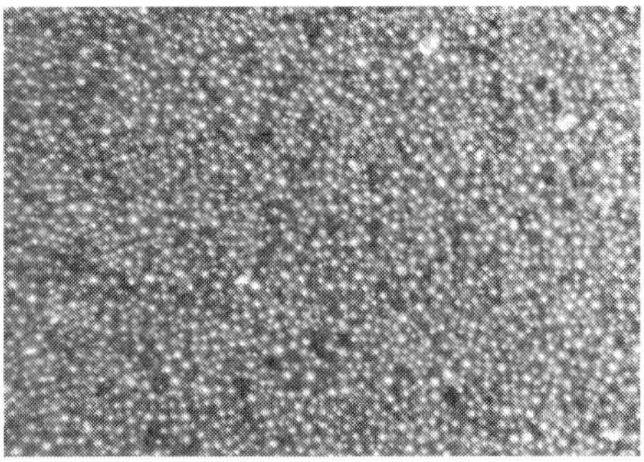

Fig. 11. Microscopic view of the used conductive rubber on a broken side (visual field is 2 mm x 1.5 mm).

This figure has been taken by an optical microscope of our Electronic Devices Laboratory. The resistivity is controlled by the contact surface area between spheroids. This area varies according to the mechanical stress, so that resistivity is very sensitive to the mechanical stress. This material did not satisfied our initial request, because it is not so strong and has a low resistivity, but the sensibility was so high that we have selected this material to develop our prototype.

We took a sample of Xilor rubber 120 mm long, 20 mm large and 0.3 mm thick that was fit in the breast belt, at the place of a piece of belt. Since the sample is not capable to stand all the belt stress, it is not feasible a full belt built only with this kind of conductive rubber. To solve this problem we have added an ordinary non conductive rubber in a mechanical parallel to this sample of Xilor rubber. We are also looking for conductive rubbers having both the sensitivity and the mechanical strength, but our actual solution with two rubbers is very satisfactory since it splits the mechanical and the electrical problem leaving us more degrees of freedom in the rubbers choice, requiring just a small amount of the more expensive conductive rubber.

Moreover, in this way we can reduce another ageing problem, due to the time variation of the rubber sensibility. Since the sensor is not expansive, we foresee a disposable use of the sensor to overcome the rubber ageing.

Two couples of small iron plates were tightened to each end of the rubber sandwich to ensure electrical connections, as shown in Fig. 10.

4.a.2 Electronic interface and experimental results

The resistance of conductive rubber, about 1 Ω, was measured with the four wires method, two wires to inject a constant current, two wires to sense the voltage. We have not used the well known Wheatstone bridge method because the sensor resistance drift, due to the ageing, could require a continuous bridge balancing and, above all, because the resistance variation is not small.

Since breathing rate ranges from 0.1 Hz to 3 Hz and chest movement signal is impulsive with frequency in the frequency range [0.4 Hz, 3 Hz] our front end amplifier was connected to the sensor through a first-order filter with a low cut off frequency at 0.4 Hz, in order to eliminate the low frequency noise of sensor, and the upper cut off frequency at 3 Hz. Moreover we have considered the low cut off frequency at 0.4 Hz because our prototype is particularly dedicated to sportsmen. Therefore we have considered the 3-Hz breathing rate, corresponding to 180 breaths per minute, to simulate also the transient breathlessness condition due to, for an example, a race. Furthermore it is possible to change the element values of the first-order filter to have a low cut off frequency at 0.1 Hz.

The amplified signal is sent to a peak detector (tuned for breathing rate frequencies), whose output pulses are sent to a peak shaper to have standard length pulses.

This output is already a good signal for breathing rate measurement, but, since we preferred to measure a voltage than a frequency, we feed the pulses in a frequency/voltage converter. A voltage signal for breathing rate measurement allows us to use the ADC of a microcontroller.

In order to have a breath by breath conversion, without contiguous period averaging, we have used the circuit shown in Fig. 12, whose key elements are an exponential-pulse generator and a Sample & Hold (S&H).

For each pulses coming from the previous circuit the exponential pulse generator is triggered, then the tail of this pulses is sampled just before the generator is re-triggered. The synchronization between the S&H and the generator is controlled by a negative edge triggered pulse generator which sends delayed pulses to the exponential generator. Since the exponential pulse is sampled before the reset, the voltage held to the output of the S&H is one to one function of the time length of the last breathing act, that is, in our case, a non linear map from [0 Hz, ∞ Hz] to [0 V, 2.5 V], as shown in Fig. 13.

As benefit no average between consecutive pulses is done and the output staircase waveform is useful for a slow ADC sampling. Since this signal is available only at the end of the breath, this is unsuited for triggering warning in case of breathing stop. Whether this warning would be needed, the output of the pulse shaper (or the output of exponential generator) would be used.

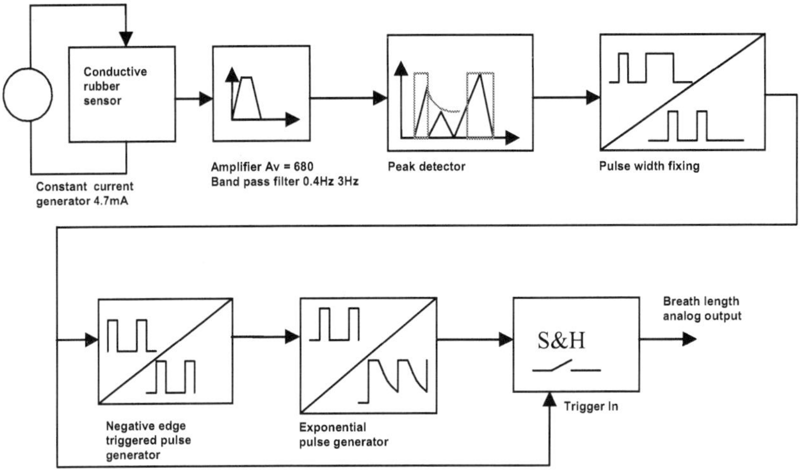

Fig. 12. Circuit used to have a frequency-voltage conversion.

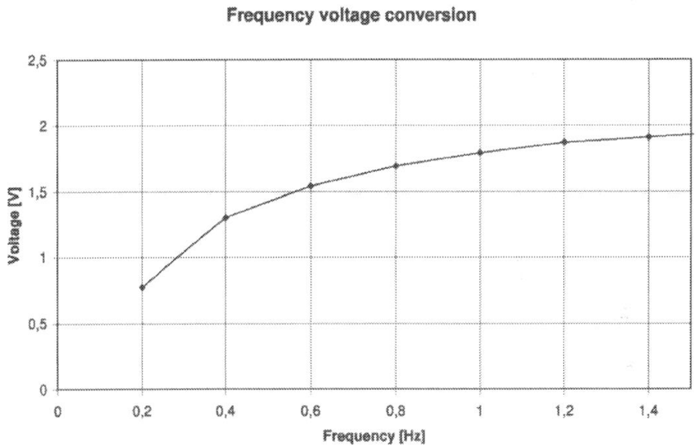

Fig. 13. Frequency voltage conversion diagram.

Using exponential generator, the map between the frequency and the voltage is nonlinear. This is not so bad, since nonlinearity could be corrected on the remote computer display and the exponential allows to map any time length to a finite voltage. Furthermore, since the output voltage is fed to an ADC, and because of the nonlinearity, the best resolution would be given at the most common breathing rate, while the uncommon rates would have lower resolution.

Of course, noise and time delay would cut off the far ends of the [0 Hz, ∞ Hz] range from the map, but the remaining interval is still wide: the system has been tested on the wide interval [0.05 Hz, 6 Hz].

Figs. 14 and Fig. 15 show the signal obtained with the described electronic set-up.

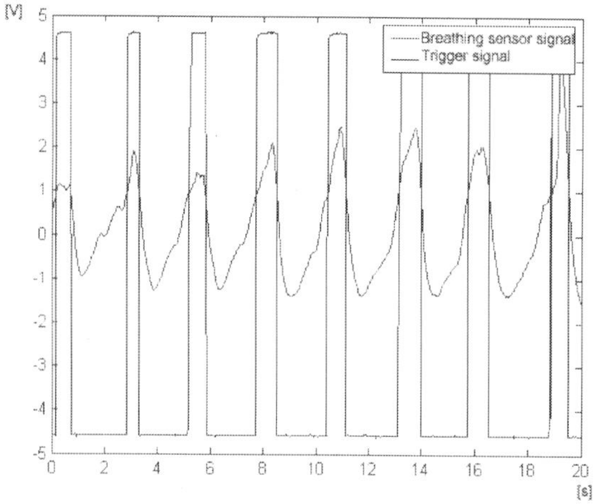

Fig. 14. Breathing act identification: the square pulses are from peak detector while the wavy signal is the amplified sensor signal.

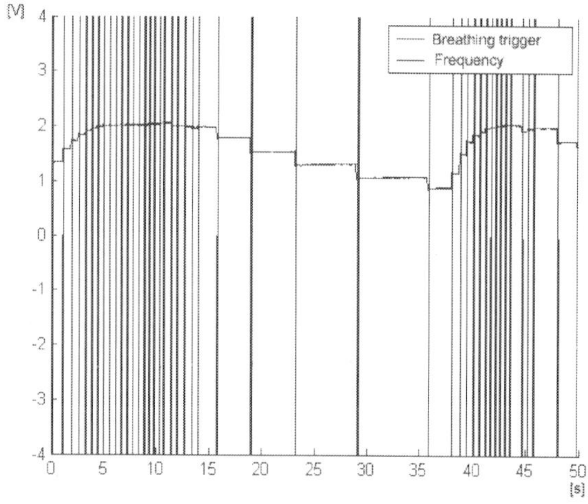

Fig. 15. Frequency measurement: the vertical pulses are trigger pulses from the pulse width fixing block, while the wavy line is the voltage converted frequency at the circuit output.

As shown in Fig. 14, the signal is clear and noiseless; it is also shown the signal from the peak detector which is well behaved.

The system has been successfully test on a wide breathing rates interval (see Fig. 15), but still the ageing problem remains.

In order to allow a test on a wider frequency range, Fig. 15 has been obtained using an electronic pulse generator whose signal was feed to the frequency voltage converter.

4.b Kinetic activity sensor monitoring

The physical activity is important also to understand the medical meaning of heart and breath dynamics. For example, let's think how the meaning of an high heart rate could be different whether the subject is running or standing.
Physical activity monitoring is also very useful to understand objectively the lifestyle of a patient to evaluate his daily energetic expenses.

4.b.1 Sensor

We have observed that root mean square (r.m.s.) values of acceleration (passed through a high pass filter) on the body surface is fully correlated with walking speed. Experimental data collected in previous experiences with other accelerometer, show that vertical acceleration on the shoulder of a running patient peaks from -1 g to 2 g, while power spectrum spans up to 20 Hz (Fig. 16). Peaks comes from each impact of feet on ground.
This signal includes a contribute coming from the gravity that is $g(\cos\theta)$ where θ is the angle between the sense direction of the accelerometer and the gravity. The variable θ is not constant at all when the accelerometer is fixed on the clothes of a patient but varies widely when a subject bows or stands up. Fortunately the power spectrum of θ is concentrated at frequency below 1 Hz, much lower than the frequencies of the acceleration of a walking or running patient. In conclusion it is necessary and also enough to use a high pass filter to cut off the gravity.

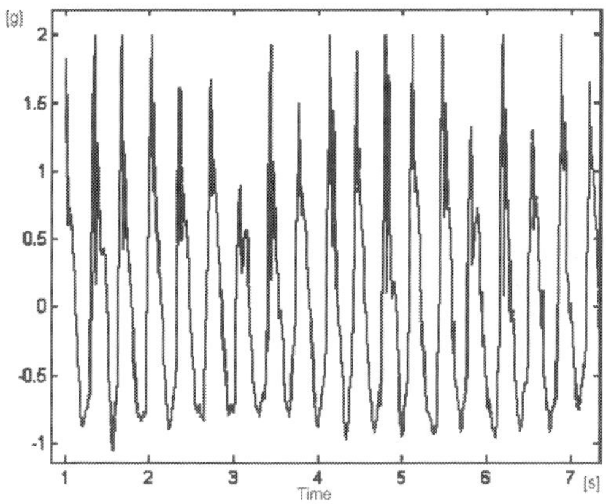

Fig. 16. Acceleration signal detected on a running man. The acceleration is measured in g = 9.81 m/s^2.

We have chosen the accelerometer ADXL103 (by Analog Devices) whose characteristics are ideal for our application. While the band is much larger than what we need (but this is not a problem), the noise density is low, 10^{-4} $g/\text{Hz}^{½}$, useful for good measurements. Its power dissipation is low, it takes 0.7 mA at 5 V, very useful since our system is battery powered. It is also quite cheap (about 9 $).
A particular explanation should be deserved to our interest in the sensitivity range: ±1.7 g. This is a bit lower than maximum measurement on a running patient, so this would cause accelerometer signal clipping and would create a progressive saturation of our circuit

output signal. We do not foresee a complete saturation, since this would happen only if the patient runs in a very heavy way.

This is not a real limitation, since a running patients could be statistically marginal and signal partial saturation would be marginal; furthermore for athletic application a new device would be used with larger sensitivity range and different tuning. On the other hand, the cut at ±1.7*g* cuts off the high acceleration peaks, up to several tens of *g*, coming from collisions of accelerometer with the environment. In absence of clipping, high *g* peaks could ruin the 24 hour averages of r.m.s. acceleration.

4.b.2 Electronic interface and experimental results

The signal chain is quite simple and requires a band pass filter to cut off low frequencies at 0.7 Hz (related to gravity) and high frequencies at 20 Hz to clean unforeseen unwanted signal outside the signal band. The upper part of Fig. 17 shows the output signal.

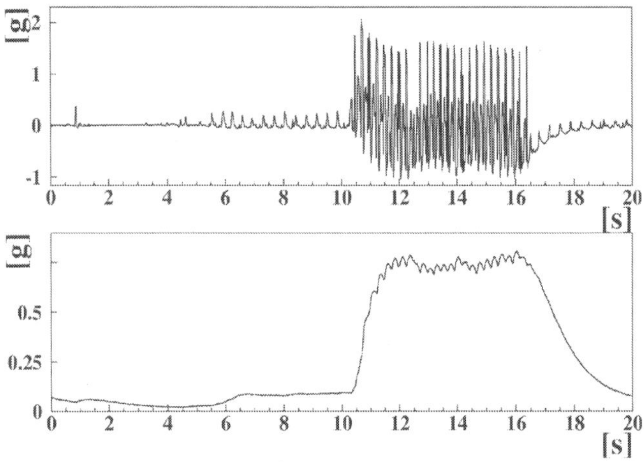

Fig. 17. Upper trace: accelerometer signal. Lower trace: r.m.s. filtered signal.

The filtered signal is passed to a cheap and effective r.m.s. converter, the AD737, whose precision is enough for our purposes. The r.m.s. converter output is filtered to cut off frequencies over 0.1 Hz to kill off the residual ripple observed on running patients. The lower part of Fig. 17 shows this signal.

The signal is clean and spanned voltage range is matched to input span of the ADC of our wearable unit.

Unfortunately the proposed system still presents some ageing problems (Marani et al., 2010).

Indeed the rubber resistivity raised tenfold after few hour of usage, when the rubber was fit in the belt with the dilatation method. While this could be compensated with an automatic gain control at the front end amplifier, it would be better to measure compression effects on rubber conductivity.

A second problem is the sensibility to the arms movements, which could trigger false breathing pulses. This is intrinsic to the belt method, but the effect is not so frequent compared to the breathing rate.

The proposed kinetic sensor, based on commercial accelerometer, has been tested on several subjects, for each patient it was clearly possible to recognized whether the subject was standing, walking or running.

The observed signal is correlated to the physical activity but also to the weight of the subject, and (we suppose) also the way subject walks. For simple qualitative analysis this is not a problem, but, if a quantitative analysis is required, a personal calibration would be performed, or simply a statistical parameterization of calibration on some biological parameter, e.g. weight, height, sex and age.

With this calibration, we hope that this physical activity measurement would allow a good quantitative estimator of the energetic expenses to what concern walking and running, and we hope that, using also other biological parameters to evaluate basic metabolism, it could be possible to estimate the daily energetic expenses.

This would be very interesting since available method that measure the CO_2, with mouth and nose tubing (Lay-Ekuakille et al., 2010) (Wei et al., 2010)., and the heat production (in a calorimetric box) are not suited for 24 hour measurements.

5. A system for holter applications with ECG transmission by Bluetooth

Today the most used tape-recorder type electrocardiographs for the long term registration provide the acquisition of two or three channels thus allowing the detection of a limited number of pathologies and missing crucial details relevant to the morphology of the heart pulse and the related pathologies, given only by a static ECG executed in the hospital or in medical centres (Carr et al., 2001) (Webster, 2004).

Moreover, the sampling frequency for the analog to digital conversion of the signal, for the best known portable ECG, is typically lower than 200 Hz, thus missing important medical data carried out by the electrocardiograph signal. Finally, the most used medical devices for long term registration (holter) of cardiac activity are generally so uncomfortable especially due to their dimensions.

Within our biomedical engineering researches, we have designed and prototyped a new medical device for holter applications intended to overcome the above mentioned limitations and to advance the state of the art.

In fact the designed device presents the following advantages:

1. data from up to 12 channels;
2. sensors, embedded in a kind elastic band;
3. possibility to place on the thorax many electrodes without reducing the movement potentials;
4. the elastic band mounting a wireless module (Bluetooth) (Senese, 2003) to send the data to the recorder/storage unit;
5. implementation of a diagnostics algorithm and/or to download, in real time, the data by UDP channel.

The system core is a microcontroller-based architecture. It is composed by: multiplexed internal ADC with a 12 bit resolution, 8K bytes Flash/EE program memory; 32 Programmable I/O lines, SPI and Standard UART. Normal, idle and power-down operating modes allow for flexible power management schemes suited to low power applications.

Fig. 18 shows the prototyped electrocardiograph recorder/storage unit.

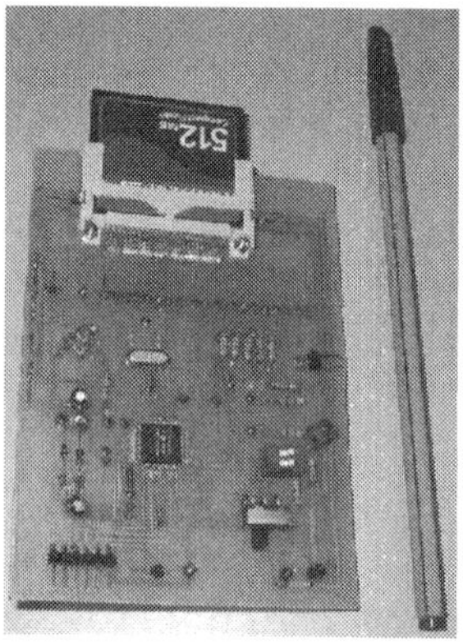

Fig. 18. Picture of the prototyped new electrocardiograph receiving unit.

The small dimensions are remarkable even if a further reduction is possible.
The management software to data-download has been properly developed by the us, being it custom for this application. It receives the data from the electrocardiograph and allows to store/plot them.
In Fig.19 a draft of an acquisition example is shown.

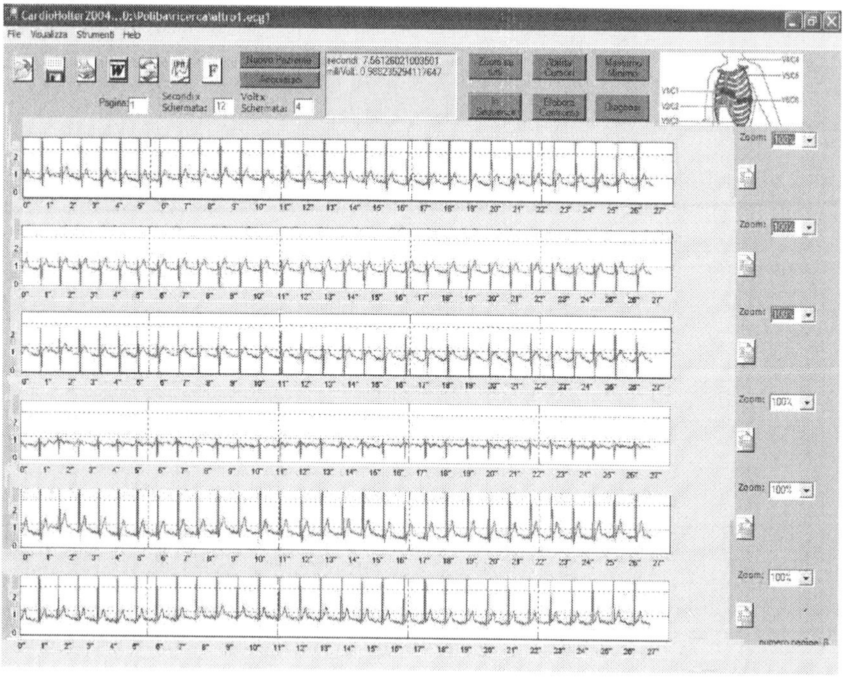

Fig. 19. An acquisition example of ECG.

The management software allows to view/plot one or more channels, to make a real-time automatic analysis of the incoming signal and to perform digital filtering. In fact the software performs the Fourier Transform of the incoming signal, useful to make a real time filtering if needed to improve the quality of the ECG. A wavelet filtering is also available. The operator has to evaluate only the frequencies to suppress, after seeing the Fourier Transform of the signal, and the software performs the signal filtering.
As regards the wireless module to send the data to the recorder/storage unit, Fig. 20 shows the relative prototype, realized at our Electronic Device Laboratory.

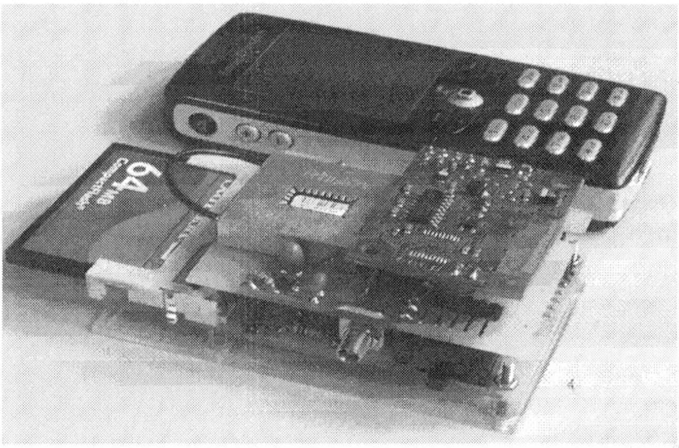

Fig. 20. System for ECG transmission by Bluetooth.

It is also equipped with GPS module for the patient location in real time.
It proves particularly useful indefinite places such as nursing homes and rest homes for elderly people.
However by using a mobile phone the system also allows transmission within a long range by GPRS/GSM.
The microcontroller permits to implement a diagnostics algorithm and/or to download, in real time, the data by UDP channel.
The tracing can be also stored on flash cards legible with any PC equipped with a reader of flash memories.

6. Conclusions

In this chapter we have presented a review of our principal projects in biomedical electronic field, developed at the Electronic Device Laboratory of the first Faculty of Engineering of Polytechnic of Bari, Italy, within a research program, with the support of national university medical centre.

Firstly we have proposed a medical electronic-computerized platform for diagnostic use, which allows the doctor to carry out a complete cardio-respiratory control on remote patients in real time. The system has been patented and has been designed to be employed also to real-time rescue in case of emergency without the necessity for data to be constantly monitored by a medical centre, leaving patients free to move.

We have also proposed a low-cost, electronic medical device, designed for the non-invasive continuous real-time monitoring of breathing functions.

Moreover we have presented a new system for acquiring simultaneously the breathing rate and the kinetic activity.

At last a new system for cardioholter applications, characterized by the possibility to send ECG by Bluetooth to 6 or 12 leads, has been described.

All proposed systems have been prototyped and tested.

7. References

She H.; Lu Z.; Zhou D.; Jantsch A.; Zheng L. (2007). A Network-based System Architecture for Remote Medical Applications. *Proceedings of the 23rd Asia Pacific Advanced Network (APAN) Meeting*, 2007, Manila, Philippines.

Prolux J.; Clifford R.; Sorensen S.; Lee D.; Archibald J. (2006). Development and evaluation of a Bluetooth EKG monitoring sensor. *Proceedings of the 19th International Symposium on Computer Based Medical Systems (CBMS)*, 2006, Salt Lake City, Utah.

Woolard M.; Pitt K.; Hayward A. J.; Taylor N.C. (2005). Limited benefits of Ambulance Telemetry in Delivering Early Thrombolysis: a Randomized Controlled Trial. *Emergency Medicine Journal*, 2005, vol. 22, pp. 209-215.

Kyriacou E.; Voskarides S.; Pattichis C. S.; Istepanian R.; Pattichis M. S.; Schizas C. N. (2002) Wireless Telemedicine Systems : a brief overview. *Proceedings of Healthcom 2002*, 2002, Nancy, France, vol.1, pp. 50-56.

Convertino A.; Marani R.; Perri A.G. (2009) Sistema di monitoraggio remoto continuo, non invasivo, della salute. Proceedings of @ITIM 2009, *Cagliari, Italy, pp. 205 - 214.*

Jovanov E.; O'Donnel Lords A.; Raskovic D.; Cox P.G.; Adhami R.; Andrasik F. (2003). Stress monitoring using a distributed wireless intelligent sensor system. *IEEE Engineering in Medicine and Biology Magazine*, 2003, vol. 1, pp. 49-55.

Pavlopoulos S.; Kyriacou E.; Berler A.; Dembeyiotis S.; Koutsouris D. (1998). A novel emergency telemedicine system based on wireless communication technology - AMBULANCE. *IEEE Transactions on Information Technology in Biomedicine*, 1998, vol. 2, no. 4, pp. 101-107.

Marani R.; Perri A.G. A New Pressure Sensor-Based Electronic Medical Device For The Analysis of Lung Sounds. *Proceedings of MELECON 2010*, Valletta, Malta, 25 - 28 April 2010.

Sovijärvi A. R. A.; Vandershoot J.; Earis J. E. (2000). Standardization of computerized respiratory sound analysis. *European Respiratory Review*, 2000, 10:77, p. 585.

Earis J. E.; Cheetham B. M. G. (2000). Future perspectives for respiratory sound research. *European Respiratory Review*, 2000, 10:77, pp. 641-646.

Kirianaki, M.V. (2002). *Data Acquisition Signal Processing for Smart Sensors*. John Wiley & sons, 2002.

Grasso S.; , Mascia L.; Trotta T.; Di Fonzio M.; Ribezzi M.; Puntillo F.; Ancona G.; Bruno F.; Fiore T.; Giunta F.; Slutsky A.; Ranieri M. (2000). Dynamic airway pressure/time curve analysis to realize lung protective ventilatory strategy in ARDS patients. *Intensive Care Medicine*, 2000.

Vena A.; Perchiazzi G.; Insolera G. M.; Giuliani R.; Fiore T. (2002). Computer analysis of acoustic respiratory signals, Modelling biomedical signals. *World Scientific Publishing*, 2002, Singapore, 60.

Kompis M.; Pasterkamp H.; Wodicka G. R. (2001). Acoustic Imaging Of The Human Chest. *Chest*, 2001, 120:1309–1321.

Charleston-Villalobos S.; Cortés-Rubiano S.; González-Camarena R.; Chi-Lem G.; Aljama-Corrales T. (2004). Respiratory acoustic thoracic imaging (RATHI): assesing deterministic interpolation techniques. *Medical & Biological Engineering & Computing*, 2004, vol. 42, No. 5, pp. 618-626.

Marani R.; Perri A.G. An Electronic Medical Device for Preventing and Improving the Assisted Ventilation of Intensive Care Unit Patients. *The Open Electrical & Electronic Engineering Journal*, 2010, ISSN:1874-1290, vol.4, pp.16 – 20.

Welkowitz W.; Deutsch S. (1976). *Biomedical Instruments: Theory and design*. Academic Press, New York, pp. 35-46.

Konno K.; Mead J. Measurement of the separate volume changes of rib cage and abdomen during breathing. *Journal of Appl. Physiol.*, 1967, vol.22(3), pp. 407-422.

Webster J. G. ed. (1998). *Medical instrumentation*. John Wiley & Sons, 1998.

Moore J.; Zouridakis ed. (2004). *Biomedical technology and devices handbook*. CRC Press, USA, 2004.

Tarassenko L.; Mason L.; Townsend N. (2002). Multi-sensor Fusion for Robust computation of breathing rate. *Electronics Letters*, 2002, vol. 38, no. 22, pp. 1314 – 1316.

Lay-Ekuakille A.; Vendramin G.; Trotta A. (2010). Spirometric Measurement Postprocessing: Expiration Data Recover. *IEEE Sensors Journal*, 2010, vol. 10, no. 1, pp. 25 – 33.

Wei C.; Lin C.; Tseng I. (2010). A Novel MEMS Respiratory Flow Sensor. *IEEE Sensors Journal*, 2010, vol. 10, no. 1, pp. 16 – 18.

P. Bonato P. (2003). Wearable sensors/systems and their impact on biomedical engineering. *IEEE Engineering in Medicine and Biology Magazine*, pp. 18-20.

Kim K.; Lee I.; Choi S.; Lee T.; Cha E. (2006). Conductive rubber belt to monitor respiratory changes. *Proceedings of IEEE SENSORS 2006*, EXCO, Daegu, Korea, pp. 74-76.

Marani R.; Gelao G.; Perri A.G. A New System for Continuous Monitoring of Breathing and Kinetic Activity. Submitted to *Journal of Sensors*, 2010.

Carr J.J.; Brown J.M. (2001). *Introduction to Biomedical Equipment Technology*, 4th Edition, Prentice Hall, 2001.

Webster J. G. (2004). *Bioinstrumentation*, John Wiley & Sons, 2004.

Senese B. (2003). Implementing Wireless Communication in Hospital Environments with Bluetooth, 802.11b, and Other Technologies. *Medical Device & Diagnostic Industry*, 2003.

28

Practical Causal Analysis for Biomedical Sensing Based on Human-Machine Collaboration

Naoki Tsuchiya and Hiroshi Nakajima
OMRON Corporation
Japan

1. Introduction

In general, human understand phenomena by considering causalities when they face any problem. In fact, many causal-based applications and solutions have been proposed in keeping with theoretical development.

For instance, in industrial domain, Furuta et al. proposed a training support system for plant operation in which trainee's knowledge is represented as two-layered model of task hierarchy and qualitative causality (1998). In medical domain, Thang et al. proposed a medical diagnosis support system based on oriental diagnosis knowledge (2006). In their approach, the causality among some subject's symptoms and their diagnostic outcome is described by using RBF neural network. Nakajima et al. proposed a generic health management framework named *Human Health Management Technology* which is applied to not only human being but also manufacturing process, energy consumption management, and so forth (2008b). In addition, Hata et al. suggested a concept named *Human Health Care System of Systems* which focus on health management, medical diagnosis, and surgical support. In the concept, the human health management technology is discussed from view point of system of systems engineering (2009). Thus, causality acquisition and its utilization among complex systems has a quite important role in optimal management.

On another front, from a viewpoint of theoretical development, lots of causal analysis theories have been proposed (Bishop, 2006). Bayesian network describes statistical causality among phenomena observed from certain managed systems, and the statistical causality provides inference and reasoning functions (Pearl, 2001). Graphical model visualizes causality among components in complex systems (Miyagawa, 1991). Fuzzy logic helps intuitive representation of causality which is experts' tacit knowledge (Zadeh, 1996).

As mentioned above, causal analysis theories and their applications and solutions in many domains have been improved for long time. However, causal analysis for designing sensors is not discussed enough yet. Thus, in this chapter, a role of causal analysis in biomedical sensing is discussed.

In the rest of this article, in section 2, the importance of human-machine collaboration in causal analysis is described. In the section, problems which we address in this chapter is defined. In section 3, a human-machine collaborative causal analysis is proposed. Then, in section 4 and 5, two kinds of biomedical sensing which employ the human-machine collaborative causal analysis are demonstrated, that is, visceral fat measurement and heart rate monitoring.

2. Problem definition and related works

In this section, the importance of human-machine collaboration in causal analysis is discussed from a viewpoint of requirements for practical biomedical sensing. And, problem definitions are discussed.

2.1 Requirements for biomedical sensing from a viewpoint of practical use

Considering practical usage, biomedical sensing has to be easy to use. In addition, it should be non-invasive, low-intrusive, and unconscious regarding consumers' home usage. For instance, X-ray CT is not available at home because of its X-ray exposure.

In addition, biomedical sensing is required to have not only measurement accuracy but also transparent measurement theory because it provides users with feeling of security besides informed consent (Marutschke et al., 2010). However, measurement accuracy becomes worse while measurement theory becomes too simplified. Thus, the satisfaction of accuracy and transparency should be considered while experts design certain biomedical sensing equipments.

Regarding the above-mentioned problem, a new designing process of biomedical sensing is proposed which employs causal analysis based on human-machine collaboration. In the next section, the human-machine collaboration is discussed, and its importance described.

2.2 Human-machine collaboration

As means for representing causality, many theories have been proposed, that is, Bayesian networks, graphical modeling, neural networks, fuzzy logic, and so forth. Additionally, as means for modeling cause-effect structure, lots of learning theories have been studied considering the characteristics of each theory (Bishop, 2006; Zadeh, 1996). Particularly, Bayesian network and graphical modeling are utilized for a variety of applications in the broad domain, due to transparency of the causality (Pearl, 2001).

These previous works show two primary approaches to causality analysis: one for generating causality based on experts' knowledge and then optimizing the causalities by using actual datasets, and the other for automatically processing a measured dataset and then modeling causalities based on the trend and statistics from the data. The former is based on experts' knowledge and has an advantage in understandability of the causality, but needs sufficient knowledge on a certain target system and much more efforts for modeling such a system with many components. Conversely, the latter provides subjective causality obtained from datasets and has an advantage of not requiring any knowledge from experts, but sometimes has difficulty in understanding the causality. Here, there could be another approach that makes use of benefits of both in order to effectively model causalities by using experts' knowledge during working with machines. This idea is considered an effort to achieve goals through human-machine collaboration (Tsuchiya et al., 2010).

2.3 Problems to be solved and related works

According to the above discussion in section 2.2, the causal representation process and its framework for causality acquisition based on human-machine collaboration has an important role in practical causality acquisition. Regarding causality acquisition process and its framework based on human-machine collaboration, a similar study has been shown in Knowledge Discovery in Databases (KDD) processes (Fayyad et al., 1996). KDD defined the process of knowledge discovery and data mining techniques. Nadkarni has proposed a

learning method with causal maps which is practically applicable in Bayesian networks, and then dividing the cause-effect structure into D-maps and I-maps considering independency among the causality (2004). Gyftodimos represented causality in a hierarchical manner and proposed a set of frameworks regarding the representation and inference for understandable relationships (2002). Tenenbaum et al. showed that a following process is effective for learning and inference in the target domain; treating the fundamental principle of the domain as something abstract, structuring it, and fitting the structure into the final measured data (2006). The authors proposed that hierarchical representation of causality among components which are obtained from certain target systems (Tsuchiya et al., 2010).
These studies have indicated that conceptualization of components is effective for acquiring significant causality. Thus, in the following section, an effective causal analysis process for practical biomedical sensing is proposed.

3. Practical causal analysis for biomedical sensing

To solve the problems which defined in the previous section, the proposed process represents a causality of target components with a conceptual model and evaluates the independency of the conceptual causality by employing experts' knowledge. Then, feature attributes and cause-effect structure are prepared in each independent subset of the causality. Finally, whole cause-effect structures of each subset are integrated, and the integrated cause-effect structure is fitted to the actual dataset. These process is executed via human-machine collaboration.

In the following, the detailed steps of the above causal analysis are determined.

Step 1. Illustration of conceptual causality based on measurement principle

The intuitive causality among components in the target system is represented by a directed graph based on experts' knowledge. The represented intuitive causality is determined conceptual causality.

Step 2. Causal decomposition based on experts' knowledge

The conceptual causality defined in Step 1 is decomposed into independent subsets by employing experts' knowledge including design information about the target system.

Step 3. Practical cause-effect structure formulation via human-machine collaboration

Firstly, in each subset of the conceptual causality, feature extraction is executed by combining components, multiplying by itself, and so forth. In the next, cause-effect structure among the prepared feature attributes is formulated. Then, the cause-effect structures are integrated according to the conceptual causality. And feature selection is conducted if necessary. At last, components in formulated cause-effect structures are optimized by using actual dataset.

In the following section 4 and 5, the proposal causal analysis process is applied to two kinds of biomedical sensing.

4. Visceral fat measurement by using bioelectric impedance

In the 21st century, declining birth rate and growing proportion of elderly people develop into more serious social problems in advanced nations. Not only solving the labor power reduction but also extending healthy life expectancy are the important challenge which human beings should address. In terms of the issue, primary prophylaxis has got lots of attention as an important activity to prevent lifestyle-related diseases.

According to such a social problems, metabolic syndrome has been recognized in advanced nations. Currently, the waist circumference, blood pressure, blood sugar, and serum lipid are evaluated for the primary screening whether the person is diagnosed with metabolic syndrome at the medical checkups. Here, the purpose of waist circumference is for screening visceral fat accumulation since it is well known that visceral fat area at abdominal level is strongly related to lifestyle-related diseases (Matsuzawa, 2002). However, the waist circumference reflect not only visceral fat but also subcutaneous fat, organs, and so forth. Thus, more accurate screening method is desired. On another front, in major hospitals, X-ray CT image processing at abdominal level is the gold standard (Miyawaki et al., 2005). However, X-ray CT has a serious problem of X-ray exposure.
Thus, non-invasive and low-intrusive visceral fat measurement is desired.

4.1 Measurement principle

Fig. 1 shows a X-ray CT image at abdominal level, and the visceral fat is located in the light grey area in Fig. 1. Therefore, the objectives of visceral fat measurement is to estimate the square of the light grey area.

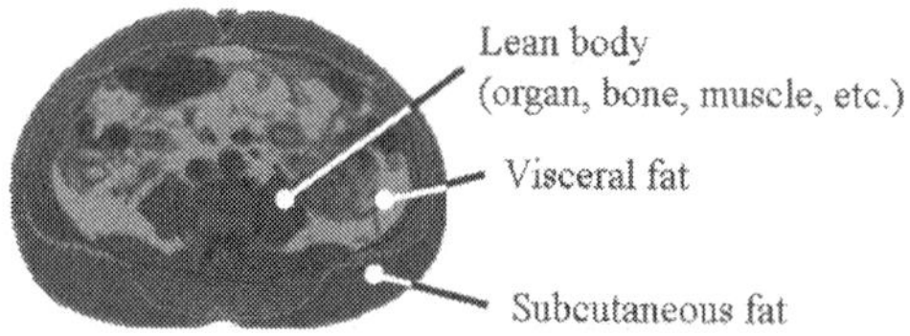

Fig. 1. Body composition at abdominal level

To measure the visceral fat area non-invasively, biomedical impedance analysis (BIA) has been employed (Gomi et al., 2005; Ryo et al., 2005; Shiga et al., 2007). BIA is famous for its consumers' healthcare application, that is, body composition meters, and has been studied by lots of researchers (Deurenberg et al., 1990; Composition of the ESPEN Working Group, 2004).
Considering each body composition in Fig. 1, the impedance of lean body is low since muscle comprised in lean body involves much water, and the impedance of visceral fat and subcutaneous fat are high. Thus, each area of body composition could be estimated independently by taking advantage of the impedance characteristics of each body composition.
The basic idea of visceral fat measurement via BIA is that the visceral fat area (VFA) S_v is estimated by reducing subcutaneous fat area (SFA) S_s and lean body area (LBA) S_l from abdominal cross-section area (CSA) S_c. This idea is illustrated in Fig. 2, and is formulated in equation (1).

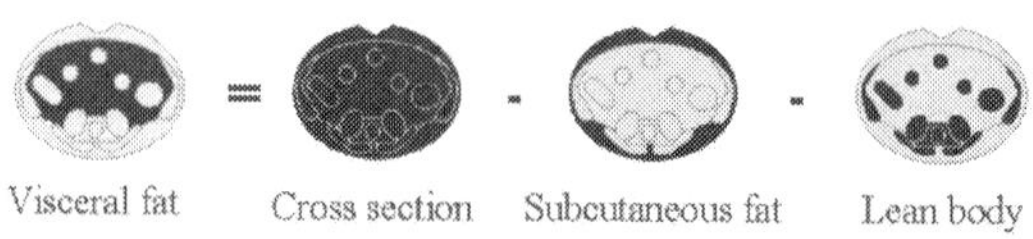

Fig. 2. Visceral fat measurement principle

$$S_v = S_c - S_s - S_l \tag{1}$$

where S_v, S_c, S_l are visceral fat area, subcutaneous fat area, and lean body area respectively.

4.2 System configuration

In accordance with the measurement principle, the visceral fat measurement equipment is implemented. The equipment obtains human's body shape and two kinds of electrical impedance at abdominal level.

At the beginning of measurement, the equipment measures human's body shape as shown in Fig. 3 and 4. Obtained a and b are body width and depth at abdominal level respectively.

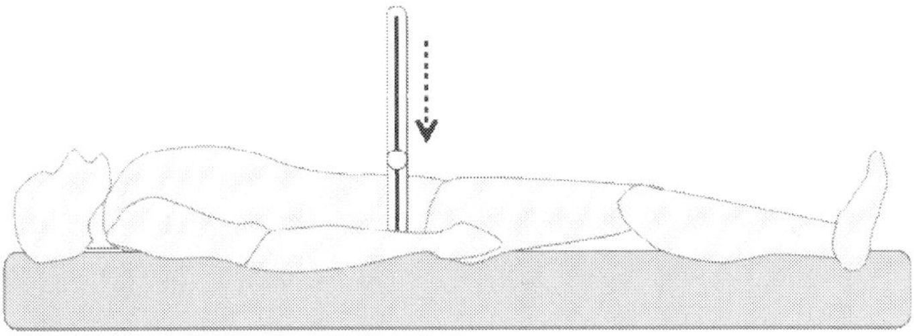

Fig. 3. Body shape measurement procedure

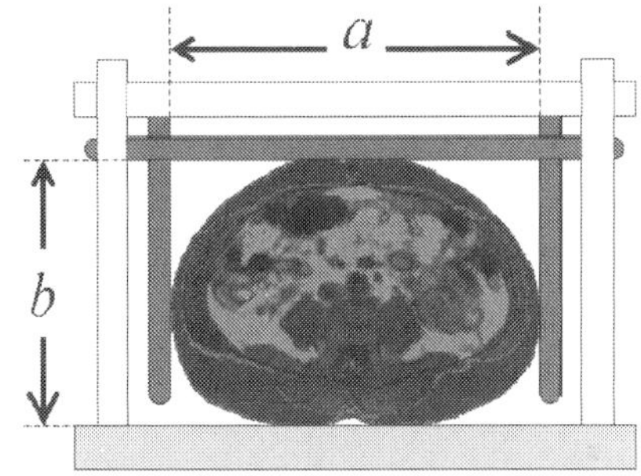

Fig. 4. Body shape information

In the next, the equipment measures two kinds of electrical impedance at abdominal level. Eight paired electric poles are placed on surroundings of the abdominal as shown in Fig. 5. And an weak current, 250 μA with 50 kHz, is turn on between subject's wrist and ankle as shown in Fig. 6. Then, eight impedances are obtained via eight paired poles, and their average is determined as Z_t.

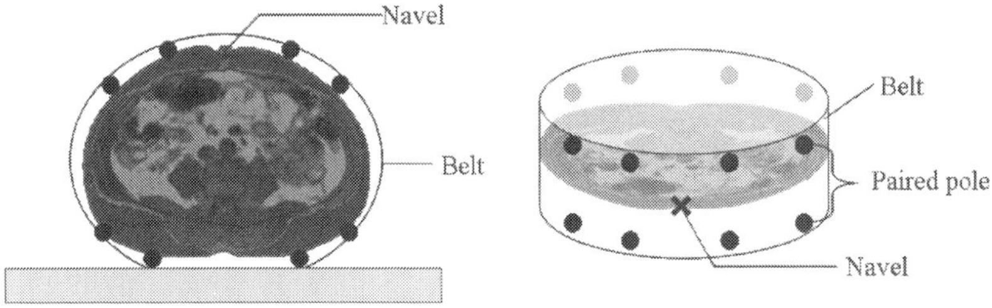

Fig. 5. Eight paired electric poles placed on surroundings of abdominal

After that, in the same manner, an weak current is turn on subject's surface at abdominal level via eight paired poles. And, eight impedances are obtained via eight paired poles as shown in Fig. 7, and their average is determined as Z_s.

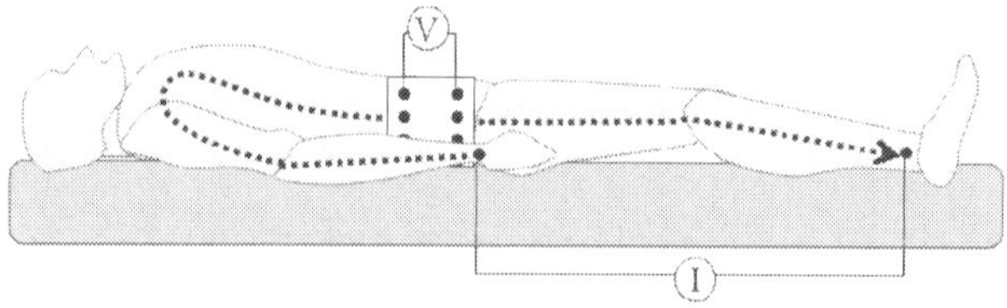

Fig. 6. Impedance Z_t measurement procedure

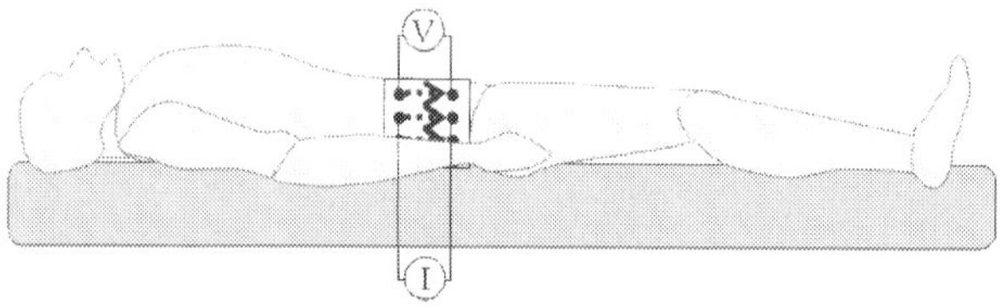

Fig. 7. Impedance Z_s measurement procedure

As a result, body shape a and b, two kinds of impedance Z_t and Z_s are acquired by using the implemented equipment.

4.3 Causal analysis via human-machine collaboration

Firstly, the actual dataset of 196 subjects was prepared before the following causal analysis. The dataset consists of 101 males and 95 females at age 49.0 ± 11.3 for males and 49.6 ± 11.3 for females. Two kinds of impedance Z_t, Z_s and body shape information a and b are calculated by using the visceral fat measurement equipment. In addition, VFA S_v , LBA S_l , SFA S_s , and CSA S_c are obtained by X-ray CT image processing as reference.

Step 1. Illustration of conceptual causality based on measurement principle

According to measurement principle and the equipment system configuration, the relationship among the set of obtained four components a, b, Z_t, Z_s and three kinds of body composition S_l, S_s, S_c is illustrated with a conceptual causality as shown in Fig. 8.

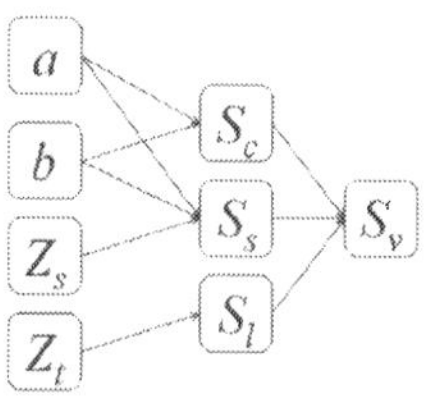

Fig. 8. Conceptual causality in visceral fat measurement

Step 2. Causal decomposition based on experts' knowledge

At first, according to the measurement principle, the causality among body composition is independent from four component obtained via the equipment. Thus, the subset consist of body composition is decomposed from conceptual causality. In the next, since S_c doesn't affect a and b directly, the subset consist of S_c, a, and b is decomposed from conceptual causality. In the same manner, the subset related to S_s and S_l is decomposed respectively. As a result, the conceptual causality is decomposed into four subsets in Fig. 9.

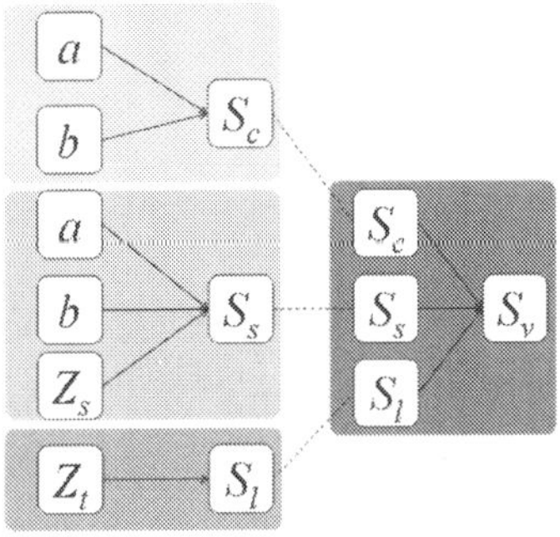

Fig. 9. Decomposed conceptual causality in visceral fat measurement

Step 3. Practical cause-effect structure formulation via human-machine collaboration
According to equitation (1) and the decomposed conceptual causality in Fig. 9, the cause-effect structure is formed in equation (2).

$$\tilde{S}_v = \alpha_1 f_c(a,b) + \alpha_2 f_l(Z_t) + \alpha_3 f_s(a,b,Z_s) + \varepsilon \tag{2}$$

Then, by assuming that the body shape at abdominal level is ellipse, feature attributes a^2, b^2, ab, $(a^2 + b^2)^{1/2}$, $1/Z_t$, $Z_s a^2$, $Z_s b^2$, and $Z_s(a^2+b^2)^{1/2}$ are prepared (Yoneda et al., 2008). By replacing the corresponding terms in equation (2) with these attributes, the following cause-effect structure can be acquired as shown in equation (3).

$$\tilde{S}_v = \beta_1 ab + \beta_2 1 / Z_t + \beta_3 Z_s a^2 + \beta_4 Z_s b^2 + \beta_5 Z_s (a^2 + b^2)^{1/2} + \varepsilon \tag{3}$$

where β_i are regression coefficients and ε is an error term. However, considering the complexity in the shape of the abdomen, it is not always true that employing all of the feature attributes included in equation (3) could result in over estimation. Thus, from the statistical viewpoint, we perform feature selection by employing Akaike Information Criterion (Akaike, 1974). As a result, the cause-effect structure in equation (4) is obtained.

$$\tilde{S}_v = \gamma_1 ab + \gamma_2 1 / Z_t + \gamma_3 Z_s b^2 + \gamma_4 Z_s ab + \varepsilon \tag{4}$$

where γ_i are regression coefficients and ε is an error term.

4.4 Experimental result and discussion

To compare performance, a experts' knowledge-based measurement model is prepared (Shiga et al., 2007), and is fitted to the sample dataset which is described in the previous section.

Table 1 shows comparison of accuracy of visceral fat measurement. In Table 1, *EM* and *ESD* indicate the mean of absolute errors and the standard deviation of estimated errors respectively, and *R* is the correlation between the X-ray CT reference and the estimated value.

According to the results, the improved estimation model provides higher performance in *EM* by 3.73 cm², in *ESD* by 5.03 cm², and *R* by 0.063. Thus, the proposed causality analysis process is proven to have enough performance to model a practical cause-effect structure.

	EM [cm²]	ESD [cm²]	R
Experts' knowledge-based model	20.369	26.702	0.826
Human-machine collaboration	16.638	21.676	0.889

Table 1. Visceral fat estimation performance comparison

5. Heart rate monitoring in sleep by using air pressure sensor

Among vital-signals, heart rate (HR) provides important information of humans' health transit such as an early stage of cardiac disease (Kitney & Rompelman, 1980). In addition, HR variability provides information of autonomic nerve activity (Kobayashi et al., 1999). Considering such values, continuous HR monitoring would have a quite important role in daily life. Thus, it is pretty important for us to measure our HR continuously to know its changes in our daily life.

Considering human's activities of livelong day, sleep has a high proportion. In addition, human being is in resting state in sleep. Thus, wealth of heart rate variability in sleep provides much information about human's health condition.

Currently, in a medical domain, an electrocardiography (ECG) is the gold standard for measuring HR variability accurately. However, ECG restricts human's free movement since many poles are put on body. Thus, ECG is hard to be used in sleep.

Thus, a low-intrusive and non-invasive continuous heart rate monitoring in sleep on lying on the bed is desired.

5.1 Measurement principle

To solve such a problem, HR monitoring equipment by using an air pressure sensor (APS) has been developed (Hata et al., 2007; Yamaguchi et al., 2007; Ho et al., 2009; Tsuchiya et al., 2009). Considering sleep condition, heartbeat causes pressure change of back. Thus, the basic idea of measuring heart rate monitoring is to extract heartbeats from pressure change of back. However, pressure change of the body is caused not only heartbeat but also roll-over, respiration, snore, and so forth. Thus, a new method to extract heartbeats from pressure change on back is required.

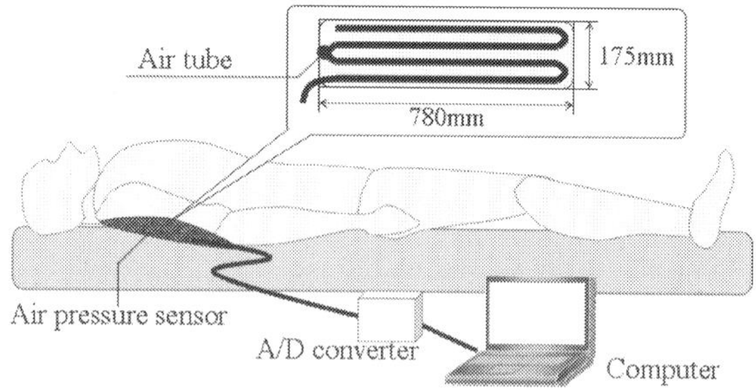

Fig. 10. Heart rate monitoring equipment

5.2 System configuration

The HR monitoring equipment measures body pressure variability x_{APS} via an APS to extract HR variability from the obtained pressure variability. Fig. 10 shows the configuration of the equipment. The APS composed of air tube, and is set under human's back on the bed. The characteristics of APS is drawn in Fig. 11. APS record pressure change at 100Hz, and quantizes pressure change into 1024 level via A/D convertor.

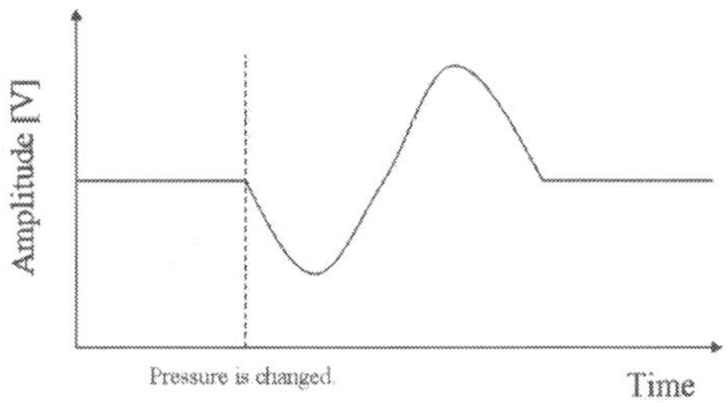

Fig. 11. Air pressure sensor characteristics

In HR monitoring, the heartbeats are detected and the HR variability x_{HR} is extracted from heartbeat intervals.

5.3 Causal analysis via human-machine collaboration

Firstly, the actual dataset of 8 subjects was prepared before the following causal analysis. The detailed profile of each subject is shown in Table 2.

Subject	Age [yrs]	Height [cm]	Weight [kg]	Gender
A	23	175	76	Male
B	23	171	68	Male
C	23	165	50	Male
D	25	171	56	Male
E	22	180	92	Male
F	22	172	55	Male
G	23	170	62	Male

Table 2. Profile of subjects

Each subject lied on bed for 10 minutes, and ECG is obtained for each subject while HR monitoring equipment measured pressure change of back.

Step 1. Illustration of conceptual causality based on measurement principle

According to the measurement principle, the conceptual causality among heartbeat x_{HB}, body movement x_{MV}, respiration x_{RSP}, obtained air pressure x_{ASP}, and heart rate x_{HR} is illustrated in Fig. 12.

In addition, according to the knowledge on heart rate that heart rate is defined by the interval of heartbeat, the conceptual causality is modified as shown in Fig. 13. It shows that HR variability is calculated from R-R interval τ_{RR} like ECG when R-waves τ_R.

Step 2. Causal decomposition based on experts' knowledge

Since the HR extraction from τ_R is generalized, the causality shown in Fig. 13 is decomposed into two parts as shown in Fig. 14. They consist of the causality for generalized HR extraction, and the causality for τ_R extracted from x_{ASP}.

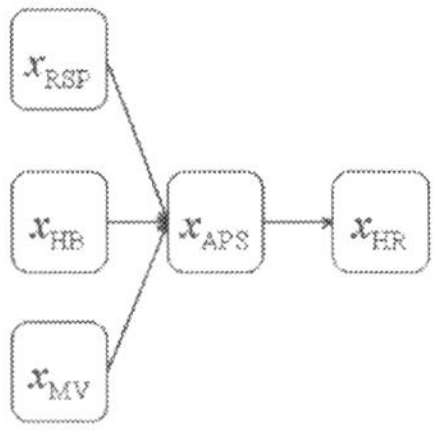

Fig. 12. Conceptual causality in heart rate monitoring via air pressure sensor

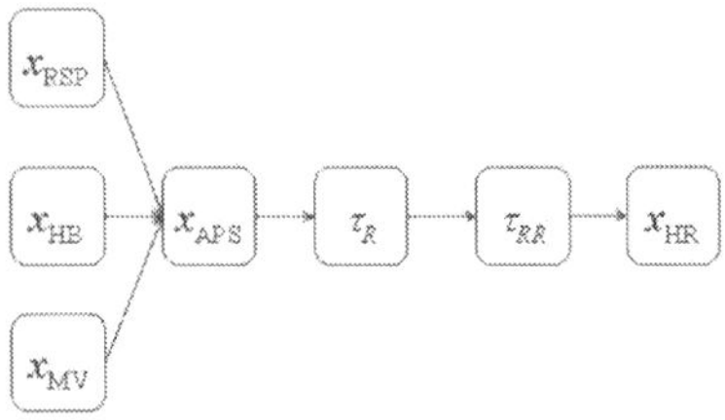

Fig. 13. Conceptual causality in heart rate monitoring

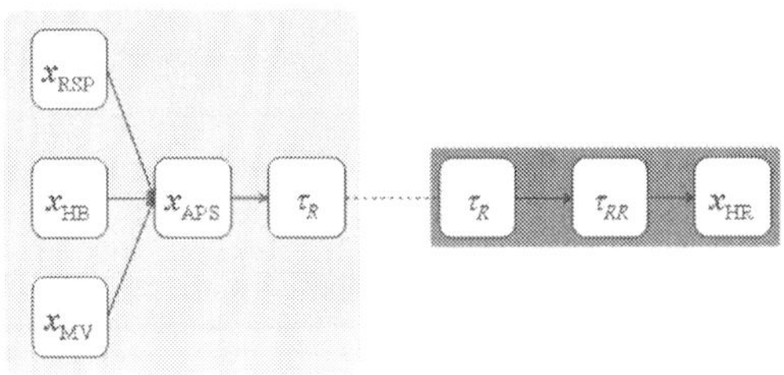

Fig. 14. Decomposed conceptual causality in heart rate monitoring

Step 3. Practical cause-effect structure formulation via human-machine collaboration
As for τ_R extraction from pressure change, the pressure change involves not only heartbeat but also respiration and body movement. Because of the nature of the signals, it could be difficult to determine the precise position of R-waves τ_R by autocorrelation function and peak detection method. In this study, fuzzy logic is employed to formulate the knowledge about heartbeat.
Firstly, full-wave rectification is applied to x_{ASP}, and the result signal is determined as x_{FRA}. Then, the fuzzy logic based on the knowledge about τ_{RR} is applied to the pre-processed pressure changes. These fuzzy rules are described in the following.

Knowledge 1 : The large pressure change is caused by heartbeat.
Knowledge 2 : Heartbeat interval does not change significantly.

According to the knowledge on heartbeat characteristics, the fuzzy rules are denoted in the following.

Rule 1 : IF x_i is HIGH, THEN the degree of heartbeat point μ_{Amp} is HIGH.
Rule 2 : IF t_i is CLOSE to $\overline{T}$, THEN the degree of heartbeat point μ_{Int} is HIGH.

Where $\mu_{Amp}(i)$ is the membership function of Rule 1, x_i is pre-processed pressure change, t_i is the sampling point of obtained pressure change, $\overline{T}$ is the average of heartbeat intervals that calculated by using previous ten heartbeats, and $\mu_{Int}(i)$ is the membership function of Rule 2. Then, the membership functions respond to the fuzzy rules are illustrated in Fig. 15 and 16, and formulae are equations (5)-(7) and (8), (9).

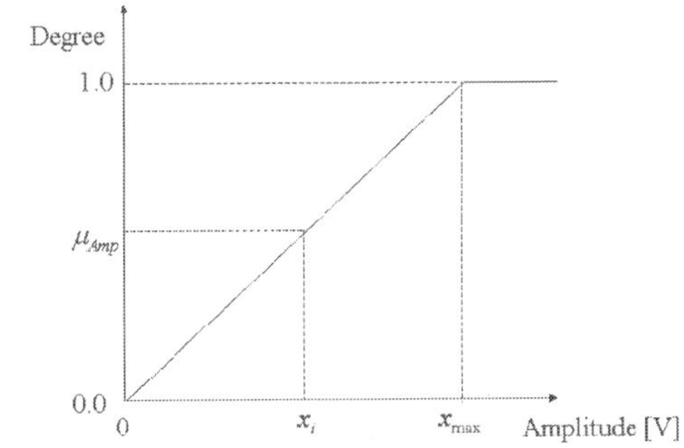

Fig. 15. Membership function for evaluating degree from viewpoint of amplitude

$$\mu_{Amp}(i) = \begin{cases} 0 & \text{if } x_i < x_{min} \\ \dfrac{x_i - x_{min}}{x_{max} - x_{min}} & \text{if } x_{min} \le x_i \le x_{max} \\ 1 & \text{if } x_i > x_{max} \end{cases} \tag{5}$$

$$x_{min} = \min(x_{FRA}) \tag{6}$$

$$x_{max} = \max(x_{FRA}) \tag{7}$$

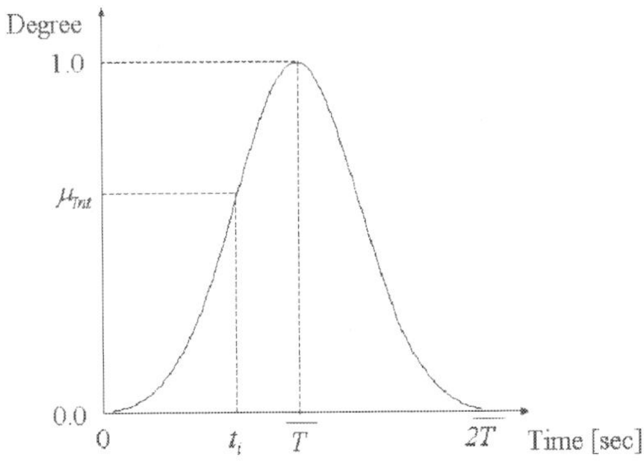

Fig. 16. Membership function for evaluating degree from viewpoint of heartbeat interval

$$\mu_{Int}(i) = \exp\left(\frac{-(t_i - \overline{T})^2}{2\sigma^2}\right) \tag{8}$$

$$\sigma = \overline{T} / 3 \tag{9}$$

Finally, μ_i is calculated by multiplying μ_{Amp} and μ_{Int} and the location with maximum μ_i is determined as heartbeat x_{HB} as formulated in equation (10).

$$\mu(i) = \mu_{\text{Amp}}(i) * \mu_{\text{Int}}(i) \tag{10}$$

5.4 Experimental result and discussion

In this experiment, the proposed heart rate monitoring based on human-machine collaboration is compared with conventional typical method that is based on autocorrelation functions and peak detection and one with proposed method by using fuzzy logic. Table 3 shows correlations between HR changes obtained from the ECG and those obtained from the heart rate monitoring equipment.

The results indicate that the method of fuzzy logic achieved higher performance for all of the subjects. In particular, the correlation to ECG for the subject A and E is over 0.97, which is extremely high.

Subject	R	
	Human-machine collaboration	Autocorrelation functions-based
A	0.973	0.703
B	0.807	0.389
C	0.754	0.621
D	0.872	0.699
E	0.972	0.658
F	0.844	0.677
G	0.737	0.346
Avg	0.851	0.585

Table 3. HR monitoring performance comparison

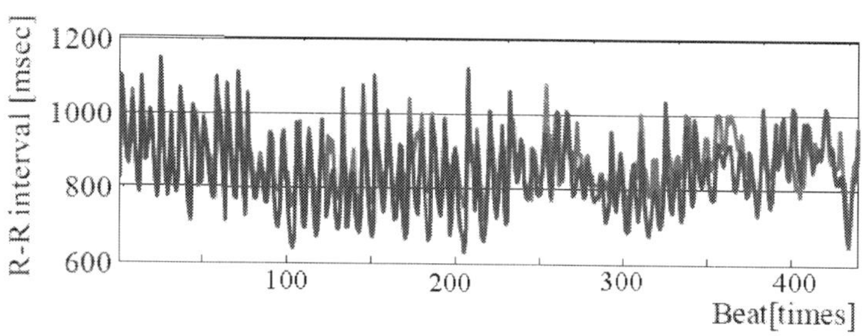

Fig. 17. Heartbeat count vs. R-R interval against subject B

In the following, the some of detailed HR monitoring results are discussed.

Fig. 15-18 shows the result for subject B and E where horizontal axis and virtual axis are heartbeat count and R-R interval respectively, and the blue line and red line is the R-R interval variability obtained by using the HR monitoring equipment and ECG respectively.
According to the results for subject B and E, the result of HR monitoring is quite similar to ECG's one. In addition, in Fig. 17, the HR monitoring could detect the significant R-R interval occurred around 200 beats.

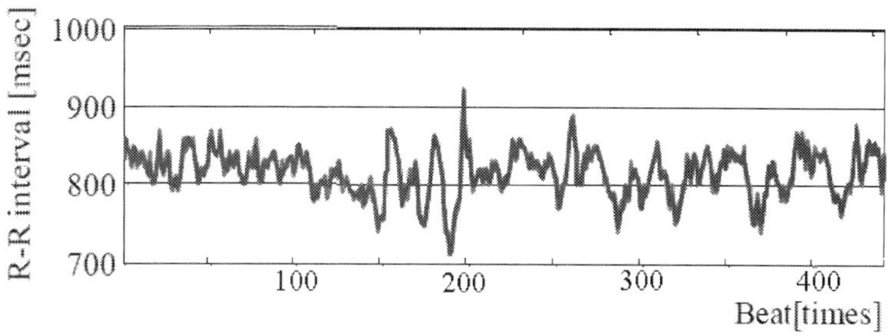

Fig. 18. Heartbeat count vs. R-R interval against subject E

6. Summaries and conclusions

This chapter has introduced a causal analysis based on human-machine collaboration for practical biomedical sensing. In the proposed method, the cause-effect structure is actualized in three steps. Firstly, experts illustrate the conceptual causality among components which are obtained from sensing target. In the next step, the conceptual causality is decomposed into independent subset by employing experts' knowledge. Then, feature attributes are prepared by using components, and each subset is formulated. At last, the formulae of each subset is integrated and optimized by using actual dataset obtained from sensing target.
Additionally, two applications of practical biomedical sensing have been presented; visceral fat measurement based on bioelectrical impedance analysis and heart rate monitoring by air pressure sensor.
In the case of visceral fat measurement, the conceptual causality was constructed by using experts' knowledge of the relationship among two kinds of bioelectrical impedance, body shape and body composition and the cause-effect structure was realized by fitting 196 subjects' dataset. According to the comparative experimental results, the measurement accuracy was improved in keeping with its measurement transparency.
In case of heart rate monitoring, the conceptual causality among air pressure sensor, R-wave, R-R interval and heart rate was constructed by using experts' knowledge on electrocardiograph. Then, the conceptual causality is decomposed into two subset, that is, the causality which describes heart rate extraction from heartbeat and the one among air pressure sensor, heartbeat, respiration, and body movement. According to the experimental result, the accuracy improvement was confirmed by comparing with the typical heart rate extraction used in the electrocardiograph.
According to the above two application, the proposal causal analysis based on human-machine collaboration is useful to realize practical biomedical sensing.

7. References

Akaike, H. (1974). A new look at the statistical model identification. *IEEE Transactions on Automatic Control*, Vol. AC-19, No. 6, pp.716-723, ISSN 00189286

Bishop, C.M. (2006). *Pattern Recognition and Machine Learning*, Springer, ISBN 0387310738, Berlin

Composition of the ESPEN Working Group (2004). Bioelectrical impedance analysisFpart I: review of principles and methods, *Clinical Nutrition*, Vol. 23, pp.1226-1243, ISSN 02615614

Deurenberg, P.; Kooij, K.; Evers, P. & Hulshof, T. (1990) Assessment of body composition by bioelectrical impedance in a population aged > 60 y, *The American Journal of Clinical Nutrition*, Vol. 51, pp.3-6, ISSN 00029165

Fayyad, U.M.; Piatetsky-Shapiro, G.; Smyth, P. & Uthurusamy, R. (1996). *Advances in Knowledge Discovery and Data Mining*, The MIT Press, ISBN 0262560976, Cambridge

Furuta, K.; Furuhama, Y.; Sakai, T. & Kondo, S. (1998) Construction method of student model for training support system of plant operation, *Journal of Japanese Society for Artificial Intelligence*, Vol. 13, No. 5, pp.811.821, ISSN 09128085

Gomi, T.; Kawawa, Y.; Nagamoto, M.; Terada, H. & Kohda, E. (2005). Measurement of visceral fat/subcutaneous fat ratio by 0.3 tesla MRI, *Radiation Medicine*, Vol. 23, No. 8, pp.584-587, ISSN 02882043

Gyftodimos, E. (2002). Hierarchical Bayesian networks: a probabilistic reasoning model for structured domains, *Proceedings of The Nineteenth International Conference on Machine Learning*, pp.23-30, ISBN 0733419348, Sydney, Australia, July 2002

Hata, Y.; Kamozaki, Y.; Sawayama, T.; Taniguchi, K. & Nakajima, H. (2007). A heart pulse monitoring system by air pressure and ultrasonic sensor systems, *Proceedings of IEEE International Conference on System of Systems Engineering 2007*, pp.1-5, San Antonio, Texas, USA, April 2007

Hata, Y.; Kobashi, S. & Nakajima, H. (2009). Human health care system of systems. IEEE System Journal, Vol. 3, No. 2, pp.231-238, ISSN 19328184

Ho, K.; Tsuchiya, N.; Nakajima, H.; Kuramoto, K.; Kobashi S. & Hata, Y. (2009). Fuzzy logic approach to respiration detection by air pressure sensor, *Proceedings of 2009 IEEE International Conference on Fuzzy Systems*, pp.911-915, Jeju Island, Korea, August 2009

Kitney, R.I. & Rompelman, O. (1980). *The Study of heart Rate Variability*, Clarendon Press, ISSN 00034819, Oxford

Kobayashi, H.; Ishibashi, K. & Noguchi, H. (1999). Heart rate variability; an index for monitoring and analyzing human autonomic activities. *Applied Human Science*, Vol. 18, No. 2, pp.53-59, ISSN 13413473

Marutschke, D.M.; Nakajima, H.; Tsuchiya, N.; Yoneda, M.; Iwami, T. and Kamei, K. (2010). Actualization of causality-based transparency and accuracy in system modeling with human-machine collaboration. *International Journal of Intelligent Computing in Medical Sciences and Image Processing*, Vol. 3, No. 2, pp. 131-141 (in press)

Matsuzawa, Y. (2002). New criteria for 'obesity disease' in Japan: the examination committee of criteria for 'obesity disease' in Japan, Japan society for the study of obesity. *Circulation Journal*, Vol. 66, No. 11, pp.987-992, ISSN 13469843

Miyagawa, M. (1991). Statistical causal inference using graphical models. *Journal of the Japan Statistical Society*, Vol. 29, No. 3, pp.327-356, ISBN 03895602

Miyawaki, T; Hirata, M.; Moriyama, K.; Sasaki, Y.; Aono, H.; Saito, N. & Nakao, K. (2005). Metabolic syndrome in Japanese diagnosed with visceral fat measurement by computed tomography, *Japan Academy, Series B*, Vol. 81, No. 10, pp.471-479, ISSN 03862208

Nadkarni, S. (2004). A causal mapping approach to constructing Bayesian networks, *Decision Support System*, Vol. 38, No. 2, pp.259-281, ISSN 01679236

Nakajima, H; Hasegawa, Y.; Tasaki, H. & Kojitani, K. (2008a). SoS aspects of health management technology in substrate manufacturing process, *Proceedings of the Third International Conference on System of Systems Engineering*, pp.1-6, ISBN 9781424421725, Singapore, June 2008

Nakajima, H.; Hasegawa, Y.; Tasaki, H.; Iwami, T. & Tsuchiya, N. (2008b). Health management technology as a general solution framework. *The Society of Instrument and Control Engineers Journal of Control, Measurement and System Integration*, Vol. 1, No. 3, pp.257-264, ISBN 9784339892031

Pearl, J. (2001). *Causality: Models, Reasoning and Inference*, Cambridge University Press, ISBN 0521773628, Cambridge

Ryo, M.; Maeda, K.; Onda, T.; Katashima, M.; Okumiya, A.; Nishida, M.; Yamaguchi, T.; Funahashi, T.; Matsuzawa, Y.; Nakamura, T. & Shimomura, I. (2005). A new simple method for the measurement of visceral fat accumulation by bioelectrical impedance, *Diabetes Care*, Vol. 28, No. 2, pp451-453, ISSN 01495992

Shiga, T.; Ohshima, Y.; Kanai, H.; Hirata, M.; Hosoda, K. & Nakao, K. (2007). A simple measurement method of visceral fat accumulation by bioelectrical impedance analysis, *Proceedings of the 13th International Conference on Electrical Bioimpedance and the 8th Conference on Electrical Impedance Tomography*, pp.687-690, ISSN 16800737, Graz, Austria, August 2007, Springer, Berlin

Tenenbaum, J.B.; Griffiths, T.L. & Kemp, C. (2006). Theory-based Bayesian models of inductive learning and reasoning, *TRENDS in Cognitive Sciences*, Vol. 10, No. 7, pp.309-318, ISSN 13646613

Thang, C.; Cooper, E.W. & Hoshino, Y. (2006). A proposed model of diagnosis and prescription in oriental medicine using RBF neural networks, *Journal of Advanced Computational Intelligence and Intelligent Informatics*, Vol. 10, No. 4, pp.458-464, ISSN 13430130

Tsuchiya, N. & Nakajima, H. (2010) Causal-effect structure transformation based on hierarchical representation for biomedical sensing. *World Review of Science, Technology and Sust. Development*, Vol. 7, Nos. 1/2, pp.116-129, ISSN 17412242

Yamaguchi, H.; Nakajima, H.; Taniguchi, K.; Kobashi, S.; Kondo, K. & Hata, Y. (2007). Fuzzy detection system of behaviour before getting out of bed by air pressure and ultrasonic sensors, *Proceedings of the IEEE International Conference on Granular Computing 2007*, pp.114-119, San Jose, California, USA, November 2007

Yoneda, M.; Tasaki, H.; Tsuchiya, N.; Nakajima, H.; Hamaguchi, T.; Oku, S. & Shiga, T. (2007). A study of bioelectrical impedance analysis methods for practical visceral fat estimation, *Proceedings of the IEEE International Conference on Granular Computing 2007*, pp.622-627, San Jose, California, USA, November 2007

Yoneda, M.; Tasaki, H.; Tsuchiya, N.; Nakajima, H.; Hamaguchi, T.; Oku, S. & Shiga, T. (2008). Development of visceral fat estimation model based on bioelectrical impedance analysis method. *Journal of Japan Society for Fuzzy Theory and Systems*, Vol. 20, No. 1, pp.90-99, ISSN 13477986 (in Japanese)

Zadeh, L.A. (1996). *Fuzzy Sets, Fuzzy Logic, Fuzzy Systems*, World Scientific Publishing, ISBN 9810224214, Singapore.

29

Design Requirements for a Patient Administered Personal Electronic Health Record

Rune Fensli[1], Vladimir Oleshchuk[1], John O'Donoghue[2] and Philip O'Reilly[2]
[1]Faculty of Engineering and Science, University of Agder, Grimstad
[2]Business Information Systems, University College Cork
[1]Norway
[2]Ireland

1. Introduction

It is anticipated that the patient's access to his/her own medical records and treatment information in the future will play an important role in managing treatment of chronic diseases and protecting patients' health as described by Coulter et al. (2008). Shared access to electronic health records will thus be important for obtaining electronic collaboration, both for the patient and also for the health care professionals.

The patient empowerment approach as defined by Anderson & Funnell (2009) implies that the patient is capable of managing necessary self-selected changes by recording daily control of (their) his/her illness and rehabilitation. The ability to enter daily recordings of clinical data by the patient will be important in future health care services, where remote home monitoring will be a normal procedure in following up hospital treatment. Such recordings and patient details need to be safely stored within the patient's Electronic Health Record (EHR) system, and they should be shared between the patient and the health care providers. When patients are monitored remotely by means of wearable sensors and communication equipments, recorded information of clinical recordings should be automatically incorporated into EHRs. Such functionality will be important for the doctors to make the more informed diagnosis of the patient's (actual) current condition, and solutions like these can be regarded as an important part of the personalized health care concept.

The Markle Foundation (2003) has defined Personal Health Records (PHR) as:

> *"An electronic application through which individuals can access, manage and share their health information, and that of others whom they are authorized, in a private, secure, and confidential environment."*

The American Medical Informatics Association's College of Medical Informatics has in a strategy for adoption of PHR elaborated on technical architecture and described organizational and behavioural barriers needed to be overcome, as described by Tang et al. (2006). They focused on potential benefits both for the patients and caregivers, but presupposed the systems must be easy to learn and easy to use in order to be used on a daily basis.

According to Hurtado et al. (2000), such patient-centric solutions can be defined as:

> *"Systems that enable a partnership among practitioners, patients, and their families (when appropriate) to ensure that procedures and decisions respect patients' needs and preferences."*

The CEN/ISSS eHealth Standardization Focus Group (2005) has finalized a report addressing future standardization and interoperability in the e-health domain, highlighting the importance of obtaining improved access to clinical records and enabling patient mobility and cross-border access to health care. One proposed action is to establish an EU Health Insurance Card containing a medical emergency data set and the use of this card to control access to the patient's medical record.

There are several barriers to overcome in designing shared PHRs, but new solutions for the patient's access to his/her own PHR are emerging within EU countries. However, in designing new solutions for shared PHR systems, functional requirements from the patient's perspective will probably be a key issue, as the patient will have to realise clear benefits from using such tools in his ongoing communication with the health care personnel. This can be comparable to perceived advantages as from using Internet solutions for private purposes like email and the use of social media.

2. Chapter outline

In this chapter, we analyse the security and privacy requirements of the patient's access to his own PHR, focusing also on patient empowerment and self-care. We analyse the European and US National Health Care strategies. Based on scenarios with a patient-centric view in establishing new services, we propose a solution for a Patient administered Personal electronic Health Record (PaPeHR) service, which would include a cross-country certification of health care personnel in order for patients to receive medical assistance when they are abroad. Some emergency access mechanisms should also be included. Finally, we will highlight some design requirements in order to define roles and support patient´s access to shared information within a collaborative health care framework.

3. Security, privacy and trust requirements

In general, the question of privacy will be one of the fundamental requirements for patients, as the actual solutions can be designed in a way that the patient can be confident in being able to take control of his own private information. Privacy can be defined as:

> *"The right of individual to determine for themselves when, how and to what extent information about them is communicated to others";* Agrawal et al. (2002).

As Tang et al. (2006) focused on the ability for the patient to define which part of the information stored in the PHR is to be shared by others, this is in fact a question of privacy regulation in the actual solution. There are several privacy-aware solutions offered on the market, such as the iHealthRecord[1], PatientSite[2], Microsoft HealthVault[3] and Google Health[4]. However, most of those solutions differ on conceptual levels and are based on proprietary standards, making trans-institutional data exchange difficult. When making a decision on which solution to choose, the patient will also have to evaluate the trustworthiness of the company offering a secure solution for life-long storage of life-critical medical information. In many countries you will probably not trust a foreign private

---

[1] http://www.ihealthrecord.org

[2] http://www.patientsite.org/

[3] http://www.healthvault.com/

[4] http://www.google.com/health/

company; however, you will trust your bank manager when it comes to your net-bank account. In the same manner, you will have to trust your net-health account, and regarding privacy you will be certain that the data storage is preserved in a safe and secure place, where you are the only person managing this account and where only you can control which persons are given access to the information stored.

It is a challenging task to define shared access to the PHR information based on concept of roles defined by Role-Based Access Control (RBAC) which typically are incorporated into the design of EHR-systems used in hospitals and health care services. RBAC is a concept where access to data is restricted to authorized users, and where the actual person's functional role within the organization will determine which part of the information he is authorized to access, as defined by the standard ANSI/INCITS 359-2004 (2004).

Such solutions will first of all require a well defined structure of information in different types, each with different needs of shared access; thus the RBAC solutions have a need of including granulated context aware RBAC. In addition, there should be possibilities of defining generic roles, as typically will be your local doctor or general practitioner, your home nurse (which will be a role shared by many nurses), your spouse/next of kin, persons in your health exercise group etc. Any solution will require the secure identification of all healthcare personnel, and many countries have established a common name-space with a central storage of this public information. However, the secure identification of informal caregivers (voluntary resources) and family members can be a challenging task.

Assuming that the patient is the owner of his/her own PHRs, he/she will need to ensure the integrity of the system; thus he/she will be the responsible person for the data integrity and confidentiality. This (will have the implications) implies that the patient will need to have the administrative privileges of assigning roles and access to the information stored within the PHRs. This will, in fact, be a Patient administered Personal Electronic Health Record (PaPeHR). In such a new concept the challenge will be to design the administrative part of the RBAC interface in a simple and intuitive way, enabling the patient to perform the role of system administrator without making any mistakes. This will be a question of human interface design, but depending on computer skills, probably not all patients can take the responsibility on their own. If a system facilitator is needed in helping the patient with the system setup and assigning roles, this facilitator role should not have access to stored medical information. Technically, this can be solved in a front-end/ back-end solution. However, the facilitator role will be crucial when it comes to privacy issues.

Many proposed solutions only slightly approach security and even less privacy issues. For example, an architecture proposed by Vogel et al. (2006) for distributed national electronic health record system in Austria stated that:

> *"The privacy of patient related data is temporary solved in a way that participating institutions are bound by contract to only access data relevant for specific treatment case"* [page 5].

This is not a technological solution. It is more a question of agreed policy, and should generally not be considered a sufficient protection of patient privacy (otherwise the privacy protection problem would already be solved, since current privacy related legislation requires similar protection of patient data in most countries). Some other approaches focus more on security issues and partly mixing them with privacy issues, and it is important to be aware of the fact that high degree of security does not necessarily protect data privacy.

From the definition of privacy, it is easy to see that perfectly secured data does not necessarily provide protection of patient privacy, as there may not be implemented solutions for the patient's access control. It should be mentioned that in a real-life situation the above definition of privacy can be ensured by claiming individual may be replaced by any entity (such other individuals or organizations) he/she has sufficient level of trust to. The relaxation was implicitly made in many approaches proposed in the literature, and is described in a global perspective by HiMSS (August 2008). However, it poses another issue associated with correctly assessing trust relations in an ad hoc setting (for example when a patient is abroad on holiday etc.). This is a reason that many proposed frameworks require the availability of a special infrastructure such as for example PKI, digital certificates, health cards, etc., and these may be difficult to implement in cross-border settings. Generally, providing privacy protection is more difficult than providing security of patient data. In some cases it can be contradictory, for example when patient privacy is based on anonymity.

4. Patient empowerment and self-care

In health care services today, there is an increased awareness of patient empowerment. The term "Patient empowerment" implies that the patient should have gained knowledge about his own health and illness, and can be able to make decisions of actual treatment and self care. This is not about "doing something for the patient", but facilitating and supporting patients to understand the consequences of their decisions. There are several relevant papers that describe the understanding of patient empowerment. One example is the WHO report written by Anderson & Funnell (2009) and Coulter et al. (2008) where the situation for patients and decision making is described.

Chronically ill patients experience a greater degree of freedom and are more involved in the treatment with daily monitoring of vital information during hospitalization in their own home, than with the traditional treatment procedures at a hospital. Introducing advanced medical technology in the patient's own home will influence the patient's situation as it makes empowerment and self-management possible as described by Barlow et al. (2002). At the same time, coordinated follow-up and new workflow procedures for the health-care services need to be implemented in order to give the patient satisfactory support by virtual visits in his/her home, which was put in focus by Wootton & Kvedar (2006). However, this support also must be integrated in the self-monitoring of vital signs information performed by the patients, with understandable interpretations of the results.

In an evaluation by Wald et al. (2007) of the physician - patient relationship, it was found that the impact of Internet use with possibilities of collaborative teamwork approach and access to the patient's own health information were effective and contributing to quality of health care. Weingart et al. (2006) evaluated patients who used the PatientSite, and they discovered a steady growth of use after the introduction, by typically younger patients with few medical problems. But to expand the use of patient portals it is important to overcome obstacles for those patients who might benefit most from this technology, as they will probably be the first users of the new system.

In a review analyzing potential benefits and drawbacks of patients' access to PHR, Ross & Lin (2003) found improved communication between patient and doctor, improved patient empowerment and improved education. However, this can require a fundamental redesign of the health care process, with full electronic integration and communication with patient-centric applications for disease management and prevention, as Demiris et al. (2008) are pinpointing. When designing such solutions, the patients will probably expect a quick feedback from the doctor to recorded event situations or messages requesting for advice; thus a reliable workflow and defined response times should be defined according to Fensli & Boisen (2008).

As the health care personnel normally will be using secure solutions within a national health care framework, there is a need to establish secure communication and exchange solutions crosswise health network borders. At the same time, the patient should be able to participate in a training group for patients with the same diseases, as the encouragement from other patients will have a positive impact. This should imply functionality known from social media, with shared training results, questions and answers, blogs. Such functionalities are well known from most weight watcher programmes found on the Internet, but are rarely used within a health care and rehabilitation domain.

Today, many athletes are using a pulse watch during their regular training. This watch enables them to share their achieved results with training partners on the web, and even as a virtual competition. Grimsmo et al. (2010) found that prevalence of atrial fibrillation is increased for middle-aged over-trained athletes, and the next thing they will have to do will be sharing their training records also with the doctor. However, being able to distinguish between different security needs can be a challenging factor for patients in their role as system administrators, defining the actual roles and access to different types of information.

5. European and US national health care strategies

5.1 Core electronic health records

Within a national health network, mechanisms for secure transfer of clinical information are in many countries established between hospitals and General Practitioners (GP), and also with the local municipal health care services, based on different infrastructure principles and secure message exchange.

In Denmark, the Danish eHealth Portal, sundhed.dk (2010), is designed to give the patients on-line access to their personal health data with the medical history from Danish hospitals, including e-Journal and Medicine profile. In addition, the health professionals can get access to a summary of the patient's electronic health record.

In Norway, a patient portal "Min journal" is established by Oslo University Hospital, in close collaboration with a number of hospitals and rehabilitation clinics. A secure electronic ID is used for authentication of the patient, and he/she will have access to secure message exchange with the health care services. The patient will also have an overview of the medical prescriptions and epicrisis from the hospital. Such solutions can be classified as a patient portal approach, with access to the health systems owned by the providers.

In Scotland, the National Health Services (NHS) has established a common Core-Electronic Health record, The Emergency Care Summary; to be accessed by all health care services within the country. However, up until now the patients are yet not given access to this solution as described in the report by The Scottish Government (2006).

Within The UK, the Healthspace portal operated by the NHS enables the patients to view their Summary Care Record (SCR) and to book a hospital appointment as described by the UK National Health Service (2008). Within the HealthSpace portal, patients can manage their own health and lifestyle information. By having an account, the patients can fill in important information about their health details; keep a record of their own medication, daily intake of alcohol, smoking and calorie, and also monitor blood pressure and fitness recordings.

In order to establish a common database of patient information to be shared between health care professionals, several European countries have focused on defining a common shared EHR, summarized by the CEN/ISSS eHealth Standardization Focus Group (2005).

Within several European countries, efforts have also been made to define a core dataset for public health, "Core-EHR", where a minimum common dataset of important clinical information can be securely stored and shared among health care professionals at different administrative levels. In the EU report "Connected Health", the European Commission (2006) has described the term Patient Summary as (p 13):

> *"A clinical document that is stored in repositories with cumulative indexing systems and secure access by authorized people. In order to achieve maximum benefit from this instrument, the structured content of patient summaries should be agreed at an international level, starting from a few generic summaries and gradually developing a series of summaries specific for each clinical context."* (Citation from an eHealth ERA coordination action deliverable)

In the report, three specific topics are considered as prioritized activities, namely a proposal of requirements of interoperability of patient summaries, patient and health practitioner identifiers and an emergency data set incorporated in the patient summary. This summary of important medical information will typically include a summary of patient history, a list of allergies, active problems still under treatment, recent test results and a medication list. In addition, the eHealth action plan as a strategy from the Commission (2004) addressed the question of ePrescribing, in the future this can give possibilities for cross-border prescriptions when patients are abroad on holiday etc.

5.2 Different approaches for patients' access

In the description of how different countries have approached the acceptance, adoption, deployment, operation and support of a national EHR solution, a HiMSS (August 2008) Steering Committee has defined four architectural models to describe how the ownership of the patient records are organized, and whether or not a country allows for EHRs to be accessed by patients.

These four approaches are as follows: 1) A Fully Federated model where the data remain in the source systems; 2) A Federated model where patient data are consolidated with source facility in a clinical document record; 3) A Service Oriented model where patient data are sent to a central EHR by messaging, and where the patient can get access to the events registered in the system, and 4) An Integrated EHR model with a single integrated hospital system where the patients can get access through embedded capabilities. To this list, a fifth model should be added as a privately owned standalone PHR as listed in Table 1.

EHR Approach	National health care strategies
#1 Fully Federated	U.S.
#2 Federated	Netherlands, Wales
#3 Service Oriented	Germany, Denmark, Israel, New Zealand
#4 Integrated EHR	England, Canada
#5 Standalone PHR	None (only private initiatives)

Table 1. Models of approaches to EHR solutions within national health care strategies based on HiMSS (August 2008), with addition of a private standalone PHR solution

In the different strategies to adopt PHR solutions, we have described the range of complexity for a PHR either as a stand-alone application or fully integrated so that patients can view their own information stored in the EHR system at the health care provider. As a minimum requirement, there is a need to export and import data from other systems in a standardized way, and in future solutions there should be seamlessly interoperable systems as described by Tang et al. (2006). In this paper, they also highlighted the potential benefits for the consumers having a PHR.

Patient's access to their doctor's EHR system has been developed as a web-based service proposed by Cimino et al. (2002), demonstrating that patients gain an improved understanding of their health and that such systems can have beneficial effects on health outcomes where patients and doctors can have a shared workload and a better communication. An e-consent based solution to share the EHR between the patient and health care personnel has been suggested by Bergmann et al. (2007) as a virtual shared EHR and with the use of an e-consent object based on digital signatures for authorized access to the patient's shared her. However, the formal requirements can be difficult to implement in cross-border solutions.

An architecture for a patient-centred shared electronic health record using a Medical Data GRIDs[5] as an open source implementation has been suggested by Vogel et al. (2006). This solution enables the patient to give a fine grained permission to access specific parts of the record. A distributed service using roles defined by the e-Health directory was implemented, and authentication was based on digital certificates. It can also be possible to establish an independent service as a health record data bank, described by Shabo (2006), into which the actual health care providers will have to submit the desired content.

An interesting show-case with two clinical scenarios was developed using a patient-centred approach which demonstrated integration of a PHR to a healthcare enterprise, based on a Cross-enterprise Document Sharing (XDS) profile implemented in a ebXML architecture, as described by Stolyar et al. (2006). In this way metadata were used as index to locate the actual health information stored within a regional health information network.

There is a need to clarify actual standards suitable for integration of information, and how patient-entered data, including vital signs recordings and fitness and lifestyle details can be shared between the patient, his/her relatives, training partners and the health care professionals. In order to adopt a solution to be used in broad scale, it can be beneficial to use open standards in the infrastructure framework, thus different vendors can easily adopt their systems to be used within a national health care data network designed to share information among different applications and clinical tools. The standardization issues are addressed in a joint project on interoperability of eHealth standards organized by NEN (2009), and a final report, M403 Phase 1, was in February 2009 submitted to the European Commission for formal approval.

However, as pinpointed by Kahn et al. (2009) the existing gap between today's PHRs solutions and what integrated services patients say they want and need, is a limiting factor in the adoption. It is also important to keep in mind that Kahn et al. (2009) unveiled that the patients are concerned about security and privacy issues. To summarise, this review reveals that no simple way exists for the patient to gain control of the consent rights given in the EHR approach models #1 to #4. Nor is a proper model for data access in emergency situations proposed.

6. Scenario with remote home monitoring

6.1 Information flow

When defining a framework for information flow, storage and retrieval, it is necessary to focus on the (actual) system users and their responsibility. Putting the patient in focus can

[5] GRID computing is combining resources from multiple of distributed computers

give a perspective where the important information flow and responsibility for the different health care professionals can be identified. A typical scenario may be the situation which is shown in Figure.1, where a patient's vital signs are monitored during his/her outdoor walk. The electrocardiogram (ECG) signals are automatically transmitted to the patients PaPeHR using secure mobile data communication (1).

If an arrhythmia situation is detected, this information can be transmitted to the local doctor/General Practitioner (2) to be prepared and preliminary evaluated by the care coordinator for a quick focus on important findings. This can be timesaving for the doctor's evaluation to determine appropriate interventions. As he may not have necessary cardiology competence, he can forward the arrhythmia event to a specialist at the hospital as a telemedicine referral (3). Depending on the epicrisis received (4), he can both send a message to the home nurse for necessary follow up (5) and inform the patient (6). All the information on the arrhythmia event recorded data, referral, epicrisis and messages should be properly stored within the patients PaPeHR (7).

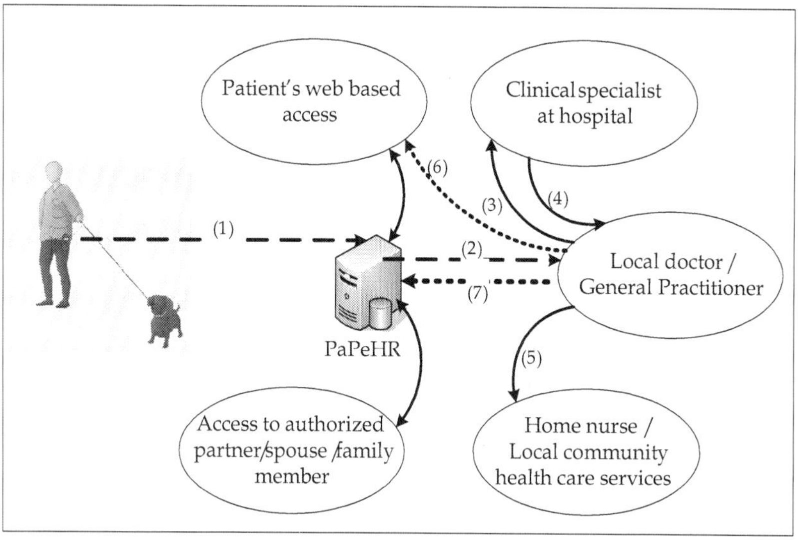

Fig. 1. The principle information flow (1-6) between the patient, the local doctor, the clinical specialist and the home nurse, in response to a detected cardiac event. The patient should also have online access to his own PaPeHR to update actual information and read the feedback from his doctor (7). In addition, the patient should have possibilities to define access to his partner/spouse/family member

Of course, a detailed log will record any access to the stored information, in order for the patient to have an overview of what has been read or evaluated by the health care personnel and other persons given access privileges. As the patient may have consented to allow family members to access actual parts of the information stored, there will be a need of RBAC mechanisms to control the privacy as described in section 3.

The patient should not need to worry about security issues; however, he/she would need to trust the organization or company offering the PaPeHR solution. Preferably, this could be a well known public service in the country, but it could be anyone offering a reliable and easy to use solution as a trusted third party. This principle is well known for security systems when it comes to offering digital ID's (normally private companies), secure net bank accounts, secure payment solutions, secure storage of private information like family photos, and others.

6.2 Integration of remote monitoring

When patients are monitored remotely by wearable sensors and communication equipments, the automatically recorded information is important for the doctors to make the correct diagnosis of the patient's current situation, and it is an important part of the personalized health care concept as described by Aziz et al. (2008). Several wearable vital signs recording solutions have been developed, with different aspects of how to record and transfer such information. In an overview and an evaluation of different telecom solutions for remote cardiac patients it is suggested by Kumar et al. (2008) that next-generation telecardiology network architecture should incorporate a signal processing module for local analysis of recorded physiological measurements. Preferably, it should only transmit to the doctor detected events where recorded data are out of defined thresholds values. The systems should be able to use multiple wireless interfaces and include location-based services.

Fensli et al. (2005) and Dagtas et al. (2008) have proposed a local signal processing solution and transmission of periodic reports with detected alerts to a central server as an entry point for the professional staff to monitor the recorded data.. Similarly, a remote diagnostic system which integrates digital telemetry using a wireless patient module, a homecare station and a remote clinical station has been developed by Kong et al. (2000). However, none of those solutions discussed how the recorded information at the central server can be stored securely within a patient EHR or PHR framework.

Telemedical solutions have been used in several interesting projects to evaluate patient outcome, and the Airmed-Cardio project described by Salvador et al. (2005) showed the importance of enabling patients with chronic heart disease perform out-of-hospital follow-up and monitoring, where they developed a dedicated platform for necessary measurements and contact between the patients and the health care agents. However, the platform used was not integrated into the patients EHR system. A clear outcome effects of a home-based tele-cardiology service has been verified by Scalvini et al. (2005), where the patients' ECG recordings automatically were transmitted to a receiving station available for trained nurses (telemonitoring), also this solution was a stand-alone receiving database.

In a report on remote monitoring, the U.S. Department of Health and Human Services has described use cases to define possible solutions for information exchange and integration of patient-monitored data into a national health information technology (U.S. Dept of Health and Human Services (2008). This report highlights the importance of a clinician to monitor patient information captured remotely in management of chronic health problems and to diagnose new conditions. Such measurements can include physiologic measurements, diagnostic measurements, medication tracking and activities of daily living measurements. However, common data standards and interoperability are necessary to establish a pathway to incorporate the remotely monitored information into EHRs and PHRs, and they defined a data intermediary into which a remote device could be able to exchange and store information and where privacy controls and restrict data access mechanisms were incorporated. One of the important problems discovered, was a lack of standardized interface and interoperable data, giving restrictions when trying to integrate remote monitored data into the EHRs and PHRs. In use cases describing exchange of measurements between patients' monitoring device and their clinicians, they described three different roles and functions: *The Clinician* (personnel who clinically evaluate the remote measurements in the EHR and determine appropriate interventions), *Care Coordinator* (clinically-trained individuals who monitor the information received from the patient's device and assist the patient and/or clinician in managing the remote monitoring information) and the *Patient* (including family caregivers who use a remote monitoring device to gather measurements). From the data intermediary, persons with the defined role could be given controlled access to information by a web-based portal, and decision support capabilities should be incorporated to generate alerts and communicate information to the EHR or PHR reaching threshold values in the remote monitored data.

6.3 Daily use of a PaPeHR solution in patient's self care

In the patient's daily use of his/her PaPeHR, he/she should have access to a variety of information like general health status, care plan, medication list, allergies, doctor's journal record documents, medical advises, vital signs recorded, a calendar with scheduled actions and visits to the doctor and health care personnel, in addition to the ability to write a medical diary to follow up the planned treatment and exercises. The vital signs can, upon the doctor's request, be a combination of physiological measurements either done automatically by wearable sensors, or manually by reading the values of the recording instrument and uploading the measurements via web-based interface. Such information can be physiological measurements (e.g. blood pressure, blood glucose, INR-values), diagnostic activities of daily living, drug intake, food, performed exercise (including use of step counters etc.). As the patient normally will have the ability to freely move around, most of the automatic recordings should preferably be based on secure mobile communication solutions. Also manually entered data should be able to be uploaded from a mobile device, and in a web-based solution this should be available from an ordinary mobile phone with secure data transfer.

One important aspect to the patient will be to have a quick response from the health care personnel in case of abnormal recordings. This could be values outside threshold limits, and may indicate an action from the patient or a health care intervention. Thus necessary alert mechanisms should be incorporated with an automated tracking of actions and responses, including a system for escalating the case to a more urgent action if needed. However, automatic escalation may involve giving access to information by other health care personnel as the emergency response team as proposed by Hansen & Fensli (2006). It can be difficult to predict such needs, thus the rescuing team may not be registered with access permissions, and there will be a need to incorporate emergency access solutions as described by Oleshchuk & Fensli (2010).

There may be a need of access from the patient's close relatives/spouse/next of kin/family members, depending on the patient's mental condition and need of help controlling his treatment and follow up. Such assistance can also be the case for patients with dementia, where the question of location tracking by use of global positioning systems (GPS) also will imply ethical issues and legal issues for this specific use of tracking persons. In order for health care personnel to access data of position, there should be an automatic logging of this access, together with a written report describing the need of access in this particular situation.

The patient's use of social media will imply sharing actual experiences with others and supporting and encouraging friends in their coping with illness. Some information can be freely shared on the web as is the case using Facebook, Twitter or similar media. However, we will recommend defining a secure social portal, where the patient easily can add friends with a proper sign-on for them to get access to the shared information. Thus, this portal can be a front-end of a PaPeHR with secure Internet access, while at the same time the back-end services should be integrated within a secure national health network.

6.4 Special attentions and emergency situations

Several emergency situations can require special attention. In an acute situation the system should automatically detect the change in the patient's situation, and perform an escalation of the access rights for the parties involved (in case of emergency event). As proposed by Ferreira et al. (2009) the "Break The Glass" policies are flexible and allow users to override the defined access policies in a controlled manner. Within health care services such "Blue Light" access situations can occur, but it can be necessary to know the exact location of the patient and a Spatial Role Based Access Control system can be useful as proposed by Hansen & Fensli (2006).

If the patient is able to control the access by others to his PHR-information, this will normally be based on informed consent. In situations where there is a change in the health care personnel normally taking care of the patient, he/she should give new permissions to new persons, either as one-time access, temporarily access (limited time) or as permanent access (shift in the staff). There might also be situations where the patient is transferred to a hospital for treatment, and where he/she will not be able to distinguish between the actual personnel/staff; so the permissions can be given to the hospital as an institution (and not defined persons). Thus it will require some infrastructure to be able to identify and authenticate the actual hospital personnel responsible for the treatment. Such role-based access can be achieved by establishing a Public Key Infrastructure (PKI) using digital IDs, and preferably there will be a public name-space within a secure national health network to identify both hospitals as organizations, as well as all registered authorized health care personnel.

In an emergency situation, the patient may be unconscious and therefore not able to give the required permissions. As such, there should be defined ad-hoc read-only access by authenticated doctors in order to get access to important life-threatening information as the Patient Summary with the medication list. In fact, this could preferably be the patient's Core-EHR, where the patient summary is safely stored within a national health network, as is the case in Scotland electronic patient record system. Furthermore, when the patient is travelling abroad, situations can occur where there is a need of local treatment; thus the access possibilities should be based on an international cross-identification infrastructure to allow cross countries data exchange.

7. Design requirements

Based on the scenario with important aspects of the PaPeHR use, some fundamental basis of requirements can be stated which should be implemented in a future solution. It can be useful to separate the list in functional and non-functional requirements as defined in Table 2 and 3, in which the necessary privacy and security mechanism are defined. As the system should be easy to use for persons with relatively low computer competence, the actual solutions will require a good interface, with universal design and according to use for persons with disabilities. The Web Content Accessibility Guidelines published by W3C

(1999), gives recommendations for how to make the web content accessible for people with disabilities, but will also be useful guidelines when developing web content for all users. In order to evaluate a web site for accessibility, a multi-page resource suite is also published by the Web Accessibility Initiative, W3C (2008).

7.1 Suggested implementations

This approach will protect patient privacy by means of providing control of access to their PaPeHR. Having control of access to his/her own PaPeHR means that the patient would be able to provide access to stored data to any nominated medical practitioner, anytime and anywhere. Therefore only systems with patient-controlled access can be considered as adequately protecting patient privacy. Thus comparing five approaches to EHR system design (presented at Table 1) we purport that at present only a Standalone PHR (Approach #5) gives adequate protection of patient privacy. Three approaches (fully federated, federated and service oriented, see Table 1) implicitly assume that a trust relation with users exist. These three approaches are mostly suitable and designed to secure the EHR solution, and not to protect patient's EHR privacy. This will also be the case for the fourth model (integrated EPR), where the patient's influence on access permissions is not implemented.

The approach based on patient-controlled access can easily be extended to give patients an opportunity to continuously update their health-related data by uploading new data collected privately by body area networks (BAN) or Body Sensors Networks (BSN) on the regular base when monitoring vital signs data in the course of daily activities, for example jogging. It will be more important in the future when such body area networks will wide-spread and can be used for continuous monitoring of patients' health conditions (especially chronic patients), and where the recorded information can be used later by medical practitioners to provide more specific health care and optimize number and time used to visits medical practitioners. It can also be related to lifelong EHR, as defined by Shabo (2006). However, handling of special emergency situations when the patient is unconscious or unable to grant access for some other reason should also be included in such system. In this case a verifiable trusted representative should be able to grant such permission.

In the following section we will describe a solution that enforces patients' control of their PaPeHR. We assume that there is a database (distributed or on a single server) that contains PaPeHRs of patients and which can be accessed via the internet. This patient wants to be able to both download and upload data to the database. The patient will need the ability to control access to these data by granting and revocation of access permissions to his PaPeHR. They want to be able to grant ad hoc access to these datasets from a specific computer, to specific records for example in the case of visit to a medical practitioner aboard, while on vacation.

We assume that a patient can securely log on the web site that is at the front-end of his/her personal PaPeHR system and can be accessed from anywhere where Internet access is available. The patient can use available authentication methods (password, smartcard, token, biometrics, etc.) to be authenticated. Through this webpage the patient can administrate permissions that other individuals can have with respect to his PaPeHR, as described by Tang et al. (2006). The patient can register new users and define their permissions with respect to their PaPeHR (such as read, write, update, print etc). Such users can for example be family members, friends, medical practitioners, etc. In this way the patient serves as a security administrator with respect to their PaPeHR.

Functional requirements	
Situations / activities	**Actual functions and requirements**
Remote monitoring from patient's vital signs data (automatically upload of recorded data)	
• Physiological measurements • Activities of daily living measurements • Automatic detection of alarms	• Secure transfer from the patient's HUB to the intermediary/Gateway for data upload • Data formats according to open standards
Patient entered vital signs data (manually upload of recorded data)	
• Medical diary information • Drug intake and medications • Follow up activities in the care plan • Feelings, behaviour, well-being	• Web-based schema incorporated into PaPeHR • Data formats according to open standards • Directly integrated into the Core-EHR database • Internet-based frontend/secure social media
Patient Privacy	
• The patient should be responsible for his own PaPeHR and permissions given • Define authorization - access to different types of information/persons	• Delegation of access based on roles • Role based delegation to authorized health care organisations (home nurse, hospitals etc) • Incorporate a "blue-light" emergency access
Sealed sensitive information	
• In situations when the patient should not be able to read his doctors evaluation	• The patient can give access permissions to other defined clinicians
Basic Core EHR information according to defined standardized regulations	
• Important info in case of emergencies • Name and address to regularly used health care services in case of more information is needed	• Personalia • Current health status Medication list • Allergies • Regular health care services used
Tele-home-care services	
• Patients self-care • e-Communication with the health care services	• Data formats according to open standards • Secure transfer from the patient's mobile phone with web-based solutions
Secure location based tracking (GPS) of patients position	
• Need of finding patients with dementia not finding their way back home • In case of emergency situations, rescue team will need to locate the patient	• Trusted services authorized only when needed • Automatic logging of events • Written reports describing the actual need of access in each cases
Limited access when change in health care personnel and in emergencies	
• Transferral to another hospital • Staying abroad /on holiday • Unconscious patient	• New limited permissions should easily be given • Cross boarder identification personnel/hospitals • Ad-hock read only permissions to Core-EHR

Table 2. Specifications of functional requirements with important situations and activities, and the corresponding functions and requirements for a future PaPeHR

Non-functional requirements	
Situations / activities	**Actual functions and requirements**
Integration of Core-EHR information with other EHR integrations	
• The Core-EHR should automatically be updated after a doctor's visit or hospital treatment	• Export and import of data to other EHR systems • Indexes to locate more detailed information stored within national health information EHRs
Patient's transparent access to Core-EHR information	
• Update personalia • View medication list etc	• Direct integration with the Core-EHR located within a national health network
Front-end / back-end solution with security	
• Internet-available front-end with secure logon for actual users • Secure back-end service for all health care personnel and institutions	• Separated database solution • Dedicated AAA for secure logon • Access to a national namespace • Transparent service for the patient
Cross country integration	
• Patients mobility and travel abroad still being able to use the PaPeHR • Need of temporary access abroad	• National namespaces should be available • Standardization of access, information, data formats, etc.
Secure authentication	
• All persons given access should be authorized based on secure authentication • Automatic functions without the need of computer skills for the patient to define	• Two-factor authentication based on a PKI infrastructure or similar solution • Establish a digital ID for patients and health care personnel according to national standards
Secure and trusted longitudinal storage of data for a patient's lifetime	
• Based on the patient's privacy issues • The patient must be the "owner" of his PaPeHR and have fully control • Several solutions should compete the market (both private and public)	• Trusted third party services authorized by national authorities • Preferably established within the security of national health networks • Encryption of stored information

Table 3. Specifications of non-functional requirements with important situations and activities, and the corresponding functions and requirements for a future PaPeHR

In the architecture presented in Fig. 2, showing principles of the security design, a patient can log on AAA (authentication, authorization and accounting) server via web-based interface to assign permissions to other users he/she wants to give access to the PaPeHR. To simplify such permission administration we propose to use Role-Based Access Control principles as described by Ferraiolo et al. (2003), Hansen & Oleshchuk (2003) and Hansen & Oleshchuk (2006). In such systems there is a set of predefined roles e.g. *general practitioner, cardiologist, wife, parents, children,* etc with permissions defined according to law and regulations. In addition, a patient may prefer to define new roles that can be applied after testing on conformance with secure identification.

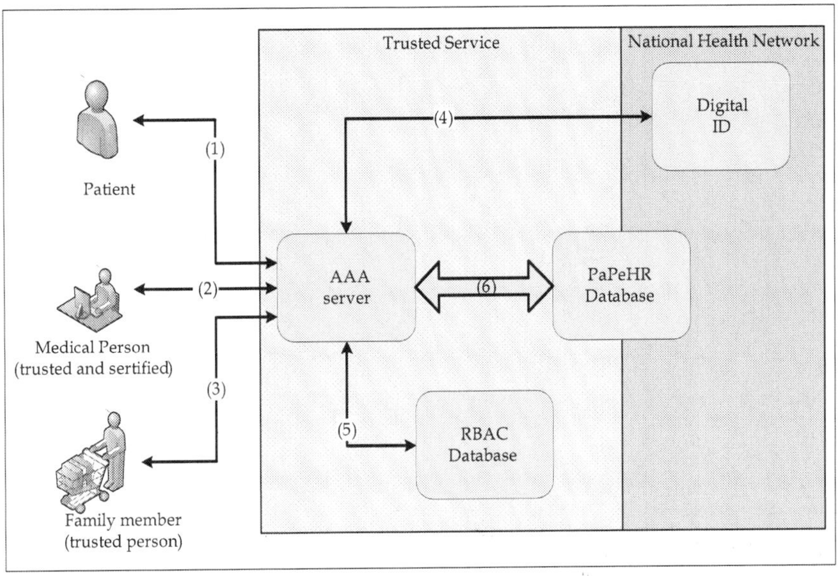

Fig. 2. Patient controlled acces to a PaPeHR, where a front-end Trusted Service is available from the Internet and with a back-end service within a secure National Health Network. The Patient (1), trusted and sertified Medical Person (2) and trusted Family Member (3) can log onto the system. After secure logon according to digital ID permissions (4) and granting the roles and access rights from the RBAC Database (5), the person is given access to the PaPeHR database (6)

As outlined in Fig. 2, the patient (1), trusted and sertified medical persons (2) and trusted family members (3) can log onto the system. After secure logon according to digital ID permissions (4) and granting the roles and access rights from the RBAC Database (5), the person is given access to the PaPeHR database (6).

By registering new users the patient will define the authentication method of these new users and their permissions and constraints with respect to his/her personal PaPeHR. It can be done by assigning corresponding roles such as MD, family member etc. The set of role templates should be pre-defined and available on AAA server. However, roles with critical permissions (for example, right to prescribe medications) should be assigned only to authorized personnel. This will be done by verifying user identity in Health personal namespace before the role will be assigned. Roles associated with limited set of permissions may be assigned on the base of the patient's trust to this user.

By registering a new user the patient selects user name and password, and their delivery method (delivered personally by the patient, via SMS to new user's mobile phone, by email, etc). After registration and role assignment all users are able to access the patient's PaPeHR directly via the Internet after authentication and according to assigned roles. Note that currently in a majority of the solutions protection of patient privacy is based on the assumption of trust by patients that their data will not be misused. However, the experience from real life shows that it is not the case (see for example a list of privacy related accidents in Appendix A in a description of Hippocratic Databases by Agrawal et al. (2002)). Therefore an approach based on patient controlled access described in this section can be considered as a sound solution that gives real privacy protection.

It should also be possible to have a dedicated role that can be used only to administrate access to the patient's PaPeHR on behalf of the patient. It can be assigned by the patient to any trusted person for some period of time (for example, due to the patient's health conditions). This administrative access should only have access to the AAA service defining permissions in the RBAC Permission Database, and not to the content stored within the PaPeHR database.

However, as the patient's PaPeHR should be securely stored for a lifelong period, integration with health care services is preferable; the PaPeHR solution should not be a stand-alone database but integrated into the national health care service. There should be a seamless integration of the patient's Core-EHR, transparent to the user, with actual access permissions.

Based on those assumptions, we recommend system architecture as shown in Fig. 3, where the Personal National Electronic Health Record (PNEHR) is securely established within a national health network service as an encrypted database. This database should consist of two different but integrated parts: the Spine/Core EHR and a database containing the raw data uploaded from the remote vital signs recording equipments. In principal, this model is based on the architecture for the English National Health Services, where the PRIMIS+ (2009) service (Primary Care Information Services) is established with defined standards for recording and exchange of health data.

7.2 Remote home monitoring

A remote Electrocardiography (ECG) monitoring system has been developed, and designed to be integrated into the PaPeHR framework as proposed by Fensli et al. (2005). The principles for a secure infrastructure with transfer of the patient's recorded information and mechanisms for exchange of information between health care professionals need to be established, in order to make the necessary interpretation and patient intervention as a response to the recorded vital signs information with detected arrhythmia events.

We will focus on how the patients can define and control access to share the recorded information with health care professionals, both on a daily basis and as ad-hoc access in case of emergencies. This solution should be an integrated part of the patient's PaPeHR and integrated in a shared "Core-EHR" solution where security and privacy issues are well defined and implemented. When measuring vital sign information, this should preferably be according to an international standard data format, and not as of today with mostly proprietary data formats used in the different products available on the market. If the remote monitoring system is measuring ECG signals, there exist several international standards. However, their capability of being used in a telemedicine context differs. For a near real-time ECG recording solution, it should be possible to record files containing a defined duration of the ECG signal sequence, and transfer these files from the patient worn HUB or mobile Hand Held Device (HHD) to the PaPeHR system.

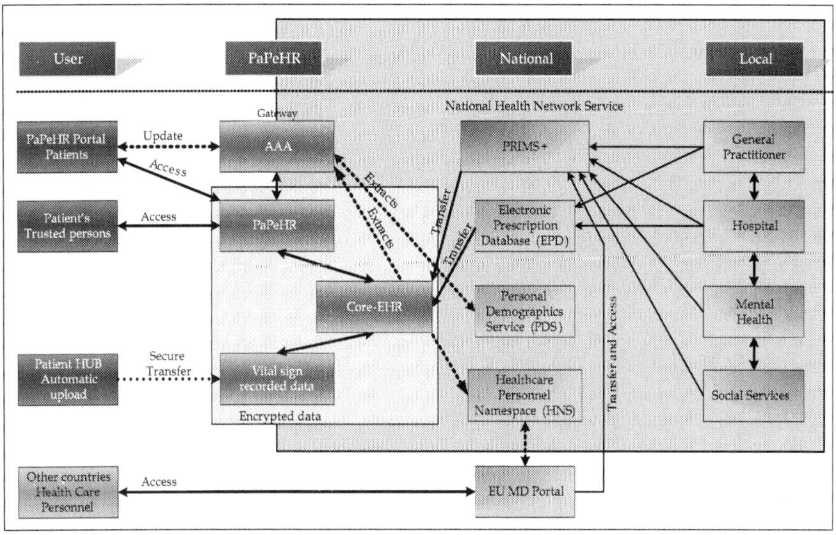

Fig. 3. Principles for a Patient administered Personal electronic Health Record (PaPeHR) service implemented within the framework of a National Health Network. In order to give emergency medical assistance for patients travelling abroad, an EU MD portal is proposed as a standardized gateway into the actual national framework

In the European drafted standard CEN ENV 1064, known as the Standard Communications Protocol for Computer - Assisted Electrocardiography (SCP-ECG), CEN/TC 251 Working Group IV (2006), specifications are given for transferring ECG reports and data from a vendor's ECG recorder to a central management system. In the specification and structure of the data content, it has the intention of being a general and interoperable standard. It is, however, not intended to be used for long-term ECG recordings as an ambulatory "Holter recorder" as may be the case for remote home monitoring solutions. The standard describes a binary file structure, and compression algorithms are used for the ECG signal representation. Because of the file compression methods used in the SCP-ECG format, the file size is relatively small, and could easily be sent from one hospital to another as a secure message within a National Health Network.

The described standard for medical waveform format encoding rules, MFER, is defined as an ISO standard, ISO/TS 11073-9201:2007 (2007). This format was developed as a universal standard description format for medical waveforms to be used for several defined types of Vital Signs. The standard describes different waveform types (electrocardiogram, sound, pulse, monitoring, magneto cardiogram, electroencephalogram etc.) which make this format open and flexible. It uses a binary format with a compact code in the header section, which gives relatively small file sizes. In the supplementary description at Level 2, tags representing waveform-related information, such as measurements, are defined to implement necessary beat annotations. It is possible to define long-term series of ECG recordings, thus this standard can be used for remote home monitoring solutions. Ideally, within a telemedical application to remotely monitor vital signs information, both actual standards SCP-ECG and MFER should be supported.

Integration of patient-entered data of daily measured vital sign information or automatically recorded information as a remote ECG recording solution, are today not defined within the Core-EHR framework. Such solutions can be established as an addendum to the Core-EHR and stored in a separate database which can be directly linked to the patient's Core-EHR. In such a solution the security and privacy issues should be combined, and necessary access to the information should be defined.

Recorded vital signs data can represent a huge amount of raw data for temporary storage to be accessed by the clinician. His signed evaluation of the data together with selected data samples should be extracted from the temporary storage and stored within the Core-EHR database for long-time storage. A remote ECG recording solution has been developed by Fensli et al. (2005), using a wireless ECG recording sensor attached to the patient's chest and communicating within a closed Body Area Network to a wearable hand held receiver or HHD. Arrhythmia detection algorithms implemented in this HHD will perform a continuous evaluation of arrhythmias, and upload detected events to the patient's vital signs database. In order to establish a secure mobile communication channel from the HHD at the patient, such solutions can be dependent of the actual services available by the telecom operator. A secure VPN channel can be established from the device either by implementing VPN software within this mobile terminal or by using encryption algorithms stores in the SIM card. This will give a secure transfer of recorded data from the HHD to an intermediary or Gateway implemented at the edge of a National Health Network. From this gateway, the transmitted recordings can be polled by a data server storing the database of recorded Vital Signs, as shown in Fig. 4.

7.3 Patient's role as administrator

Within a PaPeHR solution, a challenging task for the patient will be to fulfil the role as system administrator, as this will include assigning access rights to other persons. There is a lack of scientific publications describing how the patient can be able to manage the required tasks, and how those systems should be designed in order to give an intuitive way of performing necessary tasks. In many countries, the use of net-bank accounts is widely adopted. However, those systems are for single users with full permissions, and you will normally not be able to give access privileges to other persons unless you share the same net-bank account with your spouse or have similar solutions defined by your net-bank.

There are several difficulties to overcome. First of all, based on principles from the RBAC approach, patient/user should be able to define/configure suitable roles with needed privileges. Roles can be your local doctor, your home nurse, your private physiotherapist, spouse/next of kin, close friends etc.

As the PaPeHR will contain different types of data, it can be difficult to have sufficient overview. In addition, it should preferably be used common names of the different parts of information that can be understandable to the patient. As medical records use many Latin words, it is challenging to use more common names familiar to the patients with a normal vocabulary.

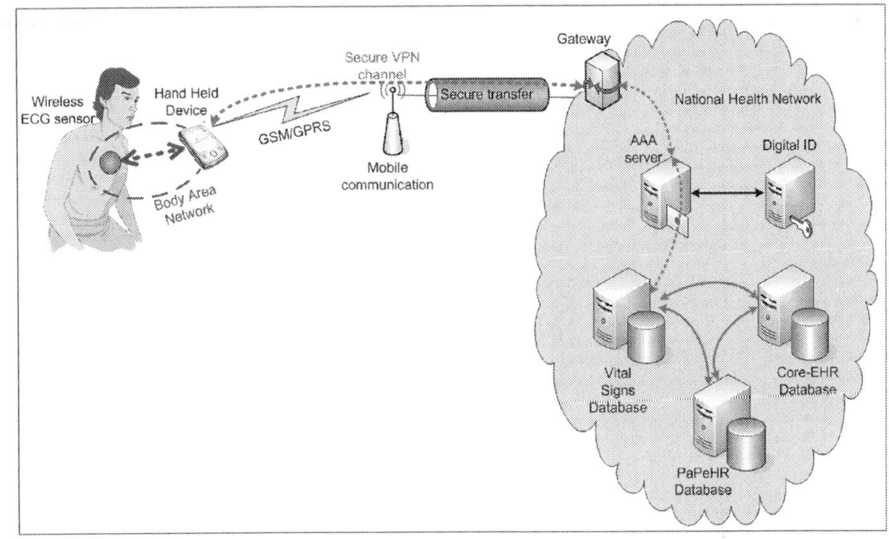

Fig. 4. Principles for secure transfer of real-time recorded ECG signals from a wireless sensor at the patient's chest to a Hand Held Device (HHD) where incorporated arrhythmia detection algorithms will store detected events. The files are transmitted via secure VPN channel to a Gateway at the edge of a National Health Network, where a Data Server can poll for the transmitted files, thus the files can be stored in a Vital Signs database, which is directly linked to the patient's PaPeHR database and also to the Core-EHR database

The problem of having an understandable format in medical documents within the PHR was also focused on in the study by Kahn et al. (2009). Access can be defined as denied, read only, permissions to write etc; however, normally no information should ever be deleted or changed after it is signed, as will be the cases for ordinary EHR solutions used within the health care services.

In Fig. 5, we have implemented a role-based interface for assigning actual persons to the required roles. As can be seen, the patient, after choosing the Access folder, can define persons being assigned to the actual roles. In this case, the patient can look up his/her doctor by entering the first name and surname, and by selecting the correct doctor from the list. It will be necessary to use digital ID's for secure login, and it can be defined a second step for the login procedure using onetime passwords transmitted to the mobile phone.

8. Discussions and conclusion

First of all, the use of patients' portals to access personal medical information and the ability to have electronic communication with health care services will obviously increase in the future, with the intention of providing the patient with higher degree of empowerment and better self-care. In order to give acceptable privacy to the patient, such solutions should preferably be based on the model of a standalone PHR; while at the same time should seamlessly integrate the access to a Core-EHR solution. The different models for a national Summary Care record or Core medical record system should be established with necessary

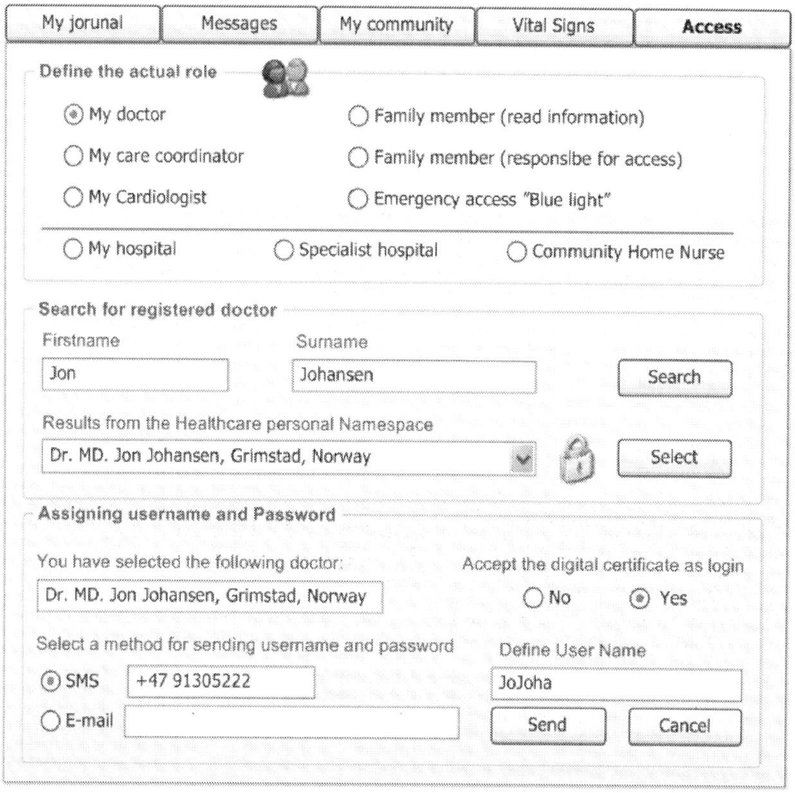

Fig. 5. Example of user interface for assigning access rights based on pre-defined roles, where the patient can select a registered doctor from the National Healthcare Namespace, and give him privileges as "My doctor". It should be incorporated possibilities for use of one-time secure password solutions, where a randomized password is sent to the person's defined mobile phone or to a defined E-mail address

security measures within the framework of a national health network. There are several models of EHR approach; however, it should be established an EU MB Portal where each national authority will be responsible for accreditation of medical personnel and with a cross-country namespace lookup.

Ongoing European initiatives focusing on interoperability and standardisation are important to obtain cross-border implementations. This can give opportunities for using open standards when developing new solutions, and there should preferably be several competing solutions available on the market offered by trusted third-party companies or organizations, where the patient can choose which PaPeHR solution he/she will use with the necessary confidence and trust.

Solutions for remote monitoring of vital signs data should not be developed as stand-alone applications, but integrated into the patient's PaPeHR system. As the amount of raw data can reach huge levels of stored information, those recordings should be stored in a separate database. From this temporarily database, the clinicians can do necessary evaluations and calculations/simulations/trend analysis/parameter estimations, and actual extracts of important findings should be imported and stored directly in the Core-EHR together with the medical epicrisis. The vital signs data should also be recorded according to defined international standards in order to exchange of data and integration into different EHR systems. Thus open viewers to show recorded and stored data should be developed and implemented into all EHR systems.

There are several challenges to overcome in the design of a Patient administered Personal electronic Health Record, and functionality requirements should be thoroughly explored in further research studies. However, the most delicate issue will probably be the question of how the patient will be able to fulfil the task as a system administrator, in managing roles and access privileges to all the persons (health care personnel and spouse/next of kin/ family members and friends/training partners, etc.) who should have different kinds of authorization to the information stored and to being able to add actual records of new information.

Taking into account the probable use of a facilitator helping the patient to perform those functions correctly, the human computer interaction in design of such new solutions should be focused on in future research projects. This focus is essential in order to develop an easy to use solution which can give the patient a feeling of usefulness helping him/her to better overcome the disease treatment and follow-up. If the obstacles we have pinpointed are overcome in a well designed solution with sufficient functionality, we believe that patients will quickly adopt the use of a secure health-care net account in the same way as electronic banking.

9. References

Agrawal, R., J. Kiernan, et al. (2002). Hippocratic databases, VLDB Endowment.

Anderson, R. M. and M. M. Funnell (2009). Patient empowerment: Myths and misconceptions. *Patient Education and Counseling*.

ANSI/INCITS 359-2004 (2004). Information Technology - Role Based Access Control. I. C. f. I. T. Standards: 56.

Aziz, O., B. Lo, et al. (2008). From computers to ubiquitous computing by 2010: health care. *Philos Transact A Math Phys Eng Sci* 366(1881): 3805-11.

Barlow, J., C. Wright, et al. (2002). Self-management approaches for people with chronic conditions: a review. *Patient Educ Couns* 48(2): 177-87.

Bergmann, J., O. J. Bott, et al. (2007). An e-consent-based shared EHR system architecture for integrated healthcare networks. *International Journal of Medical Informatics* 76(2-3): 130-136.

CEN/ISSS eHealth Standardization Focus Group. (2005). Current and future standardization issues in the eHealth domain: Achieving interoperability. Executive Summary. Retrieved 10 06, 2008, from ftp://ftp.cenorm.be/PUBLIC/Reports/eHealth/eHealthStandardizationExecutive%20summaryFinalversion2005-03-01.pdf.

CEN/TC 251 Working Group IV (2006). prEN 1064: 2005 (SCP-ECG) - Amendment

Cimino, J. J., V. L. Patel, et al. (2002). The patient clinical information system (PatCIS): technical solutions for and experience with giving patients access to their electronic medical records. *International Journal of Medical Informatics* 68(1-3): 113-127.

Commission, E. (2004). Commission Communication on "eHealth - making healthcare better for European citizens: An action plan for a European eHealth Area". COM(2004) 356 final.

Coulter, A., S. Parsons, et al. (2008). Where are the patients in decision-making about their own care? *World Health Organization.*

Dagtas, S., G. Pekhteryev, et al. (2008). Real-Time and Secure Wireless Health Monitoring. *International Journal of Telemedicine and Applications* Article ID 135808: 10p.

Demiris, G., L. B. Afrin, et al. (2008). Patient-centered Applications: Use of Information Technology to Promote Disease Management and Wellness. A White Paper by the AMIA Knowledge in Motion Working Group. *Journal of the American Medical Informatics Association* 15(1): 8-13.

European Commission (2006). Connected Health: Quality ans Safety for European Citizens. Report of the Unit ICT for Health in collaboration with the i2010 sub-group on eHealth and the eHealth stakeholders' group: 36.

Fensli, R. and E. Boisen (2008). How to evaluate human factors of wireless biomedical sensors. Identifying aspects of patient acceptance based on a preliminary clinical trial. *International Conference on Health Informatics, HEALTHINF*, Funchal, Madeira-Portugal.

Fensli, R., E. Gunnarson, et al. (2005). A wearable ECG-recording System for Continuous Arrhythmia Monitoring in a Wireless Tele-Home-Care Situation. *Proceedings. 18th IEEE Symposium on Computer-Based Medical Systems*, Dublin, Ireland.

Ferraiolo, D. F., D. R. Kuhn, et al. (2003). Role-Based Access Control. *Computer Security Series.*

Ferreira, A., D. Chadwick, et al. (2009). How to Securely Break into RBAC: The BTG-RBAC Model. *2009 Annual Computer Security Applications Conference (ACSAC)*, Honolulu, Hawaii, USA, IEEE.

Grimsmo, J., H. Arnesen, et al. (2010). Changes in cardiorespiratory function in different groups of former and still active male cross-country skiers: a 28–30-year follow-up study. *Scandinavian Journal of Medicine and Science in Sports* 20(1): e151-e161.

Hansen, F. Ø. and R. Fensli (2006). Method for Automatic Escalation of Access Rights to the Electronic Health Record. *MIE 2006 The 20th International Congress of the European Federation for Medical Informatics*, Maastricht, Netherlands, IOS Press.

Hansen, F. Ø. and V. Oleshchuk (2003). Application of Role-Based Access Control in Wireless Healthcare Information Systems. *Scandinavian Conference on Health Informatics*, Arendal, Norway, Agder University College.

Hansen, F. Ø. and V. Oleshchuk (2006). Location-based Security Framework for use of Handheld Devicces in Medical Information Systems. *4th IEEE Conference on Pervasive Computing and Communications Workshop (PerCom 2006 Workshops*, Pisa, Italy, IEEE Computer Society.

HiMSS (August 2008). Electronic Health Records: A Global Perspective. A Work Product of the HIMSS Enterprise Systems Steering Committee and the Global Enterprise Task Force.

Hurtado, M. P., E. K. Swift, et al. (2000). Institute of Medicine (IOM) Committee on the National Quality Report on Health Care Delivery, Board on Health Care Services. Envisioning the National Health Care Quality Report. Washington DC, National Academic Press.

ISO/TS 11073-9201:2007. (2007). Health informatics – Medical waveform format – Part 92001:Encoding rules (MFER). Retrieved 15 October, 2008, from http://webstore.ansi.org/RecordDetail.aspx?sku=ISO%2fTS+11073-92001%3a2007.

Kahn, J. S., V. Aulakh, et al. (2009). What It Takes: Characteristics Of The Ideal Personal Health Record. *Health Aff* 28(2): 369-376.

Kong, K. Y., C. Y. Ng, et al. (2000). Web-Based Monitoring of Real-Time ECG Data. *Computers in Cardiology* 27: 189-192.

Kumar, S., K. Kambhatla, et al. (2008). Ubiquitous Computing for Remote Cardiac Patient Monitoring: A Survey. *International Journal of Telemedicine and Applications* Article ID 459185.

Markle Foundation (2003). Connecting for Health. The personal health working group final report.

NEN. (2009). E-HEALTH-INTEROP. Retrieved 04,09, 2010, from http://www.ehealth-interop.nen.nl.

Oleshchuk, V. and R. Fensli (2010). Remote Patient Monitoring Within a Future 5G Infrastructure. *Wireless Personal Communications*: 1-9.

PRIMIS+. (2009). What is PRIMIS+. Retrieved 06.09, 2010, from http://www.primis.nhs.uk/index.php/about-us.

Ross, S. E. and C. T. Lin (2003). The Effects of Promoting Patient Access to Medical Records: A Review. *Journal of the American Medical Informatics Association* 10(2): 129-138.

Salvador, C. H., M. P. Carrasco, et al. (2005). Airmed-Cardio: A GSM and Internet Services-Based System for Out-of-Hospital Follow-Up of Cardiac Patients. *IEEE Trans Inf Technol Biomed* 9(March): 73-85.

Scalvini, S., S. Capomolla, et al. (2005). Effect of home-based telecardiology on chronic heart failure: costs and outcomes. *Journal of Telemedicine & Telecare* 11(S1): 16-18.

Shabo, A. (2006). A global socio-economic-medico-legal model for the sustainability of longitudinal electronic health records. Part 1. *Methods of Information in Medicine* 45(3): 240-5.

Stolyar, A., W. B. Lober, et al. (2006). A Patient-Centered Health Record in a Demonstration Regional Health Information Network. *The 1st Distributed Diagnosis and Home healthcare (D2H2) Conference*, Arlington, Virginia, USA.

sundhed.dk. (2010). The Danish eHealth Portal. Retrieved 04.09, 2010, from https://www.sundhed.dk/profil.aspx?id=11062.105

Tang, P. C., J. S. Ash, et al. (2006). Personal Health Records: Definitions, Benefits, and Strategies for Overcoming Barriers to Adoption. *Journal of the American Medical Informatics Association* 13(2): 121-126.

The Scottish Government. (2006). Your Emergency Care Summary: What does it mean for you? Retrieved 04,09, 2010, from http://www.scotland.gov.uk/Publications/2006/08/16152132/0.

U.S. Dept of Health and Human Services (2008). Remote Monitoring. Draft Details Use Case. http://library.ahima.org/xpedio/groups/public/documents/government/bok1_036413.pdf#page%3D1, Office of the National Coordinator for Health Information Technology: 34.

UK National Health Service. (2008). HealthSpace. Retrieved 10 04, 2008, from https://www.healthspace.nhs.uk/.

Vogel, R., F. Wozak, et al. (2006). Architecture for a Distributed National Electronic Health Record System in Austria. Retrieved 10.05, 2008, from http://www.europacs.net/Extended%20abstracts/Integration%20of%20PACS%20RIS%20and%20EPR/Raimund%20Vogel%20Full_Paper_DistEHR_RVo_EuroPACS2006.pdf.

W3C. (1999). Web Content Accessibility Guidelines 1.0. Retrieved 04,09, 2010, from http://www.w3.org/TR/WAI-WEBCONTENT/.

W3C. (2008). Evaluating Web Sites for Accessibility: Overview. Retrieved 04,09, 2010, from http://www.w3.org/WAI/eval/Overview.html.

Wald, H. S., C. E. Dube, et al. (2007). Untangling the Web—The impact of Internet use on health care and the physician-patient relationship. *Patient Education and Counseling* 68(3): 218-224.

Weingart, S. N., D. Rind, et al. (2006). Who Uses the Patient Internet Portal? The PatientSite Experience. *Journal of the American Medical Informatics Association* 13(1): 91-95.

Wootton, R. and J. C. Kvedar (2006). Home Telehealth: Connecting Care Within the Community, RSM Press.

30

Nonparametric Variable Selection Using Machine Learning Algorithms in High Dimensional (Large P, Small N) Biomedical Applications

Christina M. R. Kitchen
University of California, Los Angeles, United States of America

1. Introduction

Biomedical data is facing an ever increasing amount of data that resist classical methods. Classical methods cannot be applied in the case of high dimensional datasets where the number of parameters greatly exceeds the number of observations, the so-called "large p small n" problem. Machine Learning techniques have had tremendous success in these realms in a wide-variety of disciplines. Often these machine learning tools are combined to include a variable selection step and model building step. In some cases the goal of the analysis may be exploratory in nature and the researcher is more interested in knowing which set of variables are strongly related to the output variable rather than predictive accuracy. For those situations, the goal of the analysis may be to provide a ranking of the input variables based on their relative importance in predicting the outcome. Other purposes for variable selection include elimination of redundant or irrelevant variables and to improve the performance of the predictive algorithm.

Even if prediction is the goal of the analysis, several machine learning algorithms require that some dimension reduction is done prior to the model building, thus variable selection is an important problem. Let Y be the outcome of interest. Y can be continuous or categorical. When Y is continuous we call this a regression problem and when Y is categorical we call this a classification problem. Let $X_1,...,X_p$ be a set of potential predictors (also called inputs). X and Y are vectors of n observations. The goal of variable selection, broadly defined, is finding the set of X's that are strongly related the outcome Y. Even for moderate values of p, estimating all possible linear models (2^p) is computationally expensive and thus there needs to be some dimension reduction. If p is large, and the set of all X's contain redundant, irrelevant or highly correlated variables, such as the case in many biomedical applications including genome wide association studies and microarray studies, then the problem can be difficult. Further complicating matters, real-world data can have X's that are of mixed type, where predictors are measured on different scales (categorical versus continuous) and the relationship between the outcome may be highly non-linear with high-order interactions.

Generally, one can consider several machine learning methods for variable selection: one is a greedy search algorithm that examines the conditional probability distribution of Y, the response variable, for each predictor variable X. However, this method is at a disadvantage when there are interactions present. Another method is best subset selection which looks at the change in predictive accuracy for each subset of predictors. When the number of parameters becomes large, examining each possible subset becomes computationally infeasible. Methods such as forward selection and backwards elimination are also not likely to yield the optimal subset in this case. The third method uses all of the *X*'s to generate a model and then use the model to examine the relative importance of each variable in the model. Random Forests and its derivatives are machine learning tools that were primarily created as a predictive model and secondly as a way to rank the variable in terms of their importance to the model. Random Forests are growing increasingly popular in genetics and bioinformatics research. They are applicable in the small n large p problems and can deal with high-order interactions and non-linear relationships. Although there are many machine learning techniques that are applicable for data of this type and can give measures of variable importance such as Support Vector Machines (Vapnik 1998; Rakotomamonjy 2003), neural networks (Bishop 1995), Bayesian variable selection (George and McCulloch 1993; George and McCulloch 1997; Kuo and Mallick 1999; Kitchen et al., 2007) and k-nearest neighbors (Dasarathy 1991), we will concentrate on Random Forests because of their relative ease of use, popularity and computational efficiency.

2. Trees and Random Forests

Classification and regression trees (Breiman et al., 1984) are flexible, nonlinear and nonparametric. They produce easily interpretable binary decision trees but can also overfit and become unstable (Breiman 1996; Breiman 2001). To overcome this problem several advances have been suggested. It has been shown that for some splitting criteria, recursive binary partitioning can induce a selection bias towards covariates with many possible splits (Loh and Shih 1997; Loh 2002; Hothorn et al., 2006). The key to producing unbiasedness is to separate the variable selection and the splitting procedure (Loh and Shih 1997; Loh 2002; Hothorn et al., 2006). The conditional inference trees framework was first developed by Hothorn et al (Hothorn et al., 2006). These trees select variables in an unbiased way and are not prone to overfitting. Let $w = (w_1,...,w_n)$ be a vector of non-negative integer valued case weights where the weights are non-zero when the corresponding observations are included in the node and 0 otherwise. The algorithm is as follows: 1) At each node test the null hypothesis of independence between any of the *X*'s and the response *Y*, that is test $P(Y \mid X_j) = P(Y)$ for all j: $j=1,\dots,p$. If the null hypothesis cannot be rejected at alpha level less than some pre-specified level then the algorithm terminates. If the null hypothesis of independence is rejected then the covariate with the strongest association to Y is selected (that is, the X_j with the lowest p-value). 2) Split the covariate into two disjoint sets using permutation test to find the optimal binary split with the maximum discrepancy between the samples. Note that other splitting criteria could be used. 3) Repeat the steps recursively. Hothorn asserts that compared to GUIDE (Loh 2002) and QUEST (Loh and Shih 1997), other unbiased methods for classification trees, conditional inference trees have similar prediction accuracy but conditional inference trees are intuitively more appealing as alpha has the more familiar interpretation of type I error instead being used solely as a tuning parameter, although it could be used as such. Much of the recent work on extending classification and regression trees have been on growing ensembles of trees. Bagging, short for bootstrap aggregation, whereupon many bootstrapped samples of the data are generated from a dataset with a separate tree grown for each sample was proposed by Breiman in 1996. This technique has been shown to reduce the variance of the estimator (Breiman 1996). The random split selection proposed by Dietterich 2000 also grows multiple trees but the splits are chosen uniformly at random from among the K best splits (Dietterich 2000). This method can be used either with or without pruning the trees. Random split selection has better predictive accuracy than bagging (Dietterich 2000). Boosting, another competitor to bagging, involves iteratively weighting the outputs where the weights are inversely proportional to their accuracy, has excellent predictive accuracy but can degenerate if there is noise in the labels. Ho suggested growing multiple trees where each tree is grown using a fixed subset of variables (Ho 1998). Predictions were made by averaging the votes across the trees. Predictive ability of the ensemble depends, in part, on low correlation between the trees. Random Forests extends the random subspace method of Ho 1998. Random Forests belong to a class of algorithms called weak learners and are characterized by low bias and high variance. They are an ensemble of simple trees that are allowed to grow unpruned and were introduced by Breiman (Breiman 2001). Random Forests are widely applicable, nonlinear, non-parametric, are able to handle mixed data types (Breiman 2001; Strobl et al., 2007; Nicodemus et al., 2010). They are faster than bagging and boosting and are easily parallelized. Further they are robust to missing values, scale invariant, resistant to over-fitting and have high predictive accuracy (Breiman 2001). Random forests also provide a ranking of the predictor variables in terms of their relative importance to the model. A single tree is unstable providing different trees for mild changes within the data. Together bagging, predictor subsampling and averaging across all trees helps to prevent over-fitting and increase stability. Briefly Random Forests can be described by the following algorithm:

1. Draw a large number of bootstrapped samples from the original sample (the number of trees in the forest will equal the number of bootstrapped samples).
2. Fit a classification or regression tree on each bootstrapped sample. Each tree is maximally grown without any pruning where at each node a randomly selected subset of size *mtry* possible predictors from the p possible predictors are selected (where $mtry < p$) and the best split is calculated only from this subset. If $mtry=p$ then it is termed bagging and is not considered a Random Forest. Note, one could also use a random linear combination of the subset of inputs for splitting as well.
3. Prediction is based on the out of bag (OOB) average across all trees. The out-of-bag (OOB) samples are the data that are not used in the test set (roughly 1/3 of the variables) and can be used to test the tree grown. That is, for each pair (x_i, y_i) in the training sample select only the trees that do not contain the pair and average across these trees.

The additional randomness added by selecting a subset of parameters at random instead of splitting on all possible parameters releases Random Forests from the small n, large p problem (Strobl et al., 2007) and allows the algorithm to be adaptive to the data and reduces correlation among the trees in the forest (Ishwaran 2007). The accuracy of a Random Forest depends on the strength of the individual trees and the level of correlation between the trees (Breiman 2001). Averaging across all trees in the forest allows for good predictive accuracy and low generalization error.

3. Use in biomedical applications

Random Forests are increasingly popular in the biomedical community and enjoy good predictive success even against other machine learning algorithms in a wide variety of applications (Lunetta et al., 2004; Segal et al., 2004; Bureau et al. 2005; Diaz-Uriarte and Alvarez de Andes 2006; Qi, Bar-Joseph and Klein-Seetharaman 2006; Xu et al., 2007; Archer and Kimes 2008; Pers et al. 2009; Tuv et al., 2009; Dybowski, Heider and Hoffman 2010; Geneur et al., 2010). Random Forests have been used in HIV disease to examine phenotypic properties of the virus. Segal et al used Random Forests to examine the role of mutations in polymerase in HIV-1 to viral replication capacity (Segal et al., 2004). Random Forests have also been used to predict HIV-1 coreceptor usage from sequence data (Xu et al., 2007; Dybowski et al., 2010). Qi et al found that Random Forests had excellent predictive capabilities in the prediction of protein interaction compared to six other machine learning methods (Qi et al., 2006). Random Forests have also been found to have favorable predictive characteristics in microarray and genomic data (Lunetta et al., 2004; Bureau et al. 2005; Lee et al., 2005; Diaz-Uriarte and Alvarez de Andes 2006). These applications, in particular, use Random Forests as a prediction method and as a filtering method (Breiman 2001; Lunetta et al., 2004; Bureau et al. 2005; Diaz-Uriarte and Alvarez de Andes 2006). To unbiasedly test between several machine learning algorithms, a game was devised where bootstrapped samples from a dataset were given to players who used different machine learning strategies specifically Support Vector Machines, LASSO, and Random Forests to predict an outcome. Model performance was gauged by a separate referee using a strictly proper scoring rule. In this setup, Pers et al found that Random Forests had the lowest bootstrap cross-validation error compared to the other algorithms (Pers et al. 2009).

4. Variable importance in Random Forests

While variable importance in a general setting has been studied (van der Laan 2006) we will examine it in the specific framework of Random Forests. In the original formulation of CART, variable importance was defined in terms of surrogate variables where the variable importance looks at the relative improvement summed over all of the nodes of the primary variable versus its surrogate. There are a number of variable importance definitions for Random Forests. One could simply count the number of times a variable appears in the forest as important variables should be in many of the trees. But this would be a naïve estimator because the information about the hierarchy of the tree where naturally the most important variables are placed higher in the tree is lost. One the other hand one could only look at the primary splitters of each tree in the forest and count the number of times that a variable is the primary splitter. A more common variable importance measure is Gini Variable Importance (GVI) which is the sum of the Gini impurity decrease for a particular variable over all trees. That is, Gini variable importance is a weighted average of a particular variables improvement of the tree using the Gini criterion across all trees. Let N be the number of observations at node j, and N_R and N_L be the number of observations of the right and left daughter nodes after splitting, and let d_{ij} be the decrease in impurity produced by variable X_i at the jth node of the tth tree. If Y is categorical, then the Gini index is given by $\hat{G} = 2\hat{p}(1-\hat{p})$, where $\hat{p}$ is the proportion of 1's in the sample. So in this case,

$d_{ij} = \hat{G} - (\frac{N_L}{N}\hat{G}_L + \frac{N_R}{N}\hat{G}_R)$; where $\hat{G}_L$ and $\hat{G}_R$ are the Gini indexes of the left and right node respectively. The Gini Variable importance of variable X_i is defined as

$$G\hat{VI}(X_i) = \frac{1}{T}\sum_{t=1}^{T} (\sum_{J} d_{ij} I_{ij})$$

where I_{ij} is an indicator variable for whether the ith variable was used to split node j. That is, it is the average of the Gini importance over all trees, T.

Permutation variable importance (PVI) is the difference in predictive accuracy using the original variable and a randomly permuted version of the variable. That is, for variable X_i, count the number of correct votes using the out-of-bag cases and then randomly permute the same variable and count the number of correct votes using the out of bag cases. The difference between the number of correct votes for the unpermuted and permuted variables averaged across all trees is the measure of importance.

$$PVI(X_i) = \frac{1}{T}\sum_{t}(errorOOB_{ti} - error\overline{OOB_{ti}})$$

Where t is a tree in the Out of Bag sample, $errorOOB_{ti}$ is the misclassification rate of the original variable X_i in tree t, and $error\,\overline{OOB_{ti}}$ is the misclassification rate on the permuted X_i variable for tree t.

Strobl et al (Strobl et al. 2008) suggested a conditional permutation variable importance measure for when variables are highly correlated. Realizing that if there exists correlation within the X's, the variable importance for these variables could be inflated as the construction of variable importance measures departures from independence of the variable X_i from the outcome Y and also from the remaining predictor variables $X_{(-i)}$, they devised a new conditional permutation variable importance measure. Here $X_{(-i)}$ reflects the remaining covariates not including X_i in other words $X_{(-i)} = \{X_1,...,X_{i-1},X_{i+1},...,X_p\}$. The new measure is obtained by conditionally permuting values of X_i within groups of covariates, $X_{(-i)}$ which are held fixed. One could use any partition for conditioning or use the partition already generated by the recursive partitioning procedure. Further one could include all variables $X_{(-i)}$ to condition on or only include those variables whose correlation with X_i exceeds a certain threshold. The main drawback of this variable importance scheme is its computational burden. Ishwaran (Ishwaran 2007) carefully studied variable importance with highly correlated variables with a simpler definition of variable importance. Variable importance was defined as the difference in prediction error using the original variable and a random node assignment after the variable is encountered. Two-way interactions were examined via jointly permuted variable importance. This method allows for the explicit ranking of the interactions in relation to all other variables in terms of their relative importance even in the face of correlation. However for large p, examining all two-way variable importance measures would be computationally infeasible. Tuv et al (Tuv et al., 2009) takes a random permutation of each potential predictor and a Random Forest is generated from this and the variable importance scores are compared to the original scores via the t-test. Surrogate variables are eliminated by the generation of gradient boosted trees. Then by iteratively selecting the top variables on the variable importance and then re-running Random Forests, they were able to obtain smaller and smaller numbers of predictors.

5. Other issues in variable importance in Random Forests

Because Random Forests are often used as a screening tool based on the results of the variable importance ranking, it is important to consider some of the properties of the variable importance measures especially under various assumptions.

5.1 Different measurement scales

In the original implementation of CART, Breiman noted that the Gini index was biased towards variables with more possible splits (Breiman et al., 1984). When data types are measured on different scales such as when some variables are continuous while others are categorical, it has been found that Gini importance is biased (Strobl et al., 208; Breiman et al., 1984; White and Liu 1994; Hothorn et al., 2006; Strobl et al., 2007; Sandri and Zuvvolotto 2008). In some cases suboptimal variables could be artificially inflated in these scenarios. Strobl et al found that using the permutation variable importance with subsampling without replacement provided unbiased variable selection (Strobl et al., 2007). In simulation studies, Strobl (Strobl et al., 2007) shows that the Gini criteria is strongly biased with mixed data types and proposed using a conditional inference framework for constructing forests. Further they show that under the original implementation of random forests, permutation importance is also biased. This difference was diminished when using conditional inference forests and when subsampling was performed without replacement. Because of this bias, permutation importance is now the default importance measure in the random forest package in R (Breiman 2002).

5.1 Correlated predictors

Permutation variable importance rankings have been found to be unstable for when filtering Single Nucleotide Polymorphisms (SNP) variable importance (Nicodemus et al., 2007; Calle and Urrea 2010). The notion of stability, in this case, is that the genes on the "important" lists remain constant throughout multiple runs of the Random Forests. Genomic data such as microarray data and sequence data often have high correlation among the potential predictor variables. Several studies have shown that high correlation among the potential predictor X's poses problems with variable importance measures in Random Forests (Strobl et al. 2008; Nicodemus and Malley 2009; Nicodemus et al., 2010). Nicodemus found that there is a bias towards uncorrelated predictors and that there is a dependence on the size of the subset sample *mtry* (Nicodemus and Malley 2009). Computer simulations have found that surrogate (highly correlated variables) are often within the set of highly ranked important variables but that these variables are unlikely to be on the same tree. In a sense, these variables compete for selection into a tree. This competition diminishes their impact on the variable importance scores. The ranking procedure based on Gini and permutation importance cannot distinguish between the correlated predictors. In simulations when the correlation between variables is less that 0.4, any variable importance measure appears to work well with the true variables being among the top listed variables in the variable importance ranking with multiple runs of the Random Forest. Using Gini variable importance, variables with correlations less than 0.5 appear to have minimal impact on the size of the variable importance ranking list that includes the variables that are truly related to the outcome. The graph below shows how large the variable importance list has to be to recover 10 true variables among 100 total variables, 90 of which are random noise and independent of the outcome variables under various levels of correlation among the predictors using Gini variable importance (GVI) and permutation variable importance (PVI).

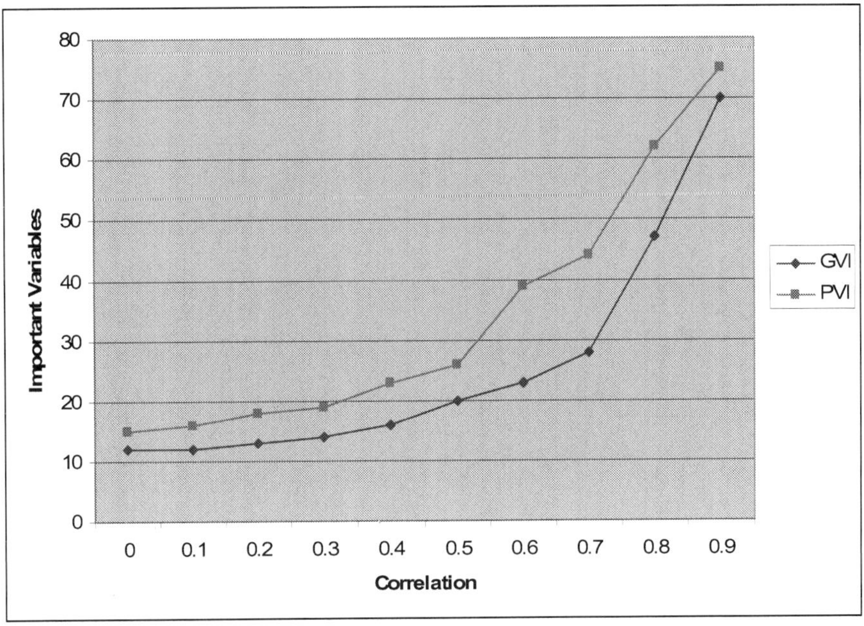

This result is similar to that found by Archer and Kimes showing that Gini variable importance is stable under moderate correlation in that the true predictor may not be the highest listed under the most important variables but will be among the set of high valued variables (Archer and Kimes 2008). This result is also consistent with the findings of Nonyane and Foulkes (Nonyane and Foulkes 2008). They found that in comparing Random Forests and Multivariate Adaptive Regression Splines (MARS) in simulated genetic data with one true effect, X_1, and seven correlated but uninformative variables and one covariate Z under six different model structures. They define the true discovery rate as: if the X_1, the true variable, is listed first or second to Z in the variable importance ranking using the Gini variable importance measure. They found that for correlation less than 0.5, the true discovery rate is relatively stable regardless of how one handles the covariate.

Several solutions for correlated variables have been proposed. Sandri and Zuccolotto proposed the use of pseudovariables as a correction for the bias in Gini importance (Sandri and Zuvvolotto 2008). In a study of SNPs in linkage disequilibrium, Meng et al restricted the tree-building algorithm to disallow correlated predictors in the same tree (Meng et al. 2009).

They found that the stronger the degree of association of the predictor to the response, the stronger the effect of the correlation has on the performance of the forest. Strobl 2008 also found that with under strong correlation, conditional inference trees using permutation variable importance also had a bias in variable selection (Strobl et al. 2008). To overcome this bias they developed a conditional permutation scheme where the variable to be permuted was permuted conditional on the other correlated variables which are held fixed. In this set up one can use any partition of the feature space such as a binary partition learned from a tree to condition on. Use the recursive partitioning to define the partition and then: 1) compute OOB prediction accuracy for each tree, 2) for all variables Z to be conditioned on, create a grid 3) permute within a grid of X_i and compute OOB prediction accuracy 4) difference the accuracy averaged across all trees. Z could be all other variables besides X_i or all variables correlated with X_i with a correlation coefficient higher than a set threshold. Similar to Nicodemus and Malley, they found that permutation variable importance was biased when there exists correlation among the X variables and this was especially true with small values of *mtry* (Nicodemus and Malley 2009). They also found that while bias decreases with larger values of *mtry*, variability increases. In simulations, conditional permutation variable importance still had a preference for highly correlated variables but less so that standard permutation variable importance. The authors suggest using different values of *mtry* and a large number of trees so results with different seeds do not vary systematically.

In another study Nicodemus found that permutation variable importance had preference for uncorrelated variables because correlated variables compete with each other (Nicodemus et al., 2010). They also found that large values of *mtry* can inflate the importance for correlated predictors for permutation variable importance. They found the opposite effect for conditional variable importance. Further they found that conditional variable importance measures from Conditional Inference Forests inflated uncorrelated strongly associated variables relative to correlated strongly associated variables. They also found that conditional permuation importance was computationally intractable for large datasets. The authors were only able to calculate this measure for n=500 and for only 12 predictors. They conclude that conditional variable importance is useful for small studies where the goal is to identify the set of true predictors among a set of correlated predictors. In studies such as genetic association studies where the set of predictors is large, original permutation based variable importance may be better suited.

In genomic association studies, often one wants to find the smallest set of non-related genes that are potentially related to the outcome for further study. One method is to select an arbitrary threshold and list the top *h* variables in the variable importance list. Another approach is to iteratively use Random Forests, feeding in the top variables from the variable importance list as potential predictors and selecting the final model as the one with the smallest error rate given a subset of genes (Diaz-Uriarte and Alvarez de Andes 2006). Geneur et al used a similar two-stage approach with highly correlated variables where one first eliminates lowest ranked variables ranked by importance and then tested nested models in a stepwise fashion, selecting the most parsimonious model with the minimum OOB error rate (Geneur et al., 2010). They found that under high correlation there was high variance on variable importance lists. They proposed that *mtry* be drawn from the variable ranking distribution and not uniformly across all variables although this was not specifically tested. Meng et al also used an iterative machine leanring scheme where the top ranked important variables were assessed using Random Forests and then used as predictors in a separate prediction algorithm (Meng et al. 2007). Specifically, Random Forests was used to narrow the parameter space and then the top ranked variables were used in a Bayesian network for prediction. They found that using the top 50SNPs in the variable importance list as the predictors for a second Random Forest resulted in good variable selection in their simulations, although the generalizability is not known (Meng et al. 2007).

6. Recommendations

For all Random Forest implementations it is recommended that one:

1. Grow a large forest with a large number of trees (*ntree* at least 5000).
2. Use a large terminal node size.
3. Try different values of *mtry* and seeds. Try setting $mtry = \sqrt{mdim}$ as an initial starting value for mtry; where *mdim* is the number of potential predictors.
4. Run algorithm repeatedly. That is, create several random forests until the variable importance list appears stable.

In using Random Forests for variable selection we can make several recommendations. These recommendations vary by the nature of the data. It is well known that the Gini variable importance has bias in its variable selection thus for most instances we recommend permutation variable importance. Indeed this is the default in the R package randomForest. If the predictors are all measured on the same scale and are independent then this default should be sufficient. If the data are of mixed type (measured on different scales), then use Conditional Inference Forests with permutation variable importance. Use subsampling without replacement instead of the default bootstrap sampling as suggested by Strobl 2007. All measures of variable importance have bias under strong correlation. It is important to test whether the variables are correlated. If there is correlation, then one must assess the goal of the study. If there is high correlation among the X's and the p is small and the goal of the study is to find the set of true predictors, then using conditional inference trees and conditional permutation variable importance is a good solution. However if there is a large p using conditional permuation importance may be computationally infeasible and either some parameter space reduction will be necessary. In that case, using permutation importance using Random Forests or iterative random Forests may be better suited for creating a list of important variables.

If there are highly correlated variables and there if p or n is large thenone can use Random Forests iteratively with permutation variable importance. In this case one selects the top h variables in the variable importance ranking list as predictors for another Random Forest. In this case h is selected by the user. Meng et al used the top 50 percent of the predictors. This scenario works best when there is a strong association of the predictors to the outcome (Meng et al., 2007).

7. References

Archer, K. and R. Kimes (2008). "Empirical characterization of random forest variable importance measures." Computational Statistics and Data Analysis 52(4): 2249-2260.

Bishop, C. (1995). Neural networks for pattern recognition. Oxford, Clarendon Press.

Breiman, L. (1996). "Bagging predictors." Machine Learning 24(2): 123-140.

Breiman, L. (2001). "Random Forests." Machine Learning 45: 5-32.

Breiman, L. (2001). "Statistical modeling: the two cultures." Stat Science 16: 199-231.

Breiman, L. (2002). "Manual on setting up, using, and understanding Random Forests V3.1." Technical Report

Breiman, L., J. Friedman, R. Olshen and C. Stone (1984). Classification and Regression Trees. Belmont, CA, Wadsworth International Group.

Bureau, A., J. Dupuis, K. Falls, K. L. Lunetta, L. B. Hayward, T. P. Keith and P. V. Eerdewegh (2005). "Identifying SNPs predictive of phenotype using random forests." Genetic Epidemiology 28: 171-182.

Calle, M. and V. Urrea (2010). "Letter to the editor: stability of random forest importance measures." Briefings in Bioinformatics 2010.

Dasarathy, B. (1991). Nearest-neighbor pattern classification techniques. Los Alamitos, IEEE Computer Society Press.

Diaz-Uriarte, R. and S. Alvarez de Andes (2006). "Gene selection and classification of microarray data using random forests." BMC Bioinformatics 7: 3.

Dietterich, T. (2000). "An experimental comparison of three methods for constructing ensembles of decision trees: bagging, boosting and randomization." Machine Learning 40: 139-158.

Dybowski, J., D. Heider and D. Hoffman (2010). "Prediction of co-receptor usage of HIV-1 from genotype." PLOS Computational Biology 6(4): e1000743.

Geneur, R., J. Poggi and C. Tuleau-Malot (2010). "Variable selection using random forests." Pattern Recognitions Letters 31: 2225-2236.

George, E. I. and R. E. McCulloch (1993). "Variable selection via gibbs sampling." Journal of the American Statistical Association 88: 881--89.

George, I. and R. E. McCulloch (1997). "Approached for Bayesian variable selection." Statistica Sinica 7: 339-373.

Ho, K. (1998). "The random subspace method for constructing decision forests." IEEE Transactions on Pattern Analysis and Machine Intelligence 20(8): 832-844.

Hothorn, T., K. Hornik and A. Zeileis (2006). "Unbiased recursive partitioning: a conditional inference frameork." Journal of Computational and Graphical Statistics 15(3): 651-674.

Ishwaran, H. (2007). "Variable importance in binary regression trees and forests." Electronic Journal of Statistics 1: 519-537.

Kitchen, C., R. Weiss, G. Liu and T. Wrin (2007). "HIV-1 viral fitness estimation using exchangeable on subset priors and prior model selection." Statistics in Medicine 26(5): 975-990.

Kuo, L. and B. Mallick (1999). "Variable selection for regression models." Sankya B 60: 65--81.

Lee, J., J. Lee, M. Park and S. Song (2005). "An extensive compairson of recent classification tools applied to microarray data." Computational Statistics and Data Analysis 48: 869-885.

Loh, W.-Y. (2002). "Regression trees with unbiased variable selection and interaction detection." Statistica Sinica 12: 361-386.

Loh, W.-Y. and Y.-S. Shih (1997). "Split slection methods for classification trees." Statistica Sinica 7: 815-840.

Lunetta, K. L., L. B. Hayward, J. Segal and P. V. Eerdewegh (2004). "Screening large-scale association study data: exploiting interactions using random forests." BMC Genetics 5: 32.

Meng, Y., Q. Yang, K. Cuenco, L. Cupples, A. DeStefano and K. L. Lunetta (2007). "Two-stage approach for identifying single-nucleotide polymorphisms associated with rheumatoid arthritis using random forests and Bayesian networks." BMC Proceedings 1(Suppl 1): S56.

Meng, Y., Y. Yu, L. Adrienne Cupples, L. Farrer and K. Lunetta (2009). "Performance of random forest when SNPs are in linkage disequilibrium." BMC Bioinformatics 10: 78.

Nicodemus, K. and J. Malley (2009). "Predictor correlation impacts machine learning algorithms: implications for genomic studies." Bioinformatics 25(15): 1884-90.

Nicodemus, K., J. Malley, C. Strobl and A. Ziegler (2010). "The behaviour of random forest permutation-based variable importance measures under predictor correlation." BMC Bioinformatics 11: 110.

Nicodemus, K., W. Wang and Y. Shugart (2007). "Stability of variable importance scores and rankings using statistical learning tools on single nucleotide polymorphisms (SNPs) and risk factors involved in gene-gene nd gene-environment interaction." BMC Proceedings 1(Suppl 1): S58.

Nonyane, B. and A. S. Foulkes (2008). "Application of two machine learning algorithms to genetic association studies in the presence of covariates." BMC Genetics 9: 71.

Pers, T., A. Albrechtsen, C. Holst, T. Sorensen and T. Gerds (2009). "The validation and assessment of machine learning: a game of prediction from high-dimensional data." PLoS One 4(8): e6287.

Qi, Y., Z. Bar-Joseph and J. Klein-Seetharaman (2006). "Evaluation of different biological data and computational classification methods for use in protein interaction prediction." Proteins 63: 490-500.

Rakotomamonjy, A. (2003). "Variable selection using SVM-based criteria." Journal of Machine Learning Research 3: 1357-1370.

Sandri, M. and P. Zuvvolotto (2008). "A bias correction algorithm for the Gini variable importance measure in classification trees." Journal of Computational and Graphical Statistics 17(3): 611-628.

Segal, M. R., J. D. Barbour and R. Grant (2004). "Relating HIV-1 sequence variation to replication capacity via trees and forests." Statistical Applications in Genetics and Molecular Biology 3: 2.

Strobl, C., A. Boulesteix, T. Kneib, T. Augustin and A. Zeileis (208). "Conditional variable importance for random forests." BMC Bioinformatics 9: 307.

Strobl, C., A. Boulesteix, T. Kneib, T. Augustin and A. Zeileis (2008). "Conditional variable importance for random forests." BMC Bioinformatics 9: 307.

Strobl, C., A. Boulesteix, A. Zeileis and T. Hothorn (2007). "Bias in random forest variable importance measures: illustrations, sources and a solution." BMC Bioinformatics 8: 25.

Tuv, E., A. Borisov, G. Runger and K. Torkkola (2009). "Feature selection with ensembles, artifical variables and redundancy elimination." Journal of Machine Learning Research 10: 1341-1366.

van der Laan, M. (2006). "Statistical inference for variable importance." International Journal of Biostatistics 2: 1008.

Vapnik, V. (1998). Statistical learning theory, Wiley.

White, A. and W. Z. Liu (1994). "Bias in information-based measures in decision tree induction." Machine Learning 15: 321-329.

Xu, S., X. Hunag, H. Xu and C. Zhang (2007). "Improved prediction of coreceptor usage and phenotype of HIV-1 based on combined features of V3 loops sequence using random forest." The Journal of Microbiology 45(5): 441-446.

31

Biomedical Knowledge Engineering Using a Computational Grid

Marcello Castellano and Raffaele Stifini
Politecnico di Bari, Bari
Italy

1. Introduction

Bioengineering is an applied engineering discipline with the aims to develop specific methods and technologies for a better understanding of biological phenomena and health solutions to face the problems regarding the sciences of life. It is based on fields such as biology, electronic engineering, information technology (I.T.), mechanics and chemistry (MIT, 1999). Methods of Bioengineering concern: the modeling of the physiological systems , the description of electric phenomena or magnetic ones ,the processing of data, the designing of medical equipments and materials or tissues, the study of organisms and the analysis of the link structure property typical of biomaterials or biomechanical structures. Technologies of Bioengineering include: biomedical and biotechnological instruments (from the elementary components to the most complex hospital systems), prosthesis, robots for biomedical uses, artificial intelligent system, sanitary management systems, information systems, medical informatics, telemedicine (J. E. Bekelman et al, 2003).

Biomedicine has recently had an innovative impulse through applications of computer science in Bioengineering field. Medical Informatics or better the Bioinformatics technology is characterized by the development of automatic applications in the biological sector whose central element is the information. There are several reasons to apply the "computer science" in many fields, such as the biomedical one. Advantages as the turn-around time and precision are among the basically improving factors for a job. For example the identification of the functions of genes has taken advantage from the application of an automatically system of analysis of database containing the result of many experiments of microarray getting information on the human genes involved in pathologies (C. Müller et al, 2009). With a such approach regions with specifically activities have been identified inside the DNA regions, different regions exist in the genome, some stretches are the actual genes, others regulates the functions of the former ones. Other research have been made through computational techniques on the Functional Genomics, Biopolymers and Proteomics, Biobank e Cell Factory (M. Liebman et al, 2008).

This chapter explores a particularly promising area of systems development technological based on the concept of knowledge. The knowledge is useful learning result obtained by an information processing activity. The **Knowledge Engineering**, regards the integration of the knowledge in computer systems in order to solve the difficult problems which typically require a high level of human specialization. (M. C. Linn, 1993)

Whereas standalone computer system have had an important impact in Biomedicine, the computer networks are nowadays a technology to investigate new opportunities of innovation. The capacity of the networks to link so many information allows both to improve the already existing applications and introduce new ones; Internet and the Web are two well know examples. Information based processes involved in the research to discovery new knowledge take advantage from the new paradigms of distributed computing systems. This chapter is focuses on the design aspects of the **knowledge-based computer systems** applied to the biomedicine field. The mission is to support the specialist or researcher to solve problems with greater awareness and precision. At the purpose, a framework to specify a computational model will be presented. As an example, an application of the method to the diagnostic process will be discussed to specify a knowledge-based decision support system. The solution here proposed is not only to create a knowledge base by the human expert (or by a pool of experts) but support it using automatic knowledge discovery process and resources enhancing data, information and collaboration in order to produce new expert knowledge over time.

Interoperability, resource sharing, security and collaborative computing will emerge and a computational model based on grid computing will be taken into account in order to discuss an advanced biomedical application. In particular in the next section it will be presented a framework for the Knowledge Engineering based on a problem solving strategy. In section 3 the biomedical diagnostic process will be analyzed using the knowledge framework. In particular the problem, the solution and knowledge resources will be carried out. In section 4 the design activity of the diagnostic process is presented. Results in terms of system specifications will be shown in terms of Decision Support System architecture, Knowledge Discovery and Grid Enable Knowledge Application. A finally discussion will be presented in the last section.

2. Method for the knowledge

Modeling is a building activity inspired by the problem solving for real problems which not have a unique exact solution. The Knowledge Engineering (K- Engineering) deals with the computer-system applications which are computational solutions of more complex problems which usually ask for a high levels of human skill. In this case the human knowledge must be encoded and embedded in knowledge based applications of computer systems. The K-Engineer build up a knowledge model useful for an algorithmic description by a structured approach or method. Three macro phases can be distinguished in the modeling process of knowledge:

1. Knowledge Identification (K- Identification);
2. Knowledge Specification (K- Specification);
3. Knowledge Refinement (K- Refinement).

These phases can be cyclical and times retroaction rings are necessary. For instance, the simulation in the third phase can cause changes in the knowledge model. (A. Th. Schreiber, B. J. Weilinga, 1992). Each phases is composed by specific activities and for each activities the K- Engineering literature proposes different techniques. The Fig. 1 shows the modeling of the knowledge based on the problem solving strategy. The proposed framework is applied at different levels of abstraction from high to low level mechanisms (top-down method).

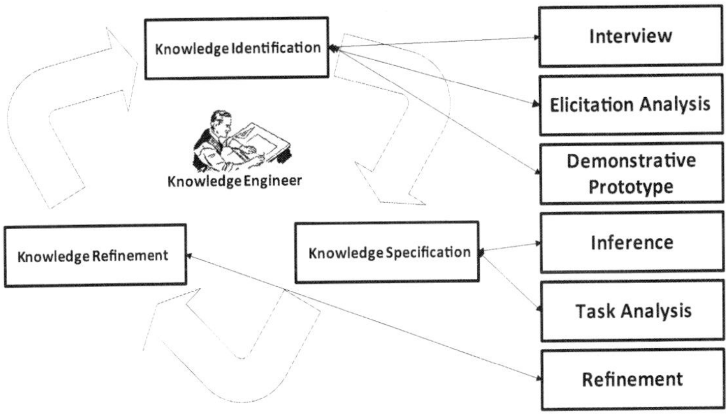

Fig. 1. The knowledge modeling framework composed by phases and activities.

The knowledge model is only an approximation of the real world, which can and must be modified during time.

2.1 Knowledge Identification

A Knowledge Based System (KBS) is a computational system specialized in applications based on knowledge, aiming at reaching a problem solving ability comparable with a human expert. The expert can describe a lot of aspects typical of his own way of reasoning but tends to neglect a significant part of personal abilities which cannot be easily explained. This Knowledge, which is not directly accessible, must, however, be considered and then drawn out. To mine the tacit knowledge an application on the elicitation techniques can be useful and it must be represented using a dynamic model.

The analysis must be inherent in the aims of the planner. On the other hand the representation of the complete domain is un-useful, so the effort is now to identify the problem, in order to finalize the domain analysis.

The approach here proposed is based on the answer to questions that must be taken in to account to develop the basic characteristics of the K-Model as shown in Table 1.

The phase of Knowledge Identification is subject to important considerations that go to better specify the system architecture. Most of a man knowledge or of a group is tacit and cannot be outspoken wholly or partly. Therefore, in a knowledge system, the human beings are not simple users, but an integrating part of the system. The representation is necessarily different from what is represented; it can capture only the most relevant aspects, chosen from the modeler. This difference can cause problems if one wants to use the model for differ purpose from the ones it quality allows. Moreover the difference between the real world and its representation should cause problems of uncertainty and approximation which will be solved showing the quality of the relevant knowledge in real way.

2.1.1 Interview

The interview is a conversation provoked by the interviewer, addressing to subjects choosen according ground of a plan of survey, aiming at the knowledge, through the conversation driven from the interviewer, using a flexible and not standardized scheme. *(Corbetta, 1999).*

What must be represented:	At the epistemological level identify what should represent aspects of knowledge that is necessary to consider the application to be addressed. In particular, what are its classes, patterns, what are the inferential processes involved and the quality of relevant knowledge.
Which is the problem:	To identify the problem to be solved is important to address the investigation about the relevant knowledge. It will be very important in the next modeling phases.
How the problem can be solved:	It indicates strategies for solving a given problem based on patterns bounded in the application domain.
How to represent:	Modeling derives from the subjective interpretation of the knowledge engineer with regards to the problem to be faced; a mistake is always possible and therefore the knowledge model must be made in a revisable way. Tools and processes for the knowledge management have been consolidated, this management can be expressed in several ways: rules, procedures, laws, mathematical formulae, structural descriptions.

Table1. Knowledge Identification guidelines.

The interviewee must have some characteristics related with his life or his belonging to a certain social group, the number of the people interviewed must however be consistent, so it is possible to obtain every possible information on the phenomenon.
The conversation between the two parts is not comparable to a normal conversation because the roles are not balanced: the interviewer drives and controls the interview respecting the freedom of the interviewer in expressing his opinions.
According to the different degree of flexibility is possible to distinguish among:

1. structured interview
2. semi-structured interview
3. not structured interview.

Usually the structured interview is used to investigate a wide phenomenon, the interview is carried out by a questionnaire supplied to a large sample of people; in this case the hypothesis must be well structured a priori.
The structured interview can be used in a standard way but at the same time the limited knowledge of the phenomenon does not allow the use of the multiple choice questionnaire. As the number of the interviewees decreases a semi-structured or a un-structured interview can be taken in to account.

2.1.2 Elicitation analysis

The elicitation analysis is an effective method used by the knowledge engineer to individuate the implicit mental patterns of the users, and categorizing them.

The knowledge engineer carry out this phase analyzing documentations about the domain under the investigation and match the information according to some well know mental model of him.

Knowing the mental patterns and the implicit categorizations makes possible the organization of the information so that it is more simple to use them, improving, in that way, the quality of the product.

Through the elicitation analysis it is possible to identify the classification criterion used by the users and to identify the content and the labels of categories they used. Possible differences in the categorization among various groups of interviewed can be seen and controlled.

2.1.3 A draft of the conceptual model

This activity establish a first formal representation of knowledge acquired up to now composed by elements and their relationships. The representation is used to check the correctness by the user. It is a formal scheme on which the K-specification phase will runs. The knowledge is represented using an high level description called conceptual model. This model is called conceptual because it is the result of a survey carried out by the literature and domain experts for the transfer of concepts considered useful in the field of study is concerned. Fundamental indications about "what is" and "how to build" the conceptual model are shown in Table 2. Some formalisms are proposed in the literature: the semantic networks are used to represent the knowledge with a graph structure; the frames are data structures which allow group, like inside a frame, the information about an entity; an object representation allows to join procedural aspects with declarative aspects, in a single formalism; and so on.

What it is not:	• it is not a basic of knowledge on paper/calculator • it is not an intermediate representation
What it is:	• it is a complete articulate and permanent representation of the structure of the knowledge of an applicative dominion both from a static point of view and a dynamic one • it is a representation independent from implementation • it is the main result of the activity of knowledge analysis and modeling.
How the conceptual model is built (some criteria)	• a formalism for the expressive conceptual representation allows to express powerfully all the concepts, the relationships and the link typical of the application • economic: synthetic, compact, readable, modifiable • communicative: easily intelligible • useful: a support for the analysis and modeling activities

Table 2. The Conceptual Model guidelines.

2.2 Knowledge specification

The goal of this stage is to get a complete specification of the knowledge. The following activities need to be carried out to build such a specification.

2.2.1 Inference

Now let is write about the inferential structures which make possible to know things starting from a codified knowledge. It is interesting, even for the inferential structures, to identify different types of structures, in order to focalize, during the construction of the conceptual pattern, the structures which are actually used in the specific application. The most general form is the one which turns into rules. However it is interesting to consider even more specific structures, as these ones help the identification of particular necessities inside an application. (Waterman [Wa86]). The main characteristics of an inference are the ability of specifying the knowledge, the ability of reasoning, the ability of interacting with the external world, the ability of explaining own behavior and the ability of learning. The inference architecture can be organized in object level and meta level. Each of them can be seen as an individual system, with an appropriate language of representation. The aim of the level object is to carry on reasoning in the domain of the system application, whereas the aim of the meta-level is to control the behavior of the object level.

2.2.2 Task analysis

The aim of the task analysis is to identify the "main task" by the analysis of the users involvement in order to understand how to they execute their work, identifying types and levels:

- How is the work carried on when more people are involved (workflow analysis);
- A single man work during a day , a week or a mouth (job analysis);
- Which tasks are executed by all the people who could use to product (task list);
- The order every uses of execution of the tasks (tasks sequences);
- Which steps and decision the user chooses to accomplish a task (procedural analysis);
- How to explode a wide task into more subtasks (hierarchies of task).

The Task analysis offers the possibility to view the needs, display the improvement areas and simplify the evaluation. It can be carried out according to: (Mager,1975; Gagnè,1970)

- rational analysis - Inside the theories of the Knowledge it is a procedure which divides a task into simpler abilities, up to reaching the activities that can be executed by every process the task is assigned to. The result of this procedure is a typical hierarchy of activities with a correspondent hierarchy of execution aims.
- empirical analysis - Inside the Knowledge Engineering it indicates a procedure which splits up the activity or task into executive process, strategies and meta-cognitive operations which the subject accomplishes during the execution of that task. The result is a sequence, not always ordered, of operations aiming at the realization of the task.

This is an activity about K-Specification. It works on the output of the K-Identification (see Table 1), that specify the resolution strategy of the problem. At the purpose the task analysis is carried out by the following specific steps: Problem specification; Activity analysis; Task modeling and Reaching of a solution.

In the **Problem Specification** phase the problem must be identified specifying one or more activities for its realization, at the conceptual level; these activities will be analyzed in the following step. In **Activity Analysis** a task is identified grouping activities which must be executed to achieve the aim of the task. There are different task hierarchies where the activities can be divided into subtask. This exercise on the task hierarchy means both to specialize every task and to study the task execution on the base of priorities and temporal lines. **Task Modeling** builds a model which precisely describes the relationships among tasks. A model is a logical description of the activities which must be executed to achieve the users goals. The model based design aims to specify and analyze interactive software applications from a more semantic level rather than from an implementative one. Methods for modeling the tasks are:

- Standard : analysis on how tasks should be made;
- Descriptive: analysis of the activities and tasks just as they are really made. Task models can be taken into accounts according to the following point of view:
- System task model. It describes how the common system implementation states the tasks must be executed;
- Envisioned task model. It describes how the users must interact with the system according to the opinion of the designer;
- User task model. It describes how the tasks must be done in order to reach the objects according to the opinion of the users.

Usability problems can arises when discrepancy occurs between the user task model and the system model. The last step in the task analysis (**Reaching of a solution**) is devoted to specify the tasks identified. That are conceptual building block of this analysis. Table 3 shows a formalism to specify the task aim, the technique used for the realization of it and the result produced on the task execution. Moreover a procedural description of the task must be carried out using conceptual building blocks based tools.

Task	Name of the task
Goal	Aim of the task
Techniques	Task descriptions and it implementation
Result	Output task

Table 3. A Task Description formalism.

2.3 Knowledge refinement

The aim of the Knowledge Refinement is to validate the knowledge model using it in a simulation process as much as possible. Moreover it is to complete the knowledge base by inserting a more or less complete set of knowledge instances.

3. Analyzing the biomedical diagnostic process building a model for knowledge based system

The case of study here presented, refers to the diagnostic process. This is a rich knowledge process prevalent in the biomedical field and to diagnostic pathologies starting from the symptoms.

3.1 Knowledge identification

The identification of knowledge in biomedicine has been here applied as described in table 4, using the framework proposed in the previous section.

Key Questions to drive the Knowledge	Methods
<What to represent>	Elicitation Analysis
<Which is the problem>	Interview
<How it can be solved>	Interview, Elicitation Analysis
<How to represent>	Semantic Network, Elicitation Analysis, Interview

Table 4. The K-Identification for the diagnostic process.

3.1.1 Elicitation analysis

In order to create the first reference model of the diagnostic process the K-Identification starts with the elicitation study. As the final aim is the development of an conceptual model could be useful to consider a process comparable where a living organism is like a perfectly working computer. If a computer problem rise, the operative system signal it to the user. To activate such a process, a warning is necessary, i.e. a message of mistake or wrong working. At this point a good computer technician put in action a diagnostic process based on the warning to individuate the problem, or in other words the error.

The diagnosis on an organism is similar at the described scenery: the occurring of a pathology is pointed out to the organism through the signal of one or more symptoms (as already described for the computer errors). The diagnostic medical process is exercised by the specialist (in analogy of the computer technician) that will study the symptom origin and its cause and hence the diseases. The arising of a problem can be due both endogen and exogenous causes and provokes an alteration which would not normally happen (for instance an alteration in the albumin level produced by the pancreas); this mutation causes a change, a working different from the mechanisms associated to that element (for example the mechanism, thanks to which the insulin makes the glucose enter into the cells for the production of vital energy, changes as an accumulation of glucose in the blood circle is met: subjects affected with diabetes). What it has been learned by the above application described on the elicitation analysis is shown in Table 5.

A stirring up cause...	Following a diminution of electric tension the computer is turned off while the hard disk is on	A strong and cold wind blows for several minutes on the patient neck
...modifies some values	The head fall and ruins the computer record	Not desired presence of Ag.VHI-A
...and a problem arises in the system	Not readable starting record	Aching eymphonodes
...and makes clear. Reveals itself.	The computer show the error	The patient has throat ache

Table 5. Some elicitation analysis results to know the Diagnostic Process.

3.1.2 Interview

Although the elicitation study supply important elements to build a conceptual model of the knowledge, the expert contribution is of the great important also. At the purpose the structured interview is here applied to extract the knowledge and the mental process of the experts when they work. In other words the interview application aims to describe the experiences of the specialists in terms of structured knowledge. By interview the Clinical Case emerges as a summary composed by: all the possible information about the patient, a list of symptoms and a set of objective and instrumental exam results. Table 6 summarizes the results carried out by interview and elicitation analysis, in terms of problem and solution.

Key Questions to drive the Knowledge	Results
Which is the problem	The diagnoses are not always easy to be identified from a set of the possible solutions, sometimes several possible investigations must be done up to individuate an optimal solution.
How it can be solved	A valuable support to the specialist in order to makes a decision is highly desirable. An automatic computer system based on biomedical knowledge should be able to support the specialist using updated information and supporting decisions using a computational formal approach.

Table 6. Interview and Elicitation Analysis Results for the Diagnostic Process.

The solution here proposed is not only to create a knowledge base directly from the human expert (or by a pool of experts) but especially to increase the own knowledge through the provision of advanced computational analysis tools capable of enhancing data, information and collaboration in order to become expert knowledge over time.

3.1.3 Semantic network

Here is applied the semantic networks representation formalism to complete the knowledge identification phase and to provide a conceptual model in input to the next phase. See Fig. 2.

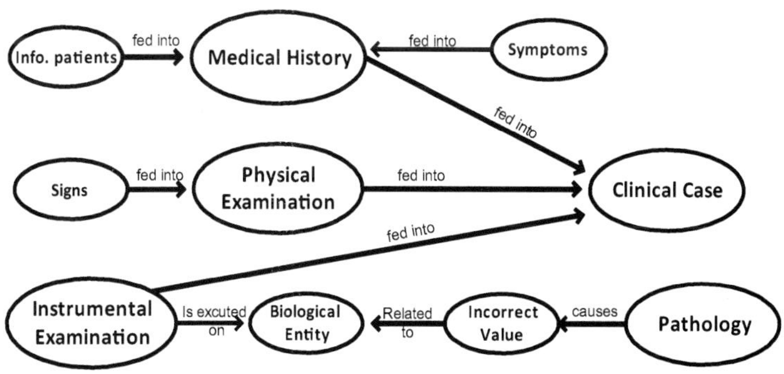

Fig. 2. Biomedical Knowledge representations using Semantic Annotations.

Nodes are objects, concepts, states while arcs, represent the relationships between nodes as carried out by knowledge identification phase. For example, the figure highlights how a pathology will lead to an alteration of the value of a biological entity and how this variation is detected by an instrumental examination. New relationships can be made clear, not only the evident ones but also those coming deducted from the father-son hereditariness. Fig. 2 suggests that the signs detected during physical examination can be directly annotated in the clinical case.

3.2 Knowledge specification

The second stage in the presented framework is to construct a specification of the k-model. In order to specify k-model of the biomedical diagnostic process it has been used an approach based on the inference and task knowledge.

3.2.1 Inference

Inference rules are used to capture the way in which a specialist reason according to the inference logical scheme. The inference rules so defined will be embedded into Decision Support System in order to develop a Knowledge-Specialist Based System. The summary of all these inferences help to develop activities that the system must make either for the development of a formal instrument describing the said inferences or the classes studied in the representative formalism. In Fig. 3 is represented the logical schema of the classes that describes some rules of inference such as "*the observation of a symptom strictly depends on the patient who is suffering from it*".

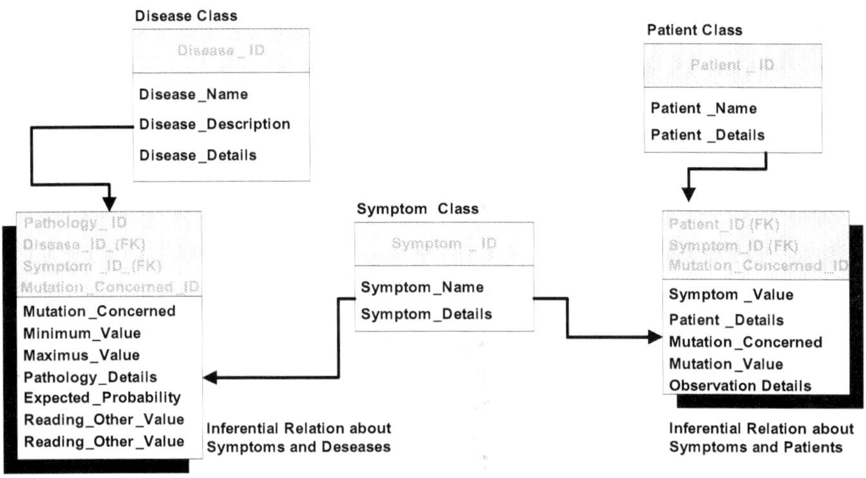

Fig. 3. Logical Schema based on Classes to represent the Inference component of the K-model.

The dependence of the activities of a system from the inferences rules can be translated both into obliged passages or into a series of guide-line on designing the activities of the system to be followed. Many informatics system translate it into an "algorithm" called "inferential engine" which can complete the design phase of the activities automatically. In some cases a prototype of the inferential engine is build up. In the implementation phase it will be possible to choose whether developing a suitable software or maintaining that engine at a conceptual level. Fig. 4 shows a conceptual description of biomedical diagnostic inferential engine, composed by the following elements:

- **Interpreter**: it decides the rule to be applied (meta-level);
- **Scheduler**: it decides the execution order of the rules (object level);
- **Job memory**: it contains a list of developed operations is (object level).

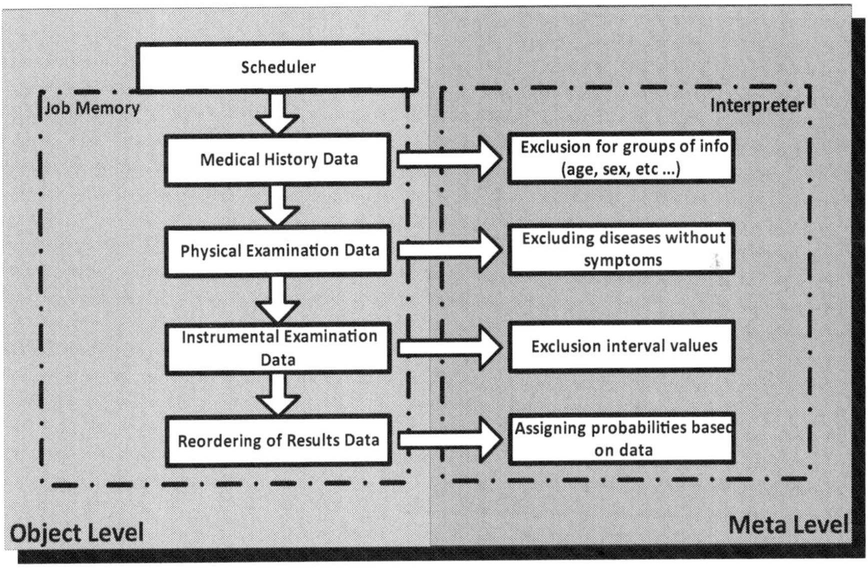

Fig. 4. A Conceptual Description of the Biomedical Diagnostic Inferential Engine.

3.2.2 Task analysis

To design an efficient and technologically advanced decisional system of support, the correctness of the applied methodology and rightness of the information must be considered. A good working system is based not only on accurately selected and organized data but also on a model epistemologically adherent to the everyday medical actions. The task design occurs at the purpose. Using the "top-down approach" the analysis and the task design starts from the macro-activity or main task designed for the solution about the problem that regard the support to the specialist decision.

The Fig. 5 shows the main task of the solution composed by both Central System and Central Db components. Different Database are referred by External and Internal Db components.

The kind of result proposes a **form** which gives back a list of pathologies with the relative probabilities from the letting in of a list of symptoms inserted by the specialist.

The solution is an automatic computer system based on biomedical knowledge that should be able to support the specialist using updated information and supporting decisions by

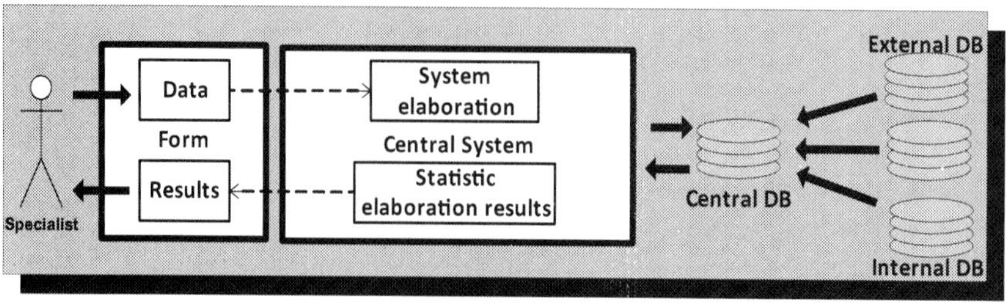

Fig. 5. A representation of the Main Task based on Functional Blocks and Components.

computational formal approach. The execution of a test implies a sequences of steps, each of them contributing to the achievement of the purpose. Task Analysis can be carried out using or the Descriptive approaches that describes the system organization in an analytical way or the Applicative approach to obtain single and simple elements, so that they can be studied. Task analysis starts from the study of the activities composing the main activity to the define the real phase, they will be translated into task system. Fig. 6 shows a scheme both to understand the succession of the activities and to determine the hierarchies.

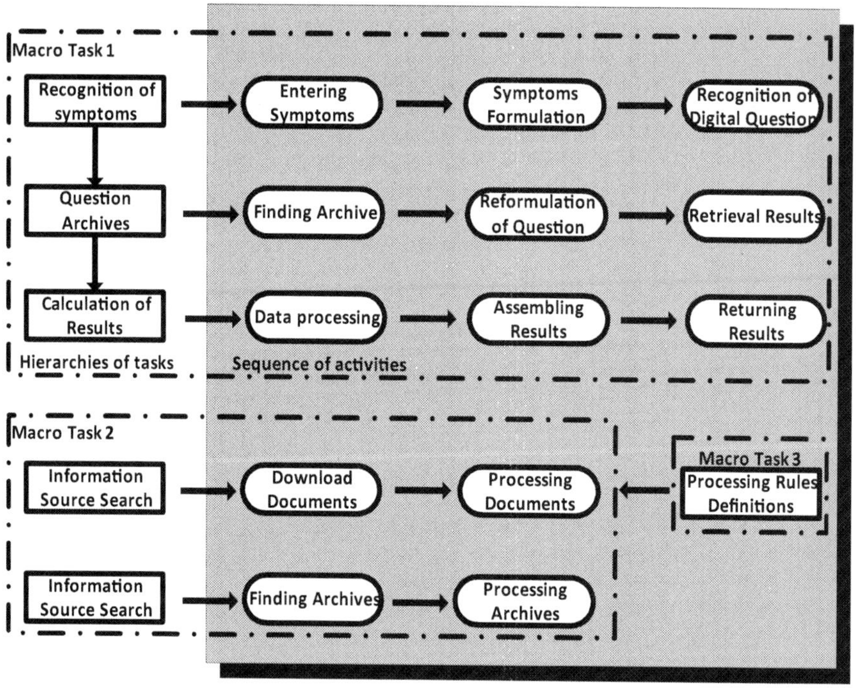

Fig. 6. Task Analysis and Design Results: hierarchies of tasks and task composition by sequences of Activities using building blocks based tools.

The results of the single task design is shown in Table 7.

Task Model	Knowledge Item Worksheet
NAME	Insert the symptom
POSSESSED BY	User terminal
USED IN	Main form
DOMAIN	It can be found both in the central system and in a remote terminal
PEOPLE	Users

Table 7. An example of Knowledge Specification for the Task Model in Diagnostic Process.

3.3 Knowledge refinement: analysis of information sources and data types

In this application the Knowledge Refinement phase is carried out to complete the Knowledge modeling. At the purpose an analysis of the additional sources of information is here presented as suggested by the task analysis. The biomedical knowledge is mainly organized in order to solve problems in the formulation of diagnosis and therapies. A problem that the specialist has to be solved can be classified according to the complexity of the diagnostic process: in the more simple case is available the useful knowledge that leads to a disease individuation directly; complex problem involves situations in progress about the disease knowledge so that not all the reasoning have been produced and some of these can be hidden in a large quantity of data. In this cases different thinking schools lead to different solutions and then the specialist makes a decision on heuristic knowledge. From the information point of view the scientific literature, medical documents, experts consultations and forums, can be cited as the main source of information. In particular the digital information can be organized in databases, glossaries and ontologies. Table 8 shows the different source of knowledge with their data types.

Information Source	Data Types
Archives of known and soluble cases	Structured data organized into databases.
Treatises of research and scientific publications	Not structured data in a textual form, with some metadata.
Social Networks and Forums	Heuristic data.

Table 8. Information Sources of Knowledge for the Diagnostic Process.

In information technology, the terms database indicates archives structured so as to allow the access and the management of the data (their insertion, delete and update) on account of particular software applications. The database is a whole of data parted according the arguments into a logical order and then these arguments are divided into categories. A database is much more than a simple list or table. It offers the possibility to manage the data allowing their recovery, arrangements, analysis, summaries and the creation of the **report** in a few minutes. However a more thorough consultation of the data can be carried out with the most advanced technologies such as data mining.

The activities of research provides large knowledge patrimonies. Several organizations works to organize patrimonies and accesses to them (i.e. **NLM, BMC**). They are available on different portals and catalogued into technical-scientific disciplines, geographical areas and, sometimes, into strategic programmers. Thanks to that cataloguing it is possible to make use of Information Retrieval techniques, which allows any system the automatically finding of scientific treatises. Nevertheless the information structures discussed up to now do not allow direct extraction of knowledge from data or among documents, at the purpose text mining technology could be used.

Another very interesting source of knowledge is the one coming from socialization of experiences in describing and persistent stores: like forum, social network, web pages, FAQ and any other place used for exchanging ideas and opinions. These tools have the ability to make explicit the tacit knowledge of individuals through socialization. In fact, these virtual places, users describe their experiences in making themselves available to compare with others, increasing their level of knowledge and acquiring new skills. The Social Knowledge is a flexible approach that support the specialist to make our decisions.

4. Designing the knowledge based system

Decision Support Systems are here considered to address the design of the solution to support the specialist in the diagnostic process.

4.1 Decision Support System

A system which aims is to support the user to make a decision, is called Decision Support System (DSS). That is a system which makes available tools in order to increase the efficiency of the decisional process (G Desanctis, RB Gallupe, 1987). Fig. 7 shows a DSS high level architecture.

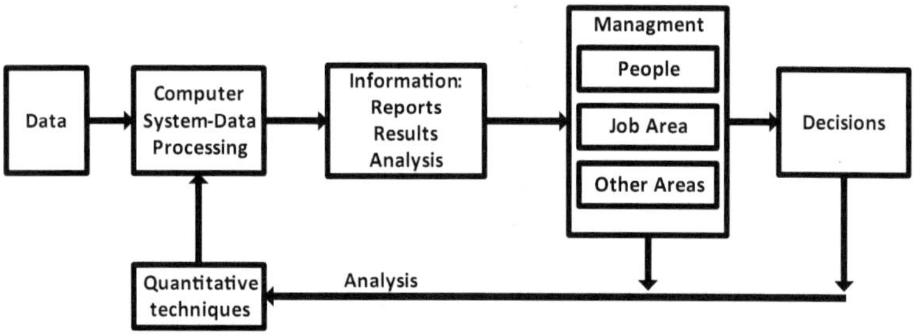

Fig. 7. A Scheme of a Computer Based DSS reference architecture.

Fig. 8 shows a structure of decision-making process over the different forms of knowledge possessed by the specialist. In particular, it describes the steps taken by decision makers from the most simple, based on data held, then the decision maker to proceed in its decision path will refer in order to other information that will acquire and then on explicit knowledge domain and finally on heuristic knowledge.
A "decision" is a definitive choice among incompatible options. The clinical decision are always temporary and can be modified as the clinical case alters. In many cases such a decision must be taken among different options and it can be often followed by further diagnostic or therapeutic decision, which have the same difficulty level of the first one.
Fig. 9 shows a decisional clinical tree. It is a schematic representation of the logical and temporal structure, of a clinical situation, in which it is necessary to take one or more decisions.
Based on the decision tree clinical model, different clinical strategies can be descrived by spefying the action which must be made for every possible situations. The analytical decisional structures so produced have a lot of advantages in comparison with the intuitive method to make clinical decisions.

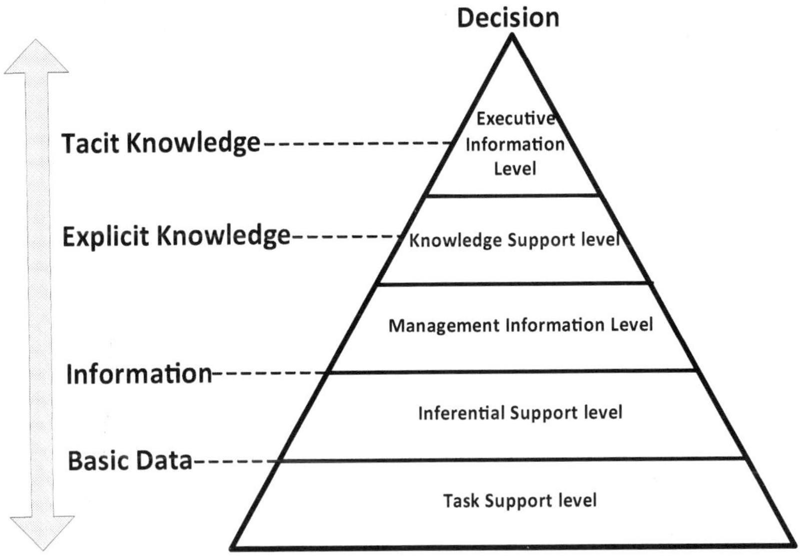

Fig. 8. Hierarchical Relationship among Information, Knowledge and Decision.

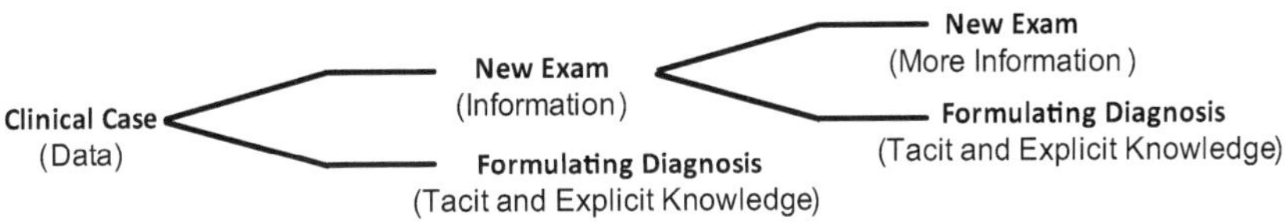

Fig. 9. A Decisional Clinical Tree Diagram to formulating Diagnosis.

Among these advantages there is the posibility to concentrate on a single aspect of the problem, always taking into account the whole. Another advantage is the analysis of the decisions which obliges the specialist to consider the relation between the acquired information and the subsequent decision. An example of analytical decisional structure is showed in Fig.10.

4.2 System structure

Fig. 11 shows the knowledge-based system architecture. The **K-Engineer** collects, analyzes and formalizes the knowledge producing a knowledge model, he is trained by the Domain Expert; the **User** (Biomedicine Specialist) will use the system and says what he would like and if he is satisfied and the **K-maintainer** provides the resources and use conceptual tools for the knowledge system updating.

The DSS examined has some functional elements which use conceptual instruments and resources, such described in Table 9. The **Knowledge Core Layer** contains all the procedures necessary to solve the problem of the user. To carry out a knowledge based system must be utilized precise procedures in order to identify the relationships between apparently

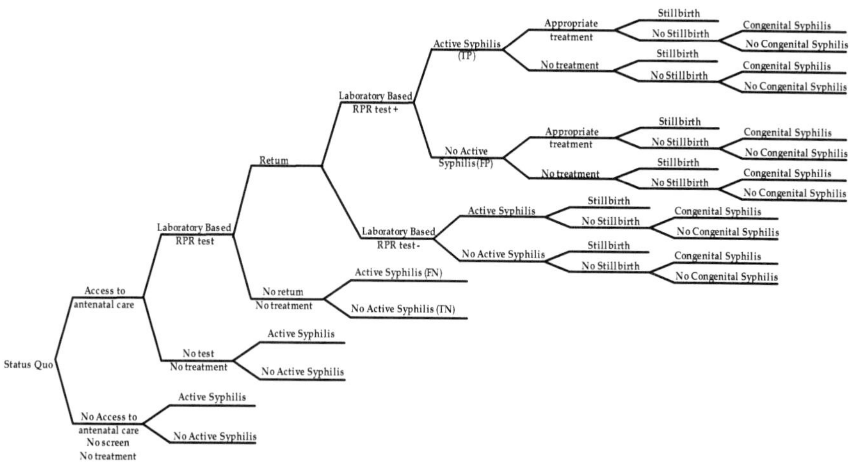

Fig. 10. An Analytical Decisional Structure.

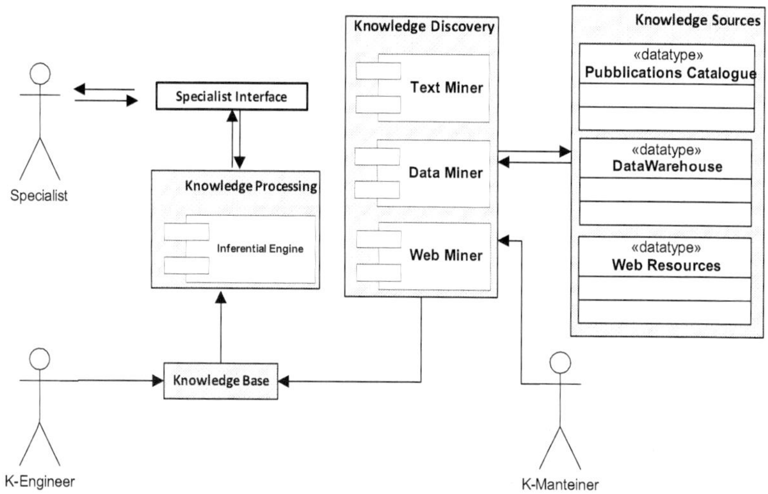

Fig. 11. DSS scheme of the organization.

independent variants, like sign and symptoms, and dependent variants like possible pathologies. The procedures can be obtained from various forms of decision tree. These relationships, stored in the **Knowledge Base,** use pre-arranged rules (if-else if-then) to drive the decision in the diagnostic process. Another functional elements are the **Knowledge Engine** whose perform automatic activities like the analysis of the texts and data; and finally the **Knowledge Sources**.

Functional elements	Conceptual Tools	Resources
Knowledge Discovery	Web mining, Data mining, Text Mining	Web Miner, Data Miner, Text Miner
Knowledge Processing	Statistical Procedures, Diagnostic Patterns	Inferential Engine
Knowledge Base	Knowledge Rules	
Knowledge Sources	Database Management Systems	Publication Catalogue, Web Resources, DataWarehouse

Table 9. List of functional elements.

The **Web Miner** is the element for the knowledge discovery from the web: it applies procedures similar to Data Mining to extract information from the resources present in the web. The computer paradigm is the Web Mining which derives from the Data Mining and deals with the discovery of resources on the web. It analyses web pages and from them extracts the resources of biomedical literature though query. The **Text Miner** has two objects: the transformation of the documents into a representation fit for the learning algorithm (the so called preprocessing phase) and the grammar analysis on the non structured text to extract the structured knowledge. As to processing phase the Text Miner draws out the meta information contained in the scientific texts and uses it to catalogue them in the Publication Catalogue where the document will wait for the analysis accomplishment according to the Text Mining algorithm . The grammar analysis starts after an K-Maintainer call which gives the Text Miner the parameters necessary to execute the analysis parameters contained in a document XML called Analysis Engine. The structured information will be memorized inside the Knowledge Repository. The **Data Miner** extracting the knowledge from the data the Text Miner got through automatic method, and elaborating them according to the K-Maintainer selected procedure. It is interfaced with the Publications Catalogue and makes use of the Data Mining Paradigm, which provides the instruments to locate, to extract and transform the data and the instruments for the management of data. The **Inferential Engine** is made by: an interpreter which decides the useful rules to request to the Knowledge Base, and a scheduler which organizes the rules to get developed and their execution order. The engine goal is to extract the rules for the problem solving according to an activation and recognition of the same, executing an exam of the rules on the ground of knowledge select the right rule. It is organized in two phases: a work memory (or blackboard) where the general plan is memorized and a workflow engine of what to do, besides a description of the solutions conjectured up to now. In the inferential engine there is also the consistence enforcer; this is a schedule which, once conjectured an hypothesis, looks for evidences to enforce or eliminate the hypothesis. Thus if the inference is a single deduction that the system can get from the premises (for example a single calculation), the inferential engine is the instrument fit to determinate the inferences complex. The **DataWarehouse** contains the information drawn out from the operations of text mining, whose structure is just like the semantic networks model one and is fit for the analysis algorithm of the Data Miner. It contains also the structured information from any external databases that the K-Maintainer wants to integrate into the system. The **Web Resources** is the database that contains the extracted information from the resources present in web. The **Publication Catalogue** is the repository of the scientific literature founded.

4.3 Grid-enabled knowledge application

In the field of the computer systems for the bio-medicine, the case studies have a long list of electronic documents about their health status, e.g. lab exams, diagnostic images, medical records, several special texts or even the letter of hospital discharge. Such data and information, since they are sector based, cannot be integrated or read by different systems tools even if digitalized, sometimes also because of the lack of appropriate communication infrastructures among the different systems. Even though they can be rebuilt or transferred on a similar computer platform, these documents cannot be reached from all researchers or specialists working on the same case study, just because such documentation has been kept in several autonomous computer systems. One of the major obstacles in their integration is the lack of a unique standard, yet also the different kinds of information products in the health world, the technological gap. The research and the agreement on a standard is even more important to the re-elaboration of the information acquired from the various information resources, balancing various elements (such as local resources, local networks, Internet) and employing various communication technologies, protocols and switching and filtering systems. Besides these drawbacks, the approaching techniques analyzed in the previous sections, such as the text mining or the statistic algorithm, when extended to a great amount of resources, require a huge computational power, a large broadcast band, and inner organization which can also make possible the interoperability. The solution proposed up to now can be really useful if an advanced technology based on computer systems is able to exceed computer networks and organizational problems that often make it difficult to share data and information. The Fig. 12 refers to a scenario of distributed resources all potentially very useful for continuous improvement of expert knowledge and indicates a solution based on grid computing. A worthy approach to use and share the resources and which includes computing power, mass memory, and a large broadcast band, comprise a network of information instruments called grid, whose main characteristic is its dynamism, i.e. the ability to re-configure itself in any moment, encompassing new knots and tolerating the loss of others, and capable to adapt to any required work every time it is necessary. All these operations are automatically performed, in a completely transparent way for the user, who will perceives the grid as a unique, stable, unchangeable, effective and always accessible system.

The grids (or computational grids) are advanced services which allow to the users to share computational resources, archival space, scientific data and instruments among different computers. They are then a valid instrument to automatically store the accomplished researches and spread the knowledge to the domain. The grid technology, indeed, facilitates data downloading, arranges documents, and periodically updates the researches.

The grids (or computational grids) are advanced services which allow to the users to share computational resources, archival space, scientific data and instruments among different computers. They are then a valid instrument to automatically store the accomplished researches and spread the knowledge to the domain. The grid technology, indeed, facilitates data downloading, arranges documents, and periodically updates the researches.

To define a grid architecture valid for the activities involved by the knowledge model, is necessary to take into account that it is not only a architectural model to provide computational resources for applications with great need of processing, but it is also an infrastructure where can connect and unify heterogeneous resources issued on local or geographical scale. The interoperability becomes the main problem to solve; indeed, it is necessary to allow the interaction among different platforms, languages, and research areas. In an interconnected zone, the interoperability implies common authentication protocols, therefore the grid to implement needs an architecture of protocols first of all. In this way it is possible to define a basic system through which users and knots can communicate.

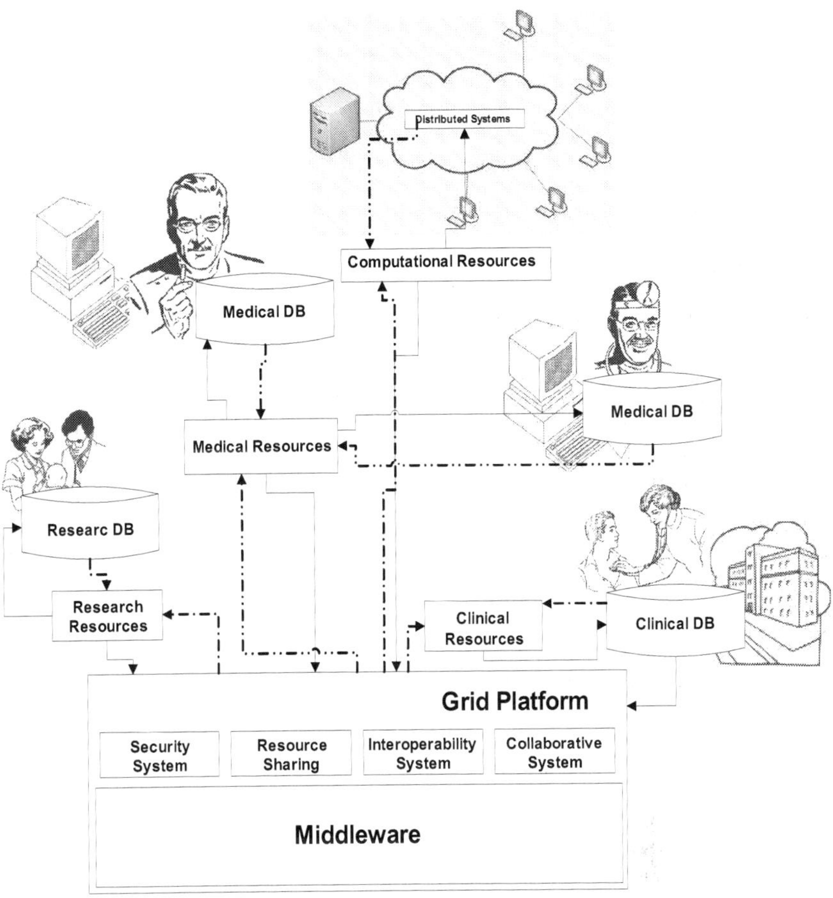

Fig. 12 Grid Computing.

A Grid system allows to manage its own resources to obtain different service qualities, such as response time, availability, security, and performance to satisfy users request. The quality of service (QoS) is a highly important parameter, but it is not the only one. An information system that has to solve highly complex problems, such as the management of the biomedical knowledge, can take other advantages of the grids. The scalability is one of these advantages: a grid can comprise millions of resources, implying a potential degradation of services. For this reason the grid-enabled application should be able to deal with connection latency on geographical distances. Dynamicity and adaptability are criteria that determine the reliability. In a grid a breakdown is a rule not an exception, since the great number of resources increases the chances of breakdown. This technology has been designed as a very promising application-level specialization and several proposals have been made of the same. (see for example Castellano at all, A bioinformatics knowledge discovery in text application for grid computing; A Workflow based Approach for Knowledge Grid Application; Intrusion Detection Using Neural Networks: A Grid Computing Based Data Mining Approach; Biomedical Text Mining Using a Grid Computing Approach)

5. Results and discussions

This chapter deals with a particular class of biomedical engineering systems such as Computer-Based Decision Support Systems. Different DSS applications are proposed in the literature to date. They highlight the system performances in the biomedical field, without examining the methodological aspects on which the investigation was based. Since these systems are of considerable complexity, their development and adoption are a problem in the field of biomedical engineering. In this chapter in response to the problem just mentioned a framework for analysis and design of these systems is discussed. It is based on a methodology of knowledge engineering. An application to a diagnostic process in the biomedical field is also presented.

Methods for problem solving vary from ad hoc to highly structured. Ad hoc approaches are often used to solve simple problems in a linear way. Highly structured methodology for studying complex problems become even more formal where it is usual to pre-specify all the system requirements. In this chapter has been used a problem solving highly structured life cycle based on the schema shown in Fig. 1. It has been used to carry out analysis and design phase: the analysis to gain an understanding of an application domain with its problem and the relative conceptual solution; the design to specify a system that meet these requirements. Although this chapter focuses on the analysis and design stages applied to the problem solving life cycle, it is said that there is a further phase of building systems in which one focuses on the actual construction of the system by an executive project.

Fig. 13 summarizes the results from the life cycle of problem solving both for the analysis and for design.

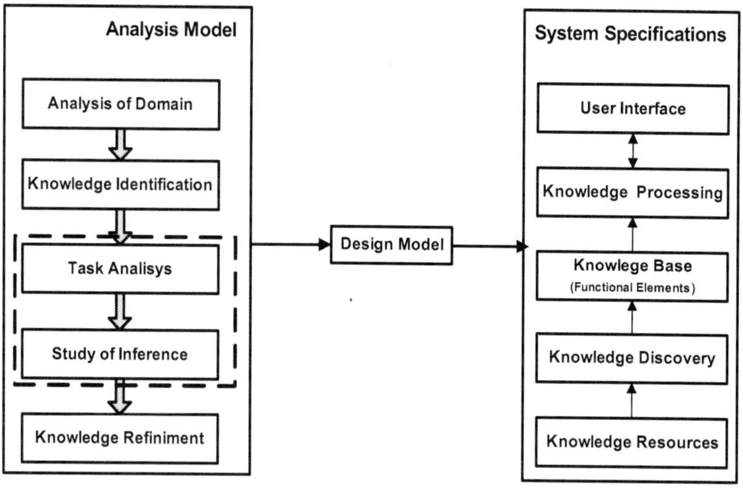

Fig. 13. Analysis and Design for the Biomedical Diagnostic Process.

The designed system is made up of any number of components. Each one carries out part of the system function. They are important because can help to handle systems complexity and then improve understanding of a system. Components communicate between them by passing messages. A good system will made up of highly independent components with minimal flows between them.
The components are identified according to the encapsulation strategy. It allows to hide the internal working of procedural elements so as to protect the other parts of the system from the changes which would occur in it, if this working was faulty, or if one decided to implement it in a different way.
From the technological solution point of view, the decision support system functional components aims to widen the human being capabilities. For example the automatic retrieval of scientific literature is important for the performances of the system. In fact the web suggest several scientific documents and that slows down the manual research. Moreover the use of automatic equipments is an advantage for the texts research, their readings and the knowledge extrapolation, which represent a study more similar to the one made by an expert, with reduced times, big quantities of examined texts and a lasting memorization. However when dividing the tasks into simple activities, it is necessary to respect the main rules of the biomedicine knowledge to develop a functional knowledge based automatic system. Algorithms and data will be effective only if the study about the knowledge domain has been clearly made.
Design decisions have specified functional blocks and their interaction needs to solve the problem. All of them can be regarded in terms of computational resources such as algorithms, data and computational power. As a consequence design phase must be specify also a computing model resource organization in order to satisfy user requirements and system performances. A grid computing based model has been discussed in order to support a knowledge based system development with high quality of services, based on interoperability, resource sharing, security and collaborative computing. Others computational aspects that are left open during analysis such as representational formats, computational methods used to computing inferences, dynamic data storage and the communication media, could be taken into account also.
Finally must be considered that the study presented in this chapter shows a methodological solution or framework focused on knowledge to develop a knowledge based system very useful in biomedical engineering and the application here presented is a case study to examine the way in which the framework works.

6. Conclusions

Different Decision Support System applications are proposed in the literature to date highlighting the system performances in the biomedical field, without examining the methodological aspects on which the investigation was based. Since these systems are of considerable complexity, their development and adoption are a problem in the field of biomedical engineering. In this chapter has been presented a tool for Biomedical Engineering based on a framework of Knowledge Engineering specialized into develop applications of decision support computer systems. The framework has been applied successfully to the Biomedical Diagnostic Process. The framework application explores technologies for knowledge applied to the processes and resources enhancing data, information, collaboration and computing models in order to produce new expert knowledge over time. The study presented in this chapter has shown that new knowledge in the digital age can also be produced automatically and that instead the knowledge produced by human processes can be effectively supported by specific digital resources (or knowledge resources). To this end, it was revealed that the application of distributed computing to these problems based on knowledge reveals structural characteristics such as interoperability, resource sharing, security and collaborative computing. At the aim the application here presented has proposed the grid computing approach.

7. References

Achuthsankar ,S. Nair, (2007). Computational Biology & Bioinformatics, A gentle Overview, Communications of Computer Society of India

Almeder, Robert, (1998). Harmless Naturalism, The Limits of Science and the Nature of Philosophy. Chicago and La Salle, Open Court.

Alston, William, (1989). Epistemic Justification, Essays in the Theory of Knowledge, Ithaca, Cornell University Press

Anderson MF, Moazamipour H, Hudson DL, Cohen ME. (1997). *The role of the Internet in medical decision making,* Int J Med Inform, University of California, VA Medical Center, USA

B. Kraft, N. Wilhelms, (2005). *Visual knowledge specification for conceptual design,* L. Soibelman, F. Pena-Mora (Eds.), Proceedings of the 2005 International Conference on Computing in Civil Engineering, pp. 1-14.

Baldi P. ,Brunak S., (2001). *Bioinformatics: The Machine Learning Approach,* MIT Press.

Barnes M.R., Gray I.C., (2003). *Bioinformatics for Geneticists, first edition.* Wiley

Berner E.S., Webster G.D. (1994) Shugerman A.A. et al. *Performances of four computer based diagnostic systems, Medical software's free future,* NEJM, pp. 1792-96

BMC, BioMed Central, The Open Access Publisher, www.biomedcentral.com

Bohem B.,(1988). *A Spiral Model of Software Development and Enhancement,* pp. 61-72.

Böhlen B., Jäger D., Schleicher A., Westfechtel B. (2005) *A Framework for Building Graph-Based Interactive Tools,* Electronic Notes in Theoretical Computer Science, Pages 91-101

Chittaro L., Guida G., Tasso C. e Toppano E., (1993). *Functional and Teleological Knowledge in the Multimodeling Approach for Reasoning about Physical Systems,* A Case Study in Diagnosis, IEEE Transaction on Systems, Man and Cybernetics

Daniel Brown. (2004), *Mastering Information Retrieval and Probabilistic Decision Intelligence Technology,* Chandos Publishing, Oxford

De Kleer J., Williams B., (1987). Diagnosing multiple faults. Artificial Intelligence pp. 97-130

Di Hai Hu,Michael Liebman,Richard J. Mural, Michael N. Liebman, (2008). *Biomedical informatics in translational research*

E. Gamma , R. Helm , R. Johnson , J. Vlissides, (1995). *Design patterns: elements of reusable object-oriented software,* Addison-Wesley Longman Publishing Co., Inc., Boston

Eisfeld M., Scherer, R. (2003) *Assisting conceptual design of building structures by an interactive description logic-based planner,* Advanced Engineering Informatics, pp. 41-57.

G Desanctis, RB Gallupe, (1987). *A foundation for the study of group decision support systems,* Management science, JSTOR

G. Carraro , Y. E. Kalay, (1994). *Knowledge-Based Computer-Aided Architectural Design,* Elsevier Science Inc., New York, NY

G. Schreiber, H. Akkermans, A. Anjewierden, R. de Hoog), N. Shadolt, W. Van de Velde, B. Wielinga. (2000), *Knowledge engineering and management: the CommonKADS methodology, he MIT Press, Cambridge, MA, 2000, ISBN: 0-262-19300-0, US*

I. Flood, (2003), *Proceedings of the Fourth International Symposium on Information Technology in Civil Engineering,* ICCC, ASCE, , pp. 1-12

K. Krauter, R. Buyya, M. Maheswaran, (2001). *A Taxonomy and Survey of Grid Resource Management System for Distributed Computing, Software, Practice and Experience*

Knowledge Engineering: Practice and Patterns, 16th International Conference,

Kraft B., Schneider G., Parameterized. (2003), *Specification of conceptual design tools in civil engineering, Proceedings of the Second International Workshop on Applications of Graph Transformation with Industrial Relevance,* AGTIVE, ser. LNCS, vol. 3062. Springer, Heidelberg. pp. 90-105.

Kraft B., Schneider G. (2007), *Semantic room objects for conceptual design support: a knowledge-based approach,* Proceedings of the 11th International Conference on Computer Aided Architectural Design Futures, pp. 207-216.

Kraft B., Wilhelm N. (2007), *Interactive distributed knowledge support for conceptual building design*

Beucke K. Firmenich B. Donath D. Fruchter R. Roddis K. (2007), *Interactive distributed knowledge support for conceptual building design,* Proceedings of the 10th International Conference on Computing in Civil and Building Engineering (ICCCBE-X), Bauhaus-Universität Weimar. pp. 1-14

M. Eisfeld, (2005). *Assistance in Conceptual Design of Concrete Structures by a Description Logic Planner,* Dissertation, TU Dresden, Kassel

Marburger, A. and Westfechtel, B., Behavioural (2003). *Analysis of telecommunications systems by graph transformations,* Proceedings of the Second International Workshop on Applications of Graph Transformation with Industrial Relevance, pp. 202-219.

M. Castellano, C. Digregorio, (2009). *A Workflow based Approach for Knowledge Grid Application,* KMIS 2009, pp. 230-235

M. Castellano, G. Mastronardi, G. Tarricone. (2009), *Intrusion Detection Using Neural Networks: A Grid Computing Based Data Mining Approach,* ICONIP, pp. 777-785

M. Castellano, G. Mastronardi, R. Bellotti, G. Tarricone. (2009), *A bioinformatics knowledge discovery in text application for grid computing,* BMC Bioinformatics

M. Castellano, G. Mastronardi, G. Decataldo, L. Pisciotta, G. Tarricone, L. Cariello (2008). *Biomedical Text Mining Using a Grid Computing Approach,*. ICIC, pp. 1077-1084

Marcia C. Linn, (1993). *Designing computer learning environments for engineering and computer science: The scaffolded knowledge integration framework,* Journal of Science Education and Technology

Maver T. (2006), *A number is worth a thousand pictures,* Automation in Construction, pp. 333-336.

Meniru, K., Bédard, C. and Rivard, H. (2002). *Early building design using computers,* Proceedings of the Conference on Distributing Knowledge in Building, Aarhaus School of Architecture, Dänemark.

Mora R. Bedard C. Rivard H. Beucke K. Firmenich B. Donath D. Fruchter R. Roddis K. (2007), *A framework for computer-aided conceptual design of building structures,* Proceedings of the 10th International Conference on Computing in Civil and Building Engineering (ICCCBE-X), Bauhaus-Universität Weimar. pp. 1-12.

NLM, U.S. National Library of Medicine, www.pubmed.org

O. Bodenreider, (2008). *Biomedical Ontologies in Action: Role in Knowledge Management, Data Integration and Decision Support*

R.D. D. Coyne , M. A. Rosenman , A. D. Radford , M. Balachandran , J. S. Gero (1989) *Knowledge-Based Design Systems,* Addison-Wesley Longman Publishing Co., Inc., Boston, MA

S. Chakrabarti. (2003), *Mining the Web: discovering knowledge from hypertext data,* Elsevier, ISBN 1558607544

Stiny, G., Gips, J. (2006), *Shape grammars and the generative specification of painting and sculpture,* Information Processing. pp. 1460-1465.

Sulaiman M.J., Weng N.K., Theng C.D., Berdu, Z. (2002), *Intelligent CAD checker for building plan approval,* Christianson, P. (Ed.), Proceedings of the Conference on Distributing Knowledge in Building, Aarhaus School of Architecture, Dänemark.

William, Douglas, Clinger, (1981). *Foundations of Actor Semantics,* Lab Technical Report

32

Efficient Algorithms for Finding Maximum and Maximal Cliques: Effective Tools for Bioinformatics

Etsuji Tomita[1], Tatsuya Akutsu[2] and Tsutomu Matsunaga[3]
[1]*The University of Electro-Communications & The Research and Development Initiative, Chuo University, Tokyo*
[2]*Kyoto University, Kyoto*
[3]*NTT DATA Corporation, Tokyo*
Japan

1. Introduction

Many problems can be formulated as graphs where a graph consists of a set of vertices and a set of edges, in which the vertices stand for objects in question and the edges stand for some relations among the objects. A clique is a subgraph in which all pairs of vertices are mutually adjacent. Thus, a maximum clique stands for a maximum collection of objects which are mutually related in some specified criterion. The so called maximum clique problem is one of the original 21 problems shown to be NP-complete by R. Karp (19). Therefore, it is strongly believed that the maximum clique problem is not solvable easily, *i.e.*, it is not solvable in polynomial-time. Nevertheless, much work has been done on this problem, experimentally and theoretically. It attracts much attention especially recently since it has found many practical applications to bioinformatics (see, e.g., (2; 15; 27; 28; 37; 3; 9; 4; 8; 14; 55; 23; 25; 22; 13)) and many others (see, e.g., excellent surveys (34; 5), and (17; 20; 31; 49; 54; 51)).
This chapter presents efficient algorithms for finding a maximum clique and maximal cliques as effective tools for bioinformatics, and shows our successful applications of these algorithms to bioinformatics.

2. Preliminaries

(1) We are concerned with a simple undirected graph $G = (V, E)$ with a finite set V of vertices and a finite set E of *unordered* pairs $(v, w) (= (w, v))$ of distinct vertices called edges. V is considered to be *ordered*, and the i-th element in V is denoted by $V[i]$. A pair of vertices v and w are said to be adjacent if $(v, w) \in E$.
(2) For a vertex $v \in V$, let $\Gamma(v)$ be the set of all vertices that are adjacent to v in $G = (V, E)$, *i.e.*, $\Gamma(v) = \{w \in V | (v, w) \in E\}$. We call $|\Gamma(v)|$, *i.e.*, the number of vertices adjacent to a vertex v, the degree of v. In general, for a set S, the number of elements in S is denoted by $|S|$.
(3) For a subset $R \subseteq V$ of vertices, $G(R) = (R, E \cap (R \times R))$ is an *induced* subgraph. An induced subgraph $G(Q)$ is said to be a *clique* if $(v, w) \in E$ for all $v, w \in Q \subseteq V$ with $v \neq w$. In this case, we may simply state that Q is a clique. In particular, a clique which is not properly contained in any other clique is called *maximal*. A maximal clique with the maximum size is called a

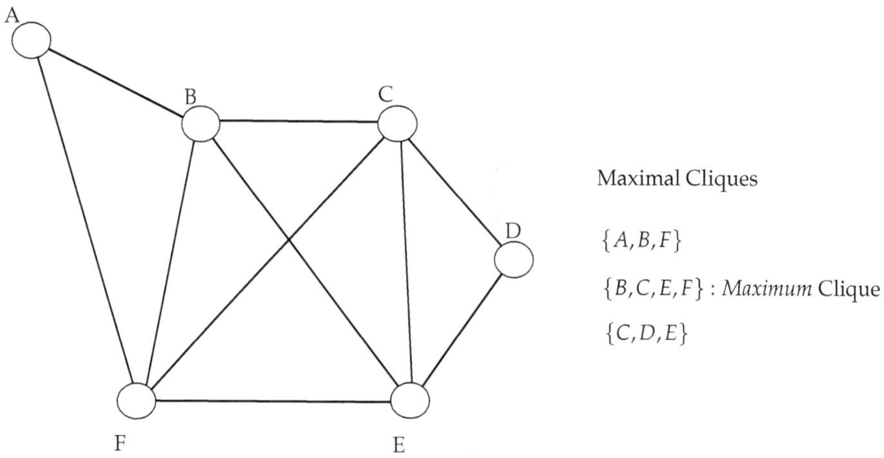

Fig. 1. Example graph

maximum clique. The number of vertices of a maximum clique in an induced subgraph $G(R)$ is denoted by $\omega(R)$.
Consider an example graph $G_0 = (V_0, E_0)$ in Fig. 1, where $V_0 = \{A,B,C,D,E,F\}$ and $E_0 = \{(A,B),(A,F),(B,C),(B,E),(B,F),(C,D),(C,E),(C,F),(D,E),(E,F)\}$. All maximal cliques are $\{A,B,F\}, \{B,C,E,F\}$ and $\{C,D,E\}$, where $\{B,C,E,F\}$ is a maximum clique of size 4. Note that $\{B,C,E\}$ is a clique, but is not a *maximal* clique since it is contained in a larger clique $\{B,C,E,F\}$.

3. Efficient algorithms for finding a maximum clique

3.1 A basic algorithm

One standard approach for finding a maximum clique is based on the branch-and-bound depth-first search method.
Our algorithm begins with a small clique, and continues finding larger and larger cliques until one is found that can be verified to have the maximum size. More precisely, we maintain global variables Q, Q_{max}, where Q consists of vertices of a current clique, Q_{max} consists of vertices of the largest clique found so far. Let $R \subseteq V$ consist of candidate vertices which may be added to Q. We begin the algorithm by letting $Q := \emptyset$, $Q_{max} := \emptyset$, and $R := V$ (the set of all vertices). We select a certain vertex p from R and add p to Q ($Q := Q \cup \{p\}$). Then we compute $R_p := R \cap \Gamma(p)$ as the new set of candidate vertices. This procedure (EXPAND()) is applied recursively while $R_p \neq \emptyset$. Note here that **if** $|Q| + |R| \leq |Q_{max}|$ **then** $Q \cup R$ can contain only a clique that is smaller than or equal to $|Q_{max}|$, hence searching for R can be pruned in this case. This is a *basic bounding condition*.
When $R_p = \emptyset$ is reached, Q constitutes a *maximal* clique. If Q is maximal and $|Q| > |Q_{max}|$ holds, Q_{max} is replaced by Q. We then backtrack by removing p from Q and R. We select a new vertex p from the resulting R and continue the same procedure until $R = \emptyset$.
This is a well known basic algorithm for finding a maximum clique (see, e.g., (12; 10)) and is shown in detail in Fig. 2 as Algorithm BasicMC. The process can be represented by a *search*

```
procedure BasicMC (G = (V,E))
begin
     global Q := ∅;
     global Q_max := ∅;
     EXPAND(V);
     output Q_max
end {of BasicMC}

procedure EXPAND(R)
begin
     while R ≠ ∅ do
          p := a vertex in R;
          if |Q| + |R| > |Q_max| then
               Q := Q ∪ {p};
               R_p := R ∩ Γ(p);
               if R_p ≠ ∅ then EXPAND(R_p)
               else (i.e., R_p = ∅) if |Q| > |Q_max| then Q_max := Q fi
               fi
               Q := Q − {p}
               else return
          fi
          R := R − {p}
     od
end {of EXPAND}
```

Fig. 2. Algorithm BasicMC

forest that is similar to Fig. 3 (b).

3.2 Algorithm MCQ

We present a very simple and efficient algorithm MCQ (46) that is a direct extension of the previous BasicMC.

3.2.1 Pruning

One of the most important points to improve the efficiency of BasicMC is to strengthen the *bounding condition* in order to prune unnecessary searching.
For a set R of vertices, let $\chi(R)$ be the chromatic number of R, *i.e.*, the *minimum* number of colors so that all pairs of adjacent vertices are colored by different colors, and $\chi'(R)$ be an *approximate* chromatic number of R, *i.e.*, a number of colors so that all pairs of adjacent vertices are colored by different colors.
Then we have that

$$\omega(R) \leq \chi(R) \leq \chi'(R) \leq |R|.$$

While obtaining $\chi(R)$ is also NP-hard, an appropriate $\chi'(R)$ could be a better upper bound of $\omega(R)$ than $|R|$, and might be obtained with low overhead. Here, we employ very simple *greedy* or *sequential* approximate coloring to the vertices of R, as introduced in (42; 12; 43). Let positive integral numbers 1, 2, 3, ... stand for colors red, green, yellow, ... *Coloring* is

also called *Numbering*. For each $p \in R$, *sequentially* from the first vertex to the last, we assign a positive integral *Number* $No[p]$ which is as small as possible. That is, when the vertices in $R = \{p_1, p_2, \ldots, p_m\}$ are arranged in this order, first let $No[p_1] = 1$, and subsequently, let $No[p_2] = 2$ if $p_2 \in \Gamma(p_1)$ else $No[p_1] = 1, \ldots,$ and so on. After *Numbers* are assigned to all vertices in R, we sort these vertices in *ascending order* with respect to their *Numbers*.
We select p as the last (rightmost) vertex in R (at the 4th line in **procedure** EXPAND(R) in Fig. 2), then $No[p] = \text{Max}\{No[q] \mid q \in R\}$, that is an approximate chromatic number of R. So, we replace the basic bounding condition:

$$\textbf{if } |Q| + |R| > |Q_{max}| \textbf{ then}$$

in Fig. 2 BasicMC, by the following *new bounding condition*:

$$\textbf{if } |Q| + No[p] > |Q_{max}| \textbf{ then}.$$

Numbering is applied every time prior to application of EXPAND().
Since the greedy Numbering to R is carried out in $O(|R|^2)$-time and is not so time-consuming, the new bounding condition can be very effective to reduce the search space with low overhead.

3.2.2 Initial sorting and simple numbering

We have shown in (12) that both search space and overall running time are reduced when one sorts the vertices in an ascending order with respect to their degrees prior to the application of a branch-and-bound depth-first search algorithm for finding a maximum clique. Carraghan and Pardalos (10) also employ a similar technique successfully. Therefore, at the beginning of our algorithm, we sort vertices in V in a descending order with respect to their degrees. This means that a vertex with the minimum degree is selected at the beginning of the **while** loop in EXPAND() in Fig. 2 since the selection of p is from the last (rightmost) to the first (leftmost). Furthermore, we initially assign *Numbers* to the vertices in V simply, so that $No[V[i]] = i$ for $i \leq \Delta(G)$, where $\Delta(G)$ is the maximum degree of G, and $No[V[i]] = \Delta(G) + 1$ for $\Delta(G) + 1 \leq i \leq |V|$. This initial *Number* has the desired property that $No[p] \geq \omega(V)$ for any p in V **while** $V \neq \emptyset$. Thus, this simple initial *Number* suffices.
This completes our explanation of the algorithm MCQ. See (46) for further details.

3.3 Algorithm MCR

Algorithm MCR (48) is an improved version of MCQ, where improvements are mainly for the *initial* sorting of the vertices. First, we alter the order of the vertices in $V = \{V[1], V[2], \ldots, V[n]\}$ so that in a subgraph of $G = (V, E)$ induced by a set of vertices $V' = \{V[1], V[2], \ldots, V[i]\}$, it holds that $V[i]$ always has the minimum degree in $\{V[1], V[2], \ldots, V[i]\}$ for $1 \leq i \leq |V|$. While the resulting order is identical to that of (10), it should be noted that time-consuming computation of the degree of vertices is carried out *only at the beginning* of MCR as in MCQ, and hence the overhead of the overall selection of vertices is *very small*, too. Here, the degrees of adjacent vertices are also taken into consideration.
Numbering of the vertices is carried out in a similar way to MCQ, but more closely. The above considerations lead to an improved clique finding algorithm MCR.
Example run We show an example run of MCR to an input graph G_1 given in Fig. 3 (a).
In the initial sorting, vertex G with the minimum degree is selected at first. Then, vertices F and E follow after G. Now the remaining vertices A, B, C, D are of the same minimum degree,

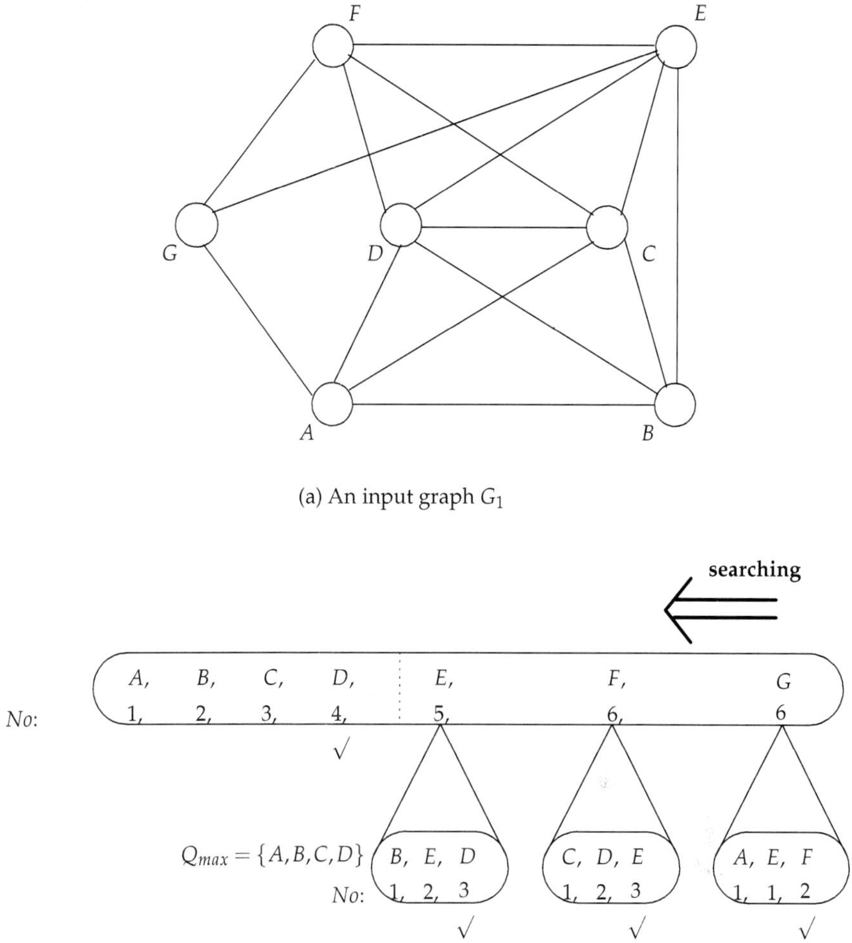

(a) An input graph G_1

(b) A search forest of G_1

Fig. 3. Example run of MCR

and then *Numbering* is applied to this set of vertices to have $No[A] = 1$, $No[B] = 2$, $No[C] = 3$, $No[D] = 4$. The other vertices are numbered as $No[E] = 4 + 1 = 5$, $No[F] = 6$ $(= \Delta(G_1) + 1)$, $No[G] = 6$. In addition, we have that $Q_{max} = \{A, B, C, D\}$ (of size 4), since every degree of the vertices in the induced subgraph $G_1(\{A, B, C, D\})$ is $3 = 4 - 1$.

The result of the initial sorting of vertices is shown at the top of Fig. 3 (b) and the corresponding numbers are just below these vertices.

Subsequently, in EXPAND( ), the rightmost vertex G is selected to have $Q = \{G\}$, $R_G = \Gamma(G) = \{A, E, F\}$. These vertices A, E, F are numbered 1,1,2 as shown in the second row of Fig. 3 (b).

Here, $|Q| + No[F] = |\{G\}| + 2 = 3 < |Q_{max}| = 4$, then prune ($\surd$: checkmark in Fig. 3 (b)). The searching proceeds from the right to the left as shown in Fig. 3 (b). As a result, the maximum clique in G_1 is $Q_{max} = \{A, B, C, D\}$.

3.4 Algorithm MCS

Algorithm MCS (39; 49; 50) is a further improved version of MCR.

3.4.1 New approximate coloring

When vertex r is selected, if $No[r] \leq |Q_{max}| - |Q|$ then it is not necessary to search from vertex r by the *bounding condition*, as mentioned in Sect. 3.2.1. The number of vertices to be searched can be reduced if the *Number* $No[p]$ of vertex p for which $No[p] > |Q_{max}| - |Q|$ can be changed to a value less than or equal to $|Q_{max}| - |Q|$. When we encounter such vertex p with $No[p] > |Q_{max}| - |Q|$ ($\stackrel{def}{=} No_{th}$) ($No_{th}$ stands for $No_{threshold}$), we attempt to change its *Number* in the following manner (16). Let No_p denote the original value of $No[p]$.

[Re-NUMBER p]

1) Attempt to find a vertex q in $\Gamma(p)$ such that $No[q] = k_1 \leq No_{th}$, with $|C_{k_1}| = 1$.

2) If such q is found, then attempt to find *Number* k_2 such that no vertex in $\Gamma(q)$ has *Number* k_2.

3) If such number k_2 is found, then change the *Numbers* of q and p so that $No[q] = k_2$ and $No[p] = k_1$.

(If no vertex q with *Number* k_2 is found, nothing is done.)

When the vertex q with *Number* k_2 is found, $No[p]$ is changed from No_p to k_1 ($\leq No_{th}$); thus, *it is no longer necessary to search from p.*

3.4.2 Adjunct ordered set of vertices for approximate coloring

The ordering of vertices plays an important role in the algorithm as demonstrated in (12; 10; 46; 48). In particular, the procedure *Numbering* strongly depends on the order of vertices, since it is a *sequential* coloring. In our new algorithm, we sort the vertices in the same way as in MCR (48) at the first stage. However, the vertices are *disordered* in the succeeding stages owing to the application of Re-NUMBER. In order to avoid this difficulty, we employ another *adjunct ordered set V_a of vertices for approximate coloring* that preserves the order of vertices appropriately sorted in the first stage. Such a technique was first introduced in (38).

We apply *Numbering* to vertices from the first (leftmost) to the last (rightmost) in the order maintained in V_a, while we select a vertex in the ordered set R for *searching*, beginning from the last (rightmost) vertex and continuing up to the first (leftmost) vertex.

An improved MCR obtained by introducing only the technique (38) in this section is named MCR*.

3.4.3 Reconstruction of the adjacency matrix

Each graph is stored as an adjacency matrix in the computer memory. Sequential *Numbering* is carried out according to the initial order of vertices in the adjunct ordered set V_a, as described in Sect. 3.4.2. Taking this into account, we *rename* the vertices of the graph and *reconstruct* the adjacency matrix so that the vertices are *consecutively ordered* in a manner identical to *the initial order of vertices* obtained at the beginning of MCR. The above-mentioned reconstruction of the adjacency matrix (41) results in a more effective use of the cache memory.

The new algorithm obtained by introducing all the techniques described in Sects. 3.4.1–3.4.3 in MCR is named MCS. Table 1 shows the running time required to solve some DIMACS

Graph	dfmax (18)	New (33)	ILOG (35)	MCQ (46)	MCR (48)	MCS (50)
brock400_1	22,051		8,401	1,783	1,771	693
block800_1	$> 10^5$		$> 10,667$	18,002	17,789	9,347
MANN_a27	$> 10^5$	$> 2,232$	14	5.4	2.5	0.8
MANN_a45	$> 10^5$		$> 10,667$	4,646	3,090	281
p_hat500-2	133	96	24	4.0	3.1	0.7
p_hat1000-2	$> 10^5$		12,478	2,844	2,434	221
san200_0.9_3	42,648		135	10	0.16	0.06
san400_0.7_2	$> 10^5$	113	50	1.0	0.3	0.1
san400_0.9_1	$> 10^5$		1,259	46.3	3.4	0.1
gen200_p0.9_44	48,262				5.39	0.47
gen400_p0.9_55					5,846,951	58,431
gen400_p0.9_65					$> 2.5 \times 10^7$	151,597
C250.9	$> 10^5$				44,214	3,257

Table 1. Comparison of the running time [sec]

benchmark graphs (18) by representative algorithms dfmax (18), New (33), ILOG (35), MCQ, MCR, and MCS, taken from (50). (10^5 seconds $\simeq$ 1.16 days).
Our user time (T_1) in (50) for DIMACS benchmark instances: `r100.5`, `r200.5`, `r300.5`, `r400.5`, and `r500.5` are 1.57×10^{-3}, 4.15×10^{-2}, 0.359, 2.21, and 8.47 seconds, respectively. (*Correction*: These values described in the Appendix of (50) should be corrected as shown above. However, other values in (50) are computed based on the above correct values, hence other changes in (50) are *not* necessary.)
While MCR* obtained by introducing the adjunct set V_a of vertices for approximate coloring in Sect. 3.4.2 is almost always more efficient than MCR (38), combination of all the techniques in Sects. 3.4.1–3.4.3 makes it much more efficient to have MCS.
The aim of the present study is to develop a faster algorithm whose use is not confined to any particular type of graphs. We can reduce the search space by *sorting* vertices in *R in descending order with respect to their degrees* before every application of approximate coloring, and hence reduce the overall running time for *dense* graphs (36; 21), but with the increase of the overall running time for *nondense* graphs. Appropriately controlled application of repeated sorting of vertices can make the algorithm more efficient for wider classes of graphs (21).
Parallel processing for maximum-clique-finding is very promising in practice (41; 53).
For practical applications, *weighted* graphs becomes more important. Algorithms for finding *maximum-weighted* cliques have also been developed. For example, see (45; 32; 30) for *vertex*-weighted graphs and (40) for *edge*-weighed graphs.

4. Efficient algorithm for generating all maximal cliques

In addition to finding only one maximum clique, generating all maximal cliques is also important and has many diverse applications.
In this section, we present a depth-first search algorithm CLIQUES (44; 47) for generating all maximal cliques of an undirected graph $G = (V, E)$, in which pruning methods are employed as in Bron and Kerbosch's algorithm (7). All maximal cliques generated are output in a tree-like form.

4.1 Algorithm CLIQUES

The basic framework of CLIQUES is almost the same as BasicMC *without the basic bounding condition.*

Here, we describe two methods to prune unnecessary parts of the search forest, which happened to be the same as in the Bron-Kerbosch algorithm (7). We regard the set $SUBG$ ($= V$ at the beginning) as an *ordered* set of vertices, and we continue to generate maximal cliques from vertices in $SUBG$ step by step in this order

First, let $FINI$ be a subset of vertices of $SUBG$ that have been already processed by the algorithm. ($FINI$ is short for *"finished"*.) Then we denote by $CAND$ the set of remaining candidates for expansion: $CAND = SUBG - FINI$. So, we have

$$SUBG = FINI \cup CAND \quad (FINI \cap CAND = \emptyset),$$

where $FINI = \emptyset$ at the beginning. Consider the subgraph $G(SUBG_q)$ with $SUBG_q = SUBG \cap \Gamma(q)$, and let

$$SUBG_q = FINI_q \cup CAND_q \ (FINI_q \cap CAND_q = \emptyset),$$

where $FINI_q = FINI \cap \Gamma(q)$ and $CAND_q = CAND \cap \Gamma(q)$. Then only the vertices in $CAND_q$ can be candidates for expanding the complete subgraph $Q \cup \{q\}$ to find *new* larger cliques.

Secondly, given a certain vertex $u \in SUBG$, suppose that *all* the maximal cliques containing $Q \cup \{u\}$ have been generated. Then every *new* maximal clique containing Q, but not $Q \cup \{u\}$, must contain at least one vertex $q \in SUBG - \Gamma(u)$.

Taking the previously described pruning method also into consideration, the only search subtrees to be expanded are from vertices in $(SUBG - SUBG \cap \Gamma(u)) - FINI = CAND - \Gamma(u)$. Here, in order to minimize $\mid CAND - \Gamma(u) \mid$, we choose such vertex $u \in SUBG$ to be the one which *maximizes* $\mid CAND \cap \Gamma(u) \mid$. This is *essential* to establish the *optimality* of the worst-case time-complexity of CLIQUES.

Our algorithm CLIQUES (47) for generating all maximal cliques is shown in Fig. 4. Here, if Q is a *maximal* clique that is found at statement 2, then the algorithm only prints out a string of characters *"clique*, instead of Q itself at statement 3. Otherwise, it is impossible to achieve the worst-case running time of $O(3^{n/3})$ for an n-vertex graph. Instead, in addition to printing "clique" at statement 3, we print out q followed by a *comma* at statement 7 every time q is picked out as a new element of a larger clique, and we print out a string of characters *"back,"* at statement 12 after q is moved from $CAND$ to $FINI$ at statement 11. We can easily obtain a tree representation of all the maximal cliques from the sequence printed by statements 3, 7, and 12.

The output in a tree-like format is also important *practically*, since it saves space in the output file.

4.2 Time-complexity of CLIQUES

We have proved that the worst-case time-complexity is $O(3^{n/3})$ for an n-vertex graph (47). This is *optimal* as a function of n, since there exist up to $3^{n/3}$ cliques in an n-vertex graph (29). The algorithm is also demonstrated to run fast in practice by computational experiments. Table 2 shows the running time required to solve some DIMACS benchmark graphs by representative algorithms CLIQUE (11), AMC (24), AMC* (24), and CLIQUES, taken from (47).

For practical applications, enumeration of *pseudo* cliques sometimes becomes more important (52).

```
procedure CLIQUES(G)
begin
  EXPAND(V,V)
end of CLIQUES

    procedure EXPAND(SUBG, CAND)
    begin
      if SUBG = ∅
        then print ("clique,")
        else u := a vertex u in SUBG which maximizes | CAND ∩ Γ(u) |;
             while CAND − Γ(u) ≠ ∅
               do q := a vertex in (CAND − Γ(u));
                  print (q, ",");
                  SUBG_q := SUBG ∩ Γ(q);
                  CAND_q := CAND ∩ Γ(q);
                  EXPAND(SUBG_q, CAND_q);
                  CAND := CAND − {q};
                  print ("back,")
               od
      fi
    end of EXPAND
```

Fig. 4. Algorithm CLIQUES

Graph	CLIQUE (11)	AMC (24)	AMC* (24)	CLIQUES (47)
brock200_2	181.4	75.2	35.9	0.7
johnson16-2-4	908	151	153	4
keller4	3,447	1,146	491	5
p_hat300-2	> 86,400	16,036	4,130	100

Table 2. Comparison of the running time [sec]

5. Applications to bioinformatics

5.1 Analysis of protein structures

In this subsection, we show applications of maximum clique algorithms to the following three problems on protein structure analysis: (i) *protein structure alignment*, (ii) *protein side-chain packing*, (iii) *protein threading*. Since there are many references on these problems, we only cite references that present the methods shown here. Most of other relevant references can be reached from those references. Furthermore, we present here only the definitions of the problems and reductions to clique problems. Readers interested in details such as results of computational experiments are referred to the original papers (1; 2; 3; 4; 8).

5.1.1 Protein structure alignment

Comparison of protein structures is very important for understanding the functions of proteins because proteins with similar structures often have common functions. Pairwise comparison of proteins is usually done via *protein structure alignment* using some scoring scheme, where an alignment is a mapping of amino acids between two proteins. Because of

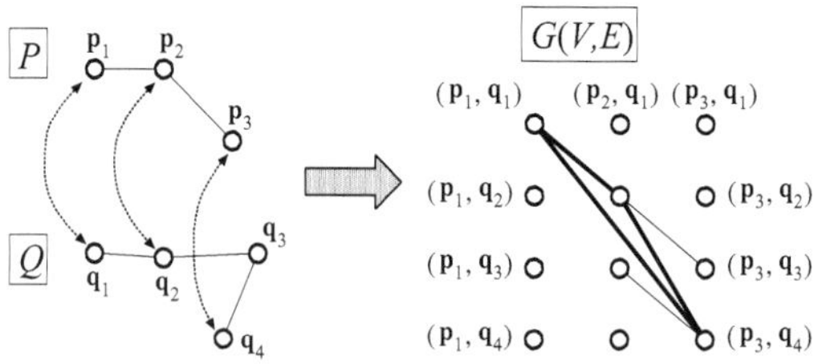

Fig. 5. Reduction from protein structure alignment to maximum clique. Maximum clique shown by bold lines (right) corresponds to protein structure alignment shown by dotted lines (left).

its importance, many methods have been proposed for protein structure alignment. However, most existing methods are heuristic ones in which optimality of the solution is not guaranteed. Bahadur et al. developed a clique-based method for computing structure alignment under some local similarity measure (2). Let $P = (\mathbf{p}_1, \mathbf{p}_2, \ldots, \mathbf{p}_m)$ be a sequence of three-dimensional positions of amino acids (precisely, positions of Cα atoms) in a protein. Let $Q = (\mathbf{q}_1, \mathbf{q}_2, \ldots, \mathbf{q}_n)$ be a sequence of positions of amino acids of another protein. For two points $\mathbf{x}$ and $\mathbf{y}$, $|\mathbf{x} - \mathbf{y}|$ denotes the Euclidean distance between x and y. Let $f(x)$ be a function from the set of non-negative reals to the set of reals no less than 1.0. We call a sequence of pairs $M = ((\mathbf{p}_{i_1}, \mathbf{q}_{i_1}), \ldots, (\mathbf{p}_{i_l}, \mathbf{q}_{i_l}))$ an *alignment* under *non-uniform distortion* if the following conditions are satisfied:

- $i_k < i_h$ and $j_k < j_h$ hold for all $k < h$,
- $(\forall k)(\forall h \neq k) \left(\dfrac{1}{f(r)} < \dfrac{|\mathbf{q}_{j_h} - \mathbf{q}_{j_k}|}{|\mathbf{p}_{j_h} - \mathbf{p}_{j_k}|} < f(r) \right)$,

where $r = \min\{|\mathbf{q}_{j_h} - \mathbf{q}_{j_k}|, |\mathbf{p}_{j_h} - \mathbf{p}_{j_k}|\}$. Then, protein structure alignment is defined as the problem of finding a longest alignment (*i.e.*, l is the maximum). It is known that protein structure alignment is NP-hard under this definition.

This protein structure alignment problem can be reduced to the maximum clique problem in a simple way (see Fig. 5). we construct an undirected graph $G(V, E)$ by

$$\begin{aligned} V &= \{ (\mathbf{p}_i, \mathbf{q}_j) \mid i = 1, \ldots, m, \ j = 1, \ldots, n \}, \\ E &= \{ \{(\mathbf{p}_i, \mathbf{q}_j), (\mathbf{p}_k, \mathbf{q}_h)\} \mid i < k, \ j < h, \ \frac{1}{f(r)} < \frac{|\mathbf{q}_h - \mathbf{q}_j|}{|\mathbf{p}_k - \mathbf{p}_i|} < f(r) \ \}. \end{aligned}$$

Then, it is straight-forward to see that a maximum clique corresponds to a longest alignment.

5.1.2 Protein side-chain packing

The *protein side-chain packing* problem is, given an amino acid sequence and spatial information on the main chain, to find *side-chain conformation* with the minimum potential energy. In most cases, it is defined as a problem of seeking a set of $(\chi_1, \chi_2, \ldots)$ angles whose *potential energy* becomes the minimum, where positions of atoms in the main chain are fixed. This problem is important for prediction of detailed structures of proteins because such prediction methods as protein threading cannot determine positions of atoms in the side-chains. It is known that protein side-chain packing is NP-hard and thus various heuristic methods have been proposed. Here, we briefly review a clique-based approach to protein side-chain packing (2; 3; 8).

Let $R = \{r_1, \ldots, r_n\}$ be the set of amino acid residues in a protein. Here, we only consider χ_1 angles and then assume that positions of atoms in a side-chain are rotated around the χ_1 axis. Let $r_{i,k}$ be the ith residue whose side-chain atoms are rotated by $(2\pi k)/K$ radian, where we can modify the problem and method so that the rotation angles can take other discrete values. We say that residue $r_{i,k}$ collides with the main chain if the minimum distance between the atoms in $r_{i,k}$ and the atoms in the main chain is less than a threshold L_1Å. We say that residue $r_{i,k}$ collides with residue $r_{j,h}$ if the minimum distance between the atoms in $r_{i,k}$ and the atoms in $r_{j,h}$ is less than L_2Å. We define an undirected graph $G(V;E)$ by

$$\begin{aligned} V &= \{\, r_{i,k} \mid r_{i,k} \text{ does not collide with the main chain} \,\}, \\ E &= \{\, \{r_{i,k}, r_{j,h}\} \mid r_{i,k} \text{ does not collide with } r_{j,h} \,\}. \end{aligned}$$

Then, it is straight-forward to see that a clique with size n corresponds to a consistent configuration of side chains (*i.e.*, side-chain conformation with no collisions). We can extend this reduction so that potential energy can be taken into account by using the *maximum edge-weighted clique* problem.

5.1.3 Protein threading

Protein threading is one of the prediction methods for three-dimensional protein structures. The purpose of protein threading is to seek for a protein structure in a database which best matches a given protein sequence (whose structure is to be predicted) using some score function.

In order to evaluate the extent of match, it is required to compute an *optimal alignment* between an amino acid sequence $S = s_1 s_2 \ldots s_n$ and a known protein structure $P = (\mathbf{p}_1, \mathbf{p}_2, \ldots, \mathbf{p}_m)$, where s_i and p_j denote the ith amino acid and the jth residue position, respectively. As in protein structure alignment, a sequence of pairs $((s_{i_1}, \mathbf{p}_{j_1}), (s_{i_2}, \mathbf{p}_{j_2}), \ldots, (s_{i_l}, \mathbf{p}_{j_l}))$ is called an *alignment* (or, a *threading*) between S and P if $i_k < i_h$ and $j_k < j_h$ hold for all $k < h$. Let $g(s_{i_k}, s_{i_h}, \mathbf{p}_{j_k}, \mathbf{p}_{j_h})$ give a score (e.g., pseudo energy) between residue positions of $\mathbf{p}_{j_k}$ and $\mathbf{p}_{j_h}$ when amino acids s_{i_k} and s_{i_h} are assigned to positions of $\mathbf{p}_{j_k}$ and $\mathbf{p}_{j_h}$, respectively. Then, protein threading is defined as a problem of finding an optimal alignment that minimizes the pseudo energy:

$$\sum_{k<h} g(s_{i_k}, s_{i_h}, \mathbf{p}_{j_k}, \mathbf{p}_{j_h}),$$

where we ignore gap penalties for the simplicity.

This protein threading problem can be reduced to the *maximum edge-weighted clique* problem (1; 4), which seeks for a clique that maximizes the total weight of edges in the clique. From an instance of protein threading, we construct an undirected graph $G(V, E)$ by

$$\begin{aligned} V &= \{\, (s_i, \mathbf{p}_j) \mid i = 1, \ldots, n, \; j = 1, \ldots, m \,\}, \\ E &= \{\, \{(s_i, \mathbf{p}_j), (s_k, \mathbf{p}_h)\} \mid i < k, \; j < h \,\}, \end{aligned}$$

where the weight of an edge is given by $-g(s_i, s_k, \mathbf{p}_j, \mathbf{p}_h)$. It is straight-forward to see that a maximum edge-weight clique corresponds to an optimal alignment. Though this clique-based approach is not necessarily the best for protein threading, the results of (1; 4) suggest that it is useful for protein threading with certain constraints.

5.2 Data mining for related genes in a biomedical database

In this subsection, we present an application of enumerating cliques. Readers interested in details are referred to the original paper (25).

Progress in the life sciences cannot be made without integrating biomedical knowledge on numerous genes in order to help formulate hypotheses on the genetic mechanisms behind various biological phenomena, including diseases. There is thus a strong need for a way to automatically and comprehensively search biomedical databases for related genes, such as genes in the same families and genes encoding components of the same pathways.

We constructed a graph whose vertices (nodes) were gene or disease pages, and edges were the hyperlink connections between those pages in the Online Mendelian Inheritance in Man (OMIM) database (25; 26). This work was based on the assumption that the structures of hyperlink connections correspond to the structural features of biological systems. Clique enumeration approach has been applied to a relational graph based on the assumption that relevant relationships are reflected in completely interconnected subgraphs (cliques) or nearly completely interconnected subgraphs (pseudo-cliques). We address the extraction of related genes by searching for densely connected subgraphs in a biomedical relational graph. Sets of related genes are detected by enumerating densely-connected subgraphs modeled as cliques (47) or pseudo-cliques (52).

We obtained over 20,000 sets of related genes (called 'gene modules') by enumerating cliques computationally. Table 3 shows gene sets included in typical large gene modules. The gene module in the first row is constituted by a family of chemokine genes, and the gene module in the second comprises NF-κB family genes (including RelA and RelB) and genes that form complexes with them (IκB). The gene module in the third row is made up of 'DNA repair'-related genes. The BRCA1-associated proteins; the BLM, MSH6, MSH2, and MLH1 proteins; and subunits of the RFC complex are involved in DNA repair. The genes in the module in the fourth row are related to general transcription factor (GTF) protein complexes. The gene module in the bottom row is associated with the signal transduction pathway of the inflammatory response. TNF receptor-associated factor 2 (TRAF2) is a protein that interacts with TNF receptors and is required for signal transduction. The MAP kinase kinase kinase 14 (MAP3K14) gene in this module encodes a protein that simulates NF-κB activity by binding to the TRAF2 gene product. The gene modules thus comprise various types of related genes including gene families, complexes, and pathways.

For applying gene modules to disease mechanism analysis, we assembled gene modules associated with the metabolic syndrome as an example of a typical multifactorial disease comprising obesity, diabetes, hyperlipidemia, and hypertension. The number of gene modules associated with diabetes, hyperlipidemia, hypertension, and obesity were 110, 16, 34, and 28, respectively. There were no overlaps among the modules. Then a total of 188 modules and 124 genes contained were identified. The 10 most frequent genes in the 188 modules are listed in Table 4 along with the numbers of times they were found in the modules (*i.e.*, cliques) of various sizes. As shown in the table, INS gene and LEP gene are

Gene module	Attribute
{ PPBP, SCYB6, GRO2, GRO3, IL8, SCYB10, IFNG, GRO1, PF4, SCYB5, MIG, SCYB11 }	Family
{ NFKBIA, NFKB1, NFKB2, RELA, REL, CHUK, MAP3K7, IKBKB, NFKBIB, MAP3K14, RELB }	Family & Complex
{ RFC4, RFC1, BRCA1, MSH2, MLH1, APC, RFC2, MSH6, MRE11A, BLM }	Complex
{ POLR2A, GTF2E1, GTF2B, GTF2F1, GTF2H1, TAF1, TAF10, GTF2A2, GTF2A1 }	Complex
{ TNFRSF5, NFKB1, TNF, TNFRSF1A, TNFRSF1B, CHUK, TRAF2, MAP3K14 }	Pathway

Table 3. Typical large gene modules computationally extracted as pseudo-cliques.

			Size					
Rank	Gene	Total	2	3	4	5	6	7
1	INS	29	2	6	2	18	1	0
2	LEP	27	2	6	4	12	3	0
3	POMC	16	1	0	3	10	2	0
4	PCSK1	13	0	1	2	9	1	0
5	IRS2	12	0	0	0	11	1	0
5	IGF1	12	0	1	0	10	1	0
5	INSR	12	3	4	1	4	0	0
8	IRS1	11	0	0	1	9	1	0
9	MC4R	10	0	0	1	7	2	0
10	FGF1	9	0	0	1	4	2	2

Table 4. The 10 most frequent genes in the 188 extracted modules associated with the metabolic syndrome.

the top and the 2nd, respectively. The modules of size 6 including INS gene or LEP gene were {Obesity,LEP,MC4R,POMC,AGRP,LEPR}, {Obesity,LEP,MC4R,POMC,AGRP,PCSK1} and {Diabetes,LEP,IGF1,IRS1,INS,IRS2}. Each module contains biologically plausible genes related to obesity or diabetes. By combining the 188 modules and 124 genes using the correspondence analysis, we obtained a coherent holistic picture helpful for interpreting relations among genes (25).

The comprehensive extraction of gene modules can be a potential aid to researchers in the biomedical sciences by providing a systematic methodology for interpreting relationships among genes and biological phenomena.

6. Conclusion

We have presented efficient algorithms for finding maximum and maximal cliques, and shown our successful application to bioinformatics. It is expected that these algorithms can be convenient and effective tools for much more problems in bioinformatics.

7. Acknowledgments

We should like to express our sincere gratitude to our many colleagues and (former) students who worked with us in this research. Many helpful comments by E. Harley are appreciated. We wish to thank P.M. Pardalos and his colleagues for reviewing our earlier works including (43), (44) in their surveys (34), (5). Our earlier works received considerable attention by their reviews. Thanks are also to D.S. Johnson and M. Trick for their efforts in organizing the Second DIMACS Implementation Challenge for Cliques, Coloring, and Satisfiability (18). They made it easier for us to compare the results of different algorithms carried out on various computers. This research was partially supported by Grants-in-Aid for Scientific Research Nos. 19500010, 21300047, 22500009, 22240009, and many others from the Ministry of Education, Culture, Sports, Science and Technology, Japan, a Special Grant for the Strategic Information and Communications R&D Promotion Programme (SCOPE) Project from the Ministry of Internal Affairs and Communications, Japan, and the Research Fund of the University of Electro-Communications to the Advanced Algorithms Research Laboratory. The research was also provided a grant by the Funai Foundation for Information Technology.

8. References

[1] Akutsu, T., Hayashida, M., Bahadur D.K.C, Tomita, E., Suzuki, J., Horimoto, K.: Dynamic programming and clique based approaches for protein threading with profiles and constraints, IEICE Trans. on Fundamentals of Electronics, Communications and Computer Sciences, E89-A, 1215-1222 (2006). The preliminary version was presented In: Akutsu, T., Hayashida, M., Tomita, E., Suzuki, J., Horimoto, K.: Protein threading with profiles and constraints, Proc. IEEE Symp. on Bioinformatics and Bioengineering (BIBE 2004), 537-544 (2004)

[2] Bahadur D.K.C., Akutsu, T., Tomita, E., Seki, T., Fujiyama, A.: Point matching under non-uniform distortions and protein side chain packing based on an efficient maximum clique algorithm, Genome Informatics, 13, 143–152 (2002)

[3] Bahadur D.K.C, Tomita, E., Suzuki, J., Akutsu, T.: Protein side-chain packing problem: A maximum edge-weight clique algorithmic approach, J. Bioinformatics and Computational Biology, 3, pp.103-126 (2005)

[4] Bahadur, D.K.C., Tomita, E., Suzuki, J., Horimoto, K., Akutsu, T.: Protein threading with profiles and distance constraints using clique based algorithms, J. Bioinformatics and Computational Biology, 4, 19–42 (2006)

[5] Bomze, I. M., Budinich, M., Pardalos, P. M., Pelillo M.: The maximum clique problem, In; Du, D.-Z., Pardalos, P.M. (Eds.), Handbook of Combinatorial Optimization, Supplement vol. A, Kluwer Academic Publishers, 1–74 (1999)

[6] Bradde, S., Braunstein, A., Mahmoudi, H., Tria, F., Weigt, M., Zecchina, R.: Aligning graphs and finding substructures by a cavity approach, Europhisics Letters, 89 (2010)

[7] Bron, C., Kerbosch, J.: Algorithm 457, Finding all cliques of an undirected graph, Comm. ACM, 16, 575–577 (1973)

[8] Brown, J.B., Bahadur, D.K.C., Tomita, E., Akutsu, T.: Multiple methods for protein side chain packing using maximum weight cliques, Genome Informatics, 17(1), 3–12 (2006)

[9] Butenko, S., Wilhelm, W.E.: Clique-detection models in computational biochemistry and genomics - Invited Review - , European J. Operational Research, 173, 1–17 (2006)

[10] Carraghan, R., Pardalos, P.M.: An exact algorithm for the maximum clique problem, Operations Research Letters, 9, 375–382 (1990)

[11] Chiba, N., Nishizeki, T.: Arboricity and subgraph listing algorithms, SIAM J. Comput., 14, 210–223 (1985)

[12] Fujii, T., Tomita, E.: On efficient algorithms for finding a maximum clique, Technical Report of IECE, AL81-113, 25–34 (1982)

[13] Fukagawa, D., Tamura, T., Takasu, A., Tomita, E., Akutsu, T.: A Clique-based method for the edit distance between unordered trees and its application to analysis of glycan structure, BMC Bioinformatics, Suppl. for APBC 2011 (to appear)

[14] Han, K., Cui, G., Chen, Y.: Identifying functional groups by finding cliques and near-cliques in protein interaction networks, Proc. 2007 Frontiers in the Convergence of Bioscience and Information Technologies, 159–164 (2007)

[15] Hattori, M., Okuno, Y. Goto, S., Kanehisa, M.: Development of a chemical structure comparison method for integrated analysis of chemical and genomic information in the metabolic pathways, J. American Chemical Society, 125, 11853–11865 (2003)

[16] Higashi, T., Tomita, E.: A more efficient algorithm for finding a maximum clique based on an improved approximate coloring, Technical Report of the University of Electro-Communications, UEC-TR-CAS5 (2006)

[17] Hotta, K., Tomita, E., Takahashi, H.: A view-invariant human face detection method

based on maximum cliques. Trans. IPSJ, 44, SIG14(TOM9), 57–70 (2003)

[18] Johnson, D.S., Trick, M.A. (Eds.): Cliques, Coloring, and Satisfiability, DIMACS Series in Discrete Mathematics and Theoretical Computer Science, vol.26, American Mathematical Society (1996)

[19] Karp, R.: Reducibility among combinatorial problems, In; Miller, R.E., Thatcher, J.W. (Eds.) *Comlexity of Computer Computations*, Plenum Press, New York, 85–103 (1972)

[20] Kobayashi, S., Kondo, T., Okuda, K., Tomita, E.: Extracting globally structure free sequences by local structure freeness. In: Chen, J., Reif, J. (Eds.), Proc. Ninth International Meeting on DNA Based Computers, 206 (2003)

[21] Kohata, Y., Nishijima, T., Tomita, E., Fujihashi, C., Takahashi, H.: Efficient algorithms for finding a maximum clique, Technical Report of IEICE, COMP89-113, 1–8 (1990)

[22] Li, X., Wu, M., Kwoh, C.-K. Ng, S.-K.: Computational approaches for detecting protein complexes from protein interaction networks: a survey, BMC Genomics, 11 (2010)

[23] Liu, G., Wong, L., Chua, H.-N.: Complex discovery from weighted PPI networks, Bioinformatics, 1891–1897 (2009)

[24] Makino, K., Uno, T.: New algorithms for enumerating all maximal cliques, SWAT 2004, Lecture Notes in Computer Science, 3111, 260–272 (2004)

[25] Matsunaga, T., Yonemori, C., Tomita, E., Muramatsu, M.: Clique-based data mining for related genes in a biomedical database, BMC Bioinformatics, 10:205 (2009)

[26] Matsunaga, T., Kuwata, S., Muramatsu, M.: Computational gene knockout reveals transdisease-transgene association structure, J. Bioinformatics and Computational Biology, 8, 843-866 (2010)

[27] Mohseni-Zadeh, S., Brézellec, P., Risler, J.-L.: Cluster-C, An algorithm for the large-scale clustering of protein sequences based on the extraction of maximal cliques, Comput. Biol. and Chemist., 28, 211-218 (2004)

[28] Mohseni-Zadeh, S., Louis, A., Brézellec, P., Risler, J.-L.: PHYTOPROT: a database of clusters of plant proteins, Nucleic Acids Res., 32 D351-D353 (2004)

[29] Moon, J.W., Moser, L.: On cliques in graphs, Israel J. Math., 3, 23–28 (1965)

[30] Nakamura, T., Tomita, E.: Efficient algorithms for finding a maximum clique with maximum vertex weight, Technical Report of the University of Electro-Communications, UEC-TR-CAS3 (2005)

[31] Nakui, Y., Nishino, T., Tomita, E., Nakamura, T.: On the minimization of the quantum circuit depth based on a maximum clique with maximum vertex weight. Technical Report of RIMS, 1325, Kyoto University, 45–50 (2003)

[32] Östergård, P.R.J.: A fast algorithm for the maximum-weight clique problem, Nordic J. Computing, 8, 424-436 (2001)

[33] Östergård, P.R.J.: A fast algorithm for the maximum clique problem, Discrete Applied Math., 120, 197–207 (2002)

[34] Pardalos, P. M., Xue, J.: The maximum clique problem, J. Global Optimization, 4, 301–328 (1994)

[35] Régin, J.-C.: Using constraint programming to solve the maximum clique problem, Principles and Practice of Constraint Programming, Lecture Notes in Computer Science, 2833, 634-648 (2003)

[36] Shindo, M., Tomita, E., Maruyama, Y.: An efficient algorithm for finding a maximum clique, Technical Report of IEC, CAS86-5, 33–40 (1986)

[37] Strickland, D.M., Barnes, E., Sokol, J.S.: Optimal protein structure alignment using maximum cliques, Operations Research, 53, 389–402 (2005)

[38] Sutani, Y., Tomita, E.: Computational experiments and analyses of a more efficient

algorithm for finding a maximum clique, Technical Report of IPSJ, 2005-MPS-57, 45–48 (2005)

[39] Sutani, Y., Higashi, T., Tomita, E. Takahashi, S., Nakatani, H.: A faster branch-and-bound algorithm for finding a maximum clique, Technical Report of IPSJ, 2006-AL-108, 79–86 (2006)

[40] Suzuki, J., Tomita, E., Seki, T.: An algorithm for finding a maximum clique with maximum edge-weight and computational experiments, Technical Report of IPSJ, 2002-MPS-42, 45–48 (2002)

[41] Takahashi, S., Tomita, E.: Parallel computation for finding a maximum clique on shared memory computers, Technical Report of the University of Electro-Communications, UEC-TR-CAS3 (2007)

[42] Tomita, E., Yamada, M.: An algorithm for finding a maximum complete subgraph, Conference Records of the National Convention of IECE 1978, 8 (1978)

[43] Tomita, E., Kohata, Y., Takahashi, H.: A simple algorithm for finding a maximum clique, Technical Report of the University of Electro-Communications, UEC-TR-C5(1) (1988)

[44] Tomita, E., Tanaka, A. Takahashi, H.: The worst-case time complexity for finding all maximal cliques, Technical Report of the University of Electro-communications, UEC-TR-C5(2) (1988)

[45] Tomita, E. Wakai, Y., Imamatsu, K.: An efficient algorithm for finding a maximum weight clique and its experimental evaluations, Technical Report of IPSJ, 1999-MPS-27, 33–36 (1999)

[46] Tomita, E., Seki, T.: An efficient branch-and-bound algorithm for finding a maximum clique, Discrete Math. and Theoret. Comput. Sci., Lecture Notes in Computer Science, 2731, 278–289 (2003)

[47] Tomita, E., Tanaka, A. Takahashi, H.: The worst-case time complexity for generating all maximal cliques and computational experiments (An invited paper in the Special Issue on COCOON 2004), Theoret. Comput. Sci., 363, 28–42 (2006) (Awarded "Theoretical Computer Science Top Cited Article 2005-2010" by Elsevier.)

[48] Tomita, E., Kameda, T.: An efficient branch-and-bound algorithm for finding a maximum clique with computational experiments, J. Global Optimization, 37, 95–111 (2007), J. Global Optimization, 44, 311 (2009)

[49] Tomita, E.: The maximum clique problem and its applications - Invited Lecture, Technical Report of IPSJ, 2007-MPS-67/2007-BIO-11, 21–24 (2007)

[50] Tomita, E., Sutani, Y., Higashi, T., Takahashi, S., Wakatsuki, M.: A simple and faster branch-and-bound algorithm for finding a maximum clique, WALCOM: Algorithms and Complexity, Lecture Notes in Computer Science, 5942, 191-203 (2010)

[51] Tomita, E.: Plenary Lecture: The maximum clique problem, Proc. 14th WSEAS International Conf. on Computers (vol. I), 19, Corfu Island, Greece (2010)

[52] Uno, T.: An efficient algorithm for solving pseudo clique enumeration problem, Algorithmica, 56, 3–16 (2010)

[53] Wakatsuki, M., Takahashi, S., Tomita, E.: A parallelization of an algorithm for finding a maximum clique on shared memory computers, Technical Report of IPSJ, 2008-MPS-71, 17–20 (2008)

[54] Yonemori, C., Matsunaga, T., Sekine, J., Tomita, E.: A structural analysis of enterprise relationship using cliques, DBSJ Journal, 7, 55-60 (2009)

[55] Zhang, B., Park, B.-H., Karpinets, T., Samatova, N.F.: From pull-down data to protein interaction networks and complexes with biological relevance, Bioinformatics, 24, 979–986 (2008)

33

A Software Development Framework for Agent-Based Infectious Disease Modelling

Luiz C. Mostaço-Guidolin[1,2], Nick J. Pizzi[2,3],
Aleksander B. Demko[2,3] and Seyed M. Moghadas[1,2]
[1]*Department of Mathematics and Statistics, University of Winnipeg,*
[2]*Institute for Biodiagnostics, National Research Council Canada,*
[3]*Department of Computer Science, University of Manitoba,*
Canada

1. Introduction

From the Black Death of 1347–1350 (Murray, 2007) and the Spanish influenza pandemic of 1918–1919 (Taubenberger & Morens, 2006), to the more recent 2003 SARS outbreak (Lingappa et al., 2004) and the 2009 influenza pandemic (Moghadas et al., 2009), as well as countless outbreaks of childhood infections, infectious diseases have been the bane of humanity throughout its existence causing significant morbidity, mortality, and socioeconomic upheaval. Advanced modelling technologies, which incorporate the most current knowledge of virology, immunology, epidemiology, vaccines, antiviral drugs, and public health, have recently come to the fore in identifying effective disease mitigation strategies, and are being increasingly used by public health experts in the study of both epidemiology and pathogenesis. Tracing its historical roots from the pioneering work of Daniel Bernoulli on smallpox (Bernoulli, 1760) to the classical compartmental approach of Kermack and McKendrick (Kermack & McKendrick, 1927), modelling has evolved to deal with data that is more heterogeneous, less coarse (based at a community or individual level), and more complex (joint spatial, temporal and behavioural interactions). This evolution is typified by the agent-based model (ABM) paradigm, lattice-distributed collections of autonomous decision-making entities (agents), the interactions of which unveil the dynamics and emergent properties of the infectious disease outbreak under investigation. The flexibility of ABMs permits an effective representation of the complementary interactions between individuals characterized by localized properties and populations at a global level.

However, with flexibility comes complexity; hence, the software implementation of an ABM demands more stringent software design requirements than conventional (and simpler) models of the spread and control of infectious diseases, especially with respect to outcome reproducibility, error detection and system management. Outcome reproducibility is a challenge because emergent properties are not analytically tractable, which is further exacerbated by subtle and difficult to detect errors in algorithm logic and software design. System management of software simulating populations/individuals and biological /physical interactions is a serious challenge, as the implementation will involve distributed (parallelized), non-linear, complex, and multiple processes operating in concert. Given these issues, it is clear that any implementation of an ABM must satisfy three objectives: reliability, efficiency, and adaptability. Reliability entails robustness, reproducibility, and validity of generated results with given initial conditions. Efficiency is essential for running numerous experiments (simulations) in a timely fashion. Adaptability is also a necessary requirement in order to adjust an ABM system as changes to fundamental knowledge occur. Past software engineering experience (Pizzi & Pedrycz, 2008; Pizzi, 2008) and recent literature (Grimm & Railsback, 2005; Ormerod & Rosewell, 2009; Railsback et al., 2006; Ropella et al., 2002) suggest several guidelines to which ABM development should adhere. These include:

i. *Spiral methodology.* ABM software systems require rapid development, with continual changes to user requirements and incremental improvements to a series of testable prototypes. This demands a spiral methodology for software development, beginning with an initial prototype and ending with a mature ABM software release, via an incremental and iterative succession of refined requirements, design, implementation, and validation phases.

ii. *Activity streams.* Three parallel and complementary activity streams (conceptual, algorithmic, and integration) will be required during the entire software development life cycle. High-level analytical ABM concepts drive the creation of functionally relevant algorithms, which are implemented and tested, and, if validated, integrated into the existing code base. Normally considered a top-down approach, in a spiral methodology, bottom-up considerations are also relevant. For instance, the choice from a set of competing conceptual representations for an ABM model may be made based on an analysis of the underlying algorithms or the performance of the respective implementations.

iii. *Version control.* With a spiral development methodology, an industry standard version control strategy must be in place to carefully audit changes made to the software (including changes in relation to rationales, architects, and dates).

iv. *Code review.* As code is integrated into the ABM system, critical software reviews should be conducted on a regular basis to ensure that the software implementation correctly captures the functionality and intent of the over-arching ABM.

v. *Validation.* A strategy must be established to routinely and frequently test the software system for logic and design errors. For instance, the behaviour of the simulation model could be verified by comparing its output with known analytical results for large-scale networks. Software validation must be relevant and pervasive across guidelines (i)–(iv).

vi. *Standardized software development tools.* Mathematical programming environments such as Matlab® (Sigmon & Davis, 2010), Mathematica® (Wolfram, 1999), and Maple® (Geddes et al., 2008) are excellent development tools for rapidly building ABM prototypes. However, performance issues arise as prototypes grow in size and complexity to become software systems. A development framework needs to provide a convenient bridge from these prototyping tools to mature efficient ABM systems.

vii. *System determinism.* In a parallel or distributed environment, outcome reproducibility is difficult to achieve with systems comprising stochastic components. Nevertheless, system determinism is a requirement even if executed on a different computer cluster.

viii. *System profiling.* It is important to observe and assess the performance of parts of the system as it is running. For instance, which components are executed often; what are their execution times; are processing loads balanced across nodes in a computer cluster?

In order to adhere to these guidelines and satisfy the objectives described above, we designed a software development framework for ABMs of infectious diseases. The next section of this chapter describes Scopira, a general application development library designed by our research group to be a highly extensible application programming interface with a wholly embedded transport layer that is fully scalable from single machines to site-wide distributed clusters. This library was used to implement the agent-based modelling framework, details of which are provided in the subsequent section. We conclude with a section describing future research activities.

2. Scopira

In the broad domain of biomedical data analysis applications, preliminary prototype software solutions are usually developed using an interpreted programming language or environment (e.g., Matlab®). When performance becomes an issue, some components of the prototype are subsequently ported to a compiled language (e.g., C) and integrated into the remaining interpreted components. Unfortunately, this process can introduce logic and design errors and the functionality of resultant hybrid system can often be difficult to extend or adapt. Further, it also becomes difficult to take advantage of features such as memory management, object orientation, and generics, which are all essential requirements for building large scale, robust applications. To address these concerns, we developed Scopira (Demko & Pizzi, 2009), an open source C++ framework suitable for biomedical data analysis applications such as ABMs for infectious diseases. Scopira provides high performance end-to-end application development features, in the form of an extensible C++ library. This library provides general programming utilities, numerical matrices and algorithms, parallelization facilities, and graphical user interface elements.

Our motivation behind the design of Scopira was to satisfy the needs of three categories of users within the biomedical research community: software architects; scientists /mathematicians; and data analysts. With the design and implementation of new software, architects typically need to incorporate legacy systems often written in interpreted languages. Coupled with the facts that end-user requirements in a research environment often change (sometimes radically) and that biomedical data is becoming ever more complex and voluminous, a software development framework must be versatile, extensible, and exploit distributed, generic, and object oriented programming paradigms. For scientists or mathematicians, data analysis tools must be intuitive with responsive interfaces that operate both effectively and efficiently. Finally, the data analyst has requirements straddling those from the other user categories. With an intermediate level of programming competence, they require a relatively intuitive development environment that can hide some of the low level programming details, while at the same time allowing them to easily set up and conduct numerical experiments that involve parameter tuning and high-level looping/decision constructs. As a result of this motivation, the emphasis with Scopira has been on high performance, open source development and the ability to easily integrate other C/C++ libraries used in the biomedical data analysis field by providing a common object-oriented application programming interface (API) for applications. This library provides a large breadth of services that fall into the following four component categories.

Scopira Tools provide extensive programming utilities and idioms useful to all application types. This category contains a reference counted memory management system, flexible/redirectable flow input/output system, which supports files, file memory mapping, network communication, object serialization and persistence, universally unique identifiers (UUIDs) and XML parsing and processing.

The *Numerical Functions* all build upon the core n-dimensional *narray* concept (see below). C++ generic programming is used to build custom, high-performance arrays of any data type and dimension. General mathematical functions build upon the *narray*. A large suite of biomedical data analysis and pattern recognition functions is also available to the developer.

Multiple APIs for *Parallel Processing* are provided with the object-oriented framework, *Scopira Agents Library* (SAL)‡, which allows algorithms to scale with available processor and cluster resources. Scopira provides easy integration with native operating system threads as well as the Message Passing Interface (MPI) (Snir & Gropp, 1998) and Parallel Virtual Machine (PVM) (Geist et al., 1994) libraries. Further, this library may be embedded into desktop applications allowing them to use computational clusters automatically, when detected. Unlike other parallel programming interfaces such as MPI and PVM, Scopira's facilities provide an object-oriented strategy with support for common parallel programming patterns and approaches.

Finally, a *Graphical User Interface* (GUI) *Library* based on GTK+ (Krause, 2007) is provided. This library provides a collection of useful widgets including a scalable numeric matrix editor, plotters, image and viewers as well as a plug-in platform and a 3D canvas based on OpenGL® (Hill & Kelley, 2006). Scopira also provides integration classes with the popular Qt GUI Library (Summerfield, 2010).

2.1 Programming utilities

Intrusive reference counting (recording an object's reference count within the object itself) provides the basis for memory management within Scopira-based applications. Unlike many referencing counting systems (such as those in VTK (Kitware, 2010) and GTK+), Scopira's system uses a decisively symmetric concept. References are only added through the *add_ref* and *sub_ref* calls – specifically, the object itself is created with a reference count of zero. This greatly simplifies the implementation of smart pointers and easily allows stack allocated use (by passing the reference count), unlike VTK and GTK+ where objects are created with a reference count and a modified reference count, respectively. Scopira implements a template class *count_ptr* that emulates standard pointer semantics while providing implicit reference counting on any target object. With smart pointers, reference management becomes considerably easier and safe, a significant improvement over C's manual memory management.

Scopira provides a flexible, polymorphic and layered input/output system. Flow objects may be linked dynamically to form I/O streams. Scopira includes *end flow* objects, which terminate or initiate a data flow for standard files, network sockets and memory buffers. *Transform flow* objects perform data translation from one form to another (e.g., binary-to-hex), buffer consolidation and ASCII encoding. *Serialization flow* objects provide an interface for objects to encode their data into a persistent stream. Through this interface, large complex objects can quickly and easily encode themselves to disk or over a network. Upon reconstruction, the serialization system re-instantiates objects from type information stored in the stream. Shared objects – objects that have multiple references – are serialized just once and properly linked to multiple references.

‡ The term "agent" used in this context refers to the software concept rather than the modelling concept. To avoid confusion, we will use the term "SAL node" to refer to the software concept.

A platform independent configuration system is supplied via a central parsing class, which accepts input from a variety of sources (e.g., configuration files and command line parameters) and present them to the programmer in one consistent interface. The programmer may also store settings and other options via this interface, as well as build GUIs to aid in their manipulation by the end user. Using a combination of the serialization type registration system and C++'s native RTTI functions, Scopira is able to dynamically (at runtime) allow for the registration and inspection of object types and their class hierarchy relationships. From this, an application plug-in system can be built by allowing external dynamic link libraries to register their own types as being compatible with an application, providing a platform for third party application extensions.

2.2 N-dimensional data arrays

The C and C++ languages provide the most basic support for one-dimensional arrays, which are closely related to C's pointers. Although usable for numerical computing, they do not provide the additional functionality that scientists and mathematicians demand such as easy memory management, mathematical operations, or fundamental features such as storing their own dimensions. Multiple dimensional arrays are even less used in C as they require compile-time dimension specifications, drastically limiting their flexibility. The C++ language, rather than design a new numeric array type, provides all the necessary language features for developing such an array in a library. Generic programming (via C++ templates, that allow code to be used for any data types at compile time), operator overloading (e.g., being able to redefine the addition "+" or assignment "=" operators) and inlining (for performance) provide all the tools necessary to build a high performance, usable array class. Rather than force the developer to add another dependent library for an array class, Scopira provides n-dimensional arrays through its *narray* class. This class takes a straightforward approach, implementing n-dimensional arrays, as any C programmer would have, but providing a type safe, templated interface to reduce programming errors and code complexity. The internals are easy to understand, and the class works well with standard C++ library iterators as well as C arrays, minimizing lock-in and maximizing code integration opportunities. Using basic C++ template programming, we can see the core implementation ideas in the following code snippet:

```
template <class T, int DIM> class narray {
T* dm_ary;                    // actual array elements
nindex<DIM> dm_size;          // the size of each of the dimensions

T get(nindex<DIM> c) const {
                assert(c<dm_size);
                return dm_ary[dm_size.offset(c)];
        }
}
```

From this code snippet we can see that an *narray* is a template class with two compile time parameters: *T*, the element data type (*int*, *float*, etc.) and *DIM*, the number of dimensions. The actual elements are stored in a dynamically allocated C array, *dm_ary*. The dimension lengths are stored in an *nindex* type, a generic class at is used to store array offsets. A generalized accessor is provided, which uses the *nindex*-offset method to convert the dimension specific index and size of the array into an offset into the C array. This generalization works for any dimension size.

Another feature shown here is the use of C's *assert* macro to check the validity of the supplied index. This boundary check verifies that the index is indeed valid otherwise failing and terminating the program while alerting the user. This check greatly helps the programmer during the development and testing stages of the application, and during a high performance/optimized build of the application, these macros are transparently removed, obviating any performance penalties from the final, deployed code. More user-friendly accessors (such as those taking an x value or an x-y value directly) are also provided. Finally, C++'s operator overloading facilities are used to override the bracket "[]" and parenthesis "()" operators to give the arrays a more succinct feel, over explicit *get* and *set* method calls.
The *nslice* template class is a virtual n-dimensional array that is a *reference* to an *narray*. The class only contains dimension specification information and is copyable and passable as function parameters. Element access translates directly to element accesses in the host *narray*. An *nslice* must always be of the same numerical type as its host *narray*, but can have any dimensionality less than or equal to the host. This provides significant flexibility; one could have a one-dimensional vector slice from a matrix, cube or five-dimensional array, for example. Matrix slices from volumes are quite common (see Figure 1). These sub slices can also span any of the dimensions/axes, something not possible with simple pointer arrays (e.g., matrix slices from a cube array need not follow the natural memory layout order of the array structure).

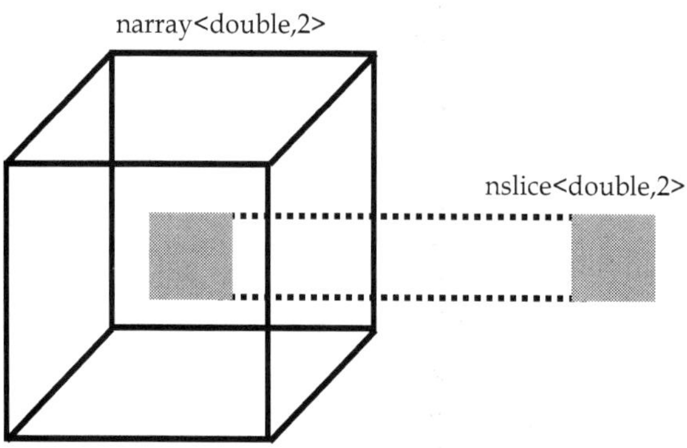

Fig. 1. An *nslice* reference into an *narray* data item.

The *narray* class provides hooks for alternate memory allocation systems. One such system is the *DirectIO* mapping system. Using the memory mapping facilities of the operating system (typically via the *mmap* function on POSIX systems), a disk file may be *mapped* into memory. When this memory space is accessed, the pages of the files are loaded into memory transparently. Writes to the memory region will result in writes to the file. This allows files to be loaded in portions and on demand. The operating system will take care of loading/unloading the portions as needed. Files larger than the system's memory size can also be loaded (the operating system will keep only the working set portion of the array in memory). The programmer must be aware of this and take care to keep the working set within the memory size of the machine. If the working set exceeds the available memory size, performance will suffer greatly as the operating system pages portions to and from disk (this excessive juggling of disk-memory mapping is called "page thrashing").

2.3 Parallel processing

With the increasing number of processors in both the user's desktops and in cluster server rooms, computationally intensive applications and algorithms should be designed in a parallel fashion if they are to be relevant in a future that depends on multiple-core and cluster computing as a means of scaling processing performance. To take advantage of the various processors within a single system or shared address space (SAS), developers need only utilize the operating system's thread API or shared memory services. However, for applications that would also like to utilize the cluster resources to achieve greater scalability, explicit message passing is used. Although applying a SAS model to cluster computing is feasible, to achieve the best computational performance and scalability results, a message passing model is preferred (Shan et al., 2003; Dongarra & Dunigan, 1997). Scopira includes support for two well established message passing interfaces, MPI and PVM, as well as a custom, embedded, object-oriented message passing interface designed for ease of use and deployment.

SAL is a parallel execution framework extension with several notable goals particularly useful to Scopira based applications. The API, which is completely object-oriented, includes functionality for: using the flow system for messaging; task movement; GUI application integration; multi-platform communication support; and, the registration system for task instantiation. SAL introduces high-performance computing to a wider audience of end users by permitting software developers to build standard cluster capabilities into desktop applications, allowing those applications to pool their own as well as cluster resources. This is in contrast to the goals of MPI (providing a dedicated and fast communications API standard for computer clusters) and PVM (providing a virtual machine architecture among a variety of powerful computer platforms).

By design, SAL borrowed a variety of concepts from both MPI and PVM. SAL, like PVM, attempts to a build a unified and scalable "task" management system with an emphasis on dynamic resource management and interoperability. Users develop intercommunicating task objects. Tasks can be thought of as single processes or processing instances, except that they are implemented as language objects and not operating system processes. A SAL node manages one or more tasks, and teams of nodes communicate with each other to form computational networks (see Figure 2). The tasks are coupled with a powerful message passing API inspired by MPI. Unlike PVM, SAL also focuses on ease-of-use: emphasizing automatic configuration detection and de-emphasizing the need for infrastructure processes. When no cluster or network computation resources are available, SAL uses operating system threads to enable multi-programming within a single operating system process and thereby embedding a complete message passing implementation within the application (greatly reducing deployment complexity). Applications always have an implementation of SAL available, regardless of the availability or access to cluster resources. Developers may always use the message passing interface, and their application will work with no configuration changes from both single machine desktop installations to complete parallel compute cluster deployments.

The mechanics and implementation of the SAL nodes and their load balancing system are built into the SAL library, and thereby, Scopira applications. Users do not need to install additional software, nor do they need to explicitly configure or set-up a parallel environment. This is paramount in making cluster and distributed computing accessible to the non-technical user, as it makes it a transparent feature in their graphical applications.

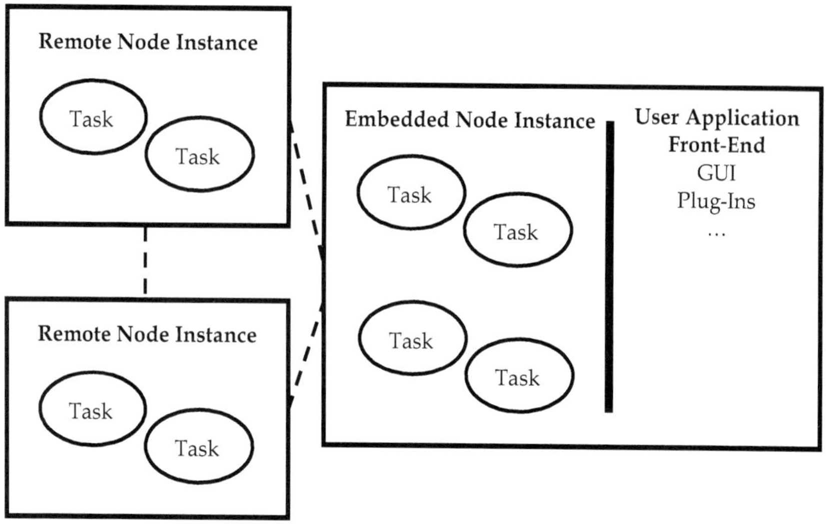

Fig. 2. SAL topology of tasks and nodes.

SAL provides an object-oriented, packet based and routable (like PVM, but unlike MPI) API for message passing. This API provides everything needed to build multi-threaded, cluster-aware algorithms embeddable in applications. Tasks are the core objects that developers build for the SAL system. A task represents a single job or instance in the SAL node system, which is analogous to a process in an operating system. However, they are almost never separate processes, but rather grouped into one or more SAL node processes that are embedded into the host application. This is unlike most existing parallel APIs, that allocate one operating system process per task concept, that, although conceptually simpler for the programmer, incurs more communication and start up overhead, as well as making task management more complex and operating system dependent. The tasks themselves are language-level objects but are usually assigned their own operating system threads to achieve pre-emptive concurrency.

A context object is a task's gateway into the SAL message passing system. There may be many tasks within one process, so each will have differing context interfaces - something not feasible with an API with a single, one-task-per-process model (as used in PVM or MPI). This class provides several facilities, including: task creation and monitoring; sending, checking and receiving messages; service registration; and group management. It is the core interface a developer must use to build parallel applications with SAL.

Developers often launch a group of instances of the same task time, and then systematically partition the problem space for parallel processing. To support this popular paradigm of development, SAL's identification system supports the concept of *groups*. A group is simply a collection of N task instances, where each instance has a *groupid*=$\{0,\ldots,N-1\}$. The group concept is analogous to MPI's communicators (but without support for complex topology) and PVM's named groups. This sequential numbering of task instances allows the developer to easily map problem work units to tasks. Similar to how PVM's group facility supplements the task identifier concept, SAL groups build upon the UUID system, as each task still functionally retains their underlying UUID for identification.

The messaging system within SAL is built upon both the generic Scopira input/output layer as well as the UUID identification system. SAL employs a packet-based (similar to PVM) message system, where the system only sends and routes complete messages, and not the individual data primitives (as MPI can and routinely does) and objects within them. Only after the sending task completes and commits a message is it processed by the routing and delivery sub-systems. A node uses operating system threads to transport the data, freeing the user's thread to continue to work.

Sending (committing) the data during the *send_msg* object's destruction (that is, via its destructor) was the result of an intentional software design decision. In C++, stack objects are destroyed as they exit scope. The user should therefore place a *send_msg* object in its own set of scope-braces, which would constitute a sort of "send block". All data transmissions for the message would be done within that send block, and the software programmer can then be assured that the message will be sent at the end of the scope block without having to remember to do a manual send commit operation. Similarly, the receiver uses a *recv_msg* object to receive, decode and parse a message packet, all within a braced "receive block." The following code listing provides an example of a task object that, via its context interface (the interface to the message network), is sending a variety data objects using the object-oriented messaging API.

```
// declare my task object and its run method
class mytask : public agent_task_i
        { public: virtual void int run(task_context &ctx); };
int mytask::run(task_context &ctx) {
        // send some data to the master task
        narray<double,2> a_matrix;
        {                           // this scope (or send) block encapsulates the sent message
        send_msg msg(ctx, 0);       // prepare the message to task #0

        msg.write_int(10);// send one integer
        msg.save(a_matrix);         // send a matrix – type safe
        msg.save(user_object);      // send a user object – via serialization

        // at this point, msg's destructor will be called (automatically)
        // triggering the sending of the message
        }
}
```

SAL currently has two types of scheduling engines, a "local" engine that uses operating system threads on a single host machine and a "network" implementation that is able to utilize a network of workstations. The "local" engine is a basic multi-threaded implementation of the SAL API. It uses the operating system's threads to implement multiprocessing within the host application process. As this engine is contained within a single-process, it is the fastest and easiest to use for application development and debugging. The programmer may fully design and test their parallel algorithm and its messaging logic before moving to a multi-node deployment. The local engine is always available and requires no configuration from the user. Developers need not write a dedicated non-message passing versions of their algorithms simply to satisfy users that may not go to the trouble of deploying a Cluster. As the local engine provides as many worker threads as active tasks, it relies on the operating system's ability to manage threads within the processors. This works quite well when the number of tasks instantiated into the system is a function of the number of physical processors, as encouraged by the API.

The network engine implements the SAL API over a collection of machines connected by an IP-based network; typically Ethernet. The cluster can be a dedicated computer cluster and/or a collection of user workstations. The engine itself provides inter-node routing and management, leaving the local scheduling decisions within each node up to a local-engine derived manager. A SAL network stack has two layers (see Figure 3). The lower transport layer contains the SAL nodes themselves (objects that manage all the tasks and administration on a single process) and their TCP/IP based links. Tasks can send messages to each other using their UUIDs, ignorant of the IP layer or the connection topology of the nodes themselves. For simplicity and efficiency, a SAL network (like PVM) has a master node residing on one process. This master node is responsible for the allocation, tracking and migration of all the tasks in the system. The network engine uses a combination of URL-like direct addressing and UDP/IP broadcast based auto-discovery in building the node network. The simplest and most popular sequence is to start an application in auto discovery mode. When a network engine starts, it searches the local network for any other node peers and, if found, joins their network. If no peers are found, then it starts a network consisting of itself as the only member and assumes the master node role. Users may also key in the master's URL directly, connecting them explicitly to a particular network. In addition to its critical routing functions, the master node is also responsible for all the task tracking and management within the network. By centralizing this information, load and resource allocation decisions can be made instantly and decisively. The master node handles all task instantiation requests. When a task within node requests the creation of more tasks, the request is routed by the hosting node to the master node. The nodes then create the actual tasks report back to the master, which in turn reports back to the initial node and task.

2.4 Graphical user interface library

This subsystem provides a basic graphical API wrapped around GTK+ and consists of widget and window classes that become the foundation for all GUI widgets in Scopira. More specialized and complex widgets, particularly useful to numerical computing and visualization, are also provided. This includes widgets useful for the display of matrices, 2D images, bar plots and line plots. Developers can use the basic GUI components provided to create more complex viewers for a particular application domain.

The Scopira graphical user interface subsystem provides useful user-interface tools (widgets) for the construction of graphical, scientific applications. These widgets complement the generic widgets provided by the GTK+ widget library with additional widgets for the visualization and inspection of numeric array data.

A matrix/spreadsheet like widget is able to view and edit data arrays (often, but not limited to matrices) of any size. This extensible widget is able to operate on Scopira *narrays* natively. The widget supports advances functionality such as bulk editing via an easy to use, stack based macro-language. This macro-language supports a variety of operations of setting, copying and filter selecting data within the array. A generic plotting widget allows the values of Scopira *narrays* to be plotted. The plotter supports a variety of plotting styles and criteria, and the user-interface allows for zooming, panning and other user customizations of the data plot. An image viewer allows fully zooming, panning and scaling of *narrays*, useful for the display of image data. The viewer supports arbitrary colour mapping, includes a legend display and supports a tiled view for displaying a collection of many images simultaneously. A simplified drawing canvas interface is included that permits software developers to quickly and easily build their own custom widgets. Finally, Scopira provides a *Lab* facility to rapidly prototype and implement algorithms that need casual graphical output. Users implement their algorithms as per usual, and a background thread handles the updating of the graphical subsystem and event loop.

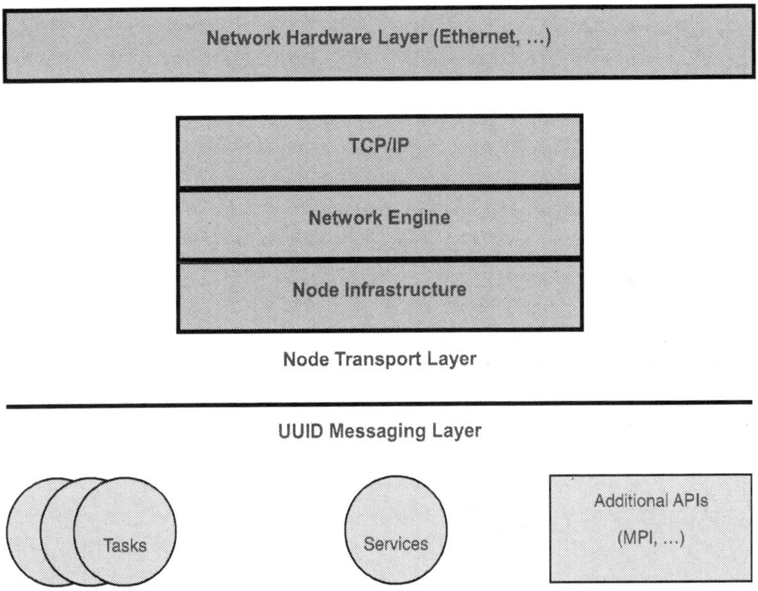

Fig. 3. The SAL network stack.

Scopira provides an architecture for logically separating models (data types) and views (graphical widgets that present or operate on that data) in the application. This view-model relationship is then registered at runtime. At runtime, Scopira pairs the compatible models and views for presentation to the user. A collection of utility classes for the easy registration of typical objects types such as data models and views are provided. This registration mechanism succeeds regardless of how the code was loaded; be it as part of the application, as a linked code library, or as an external plug-in.

Third parties can easily extend a Scopira application that utilizes models and views extensively. Third party developers need only register new views on the existing data models in an application, then load their plug-in alongside the application to immediately add new functionality to the application. The open source C++ image processing and registration library ITK (Ibáñez & Schroeder, 2005) has been successfully integrated into Scopira applications at run time using the registration subsystem.

A *model* is defined as an object that contains data and is able to be *monitored* by zero or more *views*. A *view* is an object that is able to bind to and listen to a model. Typically, views are graphical in nature, but in Scopira non-graphical views are also possible. A *project* is a specialized model that may contain a collection of models and organize them in a hierarchical fashion. Full graphical Scopira applications are typically project-oriented, allowing the user to easily work with many data models in a collective manner. A basic project-based application framework is provided for developers to quickly build GUI applications using *models* and *views*.

A complementary subsystem provides the base OpenGL-enabled widget class that utilizes the GTKGLExt library (Logan, 2001). The GTKGLExt library enables GTK+ based applications to utilize OpenGL for 2D and 3D visualization. Scopira developers can use this system to build 3D visualization views and widgets, which allows for greater data exploration and processing. Integration with more complete visualization packages such as VTK (Schroeder et al., 2006) is also possible.

3. Agent based modelling framework

3.1 Agent based models

ABM simulations consists of emulating real-world systems in which collections of autonomous decision-making entities, distributed in a grid or lattice, interact with each other unveiling the dynamics of the system under investigation (Bonabeau, 2002; Sokolowski & Banks, 2010). This kind of simulation has emerged from the need to analyse and model systems that are becoming more complex in terms of their interdependencies, at the same time that data are becoming more organized into databases at finer levels of granularity. This type of modelling and simulation originated in the field of multi-agent systems, which derived from research in distributed artificial intelligence. The idea behind distributed artificial intelligence is to solve problems (or a related set of sub-problems) by distributing them amongst a number of relatively simple programs or agents, each with its own particular type of knowledge or expertise (Gilbert & Terna, 2000; Epstein, 2007). Additionally, ABM research draws from several related fields including computer science, management science, social science, system dynamics, complexity theory, complex networks, and traditional modelling and simulation (Macal & North, 2005; Shoham & Leyton-Brown, 2008).

The first step in defining an ABM is to establish the meaning of the term "agent". Although there is not one universally accepted definition, a good characterization may be given as:

"An agent is an encapsulated computer system that is situated in some environment and that is capable of flexible, autonomous action in that environment in order to meet its design objectives." (Wooldridge, 1997). The most fundamental feature of an agent is the capability of making independent decisions and relating itself with other agents and their environment. From a practical modelling standpoint, an agent is a discrete individual, identifiable and located; goal-directed and autonomous; lives in an environment; has a set of intrinsic characteristics (properties), decision-making capabilities, a system of rules that govern its behaviour, and the ability to learn and adapt based on experience (which requires some kind of internal memory); can interact with other agents, and respond to the environment.

Depending on the subject under investigation, there may be different types of agents, for example trees, bugs, humans, viruses, bacteria, or cells. Even sub-types are possible, like tissue cells, immunological system cells, stem cells, or nerve cells. Considering the vast gamut of possible agents and situations, a system may be composed of more than one type of agent at the same time. For instance, assuming an infectious disease in a population of susceptible individuals, the variability of the species may be included considering that each agent may present different levels of susceptibility to the specific disease caused by differences in their immune system, lifestyle, prior health conditions, specific health risk factors, and so on.

The uniqueness of every agent is established by its state variables, or attributes, such as an identity number (desirably unique and immutable so that the agent can be traced during all the pertinent simulations), age, gender, location, size, weight, energy reserves, political opinion, disease stage, etc. These attributes distinguish an entity from others of the same kind, trace how the agent changes over time and guide its behaviour. In addition, these state variables may be saved allowing re-starting the simulation once interrupted. It is from the heterogeneity of agents, and consequent variety of behaviours, that the collective aspects of interest concerning the real-world system being modelled and simulated emerge.

From the uniqueness and autonomous nature of the agents, it becomes quite clear that adopting an agent-based approach demands multiple agents in order to represent the decentralized perspective of the problem. Moreover, the agents must interact with one another and with the environment. For this purpose, the agents must be spatially located in some type of grid or lattice in which they can come into contact with other agents based on defined rules and assumptions.

The agent lattice awareness is limited and localized. Agents are always placed in some position of the grid and have limited visibility of their surroundings, implying that only a few other agents are in the agent's domain of influence. This is in contrast with a typical two-dimensional cellular automata, in which every position of the grid consists of a cell; each cell can assume different states that may be updated according to some rules based only on its immediate neighbours. In an ABM, there can be more than one agent per location of the lattice at the same time. The agents are not static, ensuring that they are free to move so their radius of interaction in the long term is not restricted to their nearest agent neighbours.

In contrast to many analytical models, which are in general easier to communicate and analyse since they are described using precise mathematical formulas, ABM descriptions are frequently incomplete and therefore less accessible to the reader. In an attempt to tackle this pertinency problem, a group of modellers in the field of ecology (Grimm et al., 2006) proposed a standard protocol for describing ABMs. The "Overview, Design Concept and Details" protocol, or simply ODD, proposes that an ABM (and its various interaction rules) be described in a standardized way making model descriptions easier to understand and complete. Achieving this objective makes ABMs reproducible and a much more reliable scientific tool for investigations.

3.2 Designing an agent based model

Before modelling a problem using an agent-based approach, a few points must be considered. First, one must consider the nature of the problems that can benefit from this method and how the simulations can provide useful information about the scenarios being investigated. An ABM can provide a realistic and flexible description of a system, and it can capture emergent phenomena (Bonabeau, 2002; Shoham & Leyton-Brown, 2008). An "emergent phenomenon" can be conceptualized as a large scale, group behaviour of a system, which does not seem to have any clear explanation in terms of the systems constituent parts (Darley, 1994; Sokolowski & Banks, 2010). These phenomena may arise due to the nonlinear nature of the behaviour of the agents, which can be described by discontinuities in agent behaviour that is difficult to capture with differential equations. In addition, agent exhibits memory (non-markovian process), path-dependence, learning and adaptation. Being so, ABMs are adequate for describing real world phenomena where agent behaviour is complex (Ferguson, 2007). Upon concluding that an ABM is appropriate for a specific case, the chart in Figure 4 offers some guidelines for the development of an ABM.

Modelling agent-based simulations requires the creation of a representation of the "sub-world" under investigation. For this representation to be realistic and accurate, there should be a set of available **data** to support the various considerations adopted for the several aspects and parts included in the agent-based model. As we go through the design process of an ABM for the spread of an infectious disease in an urban centre, we are going to illustrate what data can be used in each step.

Considering the spread of an infectious disease in a population, data regarding the age-gender structure of the population can be obtained and used to create the *in silico* population. However, the lack of detailed information regarding the actual event (e.g., estimates of epidemiological parameters for an emerging infectious disease) often poses significant challenges for modelling agent-based simulations. On the other hand, experimenting with the model under various assumptions (for instance, different intervention strategies) may reveal emergent phenomena that lead to a better understanding of the system and its behaviour. It is this circular dependency relationship that makes ABMs powerful and challenging at the same time.

Although this modelling framework was built to be generic for major types of ABMs, it is possible that some aspects of very specific cases have not been included. Nevertheless, with this framework, the reader should have a starting point for designing an ABM and performing simulations by adding specific characteristics of the system. As with any software development project, the main point to be defined is the **purpose** of the application. In our example, the purpose of the model is to understand what are the key characteristics of a population, with its social interaction patterns, that influences the spread of an infectious disease and leads to epidemic scenarios. In this stage, the appropriate **disease model** for the specific disease must be chosen. Unless the disease under investigation is completely new and uncharted, it is possible to choose whether a simple susceptible-infectious-recovered (SIR) model suffices or if a more refined one, including other intermediate states, is required. It is important to note that the assumptions based on **global community parameters** influence some of the **local individual parameters**. In this example, choosing an SIR model implies that, in terms of the disease, the agents can be in only one of the three (susceptible, infective, or recovered) states. From the perspective of the local individual parameters, aspects such as pregnancy, aspirin treatment, and so on, can be taken into account.

This description gives the general idea of what is going to be simulated. At this point it is important to know the exact questions the model is aimed to answer. This way it will be clearer what data resulting from the simulation should be stored for analysis. Once the purpose is established, we will have a clear idea of what the agents in our simulation are going to be. In general, simulations will involve different kinds of agents. In a typical spread of some virus in a population, as with the 2009 H1N1 influenza pandemic, there is only one type of agent involved, namely humans. These agents are either affected by the disease or not. When infected, they can transmit the disease to a susceptible agent if they come to a close contact range (the definition of close contact is all interactions that can result in infection). In this case, there is no need to have more than one agent since the infectious disease may be considered as a property of the agent. Conversely, if the interest is to investigate the pattern of transmission of a disease from pigs to humans, then two types of agents may be involved (pigs and humans). In more specific scenarios, the interest may be in the virus population itself. In this case, there can be sub-types of agents, i.e. virus strains, which are all sub-types of a broader class of a specific virus.

Regardless of the type of agents, they will have features (state variables) that define them as individuals. For all agents, the modeller will need to list all the state variables including not only those that define their characteristics (like age, weight, and temperature), but also those that describe the agent's behavioural traits, such as velocities, strategies, probabilities, susceptibility, etc. In addition, it is important to define how the agents interact with the environment within specified time periods. Demographic data is used to create the agents so that the resulting *in silico* population follows the same distributions as the real population. In this sense, the state variables are defined as the primitive characteristics of the individuals that can be later described in terms of demographic information, such as age and gender profiles. Additionally, several other, non-demographic specific, variables must be defined. Some of these variables relate to the disease, such as symptoms duration, susceptibility, etc. Other kinds of variables relate to behavioural traits. Based on these variables and relevant information acquired from the environment and other agents, an agent can have its state altered and make decisions regarding its next steps. In short, the state variables are the most important part of the model, given that they define the agents and provide the relevant information for them to act in an autonomous fashion.

Once agents are defined, the next step is to determine where they are placed, thus defining their **environment**. If the relationship between the agent and the environment is not important for simulation purposes, the environment should be only a place that facilitates the interactions between agents. In some cases, this relationship may be important, as in the case when the demographic distribution may play an important role in the spread of an infectious disease. Once the environment is defined, its scales must be determined to establish its dimension and the size of each dimension. Additionally, the representation of the environment is not restricted to an n-dimensional space but rather defined as a complex network or some other data structure, and may contain other properties that influence the agents' decisions and behaviour. In epidemic scenarios, urban centre characteristics such as commuting distance, demographic density, and city boundaries, may affect the spread of the infectious disease, as well as agent behaviour. Being so, data regarding mobility patterns can be used to define lattice properties, which in turn can be used by the agents in its decisions and actions.

The planning of the agents and environment is not complete until the **processes** associated with them are defined, which leads us to the next block in the flowchart in Figure 4. The set of processes are the kernel of the simulation. At this stage, it should be pointed out that all actions that each agent takes are in terms of updating its state, interacting with other agents, and interacting with the environment. Likewise, all the mechanisms for updating the environment should be listed.

In terms of updating the state of an agent, several steps may be considered, such as deciding if the agent's objective has been achieved, or identifying the best course of action for achieving the objective. As an example, considering the case of an infectious disease, it must be verified if the agent is infected and, if so, to decide if it is time to seek medical care. Performing agent-to-agent (or agent-to-environment) interactions requires communication between the agents (or with the environment), so that the entities involved can access each other's information and choose their next action. In the case of a susceptible agent interacting with an infective agent, it must be determined whether the susceptible individual will become infected.

Once all the associated processes are defined, a natural question that arises is the timing at which these actions take place. This issue is represented by the **scheduling** box in Figure 4. Here, a flowchart of the processes will be useful for determining the order that the processes are performed. Several processes may occur concurrently, while others may depend on other processes. Knowing the overall picture of the events, it is possible to identify if the state variables are updated synchronously or asynchronously. Moreover, the type of time-scheme should be determined in terms of being discrete, continuous, or both.

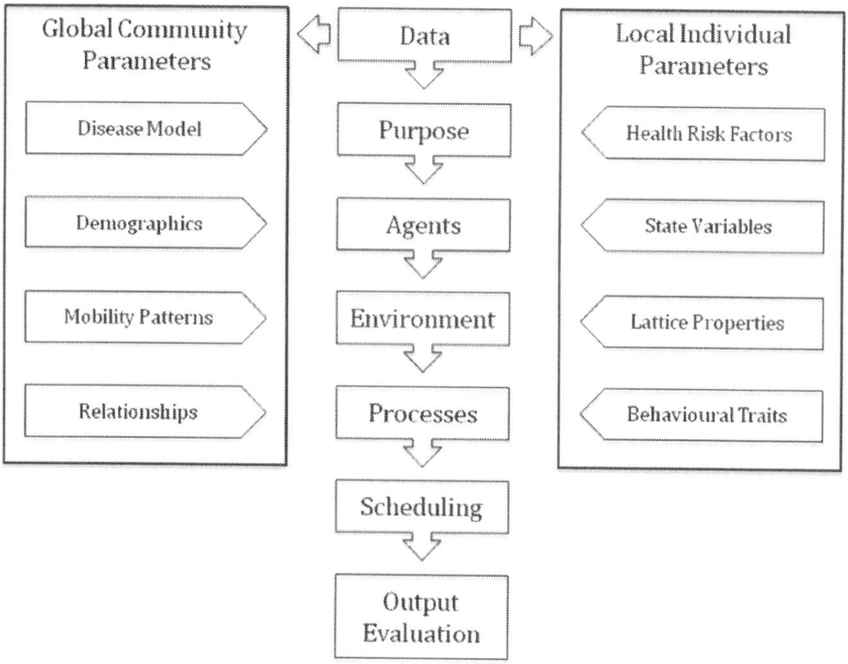

Fig. 4. Development cycle for an agent-based infectious disease model.

In the context of parallel computing, the relationship among processes will determine the ease with which to parallelize the code (for example, tightly coupled or spatially proximal relationships are more difficult to parallelize compared to loosely coupled or spatially distant relationships). ABMs may start with small and simple simulations. However, as the ABM evolves over time, it can become large and computationally complex, thus requiring the parallelization of the execution of the code. In this way, structuring the model before coding, and choosing the right tools for the task, will certainly save time in the end.

3.3 Building an agent-based simulation

In this section, we describe an ABM software framework for simulating the spread of a contagious disease in human populations. The agents in this model are a simplified representation of the real inhabitants of an urban centre in which an infectious pathogen was introduced. In this system, the three main components of simulations are: the agents, the lattice (or grid) in which these agents are placed, and the rules of between-agent and agents-environment interactions. Considering that ABM simulations rely on the interactions between agents that are similar in characteristics but have different behaviours, it is natural to choose any object oriented programming (OOP) language to run such simulations. Using OOP, each agent may be created as a representation of a common class of agents in which every software object has the same set of properties, or state variables. Assuming a different set of values for the properties of each agent, the uniqueness of each agent is established, and the variability of the species is taken into account (Grimm et al., 2006; Epstein, 2007).

In the context of an ABM, the unit of simulations is the agent (often referred to as an individual), and in the context of OOP, this unit is the object of a defined class. It is, however, important to note that agents and software objects are different components of the ABM. A software object is an appropriate way to represent agents in the sense that objects encapsulate both agent state (as data members) and agent behaviour (as methods), and communicate via message passing. But agents, on the other hand, are "rational decision making systems" that are able to react and behave according to the situation (Wooldridge, 1997).

Depending on the particular problem being modelled, the agents' properties of interest may vary. For an epidemic spread in a population of susceptible agents, some of the relevant characteristics of these agents include age, gender, susceptibility to the disease, state of the disease, among several other properties pertinent to the nature of disease in infectious agents. In such a scenario, investigating the dynamics and evolution of the contagious disease requires the development of a realistic model of the population with a significantly large number of agents (as given in pertinent demographic data) whose properties render the age-gender distribution of that specific location. Hence, the performance of the simulation framework becomes an important issue when choosing the proper tools for building the simulation.

As with every software engineering project, choosing the appropriate programming language and libraries to build the ABM application is crucial to produce reliable, efficient, and adaptable software code as described in Section 1. In an ABM, the use of OOP is an appropriate simplifying approach for the logic of simulations and coding processes. Furthermore, the choice of the right model data and libraries will impact the performance and resource utilization, reflecting in the last instance in the running time of the simulation. Keeping in mind these requirements, we adopted C++ as the most suitable programming language for the ABM described here. In terms of performance and versatility, the C++ language is comparable to the C language with the addition of some OOP specializations. Moreover, using the Scopira framework (see Section 2) functionalities and data structures like smart pointers, *narrays* and its distributed computing tools, simplifies the software development of ABM applications especially with respect to code parallelization.

Another important characteristic of ABMs is related to the stochasticity present in every part of the simulation. The variability among agents may arise from sampling, for example, an age-gender distribution, a susceptibility distribution, or distribution of infectious period. The state of an agent can be altered by means of interactions with other agents, where the outcome of these interactions depends on the value of parameters sampled from some prescribed distribution. As a result, the random number generators must be chosen carefully. For the generation of random numbers, a good choice of numerical library is the *GNU Scientific Library*, which has been widely adopted in scientific and engineering applications and which has the additional advantage of being open source, thread safe, well tested, and portable (Gough, 2009).

3.4 Simulation framework design

Agents are modelled as objects of a class named *Agents* in which the member variables represent the characteristics of the agents, such as age, gender, susceptibility to the disease, and state of the disease. The methods of this class are simple manipulators that change the values of these member variables. In this way, every agent represents a person with the same basic characteristics that may assume different values. Using age-gender distributions for a specific population, variability in age and gender is introduced. In an epidemic disease

scenario, an agent may assume different states regarding its epidemiological status, which may be one of the following: susceptible, exposed (but not yet infectious), infectious and recovered (immune against re-infection). Since the number of agents in a simulation may range from a few thousands to millions, it is important to save memory whenever possible. Considering that these states of infectious may assume only two values (*true* or *false*), stating whether the agent is in the specific state or not, the best way to store this information is to use one *unsigned int* as a bit set (or alternatively to use the *bitset* class from the C++ standard library), in which every bit represents one of the possible states. Furthermore, the state of the agent may be assessed by using bitwise operations testing only the specific bits of interest, saving in this way, a few processor operations per agent per cycle.
Similar to a real world scenario, agents, in general, live in a city (or community) in which they must be located somewhere and are free to move to different locations. Therefore, the city is modelled as another class, named *Lattice*, in which a 2-dimensional n-array is used to represent the city map and is a container to hold agents. The simplest way to build ABM simulations is to consider only one agent per site that interacts with its adjacent neighbours, as in a cellular automaton, or even with distant neighbours, but carrying these interactions without moving from its position. Another approach, which is used in the model presented here, is to consider several free-to-move agents at the same position. This model tries to mimic the behaviour of people in a city, where it is possible for people to interact with others in the same location, as would be the case in a house, office, or a shopping mall.
Considering that several agents may be in the same *x-y* position of the city grid at the same time, and that these agents may move through the map, every site in the lattice holds a standard vector of Scopira's smart pointers to agents, that is, the lattice is a two-dimensional n-array of standard vectors of pointers to agents as shown in the left panel in Figure 5. Based on this scheme, moving an agent from one location to another is done by assigning a pointer to the agent being moved to the vector at the destination location, and then removing the pointer to this agent from the vector at the initial position, as shown in the right panel in Figure 5.
Using this smart pointer strategy, there would be no additional overhead of moving or copying the agent's data into memory. Another advantage with smart pointers is that there is no need to manually free the memory at the end of the application, since it is refreshed as soon as the smart pointer goes out of the scope. Furthermore, it is possible to test if the software object is alive, which dramatically reduces the number of segmentation faults during the software development phase due to access attempts to memory pages that have already been released. Additionally, by using scope as a way to control the life cycle of the software objects, the resulting application is better structured, robust and extensible.

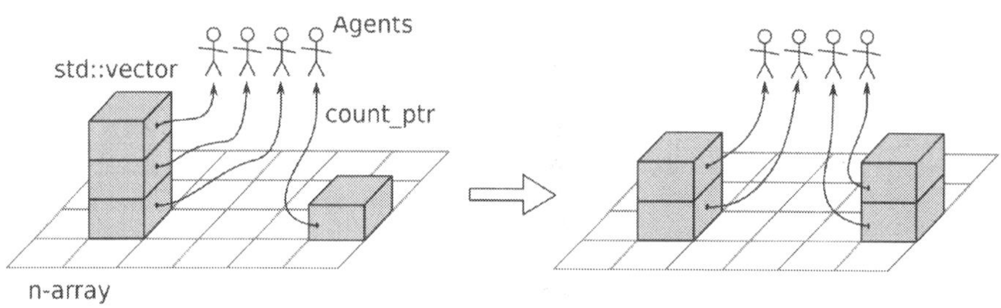

Fig. 5. Representation of agent movements in the lattice.

The methods of the *Lattice* class are used to control the access to the map locations and to the agents located in each position. Using, for example, the map of a city in which its boundaries and demographic distribution is specified, the lattice representation will define all the sites (that is, x-y positions) according to the city boundaries, and the number of agents allowed in each site according to the demographic density. In this approach, the agents are placed in the lattice but they may not be directly related. The agent-to-agent and agent-to-lattice relationships are stored in another class called *Simulation*. In this class, a smart pointer to the lattice is used, and the rules concerning the movement of the agents in the lattice and interaction between agents are considered as methods of this class. Furthermore, this class is responsible for updating counters that keep track of the number of agents in each state in the simulation, and for writing reports to files on the computer system's hard disk drive. For these two tasks, the *Counters* and *Reports* classes are generated.

Since the simulation has been built to be able to use more than one processor using threaded programming, *Counters* and *Reports* classes need to be built in order to be thread safe, thereby supporting concurrency. When working with multiple threads, it is possible that different threads will try to access the same memory area simultaneously; for example, to increment the value of the same variable at the same time; this may cause unpredictable results. One way to avoid data inconsistencies is to use mutual exclusion locks, or mutexes. Before a thread operates with a variable, it must acquire the lock on this variable in order to prevent other threads from operating on the same variable at the same time. This ensures serialization of access to the specific data area. After the thread has performed the desired operations, it needs to unlock this variable for other threads to access it. Determining what resources should be locked and unlocked, and in what order, are fundamental considerations when parallel programming. Moreover, a strategy must be adopted for interacting with these shared resources in order to minimize the number of simultaneous accesses to the same shared area. Otherwise, it will slow down the simulation considering that when a thread is waiting to acquire the lock, it stops its other operations. Although it is possible to tackle this situation in different ways, it makes the problem more complex and might introduce other unnecessary synchronization issues.

The *Counters* and *Reports* classes both perform actions on areas of common access by threads. The member variables of the *Counters* class, keep track of several aspects of the simulation, like the current time step in which the simulation is run, the total number of susceptible agents, and the number of infectious agents. Scopira provides several methods for parallel programming in SAL that simplifies this process. In the case of protecting certain data areas like variables, it defines a *shared_area* class to which is associated a mutex that can be later accessed by objects of the *lock_ptr* class. Auxiliary to the *Counters* class, it defines a data structure called *SimulationCounters* that holds all the counter variables that may be accessed by more than one thread at the same time. In the *Counters* class, an instance of the *shared_area* class associated with the *SimulationCounters* data structure is created. The methods of the *Counters* class, when manipulating these variables, call them through an object of the *lock_ptr* class associated with the object of the shared area. When the lock pointer is created, it automatically locks the shared area with which it is associated, and when it moves out of scope, it is automatically destroyed, thereby unlocking the associated shared area. Likewise, when the method is called, it creates the lock pointer and acquires the lock, then the desired operations are performed, and at the end of execution of the method, the lock pointer is destroyed automatically, hence unlocking the shared area. With this method, the programmer does not need to manually lock and unlock the variables, but rather needs to define the lock pointer inside the scope targeted for manipulation of the shared area.

Following the same idea, the *Reports* class is used to write information about the simulation into files. If two threads try to access the same file at the same time, the message may become garbled, and therefore mutexes must be used. For this purpose, Scopira provides the *fileflow* class that in turn provides methods for manipulating files and also includes mutexes. An object instance of the *Reports* class is associated with each file. It is basically responsible for opening and closing files, and overloads the stream insertion operator "<<". In this way, every time the insertion operator is called on a *Reports* object, it calls the *fileflow::write_lock()* method, passes the message to the *fileflow* object, and then unlocks it through the *fileflow::unlock()* method.
Figure 6 shows a diagram of the simulation environment with its several components. In this representation, the *Simulation* class aggregates *Lattice*, *Reports*, and *Counters* classes. These three classes are included in the *Simulation* class via smart pointers to the appropriate objects of each class. Since the *Lattice* class contains smart pointers to all the agents in the simulation that can be accessed through the *Lattice* object, the rules concerning the agent-to-agent and agent-to-lattice interactions are methods of the *Simulation* class.

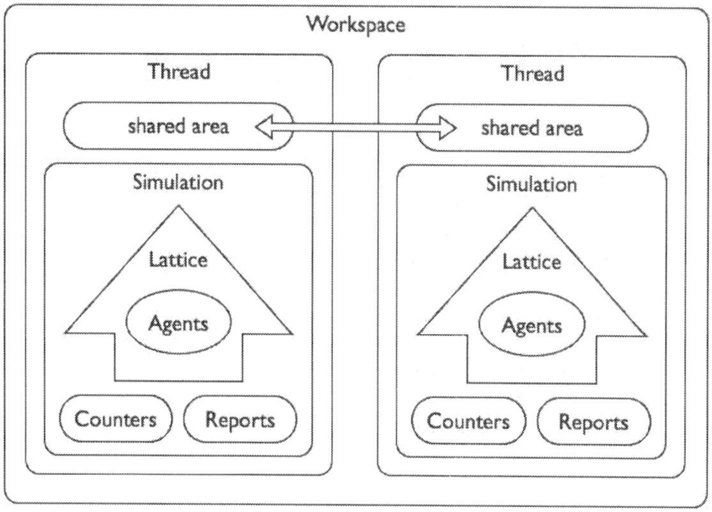

Fig. 6. Simulation environment showing the interaction of two threads.

For the agent-based simulation infrastructure proposed here, we now present the mechanisms for parallelizing the simulations. The parallelism strategy adopted in this example was to divide the lattice into chunks and assign them to different processing threads. To balance the amount of work performed by each thread, the *narray* that represents the lattice was divided into an approximately equal number of active sites, which correspond to the defined locations in the city map. Agents are allowed to move between sites in the map but the location of the destination site may be out of the scope of control for the actual processing thread. As a result, it is necessary for all threads to be equipped with a shared area to which other threads can send the moving agents (see Figure 6). The *Threads* class inherits the basic functionality of the *scopira::thread* class, which provides the mechanisms for creating the parallel environment and controlling all aspects of the threads independent of the operational system. As a result, only a few methods concerning the particular problem being investigated and a shared area for exchanging agents between threads need to be implemented in the *Threads* class. The most important method, from the simulation point of view, is the *Threads::run()* method, which is an overload of the Scopira's *thread::run()* method, where the actual simulation takes places. The pseudo-code for this method is given below.

```
Threads::run() {
        CheckSharedArea()

        foreach site:
                simulation.InteractAgentsToAgents( site )
                simulation.InteractAgentsWithLattice( site )
                simulation.MoveAgents( site )

        CheckSharedArea()
        }
```

In this case, every thread iterates over all the sites under its control, and performs the tasks required by the simulation. In a simple case, it will perform the agent-to-agent and agent-to-lattice interactions, and move the agents if necessary. The latter step of moving agents is the most critical task in terms of distributed programming, as it involves other threads and synchronization issues.

As mentioned before, an agent may move to a location out of the scope of control for its current assigned thread. For this reason, the controlling thread must verify if the agent is moving out of its domains and send it to the shared area of the responsible thread. Consequently, additional steps in the *run()* method are required, including verification of its own shared area, which is performed by the *CheckSharedArea()* method, and attribution of the moving agent to its new location, performed by the *MoveAgents()* method. At this point, synchronization issues emerge requiring strict control over the time step of the agents.

Although threads share the same address space, they are not aware of other threads and should be controlled from a central location, namely the parent process. The *Workspace* class is responsible for creating, control, destroying, and keeping track of the threads and their domains, as well as facilitating their communication. In order to perform these activities, each thread must have a reference to the instance of the *Workspace* that can be used as a mediator between all active threads.

4. Concluding remarks and outlook

The current spectacular interest in agent-based modelling has gradually built up over the last twenty years, in particular for understanding the social aspects of human populations and simulating the spread of infectious diseases within and between communities. The use of agent-based models, in general, requires a more comprehensive incorporation of agents' characteristics both individually and group-wise, detailed information of the pertinent environment and the relationship between the system's various components. Despite the rapid evolution of ABM-based software applications and development of more sophisticated simulation approaches, the study of ABMs of any kind lacks a comprehensive and flexible software development framework. While some efforts have been made on developing such simulation models more consistent with the nature of the systems under investigation, and on designing computer software algorithms for their rapid implementation, the literature on general theoretical aspects of agent-based models is, as yet, quite small.

In this chapter, we reported our attempts in developing a software simulation framework for agent-based infectious disease modelling. Models implemented using this development framework will satisfy the software objectives of reliability, efficiency, and adaptability as fully described in Section 1. This framework has already been used to implement an agent-based model to evaluate mitigation strategies applied during the 2009 influenza pandemic in urban centres. An important aspect of this development framework is its flexibility to be adopted for simulating interconnected populations with distinctly different mobility patterns and demographic structures. Strategies for implementing this framework to simulate the spread of a disease in remote and isolated populations are being currently investigated.

The agent-based modelling framework described has several advantages that go beyond computer simulation experiments, providing a platform for addressing important aspects of modern world with global connectivity. We plan to use this framework to develop desktop decision-support systems for use in public health to address critical issues arising in the acute management of public health crises. Incorporating agent-based models into these software systems can provide an essential tool for public health experts to perform preliminary analysis, which can inform the formulation of optimal mitigation strategies in the face of substantial uncertainty regarding epidemiological aspects of a novel disease. Such decision support systems will require rapid development and deployment, an intuitive graphical user interface, and must quickly produce scenario outcomes. Such requirements can be satisfied using the framework presented here.

In the context of software design and engineering, future research activities will include the development of fault-tolerant distributed agent-based modelling systems as well as a comprehensive model description markup language to generate efficient software. The end results of these activities must satisfy the requirements of both modellers and public health officials in simulating the outcomes of infectious disease transmission, as well as prevention and control strategies.

5. Acknowledgment

The research activities and software engineering described in this chapter were supported by the Natural Sciences and Engineering Research Council of Canada (NSERC), the Mathematics of Information Technology and Complex Systems (MITACS), Canadian Institutes of Health Research (CIHR), and the Department of Foreign Affairs and International Trade of Canada, Emerging Leaders of the Americas Program.

6. References

Bernoulli, D (1760). Essai d'une nouvelle analyse de la mortalité causée par la petite verole, *Histoire de l'Académie Royale des Sciences, Memoires, Année*, 1–45

Bonabeau, B. (2002). Agent-based modeling: methods and techniques for simulating human systems. *Proceedings of the National Academy of Sciences*, Vol. 99, Supplement 3, 7280–7287, ISSN: 1091-6490

Darley, V. (1994). Emergent phenomena and complexity, In: *Artificial life IV, Proceedings of the 4th International Workshop on the Synthesis and Simulation of Living Systems*, Brooks, R. & Maes, P. (Ed.), 411–416, MIT Press, ISBN: 0262521903, Cambridge

Demko, A. B. & Pizzi, N. J. (2009). Scopira: an open source C++ framework for biomedical data analysis applications. *Software: Practice and Experience*, Vol. 39, No. 6, 641–660, ISSN: 1097-024X

Dongarra, J. J. & Dunigan, T. (1997). Message-passing performance of various computers. *Concurrency and Computation: Practice & Experience*, Vol. 9, No. 10, 915–926, ISSN: 1532-0634

Epstein, J. M. (2007). *Generative Social Science: Studies in Agent-Based Computational Modeling*, Princeton University Press, ISBN: 0691125473, Princeton

Ferguson, N. M. (2007). Connections capturing human behaviour, *Nature*, Vol. 446, 733, ISSN: 0028-0836

Geddes, K.; Labahn, G. & Monagan, M (2008). *Maple 12 Advanced Programming Guide*, Maplesoft, ISBN: 9781897310472, Waterloo

Geist, A.; Beguelin, A.; Dongarra, J.; Jiang, W.; Manchek, R. & Sunderam, V. S. (1994). *PVM: Parallel Virtual Machine: A Users' Guide and Tutorial for Network Parallel Computing*, MIT Press, ISBN:0262571080, Cambridge

Gilbert, N. & Terna, P. (2000). How to build and use agent-based models in social science. *Mind & Society*, Vol. 1, No. 1, 57–72, ISSN: 1593-7879

Gough, B. (2009). *GNU Scientific Library Reference Manual*, Network Theory Ltd., ISBN: 0954612078

Grimm, V.; Berger, U.; Bastiansen, F.; Eliassen, S.; Ginot, V.; Giske, J.; Goss-Custard, J.; Grand, T.; Heinz, S. K. & Huse, G. (2006). A standard protocol for describing individual-based and agent-based models. *Ecological Modelling*, Vol. 198, No. 1–2, 115–126, ISSN: 0304-3800

Grimm, V. & Railsback, S. F. (2005). *Individual-based Modeling and Ecology*, Princeton University Press, ISBN: 069109666X, Princeton

Hill, F. S. &, Kelley, S. M. (2006). *Computer Graphics Using OpenGL (3rd Edition)*, Prentice Hall, ISBN: 0131496700, Upper Saddle River

Ibáñez, L. & Schroeder, W. (2005). *The ITK Software Guide: The Insight, Segmentation and Registration Toolkit*, Kitware, Inc., ISBN: 1930934157, Clifton Park

Kermack, W. O. & McKendrick, A. G. (1927). A contribution to the mathematical theory of epidemics, *Proceedings of the Royal Society London A*, Vol. 115, 700–721, ISSN: 1471-2946

Kitware, Inc. (2010). *VTK User's Guide: Install, Use and Extend the Visualization Toolkit*, Kitware, Inc., ISBN: 1930934238, Clifton Park

Krause, A. (2007). *Foundations of GTK+ Development*, Springer-Verlag, ISBN: 1590597931, New York

Lingappa, J. R.; McDonald, L. C.; Simone, P. & Parashar, U.D. (2004). Wresting SARS from uncertainty. *Emerging Infectious Diseases*, Vol. 10, No. 2, 167–170, ISSN: 1080-6059

Logan, S. (2001). *GTK+ Programming in C*, Prentice Hall, ISBN: 0130142646, Upper Saddle River

Macal, C. M. & North, M. J. (2005). Tutorial on agent-based modeling and simulation, *Proceedings of the 37th Winter Simulation Conference*, pp. 2–15, ISBN: 0780395190, Orlando, USA, December 4–7, Winter Simulation Conference, Orlando

Moghadas, S. M.; Pizzi, N. J.; Wu, J. & Yan, P (2009). Managing public health crises: the role of models in pandemic preparedness. *Influenza and Other Respiratory Viruses*, Vol. 3, No. 2, 75–79, ISSN: 1750-2659

Murray, J. D. (2007). *Mathematical Biology: Vol. I. An Introduction (3rd Edition)*, Springer-Verlag, ISBN: 0387952233, Heidelberg

Ormerod, P. & Rosewell, B. (2009). Validation and Verification of Agent-Based Models in the social sciences, In: *Epistemological Aspects of Computer Simulation in the Social Sciences*, Squazzoni, F. (Ed.), 130–140, Springer, ISBN: 364201108X, Berlin

Pizzi, N.J. (2008). Software quality prediction using fuzzy integration: a case study. *Soft Computing Journal*, Vol. 12, No. 1, 67–76, ISSN: 1432-7643

Pizzi, N. J. & Pedrycz, W. (2008). Effective classification using feature selection and fuzzy integration. *Fuzzy Sets and Systems*, Vol. 159, No. 21, 2859–2872, ISSN: 0165-0114

Railsback S. F.; Lytinen, S. L. & Jackson, S.K. (2006). Agent-based simulation platforms: review and development recommendations, *Simulation*, Vol. 82, No. 9, 609–623, ISSN: 0037-5497

Ropella, G. E. P.; Railsback, S. F. & Jackson, S. K. (2002). Software engineering considerations for individual-based models. *Natural Resource Modelling*, Vol. 15, No. 1, 5–22, ISSN: 1939-7445

Schroeder, W.; Martin, K. & Lorensen, B. (2006). *Visualization Toolkit: An Object-Oriented Approach to 3D Graphics*, Prentice Hall, ISBN: 0139546944, Upper Saddle River

Shan, H.; Singh, J. P.; Oliker, L. & Biswas, R. (2003). Message passing and shared address space parallelism on an SMP cluster. *Parallel Computing*, Vol. 29, No. 2, 167–186, ISSN: 0167-8191

Shoham, Y. & Leyton-Brown, K. (2008). Multiagent Systems: Algorithmic, Game-Theoretic, and Logical Foundations, Cambridge University Press, ISBN: 0521899435, Cambridge

Sigmon K. & Davis, T.A. (2010). *Matlab Primer (8th Edition)*, Chapman & Hall/CRC Press, Inc., ISBN: 1439828628, Boca Raton

Snir, M. & Gropp, W. (1998). *MPI: The Complete Reference (Volume 1: The MPI Core)*, MIT Press, ISBN: 0262692163, Cambridge

Sokolowski, J. A. & Banks, C. M. (2010). *Modeling and Simulation Fundamentals: Theoretical Underpinnings and Practical Domains*, John Wiley & Sons, Inc., ISBN: 0470486740, Hoboken

Summerfield, M. (2010). *Advanced Qt Programming: Creating Great Software with C++ and Qt 4*, Prentice Hall, ISBN: 0321635906, Upper Saddle River.

Taubenberger, J. K. & Morens, D.M. (2006). 1918 influenza: The mother of all pandemics. *Emerging Infectious Diseases*, Vol. 12,No. 1, 15–22, ISSN: 1080-6059

Wolfram S. (1999). *The Mathematica Book*, Cambridge University Press, ISBN: 0521643147, Cambridge

Wooldridge, M. (1997). Agent-based software engineering. *IEE Proceedings: Software Engineering*, Vol. 144, No. 1, 26–37, ISSN: 1364-5080

34

Personalized Biomedical Data Integration

Xiaoming Wang, Olufunmilayo Olopade and Ian Foster
University of Chicago,
USA

1. Introduction

Translational research is a growing field of science that seeks to discover the molecular underpinnings of diseases and treatment outcomes in any individual patient (Horig, Marincola et al. 2005). The mission has driven researchers out of isolated and discipline-oriented studies into collaborative and trans-disciplinary research efforts known as team science (Guimerà, Uzzi et al. 2005). In this new scientific arena, the ability to search for an individual's biomedical data across various domains and sources via a common computational platform is a vital component for the formulation of sophisticated hypotheses and research decisions.

Biomedical data is composed of records from both clinical practice and basic research. Each sector has distinct data governance policies and database management rules. While basic biological research data sources are open— some 1,230 curated databases are available in the public domain and accessible through the Internet (Cochrane and Galperin 2010), all primary clinical data sources are kept private with rigorous data access controls, due to *Health Insurance Portability and Accountability Act* (HIPAA) regulations (Faddick 1997). Furthermore, while basic biological research data sources frequently make data elements, database schemas, metadata information and *application programming interface* (API) available to the public, the majority of clinical data sources are hosted by proprietary commercial software. The vendors (or developers) of these tools usually disclose little information about schema and metadata to third-parties. Finally, while most basic research (e.g., biological molecule or pathway) data sources must have data integrity at the species level, translational research requires data integrity at the individual patient level. Indeed, integrated and individualized biomedical data sources will need to make a significant contribution to translational research in order to truly achieve personalized medicine. However, generating such data sources is a more difficult task than the already challenging mission of integrating basic biological research data (Stein 2008).

Data integration is the process of combining data from different sources into a unified format with consistent description and logical organization. After more than two decades of research, the topic continues to become more challenging due to increasing demands and persistent obstacles (Batini, Lenzerini et al. 1986; Bernstein and Haas 2008; Agrawal, Ailamaki et al. 2009). In this chapter, we focus on the issues that must be addressed to fulfil the demands for individualized biomedical data integration and introduce a customized warehousing approach for this particular purpose.

2. Background

2.1 Current status of biomedical data

To illustrate the demand of integrating individualized biomedical data, we start with an example: for a cancer translational researcher to assess the association between the genetic background and the occurrence of a particular cancer and its treatment outcomes, she likely needs to:

1) screen family history through medical surveys on a selected cohort; 2) read pathology report about each individual's histological diagnosis; 3) check surgical, chemo, and radiation records in the clinics; 4) follow the outcomes and adverse events of the treatments; 5) record dates and evidences of the cancer recurrence and metastasis; 6) find DNA samples from specimen bank; and 7) conduct genotyping experiments and link the genotype results back to the phonotypical records.

In order to extract meaningful information from these data, the researcher needs to have these data distinguishably aligned to individual persons, but linking these data together, even in a modest number of subjects, often fails due to data heterogeneity and discontinuity. Combining biomedical data with integrity at individual level frequently encounters four distinct challenges.

The first challenge is caused by source heterogeneity. Data elements and/or schemas for the same domain data that are designed by independent parties will normally be semantically different. Such heterogeneity may also exist in different (or the same) versions of software developed by the same party. To further complicate matters, many data sources are subject to dynamic change in all aspects, including data structures, ontology standards, and instance data coding methods. These sources customarily do not provide metadata or mapping information between datasets from previous and newer versions.

The second challenge stems from data descriptor inconsistencies. Many biomedical domains do not have established ontologies and others have more than one set of standard taxonomies. For example, one can find official taxonomies for describing cancers in SNOMED (Cote and Robboy 1980), *International Classification of Disease* (ICD) (Cimino 1996), and the NCI-thesaurus (Sioutos, de Coronado et al. 2007).

The third challenge comes from data source management styles. Most data sources are isolated and autonomously operated. These sources typically neither map nor retain the primary identifiers (of a person or the specimens that originated from the person) created in the other sources. The silo settings of the data sources not only generate segregated datasets but often require repetitive re-entry of the same records (e.g., patient demographic data) by hand into different sources. This practice increases the risk of human error.

The fourth challenge is due to low data source interoperability. The majority of clinical data sources are neither programmatically accessible (syntactic interoperability) nor have metadata available for the source data (semantic interoperability).

Many of these problems have been continual to date and will linger for the foreseeable future. As a consequence, biomedical source data are typically heterogeneous, inconsistent, fragmented, dirty and difficult to process. Valuable information embedded within the data cannot be consumed until the data are cleansed, unified, standardized, and integrated.

2.2 Related data integration regimes

The purpose of data integration is to deliver integrated information. This purpose can be realized via either permanent (physical) or transient (view) data integration. Among the various information integration approaches, data warehousing, view integration, and information mashup are popular regimes that are actively discussed in IT and informatics publications (Halevy 2001; Jhingran 2006; Goble and Stevens 2008). Each regime has its own distinct design principle and system architecture.

2.2.1 Data warehousing

While describing the architecture of a data warehousing solution, many focus on a multidimensional database (Louie, Mork et al. 2007; Goble and Stevens 2008). This database-centred approach is widely used across multiple fields and has a well-documented history in regards to its evolution. A warehouse delivers integrated information by organizing and storing data from various sources within a physical schema so that the integrated data can be reused for a variety of applications. Since the basic requirement for a database to function is data availability, the warehousing approach appears to be more tolerant to various data source conditions than its counterpart solutions which all require data sources to be interoperable and accessible. Warehousing is generally considered most suitable for historical data accumulation, quality data integration, and post-integration data curation and annotation (Halevy, Ashish et al. 2005). In biomedical informatics, the warehousing approach is considered most suitable for personalized biomedical data integration (Louie, Mork et al. 2007; Wang, Liu et al. 2009).

The major drawbacks of the warehousing approach are its association with stale data and the resource-consuming nature of system maintenance. These negative aspects reveal a simple truth about warehousing: data supply issues are the biggest obstacle and financial drain to the ultimate success of the strategy. These issues demonstrate the need for a data *extraction-transformation-loading* (ETL) process that determines the quality and freshness of integrated data. Thus, we discuss in greater depth of both the database and the ETL process.

2.2.1.1 Multidimensional database modelling

The database in a warehousing strategy must store multidimensional data. Three distinct conceptual modelling methods are often employed for database design: 1) the Entity-Relationship (ER) model (Chen 1976; Kamble 2008); 2) Entity-Attribute-Value representation with classes and relationships (EAV/CR) model (Dinu and Nadkarni 2007; Lowe, Ferris et al. 2009); and 3) Object-Oriented Database (OODB) (Trujillo, Palomar et al. 2001). Although no consensus has been reached concerning modelling standards, we prefer the ER model due to its solid mathematic foundation, data structure semantic clarity, and data presentation transparency. These features not only benefit high-throughput data deployment at the database layer for integration but also support satisfactory query performance at the user-application interface. In addition, since the ER model requires semantic clarity and consistency for each attribute element during cross-source data processing, the delivery of useful data and consumable information is better ensured.

At the implementation level, a data warehouse is suggested to have a star schema (a single large fact table and many smaller dimension tables) to improve application performance by reducing the time required to join multiple tables to answer a query (Kimball, Reeves et al. 1998). However, a highly de-normalized schema, like a star schema, also increases cost of database maintenance. With materialized-view technology being well-developed, the de-normalization of data entities at the primary schema level is no longer critical. Materialized-view technology is capable of flexibly aggregating data into any combination.

2.2.1.2 *ETL modelling and tools*

A warehouse relies on an ETL process to refill and refresh data from heterogeneous sources into a predefined schema for data integration. The history of developing and optimizing ETL is directly tied to the history of data warehouse systems. Yet, a significant technological breakthrough for ETL remains to be seen. In general, the process remains error-prone and labour-intensive (Rizzi, Abello et al. 2006). The methods related to the different stages of an ETL process can be briefly categorized into the following: 1) schema mapping (Bernstein and Rahm 2001); 2) metadata collection and management (Kolaitis 2005); 3) error detection and data cleansing (Kalashnikov and Mehrotra 2006); and 4) systematic modelling of the entire ETL process (Vassiliadis, Simitsis et al. 2002).

The pressing demand for data integration has spurred the development of commercial ETL software packages. Examples include DataStage (Oracle), Informix (IBM), and products from smaller vendors. To date, all ETL strategies still involve human intervention, albeit at different levels. Many approaches appear to be exhaustive and obsessive in the hierarchical levels of schema mapping while paying insufficient attention to data value integration. Some are inherently brittle, often without a clear measure of success for an ETL workflow in the real world. In the field of biomedical informatics, which fiercely promotes interoperable data integration (Komatsoulis, Warzel et al. 2008), ETL remains an autonomous in-house activity and formal reports on the topic are seldom seen.

2.2.2 View integration

The architecture behind view integration consists of an interoperable data grid with constituent primary databases that are autonomous, disparate, and heterogeneous. Yet, data from these databases need to be aligned to a common virtual schema during integration (Halevy 2001; Stein 2002). In this regime, queries issued by users are posed to the virtual schema and then translated into various customized queries against disparate data sources. Extracted source data is then transformed on the fly to meet the definitions of the common schema. Finally, unified data is presented to users as integrated information.

Because view integration combines data dynamically, without any persistent physical data aggregation, it can provide real time information. However, its effectiveness depends critically on the interoperability and network accessibility of every data source of interest, which (at least at the current time) seems unlikely to occur in practice. In addition, because view integration requires the entire data aggregation process from disparate sources to the view to be fully automated, it provides less control of data quality than data warehousing approaches in which manual curation steps can be included in the ETL process. This lack of sufficient data quality control is a serious concern for biomedical informatics researchers (Goble, Stevens et al. 2008; Galperin and Cochrane 2009).

To date, view integration systems with production level maturity are not commonly seen in the real world. However, the design concepts utilized in view integration, including global-as-view (GAV) and local-as-view (LAV), are valuable principles to all data integration efforts (Lenzerini 2002). In GAV, the virtual schema is made adjustable to accommodate all source data elements. In LAV, each source data is individually managed to be transformed to align to this global view.

2.2.3 Information mashup

The architecture behind the information mashup approach comprises of an open fabric which augments information from different sources that allow their API accessible through the

Internet. Although having some similarities to ETL, mashup is advantageous both in its ability to be light-weight and its utilization of a service model that is easily extensible via Web 2.0 techniques, e.g., *representational state transfer* (REST) technology (Fielding and Taylor 2002). The prerequisite for a mashup fabric to consistently present (overlay) different messages on a web interface is standardized information formats in the atomic data elements that carry instance data. These data feeds are either staged within the sources (or at a middleware) or converted to have consistent data interpretation, e.g., geographic code, and formats on the fly. For example, a (subject-predicate-object) triplet expressed in the W3C-standard *resource description framework* (RDF) carries metadata information for related atomic data elements. Therefore, RDF can be easily converted into an ER model and vice versa.

Unlike view integration, which has a predefined schema, a mashup fabric uses structured basic data elements to form information presentations that are not rigorously structured, e.g., information situational display overlay (Jhingran 2006). Therefore, a mashup strategy becomes more implementable and as a result, has been used in many information integration-*lite* tasks (Franklin, Halevy et al. 2005; Goble and Stevens 2008). Examples include Google maps (Wong and Hong 2007) and Avian Flu maps (Butler 2006).

However, the openness of the mashup fabric along with its integration *lite* nature limits its application as the first layer technology option for personalized biomedical data integration. At this layer, the integration framework must manipulate primary source data in a secluded network because the data contain *protected health information* (PHI). Furthermore, data integration with individualized integrity from longitudinal records is an integration-heavy task, which is better handled by a relational database in a secure environment alleviating HIPAA concerns. However, the mashup strategy may still be suitable for higher-level (anonymous) biomedical data integration for population studies that require evidence from a significant number of individuals in a particular domain or against a geographic background.

2.3 Related human-intensive efforts

In addition to computationally heavy informatics solutions, human-developed information research is also a crucial component in overall information delivery (Bernstam, Smith et al. 2010). These efforts include domain ontology creation (Yu 2006) and mapping for multiple standards in the same domain, e.g., *unified medical language system* (UMLS) (Bodenreider 2004) for SNOMED and ICD. However, despite the challenge of mapping between existing standards, newer standards keep emerging. Mapping concepts between different ontologies in the same domain or different versions within the same ontology requires good mapping references, which are usually either inadequate or not computable, e.g., cancer registry coding schema (Edge, Byrd et al. 2010). Nevertheless, discussions concerning how to best use human effort in the field of informatics are rare. It is evident that these efforts can either benefit or hinder data integration efficiency.

3. Methods

3.1 Conceptual design of the warehousing framework

Based on our analysis of existing data integration regimes, biomedical data statuses, and conditions of data sources in the real world, we adopted a warehousing strategy to address the general need for personalized data integration. The purpose of our approach is to provide a computation framework aimed at data *unification for integration* (UNIFIN). By design, the UNIFIN framework contains two essential technical components: a multidimensional database, the *Translational Data Mart* (TraM), and a customized ETL process, the *Data Translation Workflow* (TraW). UNIFIN also includes an interoperable information integration mechanism, empowered by REST and SOA technologies for data that do not need manipulation during the integration process. Examples of such data include homogeneous molecular sequence records and binary image datasets.

In this chapter, we focus on describing the semi-automated ETL workflow for heterogeneous text data processing. We explain data processing, integration and ontology issues collectively, with the intent of drawing a systematic picture describing a warehousing regime that is customized for personalized data integration. Although TraM and TraW have been developed by the same team, each is designed to be independently portable, meaning that TraM can readily accept data from other ETL tools and TraW, after customization, can supply data to target databases other than TraM.

3.2 Data warehouse TraM

3.2.1 Domain ontology integrated ER conceptual model

We used the top-down design method to model the TraM database. The modelling is based on our analysis of real world biomedical data. The results of the analysis are depicted in a four-dimensional data space (Fig 1A). The first dimension comprises study objects, which can range from human individuals to biomaterials derived from a human body. Restrictively mapping these objects according to their origins (unique persons) is essential to assure personalized data continuity across domains and sources.

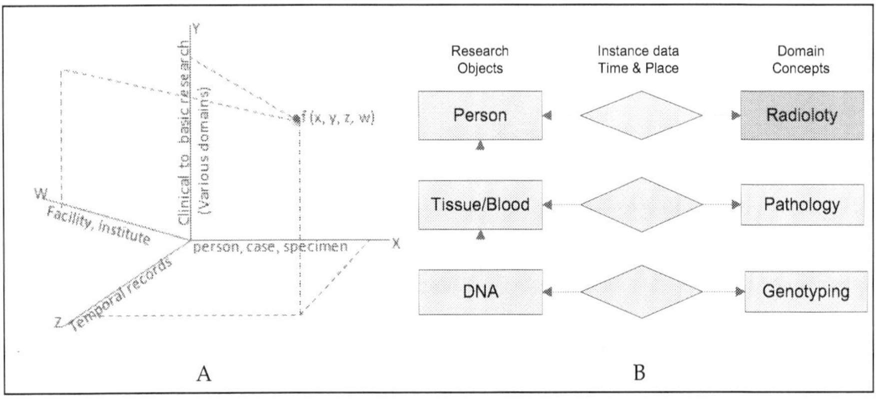

Fig. 1. Data warehouse modelling: A) Biomedical data anatomy; B) DO-ER conceptual model for the TraM database. The square shapes in panel B indicate data entities and the diamond shapes indicate relationships between the entities. The orange colour indicates that the entity can be either a regular dictionary lookup table or a leaf class entity in a domain ontology.

The second dimension is positioned with a variety of domain concepts that are present in an extensive biomedical practice and research field. Domain concepts can either be classified in domain ontologies or remain unclassified until classification takes place during integration. There are no direct logical connections between the different domain ontologies in an evidence-based data source. The associations among domain concepts will be established when they are applied to study objects that are derived from the same individual.

The other two dimensions concern the times and geographic locations at which research or clinical actions take place, respectively. These data points are consistent variables associated with all instance (fact) data and are useful to track instances longitudinally and geographically. This analysis is the foundation for TraM database modelling.

We then create a unique *domain-ontology integrated entity-relationship* (DO-ER) model to interpret the data anatomy delineated in Fig 1A with the following consistency. (See Fig 1B for a highly simplified DO-ER model.)

1. The instance data generated between DO and study objects are arranged in a many-to-many relationship.
2. Domain concept descriptors are treated as data rather than data elements. Descriptors are either adopted from well-established public ontology data sources or created by domain experts with an ontology data structure provided by TraM, assuming that there is no reputable ontology existing within that domain. Thus, domain concepts are either organized as simply as a single entity for well-defined taxonomies or as complex as a set of entities for classification of concepts in a particular domain.
3. Study objects (a person or biomaterials derived from the person) are forced to be linked to each other according to their origins regardless of the primary data sources from which they come.

There are three fuzzy areas that need to be clarified for the DO-ER model. The first is the difference between an integrated DO in the DO-ER model versus a free-standing DO for sophisticated DO development. The DO development in the DO-ER model needs to be balanced between its integrity in concept classification (meaning the same concept should *not* be described by different words and vice versa) and its historical association with the instance data (meaning some DO terms might have been used to describe instance data). The data values between the DO and ER need to be maintained regularly to align the instance data descriptors to the improved DO terms. For this purpose, we suggest that concept classification be rigorously normalized, meaning to make concept of an attribute not divisible in the leaf class of the DO, because merging data with unified descriptor is always easier than splitting data into two or more different data fields. The advantage of the DO-ER model is that these changes and alignments usually do not affect the database schema. The latter remains stable so there is no need to modify application programs.

The second is the conceptual design underlying the DO structures in the DO-ER model. In fact, the DO under this context is also modelled by ER technique, which is conceptually distinct from the popularly adopted EAV modelling technique in the biomedical informatics field (Lowe, Ferris et al. 2009) . The major difference is that the ER underlying the DO has normalized semantics for each attribute, while the EAV does not.

The third is determining the appropriate extent of DO development that should go into an evidence-based database. We believe that TraM users in general have neither the intention nor the resources to make TraM a DO producer. Thus, our purpose in allowing for DO development within TraM is solely to satisfy the minimal requirement of harmonizing highly heterogeneous data with controlled vocabulary, so that the DO is developed as needed. The resulting standardization of data concept abstractions, classifications, and descriptions will make it easier to merge data with future reputable DO standards as they (hopefully) emerge. Under this context, we further explain a use case underlined with DO-ER transformation-integration mechanism in section 4.2, and detail how an evolving DO may affect data integration workflow in section 3.3.4.

3.2.2 Enforcing personalized data integrity

Personalized data integrity is enforced throughout the entire TraM schema. To achieve this level of quality control, the first required condition is to identify uniqueness of a person in the system. HIPAA regulations categorize a person's demographic information and medical administrative identifiers and dates as PHI that should not be disclosed to researchers or transferred between databases without rigorous legal protections. However, as a person is mobile, an individual's medical records are often entered into multiple databases in more than one medical institution or clinic. Without PHI, it is almost impossible to reliably identify the uniqueness of a person unless 1) the person's identifiers are mapped across all data sources or 2) there is a universal identifier used in all healthcare and research domains. Neither condition currently exists. Therefore, a data warehouse often must be HIPAA-compliant to contain PHI data to verify the uniqueness of a person. This is the case in the TraM operation. Once the uniqueness of a person is identified, TraM has a built-in mechanism that automatically unlinks the PHI records to form the materialized view. Since the materialized view is the schema that answers queries, the application program can only access de-identified data, and therefore, regular users do not see PHI but can still receive reliable individualized information.

3.3 ETL process TraW

The TraM data model reflects one particular interpretation (our interpretation) of biomedical data in the real world. Independent parties always have different opinions about how a warehouse database should be constructed. Different data sources also interpret the same domain data differently both among themselves and from a warehouse. To bridge these gaps, TraW is designed to be configurable to adapt to different sources and targets. Since most medical data sources do not disclose database schema or support interoperability, we have focused in designing TraW on gathering the basic data elements that carry data and performing data extraction from available electronic data forms (Free text is not included in this discussion.). Unlike TraM, which has a relatively free-standing architecture, TraW is an open fabric with four essential highly configurable components:

1. A mechanism to collect metadata—routinely *not* available in source data deliveries. A web-based data element registration interface is required to collect metadata across all sources.
2. A set of systematically designed and relatively stable domain data templates, which serve as a data processing workbench to replace numerous intermediate tables and views that are usually autonomously created by individual engineers in an uncontrolled ETL process.
3. A set of tools that manipulate data structures and descriptions to transform heterogeneous data into an acceptable level of uniformity and consistency as required by the target schema.
4. A set of dynamically evolving domain ontologies and data mapping references which are needed for data structure unification and descriptor standardization.

Behind these components is a relational database schema that supports TraW and records its data processing history.

3.3.1 Metadata collection

TraW treats all data sources as new by collecting their most up-to-date metadata in each batch data collection through a web-based application interface. If the existing sources do not have any changes since the previous update, the source data managers are required to sign an online confirmation sheet for the current submission. To avoid another level of heterogeneity as generated by metadata description, TraW provides a pre-defined metadata list for data providers to choose from through the registration interface. These metadata are defined based on the TraW domain templates (the differences between domain templates and target schema are detailed in section 3.3.2). These metadata will not completely cover all source data elements, not necessarily because they do not represent the meanings of those data, but because they do not share the same semantic interpretations for the same kinds of data. Thus, TraW allows data providers to create their own metadata for unmatched data fields.

3.3.2 Domain data template

In section 2.2.2, we described the GAV and LAV concepts. The TraW domain template is derived from the GAV concept. The difference is that the GAV in *view* integration is a virtual schema that responds directly to query commands, while the domain template in TraW both carries physical data and serves as a workbench to stage data before integration. Unlike a target schema, which has normalized domain entities and relationships governed by rigorous rules to assure data integrity, domain templates in TraW do not have entity level data structures, nor do they have relationship and redundancy constraints. Instead, since there are no concerns about the user application interface, the templates can simply be frequently edited in order to accommodate the new source data elements. However, these templates must have three essential categories of data elements.

First, a template must contain elements that support *minimal information about data integration* (MIADI). MIADI is presented by a set of primary identifiers from different sources and is required for cross-domain data integration. These identifiers, which come from independent sources, should be capable of being mapped to each other when study objects are derived from the same person. If the mapping linkage is broken, PHI will be required to rebuild data continuity and integrity for one person may have multiple identifiers if served in different medical facilities.

Second, a template must contain the domain *common data element* (CDE), a set of abstracted data concepts that can represent various disciplinary data within a domain. For example, cancer staging data elements are required for all types of cancers so they are the CDE for evidence oncology data. Elements for time stamps and geographic locations are also CDEs for cross-domain incidence data. Domain CDEs are usually defined through numerous discussions between informaticians and domain experts if there is no available CDE that is widely accepted in the public domain.

Third, the template must contain elements that carry data source information, e.g., source database names, owner names of the databases, data versions, submission times, and etc, which are collectively called data provenance information. This information is required for data curation and tracking.

ETL workers continue to debate what exactly constitutes domain CDE, despite significant efforts to seek consensus within or across biomedical domains (Cimino, Hayamizu et al. 2009). Each ETL often has its own distinct semantic interpretation of data. Therefore, TraW should only provide templates with the three specified element categories in order to give ETL workers flexibility in configuring their own workbench.

Generally speaking, domain templates have looser control on CDE formulation than do target schemas because they are intended to cover all source data elements, including those that have a semantic disparity on the same domain data. For this reason, a domain template actually serves as a data transformation medium which in principle, has a consistent data structure as the target schema while simultaneously containing both an original (O-form) and a standardized (S-form) form for each data element. Data need to be in a semantically consistent structure before they can be standardized. Data in S-form are completely consistent in both structure and description to the target schema. Reaching semantic consistency relies on a set of data transformation algorithms and semantic mapping references.

3.3.3 Data transformation algorithms

Data transformation is a materialized process of LAV (refer to section 2.2.2), meaning that it converts data from each source to a common data schema with consistent semantic interpretations. Since we focus mainly on basic data element transformation, we mashup these elements from different sources and rearrange them into different domain templates. Because each domain template contains a data provenance element, we can trace every single record (per row) by its provenance tag through the entire data manipulation process. The transformation of a data element proceeds in two steps: data structure unification and then data value standardization. The algorithms behind these two steps are generic to all domain data but depend on two kinds of references to perform accurately. These references are the domain ontologies and the mapping media between sources and target schema (more details in 3.3.4). In this section, we mainly explain data transformation algorithms.
In our experience with integrating data from more than 100 sources, we have found that about 50% of source data elements could not find semantic matches among themselves or to the target schema even when they carried the same domain data. Within these semantically unmatched data elements, we consistently found that more than 80% of the elements are generated through hard-coding computation, meaning that data instances are treated as variable carriers, or in other words, as attribute or column names (Fig 2.I). This practice results in data elements with extremely limited information representation and produces an enormous amount of semantically heterogeneous data elements. It is impossible to standardize the data description in such settings unless instance values are released from the name domains of the data elements. The algorithm to transform this kind of data structure is quite straightforward, unambiguous, and powerful. The process is denoted in the formula:

$$f\{x_{(1)}, y_{(i)}\} \Rightarrow f\{x_{(i)}, y_{(specified)}\}$$

In this formula, a data table is treated as a two dimensional data matrix. x represents rows and y represents columns. Column names (left side of arrow) are treated as data values in the first row. They are transposed (repositioned) into rows under properly abstracted variable holders (columns). The associated data with those column names are rearranged accordingly (Fig 2.II). The decision as to which column names are transposed into which rows and under which columns is made with information provided by a set of mapping references. Since this process often transforms data from a wide form data matrix into a long form, we refer to it as a wide-to-long transformation. The fundamental difference between this long form data table versus an EAV long form data table is that the data table in our system is composed with semantically normalized data elements while EAV data table is not.
Once data values are released from data structures under properly abstracted data elements, normalization and standardization of the value expression can take place. This process is

called data descriptor translation and relies on a mapping reference that specifies which specific irregular expressions or piece of vocabulary are to be replaced by standardized ones. At the same time, further annotation to the instance data can be performed based on the metadata. For example, the test values in Fig 2.II are measured from two different test methods for the same testing purpose. In this circumstance, unless the test methods are also annotated, the testing results cannot be normalized for an apple-to-apple comparison. In addition, the assessment (asmt) field is added to justify the score values read from different testing methods (Fig 2.III).

There are other complex data structure issues besides hard-coded data elements requiring significant cognitional analysis to organize data. We discuss these issues in section 5.

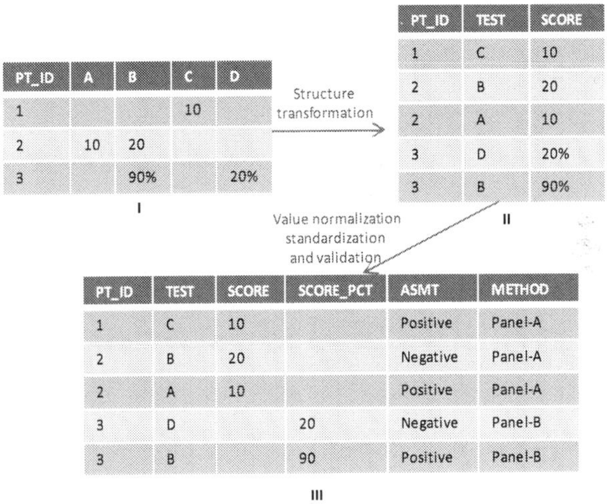

PT_ID	A	B	C	D
1			10	
2	10	20		
3		90%		20%

PT_ID	TEST	SCORE
1	C	10
2	B	20
2	A	10
3	D	20%
3	B	90%

PT_ID	TEST	SCORE	SCORE_PCT	ASMT	METHOD
1	C	10		Positive	Panel-A
2	B	20		Negative	Panel-A
2	A	10		Positive	Panel-A
3	D		20	Negative	Panel-B
3	B		90	Positive	Panel-B

Fig. 2. An example of data transformation: I) Hard-coded data elements; II) Semantically unified data structure; and III) Standardized and normalized data values with additional annotation based on metadata and data mapping references

3.3.4 Domain ontology and mapping references

Domain ontology and mapping references are human-intensive products that need to be designed to be computable and reusable for future data processing. In general, it is simpler to produce mapping references between irregular data descriptors and a well-established domain ontology. The problem is how to align heterogeneous source data elements and their data value descriptors to a domain ontology that is also under constant development. Our solution is to set several rules for domain ontology developers and provide a backbone structure to organize the domain ontology.

1. We outline the hierarchy of a domain ontology structure with root, branch, category and leaf classes, and allow category classes to be further divided into sub-categories.
2. We pre-define attributes for the leaf class, so that the leaf class property will be organized into a set of common data elements for this particular ontology.
3. Although domain concept descriptors are treated as data values in ontology, they should be in unique expressions as each should represent a unique concept.

We train domain experts with these rules before they develop ontologies, as improper classification is difficult to detect automatically. We maintain data mapping references in a key-value table, with the standardized taxonomy as the key and irregular expressions as values. Both in-house domain ontologies and mapping references should be improved, validated, maintained, and reused over time.

3.3.5 Data transformation process

Here, we describe a snapshot of the data transformation process. Typically, this process requires a set of leaf class attributes for a domain ontology, a mapping table that connects the leaf class data elements and the source data elements, a data structure transformation program, and a set of source data (Fig 3). At the end of this process, the source data structures and values are all transformed according to the concept descriptor classification in the domain ontology. The original source data attribute name is now released from the name domain (red boxes in Fig 3) of a data element and becomes a piece of value record (purple box in Fig 3) that is consistent to the taxonomy in the domain ontology.

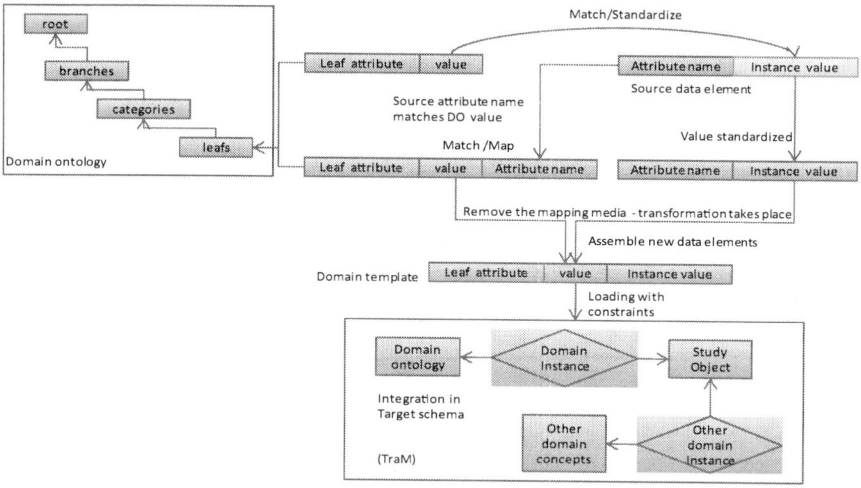

Fig. 3. A generalized data transformation processs using dynamically evolved domain ontology and mapping media.

4. Results

4.1 UNIFIN framework overview

UNIFIN is implemented through the TraM and TraW projects. TraM runs on an Oracle database server and a TomCat web application server. TraW also runs on an Oracle database, but is operated in a secluded intranet because it processes patient PHI records (Fig 4). TraM and TraW do not have software component dependencies, but are functionally interdependent in order to carry out the mission of personalized biomedical data integration. Fig 4 shows the UNIFIN architecture with notations about its basic technical components.

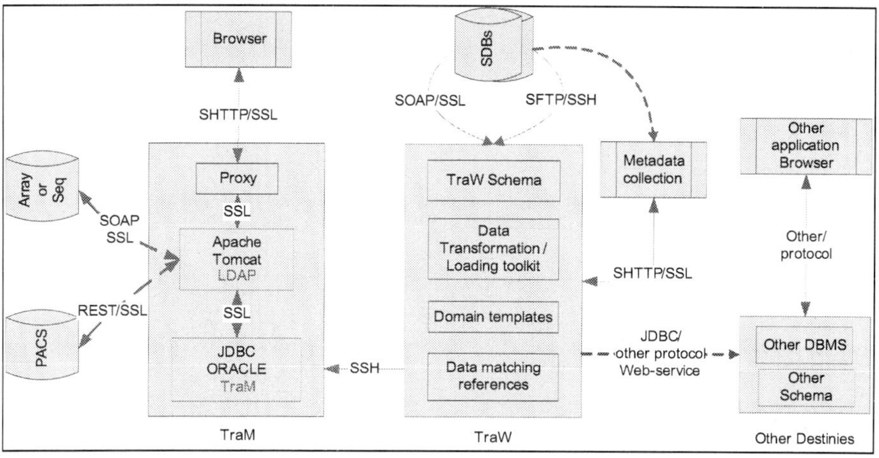

Fig. 4. UNIFIN overview: Dashed lines for the panel on the left indicate the workflow that does not route through TraW but is still a part of UINFIN. Red lines indicate secured file transmission protocols. Areas within the red boxes indicate HIPAA compliant computational environments. The right side panel of TraW indicates other data integration destinations other than TraM.

Whereas the web application interface of TraM provides user friendly data account management, curation, query and retrieving functions for biomedical researchers, TraW is meant for informaticians, who are assumed to have both domain knowledge and computation skills.

4.2 A use case of TraM data integration

We use the example of medical survey data, one of the least standardized and structured datasets in biomedical studies, to illustrate how domain ontology can play an important role in TraM. It is not uncommon to see the same survey concept (i.e., question) worded differently in several questionnaires and to have the data value (i.e., answer) to the same question expressed in a variety of ways. The number of survey questions per survey subject varies from fewer than ten to hundreds. Survey subject matter changes as research interest shifts and no one can really be certain as to whether a new question will emerge and what the question will look like. Therefore, although medical survey data is commonly required for a translational research plan (refer to the example in 2.1), there is little data integration support for this kind of data and some suggest that survey data does not belong in a clinical conceptual data model (Brazhnik and Jones 2007).

To solve this problem, we proposed an ontology structure to manage the concepts in the questionnaires. Within the DO, the questions are treated as data in the leaf class of the questionnaire and organized under different categories and branches. Each question, such as what, when, how, and why, has a set of properties that define an answer. These properties include data type (number or text), unit of measure (cup/day, pack/day, ug/ml), and predefined answer options (Fig 5A).

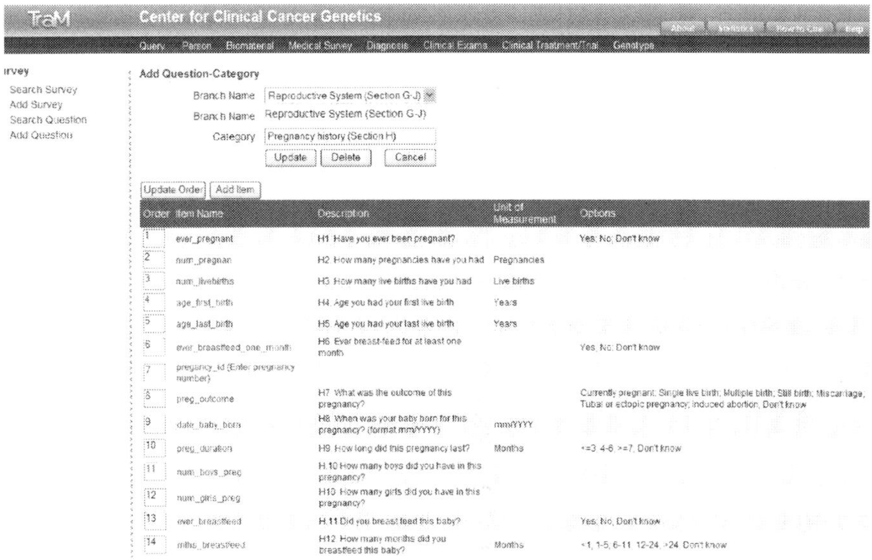

A

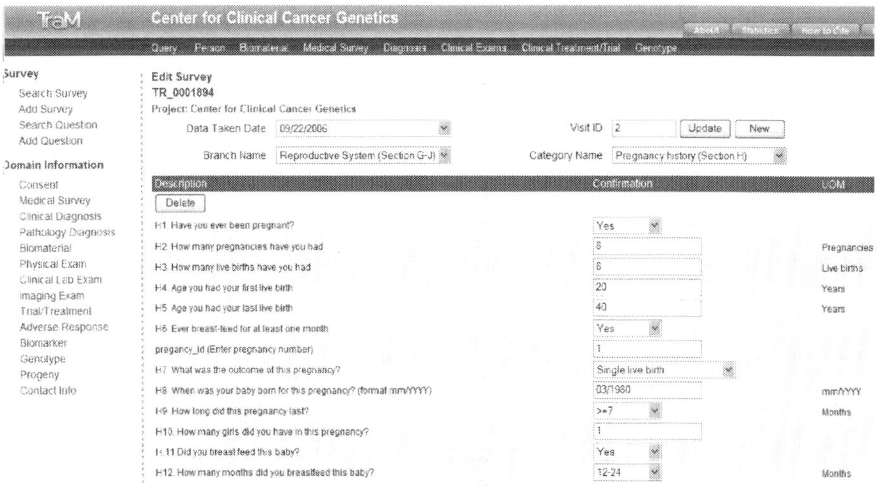

B

Fig. 5. Domain ontology and data integration: A) Leaf class attributes of the questionnaire; B) Instance data described by domain ontology. Both A and B are screenshots from the TraM *curator interface* (explained in 4.4). The left hand panel of screen B shows hyperlinks to the other domains that can also be associated with the individual (TR_0001894). The data shown is courtesy from the account of centre for clinical cancer genetics

Since a new question and its properties are treated as a new record (a new row in the leaf class table), the overall database structure stays the same. Since the possible answers in the survey are pre-defined with controlled vocabulary, the answers will be recorded in a relationship between the person entity and the question item entity. The survey results are also instantly and seamlessly integrated with the other domain data (Fig 5B). This underlying mechanism is meant to allow for the new question to play a double role: first, as a record (value) in the questionnaire ontology and second, as a question concept to recruit the survey result. In this way, the TraM system gains enormous flexibility in recruiting new concepts and is able to annotate data with controlled vocabularies.

4.3 A life-cycle of TraW process

Running a life-cycle of TraW takes four steps: 1) extract atomic data elements from various source data files; 2) unify (transform) data structure at the atomic data element level and mashup data into proper intermediate domain templates; 3) standardize (translate) and validate data values upon mixed data elements on the domain templates; 4) load and restructure data from domain templates into a target schema and complete integration.
We have yet to gain much experience in extracting data directly from sources since most of the medical data sources that we work with deny programmatic data access. The source data files we obtained are in table or XML formats delivered through a secured file transport process (SFTP).
The person(s) who operates TraW is also responsible for customizing and maintaining the essential constituent components. This responsibility includes editing domain templates, maintaining data mapping references and modifying programs in the toolkit. As a high-throughput computation process, TraW may drop a list of disqualified data at each step and keep moving forward. Disqualified data will be sent to a curator for further validation. Recovered data may rejoin the workflow after verification to be processed with other data (Fig 6). Unified and standardized data on the domain templates (in the S-forms, refer section 3.3.2) are in a mashup status but not integrated. Integration is realized through the loading procedure which resumes ER structures and constraints in the destination. Since domain templates provide a standardized and stabilized data inventory, loading procedures can be highly automated between domain templates and the target schema.

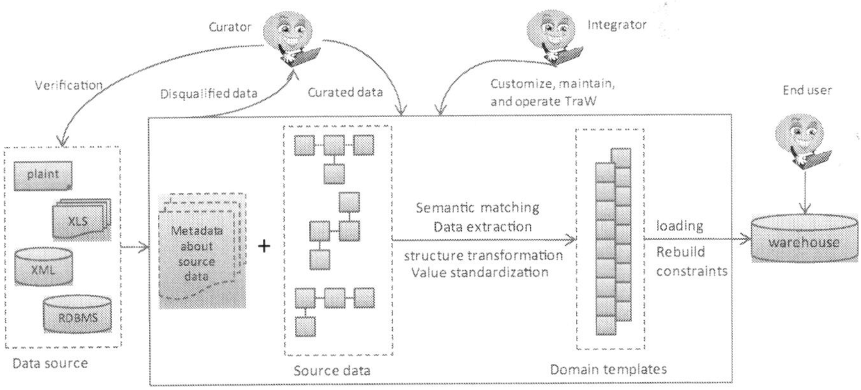

Fig. 6. Semi-automated TraW process

4.4 Information delivery

Evaluation of the success of the UNIFIN approach is assessed by its final products: personalized biomedical data and the applications that deliver these data. The quality of TraM data reflects the integration capacity of the TraM schema and efficiency of the TraW process and is measured by data uniformity, cleanness and integrity. A researcher who demands individualized cross-domain data (as described in the example in 2.1) should be able to query through the TraM application interface to obtain satisfactory information. Specifically, quality data should have the following features: 1) the same domain data should have consistent data elements (e.g., domain CDEs) and data descriptors; 2) all specimens, which are the linkage between clinical and basic science records, should be bar-coded and annotated with at minimum, the person's demographic information; 3) various domain data derived from the same person should be interlinked regardless of their disparate sources; 4) redundancies and discrepancies in the data are rigorously controlled at all hierarchical levels of schema and domains. Fig 7 displays some of these features of the TraM data in a breast cancer translational research account.

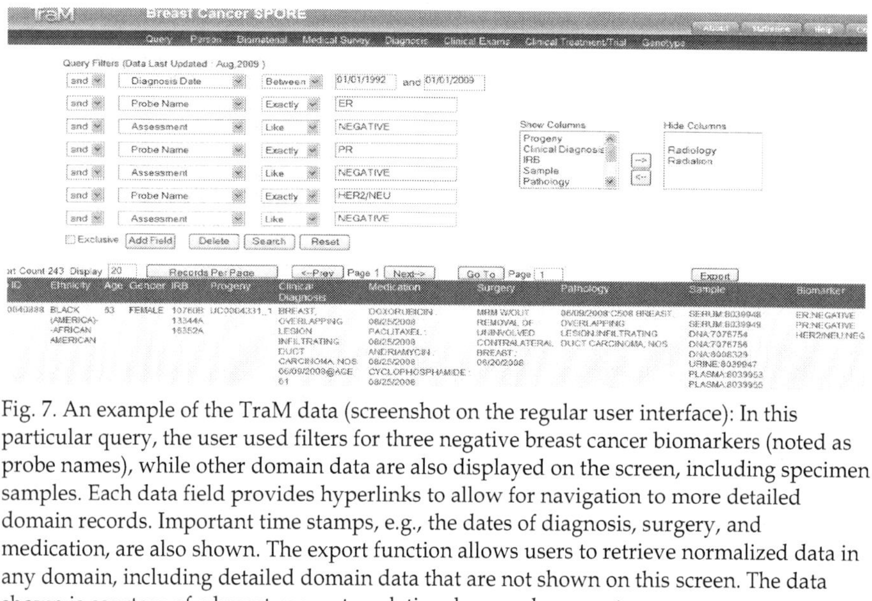

Fig. 7. An example of the TraM data (screenshot on the regular user interface): In this particular query, the user used filters for three negative breast cancer biomarkers (noted as probe names), while other domain data are also displayed on the screen, including specimen samples. Each data field provides hyperlinks to allow for navigation to more detailed domain records. Important time stamps, e.g., the dates of diagnosis, surgery, and medication, are also shown. The export function allows users to retrieve normalized data in any domain, including detailed domain data that are not shown on this screen. The data shown is courtesy of a breast cancer translational research account.

On average, when data are collected from more than 10 independent sources (batch data processing usually contains data from 10-30 disparate sources), around 50% of the distinct individual counts from these sources will be eliminated after data descriptor standardization and error correction, which means that about 50% of the person counts in the raw data are redundant because of heterogeneous descriptions and errors generated by humans in disparate sources. Furthermore, 50%-60% of source data elements do not match the target schema or among themselves because of semantic heterogeneity (detailed in section 3.3), which means that these elements need to go through a data structure transformation in order to retain the data carried by these elements. Although these simple statistics only reflect the situation of the ETL executed between our data sources and our particular target schema, it delivers a piece of important information: complicated data transformation and curation are required to achieve personalized biomedical data integrity in the real world.

For a biomedical data source that contains detailed patient data with records of time stamps, even de-identified, the data source usually is not freely accessible because of HIPAA concerns. Therefore, the application of the TraM data is quite different from a conventional biological data source in the way how data is accessed. First, the TraM data that contains healthcare administrative dates can only be viewed through project accounts. Each account usually contains at least one *institutional research board* (IRB) protocol (Fig 7). Researchers need to be approved by the same IRB protocol that patients have consented to in order to view the data within the account.

Under each project account, TraM offers four kinds of user interfaces and each allows a specified user role to access data with a uniquely defined privilege. 1) The role of account administrator has the highest privilege within an account and the person manages users within the account by assigning them different roles. 2) The role of curator has write privileges so the person can edit data even after the data have been loaded into the TraM system (Fig 5). 3) The role of power uses, usually a physician, under IRB approval, has privileges to view the patient's medical record number which is considered as PHI, but has no right to edit data. Finally 4) the role of regular user can view all de-identified TraM data (Fig 7). Although unlimited accounts are allowed to access the TraM data based on IRB protocols, there is only one copy of integrated data in the database. If the IRB protocols that a patient has consented to happen to be in different accounts, the patient's records will be shared by these accounts without duplicate records in database.

5. Discussions

Personalized biomedical data integration is a complicated and perpetual challenge in biomedical informatics. Simply utilizing a single method, technology, or system architecture may not solve all of the problems associated with the process. In comparison to the other software products available in this line of work, the focus of UNIFIN is on data processing for integration, a goal that the system has achieved utilizing current real-world data. The architecture of UNIFIN is supported by a highly abstracted data modelling strategy which provides a solid foundation to be modified, extended, and improved for future and presumably improved source data environments without altering its backbone structure. Issues related to UNIFIN are the following:

Ad hoc versus sustainable solutions: Personalized biomedical data integration is on the frontier of scientific challenges on a day-to-day basis. Rapidly evolving research has forced many to adopt ad hoc data capture solutions to keep the records. These solutions usually capture data in as-is formats and the data, along with its descriptors, are not synthesized with concept abstraction, semantic normalization and vocabulary standardization. Some ad hoc approaches are unavoidable, especially when users who create ad hoc data are not computer professionals. However, we believe that the ad hoc solutions should be limited to raw data capture but not be promoted for multiple source data integration or integrated data management. Considering the cost, scope, and endeavour of a warehousing project, making an effort up front in the design stage to separate data concepts (variable carriers) from data values (instance data) will be rewarded with long term software architecture stability and function flexibility. A software product produced with such planning should be suitable to ad-hoc events and sustainable in a constantly evolving data source environment. Here, sustainability does not mean that software is static and does not need to be modified. Instead, it means that if required, software can be modified at minimal cost to gain a significant improvement in capacity.

Reuse and impact of human efforts: TraW is a workflow that requires human-intervention. The products of human intervention are data mapping references and domain ontologies. After about three years of effort, we have reduced the time needed for a life-cycle of data processing of the same scope of data from several months to a few weeks while gaining much improved quality consistency in the final product. Yet, one of the major reasons for us not able to further significantly reduce the ETL time at present is semantic heterogeneity of source data and high modification frequency of data sources (minimal 3 times a year in some major data sources). These changes often require human cognitive attention to validate data matching, mapping, and transformation processes. In some cases (e.g., source data elements designed with implied or multiple overloaded meanings) off-line human research is required to form a data processing solution before proceeding. Therefore, it is important to design and maintain these mapping references to make the human-intensive products computable, so that they can be reused in data processing with a high-throughput manner. When these mapping references become more sophisticated, improved automation should be possible. At the current stage, the need of human intervention reveals a major limitation of the UNIFIN approach: TraW needs to be operated by experts in biomedical informatics, which not only slows down a process that was intended to be streamlined, but also has the potential to produce data with uneven quality due to the uncertainty of human behaviour.

Position and contribution of warehousing solution in a biomedical data space: If there is a spectrum for data integration strategies based on their product integrity, warehousing solution appears to fall at the top of the spectrum as the most integrated while mashup at a position of less integrated. However, the two can be successfully interlinked when individualized studies need to be transformed into population studies, e.g., medical census. UNIFIN-like approaches will potentially become conduits that allow for significant amounts of information mashup by providing standardized quality data. In order to form a harmonized ecosystem in the data-space, warehouse data sources need to work towards using interchangeable domain ontologies and CDEs to process data and making these data available for interoperable sharing. If this does not occur, the sprawling warehouses, which usually collect regional biomedical data, may contribute to yet another layer of data heterogeneity.

6. Conclusion

We have created and tested a warehousing framework consisting of a unique database conceptual model and a systematically adjusted and enhanced ETL workflow for personalized biomedical data integration. The result is a real-world tested solution that is capable of consistently and efficiently unifying data from multiple sources for integration and delivering consumable information for use by translational researchers. The UNIFIN is a work-in-progress in the field that demands new knowledge and innovative solutions to this line of work.

7. References

Agrawal, R., A. Ailamaki, et al. (2009). The Claremont report on database research. *Commun. ACM* 52(6): 56-65.

Batini, C., M. Lenzerini, et al. (1986). A comparative analysis of methodologies for database schema integration. *ACM Comput. Surv.* 18(4): 323-364.

Bernstam, E. V., J. W. Smith, et al. (2010). What is biomedical informatics? *J Biomed Inform* 43(1): 104-110.

Bernstein, A. P. and E. Rahm (2001). A survey of approaches to automatic schema matching. *The VLCB Journal* 10: 334-350.

Bernstein, P. A. and L. M. Haas (2008). Information integration in the enterprise. *Commun. ACM* 51(9): 72-79.

Bodenreider, O. (2004). The Unified Medical Language System (UMLS): integrating biomedical terminology. *Nucleic Acids Res* 32(Database issue): D267-70.

Brazhnik, O. and J. F. Jones (2007). Anatomy of data integration. *J Biomed Inform* 40(3): 252-69.

Butler, D. (2006). Mashups mix data into global service. *Nature* 439: 6-7.

Chen, P. (1976). The entity-relationship model-toward a unified view of data. *ACM Traslation on Database Systems* 1(1): 9-36.

Cimino, J. J. (1996). Review paper: coding systems in health care. *Methods Inf Med* 35(4-5): 273-84.

Cimino, J. J., T. F. Hayamizu, et al. (2009). The caBIG terminology review process. *J Biomed Inform* 42(3): 571-580.

Cochrane, G. R. and M. Y. Galperin (2010). The 2010 Nucleic Acids Research Database Issue and online Database Collection: a community of data resources. *Nucleic Acids Res 38(Database issue): D1-4.*

Cote, R. A. and S. Robboy (1980). Progress in medical information management. Systematized nomenclature of medicine (SNOMED). *JAMA* 243(8): 756-62.

Dinu, V. and P. Nadkarni (2007). Guidelines for the effective use of entity-attribute-value modeling for biomedical databases. *Int J Med Inform* 76(11-12): 769-79.

Edge, S. B., D. R. Byrd, et al., Eds. (2010). *AJCC Cancer Staging Handbook.* 7th Edition, Springer.

Faddick, C. M. (1997). Health care fraud and abuse: new weapons, new penalties, and new fears for providers created by the Health Insurance Portability and Accountability Act of 1996 (HIPAA). *Ann Health Law* 6: 77-104.

Fielding, R. T. and R. N. Taylor (2002). Principled Design of the Modern Web Architecture. ACM Transactions on Internet Technology 2 (2): 115-150.

Franklin, M., A. Halevy, et al. (2005). From databases to dataspaces: a new abstraction for information management. *SIGMOD Rec.* 34(4): 27-33.

Galperin, M. Y. and G. R. Cochrane (2009). Nucleic Acids Research annual Database Issue and the NAR online Molecular Biology Database Collection in 2009. *Nucleic Acids Res* 37(Database issue): D1-4.

Goble, C. and R. Stevens (2008). State of the nation in data integration for bioinformatics. J *Biomed Inform* 41(5): 687-93.

Goble, C., R. Stevens, et al. (2008). Data curation + process curation=data integration + science. *Brief Bioinform* 9(6): 506-517.

Guimerà, R., B. Uzzi, et al. (2005). Team assembly mechanisms determine collaboration network structure and team performance. *Science* 308: 697-702.

Halevy, A. Y. (2001). Answering queries using views: A survey. *The VLDB Journal* 10(4): 270-294.

Halevy, A. Y., N. Ashish, et al. (2005). Enterprise Information Integration: Successes, Challenges and Controversies. *SIGMOD '05* June: 778-787.

Horig, H., E. Marincola, et al. (2005). Obstacles and opportunities in translational research. Nat Med 11(7): 705-8.

Jhingran, A. (2006). Enterprise information mashups: integrating information, simply. *Proceedings of the 32nd international conference on Very large data bases.* Seoul, Korea, VLDB Endowment: 3-4.

Kalashnikov, D. V. and S. Mehrotra (2006). Domain-independent data cleaning via analysis of entity-relationship graph. *ACM Trans. Database Syst.* 31(2): 716-767.

Kamble, A. S. (2008). A conceptual model for multidimensional data. *Proceedings of the fifth on Asia-Pacific conference on conceptual modelling - Volume 79.* Wollongong, NSW, Australia, Australian Computer Society, Inc.

Kimball, R., L. Reeves, et al. (1998). *The Data Warehouse Lifecycle Toolkit: Expert Methods for Designing, Developing and Deploying Data Warehouses* with CD Rom, John Wiley & amp; Sons, Inc.

Kolaitis, P. G. (2005). Schema mappings, data exchange, and metadata management. *Proceedings of the twenty-fourth ACM SIGMOD-SIGACT-SIGART symposium on Principles of database systems.* Baltimore, Maryland, ACM: 61-75.

Lenzerini, M. (2002). Data Integration: A Theoretical Perspective. ACM PODS June: 233-246.

Louie, B., P. Mork, et al. (2007). Data integration and genomic medicine. *J Biomed Inform* 40(1): 5-16.

Lowe, H. J., T. A. Ferris, et al. (2009). STRIDE--An integrated standards-based translational research informatics platform. *AMIA Annu Symp Proc* 2009(5): 391-5.

Rizzi, S., A. Abello, et al. (2006). Research in Data Warehouse Modeling and Design: Dead or Alive? *DOLAP'06* November 10, 2006: 3-10.

Sioutos, N., S. de Coronado, et al. (2007). NCI Thesaurus: a semantic model integrating cancer-related clinical and molecular information. *J Biomed Inform* 40(1): 30-43.

Stein, L. (2002). Creating a bioinformatics nation. *Nature* 417(6885): 119-20.

Stein, L. D. (2008). Towards a cyberinfrastructure for the biological sciences: progress, visions and challenges. *Nat Rev Genet* 9(9): 678-88.

Trujillo, J., M. Palomar, et al. (2001). Designing Data Warehouses with OO Conceptual Models. *Computer* 34(12): 66-75.

Vassiliadis, P., A. Simitsis, et al. (2002). Conceptual modeling for ETL processes. *Proceedings of the 5th ACM international workshop on Data Warehousing and OLAP.* McLean, Virginia, USA, ACM: 14-21.

Wang, X., L. Liu, et al. (2009). Translational integrity and continuity: Personalized biomedical data integration. *J Biomed Inform* Feb;42(1): 100-12.

Wong, J. and J. I. Hong (2007). Making mashups with marmite: towards end-user programming for the web. *Proceedings of the SIGCHI conference on Human factors in computing systems.* San Jose, California, USA, ACM.

Yu, A. C. (2006). Methods in biomedical ontology. *J Biomed Inform* 39(3): 252-66.

35

Smart Data Collection and Management in Heterogeneous Ubiquitous Healthcare

Luca Catarinucci, Alessandra Esposito, Luciano Tarricone, Marco Zappatore and Riccardo Colella
University of Salento, Italy

1. Introduction

The increasing availability of network connection and the progress in information technology and in hardware miniaturization techniques, are determining new computing scenarios, where software applications are able to "configure themselves" based on information coming from heterogeneous sources (sensors, RFID, GPS, databases, user input, etc.) which form the so called "context". In other terms, such applications are based on the representation and codification of different kinds of data, such as biomedical parameters, environmental data, device location, user preferences, resource availability, every time, from every location and through different modalities (pervasiveness), and on the provision of services and contents adapted to current context (context-awareness). Such computing scenarios find application in a large number of real-life domains, as environment monitoring, supply-chain management and so on. Health-care is perhaps one of the most relevant and promising. Indeed, the perspectives opened by such technologies are wide and variegate: they range from the home-care of mobility-impaired people to the harmonization and presentation to hospital workers of information gathered from distributed heterogeneous sources.

The implementation of context-aware systems is based on two distinct but strongly interlaced tasks: 1) monitoring and collection of sensorial data, with the related issues concerning data transmission, costs, enabling technologies as well as the heterogeneity and the number of data to be collected 2) processing and integration of data with available context information in order to activate decision processes which are in many cases not trivial.

Key points are the selection of the enabling technologies for the collection, transmission and smart management of data gathered from heterogeneous sources, and the design of a system architecture having the following characteristics:

a. simple to use;
b. low-cost and low-power consumption in order to make possible the implementation of systems with a high number of nodes;
c. interoperable with any type of sensors;
d. customizable to different kinds of application domains with a limited effort;
e. scalable with the number of nodes;

f. suitable response times so to be adopted also in emergency situations.

Based on the above considerations, we developed a cost-effective RFID-based device for the monitoring and collection of sensorial data, and a pervasive and context-oriented system which operates on sensor data and is based on an innovative, flexible and versatile framework. The description of the RFID device and of the software framework is provided in this chapter, which starts with an introduction to potential applications for healthcare and to emerging techniques for both data collection and smart data management, and concludes with the validation of both hardware and software solutions in the real-life use-case of patient remote assistance.

2. Potential applications

This paragraph proposes an overview of the possible applications of emerging technologies for data sensing, gathering and smart data elaboration with a special focus to the healthcare domain. We partition applications into four groups, even though some overlapping between such groups exist.

2.1 Knowledge sharing, availability and integration

Management and delivery of healthcare is critically dependent on access to data. Such data are normally provided by several heterogeneous sources, such as physiological sensors, imaging technology or even handwriting and often spans different organisations. Moreover they are generally stored by using different formats and terminologies, such as electronic health records, clinical databases, or free-text reports. If such a rich collection of health and community data could be linked together, we would improve enormously our capability of finding answers to health and social questions and of tackling complex diseases (Walker, 2005). Unfortunately, sharing such a complex aggregate of information and deriving useful knowledge from it is currently very difficult.

A very promising answer to this need is provided by the enabling technologies for smart data collection and management which are named "ontologies" [Section 3.4]. Ontologies define a formal semantically rich machine-readable specification of concepts and relationships which is unique and sharable among dispersed consumers. They provide coherent representations of biomedical reality thus enabling wide-area multi-organizational sharing of data by supporting publishing, retrieving and analysis of data in large-scale, diverse and distributed information systems.

Moreover, when integrated with other enabling technologies (such as those listed in Section 3.3 and 3.5) ontologies allow the identification of the correct information to be forwarded to health care professional depending on available information about context, such as time, place, patient current state, physiological data, and so on.

2.2 Independent living

The combination of sensors, RFID, wireless protocols and software solutions, is going to enhance aging population and impaired people capability of conducting a possibly *autonomous independent living*. Indeed, pervasive and context-aware applications are more and more recognized as promising solutions for providing continuous care services, while improving quality of life of people suffering from chronic conditions.

Support to independent living encompasses a wide range of applications ranging from the telemonitoring of vital parameters to scenarios involving home automation and domotics. In the former case (Paganelli, 2007), the system allows chronic patients, such as epileptics or persons with *chronic* mental illness, to conduct a substantially normal life as it makes a continuous measurement of vital data and/or of the activities of daily living and social interactions. An immediate assistance is provided in emergency situations, when patients may be unconscious and unable to react. Indeed, the system is able to autonomously alert the best suited care giver and to forward her/him a meaningful synthesis of real-time (e.g. physiological data) and static data (e.g. historical patient information).

Smart homes (SM4ALL, 2010), instead, consist in homes augmented with networked sensors, communicating objects, and information appliances. Ambient sensors acquire information about the home environment, body near sensors acquire information about the habitant. The combination of these sensors enables the creation of activity profiles which allow the constant monitoring of patient daily life. Also in these cases, adverse events are recognized by the system ("the habitant leaves the home while the cooker is still switched on", or "the patient has a fall") and specific assistance is quickly provided.

2.3 Tracking

The capability to trace, localize and identify a large number of heterogeneous objects in a complex and dynamic environment is essential in many sectors, including the healthcare one (Bacheldor, 2008, 2009), (Swedberg, 2010). Moreover, the widespread diffusion of the object/people to be traced, forces the use of flexible, easy to use and inexpensive technologies. Such requirements are typical of RFID systems. The joint use of RFID tags and smart software infrastructures in identification badges for health care professionals, patients, and fixed assets, therefore, is more and more gaining momentum. Thanks to these technologies, physicians and nurses are tracked in real-time or near real-time, and contacted in case of emergencies, whilst specific medical devices, such as multi-channel infusion pumps, are associated with patients.

Tracking is also of utmost importance to control drug dispensation and laboratory results. Medical dosages and patient samples are validated, together with blood supplies and blood type matching.

In the pharmaceutical supply chain, where security and safety are required to prevent compromising the health of patients, smart labels and sensors are fundamental. Smart labels are attached to drugs, in order to track them through the overall supply chain. Sensors continuously monitor the status of items requiring specific storage conditions and discard them if such conditions are violated. Drug tracking and e-pedigrees also support the detection of counterfeit products and for keeping the supply chain free of fraudsters.

The smart labels on the drugs can also directly benefit patients in several manners, e.g. by storing the package insert, informing consumers of dosages and expiration date, by reminding patients to take their medicine at appropriate intervals and monitoring patient compliance, etc...

2.4 Smart hospitals

With the ability of capturing fine grained data pervasively, wireless sensors and RFID tags have numerous available and potential applications in hospitals (Wang, 2006). The quality

of patient care at the bedside is improved and errors reduced. This is accomplished by integrating the physical process of care delivery with medication information and software applications that provide clinical decision support, and quality and safety checks.
Without such systems, healthcare providers traditionally use a paper-based "flow chart" to store patient information during registration time, which is updated by different professionals and forwarded to the incoming staff at the end of each shift. As a result the paper report is not always accurate. RFIDs allow for transmitting and receiving data from patient to health professionals without human intervention. RFID wristbands are used to identify patients during the entire hospitalization period. They are used to store patient data (such as name, patient ID, drug allergies, blood group, and so on) in order to constantly keep staff informed. Medical professionals can easy access and update patient's records remotely via Wi-Fi connection using mobile devices.

3. Emerging technologies

Pervasive platforms derive from the merging of several technologies which recently had an impressive improvement, such as wireless communications and networking, mobile computing and handheld devices, embedded systems, etc.
As a result, a review of the emerging technologies which enable the development of pervasive systems may reveal a hard and tedious task. The focus of this section is therefore restricted on a subset of such technologies. We substantially concentrate on the technologies which will be cited in the course of the chapter and which we believe actually constitute, and will probably still constitute in the future, the core of pervasive context-aware systems.
Computing environments are inherently distributed and heterogeneous. They are made of components which can be mobile, embedded in everyday objects or in general hidden in the infrastructure surrounding the user (Weiser, 1991). The context data to be computed must be collected by spread, inexpensive and easy to use data collectors. Those based on the *RFID technology* (Section 3.1) guarantee both identification and localization. The *integration of sensors on traditional RFID tags* (Section 3.2) assure also the interaction with other physical values, mandatory for a realistic context reconstruction. Such heterogeneous and dispersed components have different requirements and capabilities and are expected to interact continuously and in a transparent manner.
"Interaction" and "transparency" in a "distributed" environment are well supported by the so-called *multi-agent paradigms*, which, as explained in Section 3.3, organize applications around the coordinated interaction of autonomous reasoning software entities, which wrap the "natural" components of the distributed system.
Pervasive systems must also exhibit some intelligent behavior in terms of context awareness, i.e. their components must be able to coordinate with one another in order to recognize and react aptly to environment modifications. "Coordination" and "reasoning" require a high level of (semantic) interoperability, i.e. the availability of a shared and agreed knowledge layer upon which agents base their inferences and cooperation.
For this purpose, *ontologies* (Section 3.4) and *rule based logic* (Section 3.5) seem the best combination of technologies for enabling knowledge representation and reasoning, the former provide a sharable, reusable model of reality, the latter efficiently support inferencing and event recognition.

3.1 RFID

Radio frequency identification is one of the emerging technologies that is having the most capillary diffusion, thanks to its low cost, its easiness and the very large number of applications where it can be crucial.

RFID can be seen as the enhanced version of the union between radio frequency (RF) anti-theft systems and bar codes.

RF anti-theft systems are based on passive devices, called tags, essentially constituted by a spiral antenna in parallel to a capacitor. If a tag is exposed to a certain electromagnetic field, such as those generated by the RF gates at the shop exits, the spiral antenna receives enough power to charge the capacitor. Once the capacitor discharges, a new signal is transmitted through the spiral antenna and received by the RF gate, generating the alert.

As well known, vice versa, a barcode is a series of bars and spaces through which information is encoded. The reading is then delegated to optical scanners which, however, work only a few centimetres away and only in line-of-sight condition.

RFID technology, therefore, combines the capability of barcodes to transmit complex information with the peculiarity of responding only when interrogated through a proper RF signal, characterizing passive anti-theft systems.

Substantially, if a book marked with an RF anti-theft tag passes through a RF gate, a nonspecific alert is generated (telling us that something has been stolen). A more detailed information about the book can be obtained only by reading its barcode through an optical scanner. When the same book is marked with an RFID tag, we can know which book is passing through the gate in terms of title, author, cost, number of pages, inventory number and so on. It is apparent, though, how this sophisticated anti-theft system is only one of the most simple applications which can take undeniable advantage from an RFID-based implementation.

A generic RFID system is, hence, mainly based on two entities: on one side there are the tags, which store in a microchip information in terms of electronic product code (EPC), and can receive and transmit signals by means of an aluminium or copper antenna. On the other side there are the readers and the reader antennas, which emit electromagnetic signals and wait for an answer. When a tag is in the region covered by a reader antenna, the tag microchip is powered and a signal containing the EPC, is sent back towards the reader antennas. The reader decodes such an identifier code (ID), telling a middleware system that a specific tag has been read by a certain reader antenna. In Fig.1 a schematization of an RFID system is reported.

The reasons for the spread diffusion of RFID technology, however, is not to be found in its working principle, but rather in its cost and its ease of use. The mere wireless transmission of an ID under certain electromagnetic solicitations, in fact, does not hide any particular technological impediment. On the contrary, the capability of using passive devices, which do not require maintenance and cost a few cents, is a peculiarity of RFID tags.

This promises a widespread use, for instance, also in applications where the cost should remain affordable and reusability is not guaranteed.

A comprehensive classification of the RFID technology in terms of working frequency, maximum working distance, tag powering method, cost, sensitivity, storage capacity etc., is certainly possible but is beyond the scope of this chapter. The interested reader is addressed to (Dobkin, 2007) for such a goal.

On the contrary, it is worth highlighting that, among the others, passive RFID systems in the ultra high frequency (UHF) band are those that provide the wider perspectives of applications.

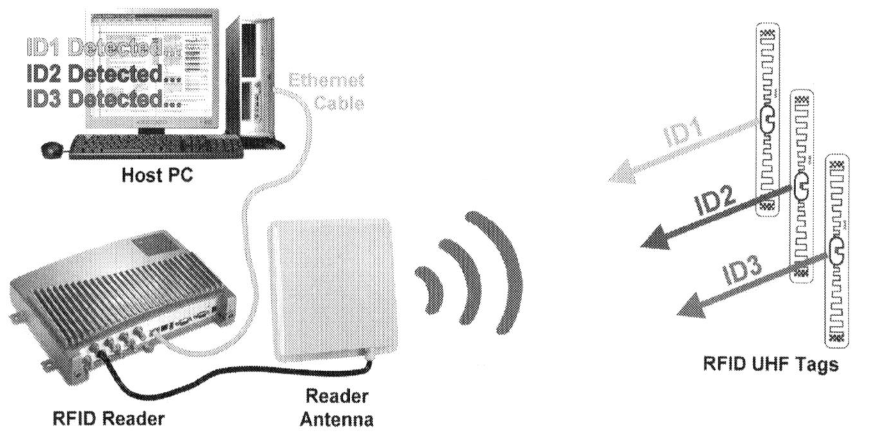

Fig. 1. Schematization of an RFID System

Their work frequency varies accordingly to individual state regulations; it ranges from a minimum of 860 MHz, for instance in Europe, to a maximum of 960 MHz, in Japan, via the 915 MHz of the United States (Dobkin, 2007). In Fig. 2 a prototype of a home-made UHF passive tag is shown. Both chip and antennas are clearly visible in the figure. RFID tags are generally bonded to a polyethylene terephthalate (PET) layer, which can be adhesive or dry. The prototype of Fig.2, on the contrary, is realized by cutting an adhesive sheet of copper by using a numerically controlled cutting plotter.

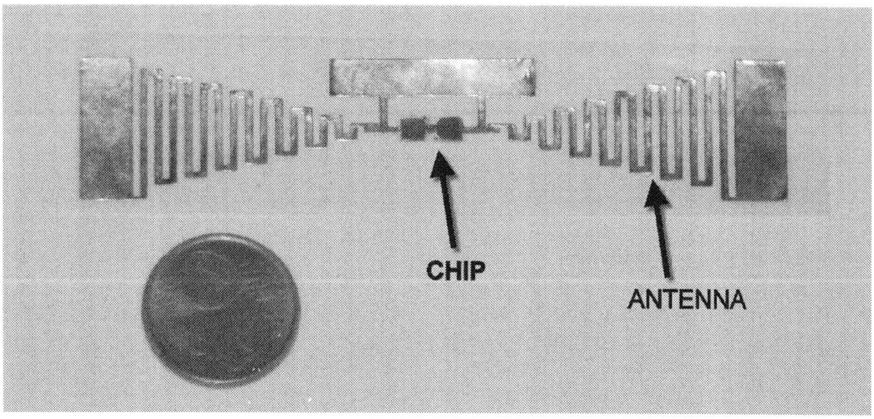

Fig. 2. Home-made prototype of a UHF RFID Tag

Although the apparent simplicity of the tag, it is important to stress that the antenna design plays a very crucial role. The chip exhibits a strong capacitive contribution, so that a conjugate matching technique, guaranteeing the maximum power transfer between chip and antenna, must be applied. Moreover, the need of a reduced size forces the use of miniaturization techniques (Dobkin, 2007). A well designed antenna guarantees reading range up to 9 m, good enough to support the use of this technology in many applications based on auto-identification. Vice versa, when an application needs the management of more complex data, such as physical values representing the context around the tag, an integration between RFID and sensors is mandatory.

3.2 RFID and sensor integration

An evolution of RFID technology is represented by its integration with sensors, so that, along with the ID code, also the value measured by the sensor is sent towards the reader. In such a way, the collection and management of heterogeneous data, similarly to canonical wireless sensor networks, is made possible, with some advances in terms of benefit/cost ratio.

Indeed, many different wireless technologies are mature for the transmission of data measured by generic sensors, much more than the inexpensive RFID. Compared with RFID technology, Wi-fi, Bluetooth, GPRS, UMTS and GSM guarantee wider transmission distances, higher bit-rates as well as larger amount of exchangeable data. Unluckily, the benefit/cost ratio of such technologies, depending on the target application, is often not so appropriate. Therefore, when a capillary diffusion of physical sources is needed, a cheaper wireless technology is desirable. Moreover, the easy interfaceability with Internet could be another added value.

So far, the integration of wireless sensor networks with RFID-based sensor systems appears to be the most practicable way. UHF RFID technology, in fact, is quite inexpensive (passive RFID tags are as cheap as few euro-cents). It is also naturally compatible with Internet, and provides a reading range adequate for many applications. It is worth mentioning that some UHF RFID tags with embedded sensors of temperature or of pressure are already available on the market (Cho et al., 2005), being often inexpensive and rather accurate. Nevertheless the study of general purpose devices that support the integration of RFID and generic sensors, independently of the size and of the cost of the sensor itself, seems to be the new tendency.

Furthermore, the ability to gather in an easy and low-cost way a large amount of identification and context data, paves the way to the solution of ambitious problems that require the smart management of data. For such a goal, though, it is necessary to complement this hardware resources with new adequate software technologies, able to smartly support the decision-making processes.

3.3 Software agents

Software agents (Bradshaw, 1997) are (semi)autonomous programs which represent objects from the real world, such as persons, devices and services. Real entities delegate to agents the capabilities which are requested by ubiquitous context-aware systems, such as the interaction with the environment and with other entities (i.e. agents).

Agents are autonomous, i.e. they are distinct entities, separated, in some sense, from the world in which they exist. They are able to correctly operate with little or no direct human input or supervision, and have control of their internal state and behavior.

Agents interaction with the environment happens in a both reactive and proactive manner. Reactivity means that the agent is able to acquire information about the operating environment - through sensors, messages or interaction with humans - and adapt to perceived changes. Pro-activity means that the agent has a number of goals and is able to take the initiative to realize them.

Agent-based systems are used in many situations. For instance, they are worth to be adopted when the knowledge required to solve a given problem is spatially distributed, when different computational entities must cooperate to reach a common goal and when a given task can be subdivided in autonomous sub-tasks. Many problems in the healthcare domain have such features: knowledge is usually distributed in different physical locations; medical problem solving strategies quite always require collaboration between different healthcare operators, structures and devices; finally medical procedures are complex and are suited to be partitioned into different sub-tasks.

According to Nealon and Moreno (Moreno, 2003) the healthcare domain is a "vast open environment, characterised by shared and distributed decision making and management... requiring the communication of complex and different forms of information between a variety of clinical and other settings, as well as the coordination between groups of healthcare professionals with very different skills and roles". As agents may tackle distributed problems, are able to communicate among each other, can partition complex problems in sub-problems, take decision autonomously and provide information to end users reactively and proactively, they represent a good choice in the healthcare domain. As a result, agents-based systems are currently used in a wide series of medical-related problems (Moreno, 2003): patient scheduling, organ and tissue transplant management, community care, information access, decision support systems, home healthcare monitoring, medicine and device management, healthcare operators scheduling.

Agents coordinate and exchange information, have a representation of their goals, and determine their course of action on the basis of a model of the environment which is shared with other agents. As explained below, ontologies are actually recognized as the best instrument for defining such a model.

3.4 Ontologies

The advent of ontologies (Gruber, 1995) in computer science in the early nineties and the current effort in their settlement and development is making the "semantic interoperability dream" come true, i.e. ontologies are more and more recognized as the best suited instrument to harmonize complex and different sources of information and to get meaningful knowledge from them.

Ontology is the branch of philosophy that provides a formal foundation for specifying, and making statements about, what exists and how the things that exist are related to each other. In computer science ontologies are used to describe the logical structure of a specified domain of interest, its concepts and the relations among them, and to present them in an explicit and standardized way.

In order to encode knowledge in the form of an ontology an appropriate language must be used. The most recent emerging standard proposed by W3C is the so called Web Ontology Language (OWL) (W3C OWL, 2005). OWL represents reality as a set of classes, properties and instances. Classes stand for the concepts which must be encoded; instances are the concrete individuals populating classes, whilst properties (relationships) assert general facts about the members of classes and/or about individuals. OWL provides also a certain number of operators (*constructors and restrictions*) for expressing complex concepts, constraints and dependencies which reflect the human model of reality.

An important feature of ontologies is that they can be processed by a reasoner, i.e. by a software tool able to extract new knowledge implied by explicitly codified knowledge. This is very interesting for context aware computing. A simple example of reasoning can be given by the exploitation of "transitive relations", which are supported by OWL. Given three entities, such relations bring the conclusion of the existence of a relation between the first and third entity, when a relation between the first and second and between the second and third occurs. For example, the 'locatedIn' relation between an 'Entity' and a 'Location' is commonly marked as "transitive". As a result, if a user is 'locatedIn' the room 'Bedroom', which is in turn 'locatedIn' the 'Home', then the reasoner concludes that the user is located in 'Home'.

Indeed, context-aware systems require more advanced reasoning mechanisms. They are expected to be able to derive higher-level, conceptual context, such as "what the user is doing" from relevant low-level context, such as "the door is moving", which is provided by context sensing. This is the reason why ontologies are normally accompanied by rule based systems.

3.5 Rule based logic

Rule-based logic (Partridge, 1994) is an expressive way to define situations. Rule-based systems (RBS) differ from standard procedural or object-oriented programs as they do not clearly define the order in which code executes. Their behaviour is embedded in a set of *rules*, each of which encodes a small piece of codified knowledge and can be executed according to the current content of the so-called *working memory* (or agenda). The working memory stores the so-called *facts*, which represent the factual knowledge of the RBS.

Rules are similar to traditional if-then-else statements, but, differently from them, they are not executed in any predetermined order. They have a left hand side (the *if* part) and a right hand side (the *then* component). The left hand side contains information about facts and *objects* which must be true in order for the rule to potentially fire (i.e. execute).

The process of firing rules is carried out by the so-called rule engine (or *inference engine*): a program (interpreter) that performs iteratively the so-called *Match-Resolve-Act* (MRA) cycle over the rule set and the working memory. In a MRA cycle, at any given time, rules are activated by matching them against the working memory elements (Match phase); then activated rules are chosen for execution according to some selection strategy (Resolve phase) and finally executed (Act or firing phase). In the Act phase, facts can be modified or deleted, and new facts can be added to the working memory as well.

In synthesis, RBSs select and execute available rules according to the current context they perceive. This makes RBSs particularly suitable for implementing context-aware architectures that must be modular and easily extensible: facts contain a symbolic and declarative description of a current situation and the rule set puts in relationship context conditions and devices' behavior and actions.

4. A real-life application: a context-aware infrastructure based on RFID sensor tags

4.1 Introduction

In this section, we propose a framework for context-aware pervasive systems built around the above mentioned technologies: RFID, sensors, ontology representation, multi-agent paradigm and rule-based logic.

The section is organized as follows. Section 4.2 introduces the general-purpose framework and its prototypal implementation. Section 4.3 synthesizes system implementation choices. Sections 4.4, 4.5 and 4.6 are centred around context modelling. First the ontology representation, then the rule-based reasoning are illustrated. Section 4.7 focuses on data collection strategies. It describes "S-tag", a novel low cost device enabling the integration of sensor networks with RFID systems. A home-health scenario in the "emergency management" domain is finally provided in Section 4.8 as specific example of application and practical result.

4.2 The Architecture

The architecture of our system (Fig. 3) follows a widely accepted abstraction (Indulska, 2003) according to which context-aware systems are organized into three layers: context sources, context management middleware and context consumer level.

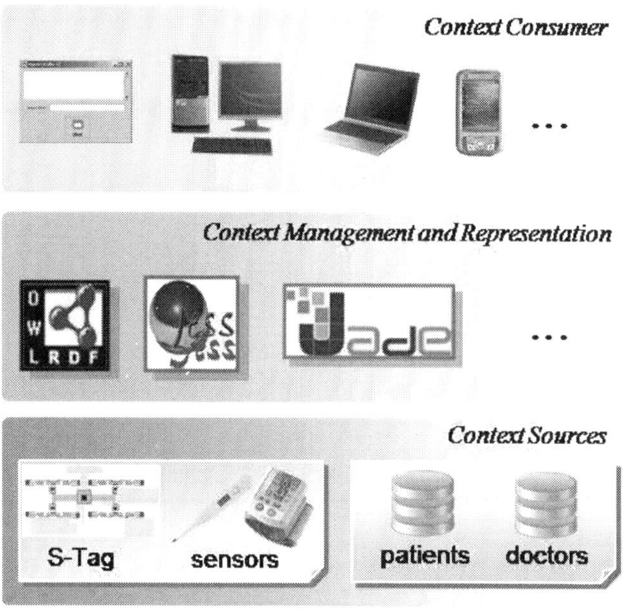

Fig. 3. Layered system architecture

Context sources include entities providing raw context data. They are conceptually partitioned into two groups: physical and virtual sources (Strang, 2004). Physical sources include hardware devices able to sense context data, such as RFID, sensors, positioning systems, etc. Virtual sources include software services able to gather context data, such as GUIs for user preferences input, databases, etc. Such data must be elaborated in an "intelligent" manner, so that the overall system reacts properly to context changes. This requires the availability of a machine-interpretable representation of context and of software components (*agents*) able to suitably process such knowledge. Both of them are conceptually situated at the intermediate level of the system architecture, the so-called middleware layer, as they provide the core building blocks of a context-aware application. Agents interoperate with one another thanks to the availability of a unified model of reality. Their behaviour is strongly influenced by data provided by context sources and substantially determines the activities to be performed at the highest layer. Indeed, the context consumer layer includes all the entities, such as mobiles, Web interfaces, laptops, which interact with final users in response to meaningful context changes, thus determining the behaviour of the context-aware application as a whole.

Fig. 4 shows the fundamental components of the prototypal implementation of the framework. The system core is a team of cooperating agents, which share an ontology-based knowledge representation and reason by means of a rule-based inference engine.

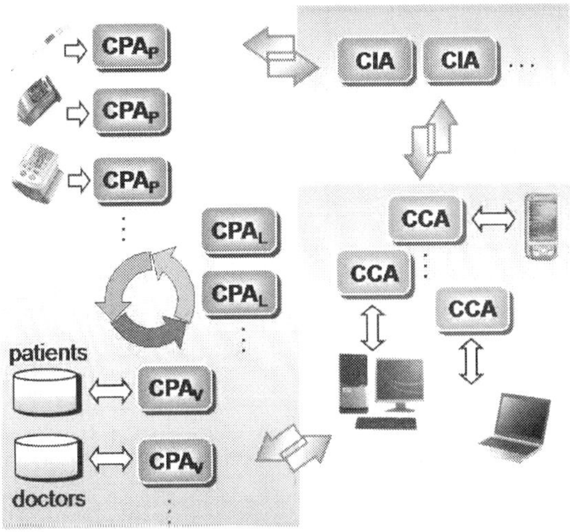

Fig. 4. The system follows a multi-agent paradigm and runs on distributed nodes connected by a local area network. Context Provider Agents (CPA) filter and integrate data provided by physical and virtual sensors. Context Interpreter Agents (CIA) identify the actions and the actors best suited for managing an emergency. Context Consumer Agents (CCA) perform the actions identified by CIAs

4.3 Implementation choices

Many ontology languages exist including Resource Description Framework Schema (RDFS) (W3C RDFS, 2004), DAML+OIL (DAML, 2010), and OWL (W3C OWL, 2005). OWL is a key to the Semantic Web and was proposed by the Web Ontology Working Group of W3C. It is much more expressive than other ontology languages such as RDFS. We chose OWL rather than DAML+OIL as the latter has been merged into OWL to become an open W3C standard. We took advantage of the Protégé (Protégé, 2010) graphical tool with the OWL plug-in and adopted Pellet (Pellet, 2010), a freeware, public domain ontology reasoner, to perform consistency checking.

The rule-based domain knowledge was implemented with Jess (Friedman-Hill, 2003) on top of OWL ontologies. Jess is a rule engine and scripting environment written in Java. Its rule engine uses the Rete algorithm (RETE, 2010) which has been shown to be fast and efficient especially for large data sets and it is widely used within a professional programmers' community.

Agents are implemented by using the Java Agent Development Environment (JADE).JADE (JADE, 2010) is a software framework to develop and run agent applications in compliance with the FIPA specifications (FIPA, 2010) for interoperable intelligent multi-agent systems. Inter-Agent communication is based on the FIPA ACL which specifies a standard message language by setting out the encoding, semantics and pragmatics of the messages.

The three technologies were glued together (Fig. 5) by taking advantage of a local adaptation of BeanGenerator (OntologyBeanGenerator, 2010), a Protégé plugin able to convert OWL codification into Java classes. As a result, the semantics of agent messages and their reasoning are built over OWL concepts and predicates, having been matched with Jess and JADE vocabulary (see next section).

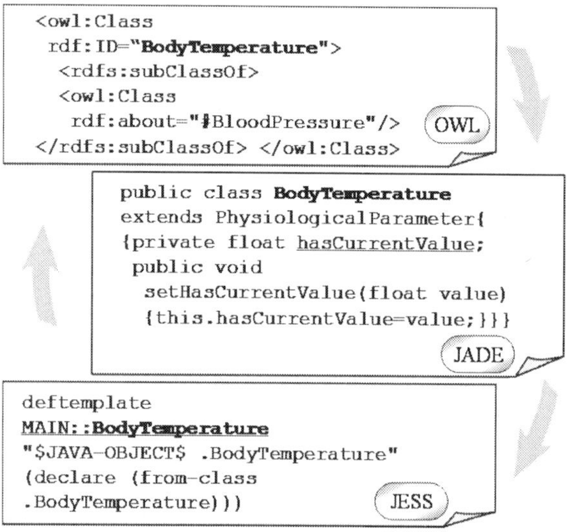

Fig. 5. The system implementation is based on the matching between OWL vocabulary with Jade agent inner context representation (in the form of Java classes) and Jess shadow facts codification

Finally, input data are provided by both physical and virtual context sources. Physical sources are obtained by integrating sensors with an RFID device (see Section 4.7), whilst virtual context sources consist in databases providing static information.

In the following sections, the system components and their way of functioning are described more in detail, with reference to a home-care giving scenario.

4.4 Context ontology

A common practise, when developing ontologies, is to adopt a *top level* (upper) shared conceptualization (Guarino, 1998) on top of which domain ontologies are built. Top level ontologies codify general terms which are independent of a particular problem or domain. Once the top level ontology is available, several *lower level* ontologies can be introduced, with the scope of incrementally specializing concepts from the high level generic point of view of the upper ontology to the low level practical point of view of the application. This way of structuring knowledge promotes sharing and reuse of ontologies in different application domains.

The hierarchical architecture of our ontology is organized into three levels (see Fig. 6, left side). Indeed, the ontology of our framework provides the knowledge representation upon which agents reason and exchange messages. Therefore, the top level concepts of our taxonomy contain terms useful for codifying the multi-agent environment, thus facilitating their interoperation. These concepts can be reused in any agent-based environment, independently from the application domain.

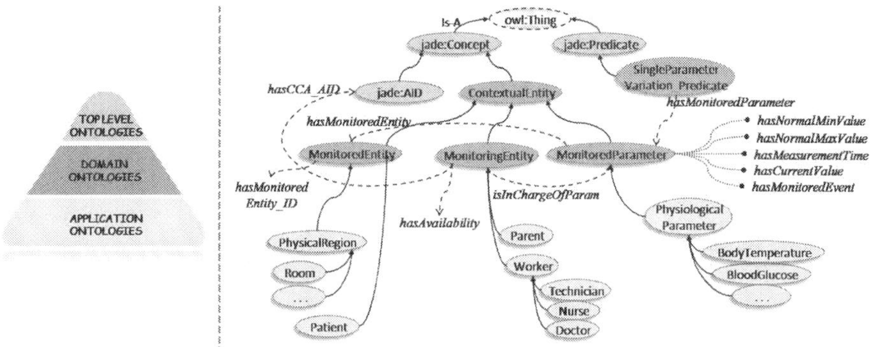

Fig. 6. A fragment (on the right) of the ontology, which is hierarchically structured in ontology modules (depicted on the left)

In order to fully exploit them in a context-aware system, a specialization is needed. In other terms, the context knowledge must be represented. This is done by implementing a "context middle level ontology" which specializes the top level ontology and codifies general concepts related to context. Terms specifically related to the application domain are introduced at the bottom level by making a further specialization. Some more details about the way our ontology is structured can be evinced by Fig. 6 (right side). Indeed, the top level ontology reflects the JADE codification of ACL message "slots", as represented in the publicly available ontology named "OWLSimpleJADEAbstractOntology" (JADE Tutorial, 2010). This ontology allows agents to give a semantics to message components. It makes a distinction between "predicates" and "terms". Predicates can assume "true" or "false" values and are used to describe the current status of codified entities (e.g. "*SingleParameterVariation_Predicate*"). Terms are specialized into "Agent Actions" (not depicted in Figure 4) and "Concepts" classes. Agent Actions codify the actions being performed by agents (such as "*NotifyAnomaly*"). Concepts are used to characterize the entities upon which predicates and actions operate (such as "*MonitoredParameter*", "*MonitoringParameter*", "*PhysicalRegion*", "*Worker*" and so on). Agents are themselves codified in the ontology by instantiating a suited subclass of the "Concepts" class, namely the "AID" class.

The vocabulary related to context entities was defined starting from the widely accepted definition of context, provided in (Dey, 1999): "Context is any information that can be used to characterize the situation of an entity." As a consequence, an entity is a person, place, computational entity, or object which is considered relevant for determining the behavior of an application. Moreover, in order to satisfy the ontology reusability requirement, the *"MonitoredEntity"*, *"MonitoredParameter"* and *"MonitoringEntity"* contextual entities have been introduced at domain level. On their turn, such entities specialize into different concepts depending on the context subdomain they belong to. For instance, a *"MonitoredEntity"* can be a patient, an object or an environment; a *"MonitoringEntity"* can be a relative of the patient or a health operator. Devices can be of different types as well.

4.5 Context rules

Jess rules are used to convert low-level information, given in a raw form by sensors, into high-level context. This is conceptually performed in an incremental fashion. When the system starts to work, the sensor network or other devices get data from physical world. Depending on the incoming events captured by sensors and context, the facts in the Jess *working memory* are updated. A set of rules determines if an alarm has to be triggered and which alarm level should be activated, according to measurement values and corresponding thresholds. Jess *rule engine* then searches automatically through the available combinations of facts to figure out which rules should be fired. Such rules, when matched, infer new facts which express the context switching to "situation of alarm". In other terms, the system acquires a sort of *anomaly awareness*, i.e. the raw data interpretation infers facts which express the occurrence of an anomaly.

In order to keep the system as general as possible (and easily customizable to different application scenarios) (Esposito, 2010), we adopted the so-called *normalized* rules (Williamson, 2010), i.e. rules that can be used in a variety of heterogeneous cases without changing their structure. For instance, rules concerning the identification of alarm events due to an anomaly behaviour of data provided by physical sensors have the same codification, independent from the specific monitored parameter.

The following example shows a rule activating an alarm when a parameter has a monitored value ("?par-c" variable) that exceeds the patient thresholds ("?par-max" and "?par-min" variables). When the rule is fired, the fact "Single Parameter Variation" ("?f-SPVp" variable) is inferred (as another predicate) and the action "notify that abnormal event" is activated ("send-single-alert" action). The "?pn" variable, finally, identifies the monitored parameter having generated the alarm.

```
(defrule verify-sensor-data
    ?f <- (SingleParameterMeasurement_Predicate
        (hasParamName ?pn)
        (hasParamCurrentVal ?par-c |: (> ?par-c ?par-max) |:
(< ?par-c ?par-min))
        (hasParamNormalMaxVal ?par-max)
        (hasParamNormalMinVal ?par-min)
        (hasParamMeasurementTime ?par-time))
      =>
; assert a Single Parameter Variation Predicate ?f-SPNp
      (send-single-alert ?f-SPVp))
```

The "anomaly awareness" facts may fire other rules, which may on their turn infer other facts. This determines the switching to the higher level context. In other terms, the context switches to a new situation, which we may call "procedure awareness", in which the activities to be performed in order to manage the alarm situation are known.

The following example shows how a rule is fired as a consequence of an abnormal status due to a couple of parameters. The rule infers the fact "Aggregated Parameter Variation" ("?f-APVp" variable) and starts the action "send-aggregate alert" in order to notify the anomaly to entities at a higher logical level.

```
(defrule aggregate-temporal-variations-for-2-params
 ?f0 <- (SingleParameterVariation_Predicate
         (hasParamName ?pn0)
         (hasParamMeasurementTime ?t0))
 ?f1 <- (SingleParameterVariation_Predicate
         (hasParamName ?pn1)
         (hasParamMeasurementTime ?t1))
 ?f-check <- (aggregation-pattern-for-2-params
        (pattern-time-width ?ptw &:
        (<= (abs(-?t0 ?t1)) ?ptw))
         (param-0 ?pn0) (param-1 ?pn1))
=>
; assert an Aggregate Parameter Variation predicate ?f-APVp
(send-aggregate-alert ?f-APVp))
```

Once that the procedures needed to manage the anomaly have been identified, the context consumers come into action by performing suited "anomaly management" actions.

As detailed in the following section, the kind of reasoning above described is carried out with the support of suited agents.

4.6. Agent-based reasoning

The following subsections respectively depict the multi agent organization of our system and an example of agents interaction.

4.6.1 The multi-agent framework

Fig. 7 shows the proposed multi-agent framework, which assigns three fundamental roles to agents:

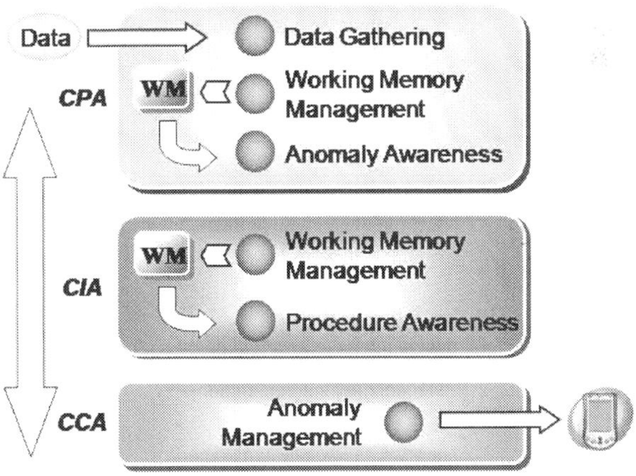

Fig. 7. The proposed multi-agent framework

Context Provider Agents (CPA). These agents wrap context sources to capture raw context data and instantiate the ontology representation. CPAs may encapsulate single sensors or multiple sources. In the former case ("single domain CPAs") they are mainly responsible for gathering and filtering data and info from sensor devices. In the latter case, (Dockorn Costa, 2005) they interact with single domain CPAs, in order to aggregate context information from various context sources (for instance sensed data must be aggregated with patient thresholds). Both kinds of CPAs are responsible also of making low level context inference and putting relevant context information into the rule engine as facts.
Context Interpreter Agent (CIA). Context Interpreter Agents are responsible for observing context changes sensed by CPAs, and, as consequence of these changes, to identify the set of actions that should be performed by context consumer agents. Substantially, they are responsible for identifying the monitoring entity best suited to manage an alarm situation, for contacting it and for forwarding context information to it.
Context Consumer Agent (CCA). Context consumer agents are responsible for performing the actions triggered by CIAs. Actions provide the application reaction to context information changes, which may assume diverse forms, such as the generation of a signal, the delivery of a notification or a web services request. Moreover, they may request further data to CPAs by contacting the suited CPA_V agent.
Registration Agents (RA). are in charge of managing agents registration and deregistration. Indeed, the system is dynamic in nature, as monitored and monitoring entities can be added and removed during its functioning. The JADE environment provides a service, namely the Directory Facilitator (DF), which supports runtime registration and service advertizing. However, DF has limited capabilities in service description and reduced performances. Therefore we implemented our own system by using the Jess virtual machine, which demonstrated to be much more efficient and supports a much richer description of agent capabilities and features.

4.6.2 Agents interaction

A simple example of agents interaction is provided in Fig. 8. A logical CPA, i.e. a CPA in

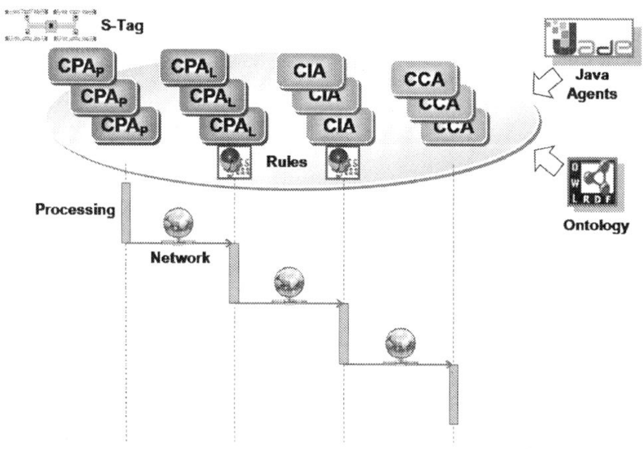

Fig. 8. A simple example of agents interaction

charge of aggregating data coming from different context sources (and their CPAs), gathers data coming from a sensor device and from the patient archive and identifies alarm events. When an alarm is issued, the CPA communicates the event to the CIA by sending an "inform" ACL message. The CIA, on its turn, requests information about the availability of physicians to the CPA being associated to the doctors archive. Finally, an "inform" ACL message is forwarded to the suited CCA in order to communicate the alarm to the selected doctor.

The code snippet below shows how ACL fields are perfectly aligned with the classes being codified in our "Ubiquitous Health-Care" (UHC) ontology (see Section 4.4). It contains an example of "inform" message sent by a physical CPA (namely "CpaP_BodyTemperature_Patient3" in the following code snippet) to a logical CPA (indicated as "CpaL_Patient3"). The UHC vocabulary is adopted to communicate sensed data of a patient (identified by his id "MonitoredEntity_ID" slot) measured at a certain timestamp ("timestamp" slot). The UHC "HasMonitoredParameter" predicate, together with its slots "NormalMinValue", "NormalMaxValue", "CurrentValue" (indicating the thresholds and the current sensed value of the monitored parameter), enrich the message with a deeper semantic meaning. Once that the message is interpreted, the identification of consequent actions is done by means of rules similar to those described in Section 4.5.

```
(INFORM
 :sender  (agent-identifier CpaP_BodyTemperature_Patient3)
 :receiver set ( agent-identifier CpaL_Patient3) )
 :content
  "( (HasMonitoredParameter (BodyTemperature
            :NormalMinValue 35.5
            :NormalMaxValue 36.5
            :CurrentValue 39.5))
    (MonitoredEntity_ID :Patient3)
    (timestamp 1205453552515) )"
:language  fipa-sl  :ontology  UHC)
```

4.7 Context sources

As previously stated, the input raw data of the proposed architecture is represented by the set of values, usually physical parameters, collected by the so-called physical sources. It has also been outlined that the realization of devices that integrate RFID technology with generic sensors has numerous advantages in terms of cost and easiness.

Indeed, the scheme proposed in Fig. 9 represents the actually designed and realized general purpose Sensor-Tag (S-Tag) connected to a generic sensor including, among the others, sensors for biomedical applications (patented). When Tag and sensor are connected one to another and are interrogated, the measured value can be read by a standard UHF RFID system and interpreted through an RFID middleware. In such a way, the system takes advantage from the standard RFID technology, preserving most of its peculiarities and maintaining the compatibility with all the devices already available and worldwide standardized.

The working principle is as easy as effective: data measured by the sensor connected to the S-Tag is used to control a set of integrated RF switches which select the appropriate IDs to be transmitted back towards the reader when the S-Tag is interrogated. Actually, as the S-

Tag is designed as a general-purpose device, the sensor signal must be preventively quantized through an ad-hoc circuit embedded in the sensor itself. Of course, the number n of bits used for the quantization must be equal to the number of available IDs on the S-Tag. As a result, the number of different combinations, excluding the one with all the bits equal to zero (which would cause interpretability problems) is $2^n - 1$.

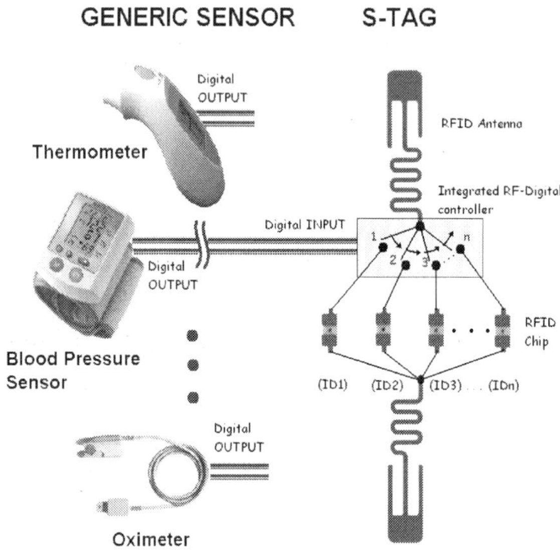

Fig. 9. A simplified scheme of the designed RFID sensor tag

Consequently, when the Tag is in the region covered by the RFID reader, it sends back a signal containing a proper combination of identity codes (IDs) depending on the value of the input itself, thus facilitating the transmission of sensor data. More specifically, the internal microwave circuit of the S-Tag samples the value at its input (which has been measured by the sensor) and quantizes it by using a number of bits equal to the number of available different IDs. For each bit with value equal to 1, the integrated micro-switch selects the corresponding ID to be transmitted; the combination of bits can be hence received by a standard RFID reader and easily decoded in order to rebuild the sensor-measured data.

For a better clarification of the working principle of the S-Tag, Fig. 10 reports a block diagram referred to a temperature sensor applied to a 4-ID S-Tag. The sensor is supposed to work in the range 35-42 °C and to be provided with a 4-bit binary digital output (15 valid combinations), guaranteeing a resolution of 0.5 °C. The measured temperature, for instance assumed to be 38.3 °C, after the quantization and the digitalization, will correspond to the binary symbol "0110", that will become, hence, the input signal of the S-Tag. Consequently, the internal logic of the S-Tag enables the transmission of the two IDs associated to the second and the third bit (those ending respectively in 752 and 753 in the figure), and disables the transmission of the others. When an RFID reader interrogates the S-Tag, hence, it receives back only the enabled IDs which are automatically associated to the logic state "1". The non-received IDs, instead, are associated to the logic state "0". The so-reconstructed

symbol is then reconverted, resulting in temperature value of 38.5 °C, slightly different from the actually measured one because of the quantization effect.
This is not the most adequate context for a more exhaustive explanation of the implementation issues of the S-Tag; we only would like to observe that, as apparent from the picture, the sensor is an external unit. In such a way, generic sensors, with the only requirement of a specific digital output, can be used. Such sensors are not integrated into the S-Tag, so that they do not influence the tag cost. Moreover, thanks to an accurate electromagnetic design of the tag antenna and of the microwave circuit (microcontroller, RF-switch and so on), also the implemented technological innovation is reasonably inexpensive.

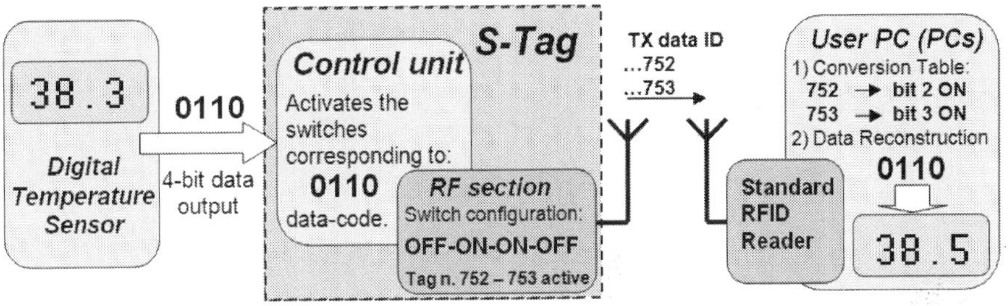

Fig. 10. Example of temperature data transmission through a 4-ID S-Tag. The binary symbol at the S-Tag input is used to discriminate the IDs to be transmitted. Vice versa, the information about whether or not an ID has been received by the RFID allows a straightforward symbol reconstruction. The difference between measured and received temperature value is due to the quantization

4.8 Results

This section provides a number of results obtained from a benchmarking phase performed to test performance and efficacy of both the S-Tag component (subsection 4.8.1) and the overall software platform fed by S-Tag data (subsection 4.8.2).

4.8.1 Benchmarking the S-Tag

In this section the proposed S-Tag is extensively tested in order to demonstrate its effectiveness and versatility. All the reported results have been obtained by using a 4-ID S-Tag receiving in input the four binary signals of the quantized measured value.
In the first presented results, the signal at the S-Tag input has been artificially generated in order to create extremely stressing conditions. Indeed, each of the four binary inputs is assumed to vary every two seconds at random. The random signal generator, hence, can generate 2^4 different uncorrelated combinations, thus covering the whole dynamic range of the S-Tag.
In such a situation, the S-Tag has been positioned at different distances (varying from 50 cm to 4 m) from a standard UHF RFID reader antenna (for instance, the Alien ALR-8610-AC). For each distance, the random signal generator has been connected to the S-Tag for a testing time of 10 minutes, in which the RFID reader has collected data and the signal has been reconstructed via an ad-hoc but very uncomplicated software. The difference between actual and received signal has then been evaluated.

In Fig.11, for instance, transmitted and received samples are compared at a Reader-Sensor distance of 3 m. It can be observed that, despite the presence of one spike, the transmitted signal is quite perfectly reconstructed. It is worth mentioning, however, that the longer is the interrogation distance, the highest is the number of recorded spikes. The spikes correspond to erroneous received samples which, obviously, should be reduced as much as possible. Because of the strong correlation between consecutively measured values in real situations, however, software filters capable to correct most of the read erroneous values can be easily implemented and applied. For a detailed quantification of the performance of the system, hence, the circled-dotted line in the graph of Fig. 12 reports, for different distances, the percentage error evaluated as ratio between number of erroneous samples and number of samples. A sample is a transmitted symbol of four bits and it is considered erroneous if at least one bit is not correctly received. Many observations result from the graph. For distances superior to 3.5 m, for instance, the measured signal cannot be correctly reconstructed.

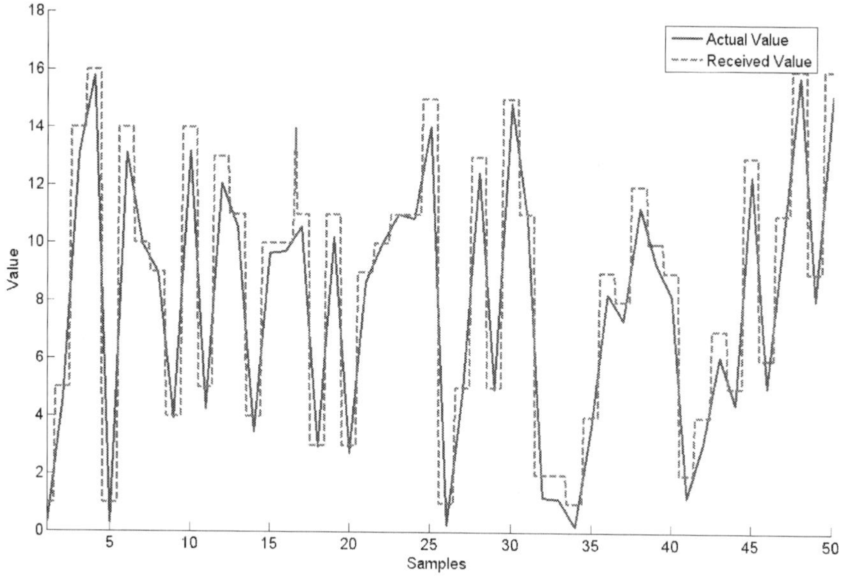

Fig. 11. Comparison between the actual random signal at the input of the S-Tag and the signal received by a RFID reader at a distance of 3 m

Even though passive RFID Tags can be read even at 9 m from the reader, in fact, the slight mismatch caused by the microwave circuits and the coupling among the S-Tag antennas, reduce the reading range. Work is in progress in order to improve such issue. For distances inferior to 3.5 m, however, the percentage error is definitely negligible, especially if it is considered that no software filter is applied to the received bits. In such a context, the squared-continuous line in the same Fig. 12 shows how the accuracy is improved after the use of a very simple filter that detects and removes the spikes. Since the RFID reader interrogates the S-Tag many times a second, the filter verifies the eventual difference among samples referred to the same transmitted value, and where only one reading differs from the others, it corrects the erroneous sample.

In order to verify that the S-Tag can be used with generic sensors, once disconnected from the random generator, it has been connected to a glucometer. In this case, it is expected an improving of the S-Tag performance. It is worth recalling, in fact, that the physical parameters potentially monitored, show much slower variation in the considered time intervals than the previously used random generator. In the same Fig. 12, for instance, the reported results refer to the blood glucose monitoring in the range 4 - 12 mmol/l. More specifically, results have been obtained by loading into the used artificial glucometer some realistic glycemia values of a diabetic patient recorded during a whole day. For such a goal, glucose values to be transmitted have been obtained from AIDA web site (AIDA, 2010), that is an on-line educational simulator designed to assist interested parties in obtaining a better understanding of how insulin and glucose interact within the body (Blanchard, 1998). More specifically, one of the sample cases proposed on the AIDA web site (the number 0015 referring to the virtual patient named "Edward Carllson"), has been chosen, and the virtual patient's blood glucose values have been charged on the artificial glucometer connected to the S-Tag. Results of Fig. 12 clearly show the optimal behavior of the system even at the maximum investigated distance both for the non-filtered and filtered received signals.

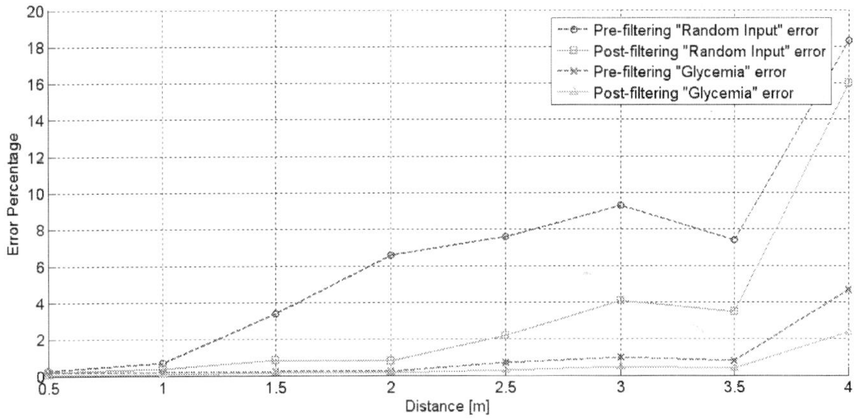

Fig. 12. Comparison among the evaluated error percentages by using two different inputs (random signal and glycemia) and by varying the distance between S-Tag and reader antenna . The same error is also reported after the software filter is applied

Finally, a more practical mobile scenario has been considered by positioning the S-Tag on a programmable robot that, moving itself in the RFID covered area, simulates patient motion. The robot has been programmed to alternate moments of stillness and moments of activity for a total test time of 24h, during which the blood glucose values are transmitted through a S-Tag each 15 minutes. After the reader has received the S-Tag signal, the blood glucose values are reconstructed both with and without the filtering process. In Fig. 13, for instance, the three reported graphs are referred to three types of signals: a) original transmitted blood glucose trend, b) reconstructed signal without filtering, and c) filtered signal.

Results show the optimum behavior of both non-filtered and filtered signals and demonstrate the very good matching between original transmitted blood glucose trend and received reconstructed signal. The slight differences among signals are due to the quantization, as described above.
In addition to the glucometer many other kinds of sensors have been tested and the S-Tag used as a source data for elementary control systems, thus showing the S-Tag capability to effectively transmit data measured by different kinds of sensors towards standard RFID readers.

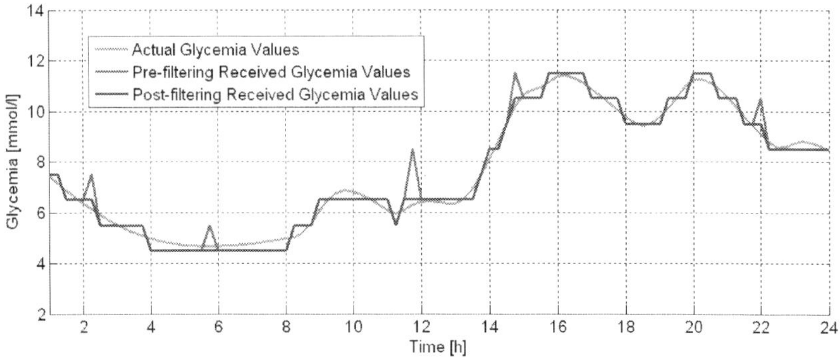

Fig. 13. Comparison of the actual glycemia values at the input of the S-Tag with the received non-filtered and filtered values

4.8.2 Benchmarking the overall system

The overall system was tested in the framework of a network of computers connected by a TCP/IP-based 100Mb/s network. Computers run under Linux operating system and have the following characteristics:

1. Intel Pentium, 3.00 GHz (single core); RAM: 512 MB;
2. AMD Athlon, 1.8 GHz (single core); RAM: 478 MB;

The experimentation consisted in collecting average alarm generation and transmission times in diverse configurations (Fig. 14). The simplest consists of a single patient monitored by one sensor and assisted remotely by four doctors. The most complex consists of 5 patients, each being monitored by 4 sensors and being assisted by 4 doctors. Results concern average times obtained over 30 runs. The system monitors data sensed by sensors, and, based on patient info (loaded once at system start-up) determines alarm events. Alarm events trigger actions which basically consist in identifying the best suited doctor and contacting him/her (via mobile). Such doctors are the ones having the appropriate specialization to tackle the out-of-range monitored parameters (i.e. cardiologists for alarms concerning heart-rate and/or blood pressure) and the ones being available in the time interval nearest to the alarm measurement time.
Measured times were taken by imposing four "stressing conditions" that simulate a real scenario: 1) each sensed parameter has always out-of-range values, 2) in the same run, all sensors send data at the same time, 3) the time-spacing between consecutive measurements is equal to two seconds, 4) only one CIA has been activated, in order to create a fictitious bottleneck in the system. Measured times consist in:

- the time elapsing at the CPA_P side between the reception of data from the sensor and the triggering of the corresponding alarm obtained by means of rule-based reasoning;
- the time elapsing at the CPA_l side between the reception of a message coming from CPA_P and the triggering of the corresponding alarm obtained by means of rule-based reasoning;
- the time elapsing at the CIA side between the reception of a message coming from CPA_l and the forwarding of a message to CCA.

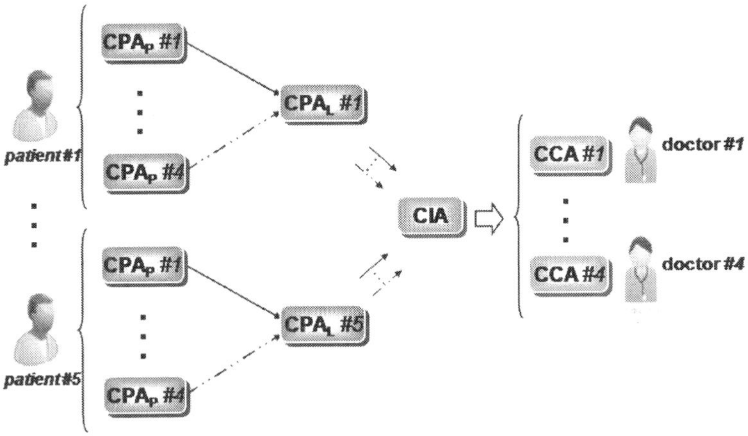

Fig. 14. Experimentation setup

As shown in Table I, CPA_P are responsible for filtering data coming from a single sensor, therefore their times do not change when the number of sensors and/or of patients change. Each CPA_l, instead, elaborates data coming from sensors connected to a single patient. In our experimentation set-up, they elaborate data coming from up to four sensors and produce two kinds of aggregate alarms: the former associates "BodyTemperature" and "BloodGlucose" patterns, the latter combines "BloodPressure" and "HeartRate" patterns. Therefore, CPA_l times increase with the number of sensors attached to single patients. CIA times, finally, depend both on the number of sensors and on the number of patients (i.e. both on the number of CPA_P and on the number of CPA_l). Table 1 also illustrates data obtained by aggregating the average times obtained for each configuration. As shown in the table, processing times are very good, thus demonstrating the amenability of the proposed approach to attach also more complex monitoring problems.

Agent	1 sensor 1 patient	2 sensors 1 patient	2 sensors 2 patients	4 sensors 1 patient	4 sensors 2 patients	4 sensors 5 patients
CPA_P	3.68	3.68	3.68	3.68	3.68	3.68
CPA_L	/	4.74	4.74	5.96	5.96	5.96
CIA	2.24	2.87	2.93	3.28	6.97	24.49
Ttot	5.92	11.29	11.35	12.92	16.61	34.13

Table 1. Performance results [ms]

5. Conclusions

Context-aware ubiquitous systems open a very large number of appealing perspectives for healthcare. They promise huge increases in performance, accuracy and availability of treatment. The range of application domains potentially benefiting from these technologies is wide and variegate, as it includes different areas, such as remote monitoring of mobility-impaired patients and support to information flow among heath-care workers.

In order to facilitate the implementation of this kind of systems, scientific community is working hard to define standards and to implement middleware solutions. In spite of that, the available systems still lack in flexibility and often are not accompanied by a well documented characterization of customization effort and/or of performance data. A number of enabling technologies seems to provide a solid building block for the design and development of flexible and robust context-aware pervasive systems. They were briefly resumed and commented in this chapter, together with a framework for context-aware computing based on such technologies.

The system harmonizes agents, ontologies and rule-based inference engines. The ontology provides the knowledge codification needed to support both agent reasoning and communication. The system elaborates data coming from heterogeneous sources, including an innovative RFID system, which embeds RFID and sensors in a reasonably inexpensive tag, thanks to an accurate electromagnetic design of the tag antenna and of the microwave circuit (microcontroller, RF-switch and so on).

The effectiveness of the system is demonstrated by reporting performance results obtained from validation in a real-life application in the home-care scenario.

The very promising results, in terms of easiness of use, reconfigurability and performance, make the proposed approach a very good candidate for the solution of even complex monitoring problems, belonging to the healthcare domain and generally to other scientific domains provided that an ontology describing them is available.

6. References

AIDA homepage: on-line free Web-based diabetes software simulator. (last accessed: 2010, September).

Bacheldor, B. (2008, February 20th). Brigham and Women's Hospital Becomes Totally RTLS-enabled". *RFID Journal* .

Bacheldor, B. (2009, May 29th). Philly Hospital Uses RTLS to Track Patient Flow, Care and Training. *RFID Journal* .

Blanchard, S., Novotny, C., DeWolf, D., Lehmann, E., Gotwals, R. J., & Rorhbach, R. (1998). AIDA On-Line: a Glucose and Insulin Simulator on the WWW. In: *Proceedings of the 20th Annual International Conference on the IEEE Engineering in Medicine and Biology Society*, 3, p. 1159-1162.

Bradshaw, J. (1997). An Introduction to Software Agents. In: *Software Agents* (p. 3-46). Cambdrige, MA, USA: MIT Press, J.M. Bradshaw Editor.

Cho, N.; Song, S.-J. et al. (2005). A 8-μW, 0.3 mm^2 RF-Powered Transponder with Temperature Sensor for Wireless Environmental Monitoring. In: *IEEE International Symposium on Circuits and Systems*, pp. 1-17.

DAML homepage. DARPA Agent Markup Language: http://www.daml.org (last accessed: 2010, July).

Dey, A. a. (1999). Toward a Better Understanding of Context and Context-Awareness. In: *GVU Techincal Report.*

Dobkin, D. (2007). The RF in RFID: Passive UHF RFID in Practice. Newton, MA, USA: Newnes.

Dockorn Costa, P., & Ferreira Pires, L. a. (2005). Architectural Patterns for Context-Aware Services Platforms. In: *2nd International Workshop on Ubiquitous Computing (IWUC2005) in conjunction with ICEIS2005.* Miami, FL, USA.

Esposito, A., & Tarricone, L. a. (2010). A Versatile Context-Aware Pervasive Monitoring System: Validation and Characterization in the Health-Care Domain. In: *Proceedings of IEEE International Symposium on Industrial Electronics (ISIE2010),* (p. 2791-2796). Bari, Italy.

FIPA repository. The Foundation for Intelligent Physical Agents: http://fipa.org/repository/index.html (last accessed: 2010, September).

Friedman-Hill, E. (2003). *Jess in Action.* Manning.

Gruber, T. (1995). Toward Principles for the Design of Ontologies Used for Knowledge Sharing. In: *International Journal of Human Computer Studies* (43), 907-928.

Guarino, N. (1998). Formal Ontology and Information System. In: *N. Guarino Editor, Proceedings of the 1st International Conference on Formal Ontologies in Information Systems* (FOIS98) (p. 3-15). Trento, Italy: IOS Press.

Indulska, J., & Sutton, P. (2003). Location Management in Pervasive Systems. CRPITS03 - In: *Proceedings of the Australasian Information Security Workshop.* 21, p. 143-151. Adelaide (Australia): Johnson, C.; Montague, P and Steketee, C.

JADE homepage. Java Agent Development Environment: http://jade.tilab.it (last accessed: 2010, September).

JADE Tutorial webpage. Application-Defined Content Language and Ontologies. From: *JADE website:* http://jade.tilab.com/doc/tutorials/CLOntoSupport.pdf (last accessed: 2010, September).

Moreno, A. a. (2003). Application of Software Agent Technology in the Health Care Domain. Basel, Switzerland. Birkäuser Verlag.

OntologyBeanGenerator webpage. From: *Protégé Wiki homepage*: http://protege.cim3.net/cgi-bin/wiki.pl?OntologyBeanGenerator (last accessed: 2010, September).

Paganelli, F. & Giuli, D. (2007). An Ontology-based Context Model for Home Health Monitoring and Alerting in Chronic Patient Care Networks, In: *21st International Conference on Advanced Information Networking and Applications Workshops (AINAW'07)* 0-7695-2847-3/07.

Partridge, D. a. (1994). Knowledge Based Information Systems. Mc-Graw Hill.

Pellet homepage. http://www.mindswap.org/2003/pellet/ (last accessed: 2010, September).

Protégé homepage. http://protege.stanford.edu (last accessed: 2010, September).

RETE Algorithm webpage. From: *JESS website:* http://herzberg.ca.sandia.gov/jess/docs/52/rete.html (last accessed: 2010, September).

SM4ALL homepage. http://www.sm4all-project.eu/ (last accessed: 2010, September).

Strang, T. a.-P. (2004, September). A Context Modeling Survey. In: *Workshop on Advanced Context Modeling, Reasoning and Management,* (p. 33-40). Nottingham, England.

Swedberg. (2010, May 28th). Nyack Hospitals Tracks Medication Compliance. *RFID Journal.*

W3C. Recommendation 10 webpage. (2004, Febraury 10th). From: *RDFS (RDF Vocabulary Description Language 1.0: RDFS Schema) webpage*: http://www.w3.org/TR/rdf-schema (last accessed: 2010, September).

W3C. Web Ontology Language Overview, W3C Recommendation webpage (2005, February 10th). http://w3.org/TR/2004/RDC-owl-features-20040210 (last accessed: 2010, September).

Walker, J., Pand, E., Johnston, D., Adler-Milstein, J., & Bates, D. a. (2005, January 19). The Value of Healthcare Information Exchange and Interoperability. In: *Health Affairs, Web Exclusive.*

Wang, S.-W. et al. (2006). RFID Application in Hospitals: a Case Study on a Demonstration RFID Project in a Taiwan Hospital. In: *Proc. of the 39th Annual Hawaii International Conference on System Sciences (HICSS'06)*, 08, p. 184-194. Kauai, Hawaii (USA).

Weiser, M. (1991). The Computer for the 21st Century. In: *Scientific American - Special Issue on Communications.*

Williamson, J. JESS Wiki: Keep Your Rules Normalized. From: *JESS website*: http://www.jessrules.com/jesswiki/view?KeepYourRulesNormalized (last accessed: 2010, September).

36

Quality of Service, Adaptation, and Security Provisioning in Wireless Patient Monitoring Systems

Wolfgang Leister[1],Trenton Schulz[1], Arne Lie[2]
Knut Grythe[2] and Ilangko Balasingham[3]
[1]*Norsk Regnesentral*
[2]*SINTEF*
[3]*Interventional Centre, Oslo University Hospital*
Dept. of Electronics & Telecommunications
Norwegian University of Science & Technology
Institute of Clinical Medicine, University of Oslo
[1,2,3]*Norway*

1. Introduction

Modern patient monitoring systems are designed to put the individual into the centre of the system architecture. In this paradigm, the patient is seen as a source of health-relevant data that are processed and transferred. Patient monitoring systems are used in health care enterprises as well as in paramedic, mobile, and home situations to foster ambient assisted living (AAL) scenarios.

There are a multitude of standards and products available to support Quality of Service (QoS) and security goals in patient monitoring systems. Yet, an architecture that supports these goals from data aggregation to data transmission and visualisation for end user has not been developed. Medical data from patient monitoring systems includes sampled values from measurements, sound, images, and video. These data often have a time-aspect where several data streams need to be synchronised. Therefore, rendering data from patient monitoring systems can be considered an advanced form of multimedia data.

We propose a framework that will fill this QoS and security gap and provide a solution that allows medical personnel better access to data and more mobility to the patients. The framework is based on MPEG-21 and wireless sensor networks. It allows for end-to-end optimisation and presentation of multimedia sensor data. The framework also addresses the QoS, adaptation and security concerns of handling this data.

In Section 2 we present background on patient monitoring systems, their requirements and how we envision communication is handled. We present communication systems in Section 3 and how to treat QoS in Section 4. A short introduction to data streaming, binary XML and how they relate to patient monitoring systems is presented in Section 5. In Section 6 we our proposed solution for the framework and present a security analysis of it in Section 7. Finally, we offer our conclusions in Section 8.

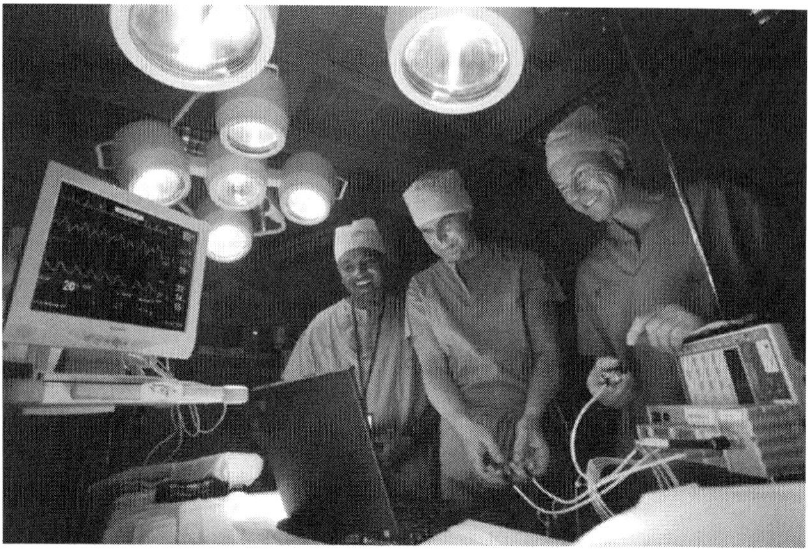

Fig. 1. Surgeons testing a patient monitoring system consisting of sensors, actuators, and communication and presentation entities.

2. Patient monitoring systems

Patient monitoring systems comprise sensors, data communication, storage, processing, and presentation of medical data. These functions are performed both near the patient, in local surgery, or remotely at a health care infrastructure, e.g., a medical centre or a hospital. An example of a patient monitoring system is shown in Fig. 1. In this figure, we see surgeons holding some sensors and actuators. On the left side of the figure, a large monitor displays the data from these devices. The information is also displayed on the laptop in the foreground of the figure.

Patient monitoring systems can be used in a variety of health care scenarios ranging from paramedic, diagnostic, surgical, post-operative, and home surveillance situations. The systems must meet a high demand of flexibility since data may be produced outside a health care enterprise. This requires specific measures in order to fulfil security, availability, privacy, and QoS demands. The properties are: *a*) mobility; *b*) outside hospital infrastructure; *c*) biomedical sensor networks in use; *d*) wireless channel.

As shown in a case study by Balasingham, Ihlen, Leister, Røe & Samset (2007), even within or between health care enterprises, the requirements that applications need to meet are strict and require specific measures or architectures. Data from patients are transferred through networks to the health care enterprise, and made available in a suitable form to the medical personnel to support the treatment of patients.

2.1 Communication levels

In order to account for the different health care scenarios, we propose the following *levels* surrounding the patient in which data are processed and transferred, as outlined in Fig. 2. These are divided into four levels — (0), (I), (II), and (III) — depending on the logical distance to the patient with Level (0) being the patient. For Level (II), usually only one type applies at a time. However, it must be possible to switch between the types in Level (II) as easily as the patient moves between them.

(0) Patient. This is the actual patient.

(I) Personal sensor network. The personal sensor network denotes the patient and the sensors measuring the medical data. These sensors are connected to each other in a biomedical sensor network (BSN). While this sensor network can be connected randomly, in most cases one special BSN node — typically one that has additional power and computational resources — is appointed to be a personal cluster head (PCH), where all data for one patient are collected. The PCH may have visualisation devices attached to be used by the patient or by medical personnel. In this case, the PCH represents all data for a patient. Other topologies are possible, including the possibility that data from other patients are transferred using the sensor nodes of another patient's BSN. However, due to resource limitations of the sensor devices, organisational and ethical issues may occur. Therefore, this possibility is disregarded.

(IIa) Paramedic. In the paramedic scenario, the BSN is connected to the medical devices of an ambulance (car, plane, helicopter) via the PCH. The devices of the ambulance can work autonomously, showing the patient status locally. Alternatively, the devices of the ambulance can communicate with an external health care infrastructure, e.g., at a hospital. Note that the ambulance needs to employ some form of long-distance communication to the external health care infrastructure.

(IIb) Smart home. The smart home scenario envisages that the patient is in a smart-home environment, where the personal sensor network is connected to the infrastructure of the smart-home. The smart home infrastructure might be connected to a health care enterprise infrastructure using long-distance data communication.

(IIc) Mobility. The mobility scenario envisages that the patient is mobile, e.g., using public or personal transportation facilities. The personal sensor network of the patient is connected to the infrastructure of a health care enterprise via a mobile device, e.g., a mobile Internet connection. Note that the mobile scenario requires temporary storage in the PCH, since communication cannot be guaranteed at all times. The application and the communication software must be aware of this.

(IId) Intensive care/surgery. During an operation the sensor data are transferred to the PCH or directly to the hospital infrastructure over a relatively short distance. The sensors are in a very controlled environment, but some sensors might be very resource limited due to their size, so extra transport nodes close to the sensors might be needed. In the operation environment, there is an increased need for QoS, so that correct data are available to the surgeons at any time during the operation.

(IIe) Pre- and postoperative. During pre- and postoperative phases of a treatment, and for use in hospital bedrooms, the sensor data are transferred from the sensor network to the PCH, and from there to the health care information system.

(III) Health care information system. The health care information system is considered a trusted environment. It comprises of the hospital network, the computing facilities, databases, and access terminals in the hospital. It should be noted that communication between Levels (II) and (III) is two-way.

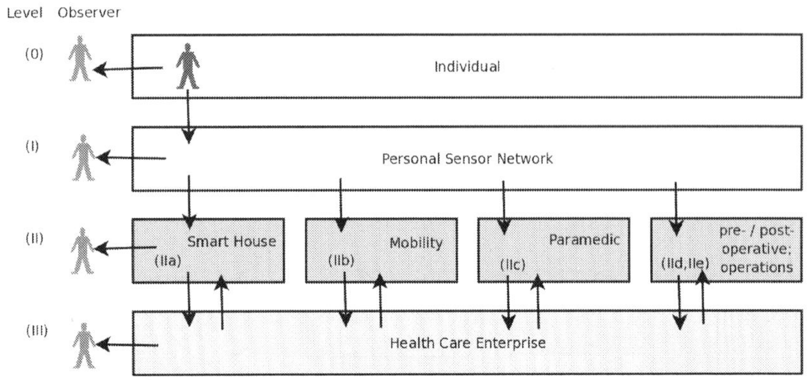

Fig. 2. Generic model of patient monitoring systems showing the data flow to the observer.

Each level may have one or more data *observers*. An observer can be either the patient, medical personnel using a suitable terminal, or a processing unit that can trigger alarms, aggregate data, create logs, etc. The observer is usually in Level (II), while the communication may, or may not go through Level (III), depending on the application. The generic model in Fig. 2 helps identify where possible technology-transitions in the line of communication appear, as well as where the levels of equal security requirements can be placed.

2.2 Medical data streams

The medical data in a patient monitoring system, regardless of which level it is in, form streams of data which can be characterised as temporal multimedia data. These data streams contain the sensor data, often sampled values, attached to time-stamps and meta data, such as type and identification of the data streams. In most cases several separate streams of different data are used to describe the situation of a patient at a given time interval. The data may also contain triggers, alarms, and video data, as the capabilities of the sensor devices increase.

Multimedia data streams have a producer—here, the biomedical sensor—and a consumer—here, a (mobile) terminal or a database. In principle, each data stream can be transferred separately from the source (producer) to the sink (consumer). However, this might be impractical for improvised situations since the assurance of requirements for QoS, availability, security, and privacy will not be possible in a unified way. Therefore, we propose to forward data in a standardised way, using the system model of a generic patient monitoring system shown in Fig. 3.

This system model is suitable for patient monitoring systems where data from sensors are transferred to an observer who retrieves these data using a terminal. The medical data may be transferred to the health care information system to be stored and processed there. Additional data from the health care information system may be used by the observer at a terminal combined with the sensor data.

This generic system model divides the communication from Channels A to D as follows: Channel A includes the sensor and the sensor network to the PCH, which acts as a gateway for the personal sensor network to a network in Levels (IIa)–(IIe), also denoted as Level (II). Channel A may involve several intermediate nodes employing both wireless or wired data transfer. Channel B describes the channel from the PCH to the observer terminal, keeping the communication in Levels (II), without going through the hospital infrastructure. Channel C

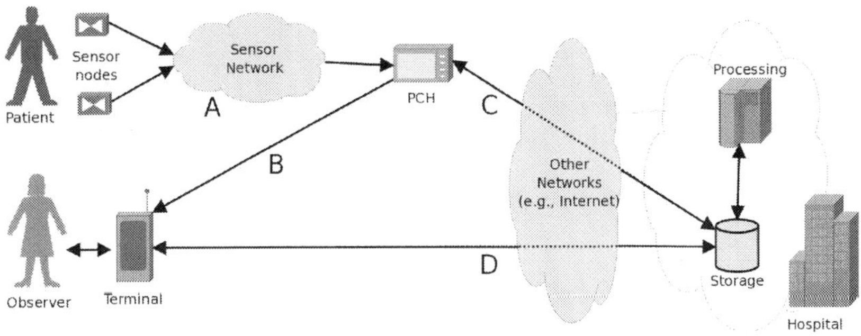

Fig. 3. System model of a generic patient monitoring system, identifying the communication channels while the patient monitoring system transfers data.

transfers data from the PCH to the hospital infrastructure in Level (III) using infrastructure like the Internet, a wired carrier or a wireless carrier. Channel D describes the data transport from the hospital information system to the observer terminal in Level (II) using infrastructure like the Internet, a wired carrier or a wireless carrier.

The generic system model in Fig. 2 shows the data flow to the observer in different health care scenarios, while Fig. 3 shows the communication channels in such a system. In this architecture, note that security functions, like establishing identities for authentication, might use different channels in advance of the phase where the medical data are transferred. The different phases are presented by Leister, Fretland & Balasingham (2009).

The generic model is not dependant on how the communication in the scenarios of Level (II) are implemented. Channels C and D can have different characteristics depending on the use case, i.e., whether an external (ambulance, mobility, smart home) or an internal (hospital-related scenarios) source is used. Note also that Channel B can meet different requirements, depending on the scenario. However, from a security perspective, a short-range wireless channel is assumed.

Using the generic system model, we are able to treat the security challenges separately for every channel, thus reducing the complexity of the security analysis. However, note that each channel is implemented using several of the communication layers in OSI model.

In our framework, we intend to provide end-to-end streaming of medical sensor data as depicted in Fig. 3: *a*) from the patient to the terminal of the medic via the PCH (using Channels A and B); *b*) from the patient to the health care infrastructure (using Channels A and C); and *c*) from the health care infrastructure to the terminal of the medic (using Channel D). This also includes data streaming using Channels A, C, and D. The characteristics of these channels vary with the scenario that is addressed.

In our concept, all medical data streams are expressed using the notion of the MDI, which in some cases, e.g., in Channel A, may be expressed as μMDI (see Section 6).

3. Communication systems

In this section, we introduce wireless sensor networks and the need for providing quality of service. We focus on the communication at Levels (I) and (II) since these are the most interesting and are in contact with the patient. At each level, we can implement a communications technology, such as ZigBee in Level (I); Bluetooth, WLAN, ZigBee or wires in

Level (IIa); Bluetooth in Level (IIc), etc. Employing only one technology in each level makes it easier to define and structure the security and QoS requirements. The medical data first must traverse Level (I), then through Level (II), and possibly arrive at the hospital infrastructure, before reaching the observer of the medical data, i.e., the medical personnel in Levels (II) or (III). It is important to have well-defined interfaces between these levels as they need to be technically implemented.

3.1 Wireless sensor networks

A wireless sensor network (WSN) is often a part of a patient monitoring system. In our reference model shown in Fig. 3, the WSN is denoted as Channel A. The WSN consists of base station receiving data from one or more tiny, low cost, low power sensor nodes that monitor information. The sensors are clustered and relay information from other sensors that may not be close enough to reach the base station.

A WSN is a good fit for a patient monitoring system since wireless technology is increasingly used in the health care industry to help eliminate cables in patient monitoring systems. Here, sensors can communicate wirelessly with a monitor that is close to the patient in a BSN. For our purposes, a BSN can be considered a special case of a WSN. The WSN can contain many small sensors that are capable of collecting vital signs and environmental information and forwarding them along to the base station; the base station can then pass this information onto the patient monitoring system. This leads, potentially, to more mobility for patients and medical staff.

While a WSN can be used in many environments and situations — for example, Römer & Mattern (2004) list applications that include herding and observing animals, checking the movement of glaciers and ocean water, and military applications — the patient monitoring systems have specific QoS and security requirements different from the other applications. For example, medical data is considered private information and wireless communication can be easily intercepted. This leads to issues in privacy, confidentiality and integrity. Also, wireless networks have their own issues with quality of service and radio interference. In addition, an attacker could alter the communication leading to threats for the patient.

The basic operations of a WSN are depicted in Fig. 4. The purpose of the deployment lies in the observation, aggregating and reporting of events in a spatio-temporal process. The communication strategies within a sensor node must support the occurrence of observed process events in various parts of the network, and possibly using distributed signal processing. Therefore, the nodes in a sensor node must cooperate to maximise the probability to fulfil their deployed mission.

There are a variety of standard solutions that are used for communication between the nodes on a wireless sensor networks. Depending upon the application and operational conditions, the most suitable is selected. ZigBee and Bluetooth are two examples out of a growing set of alternative solutions.

3.2 Quality of service provisioning

The observations made by the sensors are processed by suitable algorithms, possibly in a distributed and collaborative fashion, before the results are conveyed from the WSN to the users via a set of external networks. This way of approaching the operations of a WSN resembles the traditional encoding and transmission of a single information source (Blahut, 1987), like voice in a mobile phone. The upper reference bound for QoS experienced by the

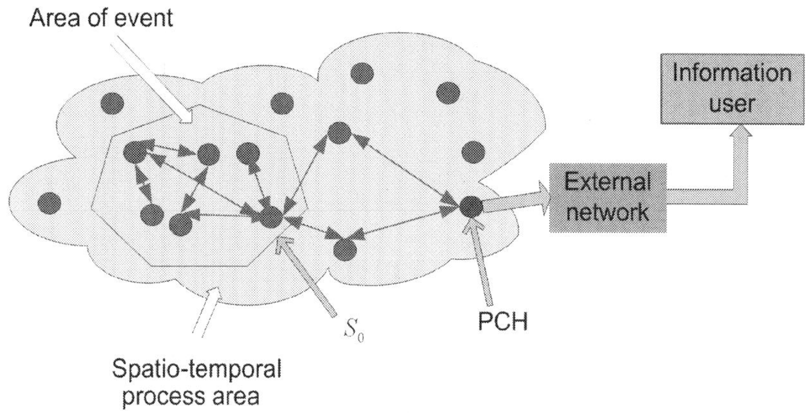

Fig. 4. Collaboration for information generation in a WSN and its transport to an external user through the WSN and external network. S_0 is the node of origin and PCH represents the patient cluster head.

user is the entropy of the source, while the delivered QoS is a result of the capabilities and degradations induced by the chosen encoding and transmission capabilities.

An overview of QoS influential factors for sensor networks are presented and discussed by Chen & Varshney (2004). These are organised into application- and network-specific factors, with emphasis on the network. A middleware for supporting QoS in WSNs is introduced by Heinzelman, Murphy, Carvalho & Perillo (2004) with examples from medical applications. This middleware integrates the application and the WSN management to respond to the required QoS and network lifetime. A protocol-independent QoS support for WSN is presented by Troubleyn, De Poorter, Ruckebusch, Moerman & Demeester (2010) where the packets between nodes are organised according to priority processing. The integration of a WSN with external networks requires these two entities to be jointly considered (Khoshnevis & Khalaj, 2007). The external transport mechanism must be mirrored in the WSN to make QoS tradeoffs at this level. Similar aspects are also discussed by Patel & Jianfeng (2010).

Although many aspects of QoS in a WSN have been given in the literature, and solutions for networks and signal processing exist, e.g., as presented by Lei & Heinzelman (2007), a structured approach for organising and balancing the tradeoffs and degradation mechanisms appears to be lacking. In the spirit of the layered QoS for IP and mobile networks (Bai, Atiquzzaman & Lilja, 2006), we include, in the following section, the layered application QoS stack presented by Grythe, Lie & Balasingham (2009). This stack organises and seperates the degradation mechanisms within a WSN for the purpose of QoS trading between the various layers. This layered approach also facilitates tradeoffs between the intra- and inter-WSN data transport.

4. Application-oriented layered QoS stack for sensor network

The purpose of the WSN deployment lies in the observation and reporting of variables or detecting events in a spatio-temporal process as indicated in Fig. 4. As such, the overall QoS to be evaluated should be oriented towards the application and end-user. The QoS experienced by the user is a result of degraded maximum theoretical information content in the event area.

The QoS degradation is due to both deployed topology and algorithmic imperfections under interaction with communication imperfections both internally and externally to the WSN.
The operations of a WSN and associated systems can be split into five different actions:

(1) Carry out the process observation by the distributed sensor nodes, each doing individual measurements.

(2) In the case of distributed signal processing, enable the nodes to collaborate under the framework of the implemented algorithms.

(3) Based upon the operations of the algorithms, the nodes finally reach a consensus called a result instance. This may be either periodically or a more random time domain operation.

(4) The result instance is transmitted to the user, initiated by a random or predetermined sensor node called the node of origin, S_0.

(5) The result instance is presented to the user via a terminal.

4.1 Layered QoS stack

The communication strategies within a sensor node must support the occurrence of observed process events in various parts of the network and possibly distributed signal processing. Therefore, the nodes in a sensor network must cooperate to maximise the probability of meeting their deployed mission. The four-layered QoS stack of Fig. 5 simplifies the organisation of the degradation tradeoffs. Generally, the user perceptual QoS evolution between the layers behave as

$$\mathrm{QoS}_{\mathrm{En}} \geq \mathrm{QoS}_{\mathrm{Dep}} \geq \mathrm{QoS}_{\mathrm{Eff}} \geq \mathrm{QoS}_{\mathrm{InTrans}} \geq \mathrm{QoS}_{\mathrm{ExTrans}} = \mathrm{QoS}_{\mathrm{UserInput}}$$

where the QoS subscripts indicate which layer they belong to. This equation of inequalities reflects that the available user experience — or perception of QoS — is decreasing through the WSN towards the user. Examples of metrics representing the user QoS are variances, signal to noise ratio (SNR) for source coding or detection probabilities for event detections. QoS metrics are derived from the specific application, representing the most proper quality criterion.
For a given WSN implementation and a given QoS metric q, the evolution of at the various levels of the layered model can be expressed as:

$$\begin{bmatrix} q_{\mathrm{En}} \\ q_{\mathrm{Dep}} \\ q_{\mathrm{Eff}} \\ q_{\mathrm{InTans}} \\ q_{\mathrm{ExTrans}} \end{bmatrix} = \begin{bmatrix} 1 & 0 & 0 & 0 \\ b_1 & 0 & 0 & 0 \\ 0 & b_2 & 0 & 0 \\ 0 & 0 & b_3 & 0 \\ 0 & 0 & 0 & b_4 \end{bmatrix} \begin{bmatrix} q_{\mathrm{En}} \\ q_{\mathrm{Dep}} \\ q_{\mathrm{Eff}} \\ q_{\mathrm{InTans}} \end{bmatrix}$$

or more compact as:

$$\mathbf{q} = \mathbf{B}\mathbf{q}^{U}$$

where $\mathbf{q}$ contains all the layer metrics while $\mathbf{q}^{U}$ contains the process and intra-WSN metrics. Associating $q_0 \equiv q_{\mathrm{En}}$ and $q_4 \equiv q_{\mathrm{ExTrans}}$, the QoS evolution is logically expressed in a product form as:

$$q_n = q_0 \prod_{i=1}^{n} b_i;\ n = 1:4$$

This expression reflects the QoS interactions and tradeoff levels of Fig. 5. Due to the statistical behaviour of the influential mechanisms, as discussed later, the parameters in the matrix $\mathbf{B}$

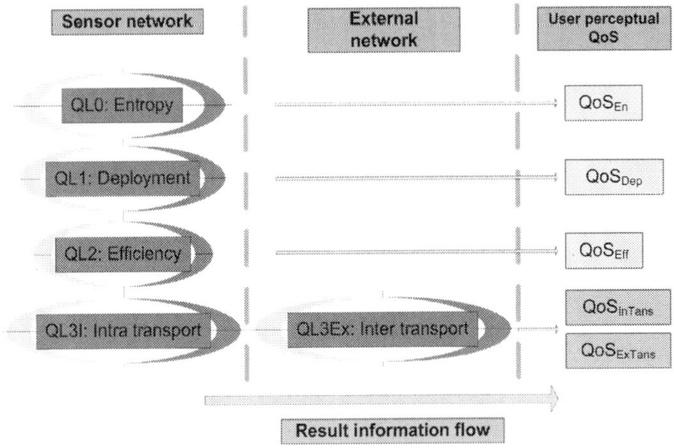

Fig. 5. The application oriented layered QoS stack for sensor networks and its association with the external network.

represent random variables, $p(\mathbf{b})$; $\mathbf{b} \equiv \{b_1, b_2, b_3, b_4\}$. Their values and quantification range depends upon the chosen metrics. Defining

$$f(\mathbf{b}^n) = \prod_{i=1}^{n} b_i;\ n = 1:4$$

the mean value of the associated value of the quality metric is expressed within the variable domain $D(\mathbf{b}^n)$ as:

$$E(q_n|q_0) = q_0 \int_{D(\mathbf{b}^n)} f(\mathbf{b}^n)p(\mathbf{b}^n)d\mathbf{b}^n$$

As is demonstrated later, for a specific application and implemented algorithm in the WSN, it is possible that not all layers are relevant.

There are many mechanisms that influence each of the four levels. We discuss a few of them below.

Level QL0 — Entropy. The Entropy level represents the maximum theoretical information content of the spatio-temporal process (STP) in the case of feature extraction (Youngchul, Poor & Heejung, 2009; Blahut, 1987) or the optimum event detection performance given the properties of the STP (Trees, 1968; Viswanathan & Varshney, 1997). These features are only related to the STP and not to any specific deployed algorithm or communication solution. As such, QL0 represents the upper performance and information bound a user can expect from the STP.

Level QL1 — Deployment. This level represents the spatial sampling of the STP performed through the topology of the specific deployed WSN and the associated implemented, possibly distributed, signal processing algorithm. Given these factors, a definition of the best performance can be done assuming that all the samples from all the sensor nodes are collected and processed in a centralised unit without transport time delays or errors. This is the maximum QoS a user or users can expect from the given WSN and does not depend upon the communication properties within or external to the WSN. The algorithm may produce a single result instance, a limited set or a continuous time discrete stream of results. In the following, we denote one quantified result as a result instance.

Level QL2 — Efficiency. Efficiency denotes the QoS degradation due to interaction between the nodes in the area of event (see Fig. 4) when executing the algorithm to obtain a result instance and how this contributes to the QoS. The factors involved may be divided into topology-related and communication-influenced. Topology-related factors include node malfunction, distributed energy consumption and saving while examples of communication-influenced factors are packet loss, bit error rate (BER), variable delays and capacity. As discussed by Bai et al. (2006); Lei & Heinzelman (2007) and others, there are several factors influencing the networking within a WSN. Cross-layer optimisation and energy efficiency are key factors in this context.

Level QL3 — Transport. Once the implemented algorithm produces a result instance, this is conveyed from a node of origin — S_0 in Fig. 4 — to the external user via intra-WSN transport and the external network. S_0 may be a fixed node or an appointed node during the algorithmic interaction. In Fig. 5, QL3 is split into QL3I and QL3Ex to separate the internal and external transport mechanisms respectively. The typical transport degradation mechanisms are delay and packet loss in addition to broken intra links due to nonfunctional nodes. Since the interaction with the external network occurs at QL3, this layer implicitly involves the issue of optimising this interaction to balance the transport QoS degradation. In the single user case, a single external, possibly heterogeneous, network is involved; with multiple users, many different external networks are possible. The transport cost functions and packet losses are factors influencing this interaction. In some cases with small losses (Khoshnevis & Khalaj, 2007), the intra- and inter-transport may be treated separately. Otherwise, a joint optimisation is necessary involving the transport statistics of all the networks, including the intra-WSN transport.

4.2 Application examples

We give three examples of signal processing in a WSN to illustrate the involvement of the different QoS layers. We apply the QoS measure at the algorithmic level and not at an information theoretical level. The latter is reflecting the STP properties.

Single sensor and one parameter. The observation is performed with one senor node. A time series, $\{z_m; m \in Z_+\}$, is generated and the samples are transmitted to the user, possibly via multiple hops, in the WSN. Here S_0 is also the sampling node. The reconstruction quality of the sequence by the user is governed by the QoS layers QL0, QL1, QL3I and QL3Ex. If the node is malfunctioning in this case, no information is conveyed and QL2 is influential. A proper algorithmic user QoS metric may be the minimum mean square error (MMSE):

$$\text{MMSE} \equiv E\left[\left(z_m - z_m^{\text{User}}\right)^2\right]$$

Uniform STP and sum aggregation. We assume that a WSN with K nodes is deployed in the STP area and that the area of event is the whole STP area, i.e., $A_{\text{Event}} = A_{\text{STP}}$. We want to calculate the spatial mean value given by the aggregation function

$$E(z_m) = \frac{1}{K}\sum_{k=1}^{K} z_m^k = \gamma_m$$

If the PCH node is identical to the node S_0, the layers involved are QL0, QL1, QL2 and QL3Ex since there is no intra-transport of the final result instants $\{\gamma_m\}$. Again MMSE is a proper user QoS metric.

Collaborative information processing (CIP). The nodes within A_{Event} is carrying out a CIP. In this case, a set of nodes use their observations and collaborate to generate a set of result instances at each time instance m. In other words:

$$\{\mathbf{Y_m}\} \underset{CIP}{\Rightarrow} \left\{\hat{\mathbf{X}}_\mathbf{m}\right\}$$

As can be seen in Fig. 4, for a deployed CIP in an event area, all the layers are contributing to the end-user QoS result. In this case, the MMSE is also applicable as an objective user QoS metric.

4.3 Local versus global optimisation

In the context of WSN for medical applications and the described variability in user terminal capabilities and heterogeneous external networks, proper QoS to each terminal is critical. Elements within a WSN influencing the QoS are briefly described by Chen & Varshney (2004). The operations of the network are governed by two modes: event reporting or queries from users. For proper operation of a medical WSN with respect to QoS and energy efficiency, external users are divided into two groups: super users and application users. Super users have access to both the PCH (Patient Cluster Head) and individual bidirectional nodes of the WSN. They can tune parameters and the performance of the WSN or initiate a deep network data query. Application users can only access the PCH and obtain streaming data from the PCH or members of parameter sets stored in the PCH. This distinction is necessary to avoid draining energy due to excessive queries and to control the access to the sensor nodes.
The general description presented previously expressed the QoS evolution in a product form as:

$$q_n = q_0 \prod_{i=1}^{n} b_i;\ n = 1:4$$

This can be considered as an expression pointing towards a single user representation or a representation for multiple users as $\mathbf{U} \equiv \left\{u_j; j = 1:J\right\}$ in the situation where all the external networks are identical. If the performance of the external networks are randomly varying or are a mix of different solutions as with heterogeneous networks, the QoS evolution for each individual user $u_j \in \mathbf{U}$ can be expressed as $q^j = b_4^j \cdot Q^0$, where the internal operations of the BAN is represented by

$$Q^0 = q_0 \prod_{i=1}^{3} b_i$$

The performance trade-offs between the internal and external behaviour of the WSN to obtain the wanted or expected user QoS can be analysed and evaluated through these mechanisms. A comment that is valid for both QL2 and QL3 is that when multiple disjoint observations areas within the WSN are active simultaneously, the wireless communication activities may

create mutual interference. Also note that a similarly layered QoS structure can be used in the situation where an actuator in a WSN is fed with an excitant signal from an external user or control algorithm.
Such a layered QoS modelling resembles the data processing theorem (Blahut, 1987) stating that, in a cascade of signal processing elements, no processing can increase mutual information. The statement puts no limit on the sophistication or complexity of the individual cascaded processing blocks.

5. Data streaming

Typically, sensor data are streamed from the source to the sink, i.e., the sensor data are consumed, e.g., presented on a terminal, while new data from the same stream are arriving; an exception might be sensors that transfer single still images on demand. For data streaming, several standards have been developed covering certain properties. Relevant Internet protocol standards include the transport protocol RTP/RTCP (Schulzrinne, Casner, Frederick & Jacobson, 2003) and session protocols like SDP (Handley, Jacobson & Perkins, 2006) and RTSP (Schulzrinne, Rao & Lanphier, 1998). Relevant media compression standards include ISO MPEG 2 Systems (ISO/IEC 13818) and MPEG 4 Systems (ISO/IEC 14496). Media content searching, filtering and transactions include MPEG 7 (ISO/IEC 15938) and MPEG-21 (ISO/IEC 21000).
The DICOM standard (*DICOM*, 2008), which is the basis for Picture Archive and Communication Systems (PACS), is not designed to support streaming of medical data. Some research has begun to add support for streaming (Dragan & Ivetic, 2009), but this is still in the preliminary stages. On the other hand, DICOM is well suited of storing and retrieving sensor data in a health care environment. So, it should be possible to import and export to DICOM.

5.1 MPEG-21

MPEG-21 (Burnett, Pereira, de Walle & Koenen, 2006) is a standard from the International Standards Organisation (ISO) that attempts to define a complete infrastructure for delivery and consumption of multimedia content. The effort was started in 2000. The ISO's introduction to Part 1 of the standard summarises the vision as, "... to define a multimedia framework to enable transparent and augmented use of multimedia resources across a wide range of networks and devices used by different communities" (International Standards Organisation, 2004, page vii). MPEG-21 currently consists of 18 parts that cover diverse issues such as defining the fundamental structures, adapting these structures between different networks, specifying creator's and user's rights, and defining testbeds and conformance suites.
The basic unit for data in MPEG-21 is the digital item (DI). Like many other parts of MPEG-21, it is defined in XML to be machine readable. The DI is a generic item that can contain components, resources, or other containers. These structures can either refer to other XML structures, included data, or reference another item by a universal resource identifier (URI). Additional parts of MPEG-21 include how to uniquely identify an item and how to process them.
MPEG-21 defines two ways of streaming information. One is by using Binary XML that was originally part of MPEG-7, but is included as Part 16 of MPEG-21. Part 18 defines digital item streaming (DIS), which is a pure XML way of streaming.
Another goal of MPEG-21 is to ensure that creators can protect their creations and that users of content have the correct rights for viewing them. Parts 4, 5, and 6 of the standard deal with

these issues. It defines the rights — Rights Data Dictionary (RDD), how to express the rights in a machine readable form — Rights Expression Language (REL), and finally, how they are enforced — Intellectual Property Management and Protection (IPMP).
Since the vision is that MPEG-21 is to be used in a variety of situations, MPEG-21 defines Part 7 — Digital Item Adaptation — for specifying how streams (i.e., the media content) should be adapted to suit different network and terminal characteristics, like bandwidth and display resolution. This is a vital mechanism in order to maximise the perceived QoS given the constraints of the network and observer equipment.

5.2 Binary XML

One of the issues with using wireless sensor networks is that the sensors cannot transfer much data in each individual packet. For example, earlier specifications of ZigBee restrict the total packet size to 128 bytes including routing information. Later versions of ZigBee allow for larger sizes, but that is dependent on the hardware in use (Daintree Networks, Inc., 2010). So, the size of the data in each packet is important. Since MPEG-21 uses XML throughout, we need to use Binary XML to compress this.
Binary XML refers to any specification which defines the compact representation of the Extensible Markup Language (XML) in a binary format (Bray, Paoli, Sperberg-McQueen, Maler, Yergeau & Cowan, 2006). While there are several competing formats, none has been accepted as a standard yet. Using a binary XML format reduces the size and eases parsing of the documents at the cost of human-readability. Binary XML is used in applications where performance or resource limitations apply. As part of this, we do not consider traditional compression methods applied to XML documents, such as using gzip, or an existing standard like ASN.1.
There are several different implementations of binary XML. For example:

- The *Fast Infoset* standard from the ISO and International Telecommunications Union (ITU) (International Standards Organisation, 2007b)
- The *Extensible XML Interchange format* from the World Wide Web Consortium (W3C) (Schneider & Kamiya, 2009; Peintner & Pericas-Geertsen, 2009)
- The *Binary MPEG format for XML (BiM)* defined by the ISO (International Standards Organisation, 2006) and is used by many ETSI standards for Digital TV and Mobile TV

There are also other binary XML formats that are defined for specific application domains.
We selected the Binary MPEG XML Format (BiM) and Efficient XML Interchange (EXI) as the most promising candidates since these were designed to work with general purpose XML, and because it was possible to get access to implementations of both.
BiM is part of the MPEG-7 standard (International Standards Organisation, 2006) and is also part of MPEG-21 (Part 16). It specifies a general method for compressing and decompressing XML documents for efficient transport and storage. It does this by examining the schemas for the document and using that information to create a separate decoder header that is used for encoding and decoding documents that use those schemas. The encoder uses this information to encode and partition the document into fragments. These fragments are then sent to the decoder. The decoder reassembles the fragments into a semantically similar document.
EXI comes from the W3C. Its purpose is to have a "...very compact, high performance XML representation that was designed to work well for a broad range of applications," (Schneider & Kamiya, 2009). It currently is a W3C Candidate Recommendation. EXI is *schema informed,* which means that it can use the schema to create a more efficient document, but a schema is not

necessary. EXI is compatible with other documents at the XML Information Set level, but not at the XML syntax level. This means that you can inter-operate with other XML documents assuming that you have everything at the Information Set level (2009). EXI does not have explicit support for fragmenting itself, instead it depends other XML technologies for this.

Ignoring the separate BiM decoding header, both EXI and BiM compress documents to comparable sizes. Therefore, other criteria were needed to figure out which method would be used. One obvious advantage that BiM has over EXI is its support for fragmentation and streaming. The BiM standard (International Standards Organisation, 2006) goes into detail about how BiM can be fragmented and reassembled, while EXI (Schneider & Kamiya, 2009) only describes that EXI fragments can exist, but not how a document could be fragmented, streamed or reassembled.

6. Proposed solution

We have experimented with a variety of different solutions and have come up with some solutions that integrate both WSN and MPEG-21 into patient monitoring systems. As the basic idea, we adapt MPEG-21 to a WSN by adapting the basic Digital Items and employing binary XML.

6.1 MPEG-21 for patient monitoring systems

MPEG-21 includes features like adaptation and security for network and users that make it a good candidate in a health care system architecture. However, most of the patient data aggregators are based on wireless sensor networks containing nodes with restricted capabilities and battery capacity. This means that they may not be able to run all of the processor intensive tasks of MPEG-21. Therefore, the MPEG-21 standard needs to be adapted to work with this restricted setup.

As mentioned in Section 5.1, a digital item (DI) is the basic unit for transferring information. Landén (2003) introduces a medical digital item (MDI) that adapts the digital item to the health care sector. The MDI also encapsulates mechanisms for adaptation and security. Since sensors have limited resources, we developed a *lightweight MDI* or μMDI for the sensors. However, to save battery capacity and processing power in some situations, the XML syntax of MPEG-21 is not employed at all.

Lie, Grythe & Balasingham (2008) present a hospital scenario where the use of digital item adaptation (DIA) is designed for sensors wirelessly connected to a PCH. The PCH is connected to the health information system. The medical personnel access the patient data using a terminal with an MPEG-21 enabled browser. After a threat analysis of patient monitoring systems (Leister, Abie, Groven, Fretland & Balasingham, 2008) we extended this architecture to include (BSNs) (Leister, Fretland & Balasingham, 2008). The architecture supports security, privacy, and authentication, by using the mechanisms of MPEG-21 in the OSI presentation layer and a carefully designed μMDI (Leister et al., 2009). It also supports content adaptation according to terminal and network capabilities, QoS, energy efficiency, and several types of session mobility. The impact of this work is currently being studied in a recently developed testbed for evaluating MPEG-21 in health care applications, which is described in Section 6.4.

Other approaches to using MPEG-21 in health care use the IPMP Part of MPEG-21 for patient records (Brox, 2005). Recently, a framework for using MPEG-21 IPMP components for a security framework for pervasive health care architectures has been presented by Fragopoulos, Gialelis & Serpanos (2009), including wireless communication between personal digital assistants (PDA). While that work introduces MPEG-21 for medical applications, our work includes the use of MPEG-21 for BSN and uses a generic model to analyse the threats.

6.2 Using binary XML

The initial plan was to use BiM since we could partition up a document into fragments, compress it, and send it all with one tool. EXI would only give us the compression. Ultimately, the final decision came down to the quality of implementations that were available since we did not have time nor resources to create our own implementation. The BiM implementation (Technische Universität München, 2007-2008) seems to be incomplete, is not documented, and has many bugs. Initially, it would not encode our μMDI document at all. After a lot of tracing and fixing, we were able to get it to encode a document similar to μMDI, but it then failed to decode it correctly. It also seems to be missing the code for partitioning the document into fragments and reassembling it.

By contrast, the EXI implementation (EXIficient) is available as an open source project (Peintner, 2010). While it is missing some documentation, it is actively developed and seems to handle all the situations we have given it. Since EXI has no built in streaming, we needed a method for streaming the items. This was solved using MPEG-21 Part 18—Digital Item Streaming.

Digital Item Streaming (DIS) works by specifying a separate XML document that defines the Bitstream Binding Language (BBL) for a document. This BBL specifies the packets or packet streams for the document, when these packets should be sent, and how the source document should be divided up. The BBL is then used by software to divide the document up and send it over arbitrary protocols. DIS also allows specifying constraints for packet streams (such as number of items, or packet size), but the standard indicates that constraints *will* be broken in order to send a packet. There is a publicly available implementation from the ISO (International Standards Organisation, 2007a). that works well. One issue with DIS is that it only works with with a "completed" document. That is, one cannot add siblings to the document after you have sent over the basic skeleton. Future packets must be children of the current elements.

6.3 The complete system

We combine μMDI, EXI, and DIS to form the following solution for a BSN using MPEG-21. We have expanded the μMDI to contain multiple entries. A portion of the new μMDI can be seen in Fig. 6. The various sensors can then send their identification information and their data as separate packets using DIS. These packets are eventually received by the base station and are attached to an already existing skeleton document. This document has a limited number of parts. After this document is done, a new skeleton is added and the sensor can then retransmit its identity and continue sending its information. The base station can transfer this information on to the patient monitoring system.

The resulting packets should be small, but we can further reduce their size by using EXI and transmitting them. The base station will receive the items as an EXI stream and will apply them to the XML document.

The packets are sent from the WSN to a PCH. The PCH takes the information and converts it from a μMDI to a real MDI, adds extra information (e.g., identifying information for the patient), and sends the information to other communication levels. This information is encrypted with strong encryption, ensuring that only medical staff with correct permissions may use it.

```
<did:DIDL xmlns:did="urn:mpeg:mpeg21:2002:02-DIDL-NS"

  xmlns:xsi="http://www.w3.org/2001/XMLSchema-instance"

  xmlns:dii="urn:mpeg:mpeg21:2002:01-DII-NS"

  xsi:schemaLocation="urn:mpeg:mpeg21:2002:02-DIDL-NS schemas/didl.xsd
                      urn:mpeg:mpeg21:2002:01-DII-NS schemas/dii.xsd">

  <did:Container>

    <did:Item id="myitem">

      <did:Descriptor>

        <did:Statement mimeType="text/xml">

          <dii:Identifier>urn:grid:a1-abcde-9873216540-f</dii:Identifier>

        </did:Statement>

      </did:Descriptor>

      <did:Descriptor>

        <did:Statement mimeType="text/xml">

          <dii:Type>urn:sensor:bloodpressure</dii:Type>

        </did:Statement>

      </did:Descriptor>
      <did:Item>

        <did:Descriptor>
          <did:Statement mimeType="text/plain">20</did:Statement>
        </did:Descriptor>

        <did:Component>
          <did:Resource mimeType="text/plain">68.300</did:Resource>
        </did:Component>

        </did:Item>

        <did:Item>
```

Fig. 6. Excerpt from a μMDI document adapted for Digital Item Streaming (DIS)

6.4 MPEG-21 testbed

A proposed architecture's performance and functionality is best verified using a dedicated software testing platform. Thus, a Java-based testbed was created to test the hospital and home-care networks. The testbed is based on an existing MPEG-21 software that was developed during the MPEG-21 standardisation work (Perkis & Drege, 2008), and then modified to support the aforementioned medical network requirements (Lie et al., 2008). The testbed design requirements had the following architecture in mind:

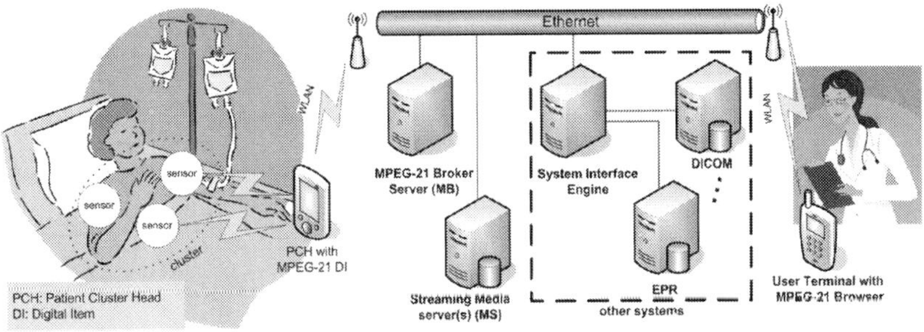

Fig. 7. The hospital network architecture envisioned for the MPEG-21 supporting testbed (Lie et al., 2008).

- Support for wireless medical sensors
- PCH bed-side terminals (optionally compatible with the NCAP—Network Capable Application Processors—architecture of the IEEE 1451 standard) (IEEE1451.0, 2007; IEEE1451.5, 2007), including WSN radio interface and WLAN radio interface
- WLAN APs and backbone network infrastructure
- User terminals equipped with MPEG-21 browsing capabilities
- An MPEG-21 Broker server (MB)
- One or several media servers (MS)
- Optional Media resource Adaptation Server (MAS)

The envisioned system is depicted in Fig. 7. The medical body sensors are communicating with the bed-side PCH terminal. This PCH includes NCAP functionality in case IEEE 1451.5 is in use, and uses short-range radio systems to communicate with the active sensors (e.g., Zigbee). Thus, the PCH will collect all the necessary meta information regarding the sensor capabilities and current status collected in MPEG-21 validated XML DIs, based on the IEEE 1451 TEDS (Transducer Electronic Data Sheets). In addition, there must be a dedicated authentication procedure to ensure that new sensors are connected to the intended PCH (the short-range radio coverage can reach other patients sensors and PCH). The principle of the *resurrecting duckling* (Stajano & Anderson, 1999) with physical imprinting between the sensor nodes and correct PCH is a viable authentication approach for exchanging symmetric secret keys.

All PCH terminals are connected to the network infrastructure, e.g., using WLAN. This helps minimise the traffic from the energy constrained sensors. A moving patient without a PCH would call for frequent handovers between the sensors and different access points.

To facilitate easy retrieval of all information available, a few centralised servers are needed. The media broker (MB) server will hold the MPEG-21 CDI (Content Description Items) that gives the updated menus on the end-users terminals, e.g., regarding patient lists. Patient and diagnosis search could be facilitated through the accompanying MPEG-7 standard and underlying meta information. Each patient will have one dedicated CDI menu system for its PCH and one for the Electronic Patient Record (EPR) system, holding all relevant EPR and pre-stored medical media. When pre-stored media is selected, it will be retrieved from the media streaming server (MS). An optional powerful adaptation server (MAS) can be used to

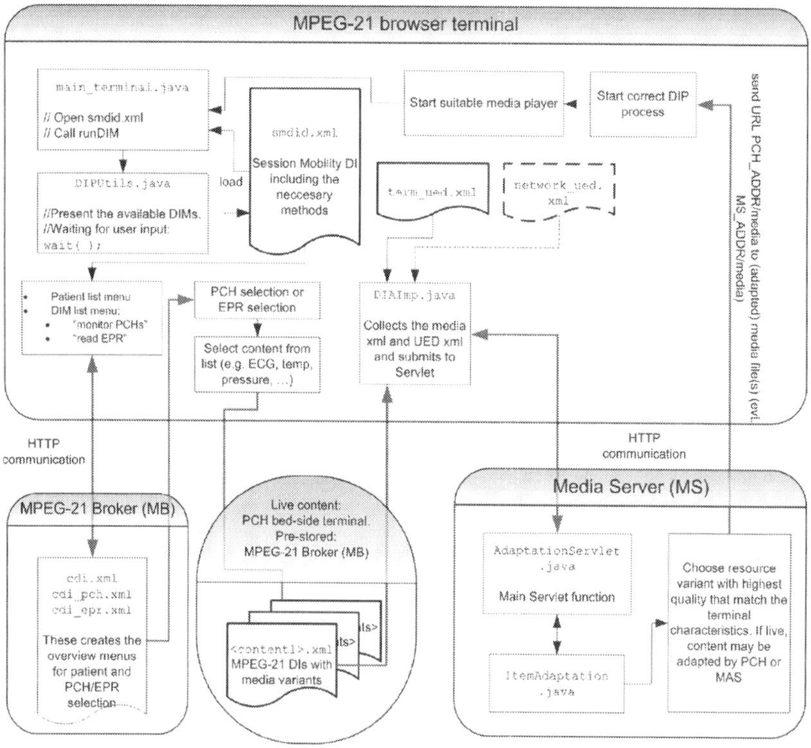

Fig. 8. The Java based MPEG-21 testbed architecture.

facilitate media format adaptation on-the-fly for both live and pre-stored media, following MPEG-21 Part 7 methodology (DIA — Digital Item Adaptation).

The observer will thus use the system via the terminal, e.g., an MPEG-21 capable browsing terminal, to access both live content streamed via the PCH, and pre-stored content from the MS. The MPEG-21 testbed also incorporates support for Session Mobility (Soma, 2007). The testbed is programmed in Java and ECMAscript, and has MPEG-21 validated XML files that format the graphical user interface menus with the supported functionality. In addition to supporting session mobility and DIA, it uses the MPEG-21 DIP — Digital Item Processing — engine to process the user activities. For example, to process media streaming it activates a Java based player named *Fobs4JMF*, which consists of Sun Java Media Framework (JMF) player enhanced with codecs from the open source package *ffmpeg* (Omnividea, 2008). Fig. 8 shows a diagram with the key software components. At top, the user terminal is shown. The initial GUI is formed by the local root DID (`smdid.xml` in this example). From this GUI the user can select the patient list CDI located at the MB. After selecting a specific patient, the user can choose either PCH or EPR. If choosing the PCH, the terminal will be given access over HTTP to the online PCH for this patient. This PCH contains the current CDI showing a list of connected wireless sensors (`cdi_pch.xml`). The user will now be able to access online data such as ECG. Available media format choices are stored in dedicated XML files (the

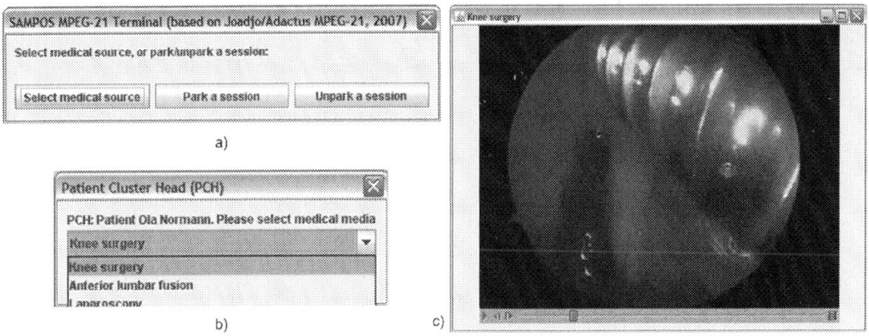

Fig. 9. Snapshots from the MPEG-21 testbed, observer terminal part: *a)* start screen with selection of source, *b)* The GUI is generated given the CDI contents, where the observer can select the particular content, and *c)* the rendering of the selected medical content.

oval object at figure mid bottom). The available media formats are checked against the UED (Usage Environment Descriptions) information, and a DIA engine located in the PCH or at a centralised MS or MAS would eventually adapt the content for optimal fidelity to the user's terminal. Finally a message will be sent to the terminal containing the URL to the possibly adapted media stream.

In Fig. 9, an example walkthrough of the user terminal functionality is displayed. The user selects a specific PCH, using IP address and path to CDI. The list of medical content described in this particular CDI is used to generate the GUI presented to the user. Behind the scenes, the selected content is adapted to the current display capabilities and network conditions, using the DIA functionality on the UED information.

7. Security analysis

In this section, we perform a security analysis of the use of MPEG-21 in patient monitoring systems. The security requirements for patient monitoring systems are given by Leister et al. (2009) as the following: (*a*) availability, (*b*) data confidentiality, (*c*) data integrity, and (*d*) data authenticity. The general threats and attacks to these security objectives are eavesdropping, denial of service, masquerading, and disclosure. Leister et al. identified the threats associated to these factors as compromised, destroyed, malfunctioning, lost or stolen components; software errors; misuse of emergency access; and denial of service attacks for the components; compromised or unstable communication infrastructure; and eavesdropping on the communication channels.

We consider these security goals separately for each of the levels introduced earlier in Section 2.1. This allows us to consider separately the threats and remedies for security, and also consider whether the particular component or channel of a patient monitoring system is within a trusted environment. Components and channels in a trusted environment can be considered secure. For components and channels outside a trusted environment, we consider the threat model by Dolev & Yao (1981), where an attacker can overhear, intercept, and synthesise any message, and is only limited by the constraints of the cryptographic methods used. Since some of the devices used may not have the resources for strong cryptographic methods, the assumption of the Dolev-Yao attacker might be not applicable in all situations, and additional measures might be necessary, especially when wireless sensor networks are a part of the patient monitoring system.

Using the Dolev-Yao threat model, availability cannot always be guaranteed since an attacker always can synthesise messages, and thus disturb or interrupt a channel. While this cannot be prevented on the OSI application layer using MPEG-21, there might be other technical measures on lower OSI layers that can be applied, such as spread spectrum technologies. The development of radio access methods based on time-hopping and frequency-hopping spread-spectrum (TH/FH-SS) addresses power-efficient signaling methods, which becomes an interesting candidate for wireless sensor networks. TH/FH-SS is preceived as an anti-jamming technique with low complexity and does not require complicated signal processing. An example of their implementation can be found in Bluetooth systems (Tsai & Chang, 1994; Salonidis et al., 2005). However, these technologies are beyond the scope of this chapter.

Some threats and vulnerabilities can be addressed on an administrative level, such as describing responsibilities for the stakeholders, educating personnel, or providing routines for keeping devices out of the hands of adversaries. These non-technical routines are not considered further in this context.

Due to the nature of the biomedical data, we consider a model where a numbered sequence of unique data packets that are on a channel are transferred from source to sink, protected by means of MPEG-21. When this data stream arrives, packets may have been lost, altered, replayed, be out of order, be subject to eavesdropping, be stored, etc. These characteristics may be the result of processes at lower OSI layers.

In patient monitoring systems, data are usually sent in packets using both connection-based or connectionless channels. Connectionless channels do not offer retransmission automatically. However, mechanisms for retransmissions on any channel might block sending of data, and thus prohibit the timely transfer of data. Ideally, short, self-contained sequences of packets are preferred to avoid the issues in retransmission.

For Level (0) the security considerations are limited to human communication patterns, such as outlined in the communication theory by Watzlawick, Beavin & Jackson (1967). The other levels can be considered more from a technical perspective, while both technical and administrative means can be used to reduce the vulnerabilities.

7.1 Security considerations for level (I)

Level (I) is usually implemented as a wired or wireless, biomedical sensor network, where most of the data traffic consists of a stream from the sensor node to the sink since we are not considering actuator networks here. Leister et al. (2009) discuss threats for biomedical sensor networks in the domains of the entity domain, the network domain, the specific protocol domain, and the routing and forwarding domain. In these domains, an adversary who has access to the medium, can eavesdrop, inject, delete and alter data packets. This can lead to incorrect data, lost data, data being attached to the wrong data stream or patient, and inferior service quality.

Eavesdropping obviously threatens confidentiality and privacy goals. Lost, delayed, and altered packets threaten the integrity and the authenticity of the data as well as the availability. As a consequence, this could cause inappropriate, delayed or missing treatment of the patient at the risk of damage to the patient's health.

MPEG-21 does not solve threats arising at the lower communication layers, but is suited to detect possible inconsistencies in the case of altered content so that wrong content can be marked or discarded. Regarding eavesdropping, MPEG-21 offers mechanisms to encrypt the content. Digital Items can be identified in MPEG-21, thus facilitating that the data belong to the correct stream and patient as long as the data source can be authenticated. Authentication is done by using the identification tags on the data and encryption. Therefore, as long as the encryption key is secret, the authentication will work. The initialisation procedure of sensor nodes shown by Leister et al. (2009) guarantees this. Here, the sensor nodes are provided with the necessary security credentials in the initialisation step, while these are used in the operation mode.

In wireless sensor networks, the data streams from the sensor to the PCH can be sent via other nodes. These nodes do not possess the capabilities to decrypt the streams from another sensor node, and cannot inject valid packets, or alter packets consistently. However, data aggregation in the sensor network is not possible in such a scenario.

Due to resource constraints in the devices, the possible cryptographic methods that can be applied are weak. Therefore, additional measures must be taken, such as restricting all data that can identify a patient in the wireless sensor network. The identifying information necessary to attach the data to the right patient must therefore be formed such that the patient is not revealed.

The architecture by Leister et al. suggests that the software loaded into the sensor nodes is tied together with the necessary credentials for encryption and authentication. Therefore, once provided with the credentials, the software in the sensor node cannot be altered unless exchanged entirely, which would be similar to an attacker providing a fake node.

7.2 Security considerations for level (II)

Compared to Level (I), there are less resource restrictions for the scenarios on Level (II). Therefore, better cryptographic methods can be applied, and the restriction on not sending identifying information is less important. The health care infrastructure can perform data aggregation if necessary, and also convert the μMDI to an MDI with data not available in the sensor network. Note, however, that identifying information should not be sent in the channel unless necessary. For other characteristics, the same mechanisms apply regarding the use of MPEG-21.

When roaming between the Levels (IIa) to (IIe) the authentication mechanism beyond MPEG-21 is responsible for establishing the trust to facilitate the communication between the PCH and the entity responsible for the respective level or scenario by using the correct keys. Note that in some scenarios the PCH can have the role of both.

7.3 Security considerations for level (III)

Devices that are in the hospital infrastructure and that can be authenticated are considered secure, and not tampered with; for these devices, no specific measures are necessary. However, note that authentication is always necessary. In Level (III), the use of MPEG-21 provides a unified method to represent the medical data, and to provide data confidentiality, data integrity, and data authenticity through the mechanisms used.

7.4 Security considerations end-to-end

While MPEG-21 can be used to provide the security goals from end-to-end, other standards might be employed in a health care enterprise, such as DICOM, ELIN XML (Christensen, 2009) or HL7 (Shaver, 2007), and make data conversions necessary for the data to be stored or

processed. The representation of medical data in a MDI data structure provides the security goals of confidentiality, data integrity, and data authenticity.
Since being placed in the presentation layer, MPEG-21 can be used in the Levels (I)-(III) and end-to-end to sustain the security goals. Functionalities of the presented architecture, such as converting the μMDI to MDI, are not necessarily performed by the PCH, i.e., Level (I), but can be performed in Level (II) or (III), before being further processed and stored. The end-to-end security is sustained as long as the entities processing MPEG-21 can be trusted, and the cryptographic methods used are strong enough.
The architecture shown here addresses the threats of devices being tampered with, eavesdropping, altered communication at several layers, in the sense that wrong data are not accepted. The limitations are in the relatively weak encryption in the sensor nodes. An adversary could eavesdrop on the traffic, break the encryption, and either introduce a fake node, or use an attack at the wireless network level. This is not considered by the Dolev-Yao attacker, but could be done in a practical case.
However, since the wireless communication using weak encryption is limited to Level (I) where the communication range is limited, an adversary needs to have access to the vicinity of the patient, or have access to communication credentials from the inside. Such threats need to be addressed on an administrative and stakeholder level, e.g., by strict control of access to areas where security is critical, rules for handling devices, measures to increase awareness among medical personnel, and so on.
The Dolev-Yao attacker sets requirements on the encryption. However, this is problematic due to limited resources in the sensors. Therefore, to avoid the risk that an attacker can get the data to the right patient, we do not include data into the stream that can be used to identify the patient, such as a personal identification number. The identity establishment must be done by routines using the mechanisms described by MPEG-21.
The security analysis shows that the communication in patient monitoring systems can be secure in principle in relation to the mentioned security goals and threats. For a concrete implementation, a formal analysis is necessary, where the involved protocols are modelled, and formally analysed using tools such as those shown by Hagalisletto, Strand, Leister & Groven (2009) in another application area. The same methods can be applied for patient monitoring systems, using concrete implementations and protocols.

8. Conclusion

We have shown a framework that includes QoS, adaptation, and security provisioning for wireless patient monitoring systems with an emphasis on a solution that integrates the patient monitoring system into the hospital infrastructure. For this, we proposed an architecture that uses the MPEG-21 standard to reach these goals. We implemented parts of the system in a testbed to show that the architecture is viable, and gained practical results.
We found that MPEG-21 is suitable for integrating a biomedical WSN with the health care infrastructure in different health care scenarios. Challenges arising from the scarce resources generally available in WSN are addressed by utilising XML compression, XML streaming, and architectural means that avoid handling XML data in its text form in the sensor nodes. One issue that remains is what should be part of the metadata in a digital item (DI) and what should be implemented in the DI adaptation engine.
We showed that security concerns can be covered by describing the scenarios and considering the different communication levels and communication channels. However, the WSN has scarce resources that result in weak cryptography and the communication medium is

accessible; the result is that not all threats can be stopped at the OSI presentation level. Therefore, in the case of certain attacks by a man in the middle, the availability might be reduced. Adaptation for a patient monitoring system is shown by the means of a testbed that also shows the integration with the information system of the healthcare enterprise.

While MPEG-21 covers security and adaptation issues, the QoS requirements are addressed in WSN by a stack-oriented approach using a degradation model in an optimisation process. How to implement these QoS structures in MPEG-21 is not investigated. However, it appears that the adaptation engine approach is more versatile than editing metadata, and permits a wider range of dynamic QoS attributes to be supported.

Future work on the architecture includes more integration and implementation on a larger scale to determine how we can adjust parameters so the architecture is suitable for a real network. These consideration about the architecture and its parameters are important for factors like power — thus battery life of sensors — achievable security, availability, and flexibility in the form of adaptation.

In the future, this work can lead to benefits for both the health care workers and patients. Using our architecture, patients are able to move around more freely, stay productive out of a hospital environment and know that their medical data is secure. At the same time, health care workers have a better overview of a patient's medical data in a variety of environments and are assured of a certain level of QoS. The result is that, in the eventuality that a patient needs it, treatment can arrive in a timely manner.

9. Acknowledgements

This research is funded by the SAMPOS and WISENET projects in the VERDIKT framework of the Norwegian Research Council.

10. References

Bai, H., Atiquzzaman, M. & Lilja, D. J. (2006). Layered view of QoS issues in IP-based mobile wireless networks, *Int. Journal on Comm. Systems* 18: 141–161.

Balasingham, I., Ihlen, H., Leister, W., Røe, P. & Samset, E. (2007). Communication of medical images, text, and messages in inter-enterprise systems: A case study in Norway, *IEEE Transactions on Information Technology in Biomedicine* 11(1): 7–13.

Blahut, R. E. (1987). *Principles and practice of information theory*, Addison-Wesley Longman Publishing Co., Inc., Boston, MA, USA.

Bray, T., Paoli, J., Sperberg-McQueen, C. M., Maler, E., Yergeau, F. & Cowan, J. (2006). Extensible Markup Language (XML) 1.1 (second edition), World Wide Web Consortium, Recommendation REC-xml11-20060816.

Brox, G. A. (2005). MPEG-21 as an access control tool for the national health service care records service, *Journal of Telemedicine and Telecare* 11 Suppl 1: 23–5.

Burnett, I. S., Pereira, F., de Walle, R. V. & Koenen, R. (eds) (2006). *The MPEG-21 Book*, John Wiley & Sons. ISBN 0-47001011-8.

Chen, D. & Varshney, P. K. (2004). QoS support in wireless sensor networks: A survey, *2004 International Conference on Wireless Networks (ICWN 2004)*.

Christensen, T. (2009). Sluttraport ELIN, *Sluttrapport*, Den norske legeforening, Pb. 7000 St. Olavs plass, NO-0130 Oslo, Norway. In Norwegian.

Daintree Networks, Inc. (2010). Zigbee specification comparison matrix. Last accessed September 2, 2010, http://www.daintree.net/resources/spec-matrix.php.

Digital Imaging and Communications in Medicine (DICOM) (2008). `http://medical.nema.org/dicom/`. Last accessed May 15, 2009.

Dolev, D. & Yao, A. (1981). On the security of public key protocols, *Proc. of the IEEE 22nd Annual Symposium on Foundations of Computer Science*, pp. 350–357.

Dragan, D. & Ivetic, D. (2009). *An Approach to DICOM Extension for Medical Image Streaming*, DAAAM International, chapter 4 in DAAAM International Scientific Book 2009, pp. 25–34.

Fragopoulos, A., Gialelis, J. & Serpanos, D. (2009). Security framework for pervasive healthcare architectures utilizing MPEG-21 IPMP components, *International Journal of Telemedicine and Applications* 2009: 1–9.

Grythe, K., Lie, A. & Balasingham, I. (2009). Interactive system design and end-to-end optimization in sensor network, *IEEE 5th Int. Workshop on Wearable Micro and Nano Technologies for Personilized Health*, Oslo.

Hagalisletto, A. M., Strand, L., Leister, W. & Groven, A.-K. (2009). Analysing protocol implementations, *in* F. Bao, H. Li & G. Wang (eds), *ISPEC*, Vol. 5451 of *Lecture Notes in Computer Science*, Springer, pp. 171–182.

Handley, M., Jacobson, V. & Perkins, C. (2006). SDP: Session Description Protocol, RFC 4566 (Proposed Standard), http://www.ietf.org/rfc/rfc4566.txt.

Heinzelman, W. B., Murphy, A. L., Carvalho, H. S. & Perillo, M. A. (2004). Middleware to support sensor network applications, *Network, IEEE* 18(1): 6–14.

IEEE1451.0 (2007). IEEE standard for a smart transducer interface for sensors and actuators - common functions, communication protocols, and transducer electronic data sheet (TEDS) formats, *IEEE Std 1451.0-2007* pp. 1–335.

IEEE1451.5 (2007). IEEE standard for a smart transducer interface for sensors and actuators wireless communication protocols and transducer electronic data sheet (TEDS formats, *IEEE Std 1451.5-2007* pp. C1–236.

International Standards Organisation (2004). Information technology—multimedia framework (MPEG-21—part 1: Vision, technologies and strategy, *Technical Report ISO/IEC TR 21000-1*.

International Standards Organisation (2006). Information technology—MPEG system technologies—part 1: Binary MPEG format for XML, *Technical Report ISO/IEC 23001-1*.

International Standards Organisation (2007a). Directory listing for /publiclyavailablestandards /iso_iec_21000-8_2008_amd_1_2009_reference_software/. Last accessed September 8, 2010, http:// standards.iso.org / ittf/ PubliclyAvailableStandards /IS_IEC_21000-8_2008_Amd_1_2009_Reference_Software/.

International Standards Organisation (2007b). Information technology—generic application of ASN.1: Fast Infoset, *Technical Report ISO/IEC 24824-1: 2007 / ITU-T Rec X891*.

Khoshnevis, B. & Khalaj, B. (2007). Optimum QoS classes in interworking of next generation networks, *Communications and networks* 9(4 (Dec)): 438–445.

Landén, M. (2003). *An MPEG-21 approach to creating the first multimedia electronic patient journal system*, Master's thesis, NTNU.

Lei, C. & Heinzelman, W. B. (2007). A survey of routing protocols that support QoS in mobile ad hoc networks, *Network, IEEE* 21(6): 30–38.

Leister, W., Abie, H., Groven, A.-K., Fretland, T. & Balasingham, I. (2008). Threat assessment of wireless patient monitoring systems, *Proc. ICTTA'08*, Damascus, Syria.

Leister, W., Fretland, T. & Balasingham, I. (2008). Use of MPEG-21 for security and authentication in biomedical sensor networks, *Proc. ICSNC'08, International Conference on Systems and Networks Communication* 0: 151–156.

Leister, W., Fretland, T. & Balasingham, I. (2009). Security and authentication architecture using MPEG-21 for wireless patient monitoring systems, *International Journal on Advances in Security* 2(1): 16–29, http://www.iariajournals.org/security/.

Lie, A., Grythe, K. & Balasingham, I. (2008). On the use of the MPEG-21 framework in medical wireless sensor networks, *Proc. of the IEEE 1st Int Symp on Applied Sciences in Biomedical and Communication Technologies (ISABEL)*, Aalborg, Denmark, 25.-28. October.

Omnividea, F. (2008). Object oriented wrapper for ffmpeg, `http://fobs.sourceforge.net/`. Last accessed August 23, 2010.

Patel, M. & Jianfeng, W. (2010). Applications, challenges, and prospective in emerging body area networking technologies, *Wireless Communications, IEEE* 17(1): 80–88.

Peintner, D. (2010). EXIFcient—Open Source Implementation of the W3C Exfficient XML Interchange (EXI) format. Last accessed September 8, 2010, http://exificient.sourceforge.net.

Peintner, D. & Pericas-Geertsen, S. (2009). Efficient XML interchange (EXI) primer, *W3C working draft*, W3C. http://www.w3.org/TR/2009/WD-exi-primer-20091208/.

Perkis, A. & Drege, P. (2008). MPEG-21 test-bed (joadjo).

Römer, K. & Mattern, F. (2004). The design space of wireless sensor networks, *IEEE Wireless Communications* 11(6): 54–61.

Salonidis, T., Bhagwat, P., Tassiulas, L. & LaMaire, R. (2005). Distributed topology construction of bluetooth wireless personal area networks, *Selected Areas in Communications, IEEE Journal on* 23(3): 633–643.

Schneider, J. & Kamiya, T. (2009). Efficient XML interchange (EXI) format 1.0, *Candidate recommendation*, W3C. http://www.w3.org/TR/2009/CR-exi-20091208/.

Schulzrinne, H., Casner, S., Frederick, R. & Jacobson, V. (2003). RTP: A Transport Protocol for Real-Time Applications, RFC 3550 (Standard), http://www.ietf.org/rfc/rfc3550.txt.

Schulzrinne, H., Rao, A. & Lanphier, R. (1998). Real Time Streaming Protocol (RTSP), RFC 2326 (Proposed Standard), http://www.ietf.org/rfc/rfc2326.txt.

Shaver, D. (2007). HL7 101: A Beginner's Guide, *For the Record* 19(1): 22.

Soma, C. W. (2007). Transparent consumption of digital items between terminals using mpeg-21 session mobility, *Technical report*, Norwegian University of Science and Technology. Master thesis.

Stajano, F. & Anderson, R. (1999). The resurrecting duckling: Security issues for ad-hoc wireless networks, *Security Protocols, 7th International Workshop Proceedings, Lecture Notes in Computer Science*.

Technische Universität München (2007-2008). MPEG-7 reference SW. Last accessed September 8, 2010, http://www.lis.ei.tum.de/index.php?id=131.

Trees, H. L. V. (1968). *Detection, estimation and modulation theory*, John Wiley and Sons.

Troubleyn, E., De Poorter, E., Ruckebusch, P., Moerman, I. & Demeester, P. (2010). Supporting protocol-independent adaptive QoS in wireless sensor networks, *Sensor Networks, Ubiquitous, and Trustworthy Computing (SUTC), 2010 IEEE International Conference on*, pp. 253–260.

Tsai, Y.-R. & Chang, J.-F. (1994). Using frequency hopping spread spectrum technique to combat multipath interference in a multiaccessing environment, *Vehicular Technology, IEEE Transactions on* 43(2): 211–222.

Viswanathan, R. & Varshney, P. K. (1997). Distributed detection with multiple sensors, I. fundamentals, *Proceedings of the IEEE* 85(1): 54–63.

Watzlawick, P., Beavin, J. H. & Jackson, M. D. D. (1967). *Pragmatics of Human Communication: A Study of Interactional Patterns, Pathologies, and Paradoxes*, W. W. Norton & Company.

Youngchul, S., Poor, H. V. & Heejung, Y. (2009). How much information can one get from a wireless sensor network over a correlated random field?, *Information Theory, IEEE Transactions on* 55(6): 2827–2847.